Therapy of Infectious Diseases

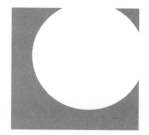

Therapy of Infectious Diseases

Larry M. Baddour, MD
Senior Associate Consultant
Department of Medicine
Division of Infectious Diseases
Mayo Clinic–Rochester

Sherwood L. Gorbach, MD
Professor of Medicine,
Microbiology, and Community Health
Tufts University School of Medicine

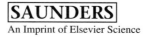

SAUNDERS
An Imprint of Elsevier Science

SAUNDERS
An Imprint of Elsevier Science

The Curtis Center
Independence Square West
Philadelphia, Pennsylvania 19106

THERAPY OF INFECTIOUS DISEASES

ISBN 0-7216-8145-X

Notice

Infectious Disease is an ever-changing field. Standard safety precautions must be followed, but as new research and clinical experience broaden our knowledge, changes in treatment and drug therapy may become necessary or appropriate. Readers are advised to check the most current product information provided by the manufacturer of each drug to be administered to verify the recommended dose, the method and duration of administration, and contraindications. It is the responsibility of the treating physician, relying on experience and knowledge of the patient, to determine dosages and the best treatment for each individual patient. Neither the Publisher nor the author assume any liability for any injury and/or damage to persons or property arising from this publication.

The Publisher

Library of Congress Cataloging-in-Publication Data

Baddour, Larry M.
    Therapy of infectious diseases / Larry M. Baddour,
Sherwood L. Gorbach.
      p. cm.
    ISBN 0-7216-8145-X
    1. Communicable diseases—Treatment. I. Gorbach, Sherwood L. II. Title.

RC111 .B33 2003
616.9′046—dc21

2002075945

Acquisitions Editor: Dolores Meloni
Production Manager: Mary Stermel

PIT / QWK
Printed in the United States of America

Last digit is the print number: 9 8 7 6 5 4 3 2 1

100318176x T

Acknowledgments

I wish to acknowledge my parents, Sam and Margaret, who have been a steady source of encouragement, Anna, my daughter, who makes me excited about the future, and Kathye, my wife, who has been my support along the way.

LMB

I want to recognize my wife, Judy, and my children, who have supported me in this and other works. In addition, I am grateful to my colleagues, fellows, and students, who have inspired me to teach and pass on whatever knowledge I have gained through our experiences on the wards and in the clinic.

SLG

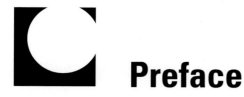

Preface

We were pleased to draft this first-edition textbook that focuses on the treatment and prevention of infectious diseases. For several reasons, it is appropriate that a textbook be dedicated to treatment and prevention. First, there has been a wealth of newer antimicrobials made available over the past few years for the treatment of a wide variety of infection syndromes. Second, antimicrobial drug resistance is at an all-time high for most organisms and this has further complicated choice of therapy. Third, busy clinicians need a detailed text that both can provide them with easy access to clinical recommendations and can supply them with thorough background knowledge and timely references if additional information is desired. Fourth, methods of infection prevention are continuously updated and this work focuses on those updated recommendations. Finally, clinicians with extensive knowledge in their respective fields of interest were identified as contributors to the text so that readers would gain valuable insight into the management and prevention of infectious diseases.

Contributors

Fredrick M. Abrahamian, DO
Assistant Professor of Medicine, UCLA School of Medicine; Director of Education and Assistant Director of Research, Department of Emergency Medicine, Olive View–UCLA Medical Center, Sylmar, CA
Animal and Human Bites

David Andes, MD
Assistant Professor, Department of Medicine, Section of Infectious Diseases, University of Wisconsin, Madison, WI
Antimicrobial Pharmacokinetics and Pharmacodynamics

Larry M. Baddour, MD
Senior Associate Consultant, Department of Medicine, Division of Infectious Diseases, Mayo Clinic, Rochester, MN
Endocarditis

Elie Berbari, MD
Assistant Professor of Medicine, Department of Medicine, Division of Infectious Diseases, Mayo Medical School, Rochester, MN
Osteomyelitis and Infectious Arthritis

William J. Burman, MD
Associate Professor of Medicine, University of Colorado Health Sciences Center; Director, Infectious Diseases Clinic, Denver Public Health, Denver, CO
Tuberculosis Treatment: Theory and Practice

Michael V. Callahan, MD, MSPH, DTM&H (UK)
Assistant Professor, International Health, Center for International Health, Boston University School of Public Health, Boston, MA
Fever of Unknown Origin

Janet R. Casey, MD
Clinical Assistant Professor, University of Rochester Medical Center, Rochester, NY
School of Medicine and Dentistry, Department of Pediatrics
Sinusitis, Otitis Media, and Mastoiditis; Tonsillopharyngitis, Bacterial Tracheitis, Epiglottitis, and Laryngotracheitis

Kevin Cassady, MD
Assistant Professor of Pediatrics, Division of Pediatric Infectious Diseases, University of Alabama at Birmingham, Birmingham, AL
Viral Infections of the Central Nervous System

Ray Y. Chen, MD
Instructor, University of Alabama at Birmingham, Birmingham, AL
Therapy and Prophylaxis for Infectious Complications of Human Immunodeficiency Virus

Anthony W. Chow, MD
Professor of Medicine, Division of Infectious Diseases, Department of Medicine; Director, MD/PhD Program, University of British Columbia, Vancouver Hospital and Health Sciences Center, Vancouver, BC, Canada
Head and Neck Infections

Theodore J. Cieslak, MD
Clinical Associate Professor of Pediatrics, E. Edward Hébert School of Medicine, Uniformed Services University of the Health Sciences, Bethesda, MD; Clinical Associate Professor of Pediatrics, University of Texas Health Sciences Center at San Antonio, San Antonio, TX
Bioterrorism: Plague, Anthrax, and Smallpox

James L. Cook, MD
Professor of Medicine, Microbiology, and Immunology, University of Illinois at Chicago College of Medicine; Chief, Section of Infectious Diseases, Department of Medicine, University of Illinois Hospital, Chicago, IL
Nontuberculous Mycobacterial Infections

Jennifer S. Daly, MD
Associate Professor of Medicine, University of Massachusetts Medical School; Clinical Chief, Infectious Diseases and Immunology, UMass Memorial Health Care, Worcester, MA
Bartonellosis

Catherine Diamond, MD, MPH
Assistant Clinical Professor, Department of Internal Medicine, University of California Irvine, Irvine, CA
Pericarditis and Myocarditis

E. Dale Everett, MD
Professor of Medicine, University of Missouri Health Sciences Center, Columbia, MO
Tularemia, Leptospirosis, Borreliosis, and Brucellosis

Durland Fish, PhD
Professor of Epidemiology and Public Health, Yale School of Medicine, New Haven, CT
Lyme Disease

Jeffrey A. Gelfand, MD
Visiting Professor of Medicine, Harvard Medical School; Professor of Medicine, Tufts University School of Medicine, Boston, MA
Fever of Unknown Origin

Robert V. Gibbons, MD, MPH
Assistant Professor of Medicine, Infectious Disease Medical Researcher, Department of Virus Diseases, Walter Reed Army Institute of Research, Silver Spring, MD
Rabies

David Glembocki, MD
Assistant Professor of Pathology, University of Virginia School of Medicine, Charlottesville, VA
Protozoal Diarrhea

John W. Gnann, MD
Professor of Medicine and Microbiology, University of Alabama at Birmingham and the Birmingham Veterans Administration Medical Center, Birmingham, AL
Viral Infections of the Central Nervous System

Yoav Golan, MD
Assistant Professor of Medicine, Tufts University School of Medicine; Attending Physician, Division of Geographic Medicine and Infectious Diseases, Tufts-New England Medical Center, Boston, MA
Candidiasis

Ellie J. C. Goldstein, MD
Clinical Professor of Medicine, UCLA School of Medicine; Director, R. M. Alden Research Laboratory, Santa Monica, CA
Animal and Human Bites

Sherwood L. Gorbach, MD
Professor of Community Health and Medicine, Tufts University School of Medicine; Attending Physician, Division of Geographic Medicine and Infectious Diseases, Tufts-New England Medical Center, Boston, MA
Skin and Soft Tissue Infections

Kenneth C. Gorson, MD
Associate Professor of Neurology, Tufts University School of Medicine; Neuromuscular Service, St. Elizabeth's Medical Center, Boston, MA
Guillain-Barré Syndrome

Lisa A. Greisman, MD
Fellow in Infectious Diseases, University of Maryland, Baltimore, MD
Protozoal Diarrhea

Susan Hadley, MD
Assistant Professor of Medicine, Division of Geographic Medicine and Infectious Diseases, Tufts University School of Medicine; Staff Physician, Tufts-New England Medical Center, Boston, MA
Candidiasis

Davidson H. Hamer, MD
Assistant Professor of Medicine and Nutrition, Tufts University School of Medicine and Friedman School of Nutrition Science and Policy; Adjunct Assistant Professor of International Health, Boston University School of Public Health; Director, Traveler's Health Service and Associate Director, Infectious Diseases Center, Tufts-New England Medical Center, Boston, MA
Bacterial and Viral Diarrhea

Alan A. Harris, MD
Professor of Medicine and Preventive Medicine, Rush Medical College; Senior Assistant Chairman and Program Director, Department of Medicine and Hospital Epidemiologist, Rush Presbyterian-St. Luke's Medical Center, Chicago, IL
Therapy of Acute Bacterial Meningitis and Focal Intracranial Bacterial Infections

Thomas M. Hooton, MD
Professor of Medicine, University of Washington School of Medicine; Medical Director, Harborview Medical Center HIV/AIDS Clinic, Seattle, WA
Urinary Tract Infections

Harold W. Horowitz, MD
Professor of Medicine, New York Medical College; Attending Physician, Westchester Medical Center, Valhalla, NY
Rickettsioses, Q Fever, and Ehrichioses

C. Robert Horsburgh Jr., MD
Professor of Epidemiology, Biostatistics and Medicine, Boston University School of Public Health and Medicine; Staff Physician, Boston Medical Center and Boston Public Health Commission Tuberculosis Clinic, Boston, MA
Tuberculosis Treatment: Theory and Practice

Raul E. Isturiz, MD
Anexo A. Consultorio 37, Centro Medico de Caracas, Sotoma 3, Caracas, Venezuela
Cysticerosis

J. Michael Kilby, MD
Associate Professor of Medicine, University of Alabama at Birmingham; Medical Director, UAB HIV Clinic, Birmingham, AL
Therapy and Prophylaxis for Infectious Complications of Human Immunodeficiency Virus

Raymond S. Koff, MD
Professor of Medicine, University of Massachusetts Medical School; Director, Clinical Hepatology Research, University of Massachusetts Memorial Medical Center, Worcester, MA
Viral Hepatitis

Mark G. Kortepeter, MD, MPH, FACP
Adjunct Assistant Professor of Pathology, F. Edward Hébert School of Medicine, Uniformed Services University of the Health Sciences, Bethesda; Chief, Medical Division, U.S. Army Medical Research Institute of Infectious Diseases (USAMRIID), Fort Detrick, MD
Bioterrorism: Plague, Anthrax, and Smallpox

Leon Lai, MD
Fellow in Infectious Diseases, Tufts–New England Medical Center, Boston, MA
Candidiasis

William J. Ledger, MD
Professor and Chairman Emeritus, Weill Medical College of Cornell University; Attending Physician, New York Presbyterian Hospital, New York, NY
Obstetric-Gynecologic Infections

Donald Y. M. Leung, MD, PhD
Professor of Pediatrics, University of Colorado Health Sciences Center; Head, Division of Allergy-Immunology, National Jewish Medical and Research Center, Denver, CO
Kawasaki Syndrome

Atul Kumar Madan, MD
Assistant Professor, University of Tennessee–Memphis, Memphis, TN
Peritonitis, Abscess, Liver Abscess, and Biliary Tract Infections

Lionel A. Mandell, MD, FRCP(C)
Professor of Medicine and Chief, Division of Infectious Diseases, McMaster University, Hamilton, Ontario, Canada
Bronchitis and Pneumonia

David S. McKinsey, MD
Clinical Professor of Medicine, University of Kansas, Kansas City, KS
Fungal Infections Other Than Candidiasis

Rima McLeod, MD
Jules and Doris Stein RPB Professor, The University of Chicago; Attending Physician, The University of Chicago Hospitals, Michael Reese Hospital and Medical Center, Chicago, IL
Toxoplasmas gondii and Toxoplasmosis

H. Cody Meissner, MD
Associate Professor of Pediatrics, Tufts University School of Medicine; Chief, Division of Pediatric Infectious Disease, Tufts-New England Medical Center, Boston, MA
Kawasaki Syndrome

Barnett Nathan, MD
Assistant Professor, Departments of Neurology and Internal Medicine, University of Virginia, Charlottesville, VA
Tetanus and Botulism

Ronald Lee Nichols, MD
William Henderson Professor of Surgery, Tulane University Health Sciences Center, New Orleans, LA
Peritonitis, Abscess, Liver Abscess, and Biliary Tract Infections

Douglas R. Osmon, MD, MPH
Associate Professor of Medicine, Department of Medicine, Division of Infectious Diseases, Mayo Medical School, Rochester, MN
Osteomyelitis and Infectious Arthritis

William A. Petri, Jr., MD, PhD
Chief, Division of Infectious Diseases, University of Virginia School of Medicine, Charlottesville, VA
Protozoal Diarrhea

Elaine Petrof, MD
Postdoctoral Fellow in Infectious Diseases, The University of Chicago, Chicago, IL
Toxoplasmas gondii and Toxoplasmosis

Michael E. Pichichero, MD
Professor of Microbiology and Immunology, Pediatrics and Medicine, Elmwood Pediatric Group, University of Rochester Medical Center, School of Medicine and Dentistry, Rochester, NY
Sinusitis, Otitis Media, and Mastoiditis; Tonsillopharyngitis, Bacterial Tracheitis, Epiglottitis, and Laryngotracheitis

Lígia Camera Pierrotti, MD
Assistant Physician, Infectious and Parasitic Disease Clinic, University of São Paulo, Brazil
Leishmaniasis and Trypanosomiasis

Mark E. Rupp, MD
Associate Professor, Division of Infectious Diseases, University of Nebraska Medical Center; Medical Director, Department of Healthcare Epidemiology, Nebraska Health System, Omaha, NE
Infections Associated with Intravascular Catheters

Francisco L. Sapico, MD
Professor Emeritus of Medicine, Keck School of Medicine at the University of Southern California, Los Angeles; Former Chief, Infectious Disease Division, Rancho Los Amigos National Rehabilitation Center, Downey, CA
Foot Infections in the Diabetic Patient and Infections Associated with Pressure Sores

John Segreti, MD
Professor, Rush Medical College; Hospital Epidemiologist, Rush Presbyterian-St. Luke's Medical Center, Chicago, IL
Therapy of Acute Bacterial Meningitis and Focal Intracranial Bacterial Infections

Jerry L. Shenep, MD
Professor of Pediatrics, University of Tennessee, Memphis, College of Medicine; Member, Department of Infectious Diseases, St. Jude Children's Research Hospital, Memphis, TN
Fever in the Neutropenic Host

Jayashri Srinivasan, MD
Assistant Professor of Neurology, Tufts University School of Medicine, Boston, MA
Guillain-Barré Syndrome

James M. Steckelberg, MD
Professor of Medicine, Department of Medicine, Division of Infectious Diseases, Mayo Medical School, Rochester, MN
Osteomyelitis and Infectious Arthritis

Dennis L. Stevens, MD, PhD
Professor of Medicine, University of Washington School of Medicine, Seattle, WA; Chief, Infectious Disease Section, Veterans Affairs Medical Center, Boise, ID
Scarlet Fever and Toxic Shock Syndromes

Jeremiah G. Tilles, MD
Professor and Associate Dean, Department of Internal Medicine, University of California Irvine, Irvine, CA
Pericarditis and Myocarditis

John F. Toney, MD
Associate Professor of Medicine, Division of Infectious Diseases and Tropical Medicine, University of South Florida College of Medicine; Medical Director, Florida STD/HIV Prevention Training Center, Tampa, FL
Sexually Transmitted Diseases

Jaime R. Torres, MD, MPH, TM
Head, Infectious Diseases Section, Tropical Medicine Institute; Universidad Central de Venezuela, Escuela de Medicina "Luis Razetti," Caracas, Venezuela
Malaria and Babesiosis

Richard J. Whitley, MD
Professor of Pediatrics, Microbiology and Medicine, Loeb Eminent Scholar Chair in Pediatrics, University of Alabama at Birmingham, Birmingham, AL
Viral Infections of the Central Nervous System

Gary P. Wormser, MD
Vice Chairman, Department of Medicine and Chief, Division of Infectious Diseases, Professor of Medicine and Pharmacology, New York Medical College; Chief, Section of Infectious Diseases, Westchester Medical Center, Valhalla, NY
Lyme Disease

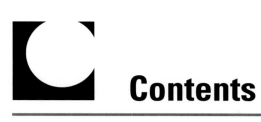

Contents

PLATE 2

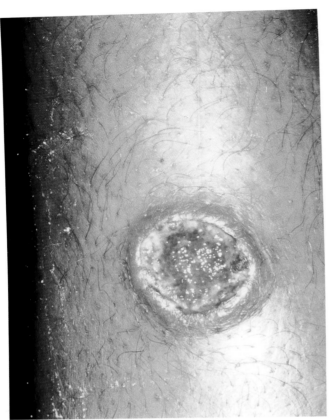

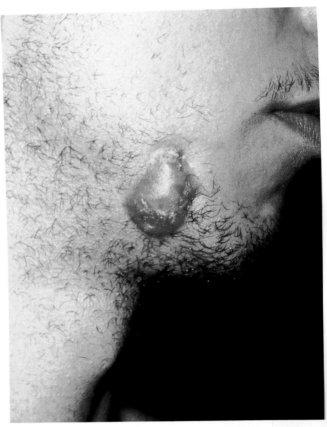

FIGURE 33–1. Localized cutaneous leishmaniasis in a Brazilian patient. An ulcer of the upper extremity caused by *Leishmania vianna brazilienses*. (Courtesy of Dr. Valdir Sabbaga Amato.)

FIGURE 33–2. Localized cutaneous leishmaniasis in a Brazilian patient. A nodular lesion mimicking tumor that was caused by *Leishmania* sp. (Courtesy of Dr. Valdir Sabbaga Amato.)

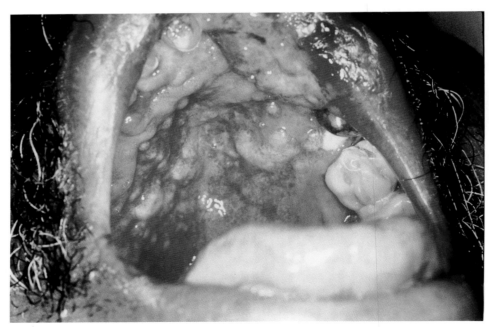

FIGURE 33–3. Mucocutaneous leishmaniasis in a Brazilian patient. A chronic lesion of the oropharyngeal mucosa caused by *Leishmania vianna brazilienses*. (Courtesy of Dr. Valdir Sabbaga Amato.)

PLATE 3

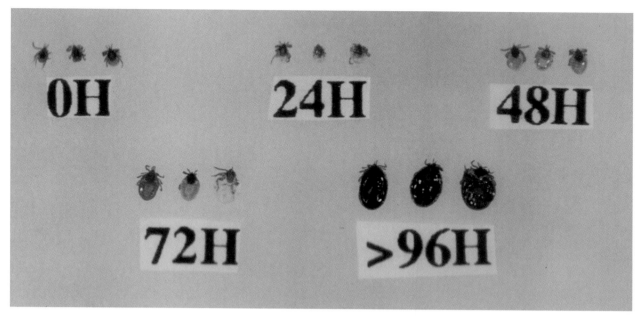

FIGURE 39–2. Nymphal *Ixodes scapularis* ticks demonstrating changes in blood engorgement after various durations of attachment to an animal host. (Photograph is a generous gift from Dr. Richard Falco.)

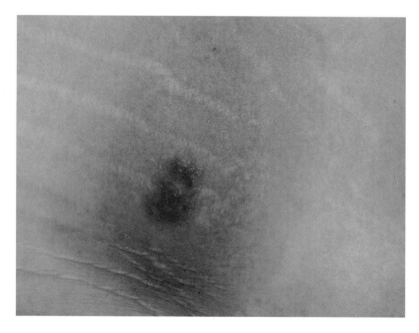

FIGURE 39–3. Example of most common clinical manifestation of Lyme disease, erythema migrans.

PLATE 4

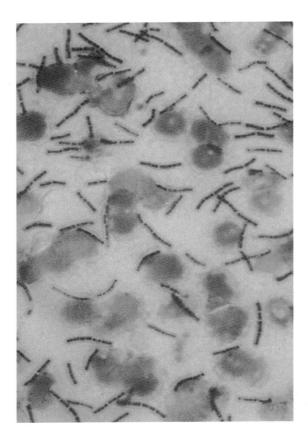

FIGURE 40–1. Peripheral blood smear from a rhesus macaque that succumbed to inhalation anthrax. (Gram stain × 1000.) (Courtesy of CoL Arthur Friedlander, MD, USAMRIID.)

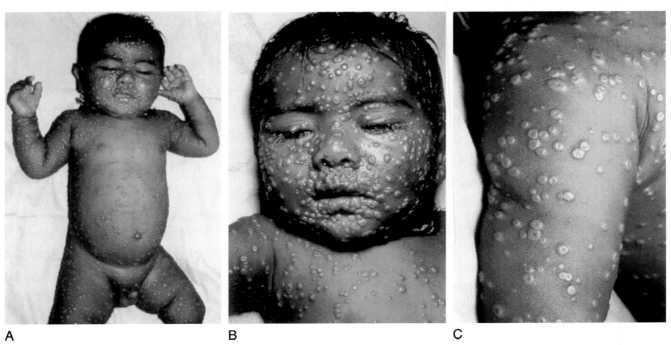

A   B   C

FIGURE 40–2. A, Full view of child with smallpox, day 7 of the rash, demonstrating more lesions on the face and extremities than on the trunk. **B**, Face of child with smallpox, day 7 of the rash, demonstrating confluence of pustules. **C**, Upper extremity of child with smallpox, day 7 of the rash, demonstrating umbilicated pustules. (From Fenner F, Henderson DA, Arita A, et al: Smallpox and its eradication. Geneva, World Health Organization, 1988.)

Antimicrobial Pharmacokinetics and Pharmacodynamics

DAVID ANDES, MD

The goal of antimicrobial therapy is to effectively eradicate pathogenic organisms while minimizing drug toxicities. Various factors affect the treatment outcomes of infectious diseases including host defense mechanisms, the site of infection, the virulence of the pathogen, and the pharmacologic properties of the antimicrobial agent used to treat the infection. The factor under the greatest control of the clinician, however, is related to the choice and dosing of antimicrobial agents. Various pharmacologic factors govern the design of an optimal antimicrobial regimen. These factors are conventionally divided into two distinct components: (1) pharmacokinetics and (2) pharmacodynamics. Examination of pharmacokinetic and pharmacodynamic relationships have been undertaken for most antibacterial drug classes and more recently for a number of antifungal and antiviral drug classes. These analyses are being recognized as increasingly important in the design of optimal antimicrobial therapies.

ANTIMICROBIAL PHARMACOKINETICS

Pharmacokinetics deals with drug disposition in the body, including the absorption, distribution, and elimination of drugs. It is these factors that determine the time course of drug concentrations in serum and tissues for a given dosing regimen. With antimicrobial agents one is particularly concerned about concentrations at the site of infection.

Kinetics at Site of Infection

Many studies have attempted to correlate antibiotic concentrations in serum with those in various tissues or sites of infection. However, several problems arise in both the measurement and the interpretation of drug concentrations in tissues. In theory, tissue concentrations consist of vascular, interstitial, and intracellular compartments. Different antimicrobial agents can vary in their ability to accumulate within these three compartments. Because most infections occur in tissues and the common pathogens are extracellular, interstitial fluid concentrations at the site of infection should be the prime determinants of efficacy. Free-drug concentrations in serum are a much better surrogate of interstitial fluid concentrations than are tissue homogenate concentrations. The majority of studies, however, have used tissue homogenates to determine antibiotic concentrations in tissue.[1–3] The relative distribution of an antibiotic within a tissue sample cannot be distinguished by this method. Tissue homogenates mix interstitial, intracellular, and vascular components together. Measurement of antibiotic concentrations in tissue homogenate tends to underestimate or overestimate interstitial fluid concentrations depending upon the ability of the antimicrobial to accumulate intracellularly. For example, one would expect that antibiotics with poor intracellular penetration, such as the β-lactams, would reach high concentrations in interstitial fluid. However, tissue homogenate methods suggest this class of drugs penetrates poorly into the interstitial space because of the dilution of samples with intracellular contents. Techniques that directly extract interstitial fluid, such as subcutaneously implanted cotton threads or more recently microdialysis methods, demonstrate high β-lactam concentrations in this tissue compartment that are similar to free drug levels in serum.[3–5]

On the other hand, since fluoroquinolones accumulate intracellularly, tissue homogenates can overestimate the concentration of drug in interstitial fluid. Not all pathogens, however, are located in the extracellular space. For example, pathogens such as *Legionella* spp. and *Chlamydia* spp. reside primarily in the intracellular space. One may then anticipate superior quinolone potency in the treatment of these infections. However, when one looks at the relationship between the amount of fluoroquinolone necessary for efficacy in the treatment of both intracellular and extracellular pathogens, no difference is seen (Fig. 1–1).[6] This may suggest that only a fraction of the amount of quinolone that is intracellular is available for antimicrobial activity. Furthermore, it is clear that not all drugs that accumulate intracellularly do so in similar intracellular compartments. For example, fluoroquinolones reside in the cytosol, whereas macrolides concentrate in phagolysosomes.[7] In the same manner, not all intracellular pathogens have the same subcellular distribution. *Legionella* spp. and *Chlamydia* spp. are found in

phagosomes, *Listeria* and *Shigella* are found in the cytosol, and *Salmonella* in phagolysosomes.[7]

Although for most antibiotics it appears that serum concentrations serve as an adequate surrogate of concentrations at the site of infection, there is growing controversy in regard to certain classes of compounds in the treatment of lower respiratory tract infections. For a few antimicrobial classes there is a large discrepancy between serum drug levels and levels in epithelial lining fluid (ELF). ELF is the fluid that bathes the respiratory epithelium, where it is believed most pathogens in bacterial pneumonia reside. For drugs such as clarithromycin and azithromycin, ELF concentrations can be 10- to 20-fold higher than in serum (Table 1–1).[8–10] Some investigators suggest that for drugs with this degree of kinetic difference, the pharmacokinetics in ELF may be better for predicting therapeutic outcomes than those in serum. However, at this time there have not been either animal model or clinical trial data supporting or disproving this hypothesis.

Impact of Protein Binding

Various pharmacologic factors can alter the activity of an antimicrobial agent. In some circumstances, protein binding can have a detrimental effect, whereas in others it may enhance dosing efficacy. The antimicrobial activity of a drug is inversely related to the extent of protein binding. Protein binding of antimicrobials in serum can interfere with biologic activity, restrict tissue distribution, and delay elimination.[11,12] For example, a drug such as phenylbutazone, known to displace penicillins from albumin-binding sites, enhances its in vitro antimicrobial activity because it is only the unbound antimicrobial fraction that is available for penetration to the site of infection for antimicrobial activity.[13] In spite of numerous investigations documenting these effects, the clinical significance of protein binding remains controversial.

A common inaccurate assumption is that a given degree of protein binding will exert a similar pharmacologic effect on all antimicrobials. On the contrary, the effects of drug protein binding on the pharmacokinetics of an antimicrobial depend on how it is eliminated by the body. Excretion of drugs into the urine occurs either by glomerular filtration or tubular secretion. Protein binding reduces the rate of elimination only of drugs cleared by glomerular filtration. In contrast, tubular secretion is largely independent of protein binding. The diverging effects of binding on drugs depending upon their route of elimination is further illustrated in Fig. 1–2, which graphs the area under the serum concentration time curve (AUC) of both total and free levels of 16 β-lactams in serum and skin blister fluid based upon the degree of protein binding.[11] In the left panel, one can see that the effect of increasing binding for drugs eliminated by tubular secretion is a progressive decline in free drug AUC in both serum and blister fluid. On the other hand, for the compounds eliminated by glomerular filtration the right

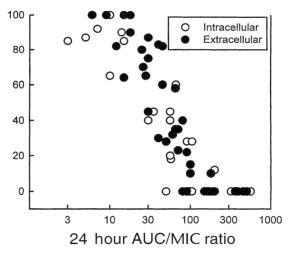

FIGURE 1–1. Relationship between the 24-hour area under the concentration curve (AUC)–to–minimum inhibitory concentration (MIC) ratio and mortality for extracellular (*hollow circles*) and intracellular (*solid circles*) pathogens in various experimental infection models in mice, rats, and guinea pigs treated with fluoroquinolones. (From Craig WA, Dalhoff A: Pharmacodynamics of fluoroquinolones in experimental animals. In Kuhlman J, Dalhoff A, Zeiler HJ, [eds]: Handbook of Experimental Pharmacology, vol 127: Quinolone Antibacterials. pp 207–232.)

24 hour AUC/MIC ratio

TABLE 1–1 ■ Comparison of Clarithromycin and Azithromycin Kinetics in Serum and ELF

Time (hours)	Clarithromycin		Azithromycin	
	Serum (μg/ml)	ELF (μg/ml)	Serum (μg/ml)	ELF (μg/ml)
4	2.0	34.5	0.08	1.0
8	1.6	26.1	0.09	2.2
12	1.2	15.1	0.04	1.0
24	0.2	4.6	0.05	1.2
24-h AUC	25	391	1.3	28

ELF, epithelial lining fluid.

AUC, area under the serum concentration–time curve;

panel demonstrates the progressive rise in AUC for total drug and the relatively constant AUC of free drug over a wide range of binding. The effect of protein binding on drugs with primarily hepatic elimination is less clear. If the drug has a low hepatic extraction ratio, however, the effect of protein binding would tend to slow elimination. On the other hand, for drugs with high extraction ratios, protein binding would affect elimination very little.

For drugs eliminated predominantly by tubular secretion or rapid hepatic extraction, the peak serum concentration level (C_{max}), the AUC, and the duration of time the serum levels exceed the minimum inhibitory concentration (MIC) expressed as the percentage of the dosing interval (T >MIC) of highly bound drugs would be reduced by high protein binding. One might predict that binding of greater than 80% would be necessary to reduce unbound free drug levels in the body enough to adversely affect antimicrobial activity. For example, in a *Staphylococcus aureus* murine peritonitis model seven penicillin antibiotics with similar in vitro activity and pharmacokinetic profiles (all eliminated by tubular secretion) with the exception of protein binding were evaluated. The amount of drug necessary to cure 50% of the mice was directly related to the degree of protein binding.[12] The higher the binding, the larger the total dose required.

For drugs eliminated predominantly by glomerular filtration, increasing binding reduces the peak level of free drug, but has no major effect on the AUC, and prolongs the duration of time free drug levels would exceed the MIC of sensitive organisms. Thus, if peak level was the important determinant of efficacy, protein binding might have a detrimental effect. On the other hand, if the duration of time serum levels exceeded the MIC were important, higher protein binding could have a beneficial effect.[14]

Pharmacokinetic Impact of Dosing Regimen Design

The pharmacokinetic parameters that characterize the time course of antibiotic concentration in serum and at sites of infection include several measures of exposure including the AUC, C_{max}, and the T >MIC (Fig. 1–3). When a drug's half-life is constant, each of these kinetic parameters will change with the dose magnitude and the frequency of drug administration. For a given total daily dose of drug the 24-hour AUC will be relatively constant regardless of the dosing regimen. Administration of large infrequent doses will result in high peak concentrations and shorter duration of time serum levels exceed a

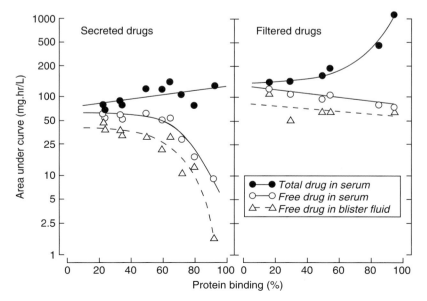

FIGURE 1–2. Relationship of the area under the concentration curve of total and free drug in serum and free drug in blister fluid with the percentage of protein bound drug for 16 β-lactams. Drugs eliminated primarily by secretion are shown in the left panel and those eliminated primarily by filtration are shown in the right panel. (From Craig WA, Suth B: Protein binding and the antimicrobial effects: Methods for the determination of protein binding. In Lorian V [ed]: Antibiotics in Laboratory Medicine, 4th ed. Baltimore, Williams & Wilkins, 1996, pp 367–402.)

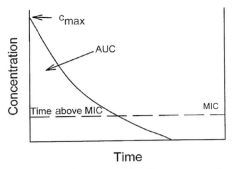

FIGURE 1–3. Antimicrobial pharmacokinetic parameters in relation to the minimum inhibitory concentration (MIC). AUC, area under the concentration curve.

threshold value such as the MIC. The converse will occur with lower drug doses administered more frequently.

PRE-PHARMACODYNAMIC DOSING TRADITIONS

Traditionally antimicrobial dosing regimens have been deduced from the relationship between some measure of drug potency in vitro such as the MIC or minimum bactericidal concentration (MBC) of an antimicrobial agent for important pathogens and the pharmacokinetics of the drug in serum. These parameters do not provide information regarding the time course activity of drugs, however. For example, the MIC does not provide information on the effect of fluctuating drug concentrations characteristically encountered in a patient, or on whether there are antimicrobial effects that can persist after drug exposure. Furthermore the MBC does not reveal the effect that higher drug concentrations have upon the extent or rate of killing. The persistent suppression of organism growth or regrowth after short antimicrobial exposures has been called the postantibiotic effect.[15] The effect of increasing concentrations upon the activity of an antimicrobial and the presence or absence of prolonged antimicrobial effects persisting after drug exposure give a much better description of the time course of activity than provided by the MIC or MBC.

The use of the MIC and MBC as predictors of antimicrobial success has led to two erroneous generalizations in dosing regimen design. One is that to achieve an optimal effect, drug concentrations must exceed the MIC for most of the dosing interval to prevent organism regrowth. Another dosing generalization has been that an increase in concentrations will invariably enhance antimicrobial efficacy.

ANTIMICROBIAL PHARMACODYNAMICS

Pharmacodynamics examines the relationships between the antimicrobial and organism over time (time course of activity), determining the effects of variations in drug kinetics on treatment outcomes. Various studies have demonstrated that the success of a drug and dosing regimen is dependent upon a measure of drug kinetics and a measure of drug potency against the infecting organism (e.g., MIC or MBC) (Fig. 1–4). Kinetic parameters, such as the C_{max}/MIC ratio, 24-hour AUC/MIC ratio, and time above MIC, have been shown to be major determinants of antimicrobial efficacy. Furthermore, studies examining the relationship between in vitro measurements (MIC and MBC) and the time course activity of various antimicrobials have demonstrated that drugs with different mechanisms of action vary in respect to the effect of increasing drug concentrations. These pharmacokinetic and pharmacodynamic analyses provide a better understanding of the relationship between drug dosing and effect. Understanding these relationships for various antimicrobial classes has proven valuable for (1) the design of appropriate dosing regimens in the treatment for both susceptible and multiply resistant pathogens, (2) the development of in vitro susceptibility breakpoints, and (3) the understanding how antimicrobial dosing relates to the emergence and spread of drug resistance.

Pharmacodynamic Determinants of Efficacy

The time course of antimicrobial activity is dependent on the drug's pharmacokinetics and two major

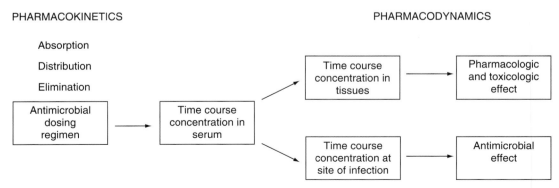

FIGURE 1–4. Overview of pharmacokinetics and pharmacodynamics in antimicrobial therapy. (From Craig WA: Pharmacokinetic/pharmacodynamic Parameters: Rationale for antibacterial dosing of mice and men. Clin Infect Dis 1998;26:1–12.)

pharmacodynamic characteristics. The first is the rate of organism killing and whether increasing drug concentrations enhances the rate and extent of killing. The second is the absence or presence of inhibitory effects on organism growth that persist after drug levels have fallen below the MIC.

Concentration-Dependent vs. Time-Dependent Killing

It is clear that progressive escalation of antimicrobial concentrations above the MIC will not enhance organism killing for all antimicrobial drug classes. For example, the killing activity of the β-lactams, macrolides, glycopeptides, clindamycin, tetracyclines, oxazolidinones, triazoles, and flucytosine is saturable with respect to the effect of drug concentration upon the rate and extent of killing.[16–24] Maximal in vitro killing with β-lactam compounds is usually observed at concentrations four to eight times the MIC.[15,25] Higher concentrations do not enhance drug activity and in fact have been demonstrated to be less active in some models (Eagle effect).[26] For agents with saturable killing with respect to drug concentration it is important to maximize the duration of time for which concentrations exceed the MIC rather than to enhance intensity of drug exposure.

On the other hand, there are a number of antimicrobial classes that do demonstrate concentration-dependent organism killing. With these drugs, higher concentrations result in more rapid and extensive organism killing. These killing characteristics have been observed with the aminoglycosides, fluoroquinolones, metronidazole, ketolides, the lipopeptide daptomycin, amphotericin B, and the new echinocandin class of antifungal.[6,15,18,19,27–31] The pharmacologic goal of dosing regimens with these agents would be to maximize concentrations by administering the total daily dose infrequently.

Persistent Effects

Prolonged persistent effects are due to various phenomena referred to as postantibiotic effects (PAE), postantibiotic sub-MIC effects, and postantibiotic-leukocyte effects.[15,25,32–34] Sub-MIC concentrations of a number of antimicrobial classes have been shown to inhibit organism growth.[35] Sub-MIC concentrations can also prolong the duration of the PAE. The postantibiotic leukocyte effect refers to the observation that organisms that have been exposed to antimicrobials are more susceptible to phagocytosis by leukocytes. This phenomenon can also prolong the duration of the PAE. Persistent suppression of growth after limited exposure was initially reported in the 1940s with penicillin.[26] These phenomena have since been demonstrated both in vitro and in animal infection models for nearly all classes of antimicrobials.[15,25] Nearly all antibacterials appear to be capable of producing persistent effects with staphylococci. For example, although cefazolin serum levels in mice remained above the MIC for only 1.6 hours, the growth of S. aureus in the thighs of treated animals was inhibited for several hours longer

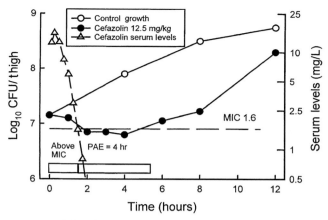

FIGURE 1–5. Cefazolin in vivo postantibiotic effect (PAE) with *Staphylococcus aureus* (American Type Culture Collection) (ATCC) 25923 in neutropenic murine thigh infection model following a 12.5 mg/kg dose. *Hollow circles* represent mean control in thighs from 3 mice. *Solid circles,* growth in thighs of treated animals. Simultaneous serum cefazolin concentrations are also shown. CFU, colony-forming units; MIC, minimum inhibitory concentration. (From Craig WA, Gudmundsson S: Postantibiotic effect. In Lorian V [ed]: Antibiotics in Laboratory Medicine, 4th ed. Baltimore, Williams & Wilkins, 1996, pp 296–329.)

(PAE 4 hours) (Fig. 1–5).[15] However, drugs that inhibit protein or nucleic acid synthesis such as the aminoglycosides, fluoroquinolones, tetracyclines, and rifampin also produce prolonged PAEs with gram-negative bacilli and streptococci.[15,25] In contrast, β-lactams produce short or no PAEs with gram-negative bacilli. The only exception is with the carbapenems, primarily with strains of *Pseudomonas aeruginosa.*

Antifungal compounds have also been shown to have prolonged persistent effects. The most pronounced effects have been observed with the polyenes such as amphotericin B.[27] The triazole compounds have not demonstrated PAEs in vitro but have demonstrated prolonged effects in vivo, probably representing significant postantifungal sub-MIC effects.[30,36,37] The pyrimidine analog flucytosine has been found to produce only modest persistent effects.[16] The new echinocandin class has also demonstrated prolonged in vitro PAEs.[30]

The clinical significance of the pharmacodynamic observation of prolonged persistent effects following a limited drug-organism interaction is related to the potential to lengthen dosing intervals. If organism growth remains suppressed after drug levels fall below the MIC, then the dosing interval could be lengthened until the beginning of organism regrowth or the end of the PAE.

Patterns of Activity

On the basis of these two time-course characteristics (effects of increasing drug concentrations and persistent effects), three patterns of antimicrobial activity have been observed. The first pattern of activity is characterized by marked concentration-dependent killing over a wide

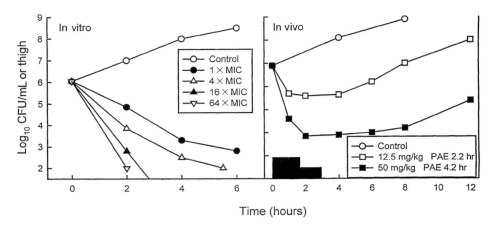

FIGURE 1–6. In vitro time-kill curves for tobramycin against *Pseudomonas aeruginosa* at escalating multiples of the minimum inhibitory concentration (MIC) (*left panel*) and bacterial counts of the same organism in vivo in neutropenic mice following single doses of tobramycin administered subcutaneously. Tobramycin MIC, 0.5 µg/mL. CFU, colony-forming units; PAE, postantibiotic effect. (From Craig WA, Gudmundsson S: Postantibiotic effect. In Lorian V [ed]: Antibiotics in Laboratory Medicine, 4th ed. Baltimore, Williams & Wilkins, 1996, pp 296–329.)

range of concentrations and prolonged persistent effects. The higher the drug concentration, the greater the extent and rate of organism killing. This is illustrated in Fig. 1–6, where the activity of tobramycin against *P. aeruginosa* is examined in vitro and in vivo.[38] In the left panel are seen marked concentration-dependent killing over a wide range of in vitro concentrations. In the right panel one can observe the prolonged dose-dependent growth suppression (PAEs) in vivo. This pattern of killing and persistent growth suppression is observed with the aminoglycosides, fluoroquinolones, metronidazole, the ketolides, daptomycin, and the polyene antifungals.[6,18,24,27,29,39–41] Since higher doses will lengthen the duration of antimicrobial effects, large infrequent doses of these agents maximizing the C_{max}/MIC ratio could enhance their activity. Furthermore, the prolonged persistent effects allow doses to be spread apart because organism regrowth will be suppressed when levels fall below the MIC.

The second pattern of activity is characterized by a saturation of the rate of killing at concentrations near the MIC and minimal-to-modest persistent effects. Thus high concentrations will not kill the organisms faster or more extensively than low concentrations. The duration of exposure rather than concentration is the major determinant of the extent of killing. This pattern of activity is

called time-dependent killing and is the pattern that characterizes the activity of all of the β-lactam antibiotics, most of the macrolides, clindamycin, the oxazolidinones, and flucytosine.[15–17,19,20,23,24,40–43] For example, Figure 1–7 shows experimental data from both an in vitro and in vivo infection model with *P. aeruginosa* examining the activity of the β-lactam, ticarcillin.[38] In both the in vitro and in vivo studies, concentrations above four times the MIC did not appreciably increase the rate of killing. Furthermore, regrowth of organisms in vivo began immediately after serum levels dropped below the MIC (no persistent effect). With these drugs the frequency of administration and the dose are both important determinants of efficacy. Time above the MIC has been the major pharmacokinetic-pharmacodynamic (PK-PD) parameter correlating with efficacy of these drugs.

The final pattern of activity is not only characterized by time-dependent killing but also by prolonged persistent effects. This unique pattern of activity characterizes the azalide azithromycin, the tetracyclines, glycopeptides, streptogramins, and the triazole antifungals.[6,19,36] The dosing frequency is usually not a major factor in determining the efficacy of these drugs. The 24-hour AUC/MIC ratio is the primary parameter correlating with in vivo efficacy because the prolonged persistent effects prevent time above MIC from becoming important.

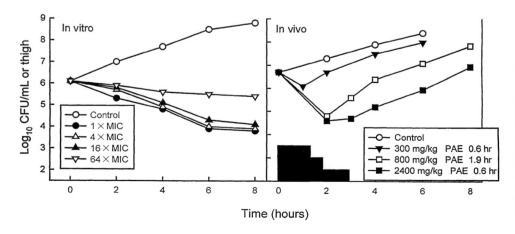

FIGURE 1–7. In vitro time-kill curves for ticarcillin against *Pseudomonas aeruginosa* at escalating multiples of the minimum inhibitory concentration (MIC) (*left panel*) and bacterial counts of the same organism in vivo in neutropenic mice following single doses of ticarcillin administered subcutaneously. Ticarcillin MIC, 16 µg/mL. CFU, colony-forming units; PAE, postantibiotic effect.

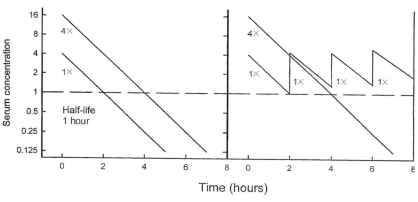

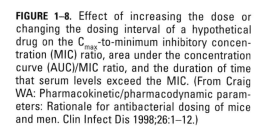

FIGURE 1–8. Effect of increasing the dose or changing the dosing interval of a hypothetical drug on the C_{max}-to-minimum inhibitory concentration (MIC) ratio, area under the concentration curve (AUC)/MIC ratio, and the duration of time that serum levels exceed the MIC. (From Craig WA: Pharmacokinetic/pharmacodynamic parameters: Rationale for antibacterial dosing of mice and men. Clin Infect Dis 1998;26:1–12.)

DETERMINATION OF PHARMACOKINETIC-PHARMACODYNAMIC PARAMETERS PREDICTING EFFICACY

The specific parameters most commonly correlated with antimicrobial treatment outcome include the C_{max}/MIC ratio, the 24-hour AUC/MIC ratio, and the T >MIC. These relationships have been examined primarily in in vitro and in vivo infection models. Investigation in human clinical trials to support or refute the observations from in vitro and animal models can be difficult because of the design of most clinical trials. Most studies are designed to determine the impact of higher doses of drug on efficacy with usually all regimens using the same dosing interval. As illustrated in the left panel of Figure 1–8, a four-fold higher dose results in a higher C_{max}/MIC ratio, a higher AUC/MIC ratio, and a longer duration of time above MIC. If a higher dose is associated with a better therapeutic outcome, it is difficult to determine which parameter is of primary importance, as all three increase to a similar extent. However, much of the interdependence among pharmacodynamic parameters can be eliminated with dosing regimens that use different dosing intervals. In the right panel of Figure 1–8 a dose administered every 2 hours is compared to a four-fold higher dose

given every 8 hours, resulting in a lower C_{max} level but a higher T >MIC. Over each 24-hour treatment regimen period the AUC/MIC ratio of the two regimens would be the same. With few exceptions, such study designs are most often not possible in human trials but are easily undertaken in animal infection models.

A study performed in the 1970s by Bodey et al did, however, vary dosing frequency comparing the efficacy of continuous vs. intermittent infusions of various antibiotics, including cefamandole, in febrile neutropenic patients.[44] For those patients infected with susceptible pathogens, continuous infusion was more efficacious than intermittent administration. Two other studies have compared continuous and intermittent infusions of ceftazidime in the treatment of gram-negative infections.[45,46] These investigations found equivalent outcomes despite the fact that less total drug was used for continuous infusion (3–4 g vs. 6 g, respectively). Both dosing regimens, however, provided concentrations that exceeded the MIC for virtually all of the dosing interval.

Although it can be difficult to vary dosing regimens in clinical trials enough to reduce the inherent parameter interrelationships, studies in animal infection models do allow dosing regimen design to eliminate much of the parameter interdependence. As shown in Figure 1–9,

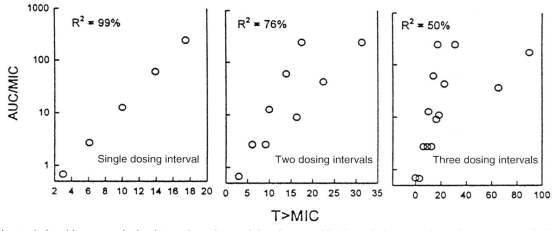

FIGURE 1–9. Interrelationship among dosing interval number and the pharmacokinetic and pharmacodynamic parameters. AUC, area under the concentration curve; MIC, minimum inhibitory concentration; R^2, percentage of variation in bacterial numbers that could be attributed to differences in each of the pharmacodynamic parameters; T > MIC, percentage of time serum concentrations exeed the MIC.

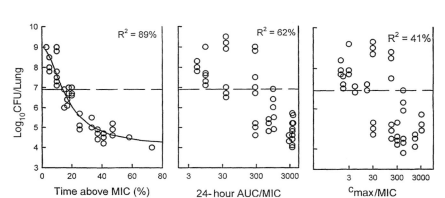

FIGURE 1–10. Relationship between three pharmacodynamic parameters (percentage of time serum levels are above minimum inhibitory concentration [MIC], the 24-hour area under the concentration curve [AUC], and the C_{max}/MIC ratio) and the number of *Pseudomonas aeruginosa* organisms in the thighs of neutropenic mice after 24 hours of therapy with meropenem. Each point represents two mice (mean of four thighs). The dotted line reflects the number of bacteria at the initiation of therapy. The R^2 value represents the percentage of variation in bacterial numbers that could be attributed to differences in each of the individual pharmacodynamic parameters. CFU, colony-forming unit.

with only a single dosing interval (frequency) there is a strong correlation between the AUC/MIC ratio and the T >MIC. With two dosing intervals the interrelationship is less significant and is even less so with three or more dosing intervals. In these experimental designs, several total daily doses and dosing intervals are used to vary the drug AUC, C_{max}, and T >MIC. Subsequent analysis of treatment endpoints in relation to each of the parameters then allows one to determine which parameter(s) best predicts antimicrobial activity.

Time above the MIC has consistently been the only PK-PD parameter that correlates with the efficacy of the β-lactams.[19] For example, Leggett et al demonstrated that the cumulative dose of several β-lactams necessary to produce 50% of the maximum bacteriologic effect (ED_{50}) increased significantly with longer dosing intervals.[23] In similar animal infection models, others have found continuous β-lactam infusion regimens to be more efficacious than those intermittently dosed.[47–49] Figure 1–10 illustrates the relationship between the treatment efficacy of the carbapenem meropenem against *P. aeruginosa* and each of the pharmacokinetic (PK) and pharmacodynamic (PD) parameters. Pairs of neutropenic mice were treated with multiple dosage regimens of meropenem that varied both in the total dose and dosing interval. Changes in organism burden after 24 hours of therapy are correlated with the C_{max}/MIC ratio, the 24-hour AUC/MIC ratio, and the

percentage of time that serum levels exceed the MIC. Regression of the data with both the AUC/MIC ratio (coefficient of determination = R^2 = 62%) and the C_{max}/MIC (R^2 = 41%) demonstrate only a modest relationship. However, regression in the percentage of time serum levels remain above the MIC (R^2 = 89%) demonstrates a strong relationship. Time above the MIC is also the parameter that correlates with the efficacy of most of the macrolides, clindamycin, oxazolidinones, and flucytosine.[16,17,19,20]

For aminoglycosides, fluoroquinolones, ketolides, streptogramins, glycopeptides, daptomycin, azithromycin, amphotericin B, and fluconazole the AUC/MIC or C_{max}/MIC ratio has been the parameter that correlate with efficacy in animal infection models.[*] Figure 1–11 demonstrates the relationship between levofloxacin efficacy and each of the PK and PD parameters in a neutropenic murine thigh infection model due to *Streptococcus pneumoniae*. The strongest parameter correlation is seen with the 24-hour AUC/MIC ratio (AUC/MIC R^2 = 88%, T >MIC R^2 = 50%, C_{max}/MIC R^2 = 45%). Several other studies have demonstrated the importance of the concentration-dependent PK and PD parameters for these drugs.[52,53] For example, Blaser et al demonstrated superior efficacy with single compared with multiple aminoglycoside and quinolone exposures, suggesting that achieving a high peak concentration is important.[28] These observations from both in vitro and in vivo models have demonstrated

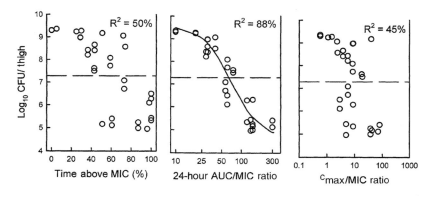

FIGURE 1–11. Relationship between three pharmacodynamic parameters (percentage of time serum levels are above minimum inhibitory concentration [MIC], the 24-hour area under the concentration curve [AUC], and the C_{max}/MIC ratio) and the number of *Streptococcus pneumoniae* organisms in the thighs of neutropenic mice after 24 hours of therapy with levofloxacin. Each point represents one mouse (mean of two thighs). The dotted line reflects the number of bacteria at the initiation of therapy. The R^2 value represents the percentage of variation in bacterial numbers that could be attributed to differences in each of the individual pharmacodynamic parameters. CFU, colony-forming unit.

*References 6,19,20,22–24,27,29,36,37,39,40,43,50,51.

that the AUC and C_{max} level are the most important dosing parameters as long as the dosing interval is not extended beyond the T >MIC and the postantibiotic effect. In these studies the major contribution of higher peak concentrations was the prevention of regrowth of resistant subpopulations.[39,54] Furthermore the toxicodynamics of the aminoglycosides would also favor optimizing the C_{max} level.[53,55–58] The aminoglycoside uptake kinetics at both of the end-organ sites of toxicity (renal tubule and organ of Corti) are saturable. Experimental animal models and human data have demonstrated that the renal cortical uptake of aminoglycosides is less with once-daily dosing than with more frequent administration (Figure 1–12).[59] Similar animal model data have also examined aminoglycoside kinetics in relation to ototoxicity.[57]

Although the glycopeptides, tetracyclines, azalides, and azoles do not exhibit concentration-dependent killing, the AUC/MIC ratio has been the major parameter correlating with therapeutic efficacy of these drugs.[19,20,36] This parameter correlation is likely related to the prolonged PAEs produced by these drug classes. For example, Louie et al demonstrated that fluconazole efficacy in a murine candidiasis model was dependent upon the total dose of drug (AUC) and not the dosing interval.[60] Subsequent evaluation demonstrated prolonged in vivo persistent effects (postantifungal effects) and confirmed the importance of the AUC in describing the activity of the azoles.[36]

Antivirals

Pharmacodynamic analysis with antivirals has been more difficult because of the lack of reproducible, standardized in vitro susceptibility testing. Various studies, however, have demonstrated the impact of dose and dosing interval upon antiviral effect and drug toxicity.[61] Drusano et al have successfully examined the effect of a variety of dosing intervals upon antiviral efficacy using an in vitro hollow fiber model.[61,62] For example, these investigations found the protease inhibitors are most efficacious when administered by continuous infusion, suggesting that the duration of time concentrations remain above a threshold level may be the most important PK-PD determinant for these compounds.[63,64] This same group of investigators found a similar dosing strategy to be important for the efficacy of zidovudine in a murine encephalitis model.[65] On the other hand, the nucleoside analog stavudine was more efficacious when dosed intermittently in the hollow fiber model.[66] Analysis of foscarnet dosing in two cytomegalovirus retinitis clinical trials have demonstrated that both efficacy and toxicity are driven by total drug exposure or the AUC.[67,68] Most recently, clinical trial analysis has demonstrated that the time to clearance of influenza is related to the AUC of the neuraminidase inhibitor.[69]

MAGNITUDE OF PHARMACOKINETIC-PHARMACODYNAMIC PARAMETER REQUIRED FOR EFFICACY AND CLINICAL IMPLICATIONS

Because PK-PD parameters can correct for differences in pharmacokinetics among species and intrinsic antimicrobial activity, it has been shown that the magnitude of these parameters necessary for efficacy is similar in different animal species including humans.[19,39,70–72] This should not be surprising since the receptor for the antimicrobial is in the pathogen and therefore is the same in both animal models and humans. Studies show that the magnitude of the PK-PD parameter required for efficacy of a drug is similar for different dosing regimens, for different drugs within the same class providing free drug concentrations are used, and for different sites of infection.[19] Furthermore, treatment of infections due to organisms with reduced susceptibility to penicillins, macrolides, and quinolones and with resistance mechanisms due to reduced target affinity also appear to require similar parameter magnitudes for efficacy.[70,73,74] Thus the results from these studies in animal infection models have been useful in the design of dosing regimens in humans.[75,76] This has been particularly helpful for the design of dosing regimens for antimicrobials under development and also for those drugs already available in clinical situations in which it is difficult to accumulate sufficient patient data, as is the case for the treatment of emerging resistant pathogens. Most recently this type of analysis has been used in the development of antimicrobial treatment guidelines for otitis media, sinusitis, and community-acquired pneumonia.[75,77–79]

β-Lactams

Studies in animal infection models and humans have demonstrated that antibiotic concentrations do not need to exceed the MIC for the entire dosing interval to exert sufficient antimicrobial activity.[43,50] For a variety

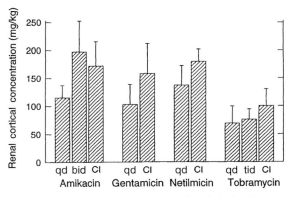

FIGURE 1–12. Renal cortical concentrations (mg/kg) of amikacin, gentamicin, netilmicin, and tobramycin following 24 hours of drug administration by continuous infusion, once daily, twice daily, or thrice daily. Cl, renal clearance. (From Urban A, Craig WA: Daily dosing of aminoglycosides. Curr Clin Top Infect Dis 1997;17:238–255.)

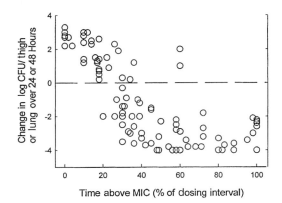

FIGURE 1–13. Relationship between time above minimum inhibitory concentration (MIC) and change in bacterial number for numerous strains of *Streptococcus pneumoniae* at 24 and 48 hours in the thighs and lungs, respectively, of neutropenic mice following treatment with amoxicillin or amoxicillin-clavulanate. CFU, colony-forming unit. (From Andes D, Craig WA: In vivo activities of amoxicillin and amoxicillin-clavulanate against *Streptococcus pneumoniae*: Application to breakpoint determinations. Antimicrob Agents Chemother 1998;42:2375–2379.)

of β-lactams, in vivo bacteriostatic efficacy in animal infection models has been observed when serum levels are above the MIC for 20% to 40% of the dosing interval, and maximal organism reductions are seen when levels are above the MIC for 60% to 70% of the interval.[19,42,70,80] Similar times above the MIC have been observed for a variety of β-lactams in several infection models and at several infection sites providing free drug levels in serum were used for comparison. Data in Figure 1–13 represent a compilation of two amoxicillin in vivo studies against *S. pneumoniae* in a thigh and lung infection model.[70] In general, the percentages of time above the MIC are slightly lower for the penicillins (30% to 40%) than for the cephalosporins (40% to 50%) and are lower yet for the carbapenems (20% to 30%).[19] These differences appear to reflect differences in the rate of killing, which is fastest with the carbapenems and slowest with the cephalosporins.

Drug kinetics in the central nervous system (CNS) are different from those in any other compartment of the body. The fluid surrounding the brain parenchyma is an ultrafiltrate of serum. Despite these clear differences in kinetics, one would expect that the patterns of antimicrobial activity predictive of efficacy outside of the CNS would also be observed in meningitis. However, the poor penetration of most antibiotics across the blood-brain barrier and the long elimination half-lives observed in cerebrospinal fluid (CSF) compared with those in serum often result in much less fluctuation in drug concentrations than is observed in other infection sites. Furthermore the goal of complete sterilization in the CSF to prevent disease relapse is with few exceptions not necessary in other infections. In general, however, the pharmacodynamic activity and relationships for the various classes of antimicrobials

do hold true in this protected site.[81–85] Here, however, it is clear that CSF levels are a much stronger predictor of efficacy than serum levels. In addition, because of the significant differences in rates of organism replication in the CSF and the lack of factors present in serum that can often contribute to prolonged PAEs, the in vitro measure with which drug kinetics are best correlated is the MBC rather than the MIC.[83] For example, the β-lactams in serum saturate killing rates with levels exceeding the MIC four or five times, whereas in the CSF maximum bactericidal activity is not observed until levels exceed the MBC by 10 to 30 times.[84] Lutsar et al found maximal killing in a rabbit meningitis model when ceftriaxone levels exceeded the MBC for 75% to 100% of the dosing interval.[85] Likewise, study of ampicillin in pneumococcal meningitis models fractionated into 8-, 12-, and 24-hour regimens showed it was successful as long as CSF ampicillin levels exceeded the MBC for about 50% of the dosing interval, similar to the relationship observed in nonmeningitis models.[79]

Although studies in animal infection models lend themselves to easily determining parameter magnitudes necessary to achieve a variety of treatment endpoints, there are obvious limitations to making similar observations in clinical trials. For prospective clinical trials there is the ethical issue regarding the design of treatment regimens thought to be potentially inferior (β-lactam regimen with T >MIC less than 40% of dosing interval). For retrospective analysis there may not be enough MIC (pathogen resistance) or drug concentration variation to produce sufficient parameter magnitude variations. However, one clinical study type that is being recognized as increasingly important for predicting pharmacodynamic outcomes in humans is the clinical trial simulation using population pharmacokinetics.[86] These investigations determine antimicrobial pharmacokinetics in patient populations representative of those who would receive antimicrobial treatments in various clinical scenarios using optimal sampling techniques. Large clinical trials of patients with varying pharmacokinetics are simulated to determine the frequency with which a specific dosing regimen would achieve a pharmacodynamic target against most (e.g., MIC$_{90}$) of the pathogens one would expect to encounter. This pharmacodynamic target is based upon results from animal model studies. The data from these studies is then related to the distribution of MICs of the target pathogens. For example, β-lactams have been shown to be effective when dosing regimens produced serum levels above the MIC for 40% to 50% of the dosing interval.

A few clinical trial investigations have lent themselves to pharmacodynamic analysis. Several investigators have performed treatment trials in acute otitis media in children and acute maxillary sinusitis in adults in which fluid at the site of infection has been sampled before and after antimicrobial therapy to determine bacteriologic cure rates.[72,87–92] Furthermore, because of the emergence of resistant *S. pneumoniae*, recent studies of this type have provided MIC fluctuation of sufficient degree to produce pharmacodynamic magnitude variation. As one would expect, the primary therapeutic agents used in these respiratory tract treatment trials have included a variety of β-lactams and macrolide antibiotics. One can estimate the time above MIC for the various antimicrobial agents based upon human pharmacokinetic data and the MICs of the organisms recovered and examine the relationship between bacteriologic treatment success and the magnitude of the T >MIC. In Figure 1–14 one sees bacteriologic cure rates in the range of 85% to 100% when β-lactam and macrolide serum levels exceeded the MIC for 40% to 50% of the dosing interval.[72] This is similar to the time above the MIC found to produce bacteriologic efficacy of β-lactam in animal models. Ambrose et al observed a similar association in the treatment of community-acquired pneumonia.[93] This study of cefuroxime therapy compared continuous infusion of 1.5 g/day (T >MIC 100%) to a lower total dose administered thrice daily (750 mg = T >MIC 50% to 60%) and found no difference in clinical endpoints. These results suggest again that serum drug levels need not exceed the MIC for the entire dosing interval and that a T >MIC magnitude of 40% to 50% may be a suitable target.

Continuous infusion is the most efficient approach for achieving serum levels above the MIC of an infecting organism. This regimen design can be convenient in the outpatient setting because of the reduction in the number of manipulations necessary. In addition, less total drug is necessary to achieve the pharmacodynamic goal. Since the rate and extent of killing with β-lactams saturates at concentrations around four times the MIC, one could choose this as a target steady state concentration for continuous infusion dosing. One could estimate the dose and rate of infusion with a simple calculation. One need only consult a common reference book to find the estimated volume of distribution and elimination half-life of the drug. Factoring in the body weight of the patient, the rate of infusion would equal (*R*):

$$R = \frac{(C_{SS})\,(V_D)\,(BW)\,(0.693)}{(t_{1/2})}$$

Where *R* is the rate of infusion (mg/h), C_{ss} is the desired steady state concentration (mg/L), V_D is the volume of distribution (L/kg), *BW* is the body weight (kg), and $t_{1/2}$ is the elimination half-life in hours. In addition to the therapeutic advantage of continuous infusion, the ability to use less total drug to achieve one's dosing goal may also reduce the incidence of dose-related adverse effects such as neutropenia. For example, a 2 g dose of ceftazidime administered every 8 hours would achieve a steady state level of 25 mg/L. On the other hand, a 3 g ceftazidime dose administered via continuous infusion would achieve a level of 29 mg/L.[45,46] Continuous infusion is best suited for β-lactam drugs with short elimination half-lives and stability at room temperature for at least 12 hours.

Macrolides

When one looks at various macrolide antibiotics, animal infection models have suggested that efficacy is achieved when serum levels are above the MIC for 50% of the dosing interval.[19,20] As with a number of β-lactams, macrolides have also been examined in double-tap otitis media trials.[72] Data in Figure 1–14 also include a number of macrolide trials. As with β-lactams, when serum levels of the macrolides exceeded the MIC 40% to 50% of the dosing interval, high rates of bacteriologic eradication are observed. For example, treatment against susceptible *S. pneumoniae* was successful in 93% and 100% of patients treated with erythromycin and clarithromycin, respectively (Table 1–2). One would anticipate this high success rate, with macrolide levels above the MIC for much more than 50% of the dosing interval. On the other hand, when examining treatment outcome against *Haemophilus influenzae* one would anticipate bacteriologic failures, as macrolide dosing would achieve levels above the MIC for far less than 50% of the dosing interval. In these trials, both erythromycin and clarithromycin resulted in bacteriologic success rates similar to those that would be observed with placebo (50% or less).

Azithromycin and Ketolides

For the azalide azithromycin and the new ketolide class of antimicrobial, the 24-hour AUC/MIC ratios have correlated best with treatment outcome. The magnitude of the azalide 24-hour AUC/MIC ratio associated with treatment efficacy in both in vivo infection models and clinical trials is near 25.[20] The clinical trial data available for azithromycin is similar to the otitis media data for the β-lactams and other macrolides. In treatment of

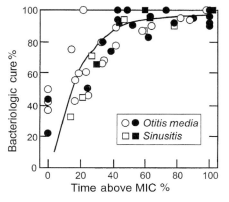

FIGURE 1–14. Relationship between the time above minimum inhibitory concentration (MIC) and bacteriologic cure for various β-lactams and macrolides against *Streptococcus pneumoniae* and *Haemophilus influenzae* in patients with otitis media and sinusitis.

TABLE 1–2 ■ **Bacteriologic Cure in Otitis Media with Macrolide Based upon Pharmacodynamic Parameter Magnitude**

	Streptococcus pneumoniae			Haemophilus influenzae		
Drug	Susceptibility	PK-PD Parameter magnitude	Bacteriologic cure	Susceptibility	PK-PD Parameter magnitude	Bacteriologic cure
Erythromycin	S	T>MIC = 88%	14/15 (93%)	R	T>MIC = 0%	3/20 (15%)
Clarithromycin	S	T>MIC = 100%	12/12 (100%)	S?	T>MIC = 0%	3/15 (20%)
Azithromycin	S	AUC/MIC = 50	15/16 (94%)	S?	AUC/MIC < 2	13/35 (37%)
	R	AUC/MIC < 0.1	1/3 (21%)	–	–	–

AUC (area under the serum concentration–time curve)/MIC (minimum inhibitory concentration) ratio; PD, pharmacodynamic; PK, pharmacokinetic; R, resistant; S, susceptible; T>MIC, percentage of time serum concentrations exceed the MIC.

azithromycin-susceptible *S. pneumoniae*, when the 24-hour AUC/MIC ratio exceeded 25, bacteriologic success was observed in 94% of patients (Table 1–2). In the treatment of resistant *S. pneumoniae* and *H. influenzae*, however, 24-hour AUC/MIC values are low (<0.1 and 2, respectively), and treatment success rates were similar to what one would expect from placebo alone (21% and 37%, respectively).[88] For treatment of pathogens in pneumonia, if ELF concentrations (24-hour AUC/MIC 25 = MIC 2 μg/mL) are more important than serum pharmacodynamics (24-hour AUC/MIC 25 = MIC 0.12 μg/mL), then one would predict being able to successfully treat infections due to organisms with MICs 16-fold higher than has been demonstrated in otitis media (Table 1–1).[10] Again, however, no studies thus far have answered this important question. Similar 24-hour AUC/MIC magnitudes may apply to the ketolides.

Fluoroquinolones

Studies against gram-negative bacilli in animals and humans have suggested that the fluoroquinolone 24-hour AUC/MIC ratio must exceed 100 to 125 to obtain high rates of bacteriologic efficacy and clinical cure.[16,24] Analyses from a variety of animal models including pneumonia, endocarditis, meningitis, and thigh infection demonstrate that the magnitude of the AUC/MIC ratio is similar regardless of the infection site.[6,19,39,40,43] Data shown in Figure 1–15 demonstrate maximal survival in a variety of gram-negative in vivo infection models when the 24-hour fluoroquinolone AUC/MIC ratio approaches a value of 100. A 24-hour AUC/MIC ratio of near 100 is essentially like maintaining serum concentrations four times above the MIC during the 24-hour dosing period. Forrest et al found a relationship between a ciprofloxacin 24-hour AUC/MIC ratio of greater than 125 and satisfactory clinical outcomes in an intensive care unit population (Fig. 1–16).[2] Lower parameter magnitudes resulted in treatment failures in nearly 50% of patients. Preston et al have also analyzed a clinical trial using levofloxacin population pharmacokinetics and demonstrated that a C_{max}/MIC ratio of greater than 12 or a 24-hour AUC/MIC ratio of 100 was predictive of treatment success.[86] However, studies using in vitro kinetic models,

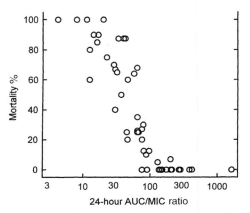

FIGURE 1–15. Relationship between the 24-hour area under the concentration curve (AUC)/minimum inhibitory concentration (MIC) ratio and mortality in various experimental infection models treated with fluoroquinolones. *Solid circles*, data from neutropenic murine thigh and lung infection models. *Hollow circles*, data from the literature using pneumonia, peritonitis, and sepsis models in mice, rats, and guinea pigs. (From Craig WA, Dalhoff A: Pharmacodynamics of fluoroquinolones in experimental animals. In Kuhlman J, Dalhoff A, Zeiler HJ [eds]: Handbook of Experimental Pharmacology, vol 127: Quinolone Antibacterial. pp 207–232.)

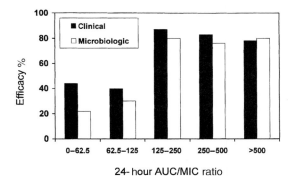

FIGURE 1–16. Relationship between the 24-hour area under the curve (AUC)/minimum inhibitory concentration (MIC) ratio and the microbiologic and clinical efficacy of ciprofloxacin in patients with serious bacterial infections. (From Craig WA: Pharmacokinetic/pharmacodynamic parameters: Rationale for antibacterial dosing of mice and men. Clin Infect Dis 1998;26:1–12.)

animal survival studies in nonimmunocompromised animals, and clinical trials suggest that the magnitude of the 24-hour AUC/MIC ratio necessary for efficacy of the quinolones in treatment of pneumococcal infections is more in the range of 25 to 35, or essentially like having levels average 1 time the MIC for the 24-hour dosing period.[6,73,94] For example, Lacy et al studied both levofloxacin and ciprofloxacin in an in vitro kinetic model of *S. pneumoniae* and observed maximal organism killing with quinolone AUC/MIC ratios of approximately 30.[95] This is also supported by studies in non-neutropenic pneumococcal infection models with a number of fluoroquinolones in which maximal survival has been observed when the 24-hour AUC/MIC ratio magnitude approaches 25 to 30 (Fig. 1–17). More recently, Ambrose et al examined the relationship between the fluoroquinolone AUC/MIC ratio and treatment outcomes in patients with pneumococcal lower respiratory tract infections. In this randomized, double-blind evaluation a fluoroquinolone 24-hour AUC/MIC ratio of 50 was associated with a 90% probability of bacterial eradication.[96] This AUC/MIC magnitude is similar to that seen in experimental models and offers an explanation for the good efficacy of the newer fluoroquinolones against *S. pneumoniae*.

Aminoglycosides

Several investigators have found a C_{max}/MIC ratio of 8 to 10 in both in vitro and in vivo models to be associated with efficacy and the prevention of the emergence of resistant subpopulations.[28,29,50,54] Recent analysis of multiple aminoglycoside animal model studies found a strong relationship between the AUC/MIC ratio and bacteriologic efficacy in meningitis.[82] In this analysis a maximal reduction in bacterial numbers was observed when the aminoglycoside AUC/MIC ratio exceeded 50. One clinical nosocomial pneumonia trial also reported a clinical response rate (reduction in fever and leukocytosis) in more than 90% of patients when the C_{max}/MIC ratio reached 8 to 10.[97] Of further interest is the fact that most patients did not achieve this dosing goal with the empiric

use of 5 mg/kg/day of the aminoglycoside. Moore et al found a similar association between C_{max}/MIC ratio and survival in the treatment of bacteremia.[98] Once-daily aminoglycoside administration is the most efficient and reliable strategy to achieve high peak concentrations. A number of other investigations have studied the impact of dosing regimens on the efficacy of aminoglycosides in clinical trials.[99,100] The results of these studies have been examined in 7 meta-analyses and suggest a small, nonsignificant trend toward better efficacy in 5 of 7 analyses and a 26% reduction in nephrotoxicity in the largest analysis with the once-daily administration of aminoglycosides.[41,101–107] Other clinical studies have demonstrated that the onset of nephrotoxicity is delayed for several days (3 vs. 7 days) when these drugs are administered once-daily rather than in multiple-daily doses.[108–111] However, once-daily dosing may not be best in all situations. Animal models of enterococcal endocarditis have demonstrated a more significant reduction in vegetation organism counts when aminoglycosides were administered in multiple rather than single daily doses.[112]

Oxazolidinones

Although the distribution of linezolid MICs have thus far been narrow, animal model studies suggest that efficacy with these compounds is observed when dosing regimens achieve serum levels above the MIC for 50% of the dosing interval.[17] The studied dosage regimen of this drug provides serum levels above an MIC of 8 μg/mL for 50% of the dosing interval and has proven effective in various comparative clinical trials.

Fluconazole

Although in vitro susceptibility testing with antifungals has only recently been standardized, data from a number of animal model studies and clinical trials suggest that triazole MICs correlate reasonably well with treatment outcomes. For fluconazole, study in animal models has found treatment success associated with 24-hour AUC/MIC ratios near 25 over a wide range of MICs.[36] This 24-hour AUC/MIC ratio correlates closely with the dose-MIC relationship recently established by the NCCLS (National Committee for Clinical Laboratory Standards).[113] As shown in Table 1–3, a fluconazole dose of 200 mg/day would produce a 24-hour AUC/breakpoint MIC (8 μg/mL) ratio of near 20. With dose escalation to 400 or 800 mg/day, a similar ratio would be seen at the susceptible-dose-dependent breakpoints (16–32 μg/mL), again similar to the parameter magnitude observed in animal infection models.

Flucytosine

Andes and van Ogtrop found maximal reduction in *Candida* burden in the kidneys of mice when flucytosine serum levels were above the MIC of the organism for

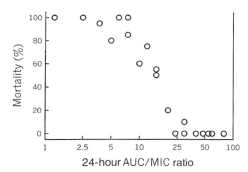

FIGURE 1–17. Relationship between the 24-hour area under the concentration curve (AUC)/minimum inhibitory concentration (MIC) ratio and survival in the neutropenic murine thigh and lung infection models infected with *S. pneumoniae* treated with fluoroquinolones.

TABLE 1–3 ■ Comparison of Fluconazole AUC/MIC Ratio to Results from Clinical Trials

NCCLS breakpoint (mg/L)	Dose (mg/day)	AUC (mg/hr/L)	AUC/Breakpoint MIC ratio	Clinical success (%)
R ≥64	800	475	7	54
S-DD 16–32	400–800	240–475	15	86
S ≤ 8	200	134	17	81

AUC, area under the serum concentration–time curve; MIC, minimum inhibitory concentration; NCCLS, National Committee for Clinical Laboratory Standards; R, resistant; S, susceptible; S-DD, susceptible-dose-dependent breakpoints.

50% of the dosing interval.[16] These studies, however, included only a single pathogen. If, however, this parameter magnitude is relevant for other organisms, it would suggest that we are currently overdosing this compound with a narrow therapeutic window. Current administration of 100 to 150 mg/kg/day in four divided doses would provide time above the MIC_{90} of commonly treated pathogens for more than 100% of the dosing interval, even if the interval were to be doubled.

PHARMACODYNAMICS OF COMBINATION ANTIMICROBIAL THERAPY

Combination therapy has been used to enhance the antimicrobial activity of two or more drugs whose activity together is either additive or synergistic. In addition, various drug combinations have also been used to reduce the emergence of resistance to one or both of the compounds and to reduce drug toxicity by occasionally allowing the administration of lower doses of drugs with a narrow therapeutic index.

A large number of in vitro studies have used a variety of techniques to examine the effects of different antimicrobial classes in combination.[91,114–116] Despite the extensive fund of pharmacodynamic knowledge available for an antimicrobial used alone, however, few studies have analyzed the in vivo pharmacodynamics of these agents used in combination. Thomas et al suggested that adding the AUC/MIC ratio of an aminoglycoside or fluoroquinolone to the AUC/MIC ratio of a β-lactam was an appropriate way to estimate their pharmacodynamic activity in combination.[117] Mouton et al however, recently demonstrated that the in vivo pharmacodynamics predictive of efficacy of β-lactams, aminoglycosides, and fluoroquinolones when used in combination is similar to that predictive of efficacy when these compounds are used alone.[118] Thus the PK-PD parameter and parameter magnitude predictive of efficacy for individual drugs are class dependent when used in combination and are similar to when they are used as single agents.

TREATMENT OF RESISTANT ORGANISMS

Studies with a number of antimicrobial classes against multiply resistant pathogens have observed similar treatment outcomes when dosing regimens are able to produce pharmacodynamic parameter magnitudes equal to those shown to be successful in the treatment of susceptible pathogens. For example, in vivo pharmacodynamic studies with amoxicillin and amoxicillin-clavulanate against a large number of strains of *S. pneumoniae*, including strains classified as penicillin-susceptible, -intermediate, and -resistant, with amoxicillin MICs varying 60-fold, demonstrated that the magnitude of the T >MIC parameter required to produce various microbiologic outcomes (static dose, ED_{50-80}, and mortality) was similar for all of the organisms (Fig. 1–18).[70] Maximal killing over 24 hours was observed when serum levels remained above the MIC for 50% to 60% of the dosing interval for both susceptible and resistant *S. pneumoniae*. In subsequent studies involving a longer course of therapy (4 days), 100% survival was achieved when dosing resulted in serum levels above the MIC for at least 40% of the dosing interval. Analysis of cefprozil therapy in this model has demonstrated similar results.[119]

In the past 5 years the NCCLS has begun to review susceptibility breakpoints for oral β-lactams. Various types of data have been factored into breakpoint determinations, including the population distribution of organism MICs, the activity of the antimicrobial in question against organisms with known mechanisms of resistance, the correlation of clinical outcome with susceptibility results, and, more recently, pharmacodynamic predictions from in vivo infection models.

In situations in which there is insufficient clinical data with various compounds against less susceptible pathogens such as β-lactam-resistant pneumococci, the NCCLS is relying upon PK-PD parameter magnitudes defined in animal infection models.[120] For example, a pharmacodynamic template for β-lactams can be based upon a pharmacodynamic goal of maintaining serum levels above the MIC of the infecting pathogen for 40% of the dosing interval. Thus susceptibility breakpoints (MICs) for various antimicrobial-organism combinations can be based upon the highest MIC that would produce levels above the MIC for 40% of the dosing interval. Table 1–4 lists the current susceptibility breakpoints for a number of oral and parenteral β-lactams and the highest MIC for which serum levels would still remain above the MIC for 40% of a standard dosing regimen. One can see that often times the current breakpoint MIC is lower than the

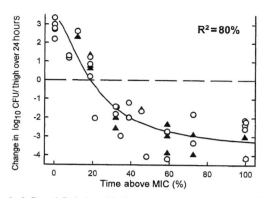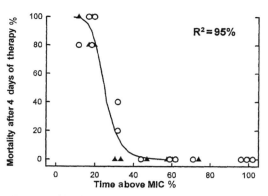

FIGURE 1–18. *Left Panel,* Relationship between change in $\log_{10}$ colony-forming units (CFU) per/thigh over 24 hours and duration of time that serum levels exceed the minimum inhibitory concentration (MIC) following doses of 2, 7, and 20 mg/kg of amoxicillin every 8 hours and doses of 7 mg/kg of amoxicillin-clavulanate every 8 hours. Each value represents the mean for two thighs. *Right Panel,* Relationship between mortality and duration of time that serum levels exceed the MIC following doses of amoxicillin at 2, 7, and 20 mg/kg and amoxicillin-clavulanate at 7 mg/kg every 8 hours. Each value represents the mean for 5 mice. R^2, percentage of variation in bacterial numbers that could be attributed to differences in each of the pharmacodynamic parameters. (From Andes D, Craig WA: In vivo activities of amoxicillin and amoxicillin-clavulanate against *Streptococcus pneumoniae*: Application to breakpoint determinations. Antimicrob Agents Chemother 1998;42: 2375–2379.)

TABLE 1–4 ■ **Accepted and Pharmacodynamic in Vitro Susceptibility Breakpoint of Selected β-Lactams**

Drug–Dosing regimen	Susceptibility breakpoint MIC (μg/mL)	Pharmacodynamic breakpoint MIC (μg/mL) (T>MIC 40%)
Amoxicillin 500 mg PO tid (40 mg/kg)	2.0*	2.0
Amoxicillin 1 g PO tid (80 mg/kg)	2.0*	4.0
Cefaclor 500 mg PO tid	1.0*	0.5
Cefuroxime 500 mg PO bid	1.0*	1.0
Cefprozil 500 mg PO bid	1.0*	1.0
Cefpodoxime 200 mg PO bid	0.5*	0.5
Cefixime 400 mg PO bid	–	0.5
Loracarbef 400 mg PO bid	–	1.0
Penicillin G 2 MU IV qid	<0.1*	4.0
Ampicillin 1 g IV qid	<0.1*	4.0
Nafcillin 2 g IV qid	1.0†	1.0
Ticarcillin-Clavulanate 3 g IV qid	8.0†	16
Cefotaxime 1 g IV tid	0.5*	2.0
Cefuroxime 0.75 g IV tid	0.5*	4.0
Ceftriaxone 1 g IV qid	0.5*	2.0
Cefepime 1 g IV bid	0.5*	4.0
Meropenem 0.5 g IV tid	4.0†	4.0
Imipenem 500 mg IV qid	4.0†	4.0

MIC, minimum inhibitory concentration; T>MIC, percentage of time serum levels remain above the MIC.

Streptococcus pneumoniae.

†Staphylococcus aureus.*

pharmacodynamic breakpoint, particularly for the parenteral agents. The susceptibility breakpoints for the parenteral compounds are almost always lower because that these values have been based upon the treatment of meningitis, where higher serum levels would be necessary to achieve adequate CSF levels. There are numerous case reports of meningitis treatment failures to support these breakpoints.[121,122] In most situations, however, these breakpoints would be too high to guide therapy of non-CNS sites such as pneumonia. A number of clinical trials in the literature have demonstrated successful outcomes when these agents have been used to treat these less sus-

ceptible pathogens in community-acquired pneumonia. Pallares et al were the first to address this issue. For a cohort of more than 500 patients with severe community-acquired pneumonia receiving both penicillins and third-generation cephalosporins, mortality rates were independent of the susceptibility of the pathogen (Table 1–5).[123] Most recently Feiken et al examined risk for mortality in more than 4000 patients with bacteremic pneumococcal pneumonia.[124] In this large analysis investigators were able to demonstrate a significant association between MIC elevation and mortality. As shown in Table 1–6 however, it was not until the penicillin MIC

TABLE 1–5 ■ Treatment Impact of Drug-Resistant Pneumococci on Mortality in Community-Acquired Pneumonia

Penicillin MIC (μg/ml)	Mortality/Patients in group (%)	
	Penicillin/Ampicillin	Ceftotaxime/Ceftriaxone
S = ≤0.06	24/126 (19)	32/127 (25)
I = 0.12–1.0	4/14 (24)	5/33 (15)
R = 2–4	6/24 (25)	13/59 (22)

I, penicillin-intermediate; MIC, minimum inhibitory concentration; R, penicillin-resistant; S, penicillin susceptible.

TABLE 1–6 ■ Risk for Mortality in Bacteremic Pneumococcal Pneumonia Based upon β-Lactam MIC

Drug MIC	Odds ratio (95% CI)
Penicillin G MIC ≥ 4.0	7.1 (1.7–30)
Penicillin G MIC = 2.0	0.7 (0.1–5.5)
Penicillin G MIC = 0.12–1.0	1.0 (0.3–3.0)
Penicillin G MIC ≤ 0.12	Referent
Cefotaxime MIC ≥ 2.0	5.9 (1.1–33)
Cefotaxime MIC = 1.0	1.5 (0.3–7.4)
Cefotaxime MIC ≤ 1.0	Referent

CI, confidence interval; MIC, minimum inhibitory concentration.

reached 4 μg/mL and the cefotaxime MIC reached 2 μg/mL that the risk of death increased. In both of these circumstances, one would have predicted treatment failure for these patients, as dosing regimens would not produce the pharmacodynamic goal of T >MIC of 40%. Re-evaluation of susceptibility breakpoints for the parenteral β-lactams in the treatment of non-CNS infections is under consideration.

Animal model studies with numerous fluoroquinolones, macrolides, and ketolides have likewise demonstrated that the pharmacodynamic parameter magnitude required to successfully treat infections due to pathogens with reduced susceptibility is most often the same as that needed against susceptible organisms.[73,74] This has been the case for all organisms whose mechanism of resistance

is due to changes in drug target affinity. This would include macrolide- and ketolide-resistant pathogens with methylase mutations and fluoroquinolone mutations in one of the gyrases. There has, however, been a general resistance mechanism for which the degree of in vitro resistance does not appear to predict the in vivo behavior. Pneumococci exhibiting resistance due to an efflux mechanism appear significantly more susceptible in vivo than the in vitro MIC testing would suggest.[73,74] For example, the magnitude of the AUC/MIC ratio required to produce a net bacteriostatic effect was twofold to sevenfold less than that required for either the susceptible organisms or those with altered ribosomal affinity (Table 1–7).[74] Similarly, in studies with the a new fluoroquinolone against susceptible organisms and those resistant because of GyrA, ParC, or ParE, a similar PK-PD parameter magnitude was required to achieve efficacy.[73] Studies with organisms overexpressing efflux pumps, however, were more susceptible than would be predicted. The magnitude of the AUC/MIC ratio necessary to achieve a bacteriostatic effect was twofold to fivefold less than that required for either the susceptible organisms or those with altered gyrase enyzmes. The reason(s) underlying this in vitro–in vivo differential with organisms expressing these efflux pumps remains unclear.

PHARMACODYNAMIC PARAMETER AND MAGNITUDE REQUIRED TO PREVENT THE EMERGENCE OF RESISTANCE

Clearly a number of factors can contribute to the development or emergence of antimicrobial resistance, including the organism inoculum and the varying mutational rates of different microbial species.[67,125,126] However, there is also a clear association between antimicrobial exposure and the selection or development of resistance. A growing knowledge base from in vitro and animal infection models has been used to examine the relationships between antimicrobial PK-PD parameters for different antimicrobials and the emergence and prevention of resistant pathogens.

TABLE 1–7 ■ Bacteriostatic Dose and Corresponding AUC/MIC Ratio of New Ketolide and Fluoroquinolone against Various Susceptible and Resistant *Streptococcus pneumoniae* Strains

Drug	MIC (mg/L)	Resistance mechanism	Bacteriostatic dose (mg/kg/day)	AUC/MIC ratio
Ketolide	0.015	Susceptible	8–20	260–826
	0.06	Decreased affinity (MLS$_B$)	73–96	660–883
	0.5	Drug efflux (Mef)	145–153	160–165
Fluoroquinolone	0.008–0.015	Susceptible	112–781	10–73
	0.06–0.5	GyrA, ParC, ParE	224–1222	10–56
	0.06–0.12	Efflux	192 (135–286)	14 (11–16)

AUC, area under the serum concentration time curve; MIC, minimum inhibitory concentration.

Resistance Mutations

In most clinical trials and in vivo animal infection models, analysis demonstrating the relationship between antimicrobial dosing and resistance mutations has been extraordinarily difficult because of the relatively low mutation rates. In a nosocomial pneumonia trial of ciprofloxacin therapy, however, in those patients infected with *P. aeruginosa*, six patients developed drug resistance during therapy.[127] In this small cohort of patients who developed resistance the ciprofloxacin C_{max}/MIC ratio was less than 8. In the group of four patients whose C_{max}/MIC ratio exceeded 8, however, only one developed resistance. Thomas et al similarly examined data from a larger cohort of 107 patients with pneumonia.[117] In this cohort, 25% of patients developed drug resistance. The incidence of resistance was highest for *P. aeruginosa* and β-lactamase (type 1)–producing gram-negative bacilli (45% and 27%, respectively). The investigators calculated the 24-hour AUC/MIC ratios from patients' serum concentrations and the organisms' MIC. The authors then determined the relationship between the magnitude of the 24-hour AUC/MIC ratio and the development of resistance. They found that quinolone AUC/MIC ratios exceeding 100 and C_{max}/MIC ratios of greater than 8 were associated with the emergence of resistance in 9% of cases, whereas resistance developed 82% of the time when these ratios were less than 100 and 8, respectively. It is not clear if the same magnitudes for the C_{max}/MIC and 24-hour AUC/MIC ratios apply to gram-positive cocci such as *S. pneumoniae*, as these studies had only a single case of infection with this organism.

In vitro models have been more successful in detecting resistant mutants following exposure to varying drug concentrations over time.[128,129] Several investigators have explored the concept of a mutation prevention concentration (MPC), defined as the lowest drug concentration in agar that prevents the growth of any colonies of resistant mutants for different organisms and for different drugs.[126] For example, the MPC_{90} for a variety of fluoroquinolones against *S. pneumoniae* has varied from 4 to 8 times the MIC_{90}.[130] One potential disadvantage of this testing system is that it only measures the effect of long-term exposure to a constant concentration and does not examine the effect of shorter term exposures to similar or higher concentrations. Further studies are necessary to examine the clinical relevance of these observations.

Selection of Resistant Mutants

Although it has been difficult for animal infection models to examine the relationship between the time course of antimicrobial exposure and the development of resistance mutations, these models have been useful for describing the relationship between antimicrobial pharmacodynamics and the selection of resistant subpopulations. For example, several animal and in vitro studies have suggested that a C_{max}/MIC ratio of at least 8 to 10 can

significantly reduce the emergence of resistant subpopulations with fluoroquinolones and aminoglycosides.[28,39,54]

Spread of Resistant Mutants

Along with eradicating the infecting pathogen from the site of infection, antimicrobial therapy for respiratory infections must aim to prevent the selection of resistant mutants, and be capable of minimizing the carriage of resistant strains in the nasopharynx.[131] The ability to achieve these pharmacologic goals depends to some extent on the PK-PD characteristics of the antibiotic and on the dosing regimen. For example, it has been theorized that long half-life drugs that provide sustained but sub-MIC concentrations may be more likely to promote selection of resistant pathogens.

Antibiotics vary in their ability to eradicate the pathogen from the nasopharynx. Times above MIC around 80% to 100% are required for β-lactams to achieve eradication, which is only possible at higher doses than are currently used for most β-lactams. Macrolides have been shown to reduce colonization in some studies, but more often macrolide therapy increases carrier status.[33,106,132–134] For example, Ghaffar et al recently examined carriage of pneumococci in the nasopharynx of children following therapy with the extra-strength formulation of amoxicillin-clavulanate and azithromycin.[135] Both amoxicillin-clavulanate and azithromycin were successful in eradicating susceptible pneumococci (10/10 [100%] and 8/10 [80%], respectively). On the other hand, amoxicillin-clavulanate eradicated intermediate and resistant pneumococci in 82% (14/17) of patients, whereas azithromycin therapy cleared resistant organisms in only 36% (5/14) of patients. Overall amoxicillin-clavulanate was superior to azithromycin for eradicating the pneumococcal carrier state ($P = 0.04$). The fluoroquinolones are generally effective at eradicating organisms from the nasopharynx.

Clearly much more information is needed to determine which PK-PD parameter and its magnitude that is necessary to prevent the emergence of resistant organisms with commonly used antimicrobials.

SUMMARY

Pharmacokinetic and pharmacodynamic parameters are the major determinants of the efficacy of antimicrobial therapy. The ability of a drug to reach the magnitude of the parameter required for efficacy against common pathogens and emerging resistant organisms should be considered in drug and dosage regimen selection for empiric therapy (Table 1–8). Antimicrobial pharmacodynamic analyses have been useful for the development of (1) in vitro susceptibility breakpoints, (2) antimicrobial treatment guidelines, (3) new drug formulations (e.g., high-dose/ratio amoxicillin-clavulanate and extended

TABLE 1–8 ■ Pharmacodynamic Activity of Antimicrobials

Drug class	Pattern of activity		Pharmacodynamics	
	Concentration dependent	Persistent effects	Parameter	Magnitude
Antibacterials				
Penicillins	No	Minimal	T>MIC	40%
Cephalosporins	No	Minimal	T>MIC	50%
Carbapenems	No	Minimal	T>MIC	25%
Macrolides	No	Modest	T>MIC	40%–50%
Azithromycin	No	Prolonged	AUC/MIC	25
Oxazolidinones (linezolid)	No	Minimal	T>MIC	40%
Trimethoprim-Sulfamethoxazole	No	Minimal	T>MIC	ND
Clindamycin	No	Minimal	T>MIC	ND
Glycylcyclines	No	Modest	T>MIC	ND
Fluoroquinolones	Yes	Prolonged	AUC/MIC	25 (G +) 100 (G –)
Aminoglycosides	Yes	Prolonged	C_{max}/MIC	8–10
Tetracyclines	No	Prolonged	AUC/MIC	ND
Ketolides	Yes	Prolonged	AUC/MIC	25–50
Streptogramins (Synercid)	No	Prolonged	AUC/MIC	ND
Daptomycin	Yes	Prolonged	AUC/MIC	ND
Glycopeptides (vancomycin)	No	Prolonged	AUC/MIC	ND
Metronidazole	Yes	Prolonged	C_{max}/MIC	ND
Antifungals				
Triazoles	No	Prolonged	AUC/MIC	25
Polyenes	Yes	Prolonged	C_{max}/MIC	ND
Flucytosine	No	Modest	T>MIC	25%–50%
Echinocandins	Yes	Prolonged	—	—
Antivirals				
Zidovudine (AZT)	ND	ND	Time > Threshold	ND
Stavudine (D4T)	ND	ND	AUC/Threshold	ND
Protease inhibitors	ND	ND	Time > Threshold	ND
Foscarnet	ND	ND	AUC/Threshold	ND
Neuraminidase inhibitors	ND	ND	AUC/Threshold	ND

AUC, area under the serum concentration–time curve; MIC, minimum inhibitory concentration; ND, no data; T>MIC, percentage of time serum concentration exceed the MIC.

release clarithromycin), and for (4) dose selection for clinical trials.

REFERENCES

1. Fish DN, Gotfried MH, Danziger LH, Rodvold KA: Penetration of clarithromycin into lung tissues from patients undergoing lung resection. Antimicrob Agents Chemother 1994;38:876–878.
2. Forrest A, Nix DE, Ballow CH, et al: Pharmacodynamics of intravenous ciprofloxacin in seriously ill patients. Antimicrob Agents Chemother 1993;37:1073–1081.
3. Ryan DM, Hodges B, Spencer GR, Harding SM: Simultaneous comparison of three methods for assessing ceftazidime penetration into extravascular fluid. Antimicrob Agents Chemother 1982;22:995–998.
4. Muller M, Stass H, Brunner M, et al: Penetration of moxifloxacin into peripheral compartments in humans. Antimicrob Agents Chemother 1999;43:2345–2349.
5. Walstad RA, Hellum KB, Thurmann-Nielsen E, Dale LG: Pharmacokinetics and tissue penetration of timentin: A simultaneous study of serum, urine, lymph, suction blister, and subcutaneous thread. J Antimicrob Chemother 1986;17(Suppl C):71–80.
6. Craig WA, Dalhoff A: Pharmacodynamics of fluoroquinolones in experimental animals. In Kuhlman J, Dalhoff A, Zeiler HJ

(eds): Handbook of Experimental Pharmacology, Vol 127. Quinolone Antibacterials. Berlin, Springer-Verlag, 1998, pp 207–232.
7. Tulkens PM: Intracellular pharmacokinetics and localization of antibiotics as predictors of their efficacy against intraphagocytic infections. Scand J Infect Dis 1990;74(Suppl):209–217.
8. Olsen KM, San Pedro G, Gann LP, et al: Intrapulmonary pharmacokinetics of azithromycin in healthy volunteers given five oral doses. Antimicrob Agents Chemother 1996;40:2582–2585.
9. Patel KB, Xuan D, Tessier PR, et al: Comparison of bronchopulmonary pharmacokinetics of clarithromycin and azithromycin. Antimicrob Agents Chemother 1996;40:2375–2379.
10. Rodvold KA, Gotfried MH, Danziger LH, Servi RJ: Intrapulmonary steady-state concentrations of clarithromycin and azithromycin in healthy adult volunteers. Antimicrob Agents Chemother 1997;41:1399–1402.
11. Craig WA, Suh B: Protein binding and the antimicrobial effects: Methods for the determination of protein binding. In Lorian V (ed): Antibiotics in Laboratory Medicine, 4th ed. Baltimore, Williams & Wilkins, 1996; pp 367–402.
12. Merrikin JJ, Briant J, Rolinson GN: Effect of protein binding on antimicrobial activity in vivo. J Antimicrob Chemother 1983;11:233–238.
13. Kunin CM: Enhancement of antimicrobial activity of penicillins and other antibiotics in human serum by competitive serum binding inhibitors. Proc Soc Exp Biol Med 1964;117:69–73.

14. Andes D, Walker R, Ebert S, Craig WA: Increasing protein binding of cefonicid enhances its in-vivo activity in an animal model. 34th Interscience Conference on Antimicrobial Agents and Chemotherapy, American Society for Microbiology, 1994.

15. Craig WA, Gudmundsson S: Postantibiotic effect. In Lorian V (ed): Antibiotics in Laboratory Medicine, 4th ed. Baltimore, Williams & Wilkins, 1996, pp 296–329.

16. Andes D, van Ogtrop ML: In vivo characterization of the pharmacodynamics of flucytosine in a neutropenic murine disseminated candidiasis model. Antimicrob Agents Chemother 2000;44:938–942.

17. Andes D, Van Ogtrop M, Craig WA: Pharmacodynamic activity of a new oxazolidinone in an animal infection model. 38th Interscience Conference on Antimicrobial Agents and Chemotherapy, American Society for Microbiology, 1998.

18. Craig WA, Andes D: Differences in the in vivo pharmacodynamics of telithromycin and azithromycin against *Streptococcus pneumoniae*. In 40th Interscience Conference on Antimicrobial Agents and Chemotherapy, American Society for Microbiology, 2000.

19. Craig WA: Pharmacokinetic/pharmacodynamic parameters: Rationale for antibacterial dosing of mice and men. Clin Infect Dis 1998;26:1–12.

20. Craig WA: Postantibiotic effects and the dosing of macrolides, azalides, and streptogramins. In Zinner SH, Young LS, Acar JF, Neu HC (eds): Expanding Indications for the New Macrolides, Azalides and Streptogramins. New York, Marcel Dekker, 1997; pp 27–38.

21. Klepser ME, Wolfe EJ, Jones RN, et al: Antifungal pharmacodynamic characterization of fluconazole and amphotericin B tested against *Candida albicans*. Antimicrob Agents Chemother 1997;41:1392–1395.

22. Knudsen JD, Fuursted K, Raber S, et al: Pharmacodynamics of glycopeptides in the mouse peritonitis model of *Streptococcus pneumoniae* and *Staphylococcus aureus* infection. Antimicrob Agents Chemother 2000;44:1247–1254.

23. Leggett JE, Fantin B, Ebert S, et al: Comparative antibiotic dose-effect relations at several dosing intervals in murine pneumonitis and thigh-infection models. J Infect Dis 1989;159:281–292.

24. Leggett JE, Ebert S, Fantin B, Craig WA: Comparative dose-effect relations at several dosing intervals for beta-lactam, aminoglycoside and quinolone antibiotics against gram-negative bacilli in murine thigh-infection and pneumonitis models. Scand J Infect Dis Suppl 1991;74:179–184.

25. Vogelman B, Gudmundsson S, Turnidge J, Craig WA: The in vivo postantibiotic effect in a thigh infection in neutropenic mice. J Infect Dis 1988;157:287–298.

26. Eagle H, Musselman AD: The slow recovery of bacteria from the toxic effects of penicillin. J Bacteriol 1949;58:475–490.

27. Andes D. In-vivo pharmacodynamics of amphotericin B against *Candida albicans*. 39th Interscience Conference on Antimicrobial Agents and Chemotherapy, American Society for Microbiology, 1999.

28. Blaser J, Stone BB, Groner MC, et al: Comparative study with enoxacin and netilmicin in a pharmacodynamic model to determine importance of ratio of antibiotic peak concentration to MIC for bactericidal activity and emergence of resistance. Antimicrob Agents Chemother 1987;31:1054–1060.

29. Craig WA, Redington J, Ebert SC: Pharmacodynamics of amikacin in-vitro and in mouse thigh and lung infections. J Antimicrob Chemother, 1991;27(Suppl C):29–40.

30. Ernst EJ, Klepser ME, Pfaller MA: Postantifungal effects of echinocandin, azole, and polyene antifungal agents against *Candida albicans* and *Cryptococcus neoformans*. Antimicrob Agents Chemother 2000;44:1108–1111.

31. Safdar N, Andes D, Craig WA: In-vivo pharmacodynamic characterization of daptomycin. 37th Annual Meeting of the Infectious Diseases Society of America, 1999.

32. Cars O, Odenholt-Tornqvist I: The post-antibiotic sub-MIC effect in vitro and in vivo. J Antimicrob Chemother 1993;31(Suppl D):159–166.

33. McDonald PJ, Wetherall BL, Pruul H: Postantibiotic leukocyte enhancement: Increased susceptibility of bacteria pretreated with antibiotics to activity of leukocytes. Rev Infect Dis 1981;3:38–44.

34. Odenholt-Tornqvist I, Lowdin E, Cars O: Postantibiotic sub-MIC effects of vancomycin, roxithromycin, sparfloxacin, and amikacin. Antimicrob Agents Chemother 1992;36:1852–1858.

35. Lorian V: Effect of low antibiotic concentrations on bacteria: Effects on ultrastructure, virulence, and susceptibility to immunodefenses. In Lorian V (ed): Antibiotics in Laboratory Medicine, 4th ed. Baltimore, Williams & Wilkins, 1996, pp 493–555.

36. Andes D, van Ogtrop M: Characterization and quantitation of the pharmacodynamics of fluconazole in a neutropenic murine disseminated candidiasis infection model. Antimicrob Agents Chemother 1999;43:2116–2120.

37. Turnidge JD, Gudmundsson S, Vogelman B, Craig WA: The postantibiotic effect of antifungal agents against common pathogenic yeast. J Antimicrob Chemother 1994;34:83–92.

38. Craig WA, Ebert SC: Antimicrobial therapy in *Pseudomonas aeruginosa* infection. In Baltch AL, and Smith RP (eds): *Pseudomonas aeruginosa* Infections and Treatment. New York, Marcel Dekker, 1994, pp 441–491.

39. Drusano GL, Johnson DE, Rosen M: Pharmacodynamics of a fluoroquinolone antimicrobial agent in a neutropenic rat model of *Pseudomonas* sepsis. Antimicrob Agents Chemother 1993;37:483–490.

40. Fantin B, Leggett J, Ebert S, Craig WA: Correlation between in vitro and in vivo activity of antimicrobial agents against gram-negative bacilli in a murine infection model. Antimicrob Agents Chemother 1991;35:1413–1422.

41. Galloe AM, Gaudal N, Christensen HR, Kampmann JP: Aminoglycosides: Single or multiple daily dosing? A meta-analysis on efficacy and safety. Eur J Clin Pharmacol 1995;48:39–43.

42. Craig WA: Interrelationship between pharmacokinetics and pharmacodynamics in determining dosage regimens for broad-spectrum cephalosporins. Diagn Microbiol Infect Dis 1995;21:1–8.

43. Vogelman B, Gudmundsson S, Leggett J, et al: Correlation of antimicrobial pharmacokinetic parameters with therapeutic efficacy in an animal model. J Infect Dis 1988;158:831–847.

44. Bodey GP, Ketchel SJ, Rodriguez N: A randomized study of carbenicillin plus cefamandole or tobramycin in the treatment of febrile episodes in cancer patients. Am J Med 1979;67:608–616.

45. Houlihan HH, Mercier RC, McKinnon PS, et al: Continuous infusion versus intermittent administration of ceftazidime in critically ill patients with gram-negative infection (abstract 42, p. 8). Abstracts of the 37th Interscience Conference on Antimicrobial, Agents and Chemotherapy, American Society for Microbiology, 1997.

46. Nenko AS, Cappelletty DM, Kruse JA, et al: Continuous infusion versus intermittent administration of ceftazidime in critically ill patients with suspected gram-negative infection. [abstract A93, page 18]. In Abstracts of the 35th Interscience Conference on Antimicrobial, Agents and Chemotherapy, American Society for Microbiology, 1995.

47. Bakker-Woudenberg IAJM, van den Berg JC, Fontijne P, et al: Efficacy of continuous versus intermittent administration of penicillin G in *Streptococcus pneumoniae* pneumonia in normal and immunodeficient rats. Eur J Clin Microbiol Infect Dis 1984; 3:131–135.

48. Craig WA, and Ebert SC: Continuous infusion of β-lactam antibiotics. Antimicrob Agents Chemother 1992;36:2577–2583.

49. Roosendaal R, Bakker-Woudenberg IA, van den Berg JC, Michel MF: Therapeutic efficacy of continuous versus intermittent administration of ceftazidime in an experimental *Klebsiella pneumoniae* pneumonia in rats. J Infect Dis 1985;152:373–378.

50. Gerber AU, Craig WA, Brugger HP, et al: Impact of dosing intervals on activity of gentamicin and ticarcillin against *Pseudomonas aeruginosa* in granulocytopenic mice. J Infect Dis 1983;147:910–917.

51. Lustar I, Friedland IR, Wubbel L, et al: Pharmacodynamics of gatifloxacin in cerebrospinal fluid in experimental cephalosporin-resistant pneumococcal meningitis. Antimicrob Agents Chemother 1998;42:2650–2655.

52. Pechere M, Letarte R, Pechere JC: Efficacy of different dosing schedules of tobramycin for treating murine *Klebsiella pneumoniae* bronchopneumonia. J Antimicrob Chemother 1987;19:487–494.

53. Powell S, Thompson W, Luthe M, et al: Once-daily vs. continuous aminoglycoside dosing: Efficacy and toxicity in animals and clinical studies of gentamicin, netilmicin, and tobramycin. J Infect Dis 1983;147:918–932.

54. Gerber AU, Vastola AP, Brandel J, Craig WA: Selection of aminoglycoside resistant variants of *Pseudomonas aeruginosa* in an in vivo model. J Infect Dis 1982; 146:691–697.

55. De Broe ME, Verbist L, Verpooten GA: Influence of dosage schedule on renal cortical accumulation of amikacin and tobramycin in man. J Antimicrob Chemother 1991;27 (Suppl C):41–47.

56. Giuliano RA, Verpooten GA, Verbist L, et al: In vivo uptake kinetics of aminoglycosides in the kidney cortex of rats. J Pharmacol Exp Ther 1986;236:470–475.

57. Tran BH, Deffrennes D: Aminoglycoside ototoxicity: Influence of dosage regimen on drug uptake and correlation between membrane binding and some clinical features. Acta Otolaryngol (Stockholm) 1988;105:511–515.

58. Verpooten GA, Giuliano RA, Verbist L, et al: Once-daily dosing decreases renal accumulation of gentamicin and netilmicin. Clin Pharmacol Ther 1989;45:22–27.

59. Urban A, Craig WA: Daily dosing of aminoglycosides. Curr Clin Top Infect Dis 1997;17:236–255.

60. Louie A, Drusano GL, Banerjee P, et al: Pharmacodynamics of fluconazole in a murine model of systemic candidiasis. Antimicrob Agents Chemother 1998;42:1105–1109.

61. Drusano GL: Pharmacodynamics of antiretroviral chemotherapy. Infect Control Hosp Epidemiol 1993;14:530–536.

62. Drusano GL, Prichard M, Bilello PA, Bilello JA: Modeling combinations of antiretroviral agents in vitro with integration of pharmacokinetics: Guidance in regimen choice for clinical trial evaluation. Antimicrob Agents Chemother 1996; 40:1143–1147.

63. Drusano GL, Bilello JA, Preston SL, et al: Hollow fiber unit evaluation of BMS232632, a new HIV-1 protease inhibitor, for the linked pharmacodynamic variable [abstract 1662, p 339]. In Abstracts of the 40th Interscience Conference on Antimicrobial Agents and Chemotherapy, American Society for Microbiology, 2000.

64. Drusano GL, D'Argenio DZ, Preston SL, et al: Use of drug effect interaction modeling with Monte Carlo simulation to examine the impact of dosing interval on the projected antiviral activity of the combination of abacavir and amprenavir. Antimicrob Agents Chemother 2000;44:1655–1659.

65. Bilello JA, Eiseman JL, Standiford HC, Drusano GL: Impact of dosing schedule upon suppression of a retrovirus in a murine model of AIDS encephalopathy. Antimicrob Agents Chemother 1994;38:628–631.

66. Bilello JA, Bauer G, Dudley MN, et al: Effect of 2,3-didehydro-3-deoxythymidine in an in-vitro hollow-fiber pharmacodynamic model system correlates with results of

67. dose-ranging clinical studies. Antimicrob Agents Chemother, 1994;38:1386–1391.

67. Drusano GL, Aweeka F, Gambertoglio J, et al: Relationship between foscarnet exposure, baseline cytomegalovirus (CMV) blood culture and the time to progression of CMV retinitis in HIV-positive patients. AIDS 1996;10:1113–1119.

68. Drusano GL, Preston SL, Berman A, et al: Relationship between foscarnet exposure and nephrotoxicity during induction therapy for CMV retinitis (abstract 499). Second National Conference on Human Retroviruses and Related Infections, Washington, DC, 1995.

69. Drusano GL, Treanor H, Fowler C, et al: Time to viral clearance after experimental infection with influenza A or B is related to baseline viral titer and the plasma area under the curve of RWJ-270201 (abstract 1391, p 29). In Abstracts of the 40th Interscience Conference on Antimicrobial Agents and Chemotherapy, American Society for Microbiology, 2000.

70. Andes D, Craig WA: In vivo activities of amoxicillin and amoxicillin-clavulanate against *Streptococcus pneumoniae*: Application to breakpoint determinations. Antimicrob Agents Chemother 1998;42:2375–2379.

71. Andes DR, Craig WA: Pharmacodynamics of fluoro-quinolones in experimental models of endocarditis. Clin Infect Dis 1998;27:47–50.

72. Craig WA, Andes D: Pharmacokinetics and pharmacodynamics of antibiotics in otitis media. Pediatr Infect Dis J 1996;15:255–259.

73. Andes D, Craig WA: Pharmacodynamics of gemifloxacin against quinolone-resistant strains of *Streptococcus pneumoniae* with known resistance mechanisms. 39th Interscience Conference on Antimicrobial Agents and Chemotherapy, American Society for Microbiology, 1999.

74. Craig WA, Andes DR: Impact of macrolide resistance on the in-vivo activity of ABT-773 on *Streptococcus pneumoniae*. 40th Interscience Conference on Antimicrobial Agents and Chemotherapy, American Society for Microbiology, 2000.

75. Dowell SF, Butler JC, Giebink GS, et al: Acute otitis media: Management and surveillance in an era of pneumococcal resistance—a report from the drug-resistant *Streptococcus pneumoniae* therapeutic working group. Pediatr Infect Dis J 1999;18:1–9.

76. Sinus and Allergy Health Partnership: Antimicrobial treatment guidelines for acute bacterial rhinosinusitis. Otolaryngol Head Neck Surg, 2000;123(Suppl 1):1–32.

77. Bartlett JG, Dowell SF, Mandell LA, et al: Practice guidelines for the management of community-acquired pneumonia in adults. Clin Infect Dis 2000;31:347–382.

78. Heffelfinger JD, Dowell SF, Jorgensen JH, et al: Management of community-acquired pneumonia in the era of pneumococcal resistance. Arch Intern Med 2000;160:1399–1408.

79. Scheld WM, Sande MA: Bactericidal versus bacteriostatic antibiotic therapy of experimental pneumococcal meningitis in rabbits. J Clin Invest 1983;71:411–419.

80. Craig WA, Ebert S, Watanabe Y: Differences in time above MIC required for efficacy of beta-lactams in animal infection models (abstract 86). In Abstracts of the 33rd Interscience Conference on Antimicrobial Agents and Chemotherapy. American Society for Microbiology, 1993.

81. Craig WA: Does the dose matter? Clin Infect Dis 2001;33(Suppl 3):5233–5237.

82. Andes DR, Craig WA: Pharmacokinetics and pharmacodynamics of antibiotics in meningitis. Infect Dis Clinics N Am 1999;13:595–618.

83. Tauber MG, Zak O, Scheld WM, et al: The postantibiotic effect in the treatment of experimental meningitis caused by *Streptococcus pneumoniae* in rabbits. J Infect Dis 1984;149:575–583.

84. Tauber MG, Doroshow CA, Hackbarth CJ, et al: Antibacterial activity of β-lactam antibiotics in experimental meningitis due to *Streptococcus pneumoniae*. J Infect Dis 1984;149:575–583.

85. Lutsar I, McCracken GH, Friedland IA: Antibiotic pharmacodynamics in cerebrospinal fluid. Clin Infect Dis 1998;27:1117–1129.

86. Preston SL, Drusano GL, Berman AL, et al: Pharmacodynamics of levofloxacin: A new paradigm for early clinical trials. JAMA 1998;279:125–129.

87. Dagan R, Abramason O, Leibovitz E, et al: Bacteriologic response to oral cephalosporins: Are established susceptibility breakpoints appropriate in the case of acute otitis media? J Infect Dis 1997;176:1253–1259.

88. Dagan R, Leibovitz E, Fliss DM, et al: Bacteriologic efficacies of oral azithromycin and oral cefaclor in treatment of acute otitis media in infants and young children. Antimicrob Agents Chemother 2000;44:43–50.

89. Gwaltney JM, Savolainen S, Rivas P, et al: Comparative effectiveness and safety of cefdinir and amoxicillin-clavulanate in treatment of acute community-acquired bacterial sinusitis. Antimicrob Agents Chemother 1997;41:1517–1520.

90. Scheld WM, Sydnor A, Farr B, et al: Comparison of cyclacillin and amoxicillin for therapy for acute maxillary sinusitis. Antimicrob Agents Chemother 1986;30:350–353.

91. Schentag JJ, Strenkoski-Nix LC, Nix DE, Forrest A: Pharmacodynamic interactions of antibiotics alone and in combination. Clin Infect Dis 1998;27:40–46.

92. Sydnor A, Gwaltney JM, Cocchetto DM, Scheld WM: Comparative evaluation of cefuroxime axetil and cefaclor for treatment of acute bacterial maxillary sinusitis. Arch Otolaryngol Head Neck Surg 1989;115:1430–1433.

93. Ambrose PG, Quintiliani R, Nightingale CH, et al: Continuous vs intermittent infusion of cefuroxime for the treatment of community-acquired pneumonia. Infect Dis Clin Prac 1997;7:463–470.

94. Lister PD, Sanders CC: Pharmacodynamics of levofloxacin and ciprofloxacin against *Streptococcus pneumoniae*. J Antimicrob Chemother 1999;43:79–86.

95. Lacy MK, Lu W, Xu X, et al: Pharmacodynamic comparisons of levofloxacin, ciprofloxacin, and ampicillin against *Streptococcus pneumoniae* in an in vitro model of infection. Antimicrob Agents Chemother 1999;43:672–677.

96. Ambrose PG, Grasella DM, Grasela TH, et al: Pharmacodynamics of fluoroquinolones against *Streptococcus pneumoniae*: Analysis of phase-III clinical trials (abstract 1387, p 28). In Programs and Abstracts from the 40th Interscience Conference on Antimicrobial Agents and Chemotherapy, American Society for Microbiology, 2000.

97. Kashuba AD, Nafziger AN, Drusano GL, Bertino JS: Optimizing aminoglycoside therapy for nosocomial pneumonia caused by gram-negative bacteria. Antimicrob Agents Chemother 1999;43:623–629.

98. Moore RD, Smith CR, Lietman PS: The association of aminoglycoside plasma levels with mortality in patients with gram-negative bacteremia. J Infect Dis 1984;149:443–448.

99. Deziel-Evans LM, Murphy JE, Job ML: Correlation of pharmacokinetic indices with therapeutic outcome in patients receiving aminoglycosides. Clin Pharm 1986;5:319–324.

100. Moore RD, Lietman PS, Smith CR: Clinical response to aminoglycoside therapy: Importance of the ratio of peak concentration to minimal inhibitory concentration. J Infect Dis 1987;155:93–99.

101. Ali MZ, Goetz MB: A meta-analysis of the relative efficacy and toxicity of single daily dosing versus multiple daily dosing of aminoglycosides. Clin Infect Dis 1997;24:796–809.

102. Bailey TC, Little JR, Littenberg B, et al: A meta-analysis of extended-interval dosing versus multiple daily dosing of aminoglycosides. Clin Infect Dis 1997;24:786–795.

103. Barza M, Ioannidis JPA, Cappelleri JC, Lau J: Single or multiple daily doses of aminoglycosides: A meta-analysis. BMJ 1996;312:338–345.

104. Ferriols-Lisart R, Alos-Alminana M: Effectiveness and safety of once-daily aminoglycosides: A meta-analysis. Am J Health Systems Pharm 1996;53:1141–1150.

105. Hatala R, Dinh T, Cook DJ: Once-daily aminoglycoside dosing in immunocompetent adults: A meta-analysis. Ann Intern Med 1996;124:717–725.

106. Hatala R, Dinh TT, Cook DJ: Single daily dosing of aminoglycosides in immunocompromised adults: A systematic review. Clin Infect Dis 1997;24:810–815.

107. Munckhof WJ, Grayson JL, Turnidge JD: A meta-analysis of studies on the safety and efficacy of aminoglycosides given either once daily or as divided doses. J Antimicrob Chemother 1996;37:645–663.

108. Maller R, Ahrne H, Holmen C, et al: Once-versus twice-daily amikacin regimen: Efficacy and safety in systemic gram-negative infections. J Antimicrob Chemother 1993;31:939–948.

109. Nordstrom L, Ringberg H, Cronberg S, et al: Does administration of an aminoglycoside in a single-daily dose affect its efficacy and toxicity? J Antimicrob Chemother 1990;25:159–173.

110. Prins JM, Buller HR, Kuijper EJ, et al: Once-versus thrice-daily gentamicin in patients with serious infections. Lancet 1993;341:335–339.

111. Rybak MJ, Abate BJ, Kang SL, et al: Prospective evaluation of the effect of an aminoglycoside dosing regimen on rates of observed nephrotoxicity and ototoxicity. Antimicrob Agents Chemother 1999;43:1549–1555.

112. Fantin B, Carbon C: Importance of the aminoglycoside dosing regimen in the penicillin-netilmicin combination for treatment of *Enterococcus faecalis*-induced experimental endocarditis. Antimicrob Agents Chemother 1990;34:2387–2391.

113. Rex JH, Pfaller MA, Galgiani JN, et al: for the NCCLS Subcommittee on Antifungal Susceptibility Testing: Development of interpretive breakpoints for antifungal susceptibility testing: Conceptual framework and analysis of in vitro–in vivo correlation data for fluconazole, itraconazole, and *Candida infections*. Clin Infect Dis 1997;24:235–247.

114. Bustamante CL, Wharton RC, Wade JC: In vitro activity of ciprofloxacin in combination with ceftazidime, aztreonam, and azlocillin against multiresistant isolates of *Pseudomonas aeruginosa*. Antimicrob Agents Chemother 1990;34:1814–1815.

115. Hallender HO, Dornbusch K, Gezelius L, et al: Synergism between aminoglycosides and cephalosporins with antipseudomonal activity: Interaction index and killing curve method. Antimicrob Agents Chemother 1982;22:743–752.

116. White RL, Burgess DS, Manduru M, Bosso JA: Comparison of three different in vitro methods of detecting synergy: Time-kill, checkerboard, and E test. Antimicrob Agents Chemother 1996;40:1914–1918.

117. Thomas JK, Forrest A, Bhavnani SM, et al: Pharmacodynamic evaluation of factors associated with the development of bacterial resistance in acutely ill patients during therapy. Antimicrob Agents Chemother 1998;42:521–527.

118. Mouton JW, van Ogtrop ML, Andes D, Craig WA: Use of pharmacodynamic indices to predict efficacy of combination therapy in vivo. Antimicrob Agents Chemother 1999;43:2473–2478.

119. Nicolau DP, Onyeji CO, Zhong M, et al: Pharmacodynamic assessment of cefprozil against *Streptococcus pneumoniae*: Implications for breakpoint determinations. Antimicrob Agents Chemother 2000;44:1291–1295.

120. National Committee for Clinical Laboratory Standards: Development of in-vitro susceptibility testing criteria and quality control parameters: Approved guideline, 2nd ed. Document M23–A2. The Committee, Jan 2000.

121. Friedland IR, Shelton S, Paris M, et al: Dilemmas in diagnosis and management of cephalosporin-resistant *Streptococcus pneumoniae* meningitis. Pediatr Infect Dis J 1993;12:196–200.

122. Kleiman MD, Wienbery GA, Reynolds JK, Allen SD: Meningitis with beta-lactam resistant *Streptococcus pneumoniae*: The need for early repeat lumber puncture. Pediatr Infect Dis J 1993;12:782–784.

123. Pallares R, Linares J, Vadillo M, et al: Resistance to penicillin and cephalosporin and mortality from severe pneumococcal pneumonia in Barcelona, Spain. N Engl J Med 1995;333:474–480.

124. Feikin DR, Schuchat A, Kolczak M, et al: Mortality from invasive pneumococcal pneumonia in the era of antibiotic resistance, 1995–1997. Am J Public Health 2000;90:223–229.

125. Fish DN, Piscitelli SC, Danziger LH: Development of resistance during antimicrobial therapy: A review of antibiotic class and patient characteristics in 173 studies. Pharmacotherapy 1995;15:279–291.

126. Martinez JL, Baquero F: Mutation frequencies and antibiotic resistance. Antimicrob Agents Chemother 2000;44:1771–1777.

127. Peloquin CA, Cumbo TJ, Nix DE, et al: Evaluation of intravenous ciprofloxacin in patients with nosocomial lower respiratory tract infections. Arch Intern Med 1989;149:2269–2273.

128. Peterson ML, Hovde LB, Wright DH, et al: Fluoroquinolone resistance in *Bacteroides fragilis* following sparfloxacin exposure. Antimicrob Agents Chemother 1999;43:2251–2255.

129. Wu YL, Scott EM, Po AL, Tariq VN: Development of resistance and cross-resistance in *Pseudomonas aeruginosa* exposed to subinhibitory antibiotic concentrations. APMIS 1999;107:585–592.

130. Blondeau JM, Zhao X, Hansen G, et al: Mutant prevention concentrations of fluoroquinolones for clinical isolates of *Streptococcus pneumoniae*. Antimicrob Agents Chemother 2001;45:433–438.

131. Schrag SJ, Beall B, Dowell SF: Limiting the spread of resistant pneumococci: Biological and epidemiologic evidence for the effectiveness of alternative interventions. Clin Microbiol Rev 2000;13:588–601.

132. Jackson M, Burry V, Olson L, et al: Breakthrough sepsis in macrolide resistant pneumococcal infection. Pediatr Infect Dis J 1996;15:1049–1051.

133. Morita JY, Kahn E, Thompson T, et al: Impact of azithromycin on oropharyngeal carriage of group A *Streptococcus* and nasopharyngeal carriage of macrolide-resistant *Streptococcus*. Pediatr Infect Dis J 2000;19:41–46.

134. Leach A, Shelgy-James T, Mayo M, et al: A prospective study of the impact of community-based azithromycin treatment of trachoma on carriage and resistance of *Streptococcus pneumoniae*. Clin Infect Dis 1997;24:356–362.

135. Ghaffar FA, Katz K, Muniz LS, et al: Effect of amoxicillin-clavulanate 14:1 vs. azithromycin on nasopharyngeal carriage and resistance of *S. pneumoniae* (abstract 98). In Abstracts of the Infectious Diseases Society of America 38th Annual Meeting, 2000.

Head and Neck Infections

chapter

2

Head and Neck Infections

ANTHONY W. CHOW, MD, FRCPC, FACP

Infections of the head and neck most commonly originate from septic complications of dental, oropharyngeal, or otorhinolaryngeal sources. From these sites, infection may extend along natural fascial planes into deep cervical spaces or vascular compartments. Suppurative infections of the head and neck are potentially life threatening. Since they have become less common in the postantibiotic era, many physicians are unfamiliar with these conditions. Furthermore, with widespread use of antibiotics and profound immunosuppression in some patients the classic manifestations of these infections are often altered. Features of systemic toxicity, such as chills and fever, and local signs, such as edema and fluctuance, may be absent. Thus physicians must be more aware and not underestimate the extent and severity of the infection. In this chapter the diagnosis and management of several odontogenic and orofacial infections as well as deep fascial "space" infections of the head and neck are discussed. The vascular and osseous complications of these suppurative infections are also highlighted.

ANATOMIC CONSIDERATIONS AND ROUTES OF SPREAD

Odontogenic infections originate from plaque: bacteria colonizing the surfaces of the tooth. Plaques located on tooth surfaces above the gingival margin (supragingival plaque) lead to dental caries that may invade the pulp (pulpitis or endodontic infection) and eventually perforate the alveolar bone (periapical abscess). Plaques located on tooth surfaces beneath the gingival margin (subgingival plaque) lead to periodontal infection (e.g., gingivitis, periodontitis, periodontal abscess, and pericoronitis) that may eventually penetrate the supporting structures and invade the deeper fascial "spaces" of the head and neck. In the mandible this is usually in the region of the molar teeth on the lingual aspect and more anterior on the buccal aspect. In the maxilla the bone is weakest on the buccal aspect throughout and relatively thicker on the palatal aspect. If pus perforates through either the maxillary or mandibular buccal plate, it will present intraorally if inside the attachment of the buccinator muscle to the maxilla or mandible and extraorally if outside this muscle attachment (Fig. 2–1). When a mandibular infection perforates lingually, it presents in the sublingual space if the apices of the involved teeth lie above the attachment of the mylohyoid muscle (e.g., mandibular incisor, canines, premolars, and first molars) and in the submandibular space if the apices of the involved teeth lie below the attachment of this muscle (e.g., second and third molars) (Fig. 2–1). Thus these local anatomic barriers of bone, muscle, and fascia predetermine the routes of spread, extent, and clinical manifestations of many orofacial infections of odontogenic origin.

The deep cervical fascial spaces intercommunicate with one another to varying extents (Fig. 2–2). Infections within deep fascial spaces of the head and neck may

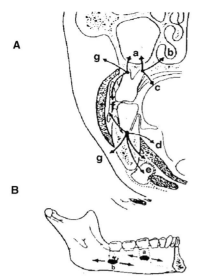

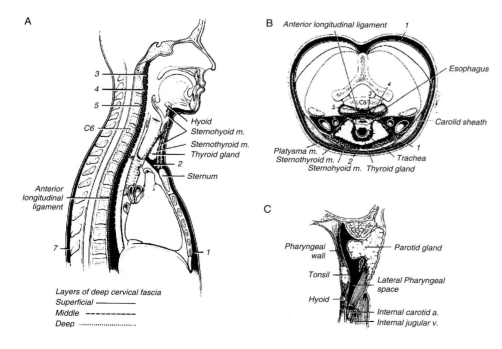

FIGURE 2–1. Routes of spread of odontogenic infections. *A,* Coronal section at first molar teeth: *a,* maxillary antrum; *b,* nasal cavity; *c,* palatal plate; *d,* sublingual space (above mylohyoid muscle); *e,* submylohyoid space; *f,* intraoral presentation with infection spreading through the buccal plates inside the attachment of the buccinator muscle; and *g,* extraoral presentation to buccal space with infection spreading through the buccal plates outside the attachment of the buccinator muscle. *B,* Lingual aspect of the mandible: *a,* tooth apices above the mylohyoid muscle with spread of infection into the sublingual space; *b,* tooth apices below the mylohyoid muscle with spread of infection into the submylohyoid space. (From Chow AW: Life-threatening infections of the head, neck, and upper respiratory tract. In Hall JB, Schmidt GA, Wood LH [eds]: Principles of Critical Care, 2nd ed. New York, McGraw-Hill, 1998, p 890.)

become life threatening either by obstruction of the airway or by direct extension to vital structures such as the mediastinum or carotid sheath. Otorhinolaryngeal infections may also cause intracranial suppuration such as cerebral or epidural abscess, subdural empyema, and cavernous or cortical venous sinus thrombosis (Fig. 2–3). A thorough knowledge of the anatomic relationships and the potential routes of spread within different fascial spaces not only will provide valuable information regarding the source and extent of infection but also will suggest the most likely microbial cause, antimicrobial treatment, and optimum approach for surgical drainage.

RADIOLOGIC INVESTIGATION OF THE HEAD AND NECK

A pantomogram may reveal the true extent of advanced periodontitis or the presence of periapical abscess. Ultrasonography, radionuclide scanning, computed tomography (CT), and magnetic resonance imaging (MRI) are particularly useful for localization of deep fascial space infections of the head and neck. Since CT can both localize a process and define its extent, particularly invasion into the cranial vault, mediastinum, or the bone, it is an invaluable tool for guiding needle aspiration or open drainage. A lateral radiograph of the neck may demonstrate compression or deviation of the tracheal air column or the presence of gas within necrotic soft tissues. The soft tissues of the posterior wall of the hypopharynx are approximately 5 mm deep, less than one-third the diameter of the fourth cervical vertebra (C4). The retropharyngeal soft tissues should be approximately two-thirds the width of C4, and the retrotracheal space slightly less (Fig. 2–4). A lateral radiograph of the cervical spine or a CT scan can determine if the soft tissue swelling or an abscess originated from the retropharyngeal space or the prevertebral space. The former suggests an odontogenic or oropharyngeal source, whereas the latter likely indi-

FIGURE 2–2. Relationship of various cervical fascial spaces to the posterior and anterior layers of deep cervical fascia: *1,* superficial space; *2,* pretracheal space; *3,* retropharyngeal space; *4,* "danger" space; *5,* prevertebral space. *A,* Cross section of the neck at the level of the thyroid isthmus. *B,* Coronal section in the suprahyoid region of the neck. *C,* Midsagittal section of the head and neck. (From Chow AW: Life-threatening infections of the head, neck, and upper respiratory tract. In Hall JB, Schmidt GA, Wood LH [eds]: Principles of Critical Care, 2nd ed. New York, McGraw-Hill, 1998, p 888.)

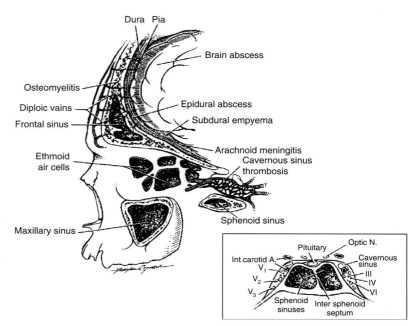

FIGURE 2–3. Major routes for intracranial extension of infection either directly or via the vascular supply. The coronal section in the inset demonstrates the structures adjoining the sphenoid sinus. (From Chow AW: Life-threatening infections of the head, neck, and upper respiratory tract. In Hall JB, Schmidt GA, Wood LH [eds]: Principles of Critical Care, 2nd ed. New York, McGraw-Hill, 1998, p 889.)

cates involvement of the cervical spine. Technetium bone scanning, used in combination with gallium- or indium-labeled white blood cells, is particularly useful for the diagnosis of acute or chronic osteomyelitis. MRI is more sensitive than CT, and probably more accurate than bone scan in detecting bone involvement.[1,2] T2-weighted images may identify and localize areas of pus for drainage or aspiration. Gadolinium enhancement is important to accurately define the soft tissue component. Finally, MRI is useful for imaging vascular lesions, such as jugular thrombophlebitis.[3]

MICROBIOLOGY

The microbial cause of head and neck infections may be anticipated from the normal resident flora of the contiguous mucosal surfaces from which the infection originated. Because of the close anatomic relationship, the resident flora of the oral cavity, upper respiratory tract, and certain parts of the ears and eyes share many common organisms[4] (Fig. 2–5). Anaerobes generally outnumber aerobes at all sites by a factor of 10:1.[5] Important differences in bacterial compositions have been noted for dental caries, gingivitis, and different forms of periodontitis when compared with cultures from healthy tissues (Table 2–1).[6,7] A causal association of *Streptococcus mutans* with dental

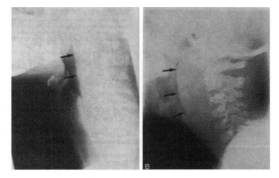

FIGURE 2–4. Lateral radiograph of the neck. *A*, Normal lateral cervical view. *B*, Expansion of the retropharyngeal soft tissues. (From Baker AS, Nau GJ: Infections of head and neck spaces and salivary glands. In: Gorbach SL, Bartlett JG, Blacklow NR [eds]: Infectious Diseases, 2nd ed. Philadelphia, WB Saunders, 1998, p 514.)

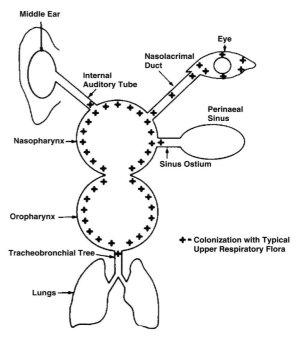

FIGURE 2–5. Anatomic relationship of head and neck structures and distribution of the indigenous microflora. (From Roscoe DL, Chow AW: Normal flora and mucosal immunity of the head and neck. Infect Dis Clin N Am 1988; 2: 5.)

TABLE 2–1 ■ Microbial Specificity and Antimicrobial Regimens in Dental Caries and Different Clinical Forms of Periodontal Disease

Clinical entity	Unique microbial species	Antimicrobial regimens
Supragingival dental plaque and dental caries	*Streptococcus mutans*, other streptococci, *Actinomyces* spp	Fluoride-containing dentifrices or oral rinses (e.g., sodium fluoride 1.1% or stannous fluoride 0.4%) Chlorhexidine 0.12% oral rinses
Subgingival dental plaque and gingivitis		Penicillin G 1–4 MU IVq4–6h Ampicillin-sulbactam 1.5–3 g IV q6h Metronidzole 500 mg PO or IV q8h Clindamycin 450 mg PO or 600 mg IV q6–8h
Simple	Streptococci, *Actinomyces* spp, spirochetes	
Acute necrotizing ulcerative	*Prevotella intermedia*, *Fusobacterium* spp, spirochetes	
Periodontitis		Doxycycline 200 mg PO or IV q12h Metronidazole 500 mg PO or IV q8h Topical application of minocycline microspheres (Aristin)
Localized juvenile	*Actinobacillus actinomycetemcomitans*	
Adult onset	Spirochetes, black-pigmented *Bacteroides* (*Porphyromonas gingivalis* and *Prevotella melaninogenica*), *A. actinomycetemcomitans*	

caries has been firmly established.[8,9] Similarly, in gingivitis and periodontitis a unique and specific bacterial composition of the subgingival plaque has been identified. In the healthy periodontium the microflora are sparse and consist mainly of gram-positive organisms such as *Streptococcus sanguis* and *Actinomyces* spp. In the presence of gingivitis the predominant subgingival flora shift to a greater proportion of anaerobic gram-negative rods, and *Prevotella intermedia* (formerly *Bacteroides intermedius*) is most commonly isolated.[10] With established periodontitis the flora further increase in complexity, with a preponderance of anaerobic gram-negative and motile organisms. *Porphyromonas gingivalis* (formerly *Bacteroides gingivalis*) is most commonly isolated. In juvenile periodontitis, a clinical variant seen primarily in adolescents, the subgingival plaque mainly consists of saccharolytic organisms, with *Actinobacillus actinomycetemcomitans* and *Capnocytophaga* spp as the most common identifiable species. *P. gingivalis* is rarely found in this condition.[11] In suppurative odontogenic infections, oral anaerobes including *Fusobacterium nucleatum*, pigmented *Prevotella* species such as *Prevotella melaninogenica* (formerly *Bacteroides melaninogenicus),* *Veillonella* spp, and *Peptostreptococcus* spp are the most common isolates[12] (Table 2–2). In contrast, suppurative infections arising from the pharynx contain both oral anaerobes and facultative streptococci, particularly *Streptococcus pyogenes*, whereas rhinogenic or otogenic infections may harbor *Streptococcus pneumoniae, Haemophilus influenzae*, and facultative gram-negative rods as well as anaerobes. Although less is known about the pathogenic potential of individual species, it is clear that as a group these organisms are structural opportunists and invade deep tissues when normal mucosal barriers are disrupted.

Invasiveness is often influenced by synergistic interactions of multiple species, both aerobic and anaerobic. Moreover, certain species or combinations may be more invasive or more resistant to therapy than others.

Most pathogens implicated in head and neck infections are sensitive in vitro to penicillin G, but an increasing number of species (e.g., 40% or more of *P. melaninogenica* in certain geographic areas) are now resistant.[13] The importance of this in vitro finding in the treatment of polymicrobial head and neck infections is largely unknown, but failure of therapy with penicillin alone in orofacial infections has been reported.[14] Although anaerobes are likely to be the predominant pathogens in most head and neck infections, a small but significant proportion of cases, particularly in immunocompromised patients, will also contain other pathogens such as *Staphylococcus aureus* and facultative gram-negative rods including *Pseudomonas aeruginosa*.

TREATMENT OF SELECTED HEAD AND NECK INFECTIONS

Antimicrobial treatment of head and neck infections should be guided by the clinical history, careful physical examination, and associated or underlying medical conditions. Because the etiologic agents are remarkably diverse, every effort should be made to narrow the differential diagnosis by pursuing a judicious but aggressive plan of investigation. Results of culture and susceptibility data, although important for establishing the etiologic diagnosis, are often not available. Thus, particularly in severely ill or immunocompromised patients, the initial choice of antimicrobial therapy is often empiric and designed to cover the most

TABLE 2–2 ■ Usual Causative Organisms and Initial Empiric Antimicrobial Regimens for Suppurative Infections of the Head and Neck

Infection	Usual causative organisms	Antimicrobial regimens	
		Normal host	**Compromised host**
Suppurative orofacial odontogenic infections including Ludwig's angina	Viridans and other streptococci, *Peptostreptococcus* spp, *Bacteroides* spp, and other oral anaerobes	Penicillin G 2–4 MU IV q4–6h *plus* metronidazole 0.5 g IV q6h *or* Ampicillin-sulbactam 2 g IV q4h *or* Clindamycin 600 mg IV q6h *or* Doxycycline 200 mg IV q12h *or* Cefoxitin 1–2 g IV q6h *or* Cefotetan 2 g IV q12h	Cefotaxime 2 g IV q6h *or* Ceftizoxime 4 g IV q8h *or* Piperacillin 3 g IV q4h *or* Imipenem 500 mg IV q6h *or* Meropenem 1 g IV q8h *or* Gatifloxacin 200 mg IV q24h
Peritonsillar abscess (Quincy)	Group A streptococcus (*Streptococcus pyogenes*), *Fusobacterium* spp, *Peptostreptococcus* spp, and other oral anaerobes	Penicillin G 2–4 MU IV q4–6h *plus* metronidazole 0.5 g IV q6h *or* Ampicillin-sulbactam 2 g IV q4h *or* Clindamycin 600 mg IV q6h *or* Cefoxitin 1–2 g IV q6h	Cefotaxime 2 g IV q6h *or* Ceftizoxime 3 g IV q8h *or* Piperacillin 3 g IV q4h
Sialadenitis and suppurative parotitis	*Staphylococcus aureus*, viridans and other streptococci, *Bacteroides* spp, *Peptostreptococcus* spp, and other oral anaerobes	Nafcillin 1.5 g IV q4–6h *plus* metronidazole 0.5 g IV q6h *or* Clindamycin 600 mg IV q6h	Vancomycin 0.5 g IV q6h *plus* cefotaxime 2 g IV q6h *or* ceftizoxime 3 g IV q8h *or* piperacillin 3 g IV q4h
Severe mucositis	Viridans and other streptococci, *Staphylococcus* spp, *Peptostreptococcus* spp, *Bacteroides* spp, and other oral anaerobes, facultative gram-negative bacilli	Penicillin G 2–4 MU IV q4–6h, *plus* metronidazole 0.5 g IV q6h *or* Ampicillin-sulbactam 2 g IV q4h *or* Clindamycin 600 mg IV q6h *or* Cefoxitin 1–2 g IV q6h	Cefotaxime 2 g IV q6h *or* ceftizoxime 4 g IV q8h *or* piperacillin 3 g IV q4h *or* imipenem 500 mg IV q6h *or* meropenem 1 g IV q8h
Cervicofacial actinomycosis	*Actinomyces israelii, Arachnia propionica, Actinobacillus actinomycetemcomitans*	Penicillin G 2–4 MU IV q4–6h, *or* Doxycycline 200 mg PO or IV q6h, *or* Clindamycin 450 mg PO or 600 mg IV q8h	Same as for odontogenic space infections
Lateral pharyngeal or retropharyngeal space infections			
Odontogenic	Viridans and other streptococci, *Staphylococcus* spp, *Peptostreptococcus* spp, *Bacteroides* spp, and other oral anaerobes	Penicillin G 2–4 MU IV q4–6h, *plus* metronidazole 0.5 g IV q6h *or* Ampicillin-sulbactam 2 g IV q4h *or* Clindamycin 600 mg IV q6h	Cefotaxime 2 g IV q6h *or* ceftizoxime 4 g IV q8h *or* piperacillin 3 g IV q4h *or* imipenem 500 mg IV q6h *or* gatifloxacin 400 mg IV q24h
Rhinogenic	*Streptococcus pneumoniae, Haemophilus influenzae,* viridans and other streptococci, *Bacteroides* spp, *Peptostreptococcus* spp, and other oral anaerobes	Penicillin G 2–4 MU IV q4–6h *or* Ciprofloxacin 0.2 g q12h, *plus* metronidazole 0.5 g IV q6h *or* clindamycin 600 mg IV q6h; *or* Gatifloxacin 400 mg IV q24h	Same as for odontogenic space infections

Continued

TABLE 2–2 ■ Usual Causative Organisms and Initial Empiric Antimicrobial Regimens for Suppurative Infections of the Head and Neck (*Continued*)

Infection	Usual causative organisms	Antimicrobial regimens	
		Normal host	**Compromised host**
Otogenic	Same as for rhinogenic space infections	Same as for rhinogenic space infections	Same as for odontogenic space infections
Septic jugular thrombophlebitis (Lemierre syndrome)	*Fusobacterium necrophorum*; same as for peritonsillar abscess or odontogenic space infections	Same as for peritonsillar abscess or odontogenic space infections	Same as for odontogenic space infections
Septic cavernous or dural sinus thrombosis	Same as for odontogenic, rhinogenic or otogenic space infections	Same as for odontogenic, rhinogenic, or otogenic space infections	Same as for odontogenic space infections
Extension of osteomyelitis from Prevertebral space infection	*S. aureus*, facultative gram-negative bacilli	Nafcillin 1.5 g IV q4–6h, *plus* tobramycin 2 mg/kg IV q8h *or* ciprofloxacin 0.2 IV q12h	Vancomycin 0.5 g IV q6h, *plus* cefotaxime 2 g IV q6h *or* cefizoxime 4 g IV q8h *or* imipenem 500 mg IV q6h
Prevertebral space infection			
Pott's puffy tumor (frontal osteitis)	Same as for rhinogenic space infections	Same as for rhinogenic space infections	Same as for odontogenic space infections
Malignant otitis media and petrous osteitis	*Pseudomonas aeruginosa*	Ciprofloxacin 200 mg IV q12h, *or* Tobramycin 2 mg/kg q8h *plus* cefatzidime 2 g IV q6h *or* piperacillin 3 g IV q4h *or* imipenem 1 g IV q6h	Ciprofloxacin 200 mg IV q12h, *or* tobramycin 2 mg/kg IV q8h *plus* cefatzidime 2 g IV q6h *or* piperacillin 3 g IV q4h *or* imipenem 1 g IV q6h
Mandibular osteomyelitis	Same as for odontogenic space infections	Clindamycin 600 mg IV q6h *or* Gatifloxacin 400 mg IV q24h	Piperacillin 3 g IV q4h *or* Imipenem 500 mg IV q6h *or* Gatifloxacin 400 mg IV q24h

likely pathogens with broad-spectrum agents. Maximum doses of systemic antimicrobials should be administered to optimize tissue penetration. Therapy should be continued for 2 to 3 weeks. Intracranial extension of infection and vascular or osseous complications may require at least 6 to 8 weeks of intravenous antibiotics.

Odontogenic and Orofacial Infections

Dental Caries and Periodontal Disease

The carious process most frequently begins in pits and fissures on the occlusal surfaces of the molars or premolar teeth. Interproximal sites and the gingival margin are the next most common locations. Demineralization of the enamel results in discoloration, the first visible evidence of dental caries. Destruction of the enamel and dentin leads to invasion of the pulp, producing a pulpitis. If drainage from the pulp is obstructed, pulpal necrosis and proliferation of endodontic microorganisms rapidly invade the periapical areas (periapical abscess) and alveolar bone (acute alveolar abscess).

Clinically the tooth is sensitive to percussion and to both heat and cold during early or reversible pulpitis, although the painful response will stop abruptly when the stimulus is withdrawn. During late or irreversible pulpitis the tooth is exquisitely painful to a hot stimulus, and

prompt relief is achieved by the application of cold. If drainage is established through the tooth before extension into the periapical region, chronic irritation from the necrotic pulp may result in periapical granuloma or cyst formation that may be relatively asymptomatic. Dental radiographs are particularly helpful for the detection of silent lesions, particularly those caused by interproximal caries, which are difficult to detect clinically.

The single most cost-effective measure for reducing dental caries is fluoridation of public water supplies.[15] Fluoride forms a complex with the apatite crystals in dentin by replacing the hydroxyl group, thereby lending strength to the entire structure. Further, fluoride promotes remineralization of the carious lesions and also exerts a bacteriostatic effect. In addition to fluoridated water, fluoride-containing dentifrices and rinses (e.g., sodium fluoride 1.1% or stannous fluoride 0.4%) and dental flossing should be encouraged after each meal.

Oral antimicrobial rinses with 0.12% chlorhexidine are also effective for the control of dental plaque bacteria (Table 1–1).[16] Chlorhexidine acts as a cationic detergent killing a wide range of bacteria and is retained on the oral surfaces for prolonged periods to prevent plaque advancement.[17] Despite this beneficial effect, it has a bitter taste and stains the enamel and tongue, and prolonged application can promote the emergence of resistant microorganisms. Among topical antibiotics, although both penicillin and tetracycline have cariostatic effects in animal models, only vancomycin has been shown to reduce dental caries with some degree of success in humans.[7] Although none of these measures is routinely applied in clinical practice, they are useful for the control of dental plaque in selected patients with rampant caries.

Periodontal disease is a general term that refers to all diseases involving the supporting structures of the teeth (periodontium), which include the gingiva, periodontal ligament, alveolar bone, and cementum. In the early phase of periodontal disease, infection is confined to the gingiva (gingivitis). Later the underlying supporting tissues are affected (periodontitis), ultimately leading to complete destruction of the periodontium and permanent loss of teeth. The destructive process proceeds insidiously, usually beginning in early adulthood. Subgingival plaque is always present, and both supragingival and subgingival calculi are usually abundant. In simple gingivitis there is a bluish red discoloration, with swelling and thickening of the free gingival margin. A tendency for bleeding of the gums after eating or toothbrushing may be one of the earliest findings. There is usually no pain, but a mild fetor oris may be noticed. In acute necrotizing ulcerative gingivitis (Vincent's disease, or trench mouth), typically the patient suddenly experiences a pain in the gingiva that interferes with normal mastication. Necrosis of the gingiva occurs mainly in the interdental papilla and has a marginated, punched-out, and eroded appearance. A superficial grayish pseudomembrane is formed, and a characteristic halitosis with altered taste sensation is present. There is usually associated fever, malaise, and regional lymphadenopathy. With the onset of periodontitis there is further destruction of the supporting tissues with the formation of periodontal pockets around the affected teeth. Frank pus can be readily expressed by digital pressure or may exude freely from the pockets. Unlike pulpal infection in which drainage is frequently obstructed, periodontal infections drain freely, and patients experience little or no discomfort. Associated sensations include pressure and an itchy feeling in the gums and between the teeth, a bad taste in the mouth, hot and cold sensitivity, and vague pains in the jaws. The gingiva is inflamed and discolored and bleeds readily. Periodontal infections tend to localize in intraoral soft tissues and seldom spread into deeper structures of the face or neck. Localized juvenile periodontitis is a particularly destructive form of periodontitis seen in adolescents and is characterized by rapid vertical bone loss affecting the first molar and incisor teeth. Plaque is usually minimal, and calculus is absent. A specific defect with impaired neutrophil chemotaxis has been demonstrated in this condition.

Acute necrotizing ulcerative gingivitis should be treated with systemic antimicrobials such as metronidazole or penicillin (Table 2–1).[18] Certain types of severe periodontitis are amenable to systemic antimicrobials in conjunction with mechanical débridement (scaling and root planing).[19] This has often obviated the need for radical surgical resection of periodontal tissues. In double-blind clinical studies of advanced periodontitis, systemic metronidazole (500 mg PO three times daily) or doxycycline (200 mg PO twice daily) for 1 or 2 weeks in conjunction with rigorous mechanical débridement of the root surfaces was found to reduce the need for radical surgery by 80% compared with débridement plus placebo.[20] A topical antibiotic approach is also feasible. The United States Food and Drug Administration recently approved Arestin, a powder containing minocycline microspheres that release controlled amounts of the antibiotic beneath the gum for use in conjunction with scaling and root planing to reduce pocket depth in adult periodontitis. In localized juvenile periodontitis, systemic tetracycline therapy directed against A. actinomycetemcomitans combined with local periodontal treatment has yielded excellent results.[19] Unfortunately, the administration of tetracycline to children under 9 years of age can stain the permanent dentition and is not generally recommended. Furthermore, tetracycline resistance among periodontal pathogens has been increasingly recognized.[21] The routine use of systemic antimicrobials prophylactically during oral or periodontal surgery in a healthy host is unwarranted, since the risk of postoperative infection following periodontal surgery is less than 1%.[20]

The need for definitive restoration or extraction of the infected tooth, the primary source of an odontogenic infection, is readily apparent. Deep periodontal scaling and endodontic treatments with root fillings are required in most instances.

The key for the prevention and control of dental caries and advanced periodontitis is the active promotion of oral hygiene, including

- Rigorous brushing and dental flossing after each meal
- Dietary counseling to reduce the ingestion of carbohydrate-rich foods or beverages
- Use of topical fluorides and oral antimicrobial rinses such as chlorhexidine for high-risk patients
- Behavioral modification of risk factors such as tobacco smoking
- Overcoming the reluctance for regular visits to dental professionals

Vaccines based upon various immunogens derived from S. mutans, the principal bacterial agent associated with dental caries, have been explored.[22,23] However, the availability of an effective and safe vaccine for clinical application is unlikely in the near future.[24]

Suppurative Orofacial Odontogenic Infections

The most important therapeutic modality for pyogenic odontogenic infections is surgical drainage and removal of necrotic tissue. Needle aspiration by the extraoral route can be particularly helpful both for microbiologic sampling and for evacuation of pus. The need for definitive restoration or extraction of the infected tooth, the primary source of infection, is usually readily apparent. Deep periodontal scaling and endodontic treatments with

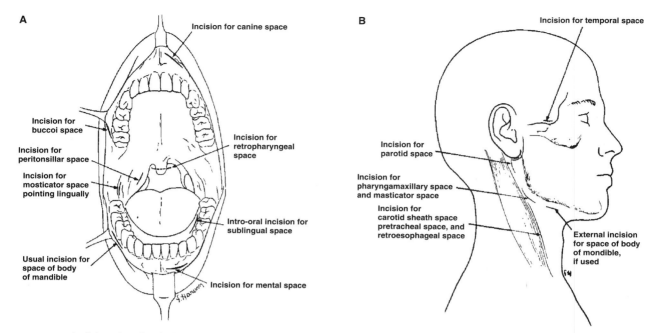

FIGURE 2–6. Incision sites for drainage of "space" infections of the head and neck. *A,* Intraoral approach. *B,* Extraoral approach. (From Echevarria J: Deep neck infections. In Schlossberg D [ed]: Infections of the Head and Neck. New York, Springer-Verlag, 1987, pp 178–179.)

root filling are required in most instances. Effective surgical management requires a thorough understanding of the most likely anatomic routes of spread. The neighboring fascial spaces should be carefully and systematically surveyed. For effective drainage the incision site should be in the most dependent location, and either an intraoral or extraoral approach may be considered (Fig. 2–6). It is equally important that the timing for incision and drainage be optimum. Premature incision into an area of cellulitis in an ill-conceived search for pus can disrupt the normal physiologic barrier and spread the infection.

Antibiotic therapy is important in halting the local spread of infection and in preventing hematogenous dissemination. Antimicrobial agents are generally indicated if fever and regional lymphadenopathy are present or if infection has perforated the bony cortex and spread into surrounding soft tissue. Severely immunocompromised patients are particularly at risk for spreading orofacial infections, and empiric broad-spectrum antimicrobial therapy in these patients is warranted. The choice of specific antibiotics is based more upon knowledge of the indigenous organisms that colonize the teeth, gums, and mucous membranes than upon the results of culture and sensitivity testing. Most organisms, including both anaerobes and aerobes, are sensitive to penicillin. Thus, penicillin monotherapy in doses appropriate for the severity of infection remains a good choice (Table 2–2). Penicillin-allergic patients can be treated usually with clindamycin (450 mg PO four times daily or 600 mg IV every 8 hours). Cefoxitin, cefotetan, or ceftizoxime are alternative choices. Erythromycin and tetracycline are not recommended because of increasing resistance to

them among some strains of streptococci and their lack of optimal anaerobic activity.[21]

The problem of β-lactamase production and penicillin resistance among *Bacteroides* spp. and *P. melaninogenica* has been increasingly recognized, and treatment failure with penicillin in odontogenic infections due to such strains has been reported.[14] Therefore in patients with life-threatening, deep fascial space infections and in patients who have had an unfavorable or delayed response to penicillin, alternative therapy with a broader spectrum against anaerobes as well as facultative gram-negative bacilli may be considered. Ambulatory patients with less serious odontogenic infections can be treated with amoxicillin with or without a β-lactamase inhibitor or with penicillin in combination with metronidazole. Metronidazole, although highly active against anaerobic gram-negative bacilli and spirochetes, is only moderately active against *Peptostreptococcus* species and is not active against aerobes, including streptococci. Except in acute necrotizing gingivitis and in advanced periodontitis, it should not be used as a single agent in odontogenic infections.

In the compromised host such as the patient with leukemia and severe neutropenia after chemotherapy, it is prudent to cover for facultative gram-negative bacilli as well, and agents with broad-spectrum activity against both aerobes and anaerobes are desirable (Table 2–2).

Aphthous Ulcers and Mucositis

Aphthous ulcers are among the most common causes of recurrent oral lesions and must be distinguished from other conditions such as herpes simplex virus or coxsackievirus infections, agranulocytosis, and Behçet's syndrome. The cause of aphthous ulcers remains uncertain, although a number of infectious agents including viruses have been implicated. Three major clinical variants are recognized: (1) minor aphthous ulcers, (2) major aphthous ulcers, and (3) herpetiform aphthous ulcers. Minor aphthous ulcers appear as a number of small ulcers on the buccal and labial mucosa, the floor of the mouth, or the tongue. The palatal soft tissues, pharynx, and tonsillar fauces are rarely involved. A prodromal stage is usually present. The ulcers appear gray-yellow, often with a raised and erythematous margin, and are exquisitely painful. Lymph node enlargement is seen only with secondary bacterial infection. The course of ulceration varies from a few days to several weeks and is followed by spontaneous healing. Major aphthous ulcers are more protracted and may last up to several months. All areas of the oral cavity including the soft palate and tonsillar areas may be involved. Prolonged periods of remission may be followed by intervals of intense ulcer activity. Herpetiform aphthous ulcers are small and multiple and characteristically affect the lateral margins and tips of the tongue. The ulcers are gray with a delineating erythematous border and are extremely painful. Despite its name, there is little clinical resemblance to an acute herpetic gingivostomatitis. The treatment of aphthous ulcers is primarily symptomatic. Strict oral hygiene should be maintained, and the use of antiseptic mouthwashes may be helpful in temporarily reducing secondary infection. Local anesthetic lozenges or gels may be used as a last resort for brief periods of pain relief. Topical or systemic steroids may be beneficial in selected patients with extensive disease, but caution must be exercised in their administration. Thalidomide (100 to 200 mg/d PO for 2 to 6 weeks) has been reported to be effective for the treatment of large aphthous lesions in patients with acquired immunodeficiency syndrome.[25]

Mucositis involving the nonkeratinized oral epithelium is a frequent complication following irradiation or during chemotherapy for acute leukemia.[26] Bacteremia with viridans streptococci is particularly common in patients with severe mucositis. Oral candidiasis, herpes simplex, varicella zoster, and cytomegalovirus infections may occur concurrently. Ulceration and pseudomembrane formation usually are evident between 4 and 7 days after the initiation of chemotherapy. The duration of lesions is often protracted. The clinical manifestations can vary. Lesions may not be associated with an inflammatory reaction, thereby masking the usual signs and symptoms of infection. Pain or tenderness may be the only abnormal finding. Since the agents causing the infection cannot be readily predicted on clinical grounds alone in such patients, specific microbiologic diagnosis by culture, histopathology, or antigen detection techniques is critical for appropriate treatment. Topical as well as systemic antimicrobial agents may be indicated along with antiseptic (e.g., chlorhexidine) and anesthetic (e.g., benzydamine or viscous lidocaine)

applications.[27] Frequent saline rinses may reduce mucosal irritation, remove thickened secretions or debris, and increase moisture in the mouth. Coating agents such as milk of magnesia or aluminum hydroxide gel (Amphojel) have been useful for the symptomatic relief of painful oral lesions. Topical or oral cytoprotective agents (e.g., sucralfate) or nonsteroidal anti-inflammatory analgesics (e.g., benzydamine or salicylates) may provide additional benefit, but further controlled clinical trials are required to assess for appropriate indications and efficacy. Meticulous oral and dental hygiene, effective management of xerostomia, selective suppression of oropharyngeal microbial colonization, and early control of reactivation by latent viral infections appear to be crucial to prevention and reduction of the overall morbidity of oromucosal infections in the severely immunocompromised.[26,28]

Sialadenitis and Suppurative Parotitis

Sialadenitis, or infection of the salivary gland, is a relatively common disease. Sialolithiasis in elderly patients (particularly calculi in Wharton's duct) often leads to ductal obstruction and secondary infection. Other predisposing factors for ductal occlusion include dehydration, sialogogic drugs, general debility, and trauma. In suppurative parotitis there is a sudden onset of firm, erythematous swelling of the preauricular and postauricular areas that extends to the angle of the mandible. This is associated with exquisite local pain and tenderness. Systemic findings of high fever, chills, and marked toxicity are generally present. Progression of the infection may lead to massive swelling of the neck, respiratory obstruction, septicemia, and osteomyelitis of the adjacent facial bones. Staphylococci have been the predominant isolates, but Enterobacteriaceae, oral anaerobes, and other facultative gram-negative rods have also been reported. Antimicrobial therapy should be directed against staphylococci and the mouth flora (Table 2–2). Early surgical drainage and decompression of the gland are generally required, since spontaneous drainage is uncommon.

Cervicofacial Actinomycosis and Botryomycosis

Actinomycosis is a chronic bacterial infection caused by *Actinomyces* species. These anaerobic or aerotolerant filamentous, branching gram-positive coccobacilli are present in high concentrations within the indigenous flora of the oral cavity and the gastrointestinal tract. Although *Actinomyces israelii* is the most common pathogen in human actinomycosis, at least 3 other *Actinomyces* species (*A. naeslundii, A. viscosus,* and *A. odontolyticus*) and *Arachnia propionica* may also be involved. The latter is morphologically indistinguishable from *Actinomyces* species and produces an identical infection. These microbes are generally of poor pathogenicity. Under special conditions that lead to tissue ischemia and lowered oxidation-reduction potential, however, these organisms may proliferate and invade surrounding healthy tissues.

Thus actinomycosis is particularly common following orofacial trauma and dental manipulations (cervicofacial actinomycosis).[29] Typically the lesion begins as a painful, indurated swelling 1 to several weeks after the initial inciting event. It frequently presents as an inflammatory mass at the angle of the jaw ("lumpy jaw") and gradually proceeds to suppurate, resulting in multiple extraoral draining sinuses. The overlying skin may become fixed to the inflammatory mass, often with a violescent discoloration. Sulfur granules may be seen in the exudate. Trismus is prominent early in the course, but cervical lymphadenopathy is uncommon. Rarely, recalcitrant osteomyelitis of the mandible may result from direct extension of infection. The most common misdiagnosis of an actinomycotic lesion is a neoplastic process.[30]

The diagnosis of actinomycosis is not difficult once the disease is clinically suspected, and the causative organism is seen on Gram stain or isolated by biopsy and culture. Since *Actinomyces* species are part of the normal oral flora, however, care must be taken during specimen collection to avoid contamination by commensal bacteria. Specimens obtained by fine needle aspiration are particularly useful for Gram stain cytologic examination and culture.[31] Although the presence of sulfur granules highly suggest actinomycosis, their presence is not diagnostic. Similar structures may be seen with nocardiosis, botryomycosis, aspergillosis, coccidioidomycosis, and lesions caused by the saprophytic fungi *Scedosporium* and *acremonium*. *Nocardia* may produce a clinical picture that is similar to actinomycosis, although subcutaneous abscesses and sinus formation are infrequent. In contrast to *Actinomyces*, *Nocardia* spp are aerobic and acid fast.

Botryomycosis is an unusual manifestation of a chronic, granulomatous infection caused by staphylococci, facultative gram-negative rods such as *Escherichia coli*, *P. aeruginosa*, and *Proteus mirabilis*, and anaerobic gram-positive rods such as *Propionebacterium acnes*.[32] The characteristic feature is the presence of funguslike granules within the suppurative foci containing many epithelioid and giant cells. Cultures, however, are negative for *Actinomyces*. The pathogenesis is thought to be a symbiotic relationship between the host and the infecting organism.[32]

Both *Actinomyces* and *Arachnia* are highly susceptible to penicillin, erythromycin, clindamycin, and minocycline. Penicillin G (2 to 4 million units every 4 hours) is the antibiotic of choice. It should be given intravenously for at least 3 to 4 weeks after the patient appears cured. Severe cases may require oral therapy of even longer duration to prevent relapse. Surgical drainage is a valuable adjunct to antimicrobial therapy.

Deep Fascial Space Infections

Peritonsillar Abscess
Peritonsillar abscess, also known as *quinsy*, is a suppurative complication of acute tonsillitis involving the peritonsillar space. Peritonsillar abscesses may affect patients of all ages but are most common among young adults between the ages of 15 and 30 years. The patient appears ill with fever, sore throat, dysphagia, trismus, pooling of saliva, and a muffled voice. The abscess is usually unilateral, with associated cervical lymphadenitis. Examination of the pharynx in most cases reveals swelling of the anterior pillar and the soft palate and, less commonly, the middle portion or lower pole of the tonsil. Initially needle drainage in the Trendelenburg position should be attempted and the patient closely monitored and managed with intravenous antibiotics alone. Failure to obtain pus is an indication for surgical incision and more formal exploration. Delays increase the risk of spontaneous rupture. Aspiration of purulent material is the main hazard, particularly in the sleeping patient. More serious complications include (1) airway obstruction, especially with bilateral disease or when laryngeal edema develops, and (2) lateral dissection (usually from infections of the middle or lower portions of the tonsil) to involve the lateral pharyngeal space (Fig. 2–2). Continued signs of sepsis after drainage of the peritonsillar space usually indicate concomitant, undrained lateral pharyngeal space infection. Fatalities associated with peritonsillar abscess (over 50% in the preantibiotic era) were largely due to this complication.

Ideally antibiotics should be tailored according to culture results from pus obtained by needle aspiration of the abscess, but this is infrequently performed. Group A ß-hemolytic streptococci (often as part of a mixed flora containing anaerobes) are most commonly isolated. Occasionally other ß-hemolytic streptococci, *H. influenzae*, *S. aureus*, or anaerobes alone are cultured. Penicillin G, however, is effective therapy in most cases. Bilateral tonsillectomy should be performed once the patient has recovered to avoid recurrences. Interim antibiotic prophylaxis should be considered in high-risk cases.

Submandibular Space Infections
Ludwig's Angina
The prototypical infection of the submandibular space is known as Ludwig's angina. It is characteristically an aggressive, rapidly spreading "woody" or brawny cellulitis involving both the sublingual space above the mylohyoid muscle and the submylohyoid space below (Fig. 2–1). Ludwig's angina most commonly follows infection of the second or third mandibular molar teeth (70% to 85% of cases), since the roots of these teeth are located below the attachments of the mylohyoid muscle to the mandible. Infection extends contiguously (rather than by the lymphatics, which would limit the infection to one side only) to involve the sublingual and thus the entire submandibular space in a symmetrical manner. Less commonly, an identical process initially involving the sublingual space can arise from infection of the premolars and other teeth or from trauma to the floor of the mouth. Once established, infection can evolve rapidly. The tongue may enlarge to two or three times its normal

size. Infection may spread directly into the lateral laryngeal space and thereby to the retropharyngeal space and the mediastinum (Fig. 2–2).

Clinically the patient is febrile and complains of mouth pain, stiff neck, drooling, and dysphagia and leans forward to maximize the airway diameter. A tender, symmetrical and indurated swelling, sometimes with palpable crepitus, is present in the submandibular area. The mouth is held open by lingual swelling. Respirations are usually difficult; stridor and cyanosis are considered ominous signs. Radiographic views of the teeth may indicate the source of infection, and lateral views of the neck will demonstrate the degree of soft tissue swelling around the airway and possibly submandibular gas. Significant asymmetry of the submandibular area should be viewed with great concern, since it may be indicative of extension to the lateral pharyngeal space. Well-timed surgical drainage will reduce the risk of spread to this space and subsequently to the superior mediastinum.

Treatment of Ludwig's angina has undergone a number of modifications since its initial description.[33] Although maintenance of the airway is the primary concern and may necessitate urgent tracheostomy, most cases can be managed initially by close observation and intravenous antibiotics. If cellulitis and swelling continue to advance rapidly or if dyspnea occurs, an artificial airway should be gained immediately before the onset of stridor, cyanosis, and asphyxia. Blind oral or nasotracheal intubation should be avoided, as it is traumatic and may precipitate severe laryngospasm. A recommended approach is to use a flexible fiberoptic scope to assess the airway and to aid in inserting an endotracheal tube. Tracheostomy is still the most widely recommended means of airway control, although cricothyrotomy is advocated by some experts because of a lower complication rate.

Penicillin G is the antibiotic of choice, but immunocompromised patients require a broader spectrum of antibiotic coverage against such organisms as facultative gram-negative rods and *S. aureus* (Table 2–2). Early surgical decompression, much advocated in the preantibiotic era, is unlikely to locate pus and at best may only moderately improve the airway. Pus collections develop relatively late (usually not present in the first 24 to 36 hours) and are sometimes difficult to detect clinically. If the patient is not responding adequately to antibiotics alone after this initial period or if fluctuance is detectable, needle aspiration or a more formal incision and drainage procedure with the patient under general anesthesia should be performed. Preferably this should be done with a cuffed tracheostomy in place. Additionally, the infected teeth implicated in the process should be extracted.

Systemic antibiotics combined with aggressive surgical intervention have lowered the mortality rate for Ludwig's angina dramatically from over 50% in the preantibiotic era to 0 to 4% currently.

Submandibular and Submental Abscesses

A submandibular abscess can result from suppuration of a submandibular lymph node or the submandibular salivary gland or from extension of a periapical abscess originating from the second or third molar tooth below the mylohyoid muscle. Fluctuance is a prominent finding, since there is no overlying musculature and the fascia is not so dense. Submental abscesses usually result from spread of a periapical abscess arising from the lower incisors. Suppuration of a submental lymph node may be another source of infection. There may be moderate elevation of the floor of the mouth, but the exuberant swelling of the soft tissues of the mouth, as seen in Ludwig's angina, is lacking. Abscesses in submandibular or submental spaces are treated by incision and drainage (Fig. 2–6).

Lateral Pharyngeal Space Infections

Lateral pharyngeal space infections are potentially life threatening because the carotid sheath, which contains several vital structures including the common carotid artery, the internal jugular vein, and the vagus nerve, is within the posterior compartment of the lateral pharyngeal space (Fig. 2–1). Since most patients are already compromised by infection elsewhere, diagnosis of lateral pharyngeal involvement is often delayed. Infections of the lateral pharyngeal space may arise from sources throughout the neck. Dental infections are most common, followed by peritonsillar abscess (postanginal sepsis) and rarely acute parotitis, otitis, or mastoiditis (Bezold's abscess). Infection of the anterior compartment is more common than infection of the posterior compartment is. The cardinal clinical features, in order of importance, are (1) trismus, (2) induration and swelling below the angle of the mandible, (3) systemic toxicity with fever and rigors, and (4) medial bulging of the pharyngeal wall. Dyspnea may be prominent as edema and swelling descend directly to involve the epiglottis and larynx. Swelling of the pharyngeal wall, if present, will be behind the palatopharyngeal arch and is easily missed. Suppuration may advance quickly to other spaces, particularly to the retropharyngeal and danger spaces, thus reaching directly to the mediastinum inferiorly or the base of the skull superiorly (Fig. 2–2). An abscess localized to the posterior neurovascular compartment of the lateral pharyngeal space is manifested by sepsis and cranial nerve involvement (e.g., Horner syndrome, hoarseness, unilateral tongue paresis) but minimal trismus. The posterior tonsillar pillar is displaced. The contiguous parotid gland is usually swollen. The source of infection is best evaluated by CT or MRI. Careful needle aspiration or more definitive incision and drainage may be required. Percutaneous drainage is contraindicated because of the proximity of the great vessels. Antimicrobial treatment depends on the primary source of infection, whether peritonsillar, odontogenic, or secondary to suppurative parotitis (Table 2–2).

Retropharyngeal Space Infections

Retropharyngeal abscesses are among the most serious of deep space infections, since infection can extend directly into the superior and posterior mediastinum via the "danger" space (Fig. 2–2B). Retropharyngeal infection is more common in young children because of lymphatic spread of infection in the pharynx or sinuses and of suppuration of regional lymph nodes within the retropharyngeal space. The onset may be insidious, with little more than fever, irritability, drooling, a muffled voice (dysphonia), or possibly nuchal rigidity. More acute symptoms include dysphagia and dyspnea. Dyspnea may be due to a local mass effect or to laryngeal edema. Generally there is little pain, but the neck may be held rigid and tilted to the unaffected side. Cervical lymphadenopathy is usually absent. Definite bulging of the posterior pharyngeal wall is usual but may need careful palpation to be appreciated. The main dangers of a retropharyngeal space infection are severe laryngeal edema with airway obstruction and rupture of the abscess with aspiration or asphyxia. Many cases will respond to antibiotic therapy alone if treatment precedes the development of frank suppuration (Table 2–2).

Retropharyngeal infection is less common in older children or adults because the retropharyngeal lymph nodes atrophy by the age of 3 or 4 years.[34] In adults, infection may reach the retropharyngeal space either by penetrating trauma to the esophagus (e.g., from chicken bones or following instrumentation) or by contiguous spread of infection from an odontogenic source or peritonsillar abscess (now a rare cause). Infection from these sources may often obscure the diagnosis because of associated trismus, which makes direct examination of the posterior pharyngeal wall difficult. Differential diagnosis includes cervical osteomyelitis, Pott's disease, meningitis, and calcific tendonitis of the long muscle of the neck.[35] In this setting, CT and radiographic views of the lateral neck are especially helpful and may demonstrate cervical lordosis with swelling and gas collections in the retropharyngeal space. The radiograph should be evaluated for increased thickness of the retropharyngeal soft tissues (Fig. 2–4), air or air-fluid levels, and the presence of foreign bodies. Radiographs may also help to differentiate this infection from cervical osteomyelitis with spread to the prevertebral space.[36,37] Treatment consists of expeditious drainage of the abscess and antimicrobial regimens selected on the basis of the most likely source of the primary infection (Table 2–2).

COMPLICATIONS OF HEAD AND NECK INFECTIONS

Vascular Infections

Carotid Sheath Infections

Involvement of the carotid sheath is a dreaded complication because of the potential for carotid artery erosion and suppurative jugular thrombophlebitis. The carotid sheath abuts all three layers of deep cervical fascia. Infection may therefore arise by spread from the lateral pharyngeal space, Ludwig's angina, or suppuration of deep cervical lymph nodes.[38] There are no characteristic symptoms or signs of carotid sheath infections. A history of sore throat, although usually present initially, is not invariable and may only be mild, unilateral, or transient. There may be a latent period of up to 3 weeks before more obvious clinical manifestations of deep infection develop. The patient presents either in a toxic or insidious condition with a fever of undetermined origin. Trismus is absent, and signs of local suppuration may be subtle because of the tight connective tissue around and within the carotid sheath. In some patients there may be diffuse swelling along the sternocleidomastoid muscle with marked tenderness and torticollis to the opposite side. Erosion of the carotid artery with rupture is a devastating complication, with a mortality of 20% to 40% irrespective of treatment.[39] The initial pathology is an arteritis caused by contiguous inflammation that eventually forms a false aneurysm. Rupture of the carotid artery may be heralded by recurrent minor hemorrhages from the nose, mouth, or ear ("herald bleeds"). This is followed by hematoma formation in the surrounding tissues of the neck, a protracted clinical course, and eventually shock due to exsanguinations. Ligation of the carotid artery may be necessary in cases of major hemorrhage, but the risk of stroke is significant.[40,41]

Septic Jugular Thrombophlebitis (Lemierre Syndrome)

Suppurative jugular thrombophlebitis (also known as Lemierre syndrome or postanginal sepsis) is the most common vascular complication of a lateral pharyngeal space infection.[42] Symptoms of jugular vein thrombosis include pain in the neck made worse by turning the head away from the involved side. This motion causes the sternocleidomastoid muscle to compress the inflamed mass. Dysphagia and dysphonia may also occur. On examination, the tonsil is displaced medially. An indurated swelling a few centimeters long may be palpable behind the sternocleidomastoid muscle or may be found more deeply behind the palatopharyngeal arch. Trismus is minimal and may be absent. Ipsilateral vocal cord paralysis or other neurologic signs representing lower cranial nerve involvement may be present. These signs are frequently missed (detected in only 20% of cases antemortem in one series) unless specifically sought and may be transient. The patient may thus present as an obscure septicemia (50% of cases). Chills and sweats may indicate blood stream infection. Septic emboli from the jugular venous system may travel to the lung, followed by hematogenous dissemination to other visceral organs.[43] There may be retrograde spread of infection with cerebral abscess or meningitis. Diagnosis and treatment may be delayed because the source of the infection is not obvious. In the absence of a demonstrable cause for sepsis, careful efforts should be

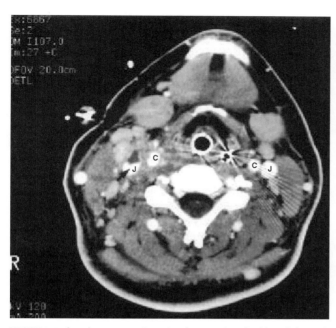

FIGURE 2–7. Jugular venous thrombosis associated with a right peritonsillar abscess in a 19-year-old. Contrast-enhanced axial CT scan showing a normal right common carotid (*C*) artery but an enlarged right internal jugular vein (*J*) (*arrow*) with a dense or enhancing wall that surrounds the more lucent intraluminal clot.

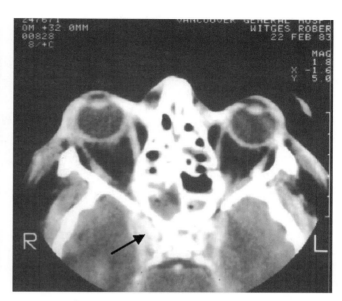

FIGURE 2–8. Cavernous sinus thrombosis associated with acute pansinusitis in a young adult. Contrast-enhanced axial CT showing opacification of the sphenoid and ethmoid sinuses and thrombus in the right cavernous sinus (*arrow*). (From Chow AW: Life-threatening infections of the head, neck, and upper respiratory tract. In Hall JB, Schmidt GA, Wood LH [eds]: Principles of Critical Care, 2nd ed. New York, McGraw-Hill, 1998, p 899.)

made to elicit a history of pharyngitis. Contrast-enhanced CT may show the normal carotid artery and an enlarged jugular venous wall surrounding a more lucent intraluminal clot (Fig. 2–7). Thrombosis of the jugular vein can also be demonstrated by magnetic resonance angiography. The organisms most frequently involved in postanginal sepsis are anaerobic streptococci and *Bacteroides* (now including *Prevotella*) spp and *Fusobacterium* spp.[42] Less common are α-hemolytic and group A β-hemolytic streptococci, *S. pneumoniae*, *S. aureus*, and *Eikenella corrodens*. Most cases of postanginal sepsis with suppurative jugular thrombophlebitis can be managed medically without the need for ligation or surgical resection of the infected vein. Prolonged courses of intravenous antibiotics (3 to 6 weeks) will be required. Since anaerobic bacteremia caused by *Bacteroides* spp or *Fusobacterium necrophorum* is frequently present and because penicillin resistance among these organisms is increasingly recognized, therapy may require the addition of metronidazole, clindamycin, or β-lactamase-stable cephalosporins (Table 2–2). Fever may be slow to resolve, even in cases successfully treated, particularly if there is metastatic involvement. Anticoagulants have sometimes been used in this setting, but efficacy is unconfirmed. Surgical ligation of the internal jugular vein, the only available therapeutic option in the preantibiotic era, is now required only in the rare patient who fails to respond to antibiotic treatment alone.

Septic Dural Sinus Thrombosis

Septic intracranial thrombophlebitis most frequently follows infection of the paranasal sinuses, middle ear, mastoid, or oropharynx. If collateral venous drainage is adequate, septic venous thrombosis may produce only transient neurologic findings or may be silent. If the thrombus outstrips collateral flow, however, progressive neurologic deficits will result with impairment of consciousness, focal or generalized seizures, and increased intracranial pressure. The clinical findings vary with the location of cortical veins or dural sinuses involved. Cavernous sinus thrombosis is characterized by abrupt onset with diplopia, photophobia, orbital edema, and progressive exophthalmos. Involvement of cranial nerves III, IV, V, and VI produces ophthalmoplegia, a midposition fixed pupil, loss of corneal reflex, and diminished sensation over the upper face. Obstruction of venous return from the retina results in papilledema, retinal hemorrhage, and visual loss. Contrast-enhanced CT (Fig. 2–8) and MRI are the imaging modalities of choice. Treatment requires early recognition, high-dose intravenous antibiotics selected on the basis of the most likely source of primary infection (Table 2–2), and surgical decompression of the underlying predisposing infection. Acute sphenoid sinusitis is the most common antecedent event. Anticoagulation and steroids are not indicated. Mortality remains high, approximately 15% to 30%. Thrombosis of the superior sagittal sinus produces bilateral leg weakness and may cause communicating hydrocephalus. It is a rare complication of chronic frontal sinusitis. Occlusion of the lateral sinus may occur as a complication of chronic mastoiditis. The patient complains of pain over the ear and mastoid and may develop edema over the mastoid (Griesinger's sign). Involvement of cranial nerves V and VI produces ipsilateral facial pain and lateral rectus weakness (Gradenigo's syndrome).

Osseous Infections

Pott's Puffy Tumor

Chronic osteomyelitis of the facial bones is a relatively rare complication of chronic sinusitis. The bone most commonly involved is the facial bone. Secondary chronic frontal sinusitis, historically known as Pott's puffy tumor, causes tenderness and frontal bossing. Diagnosis is made by physical examination that reveals local tenderness and dull pain. Definitive diagnosis is made by CT and radionuclide scanning. A surgical procedure usually is required to obtain adequate cultures of the sinus mucosa and bone. Treatment consists of intravenous antibiotics for at least 6 weeks (Table 2–2) and surgical débridement of nonviable bone if present. Close monitoring for intracranial suppurative complications such as subdural empyema or cranial epidural abscess is necessary.[44]

Malignant Otitis Externa and Petrous Osteitis

Malignant otitis externa is a progressive necrotizing infection of the external ear caused by *P. aeruginosa* that spreads through the cartilage and bony canal to the base of the skull. Affected patients usually are debilitated and often have poorly controlled diabetes mellitus. The infection is associated with severe otalgia, hearing loss, purulent discharge, edema, and granulation tissue or "polyp" in the cartilaginous portion of the external ear canal. Three stages of progression are recognized clinically: (1) locally invasive disease, (2) disease associated with facial palsy, and (3) disease associated with multiple cranial nerve palsies. In the latter stages, infection may involve the infratemporal fossa by extension into the temporal bone (petrous osteitis). Ciprofloxacin is the preferred antibiotic because of its excellent penetration into bone (Table 2–2). The combination of an aminoglycoside and an antipseudomonal β-lactam (e.g., ceftazidime, piperacillin, or imipenem) is a suitable alternative. Prolonged medical therapy in conjunction with local débridement of granulation tissue and infected cartilage is effective in most patients. In patients with more extensive disease involving the base of the skull and multiple cranial nerve palsies, results of therapy are not so successful, and up to 20 months of antimicrobial treatment may be required to eradicate infection without relapse.

Mandibular Osteomyelitis

Odontogenic infections can spread contiguously to cause osteomyelitis of the jaws. The mandible is much more susceptible to osteomyelitis than the maxilla is, mainly because the cortical plates of the mandible are thin, and vascular supply to the medullary tissues is relatively poor. Despite this, osteomyelitis secondary to odontogenic infection is relatively uncommon. When it does occur, there is usually a predisposing condition such as compound fracture, irradiation, diabetes mellitus, or steroid therapy. With initiation of infection the intramedullary pressure markedly increases, further compromising blood supply, which leads to bone necrosis. Pus travels through the Haversian and perforating canals, accumulates beneath the periosteum, and elevates it from the cortex. If pus continues to accumulate, the periosteum is eventually penetrated, and mucosal or cutaneous abscesses and fistulas can develop. When the inflammatory process persists, granulation tissue is formed. Spicules of necrotic and nonviable bone may become either totally isolated (sequestrum) or encased in a sheath of new bone (involucrum).

Severe mandibular pain is a common symptom that can be accompanied by anesthesia or hypoesthesia on the affected side. In protracted cases, mandibular trismus may develop. A clinical variant is Garré's chronic sclerosing osteomyelitis or proliferative periostitis. This entity is characterized by a localized, hard, nontender swelling over the mandible. Actinomycosis and radiation necrosis are two common causes of this form of osteomyelitis of the jaws.[45] Treatment of mandibular osteomyelitis is complicated by the presence of teeth and persistent exposure to the oral environment. Antibiotic therapy needs to be prolonged, often for weeks to months (Table 2–2). Adjuvant therapy with hyperbaric oxygen may prove beneficial in hastening the healing process.[45] In one study of 33 patients with early chronic osteomyelitis of the jaw, 79% were free of symptoms 10 to 34 months after hyperbaric oxygen therapy combined with surgical débridement.[46] Surgical management, including sequestrectomy, saucerization, decortication, and closed-wound suction irrigation, occasionally may be necessary. Rarely, in advanced cases, the entire segment of the infected jaw may have to be resected.

REFERENCES

1. Chong VF, Fan YF: Comparison of CT and MRI features in sinusitis. Eur J Radiol 1998;29:47–54.
2. Dessi P, Champsaur P, Paris J, et al: Imaging of adult sinusitis: Indications for using conventional techniques, CT scan and MRI. Rev Laryngol Otol Rhinol 1999;120:173–176.
3. Latchaw RE, Hirsch WL Jr, Yock DH Jr: Imaging of intracranial infection. Neurosurg Clin N Am 1992;3:303–322.
4. Todd JK: Bacteriology and clinical relevance of nasopharyngeal and oropharyngeal cultures. Pediatr Infect Dis 1984;3:159–163.
5. Roscoe DL, Chow AW: Normal flora and mucosal immunity of the head and neck. Infect Dis Clin N Am 1988;2:1–19.
6. Darveau RJP, Tanner A, Page RC: The microbial challenge in periodontitis. Periodontol 2000 1997;14:202–215.
7. Moore WEC, Moore LVH: The bacteria of periodontal diseases. Periodontol 2000 1994;5:66–77.
8. Shaw JH: Causes and control of dental caries. N Engl J Med 1987;317:996–1004.
9. Loesche WJ: Role of *Streptococcus mutans* in human dental decay. Microbiol Rev 1986;50:353–380.
10. Johnson TC, Reinhardt RA, Payne JB, et al: Experimental gingivitis in periodontitis-susceptible subjects. J Clin Periodontol 1997;24:618–625.

11. Rams TE, Flynn MJ, Slots J: Subgingival microbial associations in severe human periodontitis. Clin Infect Dis 1997; 25(Suppl. 2):S224–S226.

12. Matto J, Asikainen S, Vaisanen ML, et al: Role of *Porphyromonas gingivalis, Prevotella intermedia,* and *Prevotella nigrescens* in extraoral and some odontogenic infections. Clin Infect Dis 1997;25(Suppl. 2):S194–S198.

13. Lewis MA, Parkhurst CL, Douglas CW, et al: Prevalence of penicillin-resistant bacteria in acute suppurative oral infection. J Antimicrob Chemother 1995;35:785–791.

14. Heimdahl A, von Konow L, Nord CE: Isolation of β-lactamase producing *Bacteroides* strains associated with clinical failures with penicillin treatment of human orofacial infections. Arch Oral Biol 1980;25:689–692.

15. Murray JJ: Appropriate use of fluorides for human health. Geneva, World Health Organization, 1986, p 131.

16. Achong RA, Briskie DM, Hildebrandt GH, et al: Effect of chlorhexidine varnish mouthguards on the levels of selected oral microorganisms in pediatric patients. Pediatr Dent 1999;21:169–175.

17. Offenbacher S: Periodontal diseases: Pathogenesis. Ann Periodontol 1996;1:821–878.

18. Shinn DLS, Squires S, McFadzean JA: The treatment of Vincent's disease with metronidazole. Dent Pract 1965; 15:275.

19. Fine DH, Hammond BF, Loesche WJ: Clinical use of antibiotics in dental practice. Int J Antimicrob Agents 1998;9:235–238.

20. Loesche WJ: Antimicrobials in dentistry: With knowledge comes responsibility [editorial]. J Dent Res 1996;75:1432–1433.

21. Olsvik B, Tenover FC: Tetracycline resistance in periodontal pathogens. Clin Infect Dis 1993;16 (Suppl 4):S310–313.

22. Gregory RL, Filler SJ: Protective secretory immunoglobulin A antibodies in humans following oral immunization with *Streptococcus mutans.* Infect Immun 1987;55:2409–2415.

23. Taubman MA, Holmberg CJ, Smith DJ: Immunization of rats with synthetic peptide constructs from the glucan-binding or catalytic region of mutans streptococcal glucosyltransferase protects against dental caries. Infect Immun 1995;63:3088–3093.

24. Bowen WH: Vaccine against dental caries—a personal view. J Dent Res 1996;75:1530–1533.

25. Jacobson JM, Greenspan JS, Spritzler J, et al: Thalidomide for the treatment of oral aphthous ulcers in patients with human immunodeficiency virus infection: National Institute of Allergy and Infectious Diseases. AIDS Clinical Trials Group in Engl J Med 1997;336:1487–1493.

26. Epstein JB, Chow AW: Oral complications associated with immunosuppression and cancer therapies. Infect Dis Clin N Am 1999;13:901–923.

27. Epstein JB, Stevenson-Moore PB: Benzydamine hydrochloride in prevention and management of pain in oral mucositis associated with radiation therapy. Oral Surg 1986;62:145–148.

28. Epstein JB: Infection prevention in bone marrow transplantation and radiation patients. NCI Monogr 1990;9:73–85.

29. Miller M, Haddad AJ: Cervicofacial actinomycosis. Oral Surg Oral Med Oral Pathol Oral Radiol Endod 1998;85:496–508.

30. Nagler R, Peled M, Laufer D: Cervicofacial actinomycosis: A Diagnostic challenge. Oral Surg Oral Med Oral Pathol Oral Radiol Endod 1997;83:652–656.

31. Sah SP, Mishra A, Rani S, et al: Cervicofacial actinomycosis: Diagnosis by fine needle aspiration cytology. Acta Cytol 2001;45:665–667.

32. Yencha MW, Walker CW, Karakla DW, et al: Cutaneous botryomycosis of the cervicofacial region. Head Neck 2001;23:594–598.

33. Busch RF: Ludwig angina: Early aggressive therapy. Arch Otolaryngol Head Neck Surg 1999;125:1283–1284.

34. Sakaguchi M, Sato S, Ishiyama T, et al: Characterization and management of deep neck infections. Int J Oral Maxillofac Surg 1997;26:131–134.

35. Haug RH, Picard U, Indresano AT: Diagnosis and treatment of the retropharyngeal abscess in adults. Br J Oral Max Surg 1990;28:34–38.

36. Jang YJ, Rhee CK: Retropharyngeal abscess associated with vertebral osteomyelitis and spinal epidural abscess. Otolaryngol Head Neck Surg 1998;119:705–708.

37. Faidas A, Ferguson JV, Nelson JE, et al: Cervical vertebral osteomyelitis presenting as retropharyngeal abscess. Clin Infect Dis 1994;18:992.

38. Alexander DW, Leonard JR, Trail ML: Vascular complications of deep neck abscesses. Laryngoscope 1968;78:361.

39. Blomquist IK, Bayer AS: Life-threatening deep fascial space infections of the head and neck. Infect Dis Clin N Am 1988;2:237–264.

40. Chow AW: Life-threatening infections of the head, neck, and upper respiratory tract. In Hall JB, Schmidt GA, Wood LDH (eds): Principles of Critical Care. New York, McGraw-Hill, 1998, pp 887–902.

41. Kono T, Kohno A, Kuwashima S, et al: CT findings of descending necrotising mediastinitis via the carotid space ('Lincoln Highway'). Pediatr Radiol 2001;31:84–86.

42. Sinave CP, Hardy GJ, Fardy PW: The Lemierre syndrome—suppurative thrombophlebitis of the internal jugular vein secondary to oropharyngeal infection. Medicine (Baltimore) 1989;68:85–94.

43. Gowan RT, Mehran RJ, Cardinal P, et al: Thoracic complications of Lemierre syndrome. Can Respir J 2000;7:481–485.

44. Chow AW: Infections of the sinuses and parameningeal structures. In Gorbach SL, Bartlett JG, Blacklow NR (eds): Infectious Diseases. Philadelphia, WB Saunders Co., 1998, pp 517–530.

45. Topazian RG: Osteomyelitis of the jaws. In Topazian RG, Goldberg MH (eds): Oral and Maxillofacial Infections. Philadelphia, WB Saunders, 1987, pp 204–238.

46. Aitasalo K, Niinikoski J, Granman R, et al: A modified protocol for early treatment of osteomyelitis and osteoradionecrosis of the mandible. Head Neck 1998;20:411–417.

section
2

Upper Respiratory Tract Infections

MICHAEL E. PICHICHERO, MD
JANET R. CASEY, MD

Sinusitis, Otitis Media, and Mastoiditis

SINUSITIS

Most cases of sinusitis are accompanied by inflammation of the nasal passages.[1,2] Therefore, the clinical condition referred to as sinusitis is actually rhinosinusitis: inflammation of the sinuses and nasal passages. Computed tomography (CT) and magnetic resonance imaging (MRI) studies have reported sinus mucosal abnormalities in 15% to 49% of patients who have no symptoms of rhinosinusitis.[3–8] Although all cases of rhinosinusitis involve inflammation of the mucosal linings, in the practice setting the focus is on those with symptoms.

Causes of Rhinosinusitis as a Basis for Therapy

Clinical diagnosis aims to identify cases that have a similar cause and presentation and would benefit from similar treatment. Inflammation of the sinuses can be caused by infectious agents, allergic conditions, systemic diseases (endocrine, metabolic, genetic), trauma, and noxious agents.[9–11] Although bacteria can be the primary cause of sinus inflammation, they also may represent a secondary infection. In these cases the initial inflammation predisposes the sinuses to infection. That is, allergic or viral rhinosinusitis may lead to bacterial rhinosinusitis.[3,4] Often a patient's symptoms are the result of several environmental and host factors working together. In clinical practice, diagnosis is undertaken with an eye toward therapeutic or preventive interventions. Therapies are directed toward current symptoms, the underlying cause, or both (Table 3–1).

Bacterial Rhinosinusitis

Infectious causes of rhinosinusitis include bacteria, viruses, and fungi. Approximately 0.5% to 2% of adults and up to 10% of pediatric cases of viral rhinosinusitis lead to secondary bacterial rhinosinusitis.[9,12–14] The rationale for identifying patients with bacterial rhinosinusitis stems from the potential use of antibiotics.

In this chapter the focus is on acute bacterial rhinosinusitis because antibiotics are beneficial. Bacterial infection of the sinuses can result in chronic sinusitis or other serious complications (e.g., meningitis, brain abscess). Antibiotics may prevent these developments. At the same time, concerns have increased about the inappropriate use of antibiotics, both for the individual (potential side effects and out-of-pocket expenses) and society (development of antibiotic resistance).[5]

In the 1970s and 1980s *Streptococcus pneumoniae* and *Haemophilus influenzae* predominated as pathogens isolated from maxillary sinus aspirate cultures.[6–9] In the

TABLE 3–1 ■ Causes and Potential Therapies for Rhinosinusitis

Bacterial: antibiotic
Viral: treat symptoms (inflammation)
Allergic: antihistamines, intranasal steroids
NARES: intranasal steroids
Inflammatory (multiple causes): decongestants, intranasal steroids
Anatomic: removal or reconstruction (surgical)

NARES, Non-allergic rhinosinusitis with eosinophilia syndrome.

1990s *Moraxella catarrhalis* was recognized as another important pathogen, especially in children.[10–13] These three organisms are now recognized as the major rhinosinusitis pathogens. Group A β-hemolytic streptococci, *Staphylococcus aureus*, and anaerobes also cause rhinosinusitis, but they are not so prevalent.[6–8,10,11,14]

Modifying Therapy Based on Patterns of Disease Presentation

In patients with bacterial rhinosinusitis, subgroups may be defined that differ in pathophysiology, and this distinction may further direct specific therapy. Subgroupings include duration of symptoms, severity of symptoms, and other patient characteristics.

Temporal Grouping: Acute, Subacute, Recurrent Acute, and Chronic Rhinosinusitis

The distinction among acute, subacute, recurrent acute, and chronic rhinosinusitis is based on temporal differences in presentation. Acute and chronic rhinosinusitis also differ in histopathologic and bacteriologic characteristics. Although somewhat arbitrary, consensus has been reached about defining these distinct but related clinical conditions on the basis of duration of symptoms and defining clinical factors.[15–19]

Acute rhinosinusitis is defined by sudden onset of symptoms lasting less than 4 weeks. Many cases of rhinosinusitis accompany viral infections of the upper respiratory tract. Because most common cold symptoms last 5 to 7 days and mimic those of bacterial rhinosinusitis, waiting for a minimal duration of symptoms (7 to 10 days) is generally recommended before a diagnosis of bacterial rhinosinusitis is made. Recurrent acute rhinosinusitis is defined by the presence of four or more episodes per year, each lasting more than 7 days, and by the absence of intervening signs or symptoms that would suggest an ongoing or chronic rhinosinusitis. Because patients with acute rhinosinusitis have symptoms for less than 4 weeks and those with chronic rhinosinusitis have symptoms for more than 12 weeks, those who have symptoms lasting between 4 and 12 weeks are considered to have a subacute infection. Some of these cases will resolve within 12 weeks, and others will progress to chronic rhinosinusitis. Rhinosinusitis is considered chronic when the symptoms

last longer than 12 weeks. Exacerbations of symptoms in patients with chronic rhinosinusitis can be acute. With treatment of the acute symptoms, these patients return to the baseline chronic rhinosinusitis condition. *S. pneumoniae*, *H. influenzae*, and *M. catarrhalis* are the predominant organisms in acute, recurrent acute, and subacute rhinosinusitis, whereas *Staphylococcus* species (especially *S. aureus*), gram-negative bacteria (e.g., Enterobacteriaceae), anaerobes, and fungi also may be seen in chronic rhinosinusitis.[10]

Patient Characteristics: Age, Symptom Severity, Prior Treatment History

Patient characteristics provide another criteria for subgrouping. In particular, studies have looked at the similarities and differences between children and adults. The age of a patient with acute bacterial rhinosinusitis helps predict, to some extent, the most likely cause of the sinus infection (Figs. 3–1 and 3–2).

Patients with acute bacterial rhinosinusitis can be further categorized as (1) those with mild or moderate disease, (2) those with a history of antibiotic exposure in the previous 4 to 6 weeks, and (3) those without a clinical response at 72 hours or longer after initiation of therapy.[17] The descriptors *mild* or *moderate* do not represent an empiric judgment of antibiotic resistance; rather they suggest the relative possibility of treatment failure. Such treatment failure is defined as the lack of response to therapy at the arbitrary cutoff time of 72 hours or longer. At this juncture the patient may be a candidate for switching therapy to an alternative antibiotic, depending upon the pathogen likely responsible for the unsuccessful clinical outcome.

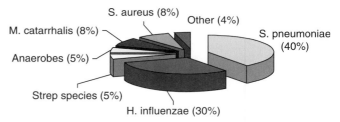

FIGURE 3–1. Prevalence of the major pathogens associated with acute bacterial rhinosinusitis in adults.

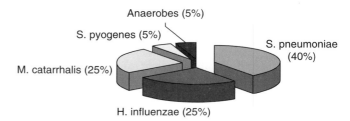

FIGURE 3–2. Prevalence of the major pathogens associated with acute bacterial rhinosinusitis in children.

Evidence-Based Analysis of Treatment Efficacy

A meta-analysis of randomized controlled trials of antibiotic treatment for acute bacterial rhinosinusitis was recently published.[19] Six studies compared any antibiotics with placebo[20–25] (Fig. 3–3). Antibiotics were significantly more effective than placebo, reducing treatment failures by almost one-half. However, symptoms improved or were cured in 69% of patients without any antibiotic treatment (95% confidence interval [CI], 57% to 79%).

A different meta-analysis of 14 trials compared amoxicillin with second-line antibiotics, most of which have an expanded spectrum of activity compared to that of amoxicillin (Fig. 3–4).[13,19,25–37] The pooled failure rate in patients treated with amoxicillin was low (11%; 95% CI, 8% to 14%). A further decrease in clinical failures with broad-spectrum antibiotics therefore was not evident. Similar results were obtained through analysis of the failure data of second-line antibiotics vs. TMP-SMX.

Thus, meta-analysis suggests about two-thirds of patients with acute bacterial rhinosinusitis appear to improve or are cured without antibiotics. In patients defined by clinical symptoms alone, without a firm radiographic or bacteriologic diagnosis, this rate may even be higher. Treatment with any antibiotic, regardless of type, reduces the rate of clinical failures by about one-half. From these data one might conclude that for uncomplicated acute bacterial rhinosinusitis, a course of first-line antibiotics is probably adequate for most patients.

In interpreting the results of the evidenced-based meta-analysis, however, one must consider the comparability of patients included in these trials with more diverse practice-based patient populations. Some of the studies were conducted before the widespread emergence of antibiotic resistance among *S. pneumoniae*, *H. influenzae*, and *M. catarrhalis*. Patients with more severe illness, secondary medical conditions, recent treatment, or recurrent disease were often excluded. Generalizability of results therefore is a concern.

Effectiveness of Ancillary Treatment

Several classes of medications are commonly used in the treatment of rhinosinusitis (of varying causes) to restore the normal sinus environment and function.[10,38] Some of the common treatments are aimed at restoring mucociliary function by increasing mucosal moisture (e.g., saline solution sprays or irrigation) and reducing the viscosity of nasal secretions (e.g., mucolytic agents). Additionally, treatments may be directed to resolving airway blockages through reducing mucosal inflammation by vasoconstriction (e.g., decongestants) or through the effect of alternative medical therapies.[39–42]

There are few reliable studies regarding ancillary treatment of acute bacterial rhinosinusitis (specifically: decongestants, steroids, antihistamines, drainage, flushing). Ten randomized controlled trials have been published (Table 3–2). Several different medication types used in these studies included a proteoltyic enzyme (bromelain), α-adrenergic agonists (xylometazoline,

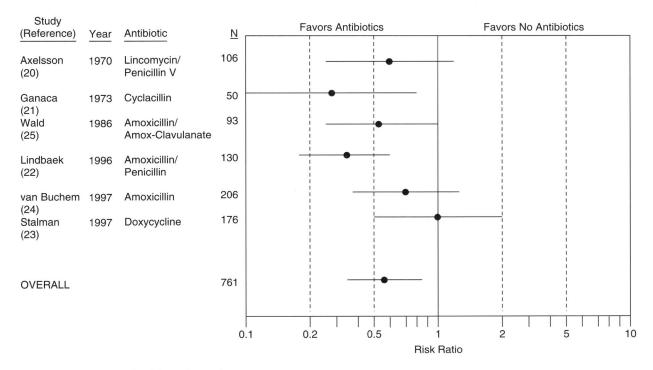

Horizontal Line is 95% Confidence Interval
AHCPR 1999 Evidence Report/Technology Assessment

FIGURE 3–3. Meta-analysis of antibiotics vs. placebo randomized controlled trials for acute rhinosinusitis.

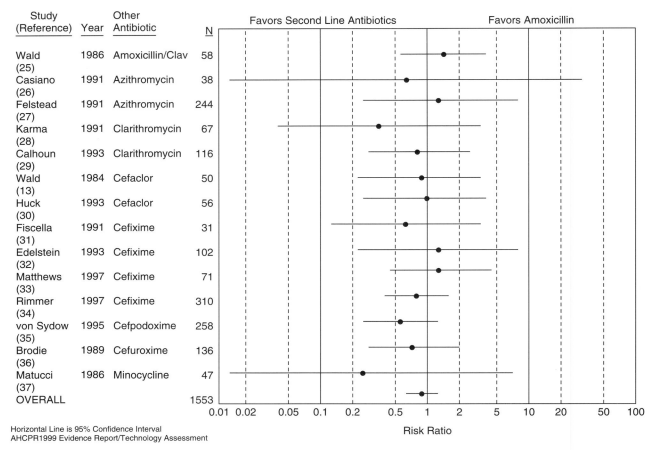

FIGURE 3–4. Meta-analysis of amoxicillin vs. second-line antibiotics for acute rhinosinusitis.

oxymetazoline), a mucolytic agent (bromhexine), glucocorticoids (budesonide, flunisolide), and an antihistamine (loratadine). In most of the studies these medications were used in conjunction with antibiotics. No randomized trials compared other nondrug treatments (e.g., sinus irrigation). The studies were carried out in both general medical and specialty clinics. Several studies combined patients with acute and those with chronic sinusitis in the study population. Two of the studies were carried out in pediatric populations.[43,44] Of the three studies that looked at bromelain compared with placebo for patients who were also given antibiotics, all three reported higher positive outcomes in the patients receiving bromelain, although the result was significant in only one study.[45] The remainder of the ancillary therapy studies looked at different treatments and reported varying efficacy.

Outcome Measures for Assessing Efficacy

Relief of Symptoms

For most patients with acute bacterial rhinosinusitis the main effects of the illness are troublesome symptoms that may keep them out of work or school. Most studies of the efficacy of treatments for rhinosinusitis have evaluated outcomes in terms of the extent of persisting symptoms at the end of treatment (typically about 10 days after the onset of treatment). Some have evaluated symptom relief at more than one interval, and a few have tracked the incidence of recurrence (relapse or reinfection) in the weeks after treatment. All these approaches yield data in the form of percentage response (cured, improved, or failure of treatment) at one or sometimes at two or three time points. Given that rhinosinusitis usually resolves spontaneously within weeks, inferring efficacy from one or two time-point "snapshots" may be insufficient to quantify the benefits of treatment.

Incidence of Serious Complications

Complications of acute bacterial rhinosinusitis are rare. The main complications of bacterial rhinosinusitis are local extension of the infection (osteitis of the sinus bones, intracranial cavity infection, and orbital cellulitis) and metastatic spread to the central nervous system (meningitis, brain abscess, and infection of the intracranial venous sinuses, including the cavernous sinus).

Relapse and Reinfection

It is well known that even when patients with allergic rhinosinusitis are excluded, some patients have frequent recurrences of presumed acute bacterial rhinosinusitis. Among these patients it is difficult to distinguish a

TABLE 3–2 ■ Randomized Controlled Trials Comparing Ancillary Treatment for Acute Bacterial Rhinosinusitis

Year	Authors	Study population	Treatment	No. patients	Clinical cure or improved (%)	
1997	Barlan et al[43]	Children	Budesonide	151	Significant improvement with budesonide	
		Adolescents	Placebo			
1997	Braun et al[139]	Adolescents	Loratadine	139	66	
		Adults	Placebo		48	
1971	Harris[140]	Adults	Bromhexine	52	96	
			Placebo		54	
1970	Lewison[141]	Adolescents	Xylometazoline	100	80	
		Adults	Phenylephrine Diphenylpyraline		67	
1996	McCormick et al[44]	Children	Oxymetazoline	68	No significant difference	
		Adolescents	Brompheniramine Phenylpropanolamine No ancillary treatment			
1993	Meltzer[142]	Adolescents	Flunisolide	180	69	
		Adults	Placebo		56	
1967	Ryan[143]	Children	Bromelain	50	87	
		Adolescents Adults	Placebo		68	
1967	Seltzer[144]	Children	Bromelain	48	80	
		Adolescents Adults	Placebo		50	
1967	Taub[145]	Adolescents	Bromelain	59	69	
		Adults	Placebo		40	
1994	Wiklund et al[146]	Adolescents		73	**DAY 7**	**DAY 28**
		Adults	Oxymetazoline (4 d)		29	57
			Placebo		34	75
			Oxymetazoline (10 d)		31	73
			Placebo		58	73
1994	Wiklund[146]	Adults		48	**DAY 7**	**DAY 14**
			Oxymetazoline		34	65
			Placebo		33	41

relapse of acute bacterial rhinosinusitis (from incomplete treatment) from multiple isolated episodes of acute bacterial rhinosinusitis (reinfection). There are no standardized criteria to assess "full recovery." The current definition of recurrent acute bacterial rhinosinusitis, based on total number of recurrences (fewer than four per year) and symptom-free intervals (at least 8 weeks), is arbitrary and not related to pathophysiologic features.[38] The effect of antibiotic or other treatment on a given episode of rhinosinusitis for prevention of subsequent recurrences is unknown.

Progression to Chronic Rhinosinusitis

A small proportion of patients with acute rhinosinusitis, especially those with multiple episodes of acute rhinosinusitis, progress to chronic rhinosinusitis. Although strong evidence is lacking, several risk factors have been implicated in the development of chronic rhinosinusitis. These risk factors include abnormalities in the normal flow of mucus and air through the sinus and nasal passages as a result of obstruction (ostial obstruction, allergic reaction, direct injury) or functional conditions (ciliary abnormalities, abnormalities in mucus secretion) or as a result of increased susceptibility to infection (immunodeficiency, or secondary to aforementioned sinus or nasal blockage).

Antibiotic Choices and Emerging Antibiotic Resistance

Before prescribing an antibiotic the physician must consider factors such as product cost, bacterial resistance patterns within the patient's community, the severity and duration of sinus infection, any recent antibiotic therapies, and any risk factors that may preclude an agent from the decision-making process. Before prescribing a second- or third-line antibiotic the physician should consider the susceptibility of the suspected pathogen as well as the patient's allergy history, drug response, and overall clinical impression.

Without direct sampling and antibiotic-sensitivity testing, antibiotic choices reflect data demonstrating effectiveness in eradication of the most likely pathogens while also taking into account compliance factors (e.g., formulation, dosing schedule) and accessibility factors (e.g., availability, cost).[46] Although studies have not reported recent significant shifts in the bacterial species and their prevalence in maxillary sinus aspirates, they have reported significant changes in the susceptibility of these organisms to various antibiotics.[47–49]

Aminopenicillins (e.g., ampicillin, amoxicillin) have long been used against *S. pneumoniae* and *H. influenzae*.[50,51] The increasing prevalence of antibiotic resistance factors, however, has changed and is continuing to change the susceptibility profiles of these bacteria (Fig. 3–5). Since the first reports of penicillin-resistant *S. pneumoniae* isolates in the United States in the 1970s, the prevalence of resistant strains has been increasing.[52,53] At the same time, increasing levels of β-lactamase-producing *H. influenzae* and *M. catarrhalis* (from 8% to 65% and up to 98%, respectively) are raising concerns about the choice of antibiotics for first-line treatment of acute bacterial rhinosinusitis.[48,51,54] Other classes of antibiotics can provide varying levels of antimicrobial activity in penicillin-resistant *S. pneumoniae* (e.g., second- and third-generation cephalosporins, clindamycin, macrolides, ketolides) and in β-lactamase-producing *H. influenzae* and *M. catarrhalis* strains (e.g., amoxicillin-clavulanate, second- and third-generation cephalosporins).[48,51,52] The finding of antibiotic-resistant strains is complicated by frequent concomitant multidrug resistance and by wide geographic variation in the prevalence of antibiotic resistance for the various bacterial species.[48,51,52,55,56] More information is needed to understand the relationships between in vitro antibiotic-susceptibility determinations and clinical responses and to fully understand the factors affecting the rise in antibiotic-resistant pathogens.[57–59]

Clinical Trials of Specific Antibiotic Regimens

Penicillin

Penicillin has been used in the treatment of acute rhinosinusitis since the 1960s. Its activity against *S. pneumoniae* even at increased doses is a concern. Penicillin has poor activity against gram-negative bacteria (*H. influenzae* and *M. catarrhalis)* and *S. aureus*. Several trials conducted in Scandinavia suggest efficacy of this agent in rhinosinusitis (Table 3–3), although it is not guideline recommended in the United States.

Aminopenicillins

Like penicillin, amoxicillin and other aminopenicillins have good activity against gram-positive organisms except *S. aureus*, which has greater gram-negative activity. Amoxicillin is susceptible to the action of β-lactamases. As the gold standard therapy, numerous clinical trials have been conducted with amoxicillin (Table 3–4), and it is guideline recommended, although usually at increased dosages (80 to 100 mg/kg/d in children and 3–3.5 g/d in adults).

Sulfonamides

Sulfonamides are most often used in patients allergic to penicillin. They have variable activity against both gram-positive and gram-negative organisms. Increasing resistance among *S. pneumoniae* and *H. influenzae* organisms has been noted. As an alternative first-line antibiotic, several trials have been conducted in the treatment of rhinosinusitis with sulfoxamides (Table 3–5), and TMP-SMX is a guideline-recommended first-line alternative antibiotic.

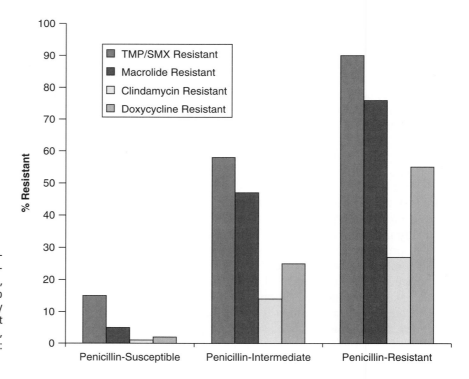

FIGURE 3–5. Cross-resistance between penicillin and other drug classes in *Streptococcus pneumoniae*. As resistance rises, resistance to other antibiotics also increases. (Data from Sinus and Allergy Health Partnership: Antimicrobial treatment guidelines for acute bacterial rhinosinusitis, Otolarynqol Head Neck Surg 2000; 123: S1–S32.)

TABLE 3–3 ■ **Randomized Controlled Trials Comparing Penicillin Treatment for Acute Bacterial Rhinosinusitis**

Year	Authors	Study population	Treatment	No. patients	Clinical cure or improved (%)
1970	Axelsson et al[20]	Adolescent Adult Sweden	Penicillin V Irrigation	156	83 81
1970	Axelsson et al[20]	Adolescent Adult Sweden	Penicillin V Lincomycin	156	83 85
1975	Quick[147]	Adolescent Adult United States	Penicillin TMP-SMX	145	84 87
1991	Soderstrom et al[148]	Children Adolescent Adult Sweden	Penicillin Erythromycin	138	90 90
1984	Von Sydow et al[149]	Adults Sweden	Penicillin V Erythromycin	100	91 98

Tetracyclines

Tetracyclines are bacteriostatic; they have modest activity against *S. pneumoniae* and *M. catarrhalis* and poor activity against *H. influenzae*. Usage in children younger than 8 years of age is contraindicated because of the risk of tooth enamel discoloration. Efficacy of this antibiotic family is shown in Table 3–6. Doxycycline is guideline recommended as an alternative first-line agent.

Amoxicillin-Clavulanate (Augmentin)

The spectrum of activity of amoxicillin-clavulanate includes gram-positive, gram-negative, and anaerobic bacteria that cause rhinosinusitis. This agent causes diarrhea more often than most other newer oral antimicrobial agents (a shortcoming that can be reduced by administration with meals). High-dose amoxicillin-clavulanate would be as effective as high-dose amoxicillin for treatment of relatively penicillin-resistant pneumococci, since resistance among pneumococci is mediated by alteration of penicillin-binding proteins. This agent is efficacious in acute, subacute, and chronic rhinosinusitis (Table 3–7); it is guideline recommended as a first- and second-line agent but generally at an increased dose for the amoxicillin component. It is available in a good-tasting suspension formulation for children.

Cephalosporins

Cephalexin (Keflex) and cefadroxil (Duricef) are first-generation cephalosporins. They have good activity against gram-positive bacteria (except penicillin-resistant pneumococci) with greater gram-negative bacteria activity than penicillin has. They are not recommended for the treatment of rhinosinusitis, unless a specific bacterial isolate has been identified and shown to be susceptible. Both of these cephalosporins come in good-tasting suspension formulations for children.

Cefaclor (Ceclor) was the first second-generation cephalosporin to be introduced in the United States. Its spectrum of activity is better than that of first-generation cephalosporins against gram-positive organisms (with marginal activity against penicillin-resistant pneumococci) with enhanced gram-negative activity. The in vitro activity of cefaclor against contemporary β-lactamase-producing strains of *H. influenzae* and *M. catarrhalis* has been inconsistent in some but not all studies. Clinical trials have demonstrated cefaclor to be efficacious for the treatment of rhinosinusitis (Table 3–8), although it is not guideline recommended. Cefaclor is rapidly and well absorbed from the gastrointestinal tract; its absorption is impaired by food, and so it is best administered as other than meal times. A suspension formulation is available. Hypersensitivity reactions, serum sickness, and erythema multiforme have been noted in children as an increased frequency following cefaclor administration.[60]

Cefuroxime axetil (Ceftin, Zinnat) is a second-generation cephalosporin; it has broad-spectrum activity against both gram-positive and gram-negative organisms. Cefuroxime axetil also has activity against selected anaerobes, which may be involved in rhinosinusitis. Its in vitro activity suggests it would be effective in eradication of relatively penicillin-resistant pneumococcal respiratory infections. This is a particularly β-lactamase-stable drug and perhaps the most β-lactamase-stable among the second-generation cephalosporins. It is effective in the treatment of rhinosinusitis (Table 3–8) and is guideline recommended as first- and second-line therapy. The half-life of cefuroxime axetil (1.2 hours) permits twice daily dosing. It is important to note that absorption of cefuroxime axetil is enhanced by administration with food. Thus patients should be advised to take it with breakfast and with their evening meal. The suspension formulation has a marginal taste to some children.

Cefprozil (Cefzil) has a spectrum of activity similar to that of cefuroxime axetil. In vitro susceptibility testing suggests this antimicrobial may not have as good stability against some β-lactamase-producing organisms

TABLE 3–4 ■ Randomized Controlled Trials Comparing Aminopenicillin Treatment for Acute Bacterial Rhinosinusitis

Year	Authors	Study population	Treatment	No. patients	Clinical cure or improved (%)
1981	Axelsson et al[150]	Adults Sweden	Amoxicillin Azidocillin	88	48 47
1981	Axelsson et al[150]	Adults Sweden	Amoxicillin Pivampicillin	88	48 41
1981	Axelsson et al[150]	Adults Sweden	Pivampicillin Azidocillin	90	41 47
1980	Christensen and Hartmann[151]	Children Adolescents Adults Norway	Pivampicillin 500 mg bid Pivampicillin 350 mg tid	155	88 91
1973	Gananca and Trabulsi[21]	Adults Brazil	Cyclacillin Placebo	50	93 55
1972	Jeppesen and Illum[152]	Children Adolescents Adults Denmark	Pivampicillin Placebo	100	91 95
1995	Kment et al[153]	Adults Austria	Amoxicillin Amoxicillin	59	No significant difference
1996	Lindbaek et al[22]	Adolescents Adults Norway	Amoxicillin Placebo	130	89 57
1996	Lindbaek et al[22]	Adolescents Adults Norway	Amoxicillin Penicillin V	130	89 82
1985	Moorehouse et al[154]	Children Adolescents Adults Ireland	Amoxicillin Pivampicillin	107	89 89
1983	Moran[155]	Adolescents Adults England	Amoxicillin Pivampicillin	463	90 93
1988	Nord[156]	Adults Europe	Amoxicillin Bacampicillin	280	77 73
1991	Nyffenegger et al[157]	Adults	Amoxicillin Brodimoprim	40	60 70
1986	Scheld et al[158]	Adolescents Adults United States	Amoxicillin Cyclacillin	80	93 89
1985	*Shenderey et al[159]	General practice Multicenter	Amoxicillin Miraxid	350	80 79
1981	Sorri et al[160]	Adults Finland	Bacampicillin 400 mg tid Bacampicillin 1200 mg bid	47	92 86
1997	Van Buchem et al[24]	Adults Dutch	Amoxicillin Placebo	214	83 77
1981	Von Sydow et al[161]	Adults Sweden	Bacampicillin bid Bacampicillin tid	148	95 97
1986	Wald et al[25]	Children Adolescents United States	Amoxicillin Placebo	136	83 60

*Miraxid, combination of pivmecillinam 200 mg and pivampicillin 250 mg.

(*H. influenzae* and *M. catarrhalis*) as cefuroxime axetil or amoxicillin-clavulanate have. Cefprozil may be effective in the treatment of relatively penicillin-resistant pneumococci. Cefprozil is effective in the treatment of rhinosinusitis (Table 3–8) and is guideline recommended as first- and second-line therapy. This agent may be dosed twice a day; its absorption is unimpaired by food; and it is available in a good-tasting suspension formulation.

Loracarbef (Lorabid) actually falls in a unique antimicrobial class called carbacephems; however, its antimicrobial activity is virtually identical to that of second-generation cephalosporins. The spectrum of activity of loracarbef is most similar to that of cefaclor. Loracarbef, however, may display greater β-lactamase stability than cefaclor does. Loracarbef is efficacious in the treatment of rhinosinusitis (Table 3–8), but it is not guideline recommended. The half-life of loracarbef (0.9 hour) permits twice

TABLE 3–5 ■ Randomized Controlled Trials Comparing Sulfonamide Treatment for Acute Bacterial Rhinosinusitis

Year	Authors	Study population	Treatment	No. patients	Clinical cure or improved (%)	
1981	Federspil and Bamberg[162]	Adults Adolescents Germany	TMP-SMX Sulfadiazine-TMP	54	95 95	
1983	Federspil and Koch[163]	Adolescents Adults Germany	TMP-SMX Erythromycin	42	75 82	
1985	Wallace et al[164]	Older Children Adolescents Adults Britain	TMP-SMX Miraxid*	318	87 84	
1995	Williams et al[165]	Adults United States	TMP-SMX 10 d TMP-SMX 3 d	80	**CURED** 19 31	**IMPROVED** 57 46

*Miraxid, combination of pivmecillinam 200 mg and pivampicillin 250 mg.

TABLE 3–6 ■ Randomized Controlled Trials Comparing Tetracycline Treatment for Acute Bacterial Rhinosinusitis

Year	Authors	Study population	Treatment	No. patients	Clinical cure or improved (%)	
1974	Agbim[166]	Adolescents Adults England	Ampicillin Doxycycline	44	35 90	
1994	Arndt et al[167]	Adults Germany	Brodimoprim Doxycycline	70	96 96	
1985	Beatson et al[168]	Adolescents Adults Britain	Tetracycline Miraxid* vs. Tetracycline†	408	90 93	
1988	Boezeman et al[169]	Adolescents Adults Netherlands	Doxycycline Spiramycin	33	**CURED** 27 25	**IMPROVED** 53 42
1986	Mattucci et al[37]	Adolescents Adults United States	Amoxicillin Minocycline	58	95 100	
1983	Otte et al[170]	Adolescents Adults Chile	Tetracycline TMP-SMX	43	65 71	
1996	Rahlfs et al[171]	Adolescents Adults Germany	Brodimoprim Doxycycline	27	100 92	
1996	Rahlfs et al[171]	Adolescents Adults Sweden	Brodimoprim Doxycycline	22	89 100	
1986	Salmi et al[172]	Adults Finland	Brodimoprim Doxycycline	60	94 100	
1997	Stalman et al[23]	Adults Netherlands	Doxycycline Placebo	175	85 85	
1975	Westerman et al[173]	Children Adolescents Adults United States	Tetracycline Clindamycin	97	78 94	

*Miraxid, combination of pivmecillinam 200 mg and pivampicillin 250 mg.
†Triple combination of tetracycline hydrochloride, chlortetracycline hydrochloride, and demeclocycline 300 mg.

daily dosing. Absorption is impaired by the presence of food, so it is best administered at other than meal times. A pleasant-tasting suspension formulation is available.

Cefixime (Suprax) was the first oral third-generation cephalosporin introduced in the United States. Typical of third-generation cephalosporins, cefixime has enhanced activity against gram-negative organisms (*H. influenzae* and *M. catarrhalis*). Cefixime has somewhat restricted activity against gram-positive bacteria and is essentially inactive against *S. aureus*. Efficacy of cefixime against *S. pneumoniae* is sometimes not comparable to that achieved with amoxicillin or the first- or second-generation

TABLE 3–7 ■ **Randomized Controlled Trials Comparing Amoxicillin-Clavulanate Treatment for Acute Bacterial Rhinosinusitis**

Year	Authors	Study population	Treatment	No. patients	Clinical cure or improved (%)
1992	Camacho et al[174]	Adults United States South America	Amoxicillin-clavulanate Cefpodoxime	317	82 85
					PATHOGENS
1992	De Abate et al[175]	United States	Amoxicillin-clavulanate Ceftibuten	35	100 100
					NO PATHOGENS
			Amoxicillin-clavulanate Ceftibuten		88 87
1993	Dubois et al[176]	Adolescents Adults North America	Amoxicillin-clavulanate Clarithromycin	497	93 97
1992	Sydnor et al[177]	Adults United States	Amoxicillin-clavulanate Loracarbef	113	88 95
1986	Wald et al[25]	Children Adolescents United States	Amoxicillin Amoxicillin-clavulanate Placebo	136	83 75 60

cephalosporins. Therefore it is not a guideline-recommended antimicrobial when pneumococci are suspected as probable pathogens. Although cefixime has shown efficacy in clinical trials (Table 3–8), its guideline-recommended use is as a second agent combined with a more effective drug for treatment of pneumococci. The half-life of cefixime (3.3 hours) permits once a day dosing. Its absorption is unimpaired by food. A pleasant-tasting suspension formulation is available. A slightly increased incidence of diarrhea has been noted with this agent compared with those of other cephalosporins.

Cefpodoxime proxetil (Vantin) has broad-spectrum activity against gram-negative bacteria and better activity against gram-positive organisms than cefixime has. Cefpodoxime proxetil is also an adequate therapy in the management of relatively penicillin-resistant pneumococci. It is effective in the treatment of rhinosinusitis (Table 3–8) and is guideline recommended as a first- and second-line therapy. The half-life of cefpodoxime proxetil permits twice daily dosing. Like cefuroxime axetil, absorption of cefpodoxime proxetil is enhanced by food, and so it is best administered with meals.[61] Some children find the lemon flavor taste of this agent in suspension formulation problematic.

Ceftibuten (Cedax) has an antimicrobial spectrum similar to that of cefixime. Clinical studies suggest this agent may be effective in patients with rhinosinusitis (Table 3–8) and could be substituted for cefixime as a combination agent with a second drug more effective in the eradication of pneumococci; it is not guideline recommended. The half-life of ceftibuten allows once or twice daily dosing. Absorption is not impaired by food, so it may be taken at meal times. A pleasant-tasting suspension formulation is available.

Cefdinir (OmniCef) has a spectrum of activity similar to that of cefuroxime axetil.[62] Cefdinir is effective in the treatment of rhinosinusitis (Table 3–8) and is guideline recommended. This agent may be taken twice a day for 5 days or once a day for 10 days. The suspension formulation is very pleasant tasting for children.

Macrolides and Azalides

Erythromycin is bacteriostatic and has moderate gram-positive and poor gram-negative activity. It is guideline recommended in mild rhinosinusitis if the patient is allergic to β-lactam antibiotics.

Clarithromycin (Biaxin) has a broad spectrum of activity that includes gram-positive and gram-negative organisms. Its activity is enhanced by a capacity to enter cells including polymorphonuclear neutrophils and respiratory epithelium. It has additive or synergistic activity with its primary metabolite, 14-hydroxy-clarithromycin, against *H. influenzae*. Clarithromycin is effective in the treatment of rhinosinusitis (Table 3–9), although it is not guideline recommended except in β-lactam-allergic patients. The half-life of clarithromycin allows twice daily dosing; absorption is unimpaired by food. Gastrointestinal intolerance occasionally can be a problem but generally is of a lesser concern than that with erythromycin. The taste of clarithromycin in suspension formulation is metallic, which children may not like.

Azithromycin (Zithromax) has a spectrum of activity similar to that of clarithromycin. Clinical trials suggest it is effective in the treatment of rhinosinusitis (Table 3–9), but it is not guideline recommended. Its half-life allows once a day dosing for an abbreviated 5-day course, which is compliance enhancing as an alternative first-line therapy in β-lactam-allergic patients. The gastrointestinal side effects can be lessened by administering it with meals. A pleasant-tasting suspension formulation is available.

TABLE 3–8 ■ Randomized Controlled Trials Comparing Cephalosporin Treatment for Acute Bacterial Rhinosinusitis

Year	Authors	Study population	Treatment	No. patients	Clinical cure or improved (%)
1994	Bockmeyer et al[178]	Adults Europe	Brodimoprim Cephalexin	49	100 95
1989	Brodie et al[36]	Adolescents Britain	Amoxicillin Cefuroxime	160	94 96
1990	Carenfelt et al[179]	Adults Norway	Cefaclor Cefixime	295	80 92
1993	Edelstein et al[32]	Adults United States	Amoxicillin Cefixime	114	96 94
1991	Fiscella and Chow[31]	Adults	Amoxicillin Cefixime	33	80 88
1990	Gauger et al[180]	Adults Switzerland	Cefaclor Cefetamet	41	95 100
1990	Gehanno et al[181]	Adults France	Cefaclor Cefpodoxime	258	93 95
1996	Gehanno and Berche[182]	Adults France	Cefuroxime Sparfloxacin	382	83 83
1993	Huck et al[30]	Adolescents Adults	Amoxicillin Cefaclor	108	86 86
1997	Matthews and Team SACS[33]	Adults United States	Amoxicillin Cefixime	182	88 84
1997	Rimmer & Team SACS[34]	Adults United Kingdom	Amoxicillin Cefixime	323	89 91
1993	Scandinavian Study Group[183]	Adolescents Adults Sweden, Finland, Iceland	Doxycycline Loracarbef	662	92 98
1999	Simon[184]	Children United States	Ceftibuten (10–15 d) Ceftibuten (20 d) Erythromycin	200	92 100 96
1998	Stefansson et al[185]	Adults Iceland	Cefuroxime Clarithromycin	370	91 93
1989	Sydnor et al[186]	Adults United States	Cefaclor Cefuroxime	106	71 95
1995	Von Sydow et al[35]	Adults Sweden, Finland, Norway	Amoxicillin Cefpodoxime	286	91 96
1984	Wald et al[13]	Children Adolescents United States	Amoxicillin Cefaclor	50	85 87
1995	Zeckel et al[187]	Adolescents Adults USA	Loracarbef 400 mg bid Loracarbef 200 mg tid	209	82 81

Fluoroquinolones

A number of fluoroquinolone antimicrobials have been introduced in the United States:

- Ciprofloxacin (Cipro)
- Ofloxacin (Floxin)
- Enoxacin (Penetrex)
- Norfloxacin (Noroxin)
- Lomefloxacin (Maxaquin)
- Levofloxacin (Levaquin)
- Moxifloxacin (Avelox)
- Gatifloxacin (Tequin)
- Gemifloxacin (Factive)

The spectrum of activity of the quinolones varies, but all are generally bactericidal against most community-acquired gram-negative organisms, e.g., *H. influenzae*, *M. catarrhalis*, *Mycoplasma pneumoniae*, and *Chlamydia pneumoniae*. Ciproflaxacin, ofloxacin, enoxacin, norfloxacin, and lomefloxacin have inconsistent activity against gram-positive organisms, and these agents poorly eradicate pneumococci. The newer fluoroquinolones (levofloxacin, gatifloxacin, moxifloxacin, and gemifloxacin) have remarkable potency against *S. pneumoniae* and are efficacious in the treatment of rhinosinusitis (Table 3–10). Although not approved for children, these newer fluoroquinolones are guideline recommended in

TABLE 3–9 ■ Randomized Controlled Trials Comparing Macrolide or Azalide Treatment for Acute Bacterial Rhinosinusitis

Year	Authors	Study population	Treatment	No. patients	Clinical cure or improved (%)
1970	Axelsson et al[20]	Adolescents Adults Sweden	Lincomycin Irrigation	156	85 81
1993	Calhoun and Hokanson[29]	Adolescents Adults United States	Amoxicillin Clarithromycin	142	89 91
1991	Casiano[26]	Adolescents Adults United States	Amoxicillin Azithromycin	78	100 100
1992	de Campora et al[188]	Adult Italy	Clarithromycin Roxithromycin	63	66 87
1991	Felstead and Daniel[27]	Adolescents Adults Europe	Azithromycin Erythromycin	142	85 75
1991	Felstead and Daniel[27]	Adolescents Adults Europe	Amoxicillin Azithromycin	258	98 97
1997	Ficnar et al[189]	Children Croatia	Azithromycin: 3 d (19 mg/kg/d) Azithromycin: 5 d (10 mg/kg/d day 1, 5 mg/kg/d days 2–5)	371	96 96
1996	Haye et al[190]	Adults Norwegian	Azithromycin Penicillin V	438	97 95
1991	Karma et al[28]	Adolescents Adults Finland, Sweden	Amoxicillin Clarithromycin	100	91 91
1993	Manzini and Caroggio[191]	Adults Italy	Brodimoprim Roxithromycin	74	86 71
1993	Muller[192]	Adolescents Adults Germany, Ireland	Azithromycin Clarithromycin	380	96 97
1996	Muller[193]	Adolescents Adults Germany	Azithromycin Roxithromycin	440	94 96
1996	O'Doherty[194]	Adolescents Adults Ireland	Azithromycin 500 mg × once daily × 3 d Cefaclor 250 mg tid × 10 d	486	93 97
1988	Wuolijoki et al[195]	Adolescents Adults Finland	Erythromycin acistrate Erythromycin base Enterocapsules Enterotablets	474	97 95 94

TABLE 3–10 ■ Randomized Controlled Trials Comparing Fluoroquinolone Treatment for Acute Bacterial Rhinosinusitis

Year	Authors	Study population	Treatment	No. patients	Clinical cure or improved (%)
1999	Adelglass et al[196]	Adults United States	Levofloxacin Amoxicillin-clavulanate	802	88 88
1999	Burke et al[197]	Adults United States	Moxifloxacin Cefuroxime	457	90 89
1999	Clifford et al[198]	Adults	Ciprofloxacin Clarithromycin	457	84 91
1999	Johnson et al[199]	Adults United States	Ciprofloxacin Cefuroxime	453	87 83
2000	Siegert et al[200]	Adults Germany	Moxifloxacin Cefuroxime	493	97 91

adults for moderate and severe rhinosinusitis as second-line agents. Most fluoroquinolones have essentially no activity against anaerobes. Because of their half-lives, the various quinolones lend themselves to once or twice a day dosing; absorption usually is unimpaired by most foods.

Guideline Recommendations

Two guidelines recently were published on rhinosinusitis treatment[16,17]; both provide similar recommendations. The guideline presented by the Sinus and Allergy Health Partnership relies on pharmacokinetic-pharmacodynamic principles to predict preferred drugs. Antibiotic classes were divided into groups according to their pharmacodynamic class and thera-

peutic goal (Table 3–11). With mathematical modeling, antibiotic efficacy was predicted for adults (Table 3–12) and children (Table 3–13), with consideration to avoidance of fluoroquinolones for children. Dosages were recommended on the basis of the manufacturer's recommendations except for amoxicillin and amoxicillin-clavulanate, for which higher dosages were advised (Tables 3–14 and 3–15).

The following drugs are recommended first-line antibiotics for adults with "mild" sinusitis who have not received antibiotic therapy in the preceding 4 to 6 weeks: amoxicillin-clavulanate, or amoxicillin (Amoxil, Trimox, Wymox; 1.5 to 3.5 g/d), or cefpodoxime proxetil, or cefuroxime axetil. If the patient is allergic to β-lactams, TMP-SMX, doxycycline, azithromycin, clarithromycin,

TABLE 3–11 ■ Antimicrobial Agents Classified by Pattern of Bactericidal Activity

Drug class	Pharmacodynamic class	Therapeutic goal
β-lactams Penicillins Cephalosporins	Concentration-independent (time-dependent)	Time above MIC >40%–50% of the dosing interval
Macrolides Erythromycin Clarithromycin Azithromycin	Concentration-independent (time-dependent)	Time above MIC >40%–50% of the dosing interval 24-h AUC/MIC ratio 25–30
Fluoroquinolones Gatifloxacin Levofloxacin Moxifloxacin	Concentration-dependent (time-independent)	24-h AUC/MIC ratio 25–30 for *Streptococcus pneumoniae*

AUC, area under curve; MIC, minimum inhibitory concentration.
From Sinus and Allergy Health Partnership: Antimicrobial treatment guidelines for acute bacterial rhinosinusitis. Otolaryngol Head Neck Surg 2000;123(Suppl 1 Pt 2):S5–S31.

TABLE 3–12 ■ Sinusitis: Antibiotic Efficacy in Adults

Efficacy rate	Antibiotic
>90%	Gatifloxacin (Tequin) Levofloxacin (Levaquin) Moxifloxacin (Avelox) Amoxicillin-clavulanate (Augmentin)
80%–90%	High dose amoxicillin (Amoxil, Trimox, Wymox) Cefpodoxime proxetil (Vantin) Cefixime (Suprax) Cefuroxime axetil (Ceftin) TMP-SMX (Bactrim, Septra)
70%–80%	Clindamycin (Cleocin) Doxycycline Cefprozil (Cefzil) Azithromycin (Zithromax) Clarithromycin (Biaxin) Erythromycin
50%–60%	Cefaclor (Ceclor) Loracarbef (Lorabid)
Spontaneous resolution: 46.6%	No treatment

Adapted from Sinus and Allergy Health Partnership: Antimicrobial treatment guidelines for acute bacterial rhinosinusitis. Executive Summary. Otolaryngol Head Neck Surg 2000;123(Suppl. 1 Pt 2):S1–S3.

TABLE 3–13 ■ Sinusitis: Antibiotic Efficacy in Children

Efficacy rate	Antibiotic
>90%	Amoxicillin-clavulanate (Augmentin) High dose amoxicillin (Amoxil, Trimox, Wymox)
80%–90%	Cefpodoxime proxetil (Vantin) Cefixime (Suprax) Cefuroxime axetil (Ceftin) Clindamycin (Cleocin) Azithromycin (Zithromax) Clarithromycin (Biaxin) Erythromycin TMP-SMX (Bactrim, Septra)
70%–80%	Cefprozil (Cefzil)
60%–70%	Cefaclor (Ceclor) Loracarbef (Lorabid)
Spontaneous resolution: 49.6%	No treatment

Adapted from Sinus and Allergy Health Partnership: Antimicrobial treatment guidelines for acute bacterial rhinosinusitis. Executive Summary. Otolaryngol Head Neck Surg 2000;123(Suppl. 1 Pt 2):S1–S3.

TABLE 3–14 ■ Oral Antibiotic Therapy for Sinusitis in Adults

Drug	Adult dose
MILD SINUSITIS, ANTIBIOTIC-NAÏVE IN PREVIOUS 4–6 WEEKS	
Amoxicillin-clavulanate (Augmentin)	1.5–2 g/d amoxicillin divided bid
Amoxicillin (Amoxil, Trimox, Wymox)	1.5–2 g/d amoxicillin divided bid
Cefpodoxime proxetil (Vantin)	200–400 mg bid
Cefuroxime axetil (Ceftin)	250–500 mg bid
β-LACTAM ALLERGIC PATIENTS	
TMP-SMX (Bactrim, Septra) or	1 DS tablet bid
Doxycycline	200 mg qd; or 100 divided bid
Azithromycin (Zithromax)	500 mg day 1; 250 mg day 2–5
Clarithromycin (Biaxin)	250–500 mg bid
Erythromycin	250–500 mg qid
MILD SINUSITIS, PREVIOUS ANTIBIOTIC THERAPY	
Amoxicillin-clavulanate (Augmentin)	3–3.5 g/d amoxicillin divided bid
Amoxicillin (Amoxil, Trimox, Wymox)	3–3.5 g/d amoxicillin divided bid
Cefpodoxime proxetil (Vantin)	200–400 mg bid
Cefuroxime axetil (Ceftin)	250–500 mg bid
β-LACTAM ALLERGIC PATIENTS	
Gatifloxacin (Tequin)	400 mg qd
Levofloxacin (Levaquin)	500 mg qd
Moxifoxacin (Avelox)	400 mg qd
MODERATE SINUSITIS, PREVIOUS ANTIBIOTIC THERAPY	
Gatifloxacin (Tequin)	400 mg qd
Levofloxacin (Levaquin)	500 mg qd
Moxifoxacin (Avelox)	400 mg qd
Amoxicillin-clavulanate (Augmentin)	1– 1.5 g/d amoxicillin divided bid
COMBINATION THERAPY WITH	
Amoxicillin (Amoxil, Trimox, Wymox) or	1.5–2.0 g/d divided bid
Clindamycin (Cleocin) *plus*	150–450 mg tid or qid
Cefpodoxime proxetil (Vantin) or	200–400 mg bid
Cefixime (Suprax)	400 mg qd

Adapted from Sinus and Allergy Health Partnership: Antimicrobial treatment guidelines for acute bacterial rhinosinusitis. Otolaryngol Head Neck Surg 2000;123(Suppl. 1 Pt 2):S4–S31.

or erythromycin may be considered, although clinical failure occurs in up to 25% of patients.

The following drugs are recommended first-line antibiotics for adults with "mild" sinusitis who have received antibiotics in the preceding 4 to 6 weeks and for antibiotic-naïve adults with moderate disease: amoxicillin-clavulanate, or amoxicillin (3 to 3.5 g/d), or cefpodoxime proxetil, or cefuroxime axetil. If the patient is allergic to ß-lactams, alternative choices include gatifloxacin, levofloxacin, and moxifloxacin.

Recommendations for first-line antibiotics for adults with "moderate" sinusitis who have received antibiotics in the preceding 4 to 6 weeks are amoxicillin-clavulanate, or gatifloxacin, or levofloxacin, or moxifloxacin, or combination therapy with amoxicillin or clindamycin (Cleocin) (gram-positive coverage) *plus* cefpodoxime proxetil or cefixime (gram-negative coverage).

If the patient's condition has not improved or has worsened after 72 hours, the physician should consider "switch" therapy to second- or third-line antibiotics. Such agents should be used when resistant pathogens are suspected. The choice of antibiotic will depend upon the organism believed responsible for the clinical failure. An anaerobic infection may be the cause of clinical failure in some patients, who may present with foul breath, a fetid odor arising from the nasal cavity, or a history of repeated courses of broad-spectrum antibiotics. Appropriate antibiotic management of such persons includes treatment with clindamycin or combination therapy with amoxicillin and metronidazole. Any concomitant dental disease that is the source of infection must be treated before sinusitis can be eradicated. Persons who remain symptomatic after appropriate antibiotic therapy may require additional evaluation by CT scan, fiberoptic endoscopy, or sinus aspiration and culture.

Because drug-resistant *S. pneumoniae* is so prevalent in many regions of the United States, it is recommended that the amoxicillin dose be increased in these locations (high-dose amoxicillin in adults: up to 100 mg/kg/d, with a maximum of 3.5 g/d; note: this dose has not received U.S. Food and Drug Administration (FDA) approval). A high-dose formulation of amoxicillin-clavulanate has recently become available. This combination will achieve a higher dose of amoxicillin without increasing the dose of clavulanate, which is a recognized gastrointestinal irritant.

The following are recommended first-line antibiotics for children with "mild" disease who have not received antibiotics in the preceding 4 to 6 weeks: amoxicillin-clavulanate, or amoxicillin (45 to 90 mg/kg/d), or

TABLE 3–15 ■ Oral Antibiotic Therapy for Sinusitis in Children

Drug	Pediatric dose
MILD SINUSITIS, ANTIBIOTIC-NAÏVE IN PREVIOUS 4–6 WEEKS	
Amoxicillin-clavulanate (Augmentin)	45–90 mg/kg/d amoxicillin divided tid or bid
Amoxicillin (Amoxil, Trimox, Wymox)	45–90 mg/kg/d amoxicillin divided tid or bid
Cefpodoxime proxetil (Vantin)	10 mg/kg/d qd or divided bid
Cefuroxime axetil (Ceftin)	250 mg bid or 30 mg/kg/d divided bid
β-LACTAM ALLERGIC PATIENTS	
Azithromycin (Zithromax)	10 mg/kg/d day 1; 5 mg/kg/d day 2–5
Clarithromycin (Biaxin)	15 mg/kg/d divided bid
Erythromycin, *or*	40 mg/kg/d divided qid
TMP-SMX (Bactrim, Septra)	8–12 mg/kg/d TMP divided bid
MILD SINUSITIS, PREVIOUS ANTIBIOTIC THERAPY, OR	
MODERATE SINUSITIS, ANTIBIOTIC-NAÏVE IN PREVIOUS 4–6 WEEKS	
Amoxicillin-clavulanate (Augmentin)	80–100 mg/kg/d amoxicillin divided bid
Amoxicillin (Amoxil, Trimox, Wymox)	80–100 mg/kg/d amoxicillin divided bid
Cefpodoxime proxetil (Vantin)	10 mg/kg/d qd or divided bid
Cefuroxime axetil (Ceftin)	250 mg bid or 30 mg/kg/d divided bid
β-LACTAM ALLERGIC PATIENTS	
Azithromycin (Zithromax)	10 mg/kg/d day 1; 5 mg/kg/d days 2–5
Clarithromycin (Biaxin)	15 mg/kg/d divided bid
Erythromycin	40 mg/kg/d divided qid
TMP-SMX (Bactrim, Septra), *or*	8–12 mg/kg/d TMP divided bid
Clindamycin (Cleocin) if *Streptococcus pneumoniae* is identified	10–20 mg/kg/d divided tid or qid
MODERATE SINUSITIS, PREVIOUS ANTIBIOTIC THERAPY	
Amoxicillin-clavulanate (Augmentin), *or*	40–45 mg/kg/d amoxicillin divided bid
COMBINATION THERAPY WITH	
Amoxicillin (Amoxil, Trimox, Wymox) *or*	40–45 mg/kg/d amoxicillin divided bid
Clindamycin (Cleocin) *plus*	8–16 mg/kg/d divided tid or qid
cefpodoxime proxetil (Vantin) *or*	10 mg/kg/d qd or divided bid
cefixime (Suprax)	8 mg/kg/d qd or divided bid
β-LACTAM ALLERGIC PATIENTS	
TMP-SMX *plus*	8–12 mg/kg/d divided bid
clindamycin	10–20 mg/kg/d divided tid or qid

Adapted from: Sinus and Allergy Health Partnership. Antimicrobial treatment guidelines for acute bacterial rhinosinusitis. Otolaryngol Head Neck Surg 2000;123(Suppl. 1 Pt 2):S4–S31.

cefpodoxime proxetil, or cefuroxime axetil. If the child is allergic to β-lactams, then alternative choices include azithromycin, clarithromycin, erythromycin, or TMP-SMX. These antibiotics are not effective against many of the major pathogens in bacterial sinusitis, however, and clinical failure is observed in up to 25% of patients. Strains of both *S. pneumoniae* and *H. influenzae* demonstrate resistance to TMP-SMX in many geographic regions. In addition, life-threatening toxic epidermal necrolysis has been associated with TMP-SMX administration. Children who experience immediate, type I hypersensitivity reactions to ß-lactams may require ancillary procedures such as desensitization and sinus cultures. Fluoroquinolones—such as gatifloxacin, levofloxacin, and moxifloxacin—are not FDA approved for use in the pediatric population.

The following drugs are recommended first-line antibiotics for children with "mild" disease who have received antibiotics in the preceding 4 to 6 weeks and for antibiotic-naïve children with "moderate" disease: amoxicillin-clavulanate, or amoxicillin (80 to 100 mg/kg/d), or cefpodoxime proxetil, or cefuroxime axetil. If the child is

allergic to β-lactams, then alternative choices include azithromycin, clarithromycin, erythromycin, or TMP-SMX. Clindamycin may be substituted if the causative organism is *S. pneumoniae*.

Recommended first-line antibiotics for children with "moderate" disease who have received antibiotics in the previous 4 to 6 weeks are high-dose amoxicillin-clavulanate (80 to 100 mg/kg/d amoxicillin) or clindamycin (gram-positive coverage) *plus* cefpodoxime proxetil or cefixime (gram-negative coverage).

If the child's condition has not improved or has worsened after 72 hours, the physician should consider "switch" therapy to second- or third-line antibiotics. Such agents should be used when resistant pathogens are suspected. The choice of antibiotic will depend upon the organism believed responsible for clinical failure. Children who remain symptomatic after appropriate antibiotic therapy may require additional evaluation by CT scan, fiberoptic endoscopy, or sinus aspiration and culture.

When amoxicillin-clavulanate is prescribed because drug-resistant *S. pneumoniae* is prevalent in the patient's community or because it is an alternative choice for switch therapy, high-dose amoxicillin/clavulanate, a new formulation of the drug, provides 80 to 100 mg/kg/d of the amoxicillin component with the amount of clavulanate in regular-strength augmentin.

A second guideline-recommended application of a clinical algorithm that based therapy on duration of illness and symptoms (Figs. 3–6 and 3–7). The specific antibiotics, dosages, and sequence of use (first-, second-, and third-line) were similar to those recommended by the other expert group.

Allergic Fungal Sinusitis

The distinct entity allergic fungal sinusitis (AFS) was first proposed by Katzenstien et al[63] in 1983. It is caused by an intense allergic and eosinophilic inflammatory response to fungal species and represents an upper airway equivalent to that of allergic bronchopulmonary aspergillosis (ABPA). The implicated fungi colonize stagnant mucus and are noninvasive. The disease appears to be more common in areas with hot, humid weather and high ambient mold spore counts.

Fungal infection of the paranasal sinuses—otherwise known as AFS—is most frequently seen in persons who are immunocompromised or diabetic. *Aspergillus* infection predominates in immunocompromised persons, whereas *Mucor* spp tend to be isolated in persons with diabetes. Other fungi identified in AFS include *Bipolaris, Candida* spp, *Rhizopus, Alternaria,* and *Curvularia.* Fungal infections may be secondary to insulin-dependent diabetes mellitus (IDDM) or immunosuppression from

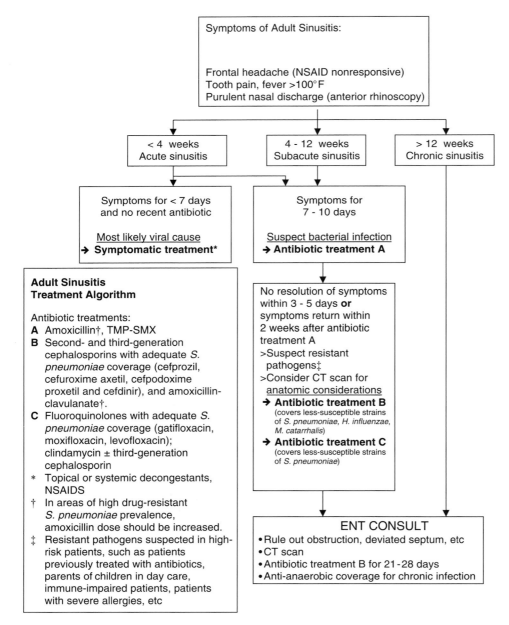

FIGURE 3–6. Algorithm for selecting antimicrobial therapy for acute sinusitis in adults.

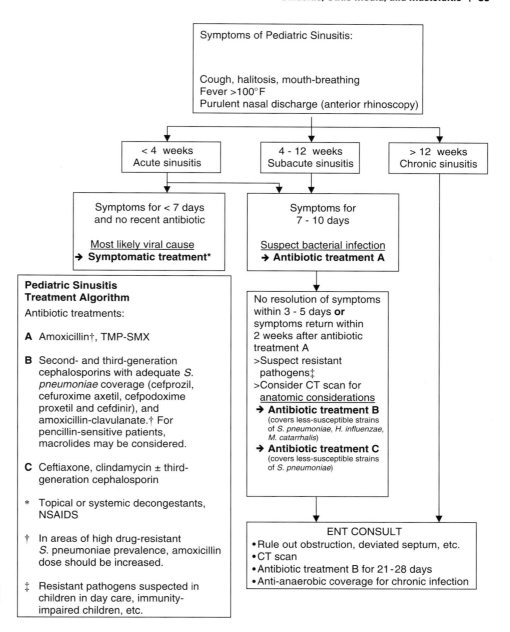

FIGURE 3–7. Algorithm for selecting antimicrobial therapy for acute sinusitis in children.

chemotherapy or bone marrow transplant or defects in cell-mediated immunity.

Treatment of AFS requires surgical removal of the allergic mucin that obstructs sinus drainage.[64] Systemic corticosteroids, however, are also essential.[64] Guidelines for the use of prednisone for adults with AFS are patterned after treatment of ABPA. Treatment is initiated with prednisone 0.5 to 1 mg/kg daily for 2 weeks, and then the same dose is given every other day for an additional 2 weeks before a gradual tapering is begun. In many cases it is necessary to continue a low daily or every-other-day dose of prednisone to control the disease. High-potency intranasal corticosteroids should also be used in AFS, preferably with the patient using the head-down-forward technique to maximize penetration of the drug into the osteomeatal and ethmoidal area.[65,66]

The total serum IgE level has been shown to be useful as a guide to steroid management of AFS.[67] Absolute blood eosinophil counts (AECs), drawn before prednisone is taken in the morning, may also be useful in this regard. AECs less than 400 µl are generally associated with control of the disease and suggest that the dose of prednisone may be tapered. The role of fungal-specific immunotherapy for AFS has gained support on the basis of a recent controlled study suggesting that it may be an important adjunct to medical and surgical therapy for AFS.[68]

Duration of Therapy

The symptoms of rhinosinusitis should abate within a few days after the initiation of treatment, and 10 days is the current standard treatment interval. Shorter courses of antimicrobial treatment lower costs, reduce side effects, increase compliance, reduce the potential for resistance, and decrease the impact on commensal flora.[69] Six studies of shortened therapy have been accomplished and are promising,[26,70–74] but further studies of short-course therapy are needed, especially in children, and clinical judgment is paramount.

Follow-up

Follow-up times vary widely according to the patient's age, risk factors, and history.[75] Additional evaluations are necessary if symptoms persist or worsen, perhaps because of resistant bacteria or poor antimicrobial coverage. Physicians should consider immunologic defects in patients who repeatedly do not respond to treatment.

When to Refer

Patients with acute rhinosinusitis rarely require surgical intervention or sinus aspiration to ventilate a sinus that is unresponsive to antimicrobial treatment.[76] Surgery should be considered when medical options have been exhausted, and it is generally reserved for patients with refractory disease or anatomic abnormalities. Evaluations by a medical specialist and a surgical specialist may be warranted because of the high complication rate of surgery. Surgery in children may interfere with normal face development.[77] The role of adenotonsillectomy in treating pediatric sinusitis is unclear. Consultation with an otolaryngologist helps determine the size of the tonsils and adenoids, their role in possible sinus obstruction, and the need for their removal.[78] Referral to an allergist is appropriate when the patient has a significant allergic history. Medical and surgical treatment of sinusitis in patients with asthma reduces the use of asthma medications.[79]

OTITIS MEDIA

Acute otitis media (AOM) and otitis media with effusion (OME) are disease entities in the otitis media continuum. There is often a transition between OME and AOM, and the two conditions sometimes may be indistinguishable from each other diagnostically.[80] It is sometimes quite difficult to diagnose accurately whether an effusion in the middle ear space is purulent (consistent with AOM) or nonpurulent (consistent with OME) and whether the effusion will be culture positive or culture negative for bacterial pathogens. As a further confounder, misdiagnosis also may occur when nasopharyngeal and eustachian tube congestion develops in a patient experiencing a viral upper respiratory tract infection. Under this circumstance it often occurs that the tympanic membrane becomes distorted (retracted), and the associated anatomic changes on otoscopic inspection mislead the practitioner to conclude that AOM or OME is present. Thus a first step in treatment decisions regarding otitis media must rely on accurate diagnosis to distinguish AOM, OME, and a retracted tympanic membrane without middle ear effusion from normal.[81,82] Principles of judicious use of antibiotics for otitis media have emphasized that episodes of otitis media should be classified as AOM or OME (Table 3–16).

Etiology of Acute Otitis Media

The microbiologic causes of AOM have been documented on the basis of results of cultures of middle ear effusions that have been obtained by tympanocentesis (needle aspiration through the tympanic membrane). Bacterial pathogens are isolated from middle ear fluids of 56% to 75% of children with AOM. Various studies from the United States, Europe, Japan, and elsewhere over the past 40 years are consistent in that they have underscored the importance of *S. pneumoniae* as the leading bacterial pathogen and nontypeable *H. influenzae* as the next most frequent pathogen (Fig. 3–8). These bacteria are also the most common causes of persistent AOM (Table 3–17). *M. catarrhalis*, group A Streptococcus, and *S. aureus* are less common causes of AOM. Respiratory viruses alone or in combination with bacterial pathogens have been identified in approximately 10% to 20% of middle ear fluids. Infection due to *M. pneumoniae* and *C. pneumoniae* is rare. The bacterial causes of AOM are often indistinguishable by history or physical examination, but some features provide clues to the cause of persistent and recurrent AOM (Table 3–18).

TABLE 3–16 ■ Principles of Judicious Use of Antimicrobial Agents for Otitis Media

Episodes of otitis media should be classified as acute otitis media (AOM) or otitis media with effusion (OME)
Antimicrobials are indicated for treatment of AOM; however, diagnosis requires documented middle ear effusion and signs or symptoms of acute local or systemic illness
Uncomplicated AOM may be treated with 5- to 7-d course of antimicrobials in certain patients
Antimicrobials are not indicated for initial treatment of OME; treatment may be indicated if effusion persists for >3 mo
Persistent middle ear effusion (OME) after therapy for AOM is expected and does not require retreatment
Antimicrobial prophylaxis should be reserved for control of recurrent AOM, defined by more than 3 distinct and well-documented episodes within 6 mo or more than 4 episodes in 12 mo

Data from Dowell SF, Marcy S, William W, et al: Otitis Media—Principles of judicious use of antimicrobial agents. Pediatrics 1998;101(Suppl 1):S165–S171.

TABLE 3–17 ■ **Bacteriology of Unresponsive, Persistent Acute Otitis Media When Organisms Are Isolated: Results Expressed as Percentage of Isolates**

Year	Authors	Streptococcus pneumoniae	Penicillin-resistant S. pneumoniae	Haemophilus influenzae or Moraxella catarrhalis	β-lactamase-positive strains	Streptococcus pyogenes or Staphylococcus aureus
1981	Teele et al[202]	17	20	58	33	12
1981	Schwartz et al[203]	24	0	76	50	0
1985	Harrison et al[204]	20	18	61	33	18
1992	Faden et al[205]	27	0	73	70	Not reported
1994	Cohen et al[85]	55	87	45	32	Not reported
1995	Block et al[206]	51	11	31	86	21
1995	Pichichero and Pichichero[86]	81	44	19	58	Not reported
1998	Leibovitz et al[108]	54	79	56	23	3
1998	Gehanno et al[87]	39	78	41	54	3

TABLE 3–18 ■ **History and Physical Examination Features Providing Clues to Etiology of Persistent and Recurrent Acute Otitis Media**

MORE LIKELY TO BE *STREPTOCOCCUS PNEUMONIAE* IF:
Increased otalgia and fever
Spontaneous perforation

MORE LIKELY TO BE RESISTANT *S. PNEUMONIAE* IF:
Therapy in preceding month was with
   Erythromycin-sulfisoxazole
   TMP-SMX
   Azithromycin
   Ampicillin
   Antibiotic prophylaxis
Epidemiologic features
   Younger than 2 years of age
   Day care attendance
   History of recurrent AOM
   Contact with individuals treated with antibiotics

LESS LIKELY TO BE *S. PNEUMONIAE* IF:
Mild symptoms
Preceding therapy was with high dose amoxicillin

MORE LIKELY TO BE *HAEMOPHILUS INFLUENZAE* IF:
Otitis-conjunctivitis syndrome

MORE LIKELY TO BE β-LACTAMASE-POSITIVE *H. INFLUENZAE* IF:
Preceding therapy was with amoxicillin

LESS LIKELY TO BE *H. INFLUENZAE* IF:
Preceding therapy was with third-generation cephalosporin

Data from Pichichero ME, Reiner SA, Brook I, et al: Controversies in the Medical Management of Persistent and Recurrent Acute Otitis Media. Recommendations of a clinical advisory committee. Ann Otol Rhinol Laryngol Suppl 2000;183:1–12.

Circumstances that Modify Therapy

Acute, Persistent, Recurrent, and Chronic OM

AOM is defined by the presence of fluid in the middle ear plus a sign of acute local or systemic illness. The patient with AOM may have signs specific to ear disease including pain, otorrhea, and hearing loss and systemic signs of fever, irritability, headache, lethargy, anorexia, or vomiting. Uncommon signs of ear infection include tinnitus, vertigo, and nystagmus. Persistent AOM is most commonly defined as the persistence of symptoms and signs of middle ear infection following one or two courses of antibiotic therapy. Recurrent AOM is most commonly defined as three or more separate episodes of AOM in a 6-month time span or four or more episodes in a 12-month time span. Chronic OM occurs when symptoms and signs persist for 3 months or longer. Uncomplicated AOM has a favorable natural history regardless of antibiotic therapy; 70% to 80% of patients will improve on a time line similar to that for antibiotic-treated patients. Patients with persistent or recurrent AOM more frequently have infections caused by antibiotic-resistant bacterial pathogens, and a combination of host, pathogen, and environmental factors result in a markedly reduced spontaneous cure rate (approximately 50% in most studies). In the absence of appropriate treatment, chronic otitis media infrequently resolves without significant hearing difficulty sequelae.

A number of factors are implicated when initial empiric treatment for AOM fails. Therapy may fail because of inadequate dosing of orally administered antibiotics, poor absorption, poor patient compliance, poor tissue penetration, or the presence of copathogens. Factors favoring development of persistent and recurrent

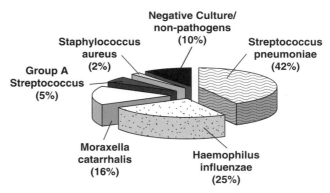

FIGURE 3–8. Bacteriology of acute otitis media infections.

AOM include an episode of AOM in the first 6 months of life, age less than 3 years, parental smoking, and day care attendance. The propensity to develop AOM has a strong genetic component.

Age

The evidence suggests that younger children, as compared with older children, have a greater likelihood of failing to meet the definitions of clinical success or resolution when they are not treated with antibiotics for AOM. The threshold appears to be sometime around 2 to 3 years of age.[83,84] This may be related to anatomic factors (delayed development of optimal eustachian tube function), exposure (especially day care attendance), or the differential incidence of resistant bacterial pathogens recovered from AOM in this age group. Children younger than 7 months tend to have a higher frequency of both penicillin-resistant *S. pneumoniae* and β-lactamase-producing gram-negative organisms than those older than 48 months of age have. Pathogens recovered from children older than 48 months are more often susceptible to traditional first-line antibiotics, such as amoxicillin and TMP-SMX.

Symptom Severity

Episodes of AOM may be classified as mild, moderate, or severe based in part on degree of otalgia and severity of systemic symptoms, for example, fever, irritability, and anorexia. Most patients who receive placebo do well if their AOM episode is uncomplicated and mild. Kaleida et al[84] described a placebo-treated resolution rate of AOM to be 63% for mild AOM and 52% for moderate AOM. Even in mild AOM, however, the benefit of antibiotic in the frequency of treatment failure and rate of effusion 2 weeks after disease onset significantly favors antibiotic therapy. Treatment with placebo and tympanocentesis (myringotomy) in patients with severe episodes has been studied in children 2 years of age or older; a benefit from tympanocentesis could not be demonstrated, and the failure rate was high in severe episodes of AOM.

Prior Treatment History

Numerous studies have indicated that antibiotic-resistant *S. pneumoniae*, *H. influenzae*, and *M. catarrhalis* are more frequently isolated in persistent and recurrent AOM. Thus recent antimicrobial exposure as a risk factor for resistant pathogens should be strongly considered in antibiotic selection and would lead to consideration of either higher dosages of a first-line agent (amoxicillin) or alternative agents for this patient population.

Some patients develop a pattern of clinical failure with first-line agents. The number of failures to be tolerated before these agents are replaced with alternative second-line antibiotics is subjective. It has been suggested that two failures with amoxicillin within a respiratory season may be sufficient to prompt the use of alternative agents in that patient. Host-specific factors

may be relevant, as absorption of amoxicillin (and amoxicillin-clavulanate) may vary, leading to variable serum concentrations and secondarily reducing tissue and middle ear levels of antibiotic.

Half of middle ear fluid cultures from patients with persistent AOM produce no bacterial growth (Table 3–19).[85–87] This finding suggests that the infecting bacteria are often eradicated by the preceding antibiotic therapy or by host defense. Symptoms and signs of inflammation may persist after bacterial eradication, causing confusion regarding persistence of infection. When a patient experiences persistent or recurrent AOM despite antibiotic therapy, the therapeutic failure is often attributed to bacterial resistance. Although bacterial resistance may account for approximately 50% of these cases of treatment failure, the bacteria isolated from patients with recurrent or persistent AOM are often susceptible to current or recent therapy (Table 3–20). These failures that are not a result of bacterial resistance may be due to inadequate dose, a dosing error, poor compliance, poor absorption, or atypical pharmacokinetics or pharmacodynamics of the antibiotic that was selected.

Day Care Attendance

The day care environment provides a circumstance in which nasopharyngeal organisms are easily transmitted from one child to the other. As a consequence of antimicrobial therapy in day care children, subsequent emergence of multiply antibiotic-resistant strains is common. Thus children attending day care more often harbor resistant AOM pathogens, and consideration should be given to this fact in antibiotic selection.

Evidence-Based Analysis of Treatment Efficacy

Observation or Placebo vs. Antibiotics

The natural history of AOM without intervention is favorable. From the few studies available, however, this is difficult to quantitate because of the lack of uniformity in the definition of outcomes, the specific outcomes monitored, and the time of measurement. In addition, most studies do not report results stratified by two major influences: age and otitis-prone state. Most studies report

TABLE 3–19 ■ Frequency of Negative Bacterial Cultures in Persistent Acute Otitis Media

Year	Author	No. patients	Cultures with no growth (%)
1994	Cohen et al[85]	293	50
1998	Gehanno et al[87]	186	32
1985	Harrison et al[204]	148	28
1998	Leibovitz et al[108]	63	32
1995	Pichichero and Pichichero[86]	137	49
1981	Schwartz et al[203]	45	18
1981	Teele et al[202]	43	57

TABLE 3–20 ■ Bacterial Susceptibility in Acute Otitis Media from 1040 Patients Unresponsive to Preceding Antibiotic Therapy

Year	Author	No. patients	Sensitive* (%)	Resistant* (%)
1995	Block et al[206]	63	67	33
1994	Cohen et al[85]	293	38	62
1992	Faden et al[205]	62	41	59
1998	Gehanno et al[87]	186	65	35
1985	Harrison et al[204]	148	62	38
1998	Leibovitz et al[108]	63	48	52
1995	Pichichero and Pichichero[86]	137	55	45
1981	Schwartz et al[203]	45	62	38
1981	Teele et al[202]	43	56	44

*Percent of bacterial isolates sensitive or resistant to the preceding antibiotic therapy given to the patient within 30 days of tympanocentesis.

follow-up of patients and clinical criteria for administering antibiotics vs. placebo or observational groups to be based on persistent or worsening symptoms or complications.

For nonsevere cases of AOM not treated with antibiotics the clinical failure rate at 24 to 48 hours was 8% in one study[84] and 26% at 24 to 72 hours in another.[88] Rosenfeld et al[89] also found a favorable difference of 12.9% (95% CI, 8.2% to 19.2%) for treatment with aminopenicillins compared to no antibiotics and a 13.7% (95% CI, 8.2% to 19.2%) favorable difference for those treated with an antibiotic compared to no antibiotic. Pooling data on failure rates at 4 to 7 days yields an estimate of 22% (three studies; 220 children; 95% CI, 10.1% to 34.3%); that is, 78% of these children not initially treated with antibiotics for AOM will have clinical resolution (Fig. 3–9).[83,84,88,90] A pooled analysis for failure from 1 to 7 days yields an estimate of 19% (five studies; 739 children; 95% CI, 9.9% to 28%); that is, 81% of these children will have clinical resolution without treatment. Rosenfeld[92] estimated that 73% of children with AOM not treated with antibiotics will have clinical resolution within 7 to 14 days after diagnosis.

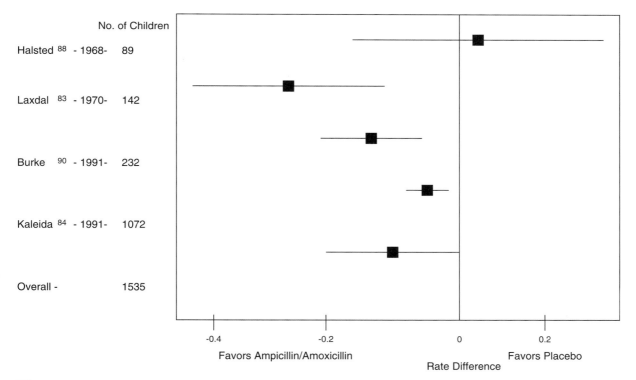

No. of Children

Halsted [88] - 1968- 89

Laxdal [83] - 1970- 142

Burke [90] - 1991- 232

Kaleida [84] - 1991- 1072

Overall - 1535

Favors Ampicillin/Amoxicillin   Favors Placebo

Rate Difference

■ Individual effect
Horizontal Line is 95% Confidence Interval
AHCPR 2001 Evidence Report/Technology Assessment

FIGURE 3–9. Meta-analysis shrinkage plot for outcome = ampicillin/amoxicillin versus placebo failure rate at 2–7 days of treatment.

The proportion with pain and fever among children with AOM not treated with antibiotics decreases rapidly, in the time periods reported, although results vary. Van Buchem et al[93] reported that 48% had pain at 2 days. Twenty-five percent reported pain at 5 to 7 days in one study,[90] whereas 10% of children still reported pain at 7 days in another.[94] Del Mar et al[95] found a 41% (95% CI, 14% to 60%) favorable rate difference in children with AOM treated with antibiotics versus no antibiotics in terms of pain at 2 to 7 days and in contralateral otitis media (43%; 95% CI, 9% to 64%), although there were no differences in pain at 24 hours, tympanic membrane perforation, 1-month tympanometry, or recurrent AOM. In another study[92] pain and fever relief at 24 hours was not related to antibiotic use in children with AOM (rate difference of 0, 95% CI, 7% to 8%), but pain and fever relief at 2 days was improved by 4% (95% CI, 2% to 7%) with antibiotic use. Clinical resolution of AOM at 7 to 14 days was 13% better (95% CI, 8% to 19%) in those given antibiotics vs. those not on antibiotics.

Similar discrepancies in findings exist for the presence of fever: 0 at 2 to 7 days by Howie and Ploussard[96] and 20% at 2 days and 11% at 5 to 7 days by Burke et al.[90] In studies reporting on pain or fever, most children with AOM are without either symptom by 3 days.[84,94,97,98] As estimated by Rosenfeld,[92] the pooled data indicate that 59% (three studies; 315 children; 95% CI, 53% to 65%) of children not treated with antibiotics do not have pain or fever within 24 hours of diagnosis of AOM, 87% (five studies; 808 children; 95% CI, 84% to 89%) of children do not have pain or fever by 4 to 7 days. Asymptomatic middle ear effusion is a common condition following AOM in children not treated with antibiotics. At 3 months, 24% to 28%[90,98] of children persist with a middle ear effusion.

Resolution of pain and fever may have a significant association with age among those not treated with antibiotics for AOM; 58% of children under 2 years of age have pain or fever at more than 3 days compared to 7% of children 2 years or older.[97] One study looked at the presence of middle ear effusion in relation to age in children with AOM not treated with antibiotics; the findings suggest a greater propensity to middle ear effusion with younger age.[84]

Other Antibiotic vs. No Antibiotic Comparisons

Other treatment regimens that have been compared to no antibiotic regimens include amoxicillin-clavulanate, penicillin G plus sulfisoxazole, penicillin V, erythromycin estolate, triple sulfonamide, and erythromycin estolate plus triple sulfonamide (Table 3–21). No statements can be made regarding the effect of age or otitis-prone status on these comparisons.

The generalizability of findings of evidence-based analysis is difficult to assess. Only two of the nine randomized controlled trials addressing natural history reported any outcome stratified as 2 years or less and older than 2 years,[84,97] and only the Kaleida et al[84] study reported early failure rate stratified in this manner. Two of the six cohort studies on natural history reported results stratified above and below 2 years of age.[99,100] These two studies reporting outcomes by age indicate that in children younger than 2 years of age clinical symptoms of AOM do not resolve as quickly as they do in older children. The studies on the clinical effectiveness of specific antibiotic regimens suffer the same problems with regard to reporting of outcomes by subject age. Three other studies also suggest that clinical failure rates are higher among children younger than 2 years receiving antibiotics.[101,102]

Most studies did not address the otitis-prone status of the child, and even fewer reported outcomes stratified by this influencing factor. In studies in which patients with recurrent otitis media[97,103] were recruited, the outcomes generally have been significantly less favorable than non–otitis-prone children.

Two other issues may be significant influencing factors: the degree of severity of AOM and increasing bacterial resistance to antibiotics. Many studies exclude those children with AOM who might be labeled high severity, i.e., those with complications, comorbid or concurrent conditions, or strong indications for antibiotic. In addition, many studies exclude children with acute or chronic perforation of the tympanic membrane. The AHCPR evidence-based analysis findings[83,84,90,91] are, therefore, most applicable to children with AOM of lesser severity without comorbidities.

The majority of studies do not explicitly address the issue of bacterial resistance. As Klein[104] notes, group A streptococci and *Streptococcus pneumoniae* developed resistance to sulfonamides in the 1940s, *Staphylococcus aureaus* to penicillins, macrolides, and tetracyclines in the 1950s, gram-negative enteric bacilli to aminoglycosides, chloramphenicol, and tetracyclines in the 1960s, *Haemophilus influenzae* to β-lactamase-susceptible penicillins in the 1970s, and more recently *S. pneumoniae* to penicillins, cephalosporins, and macrolides in the 1980s. Bacterial resistance may have an effect on outcome of AOM. The prevalence of bacterial resistance differs based on locale.[105] In 1993, Klein reviewed the data from placebo and placebo equivalent studies for AOM in children and concluded that 60% of all episodes resolve spontaneously. In all studies the average rate of spontaneous resolution varied by organism: 16% for *S. pneumoniae*-, 50% for *H. influenzae*-, and 80% for *M. catarrhalis*-induced AOM. The benefit of antibiotic therapy was most apparent when pathogenic bacteria were isolated from middle ear fluid by tympanocentesis, when bacterial eradication on day 4 to 5 was used to assess outcome or when clinical outcome was assessed at 2 to 3 days rather than 7 to 14 days.

In summary, evidence-based analysis shows that antibiotics produce a short-term benefit in more rapid resolution of symptoms of AOM and an intermediate-term

TABLE 3–21 ■ Use of Placebo in Treatment of Acute Otitis Media

Year	Authors	Study population	Treatment	No. patients	Clinical cure or improved (%)	
1991	Appleman et al[97]	Children	Placebo	121	82	
			Amoxicillin-clavulanate		84	
1991	Burke et al[90]	Children	Placebo	232	86	
			Amoxicillin		98	
2000	Damoiseaux et al[207]	Children	Placebo	240	30	
			Amoxicillin		36	
1989	Engelhard et al[208]	Children	Placebo + myringotomy	105	23	
			Amoxicillin-clavulanate ± myringotomy		60	
1990	Froom et al[99]	Children	Placebo	2982	91	
			Antibiotic (unspecified)		82	
1968	Halstead et al[88]	Children	Placebo	89	74	
			Ampicillin		67	
			Penicillin		78	
1972	Howie et al[96]	Children	Placebo	280	28	
			Triple sulfonamide		57	
			Erythromycin estolate		56	
			Ampicillin		83	
			Erythromycin estolate–triple sulfonamide		81	
1970	Laxdal et al[83]	Children Adolescents	Placebo	142	62	
			Penicillin		76	
			Ampicillin		90	
1991	Kaleida et al[84]	Children	Placebo	1072	72	
			Amoxicillin			
			Placebo + myringotomy		72	
			Amoxicillin ± myringotomy		52	
1991	Mandel et al[209]	Children	Placebo	331	No significant differences among the groups	
			Amoxicillin			
			Cefaclor			
			Erythromycin-sulfisoxazole			
1981	Mygind et al[98]	Children	Placebo	149	69	
			Penicillin		86	
1997	Tilyard et al[100]	Children Adolescents	Placebo vs. antibiotic	2367	90	
1985	Thalin et al[210]	Children Adolescents	Placebo	317	92	
			Penicillin		97	
1990	Thomsen[211]	Children	Amoxicillin-clavulanate	221	61	
			Placebo		30	
					7 D	**14 D**
1981	VanBuchem et al[94]	Children	Placebo ± myringotomy	171	51	74
			Amoxicillin ± myringotomy		58	90
1985	VanBuchem et al[93]	Children	Placebo	490	95	

benefit in more rapid resolution of middle ear effusion. Antibiotics reduce the risk that bacteremia will progress to focal, severe infection (e.g., meningitis); 2% to 4% of children younger than 3 years of age with AOM and fever have concurrent bacteremia. Antibiotics may prevent focal infections such as mastoiditis, which occur in approximately 1 in 400 untreated children. Additional advantages of antibiotic treatment include avoidance of sequential visits for patients who are not improving, as well as possibly decreasing litigation risks. Clearly there is debate about the necessity to treat all children who have AOM with antibiotics. Yet a careful examination of the published literature would suggest that younger febrile children are at increased risk for complications. This would apply specifically to children younger than

2 years of age. This is the age when AOM is most prevalent. If antibiotic therapy is to be withheld, perhaps it would be more appropriate for afebrile children older than 3 years of age.

Outcome Measures Assessing Efficacy

Microbiologic and Clinical Efficacy

Management of AOM focuses on the choice of an appropriate antibiotic. The antibiotic should have documented microbiologic and clinical efficacy. Microbiologic efficacy should be defined for each bacterial pathogen by the assessment of pretreatment tympanocentesis specimens and assessment of efficacy by clinical criteria. Cultures of middle ear aspirates obtained before initiation and 3 to 6 days after initiation of therapy provide data about the efficacy of the drug used for sterilizing middle ear fluid. Clinical efficacy should be measurable based on substantial resolution of signs and symptoms within 72 hours and prevention of relapse, recurrence, and suppurative sequelae.

Differences in microbiologic efficacy are apparent among the various antibiotics. Examination of sequential aspirates following administration of placebo and various antibiotics is presented in Table 3–22.

Relief of Symptoms

Symptoms of AOM consist mainly of pain and systemic illness. The pain is caused by pressure on the tympanic membrane. After the inflammation subsides, the consequent residual hearing loss caused by fluid retained in the middle ear space may take several weeks to resolve. Evidence regarding the impact of antibiotic therapy on pain and fever is presented earlier in this chapter. Antibiotics also reduce contralateral AOM by 43%.

Persistent Middle Ear Effusion

Impairment of hearing is associated with the presence of middle ear fluid. Current data on outcomes from medical treatments for middle ear fluid are inconclusive. Incision and drainage with placement of a ventilating tube provides immediate improvement, but the criteria for the procedure are controversial. Topical or systemic decongestants or antihistamines are of no value in clearing middle ear effusion. These agents may be effective in reducing the congestion resulting from allergic rhinitis that causes eustachian tube dysfunction and may provide symptomatic relief for patients with nasal congestion. A 2-week course of an antibiotic may resolve middle ear effusion in a limited number of cases. An analysis of

controlled studies identified a 14% increase in resolution rate when antibiotics are given. There is limited evidence suggesting that a short course of systemic corticosteroid therapy (5 to 7 days) combined with an antibiotic agent may be of value. Recent studies show a modest but significant reduction in the morbidity of OME following adenoidectomy. A 1999 report from the Agency for Health Care Policy and Research[106] provided an algorithm for treatment. They recommended for pediatric OME that follow-up visits occur 1 to 2 months after AOM resolution. When the effusion persists for 3 months or longer, treatment with a 2-week course of antibiotics alone or in conjunction with a 7-day regimen of prednisone may be indicated. Children who have had fluid in both middle ears for a total of 3 months should undergo a hearing evaluation, and if the effusion fails to resolve with medical management, they should be referred for consideration of placement of tympanostomy tubes.

Clinical Trials of Various Antibiotic Regimens

Clinical efficacy of various antibiotics in AOM is described in Tables 3–23 to 3–27. Clinical trials of antibiotics almost always reveal successful clinical outcomes. The high cure rates, however, are often unreliable because of study design flaws. Explanations for overly positive results include (1) over diagnosis of AOM at study entry, (2) inclusion of patients with only mild AOM, (3) exclusion of moderate-to-severe and difficult-to-treat cases, and (4) use of overly broad criteria (symptom resolution only) to define clinical cure or improvement.

Guideline Recommendations

The Centers for Disease Control has made recommendations with regard to treatment of AOM with consideration to bacterial resistance[107] as summarized in Table 3–28. Antibiotic selection for persistent and recurrent AOM (otitis-prone) and for children below 2 years of age must be more precise because resistant organisms are more often involved and host defense alone already has been proven suboptimal clinically. Consideration should be given to antibiotic concentration achievable in middle ear fluid relative to the concentration necessary to kill the relevant pathogens. Two selection criteria are recommended: (1) the antibiotic should be effective against most drug-resistant *S. pneumoniae* and (2) the antibiotic should be effective against β-lactamase-producing *H. influenzae* and *M. catarrhalis*. A treatment algorithm based on these criteria has been developed (Fig. 3–10). In the formation of these recommendations, trials in which tympanocentesis was performed were most prominently considered to avoid the problem of basing recommendations on patients who have been inaccurately diagnosed.

Important elements in current treatment guidelines include recommendations to start with amoxicillin for

TABLE 3–22 ■ Persistence of Bacterial Pathogens in Middle Ear Fluids after Therapy for Acute Otitis Media

| Drug | Persisting organism (%)* | |
	Streptococcus pneumoniae	*Haemophilus influenzae*
Placebo	81	52
Amoxicillin	5	13†
		64‡
Amoxicillin-clavulanate	3	19
TMP-SMX	12	25
Cefaclor	18	33
Cefixime	26	6
Cefpodoxime	17	5
Ceftriaxone (1 dose, IM)	0	0
Erythromycin	7	65

*Aspirates examined prior to and 2 to 10 days following therapy.

†β-lactamase negative.

‡β-lactamase positive.

Adapted from Klein JO: Microbiologic efficacy of antibacterial drugs for acute otitis media. Pediatr Infect Dis J 1993;12:973–975.

TABLE 3–23 ■ Aminopenicillin Treatment of Acute Otitis Media

Year	Author	Study population	Treatment	No. patients	Clinical cure or improved (%)	
1967	Bass et al[213]	Children	Oxytetracycline	400	72	
			Procaine penicillin + benzathine		82	
			Penicillin G + sulfisoxazole			
			Penicillin V + sulfisoxazole		76	
			Ampicillin		79	
1973	Bass et al[214]	Children	Penicillin V	400	82	
			Penicillin V + sulfa		83	
			Erythromycin estolate		89	
			Ampicillin		81	
1973	Bass et al[214]	Children Adolescents	Phenoxymethyl-penicillin	400	62	
			Penicillin + sulfisoxazole		73	
			Erythromycin estolate		80	
			Ampicillin trihydrate		74	
1973	Feigin et al[215]	Children	Ampicillin	171	88	
			Clindamycin		86	
88	Halsted, 1968	Children	Ampicillin	89	92	
			Penicillin G + sulfisoxazole		92	
			Placebo		100	
					S. PNEUMONIAE	HIB
1976	Howard et al[216]	Children	Penicillin V 10 d	386	75	72
			Amoxicillin 10 d		92	93
			Erythromycin estolate		72	61
			Erythromycin estolate + trisulfapyrimidines		74	93
					S. PNEUMONIAE	HIB
1974	Howie et al[217]	Children	Amoxicillin 10 d	123	59	47
			Ampicillin 10 d		70	56
1986	Kaleida et al[218]	Children	Sultamicillin	50	100	
1983	Kim & Anthony[219]	Children	Amoxicillin 10 d	109	88	
			Bacampicillin 10 d		88	
1970	Laxdal[83]	Children Adolescents	Ampicillin	142	90	
			Penicillin		76	
			Placebo		62	
1968	Lenoski et al[220]	Not specific	Erythromycin	39	95	
			Erythromycin + sulfonamide		67	
			Triple sulfonamide		61	
			Ampicillin		71	
1982	McLinn et al[221]	Children Adolescents	Amoxicillin 10 d	363	98	
			Cyclacillin 10 d		98	
1983	McLinn & Serlin[222]	Children	Amoxicillin 10 d	240	96	
			Cyclacillin 10 d		96	
1983	Moran[155]	Adolescents Adult	Amoxicillin	84	91	
			Pivampicillin		92	
1993	Murph et al[223]	Children	Amoxicillin qd + placebo bid	67	82	
			Amoxicillin tid × 10 d		68	
			40 mg/kg/d all subjects			
1969	Nilson et al[224]	Children	Ampicillin	306	75	
			Penicillin V		72	
			Penicillin V + sulfonamide		82	
1986	Principi et al[225]	Children	Amoxicillin bid 10 d	110	89	
			Amoxicillin tid 10 d		93	
1989	Puhakka et al[226]	Children	Amoxicillin 10 d	97	90	
			Bacampicillin 10 d		90	
1985	Rodriguez et al[227]	Children Adolescents	Amoxicillin	153	89	
			Erythromycin sulfate		89	
1990	Rodriguez et al[228]	Children Adolescents	Amoxicillin 10 d	86	92	
			Sultamicillin 10 d		97	
1998	Scholtz & Noack[229]	Children	Amoxicillin	302	96	
			Erythromycin estolate		94	
1986	Valtonen et al[230]	Children	Amoxicillin tid	367	86	
			Amoxicillin bid		82	

Hib, *Haemophilus influenzae* type b; *S. pneumoniae*, *Streptococcus pneumoniae*.

TABLE 3–24 ■ **Sulfonamide Treatment for Acute Otitis Media**

Year	Authors	Study popluation	Treatment	No. patients	Clinical cure or improved(%)	
					<25 KG	>25 KG
1975	Cameron et al[231]	Children	Ampicillin	79	54	60
			TMP-SMX		47	71
1976	Cooper et al[232]	Children Adults	Amoxicillin Co-trimoxazole	61	No statistical difference in efficacy	
1988	Feldman et al[233]	Children	Amoxicillin	221	88	
			TMP-SMX		87	
1990	Feldman et al[234]	Children Adolescents	TMP-SMX	202	93	
			Amoxicillin		82	
					CURE	IMPROVED
1980	Shurin et al[235]	Children	TMP-SMX	132	85	75
			Ampicillin		86	90

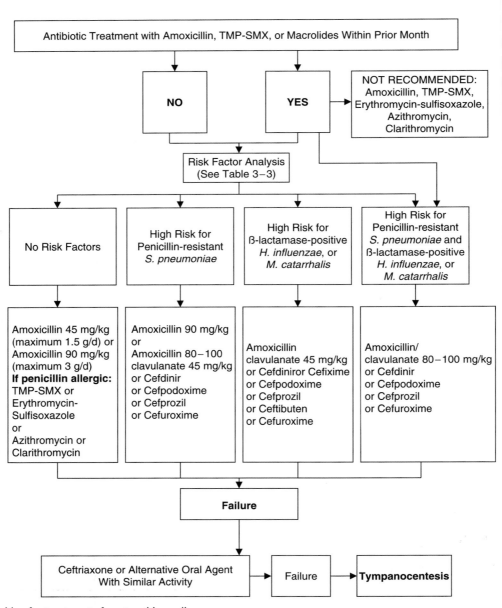

FIGURE 3–10. Algorithm for treatment of acute otitis media.

TABLE 3–25 ■ Amoxicillin-Clavulanate Treatment of Otitis Media

Year	Authors	Study population	Treatment	No. patients	Clinical cure or improved (%)
1997	Adler et al[236]	Children	Amoxicillin-clavulanate 10 d	752	90
			Cefdinir (7 mg)		91
			Cefdinir (14 mg)		89
1991	Arguedas et al[237]	Children	Amoxicillin-clavulanate 10 d	122	77
		Adolescents	Cefprozil 10 d		92
1992	Aronovitz[237a]	Children	Amoxicillin-clavulanate 10 d	323	81
			Cefprozil 10 d		85
1994	Aspin et al[238]	Children	Amoxicillin-clavulanate 10 d	180	95
			Clarithromycin 10 d		93
1997	Behre et al[239]	Children	Amoxicillin-clavulanate bid 10 d	463	92
			Amoxicillin-clavulanate tid 10 d		91
2000	Block et al[240]	Children	Amoxicillin-clavulanate 10 d	303	83
			Cefdinir qd 10 d		85
			Cefdinir bid 10 d		82
1995	Boulesteix et al[241]	Children	Amoxicillin-clavulanate 10 d	501	87
			Cefixime 10 d		88
1993	Careddu et al[242]	Children	Amoxicillin-clavulanate	50	64
		Adolescents	Brodimoprim		88
1988	Chan et al[243]	Children	Amoxicillin-clavulanate 10 d	106	52
			Amoxicillin 10 d		32
1993	Chan et al[244]	Children	Amoxicillin-clavulanate	144	Efficacy not statistically different at 10 d or 30 d
			Sultamicillin		
2000	Dagan et al[245]	Children	Amoxicillin-clavulanate	238	86
			Azithromycin		70
2000	Damrikarnlert et al[246]	Children	Amoxicillin-clavulanate bid	324	78
			Amoxicillin-clavulanate tid 7 or 10 d		85
1991	Gan et al[247]	Children	Amoxicillin-clavulanate	92	98
			Loracarbef		91
1994	Gehanno et al[248]	Children	Amoxicillin-clavulanate 10 d	92	87
			Cefprozil 10 d	99	84
1994	Gehanno et al[249]	Children	Amoxicillin-clavulanate 8 d	160	96
			Cefpodoxime proxetil 8 d		98
1998	Goldblatt et al[250]	Children with tubes	Amoxicillin-clavulanate 10 d	286	67
			Ofloxacin topical 10 d		96
1995	Gooch et al[251]	Children	Amoxicillin-clavulanate 10 d	477	95
			Cefuroxime axetil 10 d		84
1988	Jacobsson et al[252]	Children	Amoxicillin-clavulanate	122	81
			Cefaclor		82
1993	Jacobsson et al[253]	Children	Amoxicillin-clavulanate bid 7 d	311	70
			Amoxicillin-clavulanate tid 7 d		70
1987	Kaleida et al[254]	Children	Amoxicillin-clavulanate 10 d	133	98
			Cefaclor 10 d		96
1988	Kaprio et al[255]	Children	Amoxicillin-clavulanate 7 d	247	88
			Cefaclor 7 d		83
1995	Mandel et al[256]	Children	Amoxicillin 10 d + Amoxicillin 10 d	267	72
			Amoxicillin 10 d + Amoxicillin-clavulanate 10 d		81
			Amoxicillin 10 d + placebo 10 d		53
1986	Marchant et al[257]	Children	Amoxicillin-clavulanate	71	97
			Cefaclor		75
1993	McCarty et al[258]	Children	Amoxicillin-clavulanate 10 d	338	92
			Clarithromycin 10 d		90
1990	Pichichero et al[259]	Children	Amoxicillin-clavulanate 10 d	377	67
			Cefuroxime axetil 10 d		74
			Cefaclor 10 d		77
1999	Ruohola et al[260]	Children with tubes	Amoxicillin-clavulanate 7 d + prednisolone 3 d	50	91
			Amoxicillin-clavulanate 7 d + placebo		30
1997	Thomsen et al[261]	Children with SOM	Penicillin V 14 d	360	23
			Penicillin V 28 d		19
			Amoxicillin-clavulanate 14 d		31
			Amoxicillin-clavulanate 28 d		44

TABLE 3–26 ■ **Cephalosporin Treatment of Acute Otitis Media**

Year	Author	Study population	Treatment	No. patients	Clinical cure or improved (%)
1988	Aronovitz[262]	Children	Cefuroxime axetil 10 d	64	90
			Cefaclor 10 d		76
1994	Asmar et al[262a]	Children	Cefpodoxime proxetil	368	88
		Adolescents	Cefixime 10 d		60
1997	Barnett et al[263]	Children	TMP-SMZ	484	82
			Ceftriaxone		80
1987	Bergeron et al[264]	Children	Erythromycin ethylsuccinate–sulfisoxazole	119	100
			Cefaclor 10 d		98
1983	Berman & Lauer[265]	Children	Amoxicillin 10 d	40	71
			Cefaclor 10 d		74
1992	Biolcati[266]	Children	Sultamicillin 10 d	60	100
			Cefaclor 11 d		97
1984	Blumer et al[267]	Children	TMP-SMZ	100	96
			Cefaclor		92
1995	Blumer et al[268]	Children	Ceftibuten 10 d	154	89
			Cefaclor 10 d		88
1996	Blumer et al[269]	Children	Ceftibuten qd 10 d	205	83
		Adolescents	Cefprozil bid 10 d		83
1990	Brodie et al[270]	Children	Amoxicillin	660	95
			Cefuroxime		94
1997	Dagan[271]	Children	Cefuroxime axetil 10 d	266	85
			Cefaclor 10 d		68
1982	Feldman et al[272]	Children	Co-trimoxazole 10 d	197	96
			Cefaclor 10 d		91
1982	Feldman et al[272]	Adolsecents	TMP-SMZ	197	96
		Adults	Cefaclor		91
1992	Foshee[273]	Children	Amoxicillin-clavulanate 10 d	284	76
			Loracarbef 10 d		68
1992	Foshee & Qvarnberg[274]	Children	Amoxicillin	291	76
			Loracarbef		68
1994	Furman et al[275]	Children	Cefetamet pivoxil 10 d	72	97
			Cefaclor 10 d		89
1984	Giebink et al[276]	Children	Amoxicillin 10–14 d	61	83
		Adolescents	Cefaclor 10–14 d		77
1993	Gooch et al[277]	Children	Clarithromycin	281	96
			Cefaclor		92
1999	Gooch et al[278]	Children	Loracarbef 10 d	334	62
			Clarithromycin 10 d		58
1997	Gooch et al[279]	Children	Amoxicillin-clavulanate 10 d	313	77
			Cefixime 10 d		76
1993	Green & Rothrock[280]	Children	Amoxicillin	233	91
			Ceftriaxone		90
1993	Harrison et al[281]	Children	Cefixime 10 d	102	83
			Cefaclor 10 d		72
1985	Howie et al[282]	Children	TMP-SMZ	200	67
			Cefaclor		55
1987	Howie & Owen[283]	Children	Amoxicillin	140	80
			Cefixime		76
1979	Jacobson et al[284]	Children	Amoxicillin	28	87
			Cefaclor		85
1983	John and Valle-Jones[285]	Children	Amoxicillin 7 d	150	92
			Cefaclor 7 d		96
1991	Johnson et al[286]	Children	Amoxicillin	126	79
		Adolescents	Cefixime		87
1998	Kara et al[287]	Children	Amoxicillin	75	92
			Cefuroxime axetil		92
			Ceftriaxone		84
1987	Kenna et al[288]	Children	Cefixime qd 10 d	135	100
			Cefixime bid 10 d		97
			Cefaclor 10 d		97
1989	Leigh et al[289]	Children	Amoxicillin	325	95

TABLE 3–26 ■ Cephalosporin Treatment of Acute Otitis Media (*Continued*)

Year	Author	Study population	Treatment	No. patients	Clinical cure or improved (%)	
		Adolescents	Cefixime		95	
1998	Ludwig[290]	Children	Cefixime qd	50	96	
1974	Nassar & Allen[291]	Children	Ampicillin	54	97	
			Cephalexin		96	
1985	Odio et al[292]	Children	Amoxicillin-clavulanate 10 d	130	100	
			Cefaclor 10 d		92	
1996	MacLoughlin et al[292a]	Children	Cefpodoxime proxetil	90	94	
			Cefaclor		92	
1996	Mandel et al[293]	Children	Amoxicillin 14 d	210	73	
			Ceftibuten 14 d		70	
1982	Mandel et al[294]	Children	Amoxicillin 14 d	203	96	
		Adolescents	Cefaclor 14 d		96	
1993	Mandel et al[295]	Children	Amoxicillin 10 d	157	94	
			Cefaclor 10 d		95	
1981	Mandel et al[296]	Children	Amoxicillin 14 d	110	91	
		Adolescents	Cefaclor 14 d		95	
1984	Marchant et al[297]	Children	TMP-SMZ 10 d	129	95	
			Cefaclor 10 d		70	
1975	McLinn et al[298]	Children	Cephalexin 10 d	97	84	
		Adolescents				
1979	McLinn[299]	Children	Amoxicillin	100	94	
		Adolescents	Cephradine		90	
1980	McLinn[300]	Children	Amoxicillin	130	91	
			Cefaclor		95	
1987	McLinn[301]	Children	Amoxicillin 10 d	120	94	
			Cefixime 10 d		93	
1995	McLinn[301a]	Children	Amoxicillin-clavulanate 10 d	219	97	
			Ceftibuten 10 d		93	
1992	Mendelman et al[302]	Children	Amoxicillin-clavulanate 10 d	146	86	
		Adolescents	Cefpodoxime 10 d		92	
					S. PNEUMONIAE	**HIB**
1978	Nelson et al[303]	Children	Cefaclor 40 mg 10 d	100	78	70
			Cefaclor 60 mg 10 d		100	88
1993	Owen et al[304]	Children	Amoxicillin 10 d	201	77	
			Cefixime 10 d		74	
1997	Pichichero et al[103]	Children	Cefprozil 10 d	262	78	
1991	Piippo et al[305]	Children	Cefaclor 7 d	396	91	
			Cefixime 7 d		94	
1984	Ploussard[306]	Children	Amoxicillin	60	86	
			Cefaclor		100	
1991	Principi & Marchisio[307]	Children	Amoxicillin 10 d	40	90	
			Cefixime 10 d		90	
1992	Pukander et al[308]	Children	Cefetamet 7 d	40	80	
		Adolescents	Cefaclor 7 d		55	
1993	Rodriguez et al[309]	Children	Cefixime	61	94	
			Cefaclor		68	
1976	Stechenberg et al[310]	Children	Ampicillin 10 d	179	92	
			Cephalexin 10 d		75	
1998	Subba Rao et al[311]	Children	Amoxicillin-clavulanate 7 d	215	97	
			Cefaclor 7 d		84	
1992	Syrogiannopoulos et al[312]	Children	Amoxicillin tid 10 d	55	100	
			Cefuroxime bid 10 d		100	
1998	Tsai et al[313]	Children	Cefpodoxime proxetil	57	95	
			Cefaclor		90	
1998	Turik & Johns[314]	Children	Cefaclor 10 d	205	92	
			Cefuroxime axetil 10 d		89	
1988	Varsano et al[315]	Children	Amoxicillin	52	86	
			Ceftriaxone		82	
1991	Wu[316]	Children	Cefixime 10 d	25,863	86	

Hib, *Haemophilus influenzae* type b; *S. pneumoniae, Streptococcus pneumoniae.*

TABLE 3–27 ■ Macrolide/Azalide Treatment for Acute Otitis Media

Year	Author	Study population	Treatment	No. patients	Clinical cure or improved (%)
1993	Pukander et al[317]	Children	Amoxicillin	79	90
			Clarithromycin		93
1983	Rosen et al[318]	Children	Phenoxymethyl penicillin	78	90
		Adolescents	Erythromycin stearate		79

TABLE 3–28 ■ Acute Otitis Media Treatment Recommendations by the Centers for Disease Control Drug-Resistant *Streptococcus pneumoniae* Therapeutic Working Group

Antibiotics in prior month	Day 0	Clinically defined treatment failure on day 3	Clinically defined treatment failure on days 10–28
No	High dose amoxicillin; *or* Usual dose amoxicillin	High dose amoxicillin-clavulanate; *or* Cefuroxime axetil; *or* Ceftriaxone IM	Same as day 3
Yes	High dose amoxicillin; *or* High dose amoxicillin-calvulanate; *or* Cefuroxime axetil	Ceftriaxone IM; *or* Clindamycin* Tympanocentesis	High dose amoxicillin-clavulanate; *or* Cefuroxime axetil; *or* Ceftriaxone IM; Tympanocentesis

*High dose amoxicillin = 80–100mg/kg/d. High dose amoxicillin-clavulanate = 80–100 mg/kg/d for the amoxicillin component. Ceftriaxone injections recommended for 3 days. Clindamycin is not effective against *Haemophilus influenzae* or *Moraxella catarrhalis*.

Data from Dowell SF, Butler JC, Giebink GS, et al: Acute Otitis Media: Management and surveillance in an era of pneumococcal resistance—a report from the Drug-resistant *Streptococcus pneumoniae* Therapeutic Working Group. Pediatr Infect Dis J 1999;18:1–9.

uncomplicated AOM. The decision to continue or switch to an alternative antibiotic should be based on clinical response on the third day of therapy, giving the selected antibiotic enough time to work or fail. Including traditional second-line antibiotics as first-line choices is appropriate when the patient has already been on an antibiotic within the previous month or is otitis prone.

Tympanocentesis

Tympanocentesis with a culture of middle ear fluid may be useful for patients in pain and those who appear toxic or who have a high fever. Diagnostic tympanocentesis is helpful to guide the choice of therapy in persistent or recurrent AOM. The CDC has recommended that physicians learn the skills required to perform tympanocentesis or have a referral source for patients who would benefit from the procedure. Evacuation (drainage) of the middle ear effusion may be beneficial in breaking the cycle of persistent and recurrent AOM. The information provided by the culture and susceptibility report may be valuable for treating persistent and recurrent AOM. If a bacterial pathogen is reported, selecting an appropriate antibiotic will reduce the likelihood of further treatment failure; if no bacterial pathogen is isolated, the patient will not require further antibiotic treatment.

Duration of Treatment

A 10-day treatment course with antibiotic is standard in the United States, although shorter regimens are frequently used in other countries. There is microbiologic and clinical evidence that shorter treatment regimens might be effective in most AOM episodes. Pediatric studies in which tympanocentesis was used to evaluate bacteria in middle ear effusion showed sterility of the middle ear space after only 3 to 6 days of antibiotic treatment. Bacterial eradication is the key determinant of treatment success; therefore 3- to 6-day courses of antibiotic therapy might be predicted to be successful on the basis of these data. Clinical evidence supporting the efficacy of shortened courses of antibiotic therapy in AOM are presented in Table 3–29.[101,102,108–110] These data examine the percentages of patients considered clinically cured or improved at the end of therapy and demonstrate that 5-day courses of therapy are as effective in the treatment of AOM as 10-day courses for various agents. Early studies suggested that a 5-day course of therapy may be less effective than a 10-day course in children who are younger than 2 years of age. Later, clinical efficacy of 5-, 7-, and 10-day antibiotic regimens for AOM according to patient age suggested that age was not the critical factor in predicting success in shortened antibiotic regimens.[111] Rather it would appear that use of antibiotic therapy within the preceding month (a known risk factor for selection of resistant pathogens) identifies a subgroup of patients who clearly benefit from longer (10-day) courses of antibiotic therapy. Regional variations to pathogens' resistance patterns therefore would be relevant in considering the duration of therapy for an individual patient. In addition, patients with tympanic membrane perforation are less likely to experience cure with a shortened course of therapy.

TABLE 3–29 ■ Short- versus Long-Term Antibiotic Therapy

Year	Author	Study population	Treatment	No. patients	Clinical cure or improved (%)	
1995	Adam[109]	Children	Cefpodoxime 5 d Cefaclor 10 d	100	100 100	
1996	Arguedas et al[319]	Children	Azithromycin 3 d Amoxicillin-clavulanate 10 d	100	100 96	
1997	Arguedas et al[320]	Children	Azithromycin 3 d Clarithromycin 10 d	97	100 96	
1996	Aronovitz[321]	Children	Azithromycin 5 d Amoxicillin-clavulanate 10 d	92	88 100	
1985	Bain et al[322]	Children	Amoxicillin 2 d Amoxicillin 7 d	243	No significant difference in efficacy	
1997	Barnett et al[263]	Children	Ceftriaxone TMP-SMX 10 d	484	80 82	
1996	Bauchner et al[323]	Children	Ceftriaxone Amoxicillin-clavulanate 10 d	648	81 90	
1995	Boulesteix et al[324]	Children	Cefpodoxime 5 d Cefixime 8 d	245	94 93	
1994	Chamberlain et al[325]	Children	Ceftriaxone Cefaclor 10 d	79	100 100	
1982	Chaput de Saintage et al[326]	Children	Amoxicillin 3 d Amoxicillin 10 d	70	88 93	
2000	Cohen et al[327]	Children	Cefpodoxime–proxetil 5 d Cefpodoxime–proxetil 10 d	450	84 92	
1999	Cohen et al[328]	Children	Ceftriaxone Amoxicillin-clavulanate 10 d	463	79 83	
1997	Cohen et al[329]	Children	Cefpodoxime 5 d Amoxicillin-clavulanate 8 d	400	84 82	
1998	Cohen et al[330]	Children	Amoxicillin-clavulanate 5 d Amoxicillin-clavulanate 10 d	382	77 88	
1993	Coles et al[331]	Children	Amoxycillin 5 d Clarithromycin 5 d	219	96 96	
1999	Dagan et al[332]	Children	Azithromycin 5 d Amoxicillin-clavulanate 10 d	163	73 85	
2000	Dagan et al[245]	Children	Azithromycin 3 d Cefaclor 10 d	122	82 85	
1993	Daniel[333]	Children	Azithromycin single dose Co-amoxiclav 10 d	159	95 98	
1997	Ficnar et al[189]	Children	Azithromycin 3 d Azithromycin 5 d	371	96 96	
1990	Gehanno et al[334]	Children	Cefotaxime 1 d Amoxicillin-clavulanate 5 d	116	No significant difference in efficacy	
					S. PNEUMONIAE	HIB
1999	Gehanno et al[335]	Children	Ceftriaxone 3 d following oral antibiotic treatment failure	186	82	88
1996	Gooch et al[336]	Children	Cefuroxime 5 d Cefuroxime 10 d Amoxicillin-clavulanate 10 d	719	82 82 90	
1993	Green & Rothrock[280]	Children	Ceftriaxone Amoxicillin 10 d	233	90 91	
1988	Hendrickse et al[337]	Children	Cefaclor 5 d Cefaclor 10 d	151	50 89	
1997	Hoberman et al[338]	Children	Amoxicillin-clavulanate 5 d bid Amoxicillin-clavulanate 10 d bid Amoxicillin-clavulanate 10 d tid	564	71 87 79	
1982	Ingvarsson & Lundgren[101]	Children	Penicillin V 5 d (2× dose) Penicillin V 10 d (normal dose)	297	79 77	
1986	Jones & Bain[339]	Children	Cefaclor 3 d Cefaclor 7 d	96	No significant difference in efficacy	
1997	Kafetzis et al[340]	Children Adolescents	Cefprozil 5 d Cefprozil 10 d	550	87 91	
1998	Kara et al[287]	Children	Ceftriaxone 1 d Amoxicillin 10 d Cefuroxime 10 d	75	84 92 92	

Continued

TABLE 3–29 ■ Short- versus Long-Term Antibiotic Therapy (*Continued*)

Year	Author	Study population	Treatment	No. patients	Clinical cure or improved (%)
1996	Khurana[341]	Children	Azithromycin 5 d	526	92
			Amoxicillin-clavulanate 10 d		90
1998	Leibovitz et al[108]	Children	Ceftriaxone 3 d following oral antibiotic treatment failure	92	95
2000	Leibovitz et al[342]	Children	Ceftriaxone 1 d	108	73
			Ceftriaxone 3 d		98
1989	Leigh et al[289]	Children Adolescents	Cefixime 5 d	325	95
			Amoxicillin 5 d		95
1996	McCarty[343]	Children Adolescents	Azithromycin 5 d	200	81
1996	McLinn[344]	Children Adolescents	Azithromycin 5 d	677	88
			Amoxicillin-clavulanate 10 d		89
1983	Meistrup-Larsen et al[345]	Children	Penicillin 2 d	95	72
			Penicillin 7 d		86
1993	Mohs et al[346]	Children	Azithromycin 3 d	154	79
			Amoxicillin 10 d		58
1996	Muller[193]	Adults	Azithromycin 3 d	107	98
			Roxithromycin 10 d		98
1999	Pessey et al[347]	Children	Cefuroxime axetil 5 d	716	86
			Amoxicillin-clavulanate 10 d		88
			Amoxicillin-clavulanate 8 d		88
1992	Pestalozza et al[348]	Children	Azithromycin 3 d	30	93
			Amoxicillin-clavulanate 10 d		40
1984	Ploussard[306]	Children	Cefaclor 5 d	60	100
			Amoxicillin 10 d		86
1995	Principi[349]	Children	Azithromycin 3 d	413	93
			Amoxicillin-clavulanate 10 d		94
1987	Puczynski et al[350]	Children	Amoxicillin single dose	17	57
			Amoxicillin 10 d		100
1995	Ramet[351]	Children	Azithromycin 5 d	147	99
			Clarithromycin 5 d		99
1996	Rodriguez[352]	Children Adolescents	Azithromycin 3 d	259	98
			Cefaclor 10 d		97
1965	Rubenstein et al[353]	Children Adolescents	Bicillin	462	95
			Bicillin + pseudoephedrine		93
			Bicillin + triple sulfonamide		99
			Bicillin + triple sulfonamide + pseudoephedrine		96
			Tetracycline		87
			Tetracycline + pseudoephedrine		92
1993	Schaad[102]	Children	Azithromycin 3 d	389	94
			Co-amoxiclav 10 d		99
1997	Simon[354]	Children Adolescents	Ceftibuten 5 d	232	78
			Ceftibuten 10 d		98
1967	Stickler et al[355]	Children Adolescents	Penicillin	414	94
			Penicillin + antihistamine		98
			Penicillin + triple sulfonamide		96
			Penicillin + antihistamine + triple sulfonamide		99
1988	Varsano et al[315]	Children	Ceftriaxone	52	82
			Amoxicillin 7 d		86
1997	Varsano et al[110]	Children	Ceftriaxone	227	95
			Amoxicillin-clavulanate 10 d		95

Antibiotic Prophylaxis

Antibiotic prophylaxis has been successful in reducing the number of new symptomatic episodes of AOM in children who have had a history of recurring infections. Various antibiotics have been used for prophylaxis, and different schemes of administration including continuous or intermittent have been tried (Table 3–30).[112–119] A meta-analysis of randomized clinical trials confirmed that all the drugs and all the schemes used for prophylaxis are effective in preventing recurrences. Despite this, many questions regarding the time to start, the mode of administration, the duration of prophylaxis, and the adverse impact on selection of resistant organisms make this strategy controversial.

TABLE 3–30 ■ Prophylactic Use of Antimicrobials in Otitis-Prone Children

Antimicrobial agent (investigator)	Study group	Duration (mo)	Effect
Sulfonamides (Ensign et al, 1960[112])	Eskimos	9	50% reduction of discharging ears
Sulfonamides, ampicillin (Maynard et al, 1972[113])	Eskimos	12	50% reduction of discharging ears
Sulfonamides, placebo (Perrin et al, 1974[114])		3 + 3	No reduction of AOM
Sulfonamides (several studies) (Schwartz et al, 1982[115]; Principi et al, 1989[116]; Sih et al, 1993[117])			60% reduction of AOM
Penicillin V (Persico et al, 1985[118])	3–30 mo	3	40% reduction of AOM
Amoxicillin, TMP-SMX, placebo (Principi et al, 1989[116])	9–60 mo	6	Recurrent AOM in 27% Recurrent AOM in 63%
Penicillin V, placebo (Prellner et al, 1994[119])	≤18 mo	6, intermittently at upper respiratory tract infection	50% reduction of AOM

AOM, acute otitis media.
From Prellner K: Clinical aspects on antibiotic resistance: Upper respiratory tract infections. Microb Drug Resist 1995, 1:143–147.

Chronic Suppurative Otitis Media

In association with AOM, particularly recurrent AOM, a chronic tympanic membrane perforation may occur. Drainage of mucus or pus from the middle ear through the perforation creates fertile ground for bacterial super-infection. Mucosal edema frequently involves the external auditory canal, and eventually a state of chronic inflammation involving the external and middle ear ensues. Most frequently *S. aureus*, *P. aeruginosa* or other gram-negative bacilli are involved in the pathogenesis. Appropriate culture and sensitivity testing should be undertaken if possible. Empiric therapy with most oral antimicrobials or topical application of antimicrobial ear drops will not be of benefit. Parenterally administered broad-spectrum antimicrobials with activity against *Pseudomonas* spp and other gram-negative bacilli may be efficacious. Oral fluoroquinolones have been evaluated and shown to be effective in some patients. Removal of cerumen exudate and other debris from the external auditory canal through careful suction and gentle irrigation is an important adjunctive therapy. If no response is observed after 6 to 8 weeks of aggressive medical management with good compliance, referral for tympanic membrane surgery is appropriate.

External Otitis Media

Topical instillation of otic (or ophthalmic) antimicrobial drops is effective in the treatment of external otitis. Acetic acid solutions (vinegar mixed with water), hydrogen per-oxide solutions, or mixtures of the two are probably as effective as antimicrobial ear drop preparations. Cleaning the external auditory canal to remove debris by irrigation with dilute (2%) acetic acid solution will enhance recovery. Oral antibiotics are usually not necessary. Oral ciprofloxacin or other fluoroquinolone antibiotics may be justified in severe cases since these antibiotics are particularly effective against *Pseudomonas* spp. The most effective prophylaxis for external otitis is instillation of dilute isopropyl alcohol immediately following swimming, bathing, or other prolonged exposure to water.

MASTOIDITIS

Acute mastoiditis is an inflammation of the mastoid process that accompanies acute or subacute otitis media. Its clinical characteristics are forward protrusion of the auricle, retroauricular erythema and tenderness, and bulging of the ipsilateral tympanic membrane or acute purulent otorrhea. When acute mastoiditis causes a subperiosteal abscess, a fluctuant mass is palpable in the postauricular area. If acute mastoiditis is left untreated or if treated inappropriately, it can progress to severe complications such as subperiosteal abscess, meningitis, brain abscess, or sigmoid sinus thrombophlebitis. In the era of antibiotics, the incidence of mastoiditis has declined significantly.[120,121] It continues to be seen, however, and in a recent retrospective review the number of cases of mastoiditis seen at a large children's hospital actually increased during the years 1983 to 1999 as compared to the years 1955 to 1979.[122] When it does occur, matoiditis requires accurate diagnosis and appropriate treatment during the initial stages of infection to prevent serious complications.

The microbiologic causes of mastoiditis have been documented on the basis of results from cultures from surgical drainage of the mastoid area. The most common causes of acute mastoiditis are *S. pneumoniae*, *S. pyogenes*, and *S. aureus*.[123,124] The number of cases of mastoiditis caused by *S. pneumoniae* has remained stable despite increasing rates of antibiotic-resistant *S. pneumoniae* strains.[125] When acute mastoiditis does not respond as expected to therapy, one must consider other possible organisms found less commonly, such as gram-negative bacteria, specifically *Pseudomonas* spp, anaerobes, and *Mycobacterium tuberculosis*.[126]

Management of Acute Mastoiditis

Prior to the antibiotic era, acute mastoiditis primarily was managed with surgical curettage. In the era of antibiotics, treatment of acute mastoiditis has shifted to conservative medical management, reserving surgical management for cases that do not respond or that have suppurative complications.[127–129] Classic acute mastoiditis is managed with one or more parenteral antibiotics that will eradicate the most common bacterial causes. Cefuroxime (100 to 150 mg/kg/d IV or IM divided every 8 hours) is a good choice. Once the exact bacteriologic cause is identified from cultures, antibiotic therapy can be targeted. Antibiotics can be changed to oral therapy once the patient has had a good clinical response. There are no systematic studies on duration of therapy; 10 to 21 days is generally recommended. Prompt relief of pressure behind the tympanic membrane by means of a wide-field myringotomy or by insertion of tympanostomy tubes is advised. If a satisfactory clinical response is not achieved within 24 to 48 hours of initation of antibiotic therapy, simple mastoidectomy should be performed. Recently acute mastoiditis complicated by subperiosteal abscesses has been successfully treated with antibiotic therapy and aspiration of the pus without necessity for mastoidectomy.[128]

Chronic Mastoiditis

Chronic mastoiditis is a more indolent disease than acute mastoiditis is. It generally develops when there has been middle ear disease over months to years. The physical findings of chronic mastoiditis differ from those of acute mastoiditis in that fever and postauricular swelling, erythema, and tenderness may or may not be present.[130] Long-standing, persistent, mucopurulent drainage from a previously perforated tympanic membrane suggests chronic mastoiditis. The symptoms of chronic mastoiditis may be mild enough to be ignored until serious intracranial complications arise.

Chronic mastoiditis has a bacteriologic spectrum different from that of acute mastoiditis. Cultures from patients with chronic mastoiditis show predominantly *S. aureus* and gram-negative rods, especially *P. aeruginosa*. Additionally a wide variety of anaerobic organisms can be isolated from a chronically infected mastoid air space. *Actinomyces* spp. and *Bacteroides melaninogenicus* are the anaerobic organisms most commonly isolated.[131] *M. tuberculosis* is an uncommon cause of chronic mastoiditis in the United States; however, it should be considered, particularly when the response to standard therapy is poor. Treatment of chronic mastoiditis reflects the need for good gram-negative and anaerobic bacterial coverage. Antibiotic choices include

Nafcillin for *S. aureus*, aminoglycosides and piperacillin or ceftazidime for *P. aeruginosa*, penicillin for *Actinomyces* spp, clindamycin for *B. melaninogenicus*, and 2 to 4 antituberculosis drugs for tuberculosis. Four to six weeks of therapy is often necessary.

Complications of Mastoiditis

Complications of mastoiditis include subperiosteal abscess, meningitis, brain abscess, cerebellar abscess, epidural and subdural abscess, labyrinthitis, venous sinus thrombophlebitis, osteomyelitis of the temporal bone, facial nerve paralysis, and hearing loss. The rate of complications ranges from 0 to nearly 19% in a number of series.[127,132–137] Although acute mastoiditis is less common than it used to be, its severe complications are relatively frequent, and they may appear soon after the first sign of disease.

REFERENCES

1. Gwaltney JM Jr, Phillips CD, Miller RD, Riker DK: Computed tomographic study of the common cold [see comments]. N Engl J Med 1994;330:25–30.
2. Lund VJ, Kennedy DW: Quantification for staging sinusitis. The Staging and Therapy Group. Ann Otol Rhinol Laryngol Suppl 1995;167:17–21.
3. Berg O, Carenfelt C, Rystedt G, Anggard A: Occurrence of asymptomatic sinusitis in common cold and other acute ENT infections. Rhinology 1986;24(3):223–225.
4. Gable C, Jones J, Floor M, et al: Chronic sinusitis: Relation to upper respiratory infections and allergic rhinitis. Pharmacoepidemiol Drug Safety 1994;3:337–349.
5. Levy SB: The challenge of antibiotic resistance. Sci Am 1998;278(3):46–53.
6. Berg O, Carenfelt C, Kronvall G: Bacteriology of maxillary sinusitis in relation to character of inflammation and prior treatment. Scand J Infect Dis 1988;20(5):511–516.
7. Gwaltney JM Jr, Sydnor A Jr, Sande MA: Etiology and antimicrobial treatment of acute sinusitis. Ann Otol Rhinol Laryngol Suppl 1981;90(3 Pt 3):68–71.
8. Jousimies-Somer HR, Savolainen S, Ylikoski JS: Bacteriological findings of acute maxillary sinusitis in young adults. J Clin Microbiol 1988;26(10):1919–1925.
9. Van Cauwenverge P, Verschraegen G, Van Renterghem L: Bacteriological findings in sinusitis (1963–1975). Scand J Infect Dis 1976;9(Suppl):72–77.
10. Benninger MS, Anon J, Mabry RL: The medical management of rhinosinusitis. Otolaryngol Head Neck Surg 1997;117(3 Pt 2):S41–S49.
11. Gwaltney JM Jr, Scheld WM, Sande MA, Sydnor A: The microbial etiology and antimicrobial therapy of adults with acute community-acquired sinusitis: A fifteen-year experience at the University of Virginia and review of other selected studies. J Allergy Clin Immunol 1992;90(3 Pt 2):457–461; discussion 462.
12. Suzuki K, Nishiyama Y, Sugiyama K, et al: Recent trends in clinical isolates from paranasal sinusitis. Acta Otolaryngol Suppl 1996;525:51–55.
13. Wald ER, Reilly JS, Casselbrant M, et al: Treatment of acute maxillary sinusitis in childhood: A comparative study of amoxicillin and cefaclor. J Pediatr 1984;104(2):297–302.
14. Brook I: Microbiology and management of sinusitis. J Otolaryngol 1996;25(4):249–256.

15. Lanza DC, Kennedy DW: Adult rhinosinusitis defined. Otolaryngol Head Neck Surg 1997;117(3 Pt 2):S1–S7.

16. Brook I, Gooch WM, Jenkins S, et al: Medical management of acute bacterial sinusitis: Recommendations of a clinical advisory committee on pediatric and adult sinusitis. Ann Otol Rhinol Laryngol 2000;109(5[Suppl 182]):1–20.

17. Sinus and Allergy Health Partnership: Antimicrobial treatment guidelines for acute bacterial rhinosinusitis. Otolaryngol Head Neck Surg 2000;123(Suppl 1 Pt 2):5–31.

18. Spector SL, Bernstein IL, Li JT, et al: Parameters for the diagnosis and management of sinusitis. J Allergy Clin Immunol 1998;102(6 Pt 2):S107–S144.

19. Subcommittee on Management of Acute Bacterial Sinusitis. Practice guideline: Management of sinusitis. Committee on quality improvement. Subcommittee on sinusitis management. 2000, pp 1–36.

20. Axelsson A, Chidekel N, Grebelius N, Jensen C: Treatment of acute maxillary sinusitis. A comparison of four different methods. Acta Otolaryngol 1970;70:71–76.

21. Gananca M, Trabulsi LR: The therapeutic effects of cyclacillin in acute sinusitis: In vitro and in vivo correlations in a placebo-controlled study. Curr Med Res Opin 1973;1(6):362–368.

22. Lindbaek M, Hjortdahl P, Johnsen UL: Randomised, double blind, placebo controlled trial of penicillin V and amoxycillin in treatment of acute sinus infections in adults [see comments]. BMJ 1996;313(7053):325–329.

23. Stalman W, van Essen GA, van der Graaf Y, de Melker RA: The end of antibiotic treatment in adults with acute sinusitis–like complaints in general practice? A placebo-controlled double-blind randomized doxycycline trial [see comments]. Br J Gen Pract 1997;47(425):794–799.

24. Van Buchem F, Knottnerus J, Schrijnemaekers V, Peeters M: Primary-care-based randomised placebo-controlled trial of antibiotic treatment in acute maxillary sinusitis. Lancet 1997;349(9053):683–687.

25. Wald ER, Chiponis D, Ledesma-Medina J: Comparative effectiveness of amoxicillin and amoxicillin-clavulanate potassium in acute paranasal sinus infections in children: A double-blind, placebo-controlled trial. Pediatrics 1986;77(6):795–800.

26. Casiano RR: Azithromycin and amoxicillin in the treatment of acute maxillary sinusitis. Am J Med 1991;91(3A):27S–30S.

27. Felstead SJ, Daniel R: Short-course treatment of sinusitis and other upper respiratory tract infections with azithromycin: A comparison with erythromycin and amoxycillin. European Azithromycin Study Group. J Int Med Res 1991;19(5):363–372.

28. Karma P, Pukander J, Penttila M, et al: The comparative efficacy and safety of clarithromycin and amoxycillin in the treatment of outpatients with acute maxillary sinusitis. J Antimicrob Chemother 1991;27(Suppl A):83–90.

29. Calhoun KH, Hokanson JA: Multicenter comparison of clarithromycin and amoxicillin in the treatment of acute maxillary sinusitis. Arch Fam Med 1993;2(8):837–840.

30. Huck W, Reed BD, Nielsen RW, et al: Cefaclor vs amoxicillin in the treatment of acute, recurrent, and chronic sinusitis. Arch Fam Med 1993;2(5):497–503.

31. Fiscella R, Chow J: Cefixime for treatment of maxillary sinusitis. Am J Rhinol 1991;5:193–197.

32. Edelstein DR, Avner SE, Chow JM, et al: Once-a-day therapy for sinusitis: A comparison study of cefixime and amoxicillin. Laryngoscope 1993;103(1 Pt 1):33–41.

33. Matthews B, Team SACS: Effectiveness and safety of cefixime and amoxicillin in adults with acute bacterial sinusitis. Postgrad Med 1997;Spec Rpt:41–49.

34. Rimmer D, Team SACS: Efficacy of cefixime and amoxicillin in adults with acute sinusitis. Postgrad Med 1997;Spec Rpt:50–57.

35. von Sydow C, Savolainen S, Soderqvist A: Treatment of acute maxillary sinusitis—comparing cefpodoxime proxetil with amoxicillin. Scand J Infect Dis 1995;27(3):229–234.

36. Brodie DP, Knight S, Cunningham K: Comparative study of cefuroxime axetil and amoxycillin in the treatment of acute sinusitis in general practice. J Int Med Res 1989;17(6):547–551.

37. Mattucci KF, Levin WJ, Habib MA: Acute bacterial sinusitis. Minocycline vs amoxicillin. Arch Otolaryngol Head Neck Surg 1986;112(1):73–76.

38. International Rhinosinusitis Advisory Board: Infectious rhinosinusitis in adults: Classification, etiology and management. Ear Nose Throat J 1997;76(12 Suppl):1–22.

39. Davies A, Lewith G, Goddard J, Howarth P: The effect of acupuncture on nonallergic rhinitis: A controlled pilot study. Altern Ther Health Med 1998;4(1):70–74.

40. Linde K, Clausius N, Ramirez G, et al: Are the clinical effects of homeopathy placebo effects? A meta-analysis of placebo-controlled trials [see comments] [published erratum appears in Lancet 1998 Jan 17;351(9097):220]. Lancet 1997;350(9081):834–843.

41. Sezik E, Yesilada E: Clinical effects of the fruit juice of Ecbalium elaterium in the treatment of sinusitis [letter; comment]. J Toxicol Clin Toxicol 1995;33(4):381–383.

42. Wiesenauer M, Gaus W, Bohnacker U, Haussler S: Efficiency of homeopathic preparation combinations in sinusitis. Results of a randomized double blind study with general practitioners. Arzneimittelforschung 1989;39(5):620–625.

43. Barlan IB, Erkan E, Bakir M, et al: Intranasal budesonide spray as an adjunct to oral antibiotic therapy for acute sinusitis in children. Ann Allergy Asthma Immunol 1997;78(6):598–601.

44. McCormick DP, John SD, Swischuk LE, Uchida T: A double-blind, placebo-controlled trial of decongestant-antihistamine for the treatment of sinusitis in children. Clin Pediatr (Phila) 1996;35(9):457–460.

45. Seltzer A: Adjunctive use of bromelains in sinusitis: A controlled study. Eye Ear Nose Throat Mon 1967;46(10):1281–1288.

46. Gwaltney JM Jr, Jones JG, Kennedy DW: Medical management of sinusitis: Educational goals and management guidelines. The International Conference on Sinus Disease. Ann Otol Rhinol Laryngol Suppl 1995;167:22–30.

47. Gwaltney JM Jr: Acute community-acquired sinusitis. Clin Infect Dis 1996;23(6):1209–1225.

48. Jorgensen JH, Doern GV, Maher LA, et al: Antimicrobial resistance among respiratory isolates of Haemophilus influenzae, Moraxella catarrhalis, and Streptococcus pneumoniae in the United States. Antimicrob Agents Chemother 1990;34(11):2075–2080.

49. Neu H: The crisis in antibiotic resistance. Science 1992;257(5073):1064–1073.

50. Chambers H, Neu H: Penicillins. In Mandell G, Bennett J, Dolin R (eds): Mandell, Douglas and Bennett's Principles and Practice of Infectious Diseases, 4th ed. New York, Churchill Livingstone, 1995, p 264.

51. Green M, Wald ER: Emerging resistance to antibiotics: Impact on respiratory infections in the outpatient setting. Ann Allergy Asthma Immunol 1996;77(3):167–175.

52. Friedland IR, McCracken GH Jr: Management of infections caused by antibiotic-resistant Streptococcus pneumoniae [see comments]. N Engl J Med 1994;331:377–382.

53. Nelson CT, Mason EO Jr, Kaplan SL: Activity of oral antibiotics in middle ear and sinus infections caused by penicillin-resistant Streptococcus pneumoniae: Implications for treatment. Pediatr Infect Dis J 1994;13(7):585–589.

54. Rodriguez WJ, Schwartz RH, Thorne MM: Increasing incidence of penicillin- and ampicillin-resistant middle ear pathogens. Pediatr Infect Dis J 1995;14(12):1075–1078.

55. Levy SB: Confronting multidrug resistance. A role for each of us. JAMA 1993;269:1840–1842.

56. Mason EO Jr, Kaplan SL, Lamberth LB, Tillman J: Increased rate of isolation of penicillin-resistant Streptococcus pneumoniae in a children's hospital and in vitro susceptibilities to

antibiotics of potential therapeutic use [see comments]. Antimicrob Agents Chemother 1992;36:1703–1707.

57. Baquero F: Trends in antibiotic resistance of respiratory pathogens: An analysis and commentary on a collaborative surveillance study. J Antimicrob Chemother 1996;38 (Suppl A):117–132.

58. Klugman K: The clinical relevance of in-vitro resistance to penicillin, ampicillin, amoxycillin and alternative agents for the treatment of community-acquired pneumonia caused by Streptococcus pneumoniae, Haemophilus influenzae, and Moraxella catarrhalis. J Antimicrob Chemother 1996;38(Suppl A):133–140.

59. Nelson JD: Clinical importance of compliance and patient tolerance. Infect Dis Clin Pract 1994;3:158–160.

60. Levine LR: Quantitative comparison of adverse reactions to cefaclor vs. amoxicillin in a surveillance study. Pediatr Infect Dis 1985;4(4):358–361.

61. Couraud L, Andrews JM, Lecoeur H, et al: Concentrations of cefpodoxime in plasma and lung tissue after a single oral dose of cefpodoxime proxetil. J Antimicrob Chemother 1990;26(Suppl E):35–40.

62. Guay DPD: Pharmacodynamics and pharmocokinetics of cefdinir, an oral extended-spectrum cephalosporin. Pediatr Infect Dis J 2000;19:S141–S146.

63. Katzenstein AL, Sale SR, Greenberger PA: Pathologic findings in allergic aspergillus sinusitis. A newly recognized form of sinusitis. Am J Surg Pathol 1983;7(5):439–443.

64. Kuhn FA, Javer AR: Allergic fungal rhinosinusitis: Our experience. Arch Otolaryngol Head Neck Surg 1998;124(10):1179–1180.

65. Mott AE, Cain WS, Lafreniere D, et al: Topical corticosteroid treatment of anosmia associated with nasal and sinus disease. Arch Otolaryngol Head Neck Surg 1997;123(4):367–372.

66. Canciani M, Mastella G: Efficacy of beclomethasone nasal drops, administered in the Moffat's position for nasal polyposis. Acta Paediatr Scand 1988;77(4):612–613.

67. Schubert MS, Goetz DW: Evaluation and treatment of allergic fungal sinusitis. II. Treatment and follow-up. J Allergy Clin Immunol 1998;102(3):395–402.

68. Folker RJ, Marple BF, Mabry RL, Mabry CS: Treatment of allergic fungal sinusitis: A comparison trial of postoperative immunotherapy with specific fungal antigens. Laryngoscope 1998;108(11 Pt 1):1623–1627.

69. Pichichero ME, Cohen R: Shortened course of antibiotic therapy for acute otitis media, sinusitis and tonsillopharyngitis. Pediatr Infect Dis J 1997;16(7):680–695.

70. Spencer R, Hannington J, Fraser S, et al: Cefpodoxime proxetil versus co-amoxiclav in the treatment of acute infections of the ear, nose and throat in children: A multicentre randomized study [Abstract 851]. 18th International Congress of Chemotherapy 1993, Stockholm, Sweden, p 264.

71. Williams JW Jr, Holleman DR Jr, Samsa GP, Simel DL: Randomized controlled trial of 3 vs 10 days of trimethoprim/sulfamethoxazole for acute maxillary sinusitis. JAMA 1995;273:1015–1021.

72. Sabater F, Larrosa F, Guirao M, et al: Cefpodoxime proxetil (5 days) vs amoxycillin/clavulanic acid (8 days) in the treatment of acute maxillo-ethmoidal sinusitis in adult outpatients. 19th International Congress of Chemotherapy 1995, Montreal, Canada.

73. Khong T: Shortened therapies in acute sinusitis. Hosp Pract 1996;31(Suppl 1):11–13.

74. Pessey JJ, Dubreuil C, Gehanno P, et al: Efficacite et tolerance du cefixime en traitment de 4 jours ou de 10 jours versus 10 jours d'amoxicilline-acide clavulanique dans les sinusites aigues de l'adulte. Med Mal Infect 1996;26:839–845.

75. Werk LN, Bauchner H: Practical considerations when treating children with antimicrobials in the outpatient setting. Drugs 1998;55(6):779–790.

76. Wald ER: Sinusitis. Pediatr Ann 1998;27(12):811–818.

77. Evans KL: Recognition and management of sinusitis. Drugs 1998;56:59–71.

78. Lusk R: Surgical management of chronic sinusitis. In Lusk R (ed): Pediatric sinusitis. New York, Raven Press, 1992, pp 77–125.

79. DeBenedictis F, Bush A: Rhinosinusitis and asthma: Epiphenomenon or causal association? Chest 1999;115:550–556.

80. Paradise JL: On classifying otitis media as suppurative or nonsuppurative, with a suggested clinical schema. J Pediatr 1987;111(6 Pt 1):948–951.

81. Pichichero ME: Acute otitis media: Part I. Improving diagnostic accuracy. Am Fam Physician 2000;61(7):2051–2056.

82. Pichichero ME: Acute otitis media: Part II. Treatment in an era of increasing antibiotic resistance. Am Fam Physician 2000;61(8):2410–2416.

83. Laxdal OE, Merida J, Jones RH: Treatment of acute otitis media: A controlled study of 142 children. Can Med Assoc J 1970;102(3):263–268.

84. Kaleida PH, Casselbrant ML, Rockette HE, et al: Amoxicillin or myringotomy or both for acute otitis media: Results of a randomized clinical trial. Pediatrics 1991;87(4):466–474.

85. Cohen R, de la Rocque F, Boucherat M, et al: Treatment failure in otitis media: An analysis. J Chemother 1994;6 (Suppl 4):17–24.

86. Pichichero ME, Pichichero CL: Persistent acute otitis media: II. Antimicrobial treatment. Pediatr Infect Dis J 1995;14(3):183–188.

87. Gehanno P, N'Guyen L, Derriennic M, et al: Pathogens isolated during treatment failures in otitis. Pediatr Infect Dis J 1998;17(10):885–890.

88. Halsted C, Lepow M, Balassanian N, et al: Otitis media. Clinical observations, microbiology, and evaluation of therapy. Am J Dis Child 1968;115:542–551.

89. Rosenfeld RM, Vertrees JE, Carr J, et al: Clinical efficacy of antimicrobial drugs for acute otitis media: Metaanalysis of 5400 children from thirty-three randomized trials. J Pediatr 1994;124(3):355–367.

90. Burke P, Bain J, Robinson D, Dunleavey J: Acute red ear in children: Controlled trial of non-antibiotic treatment in general practice. BMJ 1991;303(6802):558–562.

91. Agency for Health Care Policy and Research: Final evidence report: Management of acute otitis media: U.S. Department of Health and Human Services, 2001.

92. Rosenfeld RM: Natural history of untreated otitis media. In Rosenfeld RM, Bluestone CD, (eds): Evidence-Based Otitis Media. St. Louis, BC Decker, 1999, pp 157–177.

93. Van Buchem F, Peeters M, Van't Hof M: Acute otitis media: A new treatment strategy. BMJ 1985;290:1033–1037.

94. van Buchem FL, Dunk JH, van't Hof MA: Therapy of acute otitis media: Myringotomy, antibiotics, or neither? A doubleblind study in children. Lancet 1981;2(8252):883–887.

95. Del Mar C, Glasziou P, Hayem M: Are antibiotics indicated as initial treatment for children with acute otitis media? A meta-analysis. BMJ 1997;314(7093):1526–1529.

96. Howie VM, Ploussard JH: Efficacy of fixed combination antibiotics versus separate components in otitis media. Effectiveness of erythromycin estolate, triple sulfonamide, ampicillin, erythromycin estolate–triple sulfonamide, and placebo in 280 patients with acute otitis media under two and one-half years of age. Clin Pediatr (Phila) 1972;11(4):205–214.

97. Appelman CL, Claessen JQ, Touw-Otten FW, et al: Co-amoxiclav in recurrent acute otitis media: placebo controlled study. BMJ 1991;303(6815):1450–1452.

98. Mygind N, Meistrup-Larsen KI, Thomsen J, et al: Penicillin in acute otitis media: A double-blind placebo-controlled trial. Clin Otolaryngol 1981;6(1):5–13.

99. Froom J, Culpepper L, Grob P, et al: Diagnosis and antibiotic treatment of acute otitis media: Report from International Primary Care Network. BMJ 1990; 300(6724):582–586.

100. Tilyard MW, Dovey SM, Walker SA: Otitis media treatment in New Zealand general practice. N Z Med J 1997; 110(1042):143–145.

101. Ingvarsson L, Lundgren K: Penicillin treatment of acute otitis media in children: A study of the duration inhibitor effects of amoxicillin plus clavulanate. Acta Otolaryngol 1982;94:283–287.

102. Schaad UB: Multicentre evaluation of azithromycin in comparison with co-amoxiclav for the treatment of acute otitis media in children. J Antimicrob Chemother 1993;31 (Suppl E):81–88.

103. Pichichero ME, McLinn S, Aronovitz G, et al: Cefprozil treatment of persistent and recurrent acute otitis media. Pediatr Infect Dis J 1997;16(5):471–478.

104. Klein JO: Protecting the therapeutic advantage of antimicrobial agents used for otitis media. Pediatr Infect Dis J 1998;17(6):571–575.

105. McCracken GH: Treatment of acute otitis media in an era of increasing microbial resistance. Pediatr Infect Dis J 1998;17(6):576–580.

106. Agency for Health Care Policy and Research: Diagnosis and treatment of acute bacterial rhinosinusitis. U.S Department of Human Services Evidence Report/Technology Assessment Number 9, 1999.

107. Dowell SF, Butler JC, Giebink GS, et al: Acute otitis media: Management and surveillance in an era of pneumococcal resistance—a report from the Drug-resistant *Streptococcus pneumoniae* Therapeutic Working Group. Pediatr Infect Dis J 1999;18(1):1–9.

108. Leibovitz E, Piglansky L, Raiz S, et al: Bacteriologic efficacy of a three-day intramuscular ceftriaxone regimen in nonresponsive acute otitis media. Pediatr Infect Dis J 1998;17(12):1126–1131.

109. Adam D: Five-day therapy with cefpodoxime versus ten-day treatment with cefaclor in infants with acute otitis media. Infection 1995;23:398–400.

110. Varsano I, Volovitz B, Horev Z, et al: Intramuscular ceftriaxone compared with oral amoxicillin-clavulanate for treatment of acute otitis media in children. Eur J Pediatr 1997;156(11):858–863.

111. Pichichero ME, Marsocci SM, Murphy ML, et al: A prospective observational study of 5-, 7-, and 10-day antibiotic treatment for acute otitis media. Otolaryngol Head Neck Surg 2001;124(4):381–387.

112. Ensign P, Urbanish E, Morgan M: Prophylaxis for otitis media in an Indian population. Am J Public Health 1960;50:195–199.

113. Maynard J, Fleshman J, Tschopp C: Otitis media in Alaskan Eskimo children. Prospective evaluation of chemoprophylaxis. JAMA 1972;219:597–599.

114. Perrin JM, Charney E, MacWhinney JB Jr, et al: Sulfisoxazole as chemoprophylaxis for recurrent otitis media. A double-blind crossover study in pediatric practice. N Engl J Med 1974;291(13):664–667.

115. Schwartz RH, Puglise J, Rodriguez WJ: Sulphamethoxazole prophylaxis in the otitis-prone child. Arch Dis Child 1982;57(8):590–593.

116. Principi N, Marchisio P, Massironi E, et al: Prophylaxis of recurrent acute otitis media and middle-ear effusion. Comparison of amoxicillin with sulfamethoxazole and trimethoprim. Am J Dis Child 1989;143(12):1414–1418.

117. Sih T, Moura R, Caldas S, Schwartz B: Prophylaxis for recurrent acute otitis media: A Brazilian study. Int J Pediatr Otorhinolaryngol 1993;25(1–3):19–24.

118. Persico M, Podoshin L, Fradis M, et al: Recurrent acute otitis media—prophylactic penicillin treatment: A prospective study. Part I. Int J Pediatr Otorhinolaryngol 1985; 10(1):37–46.

119. Prellner K, Fogle-Hansson M, Jorgensen F, et al: Prevention of recurrent acute otitis media in otitis-prone children by intermittent prophylaxis with penicillin. Acta Otolaryngol 1994;114(2):182–187.

120. Palva T: Mastoiditis in Children. Laryngoscope 1962; 72:353–360.

121. Palva T, Virtanen H, Makinen J: Acute and latent mastoiditis in children. J Laryngol Otol 1985;99(2):127–136.

122. Ghaffar F, Wordeman M, McCracken GH: Acute mastoiditis in children: A seventeen-year experience in Dallas, Texas. Pediatr Infect Dis J 2001;20:376–380.

123. Hawkins DB, Dru D, House JW, Clark RW: Acute mastoiditis in children: A review of 54 cases. Laryngoscope 1983;93(5):568–572.

124. Ogle JW, Lauer BA: Acute mastoiditis: Diagnosis and complications. Am J Dis Child 1986;140(11):1178–1182.

125. Kaplan SL, Mason EO Jr, Wald ER, et al: Pneumococcal mastoiditis in children. Pediatrics 2000;106(4):695–699.

126. Lee ES, Chae SW, Lim HH, et al: Clinical experiences with acute mastoiditis—1988 through 1998. Ear Nose Throat J 2000;79(11):884–892.

127. Luntz M, Keren G, Nusem S, Kronenberg J: Acute mastoiditis—revisited. Ear Nose Throat J 1994;73(9):648–654.

128. Khafif A, Halperin D, Hochman I, et al: Acute mastoiditis: A 10-year review. Am J Otolaryngol 1998;19(3):170–173.

129. Bahadori RS, Schwartz RH, Ziai M: Acute mastoiditis in children: An increase in frequency in Northern Virginia. Pediatr Infect Dis J 2000;19(3):212–215.

130. Holt GR, Gates GA: Masked mastoiditis. Laryngoscope 1983;93(8):1034–1037.

131. Brook I: Aerobic and anaerobic bacteriology of chronic mastoiditis in children. Am J Dis Child 1981;135(5):478–479.

132. Zoller H: Acute mastoiditis and its complications: A changing trend. South Med J 1972;65(4):477–480.

133. Ronis BJ, Ronis ML, Liebman EP: Acute mastoiditis as seen today. Eye Ear Nose Throat Mon 1968;47(10):502–507.

134. Ginsburg CM, Rudoy R, Nelson JD: Acute mastoiditis in infants and children. Clin Pediatr (Phila) 1980; 19(8):549–553.

135. Prellner K, Rydell R: Acute mastoiditis. Influence of antibiotic treatment on the bacterial spectrum. Acta Otolaryngol 1986;102(1–2):52–56.

136. Holt GR, Young WC: Acute coalescent mastoiditis. Otolaryngol Head Neck Surg 1981;89(2):317–321.

137. Rosen A, Ophir D, Marshak G: Acute coalescent mastoiditis. Otolaryngol Head Neck Surg 1981;89:317–321.

138. Sinus and Allergy Health Partnership: Antimicrobial Treatment Guidelines for Acute Bacterial Rhinosinusitis. Otolaryngol Head Neck Surg 2000;123:S1–S32.

139. Braun JJ, Alabert JP, Michel FB, et al: Adjunct effect of loratadine in the treatment of acute sinusitis in patients with allergic rhinitis. Allergy 1997;52(6):650–655.

140. Harris PG: A comparison of 'bisolvomycin' and oxytetracycline in the treatment of acute infective sinusitis. Practitioner 1971;207(242):814–817.

141. Lewison E: Comparison of the effectiveness of topical and oral nasal decongestants. Eye Ear Nose Throat Mon 1970;49(1):16–18.

142. Meltzer EO: The prevalence and medical and economic impact of allergic rhinitis in the United States. J Allergy Clin Immunol 1997;99(6 Pt 2):S805–S828.

143. Ryan RE: A double-blind clinical evaluation of bromelains in the treatment of acute sinusitis. Headache 1967;7(1):13–17.

144. Seltzer AP: Adjunctive use of bromelains in sinusitis: A controlled study. Eye Ear Nose Throat Mon 1967; 46(10):1281–1288.

145. Taub SJ: The use of bromelains in sinusitis: A double-blind clinical evaluation. Eye Ear Nose Throat Mon 1967; 46(3):361–362.

146. Wiklund L, Stierna P, Berglund R, et al: The efficacy of oxymetazoline administered with a nasal bellows container and combined with oral phenoxymethyl-penicillin in the treatment of acute maxillary sinusitis. Acta Otolaryngol Suppl 1994;515:57–64.

147. Quick CA: Comparison of penicillin and trimethoprim-sulfamethoxazole in the treatment of ear, nose and throat infections. Can Med Assoc J 1975;112(13 Spec No):83–86.

148. Soderstrom M, Blomberg J, Christensen P, Hovelius B: Erythromycin and phenoxymethylpenicillin (penicillin V) in the treatment of respiratory tract infections as related to microbiological findings and serum C-reactive protein. Scand J Infect Dis 1991;23(3):347–354.

149. von Sydow C, Axelsson A, Jensen C: Treatment of acute maxillary sinusitis. Erythromycin base and phenoxymethyl-penicillin (penicillin V). Rhinology 1984;22(4):247–254.

150. Axelsson A, Jensen C, Melin O, et al: Treatment of acute maxillary sinusitis. V. Amoxicillin azidocillin, phenyl-propanolamine and pivampicillin. Acta Otolaryngol 1981;91(3–4):313–318.

151. Christensen CH, Hartmann E: Treatment of sinusitis and otitis media with pivampicillin. Pharmatherapeutica 1980; 2(7):469–474.

152. Jeppesen F, Illum P: Pivampicillin (Pondocillin) in the treatment of maxillary sinusitis. Acta Otolaryngol 1972; 74(5):375–382.

153. Kment G, Georgopoulos A, Ridl W, Muhlbacher J: Amoxicillin concentrations in nasal secretions of patients with acute uncomplicated sinusitis and in paranasal sinus mucosa of patients with chronic sinusitis. Eur Arch Otorhinolaryngol 1995;252(4):236–238.

154. Moorehouse E, Hickey M, O'Hanrahan M, Clarke P: General practice studies with combined pivampicillin/pivmecillinam (Miraxid). Ir Med J 1985;78(11):314–317.

155. Moran DG: A multicentre general practice study comparing pivampicillin (Pondocillin) and amoxycillin (Amoxil) in respiratory tract infections. J Int Med Res 1983;11(6):370–374.

156. Nord CE: Efficacy of penicillin treatment in purulent maxillary sinusitis. A European multicenter trial. Infection 1988;16(4):209–214.

157. Nyffenegger R, Riebenfeld D, Macciocchi A: Brodimoprim versus amoxicillin in the treatment of acute sinusitis. Clin Ther 1991;13(5):589–595.

158. Scheld W, Sydnor A, Farr B, et al: Comparison of cyclacillin and amoxicillin for therapy for acute maxillary sinusitis. Antimicrob Agents Chemother 1986;30(3):350–353.

159. Shenderey K, Marsh BT, Talbot DJ: A multi-centre general practice comparison of a fixed-dose combination of pivmecillinam plus pivampicillin with amoxycillin in respiratory tract infections. Pharmatherapeutica 1985;4(5):300–305.

160. Sorri M, Peltomaki E, Jokinen K: Bacampicillin in acute maxillary sinusitis: Concentration in sinus secretion and clinical effect. A randomized, double-blind study of two dosage regimens. Scand J Infect Dis 1981;13(4):277–280.

161. von Sydow C, Einarsson S, Grafford K, et al: Bacampicillin twice daily in acute maxillary sinusitis: An alternative dosage regimen. J Antimicrob Chemother 1981;8(Suppl C):109–114.

162. Federspil P, Bamberg P: Sulphadiazine/trimethoprim once daily in maxillary sinusitis: A randomized double-blind comparison with sulphamethoxazole/trimethoprim B.I.D. J Int Med Res 1981;9(6):478–481.

163. Federspil P, Koch J: Double-blind comparative trial of trimethoprim/sulfamethopyrazine once daily vs erythromycin 4 × daily in patients with ENT infections. Int J Clin Phamacol Ther Toxicol 1983;21(10):535–539.

164. Wallace RB, Marsh BT, Talbot DJ: A multi-centre general practice clinical evaluation of pivmecillinam plus pivampicillin ('Miraxid') and co-trimoxazole ('Septrin') in respiratory tract infections. Curr Med Res Opin 1985;9(10):659–665.

165. Williams JW Jr, Holleman DR Jr, Samsa GP, Simel DL: Randomized controlled trial of 3 vs 10 days of trimethoprim/sulfamethoxazole for acute maxillary sinusitis (see comments). JAMA 1995;273(13):1015–1021.

166. Agbim OG: A comparative trail of doxycycline ('Vibramycin') and ampicillin in the treatment of acute sinusitis. Curr Med Res Opin 1974;2(5):291–294.

167. Arndt J, Riebenfeld D, Maier H, Weidauer H: Therapeutic efficacy and tolerability of brodimoprim in comparison with doxycycline in acute sinusitis in adults. J Chemother 1994;6(5):322–327.

168. Beatson JM, Marsh BT, Talbot DJ: A clinical comparison of pivmecillinam plus pivampicillin (Miraxid) and a triple tetracycline combination (Deteclo) in respiratory infections treated in general practice. J Int Med Res 1985;13(4):197–202.

169. Boezeman AJ, Kayser AM, Siemelink RJ: Comparison of spiramycin and doxycycline in the empirical treatment of acute sinusitis: preliminary results. J Antimicrob Chemother 1988;22 (Suppl B):165–170.

170. Otte J, Viada JA, Buchi MD, Salgado O: Treatment of acute sinusal processes of adults with tetracycline and a combination of sulfamethopyrazine-trimethoprim. Rev Med Chil 1983;111(11):1157–1161.

171. Rahlfs V, Macciocchi A, Monti T: Brodimoprim in upper respiratory tract infections. Clin Drug Invest 1996;11(2):65–76.

172. Salmi HA, Lehtomaki K, Kylmamaa T: Comparison of brodimoprim and doxycycline in acute respiratory tract infections. A double-blind clinical trial. Drugs Exp Clin Res 1986;12(4):349–353.

173. Westerman T, Panzer JD, Atkinson WH: Comparative efficacy of clindamycin HCl and tetracycline HCl in acute sinusitis. Eye Ear Nose Throat Mon 1975;54(6):236–238.

174. Camacho AE, Cobo R, Otte J, et al: Clinical comparison of cefuroxime axetil and amoxicillin/clavulanate in the treatment of patients with acute bacterial maxillary sinusitis. Am J Med 1992;93(3):271–276.

175. De Abate C, Perrotta R, Dennington M, Ziering R: The efficacy and safety of once-daily ceftibuten compared with co-amoxiclav in the treatment of acute bacterial sinusitis. J Chemother 1992;4(6):358–363.

176. Dubois J, Saint-Pierre C, Tremblay C: Efficacy of clarithromycin vs. amoxicillin/clavulanate in the treatment of acute maxillary sinusitis. Ear Nose Throat J 1993; 72(12):804–810.

177. Sydnor TA Jr, Scheld WM, Gwaltney J Jr, et al: Loracarbef (LY 163892) vs amoxicillin/clavulanate in bacterial maxillary sinusitis. Ear Nose Throat J 1992;71(5):225–232.

178. Bockmeyer M, Riebenfeld D, Clasen B: Controlled study of brodimoprim and cephalexin in the treatment of patients with acute sinusitis in general practice. Clin Ther 1994;16(4):653–661.

179. Carenfelt C, Melen I, Odkvist L, et al: Treatment of sinus empyema in adults. A coordinated Nordic multicenter trial of cefixime vs. cefaclor. Acta Otolaryngol 1990; 110(1–2):128–135.

180. Gauger U, Inoka P, Germano G, Kissling M: Cefetamet in the treatment of acute sinusitis in adult patients. J Int Med Res 1990;18(3):228–234.

181. Gehanno P, Depondt J, Barry B, et al: Comparison of cefpodoxime proxetil with cefaclor in the treatment of sinusitis. J Antimicrob Chemother 1990;26(Suppl E):87–91.

182. Gehanno P, Berche P: Sparfloxacin versus cefuroxime axetil in the treatment of acute purulent sinusitis. Sinusitis Study Group. J Antimicrob Chemother 1996;37(Suppl A):105–114.

183. Scandinavian Study Group: Loracarbef versus doxycycline in the treatment of acute bacterial maxillary sinusitis. J Antimicrob Chemother 1993;31(6):949–961.

184. Simon MW: Treatment of acute sinusitis in childhood with ceftibuten. Clin Pediatr (Phila) 1999;38(5):269–272.

185. Stefansson P, Jacovides A, Jablonicky P, et al: Cefuroxime axetil versus clarithromycin in the treatment of acute maxillary sinusitis. Rhinology 1998;36(4):173–178.

186. Sydnor A Jr, Gwaltney JM Jr, Cocchetto DM, Scheld WM: Comparative evaluation of cefuroxime axetil and cefaclor for treatment of acute bacterial maxillary sinusitis. Arch Otolaryngol Head Neck Surg 1989;115(12):1430–1433.

187. Zeckel ML, Johns D Jr, Masica DN, Farlow D: Twice-daily dosing of loracarbef 200 mg versus 400 mg in the treatment of patients with acute maxillary sinusitis. Clin Ther 1995;17(2):214–230.

188. de Campora E, Camaioni A, Leonardi M, et al: Comparative efficacy and safety of roxithromycin and clarithromycin in upper respiratory tract infections. Diagn Microbiol Infect Dis 1992;15(4 Suppl):119S–122S.

189. Ficnar B, Huzjak N, Oreskovic K, et al: Azithromycin: 3-day versus 5-day course in the treatment of respiratory tract infections in children. Croatian Azithromycin Study Group. J Chemother 1997;9(1):38–43.

190. Haye R, Lingaas E, Hoivik H, Odegard T: Efficacy and safetey of azithromycin versus phenoxymethylpenicillin in the treatment of acute maxillary sinusitis. Eur J Clin Microbiol Infect Dis 1996;15(11):849–853.

191. Manzini M, Caroggio A: Efficacy and tolerability of brodimoprim and roxithromycin in acute sinusitis of bacterial origin in adults. J Chemother 1993;5(6):521–525.

192. Muller O: Comparison of azithromycin versus clarithromycin in the treatment of patients with upper respiratory tract infections. J Antimicrob Chemother 1993;31 (Suppl E):137–146.

193. Muller O: An open comparative study of azithromycin and roxithromycin in the treatment of acute upper respiratory tract infections. J Antimicrob Chemother 1996;37(Suppl C):83–92.

194. O'Doherty B: An open comparative study of azithromycin versus cefaclor in the treatment of patients with upper respiratory tract infections. J Antimicrob Chemother 1996;37 (Suppl C):71–81.

195. Wuolijoki E, Flygare U, Hilden M, et al: Treatment of respiratory tract infections with erythromycin acistrate and two formulations of erythromycin base. J Antimicrob Chemother 1988;21 (Suppl D):107–112.

196. Adelglass J, DeAbate CA, McElvaine P, et al: Comparison of the effectiveness of levofloxacin and amoxicillin-clavulanate for the treatment of acute sinusitis in adults. Otolaryngol Head Neck Surg 1999;120(3):320–327.

197. Burke T, Villanueva C, Mariano H Jr, et al: Comparison of moxifloxacin and cefuroxime axetil in the treatment of acute maxillary sinusitis. Sinusitis Infection Study Group. Clin Ther 1999;21(10):1664–1677.

198. Clifford K, Huck W, Shan M, et al: Double-blind comparative trial of ciprofloxacin versus clarithromycin in the treatment of acute bacterial sinusitis. Sinusitis Infection Study Group. Ann Otol Rhinol Laryngol 1999;108(4):360–367.

199. Johnson PA, Rodriguez HP, Wazen JJ, et al: Ciprofloxacin versus cefuroxime axetil in the treatment of acute bacterial sinusitis. Sinusitis Infection Study Group. J Otolaryngol 1999;28(1):3–12.

200. Siegert R, Gehanno P, Nikolaidis P, et al: A comparison of the safety and efficacy of moxifloxacin (BAY 12–8039) and cefuroxime axetil in the treatment of acute bacterial sinusitis in adults. The Sinusitis Study Group. Respir Med 2000;94(4):337–344.

201. Dowell SF, Marcy S, William W, et al: Otitis media—principles of judicious use of antimicrobial agents. Pediatrics 1998;101(Suppl 1):S165–S171.

202. Teele DW, Pelton SI, Klein JO: Bacteriology of acute otitis media unresponsive to initial antimicrobial therapy. J Pediatr 1981;98(4):537–539.

203. Schwartz R, Stool SE, Rodriguez W, Grundfast K: Acute otitis media: Towards a more precise definition. Clin Pediatr 1981;20:549–554.

204. Harrison CJ, Marks MI, Welch DF: Microbiology of recently treated acute otitis media compared with previously untreated acute otitis media. Pediatr Infect Dis 1985;4(6):641–646.

205. Faden H, Bernstein J, Brodsky L, et al: Effect of prior antibiotic treatment on middle ear disease in children. Ann Otol Rhinol Laryngol 1992;101(1):87–91.

206. Block SL, Harrison CJ, Hedrick JA, et al: Penicillin-resistant *Streptococcus pneumoniae* in acute otitis media: Risk factors, susceptibility patterns and antimicrobial management. Pediatr Infect Dis J 1995;14(9):751–759.

207. Damoiseaux RA, van Balen FA, Hoes AW, et al: Primary care based randomised, double blind trial of amoxicillin versus placebo for acute otitis media in children aged under 2 years. BMJ 2000;320(7231):350–354.

208. Engelhard D, Cohen D, Strauss N, et al: Randomised study of myringotomy, amoxycillin/clavulanate, or both for acute otitis media in infants. Lancet 1989;2(8655):141–143.

209. Mandel EM, Rockette HE, Paradise JL, et al: Comparative efficacy of erythromycin-sulfisoxazole, cefaclor, amoxicillin or placebo for otitis media with effusion in children. Pediatr Infect Dis J 1991;10(12):899–906.

210. Thalin A, Densert O, Larsson A, et al: Is penicillin necessary in the treatment of acute otitis media? Proceedings of the International Conference on Acute and Secretory Otitis Media 1985, Jerusalem, pp 441–446.

211. Thomsen J: Antibiotic treatment of children with secretory otitis media. Arch Otolaryngol Head Neck Surg 1990;116(8):978.

212. Klein JO: Microbiologic efficacy of antibacterial drugs for acute otitis media. Pediatr Infect Dis J 1993;12(12):973–975.

213. Bass J, Cohen S, Corless J, Mamunes P: Ampicillin compared to other antimicrobials in acute otitis media. JAMA 1967;202(8):697–702.

214. Bass J, Cashman T, Frostad A, et al: Antimicrobials in the treatment of acute otitis media: A second clinical trial. Am J Dis Child 1973;125:397–402.

215. Feigin RD, Keeney RE, Nusrala J, et al: Efficacy of clindamycin therapy for otitis media. Arch Otolaryngol 1973;98(1):27–31.

216. Howard JE, Nelson JD, Clahsen J, Jackson LH: Otitis media of infancy and early childhood. A double-blind study of four treatment regimens. Am J Dis Child 1976;130(9):965–970.

217. Howie VM, Ploussard JH, Sloyer J: Comparison of ampicillin and amoxicillin in the treatment of otitis media in children. J Infect Dis 1974;129(Suppl):S181–S184.

218. Kaleida PH, Bluestone CD, Blatter MM, et al: Sultamicillin (ampicillin-sulbactam) in the treatment of acute otitis media in children. Pediatr Infect Dis 1986;5(1):33–38.

219. Kim KS, Anthony BF: Use of penicillin-gradient and replicate plates for the demonstration of tolerance to penicillin in streptococci. J Infect Dis 1983;148(3):488–491.

220. Lenoski EF, Wingert WA, Wehrle PF: Drug trials in acute otitis media. Curr Ther Res Clin Exp 1968;10(12):631–639.

221. McLinn SE, Goldberg F, Kramer R, et al: Double-blind multicenter comparison of cyclacillin and amoxicillin for the treatment of acute otitis media. J Pediatr 1982;101(4):617–621.

222. McLinn SE, Serlin S: Cyclacillin versus amoxicillin as treatment for acute otitis media. Pediatrics 1983;71(2):196–199.

223. Murph JR, Dusdieker LB, Booth B, Murph WE: Is treatment of acute otitis media with once-a-day amoxicillin feasible? Results of a pilot study. Clin Pediatr (Phila) 1993; 32(9):528–534.

224. Nilson BW, Poland RL, Thompson RS, et al: Acute otitis media: Treatment results in relation to bacterial etiology. Pediatrics 1969;43(3):351–358.

225. Principi N, Marchisio P, Bigalli L, Massironi E: Amoxicillin twice daily in the treatment of acute otitis media in infants and children. Eur J Pediatr 1986;145(6):522–525.

226. Puhakka HJ, Haapaniemi J, Tuohimaa P, Bondesson G: Clinical efficacy and tolerance of bacampicillin and amoxycillin suspensions in children with acute otitis media. J Int Med Res 1989;17(1):41–47.

227. Rodriguez WJ, Schwartz RH, Sait T, et al: Erythromycin-sulfisoxazole vs amoxicillin in the treatment of acute otitis media in children. A double-blind, multiple-dose comparative study. Am J Dis Child 1985;139(8):766–770.

228. Rodriguez WJ, Khan WH, Sait T, et al: Sultamicillin (sulbactam/ampicillin) versus amoxycillin in the treatment of acute otitis media in children. J Int Med Res 1990;18(Suppl 4): 78D–84D.

229. Scholz H, Noack R: Multicenter, randomized, double-blind comparison of erythromycin estolate versus amoxicillin for the treatment of acute otitis media in children. AOM Study Group. Eur J Clin Microbiol Infect Dis 1998; 17(7):470–478.

230. Valtonen M, Piippo T, Pitkajarvi T, Pyykonen ML: Comparison of amoxycillin given two and three times a day in acute respiratory tract infections in children. Scand J Prim Health Care 1986;4(4):201–204.

231. Cameron GG, Pomahac AC, Johnston MT: Comparative efficacy of ampicillin and trimethoprim-sulfamethoxazole in otitis media. CMAJ 1975;112(13 Spec No):87–88.

232. Cooper J, Inman JS, Dawson AF: A comparison between co-trimoxazole and amoxycillin in the treatment of acute otitis media in general practice. Practitioner 1976; 217(1301):804–809.

233. Feldman W, Momy J, Dulberg C: Trimethoprim-sulfamethoxazole v. amoxicillin in the treatment of acute otitis media. CMAJ 1988;139(10):961–964.

234. Feldman W, Sutcliffe T, Dulberg C: Twice-daily antibiotics in the treatment of acute otitis media: Trimethoprim-sulfamethoxazole versus amoxicillin-clavulanate. CMAJ 1990;142(2):115–118.

235. Shurin PA, Pelton SI, Donner A, et al: Trimethoprim-sulfamethoxazole compared with ampicillin in the treatment of acute otitis media. J Pediatr 1980;96(6):1081–1087.

236. Adler M, McDonald PJ, Trostmann U, et al: Cefdinir versus amoxicillin/clavulanic acid in the treatment of suppurative acute otitis media in children. Eur J Clin Microbiol Infect Dis 1997;16(3):214–219.

237. Arguedas AG, Zaleska M, Stutman HR, et al: Comparative trial of cefprozil vs. amoxicillin clavulanate potassium in the treatment of children with acute otitis media with effusion. Pediatr Infect Dis J 1991;10(5):375–380.

237a. Aronovitz GH, Doyle CA, Durham ST, et al: Cefprocil vs. Amoxycillin/clavulanate in the treatment of acute otitis media. Infect Med 1992;9:(Suppl 19–32).

238. Aspin MM, Hoberman A, McCarty J, et al: Comparative study of the safety and efficacy of clarithromycin and amoxicillin-clavulanate in the treatment of acute otitis media in children. J Pediatr 1994;125(1):136–141.

239. Behre U, Burrow H, Quinn P, et al: Efficacy of twice-daily dosing of amoxycillin/clavulanate in acute otitis media in children. Infection 1997;25(3):163–166.

240. Block SL, McCarty JM, Hedrick JA, et al: Comparative safety and efficacy of cefdinir vs amoxicillin/clavulanate for treatment of suppurative acute otitis media in children. Pediatr Infect Dis 2000;19(12 Suppl):S159–S165.

241. Boulesteix J, Begue P, Dubreuil C, et al: Acute otitis media in children: A study of nasopharyngeal carriage of potential pathogens and therapeutic efficacy of cefixime and amoxi-cillin-clavulanate. Infection 1995;23(Suppl 2):S79–S82.

242. Careddu P, Bellosta C, Tonelli P, Boccazzi A: Efficacy and tolerability of brodimoprim in pediatric infections. J Chemother 1993;5(6):543–545.

243. Chan KH, Mandel EM, Rockette HE, et al: A comparative study of amoxicillin-clavulanate and amoxicillin. Treatment of otitis media with effusion. Arch Otolaryngol Head Neck Surg 1988;114(2):142–146.

244. Chan KH, Bluestone CD, Tan LS, et al: Comparative study of sultamicillin and amoxicillin-clavulanate: Treatment of acute otitis media. Pediatr Infect Dis J 1993;12(1):24–28.

245. Dagan R, Leibovitz E, Fliss DM, et al: Bacteriologic efficacies of oral azithromycin and oral cefaclor in treatment of acute otitis media in infants and young children. Antimicrob Agents Chemother 2000;44(1):43–50.

246. Damrikarnlert L, Jauregui AC, Kzadri M: Efficacy and safety of amoxycillin/clavulanate (Augmentin) twice daily versus three times daily in the treatment of acute otitis media in children. The Augmentin 454 Study Group. J Chemother 2000;12(1):79–87.

247. Gan VN, Kusmiesz H, Shelton S, Nelson JD: Comparative evaluation of loracarbef and amoxicillin-clavulanate for acute otitis media. Antimicrob Agents Chemother 1991;35(5):967–971.

248. Gehanno P, Berche P, Boucot I, et al: Comparative efficacy and safety of cefprozil and amoxicillin/clavulanate in the treatment of acute otitis media in children. J Antimicrob Chemother 1994;33(6):1209–1218.

249. Gehanno P, Barry B, Bobin S, Safran C: Twice daily cefpodoxime proxetil compared with thrice daily amoxicillin/clavulanic acid for treatment of acute otitis media in children. Scand J Infect Dis 1994;26(5):577–584.

250. Goldblatt EL, Dohar J, Nozza RJ, et al: Topical ofloxacin versus systemic amoxicillin/clavulanate in purulent otorrhea in children with tympanostomy tubes. Int J Pediatr Otorhinolaryngol 1998;46(1–2):91–101.

251. Gooch WM, Blair E, Puopolo A, et al: Clinical comparison of cefuroxime axetil suspension and amoxicillin/clavulanate suspension in the treatment of pediatric patients with acute otitis media with effusion. Clin Ther 1995; 17(5):838–851.

252. Jacobsson S, Rigner P, von Sydow C, Bondesson G: Clinical and bacteriological efficacy of amoxycillin/clavulanate (Spektramox) and cefaclor (Kefolor) in children with recurrent AOM or therapy failure. Acta Otolaryngol Suppl 1988;449:43–44.

253. Jacobsson S, Fogh A, Larsson P, Lomborg S: Evaluation of amoxicillin clavulanate twice daily versus thrice daily in the treatment of otitis media in children. Danish-Swedish Study Group. Eur J Clin Microbiol Infect Dis 1993; 12(5):319–324.

254. Kaleida PH, Bluestone CD, Rockette HE, et al: Amoxicillin-clavulanate potassium compared with cefaclor for acute otitis media in infants and children. Pediatr Infect Dis J 1987;6(3):265–271.

255. Kaprio E, Haapaniemi J, Bondesson G: Clinical efficacy of amoxycillin/clavulanic acid and cefaclor in acute otitis media. Acta Otolaryngol Suppl 1988;449:45–46.

256. Mandel EM, Casselbrant ML, Rockette HE, et al: Efficacy of 20- versus 10-day antimicrobial treatment for acute otitis media. Pediatrics 1995;96(1 Pt 1):5–13.

257. Marchant CD, Shurin PA, Johnson CE, et al: A randomized controlled trial of amoxicillin plus clavulanate compared with cefaclor for treatment of acute otitis media. J Pediatr 1986;109(5):891–896.

258. McCarty JM, Phillips A, Wiisanen R: Comparative safety and efficacy of clarithromycin and amoxicillin/clavulanate in the treatment of acute otitis media in children. Pediatr Infect Dis J 1993;12(12 Suppl 3):S122–S127.

259. Pichichero M, Aronovitz GH, Gooch WM, et al: Comparison of cefuroxime axetil, cefaclor, and amoxicillin-clavulanate potassium suspensions in acute otitis media in infants and children. South Med J 1990;83(10):1174–1177.

260. Ruohola A, Heikkinen T, Jero J, et al: Oral prednisolone is an effective adjuvant therapy for acute otitis media with discharge through tympanostomy tubes. J Pediatr 1999; 134(4):459–463.

261. Thomsen J, Sederberg-Olsen J, Balle V, Hartzen S: Antibiotic treatment of children with secretory otitis media. Amoxicillin-clavulanate is superior to penicillin V in a double-blind randomized study. Arch Otolaryngol Head Neck Surg 1997;123(7):695–699.

262. Aronovitz GH: Treatment of otitis media with cefuroxime axetil. South Med J 1988;81(8):978–980.

262a. Asmar BI, Dajani AS, Del Beccaro MA, Mendelman PM: Comparison of cefpodoxime proxetil and cefixime in the treatment of acute otitis media in infants and children. Otitis Study Group, Pediatrics 1994;94(6 pt 1):847–852.

263. Barnett ED, Teele DW, Klein JO, et al: Comparison of ceftriaxone and trimethoprim-sulfamethoxazole for acute otitis media. Greater Boston Otitis Media Study Group. Pediatrics 1997;99(1):23–28.

264. Bergeron MG, Ahronheim G, Richard JE, et al: Comparative efficacies of erythromycin-sulfisoxazole and cefaclor in acute otitis media: a double blind randomized trial. Pediatr Infect Dis J 1987;6(7):654–660.

265. Berman S, Lauer BA: A controlled trial of cefaclor versus amoxicillin for treatment of acute otitis media in early infancy. Pediatr Infect Dis 1983;2(1):30–33.

266. Biolcati AH: An open comparative study of the efficacy and safety of sultamicillin versus cefaclor in the treatment of acute otitis media in children. J Int Med Res 1992;20(Suppl 1):31A–43A.

267. Blumer JL, Bertino JS, Husak MP: Comparison of cefaclor and trimethoprim-sulfamethoxazole in the treatment of acute otitis media. Pediatr Infect Dis 1984;3(1):25–29.

268. Blumer JL, McLinn SE, Deabate CA, et al: Multinational multicenter controlled trial comparing ceftibuten with cefaclor for the treatment of acute otitis media. Members of the Ceftibuten Otitis Media International Study Group. Pediatr Infect Dis J 1995;14(7 Suppl):S115–S120.

269. Blumer JL, Forti WP, Summerhouse TL: Comparison of the efficacy and tolerability of once-daily ceftibuten and twice-daily cefprozil in the treatment of children with acute otitis media. Clin Ther 1996;18(5):811–820.

270. Brodie DP, Griggs JV, Cunningham K: Comparative study of cefuroxime axetil suspension and amoxycillin syrup in the treatment of acute otitis media in general practice. J Int Med Res 1990;18(3):235–239.

271. Dagan R: Bacteriologic response to oral cephalosporins: Are established susceptibility breakpoints appropriate in the case of acute otitis media? J Infect Dis 1997; 176:1253–1259.

272. Feldman W, Richardson H, Rennie B, Dawson P: A trial comparing cefaclor with co-trimoxazole in the treatment of acute otitis media. Arch Dis Child 1982;57(8):594–596.

273. Foshee WS: Loracarbef (LY163892) versus amoxicillin-clavulanate in the treatment of bacterial acute otitis media with effusion. J Pediatr 1992;120(6):980–986.

274. Foshee WS, Qvarnberg Y: Comparative United States and European trials of loracarbef in the treatment of acute otitis media. Pediatr Infect Dis J 1992;11(8 Suppl):S12–S19.

275. Furman S, Berkowicz L, Dippenaar J, et al: Cefetamet pivoxil vs cefaclor in the treatment of acute otitis media in children. Drugs 1994;47(Suppl 3):21–26.

276. Giebink GS, Batalden PB, Russ JN, Le CT: Cefaclor v amoxicillin in treatment of acute otitis media. Am J Dis Child 1984;138(3):287–292.

277. Gooch WM III, Gan VN, Corder WT, et al: Clarithromycin and cefaclor suspensions in the treatment of acute otitis media in children. Pediatr Infect Dis J 1993;12(12 Suppl 3):S128–S133.

278. Gooch WM, Adelglass J, Kelsey DK, et al: Loracarbef versus clarithromycin in children with acute otitis media with effusion. Clin Ther 1999;21(4):711–722.

279. Gooch WM, Philips A, Rhoades R, et al: Comparison of the efficacy, safety and acceptability of cefixime and amoxicillin/clavulanate in acute otitis media. Pediatr Infect Dis J 1997;16(2 Suppl):S21–S24.

280. Green SM, Rothrock SG: Single-dose intramuscular ceftriaxone for acute otitis media in children. Pediatrics 1993; 91(1):23–30.

281. Harrison CJ, Chartrand SA, Pichichero ME: Microbiologic and clinical aspects of a trial of once daily cefixime compared with twice daily cefaclor for treatment of acute otitis media in infants and children. Pediatr Infect Dis J 1993;12(1):62–69.

282. Howie VM, Dillard R, Lawrence B: In vivo sensitivity test in otitis media: Efficacy of antibiotics. Pediatrics 1985;75(1):8–13.

283. Howie VM, Owen MJ: Bacteriologic and clinical efficacy of cefixime compared with amoxicillin in acute otitis media. Pediatr Infect Dis J 1987;6(10):989–991.

284. Jacobson JA, Metcalf TJ, Parkin JL, et al: Evaluation of cefaclor and amoxycillin in the treatment of acute otitis media. Postgrad Med J 1979;55(Suppl 4):39–41.

285. John WR, Valle-Jones JC: Treatment of otitis media in children. A comparison between cefaclor and amoxicillin. Practitioner 1983;227(1386):1805–1809.

286. Johnson CE, Carlin SA, Super DM, et al: Cefixime compared with amoxicillin for treatment of acute otitis media. J Pediatr 1991;119(1 [Pt 1]):117–122.

287. Kara C, Ozuer M, Kilic I, et al: Comparison of amoxicillin with second and third generation cephalosporins in the treatment of acute otitis media. Infez Med 1998;6(2):93–95.

288. Kenna MA, Bluestone CD, Fall P, et al: Cefixime vs. cefaclor in the treatment of acute otitis media in infants and children. Pediatr Infect Dis J 1987;6(10):992–996.

289. Leigh AP, Robinson D, Millar ED: A general practice comparative study of a new third-generation oral cephalosporin, cefixime, with amoxycillin in the treatment of acute paediatric otitis media. Br J Clin Pract 1989;43(4):140–143.

290. Ludwig E: Cefixime in the treatment of respiratory and urinary tract infections. Chemotherapy 1998;44(Suppl 1):31–34.

291. Nassar WY, Allen BM: A double-blind comparative clinical trial of cephalexin and ampicillin in the treatment of childhood acute otitis media. Curr Med Res Opin 1974; 2(4):198–203.

292. Odio CM, Kusmiesz H, Shelton S, Nelson JD: Comparative treatment trial of Augmentin versus cefaclor for acute otitis media with effusion. Pediatrics 1985;75(5):819–826.

292a. MacLoughlin GJ, Barreto DG, de la Torre C, et al: Cefpodoxime proxetil suspension compared with cefaclor suspension for treatment of acute otitis media in paediatric patients. J Antimicrob Chemother 1996;37(3):565–573.

293. Mandel EM, Casselbrant ML, Kurs-Lasky M, Bluestone CD: Efficacy of ceftibuten compared with amoxicillin for otitis media with effusion in infants and children. Pediatr Infect Dis J 1996;15(5):409–414.

294. Mandel EM, Bluestone CD, Rockette HE, et al: Duration of effusion after antibiotic treatment for acute otitis media: Comparison of cefaclor and amoxicillin. Pediatr Infect Dis 1982;1(5):310–316.

295. Mandel EM, Kardatzke D, Bluestone CD, Rockette HE: A comparative evaluation of cefaclor and amoxicillin in the treatment of acute otitis media. Pediatr Infect Dis J 1993;12(9):726–732.

296. Mandel EM, Bluestone CD, Cantekin EI, et al: Comparison of cefaclor and amoxicillin for acute otitis media with effusion. Ann Otol Rhinol Laryngol Suppl 1981;90(3 Pt 3):48–52.

297. Marchant CD, Shurin PA, Turcyzk VA, et al: A randomized controlled trial of cefaclor compared with trimethoprim-sulfamethoxazole for treatment of acute otitis media. J Pediatr 1984;105(4):633–638.

298. McLinn SE, Daly JF, Jones JE: Cephalexin monohydrate suspension. Treatment of otitis media. JAMA 1975; 234(2):171–173.

299. McLinn SE: Recurrence of otitis media after antibiotic therapy: comparison of cephradine and amoxycillin. J Int Med Res 1979;7(6):546–550.

300. McLinn SE: Cefaclor in treatment of otitis media and pharyngitis in children. Am J Dis Child 1980;134(6):560–563.

301. McLinn SE: Randomized, open label, multicenter trial of cefixime compared with amoxicillin for treatment of acute otitis media with effusion. Pediatr Infect Dis J 1987;6(10):997–1001.

301a. McLinn SE, McCarty JM, Perrotte R, Pichichero ME, members of the Ceftibuten Otitis Media US Study Group: Multicenter controlled trial comparing ceftibuten with Amoxicillin-clavulanate in the empiric treatment of acute otitis media. Pediatr Infect Dis J 1995;14:S108–S114.

302. Mendelman PM, Del Beccaro MA, McLinn SE, Todd WM: Cefpodoxime proxetil compared with amoxicillin-clavulanate for the treatment of otitis media. J Pediatr 1992; 121(3):459–465.

303. Nelson JD, Ginsburg CM, Clahsen JC, Jackson LH: Treatment of acute otitis media of infancy with cefaclor. Am J Dis Child 1978;132(10):992–996.

304. Owen MJ, Anwar R, Nguyen HK, et al: Efficacy of cefixime in the treatment of acute otitis media in children. Am J Dis Child 1993;147(1):81–86.

305. Piippo T, Stefansson S, Pitkajarvi T, Lundberg C: Double-blind comparison of cefixime and cefaclor in the treatment of acute otitis media in children. Scand J Infect Dis 1991;23(4):459–465.

306. Ploussard JH: Evaluation of five days of cefaclor vs. ten days of amoxicillin therapy in acute otitis media. Curr Ther Res 1984;36:641–645.

307. Principi N, Marchisio P: Cefixime vs amoxicillin in the treatment of acute otitis media in infants and children. Drugs 1991;42(Suppl 4):25–29.

308. Pukander JS, Paloheimo SH, Sipila MM: Cefetamet pivoxil in pediatric otitis media. Chemotherapy 1992;38(Suppl 2):25–28.

309. Rodriguez WJ, Khan W, Sait T, et al: Cefixime vs. cefaclor in the treatment of acute otitis media in children: a randomized, comparative study. Pediatr Infect Dis J 1993; 12(1):70–74.

310. Stechenberg BW, Anderson D, Chang MJ, et al: Cephalexin compared to ampicillin treatment of otitis media. Pediatrics 1976;58(4):532–536.

311. Subba Rao SD, Macias MP, Dillman CA, et al: A randomized, observer-blind trial of amoxicillin/clavulanate versus cefaclor in the treatment of children with acute otitis media. Augmentin 415 Study Group. J Chemother 1998; 10(6):460–468.

312. Syrogiannopoulos GA, Goumas PD, Haliotis FA, et al: Cefuroxime axetil in the treatment of acute otitis media in children. J Chemother 1992;4(4):221–224.

313. Tsai HY, Huang LM, Chiu HH, et al: Comparison of once daily cefpodoxime proxetil suspension and thrice daily cefaclor suspension in the treatment of acute otitis media in children. J Microbiol Immunol Infect 1998;31(3):165–170.

314. Turik MA, Johns D: Comparison of cefaclor and cefuroxime axetil in the treatment of acute otitis media with effusion in children who failed amoxicillin therapy. J Chemother 1998;10(4):306–312.

315. Varsano I, Frydman M, Amir J, Alpert G: Single intramuscular dose of ceftriaxone as compared to 7-day amoxicillin therapy for acute otitis media in children. A double-blind clinical trial. Chemotherapy 1988;34(Suppl 1):39–46.

316. Wu DH: Efficacy and tolerability of cefixime in otitis media. A multicentre study in over 25,000 children. Drugs 1991;42(Suppl 4):30–32.

317. Pukander JS, Jero JP, Kaprio EA, Sorri MJ: Clarithromycin vs. amoxicillin suspensions in the treatment of pediatric patients with acute otitis media. Pediatr Infect Dis J 1993;12(12 Suppl 3):S118–S121.

318. Rosen C, Forsgren A, Lofkvist T, Walder M: Acute otitis media in older children and adults treated with phenoxymethyl penicillin or erythromycin stearate. Bacteriological and immunological aspects. Acta Otolaryngol 1983;96(3–4):247–253.

319. Arguedas A, Loaiza C, Herrera ML, et al: Comparative trial of 3-day azithromycin versus 10-day amoxicillin/clavulanate potassium in the treatment of children with acute otitis media. Int J Antimicrob Agents 1996;6:233–238.

320. Arguedas A, Loaiza C, Rodriguez F, et al: Comparative trial of 3 days of azithromycin versus 10 days of clarithromycin in the treatment of children with acute otitis media with effusion. J Chemother 1997;9(1):44–50.

321. Aronovitz G: A multicenter, open label trial of azithromycin vs. amoxicillin/clavulanate for the management of acute otitis media in children. Pediatr Infect Dis J 1996;15(9 Suppl):S15–S19.

322. Bain J, Murphy E, Ross F: Acute otitis media: Clinical course among children who received a short course of high dose antibiotic. BMJ (Clin Res Ed) 1985; 291(6504):1243–1246.

323. Bauchner H, Adams W, Barnett E, Klein J: Therapy for acute otitis media. Preference of parents for oral or parenteral antibiotic. Arch Pediatr Adolesc Med 1996;150(4):396–399.

324. Boulesteix J, Dubreuil C, Moutot M, et al: Cefpodoxime proxetil five days versus cefixime eight days in the treatment of acute otitis media in children. Medecine Maladies Infectieuses 1995;25:534–539.

325. Chamberlain JM, Boenning DA, Waisman Y, et al: Single-dose ceftriaxone versus 10 days of cefaclor for otitis media. Clin Pediatr (Phila) 1994;33(11):642–646.

326. Chaput de Saintonge D, Levine D, Savage I, et al: Trial of three-day and ten-day courses of amoxycillin in otitis media. BMJ 1982;284:1078–1081.

327. Cohen R, Levy C, Boucherat M, et al: Five vs. ten days of antibiotic therapy for acute otitis media in young children. Pediatr Infect Dis J 2000;19(5):458–463.

328. Cohen R, Navel M, Grunberg J, et al: One dose ceftriaxone vs. ten days of amoxicillin/clavulanate therapy for acute otitis media: Clinical efficacy and change in nasopharyngeal flora. Pediatr Infect Dis J 1999;18(5):403–409.

329. Cohen R, Bingen E, Varon E, et al: Change in nasopharyngeal carriage of *Streptococcus pneumoniae* resulting from

antibiotic therapy for acute otitis media in children. Pediatr Infect Dis J 1997;16(6):555–560.

330. Cohen R, Levy C, Boucherat M, et al: A multicenter, randomized, double-blind trial of 5 versus 10 days of antibiotic therapy for acute otitis media in young children. J Pediatr 1998;133(5):634–639.

331. Coles SJ, Addlestone MB, Kamdar MK, Macklin JL: A comparative study of clarithromycin and amoxycillin suspensions in the treatment of pediatric patients with acute otitis media. Infection 1993;21(4):272–278.

332. Dagan R, Johnson CE, McLinn S, et al: Bacteriologic and clinical efficacy of amoxicillin/clavulanate vs. azithromycin in acute otitis media. Pediatr Infect Dis J 2000;19(2):95–104.

333. Daniel RR: Comparison of azithromycin and co-amoxiclav in the treatment of otitis media in children. J Antimicrob Chemother 1993;31(Suppl E):65–71.

334. Gehanno P, Taillebe M, Denis P, et al: Short-course cefotaxime compared with five-day co-amoxiclav in acute otitis media in children. J Antimicrob Chemother 1990;26 (Suppl A):29–36.

335. Gehanno P, Nguyen L, Barry B, et al: Eradication by ceftriaxone of *Streptococcus pneumoniae* isolates with increased resistance to penicillin in cases of acute otitis media. Antimicrob Agents Chemother 1999;43(1):16–20.

336. Gooch WM, Blair E, Puopolo A, et al: Effectiveness of five days of therapy with cefuroxime axetil suspension for treatment of acute otitis media. Pediatr Infect Dis J 1996;15(2):157–164.

337. Hendrickse WA, Kusmiesz H, Shelton S, Nelson JD: Five vs. ten days of therapy for acute otitis media. Pediatr Infect Dis J 1988;7(1):14–23.

338. Hoberman A, Paradise JL, Burch DJ, et al: Equivalent efficacy and reduced occurrence of diarrhea from a new formulation of amoxicillin/clavulanate potassium (Augmentin) for treatment of acute otitis media in children. Pediatr Infect Dis J 1997;16(5):463–470.

339. Jones R, Bain J: Three-day and seven-day treatment in acute otitis media: a double-blind antibiotic trial. J R Coll Gen Pract 1986;36(289):356–358.

340. Kafetzis DA, Astra H, Mitropoulos L: Five-day versus ten-day treatment of acute otitis media with cefprozil. Eur J Clin Microbiol Infect Dis 1997;16(4):283–286.

341. Khurana CM: A multicenter, randomized, open label comparison of azithromycin and amoxicillin/clavulanate in acute otitis media among children attending day care or school. Pediatr Infect Dis J 1996;15(9 Suppl):S24–S29.

342. Leibovitz E, Piglansky L, Raiz S, et al: Bacteriologic and clinical efficacy of one day vs. three day intramuscular ceftriaxone for treatment of nonresponsive acute otitis media in children. Pediatr Infect Dis J 2000;19(11):1040–1045.

343. McCarty J: A multicenter, open label trial of azithromycin for the treatment of children with acute otitis media. Pediatr Infect Dis J 1996;15(9 Suppl):S10–S14.

344. McLinn S: A multicenter, double blind comparison of azithromycin and amoxicillin/clavulanate for the treatment of acute otitis media in children. Pediatr Infect Dis J 1996;15(9 Suppl):S20–S23.

345. Meistrup-Larsen KI, Sorensen H, Johnsen NJ, et al: Two versus seven days penicillin treatment for acute otitis media. A placebo controlled trial in children. Acta Otolaryngol 1983;96(1–2):99–104.

346. Mohs E, Rodriguez-Solares A, Rivas E, el Hoshy Z: A comparative study of azithromycin and amoxycillin in paediatric patients with acute otitis media. J Antimicrob Chemother 1993;31 (Suppl E):73–79.

347. Pessey JJ, Gehanno P, Thoroddsen E, et al: Short course therapy with cefuroxime axetil for acute otitis media: Results of a randomized multicenter comparison with amoxicillin/clavulanate. Pediatr Infect Dis J 1999;18(10):854–859.

348. Pestalozza G, Cioce C, Facchini M: Azithromycin in upper respiratory tract infections: A clinical trial in children with otitis media. Scand J Infect Dis Suppl 1992;83:22–25.

349. Principi N: Multicentre comparative study of the efficacy and safety of azithromycin compared with amoxicillin/clavulanic acid in the treatment of paediatric patients with otitis media. Eur J Clin Microbiol Infect Dis 1995;14(8):669–676.

350. Puczynski MS, Stankiewicz JA, O'Keefe JP: Single dose amoxicillin treatment of acute otitis media. Laryngoscope 1987;97(1):16–18.

351. Ramet J: Comparative safety and efficacy of clarithromycin and azithromycin suspensions in the short course treatment of children with acute otitis media. Clin Drug Invest 1995:961–966.

352. Rodriguez AF: An open study to compare azithromycin with cefaclor in the treatment of children with acute otitis media. J Antimicrob Chemother 1996;37(Suppl C):63–69.

353. Rubenstein M, McBean JB, Hedgecock LD, Stickler GB: The treatment of acute otitis media in children. III. A third clinical trial. Am J Dis Child 1965;109:308–313.

354. Simon M: Five- vs 10-day treatment of acute otitis media with ceftibuten in infants and children. Adv Ther 1997;14(6):312–317.

355. Stickler GB, Rubenstein MM, McBean JB, et al: Treatment of acute otitis media in children. IV. A fourth clinical trial. Am J Dis Child 1967;114(2):123–130.

chapter 4

Tonsillopharyngitis, Bacterial Tracheitis, Epiglottitis, and Laryngotracheitis

MICHAEL E. PICHICHERO, MD
JANET R. CASEY, MD

TONSILLOPHARYNGITIS

Viruses are the most common cause of tonsillopharyngitis in children and adults (Table 4–1).[1] Group A β-hemolytic streptococci (GABHS) account for 28% to 40% of cases of tonsillopharyngitis in young children and for 5% to 9% of cases in adults.

Other causes of tonsillopharyngitis include group C, G, or F streptococci, *Neisseria gonorrhoeae*, and *Arcanobacterium haemolyticum*.[2–9] These other bacteria are responsible for sore throat more often in adolescents and young adults than in children. Tonsillopharyngitis can result from *Mycoplasma pneumoniae* and *Chlamydia pneumoniae* infection, but cough is usually present as well.[10] Anaerobes produce peritonsillar and retropharyngeal abscesses, but they do not cause exudative tonsillopharyngitis.

Staphylococcus aureus and *Haemophilus influenzae* may cause tonsillopharyngitis. Because these organisms are common colonizers of the tonsillopharynx, it is difficult to definitively establish that they are the pathogens. The resurgence of *Corynebacterium diphtheriae* infection in Europe and Russia reminds us to consider that possibility, since the organism can cause tonsillopharyngitis before the classic membrane of diphtheria forms.

In many cases the cause of sore throat cannot be definitively identified. Possible explanations for symptoms include allergy, postnasal drip, and cigarette smoking. In the consideration of treatment of tonsillopharyngitis the focus is on GABHS because it is the main treatable pathogen (Table 4–1). The physician is faced with a large number of generic and proprietary antibiotics with wide ranges in efficacy, adverse effects, and cost. Treatment following the recommendations of the American Heart Association (Table 4–2) will have bacteriologic and clinical success in most cases.[11] However, failures do occur.

Antibiotic Susceptibility

GABHS are highly susceptible to penicillins and cephalosporins (β-lactams) (Table 4–3).[12–15] GABHS are usually susceptible to erythromycin, clarithromycin, azithromycin, lincomycin, and clindamycin.[16] GABHS resistance to the macrolides, however, has occurred[17–20] and may develop in a community or country as a consequence of extensive macrolide use.[20–22] Cross-resistance among macrolides is usually seen; concurrent resistance to penicillin does not occur. Most fluoroquinolones are

TABLE 4–1 ■ Causes of Pharyngitis

Cause	Peak incidence (%) Children	Peak incidence (%) Adults
Bacterial	30–40	5–10
Group A β-hemolytic streptococci	28–40	5–9
Group C, G, or F streptococci	0–3	0–18
Neisseria gonorrhoeae	0–0.01	0–0.01
Arcanobacterium haemolyticum	0–0.05	0–10
Mycoplasma pneumoniae	0–3	0–10
Chlamydia pneumoniae	0–3	0–9
Viral	15–40	30–60
Idiopathic	22–55	30–65

From Pichichero ME: Group A streptococcal tonsillopharyngitis: cost-effective diagnosis and treatment. Ann Emerg Med 1995;25:390–403.

bactericidal against GABHS, but there are no clinical trials demonstrating efficacy.

Sulfonamides (e.g., TMP-SMX and tetracycline) are of limited value in the treatment of GABHS tonsillopharyngitis. Sulfadiazine is acceptable for secondary prophylaxis in rheumatic fever.[23] This reflects the difference between antibiotic efficacy when bacterial colonization first begins (prophylactic drugs might be effective) vs. when active infection is established (agents effective in treatment are required). Group C, G, and F streptococci and *A. haemolyticum* have antibiotic susceptibility patterns almost identical to that of GABHS.[24] *M. pneumoniae* and *C. pneumoniae* are not susceptible to β-lactam antibiotics but are susceptible to macrolides (erythromycin, clarithromycin, azithromycin), tetracycline, and the fluoroquinolones. *N. gonorrhoeae* is susceptible to fluoroquinolones and ceftriaxone but has variable susceptibility to other cephalosporins and macrolides; this organism is usually resistant to penicillin.

In vivo activity of these antibiotics is significantly influenced by the level of drug achieved at the site of infection. Antibiotics may have variable absorption, absorption influenced by food, or action mitigated by enzymatic breakdown through microbial resistance mechanisms.

Antibiotic Tolerance

Penicillin tolerance among GABHS strains has been studied in the laboratory and clinically over the past decade. A ratio of the minimum inhibitory concentration (MIC) to the minimum bactericidal concentration (MBC) of 32 or higher defines tolerant bacterial strains[25]; other definitions have been employed.[26–30] Surveys for GABHS tolerant strains have given a range of 0 to 30%[31–33]; in large part these differences can be attributed to laboratory technique. A high prevalence of penicillin-tolerant GABHS has been described in epidemics among closed or semiclosed populations.[34–37] Clinical observations on the relevance of tolerant GABHS strains have been conflicting. Some outbreaks have occurred in which all strains were penicillin tolerant and all patients were penicillin treatment failures.[36,37] In other studies, penicillin treatment failures occurred no more frequently in tolerant than in susceptible strains.[34] Macrolides have been useful in halting epidemics caused by penicillin-tolerant strains.

Tissue and Blood Levels

For penicillins and the cephalosporins (β-lactam antibiotics) the duration of effective drug levels is much more important than the height of the peak serum concentration. Increasing blood levels by concurrent administration of probenecid or the addition of procaine penicillin to

TABLE 4–2 ■ Therapeutic Recommendations of the American Heart Association for the Primary Prevention of Rheumatic Fever in the Treatment of Group A β-Hemolytic Streptococci Tonsillopharyngitis

Agent*	Dose	Route	Duration
Benzathine penicillin G			
Patients <27.3 kg (60 lb)	600,000 U	IM	Once
Patients ≥27.3 kg (60 lb)	1,200,000 U	IM	Once
Penicillin V (Phenoxymethyl penicillin)		PO	10 d
Children	250 mg bid or tid		
Adolescents and adults	500 mg bid or tid		
Erythromycin†			
Estolate	20–40 mg/kg/d; divided bid, tid, or qid (max 1 g/d)	PO	10 d
or			
Ethylsuccinate	40 mg/kg/d; divided bid, tid, or qid (max 1 g/d)	PO	10 d

*Acceptable agents: amoxicillin, azithromycin, dicloxacillin, oral cephalosporins, and clindamycin; unacceptable agents: sulfonamides, trimethoprim, tetracycline, and chloramphenicol.

†For penicillin-allergic individuals.

From Dajani A, Taubert K, Ferrieri P, et al: Treatment of acute streptococcal pharyngitis and prevention of rheumatic fever: A statement for health professionals. Committee on Rheumatic Fever, Endocarditis, and Kawasaki Disease of the Council on Cardiovascular Disease in the Young, the American Heart Association. Pediatrics 1995;96: 754–764.

TABLE 4–3 ■ In vitro Antibiotic Susceptibility of Group A β-Hemolytic Streptococci

	Minimum inhibitory concentration (MIC$_{90}$)	
	Range (µg/ml)	Median (µg/ml)
Penicillins		
Benzylpenicillin G	0.005–0.01	0.005
Phenoxymethyl penicillin	0.005–0,02	0.01
Ampicillin	0.01–0.01	0.04
Amoxicillin	0.005–0.002	0.01
Amoxicillin/clavulanate	0.06–0.15	0.01
Carbenicillin	0.02–0.8	0.2
Ticarcillin	0.2–0.8	0.4
Methicillin	0.1–0.8	0.2
Oxacillin	0.02–0.2	0.04
Cloxacillin	0.02–0.2	0.04
Dicloxacillin	0.02–0.1	0.04
Nafcillin	0.01–0.2	0.02
Cephalosporins		
Cephalothin	0.02–0.4	0.2
Cephradine	0.25–0.5	0.5
Cefadroxil	0.01–6.25	0.4
Cefazolin	0.1–0.4	0.2
Cefuroxime	0.06–0.12	0.1
Cefaclor	0.06–1	0.5
Cefprozil	0.02–0.1	0.06
Loracarbef	0.06–2	0.5
Cefixime	0.008–0.5	0.5
Cefpodoxime	0.004–0.062	0.02
Ceftibuten	0.5–2	1
Cefdinir	0.008–0.015	0.01
Cefotaxime	0.01–0.1	0.1
Ceftizoxime	0.01–0.1	0.03
Ceftriaxone	0.01–0.1	0.03
Macrolides		
Lincomycin	0.02–0.4	0.2
Clindamycin	0.02–>4	0.04
Erythromycin	0.01–>8	0.04
Clarithromycin	0.004–0.5	0.02
Azithromycin	0.008–>0.5	0.03
Quinolones		
Ciprofloxacin	0.25–0.5	0.5
Ofloxacin	1–4	1
Sparfloxacin	0.25–0.5	0.5
Lomefloxacin		
Perfloxacin		
Levofloxacin	0.5–2	1
Trovafloxacin		
Gatifloxacin	0.1–0.5	0.25
Moxifloxacin		
Others		
Rifampin	0.01–0.4	0.1
Vancomycin	0.8–3.1	1.6
Trimethoprim (TMP)	0.02–0.8	0.1
Sulfamethoxazole (SMX)	3.1–1000	12.5
TMP-SMX	0.02–>50	0.4
Chloramhenicol	1.6–25	6.3
Tetracycline	0.2–>16	1
Aminoglycosides	3.1–400	NA

benzathine penicillin does not produce better bacteriologic or clinical efficacy. Once a concentration of β-lactam antibiotic is reached that ensures bactericidal activity, increased concentrations of the drug will not eradicate GABHS more effectively. β-lactam antibiotics work against actively growing bacteria. After initial bactericidal activity, there is a period of treatment before active bacterial growth resumes in which the antibiotic is not essential. This makes intermittent oral therapy feasible. Tonsillar inflammation enhances penetration of β-lactam antibiotics; bactericidal levels of penicillin sometimes are achieved only in the presence of acute infection.

Symptom Response to Antibiotic Therapy

For many years it was thought that antibiotics had only a minimal effect on ameliorating the symptoms of GABHS tonsillopharyngitis.[38–40] This tenet was refuted by several double-blind evaluations and re-examination of historic data, which showed greater clinical improvement in patients receiving β-lactam antibiotics than in those receiving placebo.[41–47] Antibiotics can relieve symptoms of GABHS tonsillopharyngitis faster than acetaminophen alone can.[46] Symptoms and signs of GABHS tonsillopharyngitis have a rapid onset and resolve spontaneously within 2 to 5 days even without treatment. Patients who seek care after they have had a sore throat lasting for more than a week usually do not have GABHS tonsillopharyngitis. It is the spontaneous resolution of symptoms but the persistence of the organism in the tonsillopharynx that sets the stage for ongoing contagion and creates the risk of acute rheumatic fever (ARF). Even though the patient's symptoms have subsided, persistence of the organism elicits an ongoing immune response. If the strain is rheumatogenic and the host genetically predisposed, ARF may follow.

The failure to observe a clinical response to antibiotic therapy within 1 to 2 days in a patient thought to have GABHS tonsillopharyngitis should lead the physician to question the diagnosis. Prompt clinical improvement is to be expected, and failure to observe it usually indicates that GABHS is not the cause of the tonsillopharyngeal infection. GABHS either is not present or is present but the patient is only a carrier. The symptom-relieving effects of antibiotic therapy are most marked if treatment is instituted early in the course of illness. If therapy is started after the first 24 to 48 hours of illness, the symptoms and signs of GABHS tonsillopharyngitis may not disappear significantly more rapidly than they would with no treatment.

Prompt antibiotic treatment is not vital to the prevention of rheumatic fever. Catanzaro et al[48] demonstrated in their study of military recruits with exudative GABHS tonsillopharyngitis that even if treatment is delayed for 9 days after onset of symptoms, ARF can be prevented. Thus after 9 days of GABHS infection, when antigenic stimulation is already near maximum, and after acute symptoms of GABHS tonsillopharyngitis have subsided, ARF can be prevented. In contrast, inappropriate antibiotic treatment (e.g., sulfa or tetracycline antibiotics) may favorably influence the acute symptoms but fail to eradicate GABHS from the respiratory tract, thereby missing an opportunity to prevent ARF.

Contagion

Appropriate, effective antibiotic treatment prevents transmission of GABHS to other susceptible individuals. Penicillin renders an infected person minimally contagious to others in about 24 hours.[49] Contagion duration when alternative antibiotics are used has not been systematically studied. If penicillin is discontinued after 3 days of therapy, there is a 50% likelihood that the patient will relapse with a GABHS infection[50] (which may be minimally symptomatic); if penicillin is stopped after 6 to 7 days of treatment, the likelihood of relapse is approximately 34%.[50] The transmission rate of GABHS is approximately 35% within a family or school setting if the patient is untreated.[50]

Prevention of Rheumatic Fever

The efficacy of penicillin for the primary prevention of ARF was established in the early 1950s.[51,52] These studies were made up of military recruits with GABHS tonsillopharyngitis who were given injectable penicillin G mixed in peanut oil or sesame oil and 2% aluminum monostearate. The penicillin-treated groups had a significant sevenfold reduction in ARF. Cephalosporins and other antibiotics effective for GABHS eradication should prevent ARF with similar efficacy; recent data from Germany support this observation.[53]

Specific Antibiotics

Benzathine Penicillin G

Benzathine penicillin G injections came into wide use between 1952 and 1960 for treatment of GABHS tonsillopharyngitis. To reduce the discomfort from injection, preparations were developed that combined the long-acting effect of benzathine with procaine penicillin in varied mixtures. Procaine penicillin diminishes injection site pain and rapidly provides a high level of penicillin in the bloodstream and tonsillopharynx. A combination of 900,000 units of benzathine penicillin G plus 300,000 units of procaine penicillin is superior to a variety of other regimens.[54–59]

Oral Penicillin G and Penicillin V

The studies of military recruits published in 1951–1952 demonstrated that GABHS eradication by penicillin prevented ARF. Thereafter acceptable treatment of GABHS tonsillopharyngitis was evaluated on the basis of bacteriologic eradication. Although oral penicillin was never shown in a prospective controlled trial to prevent ARF, the logical presumption successfully applied to GABHS tonsillopharyngitis treatment since 1951–1952 has been to equate bacteriologic elimination of GABHS from the tonsillopharynx with likely prevention of ARF. The low incidence of ARF in patients given oral penicillin validates this hypothesis. Comparisons of penicillin in oil, benzathine penicillin G, and oral penicillin G were undertaken between 1953 and 1960 when oral therapy became available.[60] Eradication rates with 10 days of oral penicillin G were shown to be the same as with intramuscular penicillin (Table 4–4).[61–75]

TABLE 4–4 ■ **Selected Studies Showing Eradication of Group A β-Hemolytic Streptococci by Treatment with Various Intramuscular vs. Oral Dosages of Penicillin**

Year	Investigators	Therapeutic regimens[*]	Route	Cure (%)[†]
1953	Breese[62]	Procaine penicillin G	IM	
		0.3 MU once		59
		0.3 MU × 2 at 3-d interval		75
		0.3 MU × 3 at 3-d interval	IM	83
		Benzathine penicillin G 0.6 MU once		93
		Penicillin G 1.2–3.6 MU/d × 10d	PO	75
1953	Wannamaker et al[61]	Procaine penicillin G in oil 0.6 MU once	IM	33
		Procaine penicillin G in oil 0.6 MU × 4 qod	IM	100
		Benzathine penicillin G 0.6 MU once	IM	70
		Benzathine penicillin G 1 MU/d × 5d	IM	82
1956	Mohler et al[67]	Benzathine penicillin G 0.6–0.9 MU once	IM	94
		Penicillin G 0.6–0.8 MU/d × 10d	PO	82
1957	Breese and Disney[63]	Benzathine penicillin G 0.6 MU once	IM	93
		Penicillin G 0.6–0.8 MU/d × 10d	PO	86
1957	Markowitz et al[68]	Benzathine penicillin G 1.2 MU once monthly	IM	100
		Penicillin G 0.2 MU/d	PO	94
1958	Breese and Disney[64]	Benzathine penicillin G 0.6 MU once	IM	93
		Benzathine penicillin G 0.6 MU/d	PO	90
		Penicillin V 0.6 MU/d × 10d	PO	89
		Penicillin G 0.6 MU/d × 10d	PO	87
		Penicillin G+ probenecid 0.75 MU/d × 10d	PO	82
1958	Miller et al[69]	Benzathine penicillin G 0.6 MU once	IM	87
		Penicillin G 0.4 MU/d × 10d	PO	80
		Penicillin G 1.2 MU/d × 10d	PO	95
1960	Stillerman et al[65]	Benzathine penicillin G 0.6 MU once	IM	84
		Benzathine penicillin G 1.2 MU once	IM	87
		Penicillin V 0.6 MU/d × 10d	PO	80
		Penicillin V 1.2 MU/d × 10d	PO	87
1969	Stillerman[70]	Benzathine penicillin G 0.8 MU once	IM	91
		Penicillin V 0.8 MU/d × 10d	PO	83
		Penicillin V 1.6 MU/d × 7d	PO	72
1971	Howie and Ploussard[71]	Benzathine penicillin G 0.6–1.2 MU once	IM	100
		Penicillin G 0.75 MU/d × 10d	PO	70
1972	Colcher and Bass[66]	Procaine+ benzathine penicillin G mixture 1.2 MU	IM	86
		Penicillin V 250 mg divided tid × 10d	PO	
		Normally informed patients		75
		Optimally informed patients		90
1973	Shapera et al[72]	Benzathine penicillin G 0.3–1.2 MU once	IM	97
		Penicillin V 0.8–1.6 MU/d × 10d	PO	94
1974	Lester et al[73]	Benzathine penicillin G 0.6–1.2 MU once	IM	94
		Penicillin V 0.8–1.6 MU/d × 10d	PO	95
1974	Matsen et al[74]	Benzathine penicillin G 0.6–1.2 MU/d once	IM	96
		Penicillin V 0.6–1.6 MU/d × 10d	PO	97
1987	Ginsberg et al[75]	Benzathine penicillin G 0.9 MU once	IM	88
		Penicillin V 24 mg/kg/d × 10d	PO	88

[*]MU, million units; 0.2 MU = 125 mg of penicillin G or V.

[†]Measured as percentage of patients with eradication of group A streptococci from tonsillopharynx up to 4 weeks after therapy (carriers excluded if possible).

Oral penicillin V was introduced in the early 1960s as an improvement over penicillin G; it is better absorbed and therefore produces higher blood and tonsillar tissue levels. Various dosing regimens with oral penicillin G and V have been assessed (Table 4–5).[60,76–87] A daily dose of 500 to 1000 mg of penicillin V is preferable. Lower doses have lower eradication rates, and higher doses are not beneficial (Table 4–5). Twice daily dosing with oral penicillin V is adequate therapy for GABHS tonsillopharyngitis;[76,81–85] once daily treatment is not.[76,86]

Nafcillin, Cloxacillin, and Dicloxacillin

The efficacy of oral penicillin G has been compared with that of oral nafcillin, and nafcillin is less effective.[81,88,89] Cloxacillin and dicloxacillin are adequate for GABHS eradication.[90,91]

Ampicillin and Amoxicillin

Oral ampicillin and amoxicillin are equivalent but not superior to oral penicillin in eradication of GABHS from the tonsillopharynx (Table 4–6).[92–98] Amoxicillin is more

TABLE 4–5 ■ Studies of Oral Dosages of Penicillin G and V in Group A β-Hemolytic Streptococci Eradication

Year	Investigators	Agent	Daily dose (mg)	Schedule	Cure (%)*
1956	Breese and Disney[78]	Penicillin V	375	tid	89
1958	Schalet et al[79]	Penicillin V	500	tid	86
		Penicillin G	375	tid	89
1964	Breese et al[80]	Penicillin G	500	tid	75
		Penicillin V	500	tid	88
1964	Stillerman and Bernstein[77]	Penicillin V	375	tid	77
		Penicillin V	750	tid	89
1965	Breese et al[76]	Penicillin G	500	qid	58
			500	bid	85
			1000	bid	84
			500	qid	86
			1000	qid	85
1968	Rosenstein et al[81]	Penicillin V	500	bid	90
1972	Vann and Harris[82]	Penicillin G	1000	bid	89
1973	Stillerman et al[83]	Penicillin V	500	bid	86
		Penicillin V	375	tid	79
1977	Spitzer and Harris[84]	Penicillin V	1000	bid	87
		Penicillin V	750	tid	86
1989	Gerber et al[86]	Penicillin V	750	tid	72
		Penicillin V	750	tid	82
1989	Gerber et al[86]	Penicillin V	750	qd	78
		Penicillin V	750	tid	92
1990	Krober et al[87]	Penicillin V	1000	qid	89
			1000	bid	94
			1000	qd	69

*Cure defined as bacteriologic eradication at end of treatment.

TABLE 4–6 ■ Ampicillin or Amoxicillin 10-Day Treatment of Group A β-Hemolytic Streptococci Tonsillopharyngitis

Year	Authors	Agent	Daily dose (divided)	Schedule	Ampicillin/amoxicillin cure (%)*	Penicillin cure (%)*
1966	Breese et al[92]	Ampicillin	10–20 mg/kg	tid	78	83
1968	Ström[93]	Ampicillin	375–750 mg	tid	85	91
1972	Stillerman et al[94]	Ampicillin	500 mg	tid	73	74
1974	Stillerman et al[95]	Amoxicillin	375 mg	tid	87	80
1974	Breese et al[96]	Amoxicillin	375 mg	tid	85	89
1977	Breese et al[97]	Amoxicillin	15–20 mg/kg	tid	91	88
1983	Shvartzman et al[98]	Amoxicillin	50 mg/kg	qd	100	94

*Cure defined as bacteriologic eradication at end of treatment.

effective than penicillin against the common pathogens that cause otitis media and middle ear infections, and these infections are seen concurrently with GABHS tonsillopharyngitis in up to 15% of pediatric patients. In patients under 4 years of age the incidence of concurrent GABHS tonsillopharyngitis and otitis media may reach 40%.[99] Amoxicillin tastes better than oral penicillin in suspension formulation, which is compliance enhancing for children. Amoxicillin may be administered twice per day,[100] and possibly once daily.[98,101]

Amoxicillin-Clavulanate

Amoxicillin is bactericidal against GABHS, and clavulanate is a potent inhibitor of β-lactamase. Thus, amoxicillin-clavulanate would be effective if copathogens were cocolonizing the tonsillopharynx in a GABHS-infected patient (discussed below). Amoxicillin-clavulanate was shown to have better outcomes than penicillin has in three comparative studies[102–104] but not in a fourth[105] in the treatment of GABHS tonsillopharyngitis.

Erythromycin

Erythromycin emerged as the suggested agent for GABHS tonsillopharyngitis for penicillin-allergic patients. Erythromycin estolate and ethylsuccinate have consistently done better than erythromycin base or stearate in comparisons with oral penicillin for bacteriologic eradication (Table 4–7).[65,92,97,106–120] Dosing-frequency studies with various erythromycin preparations have shown that two, three, and four times daily administration produce equivalent bacteriologic eradication rates.

TABLE 4–7 ■ **Erythromycin Treatment of Group A β-Hemolytic Streptococci Tonsillopharyngitis in Children**

Year	Investigators	Formulation	Daily dose (mg/kg)	Schedule	Erythromycin cure (%)*	Penicillin cure (%)*
1960	Stillerman et al[65]	Proprionate	30–40	qid	48	82
1961	Breese et al[107]	Proprionate	30–40	qid	64	73
1963	Stillerman et al[108]	Proprionate	30–40	qid	78	72
1963	Moffett et al[109]	Estolate	15–30	qid	78	77
1966	Breese et al[299]	Estolate	20	qid	85	80
1969	Hughes et al[110]	Ethylsuccinate	40	qid	85	NA
1972	Howie and Ploussard[106]	Ethylsuccinate	40–50	tid	92	88
		Estolate	20–40	tid	92	
1972	Levine and Berman[111]	Estolate	30	tid	85	NA
1973	Shapera et al[72]	Estolate	40	qid	91	97
1973	Ryan et al[112]	Estolate	30–50	qid	92	NA
		Stearate		qid	90	
1974	Lester et al[73]	Stearate	15–30	qid	91	87
1974	Breese et al[113]	Estolate	30	tid	92	88
		Ethylsuccinate	50	tid	94	
1975	Janicki et al[114]	Estolate	23–38	tid	95	NA
		Stearate	23	tid	100	
1976	Derrick and Dillon[115]	Estolate	20	bid	86	NA
1977	Breese et al[97]	Estolate	30	tid	98	95
1979	Derrick and Dillon[116]	Estolate	20	bid	87	NA
		Ethylsuccinate	40	bid	86	
1982	Ginsburg et al[75]	Estolate	30	bid	92	NA
1982	Ginsburg et al[117]	Ethylsuccinate	30	bid	75	NA
		Estolate	30	bid	95	
1984	Ginsburg et al[118]	Estolate	15	bid	94	NA
		Ethylsuccinate	25	bid	65	
1990	Disney et al[119]	Ethylsuccinate	30	qid	76	NA
1991	Milatovic[120]	Ethylsuccinate	20	bid	80	NA
1996	Adam and Scholz[209]	Estolate	40	bid × 5d	83	88

*Cured defined as bacteriologic eradication at end of treatment.

Clindamycin and Lincomycin

Clindamycin and lincomycin have a spectrum of activity against organisms that include GABHS, some potential β-lactamase-producing copathogens, *S. aureus*, and anaerobic bacteria. Clindamycin and lincomycin have been evaluated as primary treatment for GABHS tonsillopharyngitis (Table 4–8).[71,73,83,92,113,121,122] Clindamycin is effective in eradication of the GABHS carrier.[122–124] Routine use of these agents for GABHS tonsillopharyngitis is not advocated because of concern for infrequent but significant side effects, that is, pseudomembranous colitis.

Clarithromycin, Azithromycin, Roxithromycin, and Dirithromycin

Clarithromycin has been assessed for treatment of GABHS tonsillopharyngitis and has shown a bacteriologic eradication rate similar[125–127] or superior[128,129] to that of penicillin (Table 4–9). Azithromycin has been evaluated for treatment of GABHS tonsillopharyngitis. As a 5-day regimen azithromycin is similar to or superior[130–132] to penicillin 10 days, but as a 3-day regimen it is inferior[133,134] to it (Table 4–10). The efficacy of roxithromycin is uncertain, but one trial with dirithromycin

showed it had a favorable clinical and bacteriologic response compared with that of penicillin.[135,136] Following use of azithromycin for GABHS treatment, macrolide-resistant *S. pneumoniae* strains are more frequently isolated from the nasopharynx.[137] All of the newer macrolides produce fewer gastrointestinal side effects than erythromycin does.

Rifampin

Rifampin in combination with oral penicillin has been studied as a potential antibiotic for the eradication of the GABHS carrier. Successful results have been observed.[138,139]

Cephalosporins

Oral cephalosporins were introduced as alternative antibiotics for the treatment of GABHS tonsillopharyngitis in the early 1970s; a superior bacteriologic eradication rate, and in many cases clinical cure, was observed consistently (Table 4–11).[70,74,75,94,140–160] In 1991 a meta-analysis was published comparing the bacteriologic and clinical cure rates achieved with various cephalosporins as compared with those of various penicillin preparations.[158] The meta-analysis included 19 studies fulfilling

TABLE 4–8 ■ **Clindamycin or Lincomycin Treatment of Group A β-Hemolytic Streptococci Tonsillopharyngitis**

Year	Investigators	Agent	Daily dose (divided mg/kg)	Schedule	Clindamycin or lincomycin cure* (%)	Penicillin cure* (%)
1963	Schaffer et al[121]	Lincomycin	30	qid	88	89
1965	Jackson et al[299]	Lincomycin	22–33	qid	93	89
1966	Breese et al[92]	Lincomycin	20–40	tid	88	75
1969	Breese et al[301]	Lincomycin	20–40	tid	84[†]	59[†]
1969	Randolph and DeHaan[301]	Lincomycin	20–40	qid	92	86
1970	Randolph et al[302]	Clindamycin	NA	tid or qid	93	79
1971	Howie and Ploussard[71]	Lincomycin	27–33	tid	88	79
1973	Stillerman et al[83]	Lincomycin	27–33	tid	88	79
1974	Breese et al[113]	Clindamycin	10–15	tid	92	88
1974	Lester et al[73]	Clindamycin	12–18	bid, tid, or qid	95	89
1975	Randolph et al[303]	Clindamycin	10–30	qid	88	76
1981	Brook and Leyva[123]	Clindamycin	20	qid	95[†]	NA
1985	Brook and Hirokawa[124]	Clindamycin	10	qid	93[†]	13[†]
1990	Raz et al[304]	Clindamycin	20	tid	98	NA
1991	Tanz et al[122]	Clindamycin	20	tid	92[†]	55[†]

*Cure defined as bacteriologic eradication at end of treatment.
[†]Group A streptococci carriers included in study group.
NA, not available.

rigid criteria of adequate study design and implementation. Approximately 1000 patients prospectively and randomly assigned to receive one of several cephalosporin antibiotics were compared to approximately 1000 patients treated with one of several penicillin formulations. Under these ideal study conditions the mean bacteriologic failure rate was significantly higher in those treated with penicillin (16%) than in those treated with cephalosporins (8%, $P<.001$). Overall, in 17 of the 19 studies analyzed the cephalosporins produced a higher bacteriologic cure rate than the penicillins did. The mean clinical failure rate was also evaluated by meta-analysis; it was 11% with various penicillin formulations as compared with 5% with the cephalosporins ($P<.001$). Numerous subsequent prospective, double-blind, randomized trials comparing first-, second-, and third-generation cephalosporin antibiotics continue to confirm the meta-analysis results (Table 4–12).[120,161–180]

Changes in Penicillin Treatment Success

An increase in the past few decades in penicillin treatment failures among patients with GABHS tonsillopharyngitis has been noted[181–183] (Table 4–13),[184] but the observation is not universally accepted.[183] One might presume that a rise in penicillin failures should be reflected in a rise in ARF, but this has not been consistently observed. Declining efficacy with penicillin (and other antibiotics) may not necessarily become manifest as an increased incidence in ARF because treatment failure must occur in the presence of rheumatogenic GABHS strains and as yet undetermined specific host susceptibility factors.

Descriptions of GABHS toxic shock syndrome and GABHS-mediated necrotizing fasciitis have increased concern that a resurgence of virulent GABHS infections may be occuring.[185–194] Penicillin treatment failure has been noted in patients experiencing severe GABHS infections.[195,196] Although the site of infection is usually cutaneous for these severe infections, the tonsillopharynx has been the source in some cases.[197–202] These penicillin failures may be due to the Eagle effect,[203,204] where virulent, toxin-producing strains of GABHS rapidly divide, reach a stationary phase of growth (perhaps as a consequence of diminished nutrients in the immediate environment of the infection), and while in the stationary phase resist the bactericidal activity of penicillin and other β-lactams. Antibiotics that inhibit bacterial protein synthesis (e.g., clindamycin) have proven useful in the eradication of such GABHS strains.[195]

Duration of Therapy

Injections of benzathine penicillin provide bactericidal levels against GABHS for 21 to 28 days.[205,206] The addition of procaine partially alleviates the discomfort of benzathine injections. GABHS is eradicated by the sustained levels of penicillin achieved with the benzathine formulation. The necessity for 10 days of oral penicillin therapy to achieve a maximum bacteriologic cure rate has been documented. Five to seven days of therapy with injectable penicillin or oral penicillin does not produce optimal GABHS eradication (Fig. 4–1). Since compliance with 10 days of therapy is often problematic, a shorter course of therapy is an attractive option. Studies suggest amoxicillin for 6 days therapy is as effective as 10 days penicillin therapy in adults[207] and children.[208] Erythromycin estolate for 5 days had an eradication rate of 83% compared with 88% following 10 days of penicillin V.[209]

TABLE 4–9 ■ Clarithromycin Compared to Penicillin V for Treatment of Group A β-Hemolytic Streptococci Tonsillopharyngitis

Year	Investigators	Patient population	Total number		Daily dose (divided)	Schedule	Bacteriologic eradication (%)				Clinical response (%)	
							End of treatment		Follow-up			
							Clarithromycin 10 d cure (%)	Penicillin 10 d cure (%)	Clarithromycin 10 d cure (%)	Penicillin 10 d cure (%)	Clarithromycin 10 d	Penicillin 10 d
1991	Levenstein[126]	Adults	125	Clarithromycin	500 mg	bid	100	97	98	98	96	98
1991	Bachand[127]	Adults	90	Clarithromycin	500 mg	bid	88	91	94	89	86	77
1992	Schrock[128]	Adults	356	Clarithromycin	500 mg	bid	95	87*	94	88	93	88
1993	Still et al[129]	Children	506	Clarithromycin	15 mg/kg	bid	92	81*	88	71	96	94

*$P<.05$, clarithromycin superior to penicillin V.

TABLE 4–10 ■ Studies of Short-Course Treatment with Azithromycin vs. 10 Days of Treatment with Penicillin in Children and Adults with Streptococcal Tonsillopharyngitis

Year	Investigators	Patient population	Total number		Days	Bacteriologic eradication (%)				Clinical response (%)	
						End of treatment		Follow-up			
						Azithromycin	Penicillin 10 d	Azithromycin	Penicillin 10 d	Azithromycin	Penicillin 10 d
1991	Hooten[130]	Adults	242(152)*	Azithromycin Once daily	5	91	96	90	88	99	99
1993	Hamill[131]	Children	96(49)	Azithromycin Once daily	3	95	95	86	92	93	93
1995	Still[132]	Children	366(176)	Azithromycin Once daily	5	95†	77	80	74	98†	87
		Children	278(148)	Azithromycin Once daily	5	95†	69	79†	67	97†	82
1996	Pacifico et al[133]	Children	154(76)	Azithromycin Once daily	3	67‡	91	75‡	92	75‡	91
1996	Schaad et al[134]	Children	343(152)	Azithromycin Once daily	3	65‡	82	55‡	80	93	89

*Numbers in parentheses represent number receiving shortened course.
†Azithromycin better than penicillin, $P <.05$.
‡Penicillin better than azithromycin, $P <.05$.

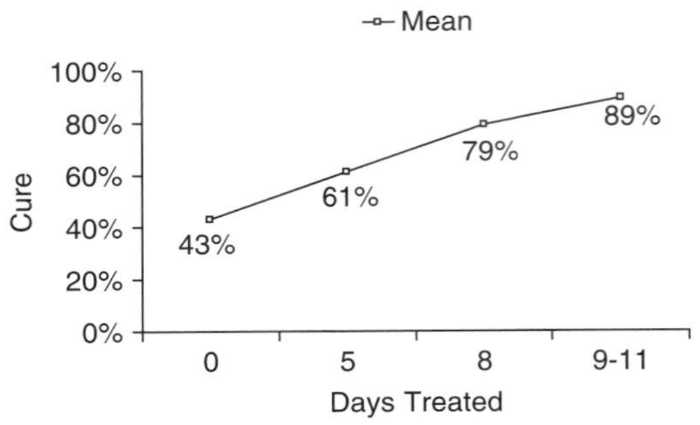

FIGURE 4–1. Bacteriologic eradication of group A β-hemolytic streptococci according to duration of penicillin therapy.

A 4- or 5-day course of therapy with several cephalosporins—cefadroxil, cefuroxime axetil, cefpodoxime proxetil, and cefdinir—has produced a similar or superior bacteriologic eradication rate than that achievable with 10 days administration of oral penicillin V (Table 4–14).[120,130–134,176,207,208,210–220]

Azithromycin may be administered for 5 days[130,132] because this antibiotic persists in tonsillopharyngeal tissues so long that bacteriostatic levels are maintained for approximately 5 to 10 days after discontinuation of the drug (total of 10 to 15 days of therapy).

Explanations for Antibiotic Failure

Antibiotic Formulation Deficiencies

The quality of benzathine penicillin G from various manufacturers in various countries may not be uniform. Benzathine penicillin G preparations that produce lower, variable, and short duration of adequate levels have been described.[221]

Compliance

For optimal absorption, oral penicillin V should be administered 1 hour before or 2 hours after meals. The inability to take doses at mealtime diminishes patient compliance. The once or twice daily dosing and the ability to take an antibiotic without regard to meals or at meal times enhances compliance.

A good-tasting suspension formulation for oral antibiotics can enhance compliance in children. On the contrary, a marginal or poor taste may lead to the child's refusing, spitting, or vomiting the drug. Penicillin V suspension does not have a good taste, whereas most children find the taste of amoxicillin and many cephalosporins quite pleasant. Taste comparisons of antibiotic suspensions have found cephalosporins to taste best.[222,223]

Patients' perception of antimicrobial side effects strongly influences compliance. All the antibiotics commonly employed to treat GABHS tonsillopharyngitis are notable for their low incidence of adverse side effects. Rash and gastrointestinal upset occurs in 1% to 2% of patients with the penicillins and cephalosporins. Macrolides, particularly erythromycin, more frequently produce gastrointestinal upset. Amoxicillin-clavulanate is associated with a higher incidence of diarrhea than other agents commonly considered for GABHS. The duration of therapy is perhaps the most important determiner of compliance. Shorter courses that are completed in 4 to 5 days are best.

TABLE 4–11 ■ Cephalosporins for Treatment of Group A β-Hemolytic Streptococci Tonsillopharyngitis, 1969–1989

Year	Investigators	Agent	Daily dose (divided)	Schedule	Cephalosporin 10 d cure (%)*	Penicillin 10 d cure (%)*
1969	Stillerman[70]	Cephaloglycin	1500 mg	tid	91	83
1970	Stillerman and Isenberg[140]	Cephalexin	1500 mg	tid	91	80
1971	Disney et al[141]	Cephalexin	30–40 mg/kg	tid	81	76
1972	Stillerman et al[94]	Cephalexin	1500 mg	tid	89	74
1972	Gau et al[142]	Cephalexin	20–40 mg/kg	tid	96	92
1973	Rabinovitch et al[143]	Cephalexin	2000 mg	qid	100	97
1974	Matsen et al[74]	Cephalexin	2000 mg	qid	97	97
1974	Derrick and Dillon[144]	Cephalexin	1125–2250 mg	tid	99	92
1976	Stillerman[145]	Ceftrazine	1125 mg	tid	96	84
1979	Disney et al[146]	Cefaclor	20 mg/kg	tid	93	87
1980	Ginsburg et al[147]	Cefadroxil	30 mg/kg	tid	93	71
1982	Ginsburg et al[75]	Cefadroxil	30 mg/kg	bid	86	80
1982	Henness[148]	Cefadroxil	30 mg/kg	bid	96	81
1986	Stillerman[149]	Cefaclor	10–31 mg/kg	tid	86	70
1986	Gerber[150]	Cefadroxil	30 mg/kg	qid	98	94
1987	Pichichero et al[152]	Cefuroxime	2–17 mg/kg	bid	85	88
1987	Pichichero et al[153]	Cefadroxil	30 mg/kg	qd	90	76
1987	Gooch et al[154]	Cefuroxime	250–500 mg	bid	92	77
1988	Stromberg et al[156]	Cefadroxil	1000–2000 mg	bid	97	94
1989	Milatovic and Knauer[157]	Cefadroxil	25 mg/kg	bid	93	81

*Cure based on bacteriologic eradication at end of therapy.

TABLE 4–12 ■ **Newer Studies Comparing 10 Days of Cephalosporin with 10 Days of Penicillin Treatment for Group A β-Hemolytic Streptococci Tonsillopharyngitis, 1990–2000**

Year	Investigators	Study population	Treatment	Number	Bacteriologic cure (%)	Clinical cure (%)
1991	Brown et al[161]	Adults	Cefpodoxime Proxetil	93	97	97
			Penicillin V		91	97
1991	Holm et al[162]	Children	Cefadroxil	176	98*	98*
			Penicillin V		86	91
1991	Reed et al[163]	Adults and children	Cefaclor	116	85	87
			Penicillin V		76	87
1991	Milatovic[120]	Children	Cefadroxil	239	93*	NA
			Penicillin		81	
1991	Holm et al[162]	Adults	Cefadroxil	489	94*	97*
			Penicillin V		88	93
1992	McCarty[165]	Adults	Loracarbef	218	90	95
			Penicillin V		92	94
1992	Disney et al[166]	Children	Cephalexin	525	93	97*
			Penicillin V		89	92
1992	McCarty & Renteria[167]	Children	Cefprozil	409	91	95*
			Penicillin		87	88
1992	Ramet et al[168]	Children	Cefetamet Pivoxil	66	94	100
			Penicillin V		91	100
1992	Disney et al[169]	Children	Loracarbef	233	87	97
			Penicillin V		82	94
1992	Block et al[170]	Children	Cefixime	110	94*	94*
			Penicillin V		77	75
1992	Muller et al[171]	Children	Loracarbef	344	95*	97
			Penicillin V		87	96
1993	Dajani et al[172]	Children	Cefpodoxime Proxetil	578	93*	92
			Penicillin V		81	87
1993	Gooch et al[173]	Children	Cefuroxime Axetil	533	94*	92*
			Penicillin V		84	81
1993	Milatovic et al[174]	Children	Cefprozil	409	91	95*
			Penicillin V		87	88
1994	McCarty[175]	Children	Cefprozil (qd)	151	89*	89*
			Penicillin V		67	74
1994	McCarty[175]	Children	Cefprozil (bid)	359	NA	94
			Penicillin V			88
1994	Pichichero et al[176]	Children	Cefpodoxime Proxetil	484	95*	96
			Penicillin V		78	91
1995	Holm et al[177]	Children	Cefuroxime Axetil	236	87*	86*
			Penicillin V		56	67
1995	Pichichero et al[178]	Children	Ceftibuten	617	91*	97*
			Penicillin V		80	89
1997	Roos and Larsson[179]	Adolescents and adults	Loracarbef	331	90*	91*
			Penicillin V		66	85
1999	Nemeth et al[180]	Children	Cefdinir (qd)	792	94*	97*
			Penicillin V		70	86

*P<.05 between treatments.

TABLE 4–13 ■ **Recurrences of Streptococcal Tonsillopharyngitis after Penicillin or Amoxicillin Therapy: Elmwood Pediatric Group 1975–1996**

Years	Episodes treated with penicillin or amoxicillin (N)	Patients with recurrence within 30 d (%)	Patients with recurrence within 60 d (%)
1975–1979	437	9	11
1980–1984	429	26	39
1985–1989	363	24	39
1990–1994	359	22	32
1995–1996	133	26	38

Adapted with permission from Pichichero ME, Green JL, Francis AB, et al: Recurrent group A streptococcal tonsillopharyngitis. Pediatr Infect Dis J 1998;17(9):809–815.

TABLE 4–14 ■ Bacteriologic Eradication Rates (Expressed as Percent of Patients) in Studies Involving Shortened Treatment Regimens for Tonsillopharyngitis

Year of publication	Study site	Percent cure	
		Shortened therapy (drug, duration)	Longer therapy (drug, duration)
		AMOXICILLIN	
1996	United States[208]	84 (amoxicillin, 6 d)	85 (penicillin, 10 d)
1996	France[207]	92 (amoxicillin, 6 d)	93 (penicillin, 10, d)
		ORAL CEPHALOSPORINS	
1990	France[212]	97 (cefpodoxime, 5 d)	94 (penicillin, 10 d)
		80 (cefuroxime, 5 d)	
1991	France[213]	96 (cefuroxime, 4 d)	96 (penicillin, 10 d)
1991	Germany[120]	84 (cefadroxil, 5 d)	88 (penicillin, 10 d)
1994	France[214]	96 (cefpodoxime, 5 d)	94 (penicillin, 10 d)
1994	United States[176]	90 (cefpodoxime, 5 d)	78 (penicillin, 10 d)
		95 (cefpodoxime, 10 d)	
1994	France[215]	94 (cefixime, 4 d)	96 (penicillin, 10 d)
1995	United States[216]	98 (cefpodoxime, 5 d)	91 (penicillin, 10 d)
		91 (cefpodoxime, 10 d)	
1995	France[217]	88 (cefuroxime, 4 d)	87 (penicillin, 10 d)
1995	Germany[218]	83 (cefotiam, 5 d)	88 (penicillin, 10 d)
1995	France[219]	84 (cefixime, 5 d)	84 (penicillin, 10 d)
1997	United States[220]	90 (cefdinir, 5 d)	72 (penicillin, 10 d)
1998	Multinational[305]	88 (cefuroxime, 5 d)	92 (cefuroxime, 10 d)
2000	Germany[306]*	90 (cefuroxime, 5 d)	84 (penicillin, 10 d)
2000	Germany[53]†	83 (cefuroxime, 5 d)	
		(ceftibuten, 5 d)	
		(loracarbef, 5 d)	
		(erythromycin, 5 d)	
		(clarithromycin, 5 d)	
		(amoxicillin-clavulanate 5 d)	

* Shortened therapy statistically superior ($P<.05$) to penicillin.

†Individual shortened course antibiotic evaluation rates not reported; the overall combined rate was 83%.

Repeated Exposure

The symptoms of GABHS tonsillopharyngitis resolve without treatment within 2 to 5 days of onset. Infected individuals remain contagious for weeks and possibly months thereafter. Crowded living conditions encourage the transmission of GABHS within the family, at work, at school, or in day care settings. After treatment, if there is a recurrence of GABHS tonsillopharyngitis and the infection involves the same serotype, patients may display milder or fewer symptoms.[224] These persons are contagious to others in their environment and are themselves susceptible to rheumatic fever. GABHS may persist on toothbrushes and removable orthodontic appliances following treatment of tonsillopharyngitis.[225]

Suppression of Immune Responses by Early Treatment

Prompt initiation of antibiotic treatment with the onset of acute symptoms may suppress the anti-streptolysin O(ASO) and anti-DNase B antibody elevations typically observed to follow GABHS infections. Antibody suppression has been associated with GABHS tonsillopharyngitis relapse and recurrence in some studies[46,226,227]

(Table 4–15) but not in all.[228] Although postponing treatment is probably not necessary in most cases of GABHS tonsillopharyngitis, it may be a useful strategy for patients who have frequent, recurrent mild-to-moderate infections. By delaying treatment for 2 or 3 days (maximum 9 days from onset of symptoms), the patient's natural immunity may be allowed to develop without risk of ARF. Such a strategy should not be considered if the patient is toxic or severely ill, or if highly virulent or rheumatogenic strains are actively circulating in a community.

Copathogens

The presence of cocolonizing bacteria in the tonsillopharynx, termed copathogens, that elaborate β-lactamase may explain some penicillin treatment failures: Penicillin is inactivated by the β-lactamase produced by the copathogens before the antibiotic can exert its bactericidal action on GABHS[158,159,229,230] (Fig. 4–2). *S. aureus, H. influenzae, M. catarrhalis,* and anaerobic spp potentially can occur as β-lactamase-producing flora in the tonsillopharynx. The prevalence of these β-lactamase-producing bacteria may be increased through selection pressure as a consequence of recent penicillin or amoxicillin treatment.

TABLE 4–15 ■ Adverse Effects of Immediate Treatment of Group A β-Hemolytic Streptococci Tonsillopharyngitis

Repeat acute group A streptococci tonsillopharyngitis	Treatment group				
	Immediate penicillin (N = 170)		Delayed (48–56 h) penicillin (N = 173)		
	Number	(%)	Number	(%)	
Early recurrence	32	(19)	14	(8)	
Late recurrence	22	(13)	5	(3)	
Total recurrence	54	(32)	19	(11)	

*Treatment groups compared by chi-square or Fisher's exact test as appropriate, 1-tailed probability.

From Pichichero ME, Disney FA, Talpey WB, et al: Adverse and beneficial effects of immediate treatment of Group A beta-hemolytic streptococcal pharyngitis with pencillin. Pediatr Infect Dis J 1987;6:635–643; and el-Daher NT, Hijazi SS, Rawashdeh NM, et al: Immediate vs. delayed treatment of Group A beta-hemolytic streptococcal pharyngitis with penicillin V. Pediatr Infect Dis J 1991;10:126–130.

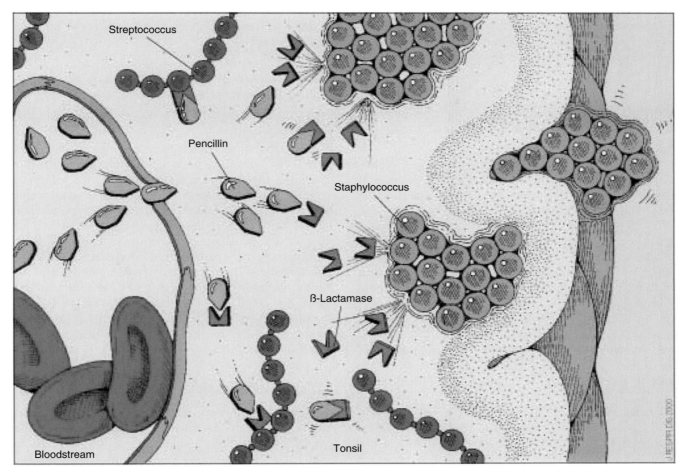

FIGURE 4–2. Penicillin may be inactivated by β-lactamase enzymes in the patient's throat. Along with the group A β-hemolytic streptococci (GABHS) that are causing the infection, a cocolonizing, nonpathogenic, β-lactamase-producing organism, such as *Staphylococcus aureus*, may be present. The copathogen or indirect pathogen prevents the penicillin molecule from reaching the GABHS, thus inactivating the agent and protecting the streptococci. (From Pichichero ME: What factors will influence treatment success? Streptococcal pharyngitis: Updating penicillin's role. Respir Dis 2000;4(2):179–186.)

Only indirect evidence supports the copathogen theory. Antibiotics that are β-lactamase stable usually are most effective at eradication of GABHS[158–160]; this is not a universal finding.[105,231] It is not necessary to eradicate the copathogens that produce β-lactamase. Rather, it is necessary for the antibiotic to remain active despite the presence of β-lactamase at the site of infection—the throat. Patients who have recurrent bouts of GABHS tonsillopharyngitis or in whom penicillin fails to eradicate GABHS might be colonized with copathogens. Selecting an alternative antibiotic that is β-lactamase stable in some cases proves an important therapeutic strategy.

Alteration of Microbial Ecology

Eradication of the normal flora, especially α-hemolytic streptococci, may enhance the susceptibility of patients to subsequent infection with GABHS; their presence has been shown to be associated with resistance to GABHS infection.[232] Antibiotics may eradicate or suppress host indigenous bacterial flora. Such alterations may result in clinical superinfections, or the alterations may be subclinical, resulting in quantitative and qualitative changes in the oropharyngeal ecosystem. Penicillin and amoxicillin treatment significantly decrease α-hemolytic streptococci in the throat, and thereby the ecologic balance is disturbed. These effects can persist weeks after therapy is completed. Elimination of α-streptococci from the throat eliminates their ability to produce bacteriocins, which are part of the natural host resistance to GABHS colonization. Cephalosporins and macrolides have lesser impact on the α-streptococci throat population, because these antibiotics are less active against these bacteria. Throat gargles of live α-streptococci possibly can prevent GABHS infection, particularly relapse or recurrent disease.[233,234]

Streptococcal Carriage

GABHS carriage is likely when a patient has a positive GABHS throat culture but shows neither symptoms nor a demonstrable rise in streptococcal titers. Unfortunately, early initiation of antibiotic therapy prevents an antibody response following GABHS infection, thereby clouding the detection of carriers. Moreover, the absence of an antibody response does not rule out a bona fide GABHS infection if treatment has been given. Patients experiencing a relapse with the same strain of GABHS (a homologous serotype) soon after a primary infection often have milder or fewer symptoms of GABHS infection, which may not be remembered, even though such patients have been shown to demonstrate an antibody rise, thus identifying them as susceptible to ARF. Among well children seen in private ambulatory practice the GABHS carrier rate is 2% to 7%.[235]

Patients are contagious to others in the early stages of this carrier state. After a period of time (1 to 2 months) the carrier has diminished numbers of GABHS organisms in the tonsillopharynx, and transmissibility to others diminishes. High rates of GABHS carriage may account for increased penicillin failures in a semiclosed community. The presence of GABHS on throat culture or as detected through rapid diagnostic testing does not distinguish between the patient with bona fide GABHS tonsillopharyngitis at risk for ARF and the patient with an acute viral sore throat who happens to be a GABHS carrier. Asymptomatic GABHS carriage may persist despite intensive antibiotic treatment. Eradication of the GABHS carrier state is infrequently achievable with penicillin; clindamycin,[122–124] penicillin plus rifampin,[138,139] or cefprozil[236] is more effective.

GABHS Strain Differences

A significantly higher incidence of GABHS relapse following penicillin therapy has been described in patients harboring certain M typable strains (especially serotypes 3 and 12) than in patients harboring nontypable strains.[77]

Disadvantages and Advantages of Penicillin Alternatives

Alternatives to penicillin for the treatment of GABHS tonsillopharyngitis have a broader spectrum of activity than traditionally considered necessary for effective eradication of GABHS, and they are more expensive. Increased use of amoxicillin-clavulanate, macrolides, or cephalosporins for treatment of sore throat often results in better GABHS eradication and fewer recurrences (Table 4–16) but also has the potential to contribute further to the escalating problem of antibiotic resistance among respiratory pathogens. Consideration of all costs of antibiotic therapy must be viewed in the light of differing bacteriologic cure rates and other consequences. Penicillin continues to be highly effective in GABHS tonsillopharyngitis treatment if the patient has been ill for longer than 2 days or if the patient is a teenager or adult (Table 4–17).

Criteria for Evaluation of New Agents

Guidelines have been developed for future studies of new agents for the treatment of GABHS tonsillopharyngitis.[237] It has been recommended that the clinical and bacteriologic assessment of patients included in

TABLE 4–16 ■ Antibiotic Treatment Failures in Group A β-Hemolytic Streptococci Pharyngitis: Elmwood Pediatric Group, 1975–1996

Medication	Number of episodes treated	Patients with recurrence within 30 d (%)	Statistical difference vs. penicillin
Penicillin	1581	21.8	NA
Amoxicillin	140	16.8	$P = .24$
Macrolides	143	14	$P = .04$
Cephalosporins	254	8.6	$P < .001$

TABLE 4–17 ■ Variables Influencing Penicillin Treatment Outcome*

Patient variables	Total number treated	Successes (%)
Number of prior days ill		
< 2	193	64[†]
≥ 2	162	82[†]
Age (y)		
2–5	71	59[‡]
6–12	254	74[‡]
13–21	34	85[‡]

*At the Elmwood Pediatric Group from 1975 to 1996.
[†]$P = .001$ using the chi-square test and the trend test.
[‡]$P = .01$ using the chi-square test and the trend test.
From Pichichero ME, Marsocci SM, Murphy ML, et al: Incidence of streptococcal carriers in private pediatric practice. Arch Pediatr Adolesc Med 1999;153:624–628.

GABHS tonsillopharyngitis trials should provide for the following:

1. Bacteriologic identification of GABHS prior to initiation of therapy
2. Repeat GABHS throat cultures performed within 4 to 7 days after conclusion of therapy and at any time clinical symptoms recur (additional cultures of throat specimens are indicated for subjects receiving antibiotics with prolonged serum or tissue concentrations)
3. Documentation of a clinical response at 3 to 5 days after initiation of therapy
4. Subsequent evaluation at weekly intervals until the patient is asymptomatic and for monitoring for relapse of disease or poststreptococcal nonsuppurative sequelae
5. Retention of all isolates for serotyping if possible
6. Adequate evaluation of medication compliance

A serologic evaluation for antibody response to the GABHS infection is not viewed as essential.

Surgical Treatment

The use of tonsillectomy for patients with repeated episodes of GABHS throat infection has declined over the past 2 decades. In children with repeated episodes of culture-documented GABHS tonsillopharyngitis (six to seven laboratory confirmed GABHS infections in a single year or five episodes in each of 2 years), however, prospective study has demonstrated the benefit of tonsillectomy.[238]

BACTERIAL TRACHEITIS

Bacterial tracheitis is an uncommon but serious respiratory tract infection in children. It is characterized by inflammation of the subcricoid and subglottic trachea with the production of copious and tenacious purulent secretions that can lead to sudden onset of airway obstruction. Varied terminology has been used to describe this entity, including membranous croup, pseudomembranous croup, bacterial croup, bacterial laryngotracheal pneumonia, and "membranous laryngotracheobronchitis. In 1979, Han et al,[239] and Jones et al[240] coined the term bacterial tracheitis.

Bacterial tracheitis is almost always a complication of viral laryngotracheobronchitis. The patient with bacterial tracheitis usually has a waning viral respiratory illness (e.g., croup, influenza, measles) when fever rises and stridor increases or worsens abruptly. *S. aureus* is the organism most commonly cultured from the trachea, followed by *H. influenzae*, α-hemolytic streptococci, and *Moraxella catarrhalis*.[240–243] Viruses also have been cultured from patients with bacterial tracheitis. The most common viruses recovered are parainfluenzae and influenzae viruses.[239,243–245] When anaerobic cultures are obtained from patients with bacterial pharyngitis, anaerobic bacteria can be isolated.[246]

Treatment of patients with bacterial tracheitis centers around airway management and the treatment of the bacterial infection. In most patients with bacterial tracheitis, progression of airway occlusion is rapid, and the need for bronchoscopy is urgent, both to confirm the diagnosis and to remove purulent material in the semiadherent membranes while an airway is secured. Endotracheal intubation with meticulous maintenance of the artificial airway and suctioning of the abundant tracheal secretion is required.

Antibiotic therapy is recommended in all patients and initially should be directed against the pathogens most commonly implicated. Cefuroxime (100 to 150 mg/kg/d IV divided every 8 hours) is an appropriate initial choice, although if the Gram stain of the tracheal secretions shows only gram-positive cocci, nafcillin or vancomycin may be appropriate. Once the tracheal cultures have returned, empiric therapy can be altered to cover the specific pathogen causing the bacterial tracheitis. Antimicrobial therapy in the immunocompromised host should be of broad spectrum to cover a wide range of pathogens including gram-negative bacilli and fungi.

The role of racemic epinephrine aerosols in the treatment of bacterial tracheitis is unclear. Many studies have found racemic epinephrine aerosols to be of no benefit in patients with bacterial tracheitis.[240,242,247,248] The lack of response to racemic epinephrine aerosols may be helpful in differentiating bacterial tracheitis from viral laryngotracheobronchitis. Others have found that racemic epinephrine aerosols may temporarily relieve respiratory distress but do not alter the course of bacterial tracheitis.[248]

There is little data on the use of glucocorticoids in bacterial tracheitis. In two series, dexamethasone was used almost exclusively to facilitate endotracheal extubation and not to help decrease the subglottic swelling that occurs in patients with bacterial tracheitis.[241,249]

With the resurgence of diphtheria in Russia, one must consider diphtheria as a possible cause of bacterial tracheitis. Infection with toxin-producing strains of diphtheria may produce systemic complications, particularly cardiac and central nervous system symptoms.[250] Appropriate therapy for diphtheria includes antitoxin and antibiotics. The only available antitoxin is of equine origin. The dosage of antitoxin is empiric, depending on the site and extent of infection. A dose ranging from 40,000 units to 120,000 units is used, with patients with more severe and extensive infections receiving the higher dose. The antitoxin is given as a one time single dose to avoid risking sensitization from repeated doses of horse serum. Penicillin and erythromycin are both effective against most strains of *C. diphtheriae*. Penicillin is given as aqueous procaine penicillin G 600,000 units intramuscularly once daily for 7 days. Patients who are allergic to penicillin can be treated with erythromycin in a dose of 40 mg/kg/d in four divided doses for 7 to 10 days. The end point of therapy is three consecutive negative cultures. Other possible choices of antibiotics include clindamycin, amoxicillin, and rifampin in appropriate dosages. The carrier state can be eradicated effectively with oral penicillin G or erythromycin. Parenteral therapy should be continued for the duration of intubation or for several days after the patient's fever has subsided. Oral antimicrobials may be used to complete a course of therapy.

EPIGLOTTITIS

Epiglottitis is a rare infection in the United States today because of the efficacy of *H. influenzae* type b (Hib) conjugate vaccines. When epiglottitis occurs in a Hib-vaccinated person, organisms to consider in selecting treatment include Hib (because of vaccine failure), untypable *H. influenzae*,[251] *Streptococcus pneumoniae*,[252,253] *S. aureus*,[251,253,254] and group A, group B and group C streptococci.[255]

Epiglottitis is a medical emergency. Most deaths due to epiglottitis occur within the first few hours after clinical presentation. Once the diagnosis is suspected, the patient should be constantly attended by persons capable of securing an airway. Nasotracheal intubation has replaced tracheostomy as the airway of choice.[256–260]

Antibiotic treatment of epiglottitis is recommended; cefuroxime 100 to 150 mg/kg/d IV divided every 8 hours, ceftriaxone 50 mg/kg/d IV given once a day, and cefotaxime 150 mg/kg/d IV divided every 8 hours are the antibiotics of choice. If a bacterium is isolated from blood cultures or direct laryngeal cultures, adjustments in the antibiotic selection can be made. In a patient with suspected cephalosporin allergy, combination therapy with clindamycin and an aminoglycoside or a second-generation fluoroquinolone (e.g., levofloxacin, gatifloxacin, moxifloxacin) are appropriate alternatives. No controlled data exist regarding the duration of therapy, but a course of 7 to 10 days is usually recommended.[261] There are no controlled data to support the use of corticosteroids or racemic epinephrine.[261]

Household and close contact prophylaxis is recommended when Hib is the cause of epiglottitis.[262] Rifampin prophylaxis (20 mg/kg/d, max dose 600 mg/dose) is recommended for the index case and for all members of the patient contact group when there is at least one contact 4 years of age or younger in the contact group who is not immunized or incompletely immunized.[263]

ACUTE LARYNGOTRACHEITIS

Acute laryngotracheitis (croup) is a common upper respiratory tract infection in young children. Parainfluenza viruses types 1, 2, and 3 account for more than 65% of croup cases. Influenza A and B viruses, adenovirus, respiratory syncytial virus (RSV), and measles also cause croup.[265]

Treatment

Mist Treatment

The tradition of using cool mist for children with viral croup began in the 19th century when physicians observed that hot steam delivered at home alleviated the symptoms. Croup kettles gave way to croup tents. There are only two studies that have tested the efficacy of humidified air in patients with viral croup, and neither of them documented a significant benefit.[265,266] Both studies had small sample sizes, and therefore the results may not be representative. A comparison of nebulized racemic epinephrine with nebulized saline solution showed a statistically significant improvement in croup symptoms after administration of the saline solution.[267] Three mechanisms of action have been proposed to explain the potential beneficial effect of humidified air:

1. Humidified air moistens secretions and thereby facilitates clearance.[268]

2. The mist may activate mechanoreceptors in the larynx that produce a reflex slowing of respiratory flow rate.[269]
3. A feeling of comfort and reassurance provided to the child by the parent who holds him or her near the humidified air source may prevent hyperventilation and resulting anxiety.[268]

Humidified air treatment is not without its possible problems: (1) It can exacerbate wheezing in a child who is having bronchospasm associated with croup, and (2) mist tents separate children from observation by parents and nursing staff. The best way to provide humidified air is by a tube held in front of the patient by the parent. Children who are experiencing bronchospasm may have a trial of cool mist; however, if wheezing increases, the treatment should be discontinued.

Nebulized Racemic Epinephrine

Racemic epinephrine administered by nebulizer with or without intermittent positive pressure breathing is frequently used to treat croup.[270] Racemic epinephrine is a 1:1 mixture of the *d* and *l* isomers of epinephrine. It is an α-adrenergic stimulant that may decrease edema in the subglottic region.[271] Five prospective double-blind, placebo-controled studies have evaluated the efficacy of racemic epinephrine (0.25 and 0.75 mg in a 2.25% solution mixed with 3 ml of normal saline) in the treatment of croup (Table 4–18). Four of the five studies concluded that racemic epinephrine decreased airway obstruction. The active *l* form of epinephrine given alone or as the racemic mixture had the same beneficial and adverse effects.[272] This is of practical importance because racemic epinephrine is not readily available outside of the United States. The *l* isomer of epinephrine may irritate the respiratory tract because of the metabisulfite contained in the solution[273]; this problem can be alleviated by diluting *l*-epinephrine in normal saline for nebulization.

Following racemic epinephrine administration there is a significant decrease in airway obstruction within 30 minutes, and by 2 hours the patient usually returns to pretreatment baseline or better. Because of this rebound phenomenon, patients requiring racemic epinephrine should be observed for 3 to 4 hours after administration or hospitalized.[274–276] A patient may be safely sent home if after 3 to 4 hours of observation there is (1) no stridor at rest, (2) normal air entry, (3) normal color, and (4) normal level of consciousness, and one dose of dexamethasone (0.6 mg/kg PO or IM) has been given.[277–279]

Severe laryngeal obstruction is an indication for the use of racemic epinephrine before intubation is attempted. Its use is also recommended in patients who have severe respiratory retractions because it may provide temporary relief while the arrival of someone skilled at intubation is awaited. Administration of nebulized racemic epinephrine to children with croup who do not have signs of respiratory distress is unnecessary.

Glucocorticoids

Systemic corticosteroids are recommended in patients with moderate or severe croup; they exert beneficial effects by decreasing edema of the laryngeal mucosa by their anti-inflammatory action. Clinical improvement is usually apparent 6 hours after treatment is started.[280]

Although various glucocorticoids have been used in treating croup, most studies have used dexamethasone or budesonide (Table 4–19). Dexamethasone is one of the most potent glucocorticoids, and it is long acting with a biologic half-life ranging from 36 to 72 hours.[281] It can be administered either by mouth or parenterally.

Dexamethasone (0.3 to 0.6 mg/kg PO or IM as a single dose) decreases (1) the severity of symptoms in the treated group as compared with those who receive placebo,[282–284] (2) the need for subsequent treatments with nebulized racemic epinephrine,[283] (3) the number of patients admitted to hospital after observation in the emergency department,[285] (4) the number of patients

TABLE 4–18 ■ **Double-Blind Randomized Trials of the Use of Epinephrine in the Treatment of Viral Croup**

Year	Investigators	Dose	Method of delivery	Significant effect*
1973	Gardner et al[307]	0.5 ml 2.25% racemic epinephrine in 3.5 ml NS	Nebulizer	–
1975	Taussig et al[274]	0.25 ml 2.25% racemic epinephrine in 1.5–2.75 ml NS, depending on weight	IPPB	+ at 10 min – at 2 h
1978	Westley et al[308]	0.5 ml 2.25% racemic epinephrine in 3.5 ml NS	IPPB	+ at 10 and 30 min – at 2 h
1982	Fogel et al[375]	0.25 ml 2.25% racemic epinephrine in 2 ml NS	IPPB vs. nebulizer	+
1988	Kuusela and Vesikari[280]	0.25 ml /5 kg body weight of 2.25% racemic epinephrine by nebulizer	IPPB	+

IPPB, intermittent positive pressure breathing; NS, normal saline solution.
*The effect of epinephrine in the treatment of viral croup had a positive (plus sign) or negative (minus sign) outcome.

TABLE 4–19 ■ **Studies of Corticosteroids in the Treatment of Croup**

Year	Study	No. patients	Setting	Intervention	Control	Outcomes	Clinical effect
1973	Massicotte et al[309]	42	Hospital	IV methylprednisolone 4 mg at 0, 4, and 8 h	Placebo	Clinical improvement, use of antibiotics, and tracheostomy	+
1992	Tibballs et al[295]	73	ICU (intubated patients)	NG prednisolone 2 mg/kg/d until 24 h after extubation	Placebo	Length of intubation, reintubation rate	+
1964	Eden & Larkin[310,311]	50	Hospital	IM methylprednisolone 4 mg/kg/d, 1 mg/kg Q6° × 24°	Placebo	Clinical improvement, use of mist tent, and antibiotics	No difference
1995	Cruz et al[284]	45	ED	IM dexamethasone 0.6 mg/kg	Placebo	Clinical improvement, MD visits, hospital admissions	+
1967	Eden et al[311]	50	Hospital	IM dexamethasone 0.1 mg/kg Q6° × 48°	Placebo	Stridor, dyspnea, retractions, and cyanosis	No difference
1969	James[312]	88	Hospital	IM dexamethasone 4–12 mg	Placebo	Use of mist tent, antibiotics, and tracheostomy	+
1979	Leipzig et al[313]	30	Hospital	IM dexamethasone 0.3 mg/kg/dose for two doses	Placebo	Stridor, cyanosis, retractions, respiratory rate, heart rate; use of epinephrine and intubation, length of stay	+
1993	Martinez[314]	66	Hospital	l-epinephrine l-epinephrine and IM dexamethasone 0.5 mg/kg, IM dexamethasone, 0.5 mg/kg	Placebo	Stridor, dyspnea, cough and cyanosis; use of mist tent	+
1966	Skowron[315]	200	Hospital	SC dexamethasone 4 or 6 mg	Placebo	Use of mist tent, antibiotics, and tracheostomy	+ No difference between doses
1989	Super et al[283]	29	Hospital	IM dexamethasone 0.6 mg/kg	Placebo	Westley croup score, clinical improvement, use of epinephrine, steroids, and mist tent; length of stay	+
1995	Geelhoed & Macdonald[284]	60	ED	PO dexamethasone 0.6 mg/kg	PO dexamethasone 0.3 mg/kg	Stridor and retractions, use of epinephrine, length of stay, admission	+ Equal effect
1995	Geelhoed & Macdonald[286]	60	ED	PO dexamethasone 0.3 mg/kg	PO dexamethasone, 0.15 mg/kg	Stridor and retractions, use of epinephrine, length of stay, admission	+ Equal effect
1996	Geelhoed et al[316]	100	ED	PO dexamethasone 0.15 mg/kg	Placebo	Return to ED for symptoms of croup	+
1982	Muhlendahl et al[315]	406	Hospital	PO dexamethasone 6 mg	Placebo	Westley croup score, clinical improvement, use of tracheostomy	+
2000	Rittichier & Ledwith[287]	277	ED	PO dexamethasone 0.6 mg/kg	IM dexamethasone 0.6 mg/kg	Resolution of symptoms and need for further evaluation	+

TABLE 4–19 ■ Studies of Corticosteroids in the Treatment of Croup (*Continued*)

Year	Study	No. patients	Setting	Intervention	Control	Outcomes	Clinical effect
1996	Fitzgerald et al[318]	67	Hospital	Nebulized budesonide 2 mg	l-epineph-rine 4 mg	Westley croup score, use of epinephrine and steroids, length of hospital stay	+
1995	Geelhoed & Mac-donald[325]	80	ED	Nebulized budesonide 2 mg PO dexamethas-one 0.6 mg/kg	Placebo	Stridor and retractions, use of epinephrine, length of stay in observation unit	+ Budesonide = dexa-metha-sone
1996	Johnson et al[320]	55	ED	Nebulized dexamethasone 10-20 mg	Placebo	Modified Westley croup score, use of mist tent and epinephrine admission rate	+ @4 hrs − at 12–24 hrs
1997	Godden et al[321]	87	Hospital	Nebulized budesonide, 2 mg initially, then 1 mg every 12 h during hospitalization	Placebo	Modified Westley croup score, use of epinephrine and intubation, length of stay	+
1993	Husby et al[291]	36	Hospital	Nebulized budesonide, 2 mg/dose for two doses 30 min apart	Placebo	Modified Westley croup score, use of antibiotics	+
1998	Johnson et al[322]	144	ED	Nebulized budesonide, 4 mg IM dexamethasone, 0.6 mg/kg	Placebo	Westley croup score, use of epinephrine and mist tent, admission rates	+ Budesonide
1998	Klassen et al[323]	198	ED	PO dexamethasone, 0.6 mg/kg and nebulized placebo PO placebo and nebulized budesonide, 2 mg PO dexamethasone, 0.6 mg/kg and nebulized budesonide, 2 mg		Westley croup score, admission rate, time spent in ED, return visits to ED, ongoing symptoms at 1 week	+ No difference between treatment groups
1994	Klassen et al[283]	54	ED	Nebulized budesonide, 2 mg	Placebo	Westley croup score, use of epinephrine and steroids, length of stay, admission rates	+
1996	Klassen et al[292]	50	ED	Nebulized budesonide, 2 mg, and PO dexamethasone, 0.6 mg/kg	PO dexa-metha-sone, 0.6 mg/kg Nebulized placebo	Westley croup score, use of epinephrine and steroids, length of stay, admission rates	+ Bud + Dex > Dex + Placebo

ED, Emergency Department; MD, medical doctor; IM, intramuscular; PO, by mouth; IV, intravenous; SC, subcutaneous; NG, Nasogastric; ICU, intensive care unit.
The Westley croup scoring system uses clinical observations of 1, Level of consciousness; 2, Cyanosis; 3, Stridor; 4, Air entry; 5, Retractions to the severity of disease.

transferred to the intensive care unit,[285] (5) the number of children requiring intubation,[282,285] and (6) the duration of hospitalization or observation in the emergency department.[285,286]

Different doses and routes of administration for glucocorticoids have been proposed and evaluated in the treatment of croup. Dexamethasone 0.15 mg/kg may be as effective as 0.3 or 0.6 mg/kg in improving symptoms of mild-to-moderate croup.[286] Oral dexamethasone usually is as effective as intramuscular administration in the outpatient treatment of mild-to-moderate croup.[287] The use of systemic corticosteroids in the treatment of croup has few complications. There is a case report of one child who developed fungal laryngotracheitis (caused by *Candida albicans*) after an 8-day course of dexamethasone and antibiotics.[288]

Nebulized Corticosteroids

Budesonide, a synthetic glucocorticoid, has twice the potency of beclomethasone and a significantly lower bioavailability because of its hepatic first-pass clearance.[289] Only 1% to 5% of a nebulized dose is delivered to the periphery of the lungs.[290] Most of the drug is deposited in the upper airway, which is the point of maximal inflammation in the patient with croup.[291] Nebulized budesonide is used at a dose of 2 or 4 mg for all children, regardless of their weight.

Nebulized budesonide may be as effective as oral dexamethasone in the management of croup symptoms.[286] The addition of nebulized budesonide (2 mg dose) to a regimen of oral dexamethasone (0.6 mg/kg) for outpatients with croup may enhance recovery as compared with oral dexamethasone alone.[292] The beneficial effects of nebulized budesonide occur within 2 to 4 hours after treatment.[289,293] This rapid onset of action is in contrast to the rather slow onset of action of systemic steroids.[280]

In the past 2 decades enough evidence has developed to support the use of corticosteroids in the treatment of patients with moderate-to-severe croup and even in some patients with mild croup. In the absence of further evidence an oral dose of dexamethasone, probably 0.6 mg/kg, should be preferred because of its safety, efficacy, and cost. In a child who is vomiting, nebulized budesonide, 2 mg, or intramuscular dexamethasone, 0.6 mg/kg, might be preferable.

Management Algorithm for Viral Croup

The level of care given to patients with viral croup depends on the severity of their symptoms (Table 4–20). Children with mild croup, as defined by stridor with crying or excitement only and no signs of respiratory distress, can be managed at home. The mainstay of therapy is mist provided for 15 to 20 minutes in a steamy bathroom or exposure to cold air outside. A cool mist humidifier in the bedroom may prove useful as well. When seeing a patient with mild croup, one might consider giving a single dose of oral or intramuscular dexamethasone 0.15 mg/kg; additional doses are unnecessary because of dexamethasone's half-life. Croup of moderate severity, defined by stridor at rest and the presence of suprasternal, intercostal, or subcostal retractions, should be treated with nebulized racemic (or l-) epinephrine with or without an oral or intramuscular dose of dexamethasone (0.3 to 0.6 mg/kg) or budesonide (2 mg). Nebulized budesonide's rapid onset of action helps the clinician evaluate a child after therapy to determine disposition.

An oxygen saturation level should be checked before and after therapy to determine if the patient needs supplemental oxygen. A child with moderate croup needs to be observed for 3 to 4 hours after a treatment is given. When stridor at rest has resolved and signs of respiratory distress are much improved, the child may be sent home. If stridor at rest persists and signs of respiratory distress do not resolve or the child needs oxygen, hospital admission is recommended.

TABLE 4–20 ■ Management of Viral Croup

Severity of disease	Management
MILD CROUP Stridor with crying or excitement, no signs of respiratory distress	Mist treatments, 15–20 min in a steamy bathroom or exposure to cold air, cool mist humidifier in bedroom +/– PO dexamethasone 0.15 mg/kg once *or* IM dexamethasone 0.15 mg/kg once Discharge to home
MODERATE CROUP Stridor at rest, suprasternal, intercostal, or subcostal retractions present	Nebulized racemic epinephrine 0.5 ml of 2.25% (or equivalent dose of l-epinephrine) And/or PO or IM dexamethasone 0.3–0.6 mg/kg once And/or nebulized budesonide 2 mg Check oxygen saturation level Observation for 3–4 h in office or emergency department Discharge to home or admit to hospital
SEVERE CROUP Severe respiratory distress, markedly decreased air entry, oxygen requirement, altered level of consciousness	Nebulized racemic epinephrine or l-epinephrine (same dose as moderate croup, but dosed more frequently according to symptoms) Admit to intensive care unit +/– Trial of helium-oxygen IM dexamethasone 0.6 mg/kg *or* Prednisolone 1 mg/kg q 12 h PO or via nasogastric tube *or* IV Solu-Medrol 1 mg/kg q 12 h Endotracheal intubation

Patients with severe croup, as defined by severe respiratory distress, markedly decreased air entry, oxygen requirement, or an altered level of consciousness, need to be managed in a hospital. Frequent treatments with nebulized racemic epinephrine should be administered. Systemic corticosteroids (intramuscular dexamethasone, oral methylprednisolone, or intravenous Solu-Medrol) should be given. A trial of a mixture of helium and oxygen before intubation could be considered. Endotracheal intubation becomes necessary if the preceding treatments have not improved the severe respiratory distress.

Endotracheal Intubation

Patients with severe croup have severe respiratory distress with marked retractions, hypoxia, severely decreased air entry, and an altered level of consciousness. These patients need to be managed in the intensive care unit. The decision to intubate is based on clinical criteria of worsening respiratory status despite maximal medical management. Endotracheal intubation has replaced tracheotomy in the patient with severe croup requiring an artificial airway.[294] A tube with a diameter of 0.5 to 1 mm less than the predicted size of the trachea for the child's age is recommended.[271] Extubation can be considered when there is a significant air leak around the tube at a positive airway pressure of 25 cm H_2O. In children who are intubated for severe croup, prednisolone 1 mg/kg every 12 hours until 24 hours after extubation reduces the duration of intubation and the need for reintubation.[295]

Helium-Oxygen Mixture

An alternative therapy to forestall intubation in patients with severe croup is the use of a helium and oxygen blended air source (70% to 80% concentration of helium).[296,297] Helium is an inert nontoxic gas. Because of its low density and viscosity, it can move through the airways, causing less turbulence and with less resistance than oxygen alone meets. Thus the effort of the respiratory muscles, which must overcome the high resistance of the stenotic subglottic space, decreases significantly. Patients with severe airway obstruction from croup who breathe a mixture of helium and oxygen become more comfortable and may avoid intubation.

REFERENCES

1. Pichichero ME: Group A streptococcal tonsillopharyngitis: Cost-effective diagnosis and treatment. Ann Emerg Med 1995; 25(3):390–403.
2. Turner JC, Hayden GF, Kiselica D, et al: Association of group C beta-hemolytic streptococci with endemic pharyngitis among college students. JAMA 1990;264(20):2644–2647.
3. Cimolai N: Beta-hemolytic non-group A streptococci and pharyngitis. Am J Dis Child 1990;144(4):452–453.
4. Gerber MA, Randolph MF, Martin NJ, et al: Community-wide outbreak of group G streptococcal pharyngitis. Pediatrics 1991;87(5):598–603.
5. Cimolai N, Elford RW, Bryan L, et al: Do the beta-hemolytic non-group A streptococci cause pharyngitis? Rev Infect Dis 1988;10(3):587–601.
6. Hayden GF, Murphy TF, Hendley JO: Non-group A streptococci in the pharynx. Pathogens or innocent bystanders? Am J Dis Child 1989;143(7):794–797.
7. Weisner P, Tronca E, Banin P, et al: Clinical spectrum of pharyngeal gonococcal infection. N Engl J Med 1978;288:181–185.
8. Waagner D: Arcanobacterium haemolyticum: Biology of the organism and diseases in man. Pediatr Infect Dis J 1991;10:933–939.
9. Karpathios T, Drakonaki S, Zervoudaki A, et al: Arcanobacterium haemolyticum in children with presumed streptococcal pharyngotonsillitis or scarlet fever. J Pediatr 1992;121(5 Pt 1):735–737.
10. Thom DH, Grayston JT, Wang SP, et al: Chlamydia pneumoniae strain TWAR, Mycoplasma pneumoniae, and viral infections in acute respiratory disease in a university student health clinic population. Am J Epidemiol 1990;132(2):248–256.
11. Dajani A, Bisno A, Chung K, et al: Prevention of rheumatic fever. A statement for health professionals by the Committee on Rheumatic Fever Endocarditis and Kawasaki Disease of the Council on Cardiovascular Disease in the Young, the American Heart Association. Circulation 1988;78:1082–1086.
12. Betriu C, Sanchez A, Gomez M, et al: Antibiotic susceptibility of group A streptococci: A 6-year follow-up study. Antimicrob Agents Chemother 1993;37(8):1717–1719.
13. Coonan KM, Kaplan EL: In vitro susceptibility of recent North American group A streptococcal isolates to eleven oral antibiotics. Pediatr Infect Dis J 1994;13(7):630–635.
14. Horn DL, Zabriskie JB, Austrian R, et al: Why have group A streptococci remained susceptible to penicillin? Report on a symposium. Clin Infect Dis 1998;26(6):1341–1345.
15. Kaplan EL, Johnson DR, Del Rosario MC, Horn DL: Susceptibility of group A beta-hemolytic streptococci to thirteen antibiotics: Examination of 301 strains isolated in the United States between 1994 and 1997. Pediatr Infect Dis J 1999;18(12):1069–1072.
16. Wittler RR, Yamada SM, Bass JW, et al: Penicillin tolerance and erythromycin resistance of group A beta-hemolytic streptococci in Hawaii and the Philippines. Am J Dis Child 1990;144(5):587–589.
17. Stingemore N, Francis GR, Toohey M, McGechie DB: The emergence of erythromycin resistance in Streptococcus pyogenes in Fremantle, Western Australia. Med J Aust 1989;150(11):626–631.
18. Holmstrom L, Nyman B, Rosengren M, et al: Outbreaks of infections with erythromycin-resistant group A streptococci in child day care centres. Scand J Infect Dis 1990;22(2):179–185.
19. Phillips G, Parratt D, Orange GV, et al: Erythromycin-resistant Streptococcus pyogenes. J Antimicrob Chemother 1990; 25(4):723–724.
20. Seppala H, Nissinen A, Jarvinen H, et al: Resistance to erythromycin in group A streptococci. N Engl J Med 1992; 326(5):292–297.
21. Seppala H, Klaukka T, Lehtonen R, et al: Outpatient use of erythromycin: Link to increased erythromycin resistance in group A streptococci. Clin Infect Dis 1995;21(6):1378–1385.
22. Seppala H, Klaukka T, Vuopio-Varkila J, et al: The effect of changes in the consumption of macrolide antibiotics on erythromycin resistance in group A streptococci in Finland. Finnish Study Group for Antimicrobial Resistance. N Engl J Med 1997;337(7):441–446.
23. Dajani A, Taubert K, Ferrieri P, et al: Treatment of acute streptococcal pharyngitis and prevention of rheumatic fever: A statement for health professionals. Committee on Rheumatic Fever, Endocarditis, and Kawasaki Disease of the Council on Cardiovascular Disease in the Young, the American Heart Association. Pediatrics 1995;96(4 Pt 1):758–764.

24. Carlson P, Korpela J, Walder M, Nyman M: Antimicrobial susceptibilities and biotypes of *Arcanobacterium haemolyticum* blood isolates. Eur J Clin Microbiol Infect Dis 1999; 18(12):915–917.

25. Asselt GV, Mouton R: Detection of penicillin tolerance in *Streptococcus pyogenes.* J Med Microbiol 1993;38:197–202.

26. Handwerger S, Tomasz A: Antibiotic tolerance among clinical isolates of bacteria. Rev Infect Dis 1985;7(3):368–386.

27. Sherris JC: Problems in in vitro determination of antibiotic tolerance in clinical isolates. Antimicrob Agents Chemother 1986;30(5):633–637.

28. Stratton C, Cooksey R: Susceptibility tests. In Balows A, Herriman KL, Isenberg HD, Shadomy HJ (eds): Manual of Clinical Microbiology, 5th ed. Washington DC, American Society of Microbiology, 1991, pp 1153–1165.

29. Kim KS, Anthony BF: Use of penicillin-gradient and replicate plates for the demonstration of tolerance to penicillin in streptococci. J Infect Dis 1983;148(3):488–491.

30. Kim KS, Kaplan EL: Association of penicillin tolerance with failure to eradicate group A streptococci from patients with pharyngitis. J Pediatr 1985;107(5):681–684.

31. Michel MF, van Leeuwen WB: Degree and stability of tolerance to penicillin in *Streptococcus pyogenes.* Eur J Clin Microbiol Infect Dis 1989;8(3):225–232.

32. Betriu C, Campos E, Cabronero C, et al: Penicillin tolerance of group A streptococci. Eur J Clin Microbiol Infect Dis 1989;8(9):799–800.

33. Krasinski K, Hanna B, LaRussa P, Desiderio D: Penicillin tolerant group A streptococci. Diagn Microbiol Infect Dis 1986;4(4):291–297.

34. Stjernquist-Desatnik A, Orrling A, Schalen C, Kamme C: Penicillin tolerance in group A streptococci and treatment failure in streptococcal tonsillitis. Acta Otolaryngol Suppl 1992;492:68–71.

35. Grahn E, Holm SE, Roos K: Penicillin tolerance in beta-streptococci isolated from patients with tonsillitis. Scand J Infect Dis 1987;19(4):421–426.

36. Dagan R, Ferne M, Sheinis M, et al: An epidemic of penicillin-tolerant group A streptococcal pharyngitis in children living in a closed community: Mass treatment with erythromycin. J Infect Dis 1987;156(3):514–516.

37. Dagan R, Ferne M: Association of penicillin-tolerant streptococci with epidemics of streptococcal pharyngitis in closed communities. Eur J Clin Microbiol Infect Dis 1989; 8(7):629–631.

38. Brink W, Rammelkamp C, Denny F, et al: Effect of penicillin and aureomycin on natural course of streptococcal tonsillitis and pharyngitis. Am J Med 1951;10:300–308.

39. Denny FW, Wannamaker LW, Hahn ED, et al: Comparative effects of penicillin, aureomycin, and terramycin on streptococcal tonsillitis and pharyngitis. Pediatrics 1953;11:7–14.

40. Peter G, Smith AL: Group A streptococcal infections of the skin and pharynx. N Engl J Med 1977;297(7):365–370.

41. Nelson JD: The effect of penicillin therapy on the symptoms and signs of streptococcal pharyngitis. Pediatr Infect Dis 1984;3(1):10–13.

42. Krober MS, Bass JW, Michels GN: Streptococcal pharyngitis. Placebo-controlled double-blind evaluation of clinical response to penicillin therapy. JAMA 1985; 253(9):1271–1274.

43. Randolph MF, Gerber MA, DeMeo KK, Wright L: Effect of antibiotic therapy on the clinical course of streptococcal pharyngitis. J Pediatr 1985;106(6):870–875.

44. Hall C, Breese B: Does penicillin make Johnny's strep throat better? Pediatr Infect Dis 1984;3:7–9.

45. Denny FW: Effect of treatment on streptococcal pharyngitis: Is the issue really settled? Pediatr Infect Dis 1985;4(4):352–354.

46. Pichichero ME, Disney FA, Talpey WB, et al: Adverse and beneficial effects of immediate treatment of group A beta-hemolytic streptococcal pharyngitis with penicillin. Pediatr Infect Dis J 1987;6(7):635–643.

47. Dagnelie CF, van der Graaf Y, De Melker RA: Do patients with sore throat benefit from penicillin? A randomized double-blind placebo-controlled clinical trial with penicillin V in general practice. Br J Gen Pract 1996;46(411):589–593.

48. Catanzaro FJ, Morris AL, et al: The role of the streptococcus in the pathogenesis of rheumatic fever. Am J Med 1954;17:749–755.

49. Snellman LW, Stang HJ, Stang JM, et al: Duration of positive throat cultures for group A streptococci after initiation of antibiotic therapy. Pediatrics 1993;91(6):1166–1170.

50. Breese B, Disney F: Factors influencing the spread of beta hemolytic streptococcal infections within the family group. Pediatrics 1956;17:834–838.

51. Denny FW, Wannamaker LW, Brink WR, et al: Prevention of rheumatic fever. Treatment of the preceding streptococcic infection. JAMA 1950;143:151–153.

52. Wannamaker LW, Rammelkamp CH, Denny FW, et al: Prophylaxis of acute rheumatic fever: By treatment of preceding pharyngitis with various amounts of depot penicillin. Am J Med 1951;10:673–695.

53. Adam D, Scholz H, Helmerking M: Short-course antibiotic treatment of 4782 culture-proven cases of group A streptococcal tonsillopharyngitis and incidence of poststreptococcal sequelae. J Infect Dis 2000;182(2):509–516.

54. Breese B, Disney F: The successful treatment of beta hemolytic streptococcal infections in children with a single injection of repository penicillin (benzathine penicillin G). Pediatrics 1955;15:516–521.

55. Stollerman G, Rusoff J: Prophylaxis against group A streptococcal infections in rheumatic fever patients. Use of new repository penicillin preparation. JAMA 1952; 150:1571–1575.

56. Diehl A, Hamilton T, Keeling I, May J: Long-acting repository penicillin in prophylaxis of recurrent rheumatic fever. JAMA 1954;155:1466–1470.

57. Chamovitz R, Catanzaro F, Stetson C, Rammelkamp C: Prevention of rheumatic fever by treatment of previous streptococcal infections. I. Evaluation of benzathine penicillin G. N Engl J Med 1954;251:466–471.

58. Stollerman G, Rusoff J, Hirschfeld I: Prophylaxis against group A streptococcal in rheumatic fever. The use of single monthly injections of benzathine penicillin G. N Engl J Med 1955;252:787–792.

59. Breese B, Disney F, Talpey W: Improvement in local tolerance and therapeutic effectiveness of benzathine penicillin. Am J Dis Child 1960;99:149–154.

60. Pichichero M: Antimicrobials for the treatment of beta-hemolytic streptococcal pharyngitis. In Tandy RRK, Narula J (eds): Rheumatic Fever. New York, Oxford University Press, 1997.

61. Wannamaker L, Denny F, Perry W, et al: The effect of penicillin prophylaxis on streptococcal disease rates and the carrier state. N Engl J Med 1953;249:1–7.

62. Breese B: Treatment of beta hemolytic streptococcic infections in the home. JAMA 1953;152:10–14.

63. Breese B, Disney F: A comparison of intramuscular and oral benzathine penicillin G in the treatment of streptococcal infections in children. J Pediatr 1957;51:157–163.

64. Breese B, Disney F: Penicillin in the treatment of streptococcal infections. A comparison of effectiveness of five different oral and one parenteral form. N Engl J Med 1958;259:57–62.

65. Stillerman M, Bernstein S, Smith M, et al: Antibiotics in the treatment of beta-hemolytic streptococcal pharyngitis: Factors influencing the results. Pediatrics 1960;25:27–34.

66. Colcher I, Bass J: Penicillin treatment of streptococcal pharyngitis: A comparison of schedules and the role of specific counseling. JAMA 1972;222:657–659.

67. Mohler D, Wallin D, Dreyfus E, Bakst H: Studies in the home treatment of streptococcal disease. II. A comparison of the efficacy of oral administration of penicillin and intramuscular injection of benzathine penicillin in the treatment of streptococcal pharyngitis. N Engl J Med 1956;254:45–50.

68. Markowitz M, Ferencz C, Bonet A: A comparison of oral and intramuscular benzathine penicillin G for the prevention of streptococcal infections and recurrences of rheumatic fever. Pediatrics 1957;191:201–207.

69. Miller J, Stancer S, Massell B: A controlled study of beta hemolytic streptococcal infection in rheumatic families. I. Streptococcal disease among healthy siblings. Am J Med 1958;25:825–844.

70. Stillerman M: Comparison of cephaloglycin and penicillin in streptococcal pharyngitis. Clin Pharmacol Ther 1969;11:205–213.

71. Howie V, Ploussard J: Treatment of group A streptococcal pharyngitis in children. Comparison of lincomycin and penicillin G given orally and benzathine G given intramuscularly. Am J Dis Child 1971;121:477–480.

72. Shapera RM, Hable KA, Matsen JM: Erythromycin therapy twice daily for streptococcal pharyngitis. Controlled comparison with erythromycin or penicillin phenoxymethyl four times daily or penicillin G benzathine. JAMA 1973;226(5):531–535.

73. Lester RL, Howie VM, Ploussard JH: Treatment of streptococcal pharyngitis with different antibiotic regimens. Clin Pediatr (Phila) 1974;13(3):239–242.

74. Matsen JM, Torstenson O, Siegel SE, Bacaner H: Use of available dosage forms of cephalexin in clinical comparison with phenoxymethyl penicillin and benzathine penicillin in the treatment of streptococcal pharyngitis in children. Antimicrob Agents Chemother 1974;6(4):501–506.

75. Ginsburg CM, McCracken GH Jr, Steinberg JB, et al: Treatment of group A streptococcal pharyngitis in children. Results of a prospective, randomized study of four antimicrobial agents. Clin Pediatr (Phila) 1982;21(2):83–88.

76. Breese B, Disney F, Talpey W: Penicillin in streptococcal infections—total dose and frequency of administration. Am J Dis Child 1965;110:125–130.

77. Stillerman M, Bernstein S: Streptococcal pharyngitis therapy. Am J Dis Child 1964;107:73–84.

78. Breese B, Disney F: Penicillin V treatment of beta-hemolytic streptococcal infections in chldren. Arch Dis Child 1956;92:20–23.

79. Schalet N, Reen B, Houser H: A comparison of penicillin G and penicillin B in treatment of streptococcal sore throat. Am J Med Sci 1958;235:183–188.

80. Breese B, Disney F, Talpey W: Beta-hemolytic streptococcal infections in children. Comparison of the therapeutic effectiveness of potassium penicillin G, tetracycline phosphate complex, and dimethylchlortetracycline. Am J Dis Child 1964;107:232–239.

81. Rosenstein B, Markowitz M, Goldstein E, et al: Factors involved in treatment failures following oral penicillin therapy of streptococcal pharyngitis. J Pediatr 1968;73:513–520.

82. Vann RL, Harris BA: Twice a day penicillin therapy for streptococcal upper respiratory infections. South Med J 1972;65(2):203–205.

83. Stillerman M, Isenberg HD, Facklam RR: Streptococcal pharyngitis therapy: Comparison of clindamycin palmitate and potassium phenoxymethyl penicillin. Antimicrob Agents Chemother 1973;4(5):514–520.

84. Spitzer TQ, Harris BA: Penicillin V therapy for streptococcal pharyngitis: Comparison of dosage schedules. South Med J 1977;70(1):41–42.

85. Gerber MA, Spadaccini LJ, Wright LL, et al: Twice-daily penicillin in the treatment of streptococcal pharyngitis. Am J Dis Child 1985;139(11):1145–1148.

86. Gerber MA, Randolph MF, DeMeo K, et al: Failure of once-daily penicillin V therapy for streptococcal pharyngitis. Am J Dis Child 1989;143(2):153–155.

87. Krober MS, Weir MR, Themelis NJ, van Hamont JE: Optimal dosing interval for penicillin treatment of streptococcal pharyngitis. Clin Pediatr (Phila) 1990;29(11):646–648.

88. Breese B, Disney F, Talpey W: The comparative ineffectiveness of nafcillin (a new antistaphylococcal drug) against beta hemolytic streptococcal infections in children. Clin Pharmacol Ther 1964;5:156–158.

89. Markowitz M: Sodium nafcillin in the treatment of group A streptococcal infections. J Pediatr 1967;71:918–919.

90. Stillerman M, Isenberg H, Bernstein S: Cloxacillin in streptococcal pharyngitis. Primary treatment and retreatment. Am J Dis Child 1966;112:408–411.

91. Aronovitz G, Morgan D, Spitzer T: Streptococcal infection in pediatric patients. Am J Dis Child 1968;116:66–69.

92. Breese B, Disney F, Talpey W: Beta-hemolytic streptococcal illness. Comparison of lincomycin, ampicilln, and potassium penicillin G in treatment. Am J Dis Child 1966;112:21–27.

93. Strom J: A comparison of the effects and side-effects of penicillin V and ampicillin in the treatment of scarlet fever. Acta Paediatr Scand 1968;57(4):285–288.

94. Stillerman M, Isenberg HD, Moody M: Streptococcal pharyngitis therapy. Comparison of cephalexin, phenoxymethyl penicillin, and ampicillin. Am J Dis Child 1972;123(5):457–461.

95. Stillerman M, Isenberg HD, Facklam RR: Treatment of pharyngitis associated with group A streptococcus: Comparison of amoxicillin and potassium phenoxymethyl penicillin. J Infect Dis 1974;129(Suppl):S169–S177.

96. Breese BB, Disney FA, Talpey WB, Green JL: Treatment of streptococcal pharyngitis with amoxicillin. J Infect Dis 1974;129(Suppl):S178–S180.

97. Breese BB, Disney FA, Green JL, Talpey WB: The treatment of beta hemolytic streptococcal pharyngitis. Comparison of amoxicillin, erythromycin estolate, and penicillin V. Clin Pediatr (Phila) 1977;16(5):460–463.

98. Shvartzman P, Tabenkin H, Rosentzwaig A, Dolginov F: Treatment of streptococcal pharyngitis with amoxycillin once a day. BMJ 1993;306(6886):1170–1172.

99. Rantz L, Maroney M, DiCaprio J: Hemolytic streptococcal infections in childhood. Pediatrics 1953;12:498–515.

100. Andrew J, Lan M, Colford JM: The impact of dosing frequency on the efficacy of 10-day penicillin or amoxicillin therapy for streptococcal tonsillopharyngitis: A meta-analysis. Pediatrics 2000;105(2):e19.

101. Feder HM Jr, Gerber MA, Randolph MF, et al: Once-daily therapy for streptococcal pharyngitis with amoxicillin. Pediatrics 1999;103(1):47–51.

102. Smith TD, Huskins WC, Kim KS, Kaplan EL: Efficacy of beta-lactamase-resistant penicillin and influence of penicillin tolerance in eradicating streptococci from the pharynx after failure of penicillin therapy for group A streptococcal pharyngitis. J Pediatr 1987;110(5):777–782.

103. Kaplan EL, Johnson DR: Eradication of group A streptococci from the upper respiratory tract by amoxicillin with clavulanate after oral penicillin V treatment failure. J Pediatr 1988;113(2):400–403.

104. Brook I: Treatment of patients with acute recurrent tonsillitis due to group A beta-haemolytic streptococci: A prospective randomized study comparing penicillin and amoxycillin/clavulanate potassium. J Antimicrob Chemother 1989;24(2):227–233.

105. Tanz RR, Shulman ST, Sroka PA, et al: Lack of influence of beta-lactamase-producing flora on recovery of group A

streptococci after treatment of acute pharyngitis. J Pediatr 1990;117(6):859–863.

106. Howie VM, Ploussard JH: Compliance dose-response relationships in streptococcal pharyngitis. Am J Dis Child 1972;123(1):18–25.

107. Breese BB, Disney F, Talpey W: Triacetyloleandomycin—a substitute for penicillin G. A comparison of the therapeutic effectiveness of triacetyloleandomycin, erythromycin propionate, and oral penicillin G in the treatment of beta hemolytic streptococcal infections. Am J Dis Child 1961;101:423–428.

108. Stillerman M, Bernstein S, Smith M, Gorvoy J. Erythromycin propionate and potassium penicillin V in the treatment of group A streptococcal pharyngitis. Pediatrics 1963;31:22–28.

109. Moffet H, Cramblett H, Black J, et al: Erythromycin estolate and phenoxymethyl penicillin in the treatment of streptococcal pharyngitis. Antimicrob Agents Chemother 1963;3:759–764.

110. Hughes WT, Collier RN: Streptococcal pharyngitis. Evaluation of erythromycin, erythromycin-sulfas, and sulfamethoxazole (possible antagonism between erythromycin and sulfas). Am J Dis Child 1969;118(5):700–707.

111. Levine M, Berman J: A comparison of clindamycin and erythromycin in beta-hemolytic streptococcal infections. J Med Assoc Ga 1972;61:108–111.

112. Ryan D, Dreher G, Hurst J: Estolate and stearate forms of erythromycin in the treatment of acute beta hemolytic streptococcal pharyngitis. Med J Aust 1973;1:20–21.

113. Breese BB, Disney FA, Talpey W, et al: Streptococcal infections in children. Comparison of the therapeutic effectiveness of erythromycin administered twice daily with erythromycin, penicillin phenoxymethyl, and clindamycin administered three times daily. Am J Dis Child 1974;128(4):457–460.

114. Janicki RS, Garnham JC, Worland MC, et al: Comparison of erythromycin ethylsuccinate, stearate and estolate treatments of group A streptococcal infections of the upper respiratory tract. Clin Pediatr (Phila) 1975;14(12):1098–1107.

115. Derrick CW, Dillon HC: Erythromycin therapy for streptococcal pharyngitis. Am J Dis Child 1976;130(2):175–198.

116. Derrick CW, Dillon HC, Jr: Streptococcal pharyngitis therapy. A comparison of two erythromycin formulations. Am J Dis Child 1979;133(11):1146–1148.

117. Ginsburg CM, McCracken GH Jr, Steinberg JB, et al: Management of group A streptococcal pharyngitis: A randomized controlled study of twice-daily erythromycin ethylsuccinate versus erythromycin estolate. Pediatr Infect Dis 1982;1(6):384–387.

118. Ginsburg CM, McCracken GH Jr, Crow SD, et al: Erythromycin therapy for group A streptococcal pharyngitis. Results of a comparative study of the estolate and ethylsuccinate formulations. Am J Dis Child 1984;138(6):536–539.

119. Disney F, Downton M, Higgins J, et al: Comparison of once-daily cefadroxil and four-times-daily erythromycin in group A streptococcal tonsillopharyngitis. Adv Ther 1990; 7:312–326.

120. Milatovic D: Evaluation of cefadroxil, penicillin and erythromycin in the treatment of streptococcal tonsillopharyngitis. Pediatr Infect Dis J 1991;10(10 Suppl):S61–S63.

121. Schaffer L, Finkelstein J, Hohn A, Djerassi I: Lincomycin—a new antibiotic. Studies in children carrying beta-hemolytic streptococci in association with acute pharyngitis, tonsillitis, or both. Clin Pediatr 1963;2:642–645.

122. Tanz RR, Poncher JR, Corydon KE, et al: Clindamycin treatment of chronic pharyngeal carriage of group A streptococci. J Pediatr 1991;119(1 [Pt 1]):123–128.

123. Brook I, Leyva F: The treatment of the carrier state of group A beta-hemolytic streptococci with clindamycin. Chemotherapy 1981;27(5):360–367.

124. Brook I, Hirokawa R: Treatment of patients with a history of recurrent tonsillitis due to group A beta-hemolytic streptococci. A prospective randomized study comparing penicillin, erythromycin, and clindamycin. Clin Pediatr (Phila) 1985; 24(6):331–336.

125. Scaglione F: Comparison of the clinical and bacteriological efficacy of clarithromycin and erythromycin in the treatment of streptococcal pharyngitis. Curr Med Res Opin 1990; 12:25–33.

126. Levenstein J: Clarithromycin versus penicillin in the treatment of streptococcal pharyngitis. J Antimicrob Chemother 1991;27:67–74.

127. Bachand RT Jr: A comparative study of clarithromycin and penicillin VK in the treatment of outpatients with streptococcal pharyngitis. J Antimicrob Chemother 1991;27(Suppl A):75–82.

128. Schrock C. Clarithromycin vs penicillin in the treatment of streptococcal pharyngitis. J Fam Pract 1992;35:622–626.

129. Still J, Hubbard W, Poole J, et al: Comparison of clarithromycin and penicillin VK suspensions in the treatment of children with streptococcal pharyngitis and review of currently available alternative antibiotic therapies. Pediatr Infect Dis J 1993;12:S134–S141.

130. Hooten T: A comparison of azithromycin and penicillin V for the treatment of streptococcal pharyngitis. Am J Med 1991;91(Suppl 3A):23S–26S.

131. Hamill J: Multicentre evaluation of azithromycin and penicillin V in the treatment of acute streptococcal pharyngitis and tonsillitis in children. J Antimicrob Chemother 1993;31(Suppl E):89–94.

132. Still J: Management of pediatric patients with group A beta-hemolytic streptococcus pharyngitis: Treatment options. Pediatr Infect Dis J 1995;14:S57–S61.

133. Pacifico L, Scopetti F, Ranucci A, et al: Comparative efficacy and safety of 3-day azithromycin and 10-day penicillin V treatment of group A beta-hemolytic streptococcal pharyngitis in children. Antimicrob Agents Chemother 1996;40(4):1005–1008.

134. Schaad UB, Heynen G: Evaluation of the efficacy, safety and toleration of azithromycin vs. penicillin V in the treatment of acute streptococcal pharyngitis in children: Results of a multicenter, open comparative study. The Swiss Tonsillopharyngitis Study Group. Pediatr Infect Dis J 1996;15(9):791–795.

135. Watkins VS, Smietana M, Conforti PM, et al: Comparison of dirithromycin and penicillin for treatment of streptococcal pharyngitis. Antimicrob Agents Chemother 1997;41(1):72–75.

136. Melcher G, Hadfield T, Gaines J, et al: Comparative efficacy and toxicity of roxithromycin and erythromycin in ethyl succinate in the treatment of streptococcal pharyngitis in adults. J Antimicrob Chemother 1988;22:549–556.

137. Morita JY, Kahn E, Thompson T, et al: Impact of azithromycin on oropharyngeal carriage of group A streptococcus and nasopharyngeal carriage of macrolide-resistant *Streptococcus pneumoniae*. Pediatr Infect Dis J 2000;19(1):41–66.

138. Chaudhary S, Bilinsky SA, Hennessy JL, et al: Penicillin V and rifampin for the treatment of group A streptococcal pharyngitis: A randomized trial of 10 days penicillin vs 10 days penicillin with rifampin during the final 4 days of therapy. J Pediatr 1985;106(3):481–486.

139. Tanz RR, Shulman ST, Barthel MJ, et al: Penicillin plus rifampin eradicates pharyngeal carriage of group A streptococci. J Pediatr 1985;106(6):876–880.

140. Stillerman M, Isenberg HD: Streptococcal pharyngitis therapy: Comparison of cyclacillin, cephalexin, and potassium penicillin V. Antimicrob Agents Chemother 1970;10:270–276.

141. Disney FA, Breese BB, Green JL, et al: Cephalexin and penicillin therapy of childhood beta-hemolytic streptococcal infections. Postgrad Med J 1971;47(Suppl):47–51.

142. Gau DW, Horn RF, Solomon RM, et al: Streptococcal tonsillitis in general practice. A comparison of cephalexin and penicillin therapy. Practitioner 1972;208(244):276–281.

143. Rabinovitch M, MacKenzie R, Brazeau M, Marks MI: Treatment of streptococcal pharyngitis. I. Clinical evaluation. Can Med Assoc J 1973;108(10):1271–1274.

144. Derrick CW, Dillon HC: Therapy for prevention of acute rheumatic fever. Circulation 1974;50:38.

145. Stillerman M: Cefatrizine and potassium phenoxymethyl penicllin in group A streptococcal pharyngitis. Antimicrob Agents Chemother 1976;16:185 (Abstract).

146. Disney FA, Breese BB, Francis AB, et al: The use of cefaclor in the treatment of beta-haemolytic streptococcal throat infections in children. Postgrad Med J 1979;55(Suppl 4):50–52.

147. Ginsburg CM, McCracken GH Jr, Crow SD, et al: A controlled comparative study of penicillin V and cefadroxil therapy of group A streptococcal tonsillopharyngitis. J Int Med Res 1980;8(Suppl):82–86.

148. Henness DM: A clinical experience with cefadroxil in upper respiratory tract infection. J Antimicrob Chemother 1982; 10(Suppl B):125–135.

149. Stillerman M: Comparison of oral cephalosporins with penicillin therapy for group A streptococcal pharyngitis. Pediatr Infect Dis 1986;5(6):649–654.

150. Gerber MA: A comparison of cefadroxil and penicillin V in the treatment of streptococcal pharyngitis in children. Drugs 1986;32(Suppl 3):29–32.

151. Gerber MA, Randolph MF, Chanatry J, et al: Once daily therapy for streptococcal pharyngitis with cefadroxil. J Pediatr 1986;109(3):531–537.

152. Pichichero ME, Disney FA, Aronovitz GH, et al: A multicenter, randomized, single-blind evaluation of cefuroxime axetil and phenoxymethyl penicillin in the treatment of streptococcal pharyngitis. Clin Pediatr (Phila) 1987;26(9):453–458.

153. Pichichero ME, Disney FA, Aronovitz GH, et al: Randomized, single-blind evaluation of cefadroxil and phenoxymethyl penicillin in the treatment of streptococcal pharyngitis. Antimicrob Agents Chemother 1987;31(6):903–906.

154. Gooch WM III, Swenson E, Higbee MD: Cefuroxime axetil and penicillin V compared in the treatment of group A beta-hemolytic streptococcal pharyngitis. Clin Ther 1987; 9(6):670–677.

155. Stromberg A, Schwan A, Cars O: Bacteriological and serological aspects of group A streptococcal pharyngotonsillitis caused by group A streptococci. Eur J Clin Microbiol Infect Dis 1988;7(2):172–174.

156. Stromberg A, Schwan A, Cars O: Five versus ten days treatment of group A streptococcal pharyngotonsillitis: A randomized controlled clinical trial with phenoxymethylpenicillin and cefadroxil. Scand J Infect Dis 1988;20(1):37–46.

157. Milatovic D, Knauer J: Cefadroxil versus penicillin in the treatment of streptococcal tonsillopharyngitis. Eur J Clin Microbiol Infect Dis 1989;8(4):282–288.

158. Pichichero ME, Margolis PA: A comparison of cephalosporins and penicillins in the treatment of group A beta-hemolytic streptococcal pharyngitis: A meta-analysis supporting the concept of microbial copathogenicity. Pediatr Infect Dis J 1991; 10(4):275–281.

159. Pichichero ME: Cephalosporins are superior to penicillin for treatment of streptococcal tonsillopharyngitis: Is the difference worth it? Pediatr Infect Dis J 1993;12(4):268–274.

160. Deeter RG, Kalman DL, Rogan MP, Chow SC: Therapy for pharyngitis and tonsillitis caused by group A beta-hemolytic streptococci: A meta-analysis comparing the efficacy and safety of cefadroxil monohydrate versus oral penicillin V. Clin Ther 1992;14(5):740–754.

161. Brown RJ, Batts DH, Hughes GS, Greenwald CA: Comparison of oral cefpodoxime proxetil and penicillin V potassium in the treatment of group A streptococcal pharyngitis/tonsillitis. The Cefpodoxime Pharyngitis Study Group. Clin Ther 1991;13(5):579–588.

162. Holm SE, Roos K, Stromberg A: A randomized study of treatment of streptococcal pharyngotonsillitis with cefadroxil or phenoxymethylpenicillin (penicillin V). Pediatr Infect Dis J 1991;10(10 Suppl):S68–S71.

163. Reed BD, Huck W, Zazove P: Treatment of beta-hemolytic streptococcal pharyngitis with cefaclor or penicillin. Efficacy and interaction with beta-lactamase-producing organisms in the pharynx. J Fam Pract 1991;32(2):138–144.

164. McCarty J, Hernon Y, Linn L, et al: Loracarbef versus penicillin VK in the treatment of streptococcal pharyngitis and tonsillitis in adults. Clin Ther 1992;14(1):30–40.

165. McCarty J: Loracarbef versus penicillin VK in the treatment of streptococcal pharyngitis and tonsillitis in an adult population. Am J Med 1992;92(6A):74S–79S.

166. Disney FA, Dillon H, Blumer JL, et al: Cephalexin and penicillin in the treatment of group A beta-hemolytic streptococcal throat infections. Am J Dis Child 1992; 146(11):1324–1327.

167. McCarty JM, Renteria A: Treatment of pharyngitis and tonsillitis with cefprozil: Review of three multicenter trials. Clin Infect Dis 1992;14(Suppl 2):S224–S232.

168. Ramet J, Pierard D, Vandenberghe P, De Boeck K: Comparative study of cefetamet pivoxil and penicillin V in the treatment of group A beta-hemolytic streptococcal pharyngitis. Chemotherapy 1992;38(Suppl 2):33–37.

169. Disney FA, Hanfling MJ, Hausinger SA: Loracarbef (LY163892) vs. penicillin VK in the treatment of streptococcal pharyngitis and tonsillitis. Pediatr Infect Dis J 1992; 11(8 Suppl):S20–S26.

170. Block SL, Hedrick JA, Tyler RD: Comparative study of the effectiveness of cefixime and penicillin V for the treatment of streptococcal pharyngitis in children and adolescents. Pediatr Infect Dis J 1992;11(11):919–925.

171. Muller O, Spirer Z, Wettich K: Loracarbef versus penicillin V in the treatment of streptococcal pharyngitis and tonsillitis. Infection 1992;20(5):301–308.

172. Dajani AS, Kessler SL, Mendelson R, et al: Cefpodoxime proxetil vs. penicillin V in pediatric streptococcal pharyngitis/tonsillitis. Pediatr Infect Dis J 1993;12(4):275–279.

173. Gooch WM III, McLinn SE, Aronovitz GH, et al: Efficacy of cefuroxime axetil suspension compared with that of penicillin V suspension in children with group A streptococcal pharyngitis. Antimicrob Agents Chemother 1993;37(2):159–163.

174. Milatovic D, Adam D, Hamilton H, Materman E: Cefprozil versus penicillin V in treatment of streptococcal tonsillopharyngitis. Antimicrob Agents Chemother 1993;37(8):1620–1623.

175. McCarty JM: Comparative efficacy and safety of cefprozil versus penicillin, cefaclor and erythromycin in the treatment of streptococcal pharyngitis and tonsillitis. Eur J Clin Microbiol Infect Dis 1994;13(10):846–850.

176. Pichichero ME, Gooch WM, Rodriguez W, et al: Effective short-course treatment of acute group A beta-hemolytic streptococcal tonsillopharyngitis. Ten days of penicillin V vs 5 days or 10 days of cefpodoxime therapy in children. Arch Pediatr Adolesc Med 1994;148(10):1053–1060.

177. Holm S, Henning C, Grahn E, et al: Is penicillin the appropriate treatment for recurrent tonsillopharyngitis? Results from a comparative randomized blind study of cefuroxime axetil and phenoxymethylpenicillin in children. The Swedish Study Group. Scand J Infect Dis 1995;27(3):221–228.

178. Pichichero ME, McLinn SE, Gooch WM III, et al: Ceftibuten vs. penicillin V in group A beta-hemolytic streptococcal pharyngitis. Members of the Ceftibuten Pharyngitis International Study Group. Pediatr Infect Dis J 1995;14 (7 Suppl):S102–S107.

179. Roos K, Larsson P: Loracarbef versus phenoxymethylpenicillin in the treatment of recurrent streptococcal pharyngotonsillitis. Scand J Infect Dis 1997;29(2):141–145.

180. Nemeth MA, McCarty J, Gooch WM III, et al: Comparison of cefdinir and penicillin for the treatment of streptococcal pharyngitis. Cefdinir Pharyngitis Study Group. Clin Ther 1999;21(11):1873–1881.

181. Kaplan EL: Benzathine penicillin G for treatment of group A streptococcal pharyngitis: A reappraisal in 1985. Pediatr Infect Dis 1985;4(5):592–596.

182. Pichichero ME: The rising incidence of penicillin treatment failures in group A streptococcal tonsillopharyngitis: An emerging role for the cephalosporins? Pediatr Infect Dis J 1991;10(10 Suppl):S50–S55.

183. Markowitz M, Gerber MA, Kaplan EL: Treatment of streptococcal pharyngotonsillitis: Reports of penicillin's demise are premature. J Pediatr 1993;123(5):679–685.

184. Pichichero ME, Green JL, Francis AB, et al: Recurrent group A streptococcal tonsillopharyngitis. Pediatr Infect Dis J 1998;17(9):809–815.

185. Stevens DL, Tanner MH, Winship J, et al: Severe group A streptococcal infections associated with a toxic shock-like syndrome and scarlet fever toxin A. N Engl J Med 1989;321(1):1–7.

186. Jackson MA, Burry VF, Olson LC: Multisystem group A beta-hemolytic streptococcal disease in children. Rev Infect Dis 1991;13(5):783–788.

187. Stevens DL: Invasive group A streptococcus infections. Clin Infect Dis 1992;14(1):2–11.

188. Rathore MH, Barton LL, Kaplan EL: Suppurative group A beta-hemolytic streptococcal infections in children. Pediatrics 1992;89(4 Pt 2):743–746.

189. Holm SE, Norrby A, Bergholm AM, Norgren M: Aspects of pathogenesis of serious group A streptococcal infections in Sweden, 1988–1989. J Infect Dis 1992;166(1):31–37.

190. Demers B, Simor AE, Vellend H, et al: Severe invasive group A streptococcal infections in Ontario, Canada: 1987–1991. Clin Infect Dis 1993;16(6):792–802.

191. Davies HD, Matlow A, Scriver SR, et al: Apparent lower rates of streptococcal toxic shock syndrome and lower mortality in children with invasive group A streptococcal infections compared with adults. Pediatr Infect Dis J 1994;13(1):49–56.

192. Bisno A, Stevens DL: Streptococcal infections of skin and soft tissue. N Engl J Med 1996;334(4):240–245.

193. American Academy of Pediatrics Committee on Infections Diseases: Severe and invasive group A streptococcal infections: A subject review. Pediatrics 1998;101(1):136–140.

194. Working Group on Prevention of Invasive Group A Streptococcal Infections: Prevention of invasive group A streptococcal disease among household contacts of case-patients. JAMA 1998;279(15):1206–1210.

195. Stevens DL, Gibbons AE, Bergstrom R, Winn V: The Eagle effect revisited: Efficacy of clindamycin, erythromycin, and penicillin in the treatment of streptococcal myositis. J Infect Dis 1988;158(1):23–28.

196. Zimbelman J, Palmer A, Todd J: Improved outcome of clindamycin compared with beta-lactam antibiotic treatment for invasive *Streptococcus pyogenes* infection. Pediatr Infect Dis J 1999;18(12):1096–1100.

197. Schwartz B, Elliott JA, Butler JC, et al: Clusters of invasive group A streptococcal infections in family, hospital, and nursing home settings. Clin Infect Dis 1992;15(2):277–284.

198. Chapnick EK, Gradon JD, Lutwick LI, et al: Streptococcal toxic shock syndrome due to noninvasive pharyngitis. Clin Infect Dis 1992;14(5):1074–1077.

199. Ichiyama S, Nakashima K, Shimokata K, et al: Transmission of *Streptococcus pyogenes* causing toxic shock–like syndrome among family members and confirmation by DNA macrorestriction analysis. J Infect Dis 1997;175(3):723–726.

200. Cockerill FR III, MacDonald KL, Thompson RL, et al: An outbreak of invasive group A streptococcal disease associated with high carriage rates of the invasive clone among school-aged children. JAMA 1997;277(1):38–43.

201. Gamba MA, Martinelli M, Schaad HJ, et al: Familial transmission of a serious disease—producing group A streptococcus clone: Case reports and review. Clin Infect Dis 1997;24(6):1118–1121.

202. Kiska D, Thiede B, Caracciolo J, et al: Invasive group A streptococcal disease in North Carolina: Epidemiology, clinical features, and genetic and serotype analysis of causative organisms. J Infect Dis 1997;176:992–1000.

203. Eagle H, Fleischman R, Masselman A: Effective schedule of administration of the therapeutic efficiency of penicillin—importance of the aggregate time penicillin. Am J Med 1950;9:280–299.

204. Stevens DL, Madaras-Kelly KJ, Richards DM: In vitro antimicrobial effects of various combinations of penicillin and clindamycin against four strains of *Streptococcus pyogenes*. Antimicrob Agents Chemother 1998;42(5):1266–1268.

205. Kaplan EL, Berrios X, Speth J, et al: Pharmacokinetics of benzathine penicillin G: Serum levels during the 28 days after intramuscular injection of 1,200,000 units. J Pediatr 1989;115(1):146–150.

206. Currie BJ, Burt T, Kaplan EL: Penicillin concentrations after increased doses of benzathine penicillin G for prevention of secondary rheumatic fever. Antimicrob Agents Chemother 1994;38(5):1203–1204.

207. Peyramond D, Portier H, Geslin P, Cohen R: 6-day amoxicillin versus 10-day penicillin V for group A beta-haemolytic streptococcal acute tonsillitis in adults: A French multicentre, open-label, randomized study. The French Study Group Clamorange. Scand J Infect Dis 1996;28(5):497–501.

208. Cohen R, Levy C, Doit C, et al: Six-day amoxicillin vs. ten-day penicillin V therapy for group A streptococcal tonsillopharyngitis. Pediatr Infect Dis J 1996;15(8):678–682.

209. Adam D, Scholz H: Five days of erythromycin estolate versus ten days of penicillin V in the treatment of group A streptococcal tonsillopharyngitis in children. Pharyngitis Study Group. Eur J Clin Microbiol Infect Dis 1996;15(9):712–717.

210. Hebblethwaite EM, Brown GW, Cox DM: A comparison of the efficacy and safety of cefuroxime axetil and augmentin in the treatment of upper respiratory tract infections. Drugs Exp Clin Res 1987;13(2):91–94.

211. Gehanno P, Pengon P, Moisy N, et al: Les angines: Enquete epidemiologique. Med Mal Infect 1987;2:75–79.

212. Portier H, Chavanet P, Gouyon JB, Guetat F: Five day treatment of pharyngotonsillitis with cefpodoxime proxetil. J Antimicrob Chemother 1990;26 (Suppl E):79–85.

213. Gehanno P, Chiche D: Traitement des angines a strotocoqui beta hemolytique due group A par le cefuroxime axetil pendant 4 jours: Etude comparative a la penicillin V pendant 10 jours. Med Mal Infect 1991;21:66–70.

214. Portier H, Chavanet P, Waldner-Combernoux A, et al: Five versus ten days treatment of streptococcal pharyngotonsillitis: A randomized controlled trial comparing cefpodoxime proxetil and phenoxymethyl penicillin. Scand J Infect Dis 1994;26(1):59–66.

215. Peyramond D, Tigand B, Bremard-Oury C, et al: Multicenter comparative trial of cefixime and phenoxymethylpenicillin for group A beta-hemolytic streptococcal tonsillitis. Curr Ther Res 1994;55(Suppl A):14–21.

216. Dajani AS: Pharyngitis/tonsillitis: European and United States experience with cefpodoxime proxetil. Pediatr Infect Dis J 1995;14(4 Suppl);S7–S11.

217. Aujard Y, Boucot I, Brahimi N, et al: Comparative efficacy and safety of four-day cefuroxime axetil and ten-day penicillin treatment of group A beta-hemolytic streptococcal pharyngitis in children. Pediatr Infect Dis J 1995;14(4):295–300.

218. Carbon C, Chatelin A, Bingen E, et al: A double-blind randomized trial comparing the efficacy and safety of a 5-day course of cefotiam hexetil with that of a 10-day course of penicillin V in adult patients with pharyngitis caused by group A beta-haemolytic streptococci. J Antimicrob Chemother 1995;35:843–854.

219. Adam D, Hostalek U, Troster K: 5-day cefixime therapy for bacterial pharyngitis and/or tonsillitis: Comparison with 10-day penicillin V therapy. Cefixime Study Group. Infection 1995;23(Suppl 2):S83–S86.

220. Tack KJ, Hedrick JA, Rothstein E, et al: A study of 5-day cefdinir treatment for streptococcal pharyngitis in children. Cefdinir Pediatric Pharyngitis Study Group. Arch Pediatr Adolesc Med 1997;151(1):45–49.

221. Zayer S, Kassem A, Abou-Sheib H, et al: Differences in serum penicillin concentrations following intramuscular injection of benzathine penicillin G (BPG) from different manufacturers. J Pharmacol Med 1992;2:17–23.

222. Ruff ME, Schotik DA, Bass JW, Vincent JM: Antimicrobial drug suspensions: A blind comparison of taste of fourteen common pediatric drugs. Pediatr Infect Dis J 1991; 10(1):30–33.

223. Demers DM, Chan DS, Bass JW: Antimicrobial drug suspensions: A blinded comparison of taste of twelve common pediatric drugs including cefixime, cefpodoxime, cefprozil and loracarbef. Pediatr Infect Dis J 1994;13(2):87–89.

224. Woodin K, Lee L, Pichichero M: Milder symptoms occur in recurrent episodes of streptococcal infection. Am J Dis Child 1991;145:389–390.

225. Brook I, Gober AE: Persistence of group A beta-hemolytic streptococci in toothbrushes and removable orthodontic appliances following treatment of pharyngotonsillitis. Arch Otolaryngol Head Neck Surg 1998;124(9):993–995.

226. el-Daher NT, Hijazi SS, Rawashdeh NM, et al: Immediate vs. delayed treatment of group A beta-hemolytic streptococcal pharyngitis with penicillin V. Pediatr Infect Dis J 1991;10(2):126–130.

227. Pichichero ME, Hoeger W, Marsocci SM, et al: Variables influencing penicillin treatment outcome in streptococcal tonsillopharyngitis. Arch Pediatr Adolesc Med 1999; 153(6):565–570.

228. Gerber MA, Randolph MF, DeMeo KK, Kaplan EL: Lack of impact of early antibiotic therapy for streptococcal pharyngitis on recurrence rates. J Pediatr 1990;117(6):853–858.

229. Brook I: Penicillin failure and copathogenicity in streptococcal pharyngotonsillitis. J Fam Pract 1994;38(2):175–179.

230. Pichichero ME, Casey JR, Mayes T, et al: Penicillin failure in streptococcal tonsillopharyngitis: Causes and remedies. Pediatr Infect Dis 2000;19:917–923.

231. Gerber MA, Tanz RR, Kabat W, et al: Potential mechanisms for failure to eradicate group A streptococci from the pharynx. Pediatrics 1999;104(4 Pt 1):911–917.

232. Roos K, Grahn E, Holm SE, et al: Interfering alpha-streptococci as a protection against recurrent streptococcal tonsillitis in children. Int J Pediatr Otorhinolaryngol 1993; 25(1-3):141–148.

233. Lilja H, Grahn E, Holm SE, Roos K: Alpha-streptococci-inhibiting beta-streptococci group A in treatment of recurrent streptococcal tonsillitis. Adv Otorhinolaryngol 1992; 47:168–171.

234. Roos K, Holm SE, Grahn E, Lind L: Alpha-streptococci as supplementary treatment of recurrent streptococcal tonsillitis: A randomized placebo-controlled study. Scand J Infect Dis 1993;25(1):31–35.

235. Pichichero ME, Marsocci SM, Murphy ML, et al: Incidence of streptococcal carriers in private pediatric practice. Arch Pediatr Adolesc Med 1999;153(6):624–628.

236. Standaert BB, Finney K, Taylor MT, et al: Comparison between cefprozil and penicillin to eradicate pharyngeal colonization of group A beta-hemolytic streptococci. Pediatr Infect Dis J 1998;17(1):39–43.

237. Peter G: Streptococcal pharyngitis: Current therapy and criteria for evaluation of new agents. Clin Infect Dis 1992;14(Suppl 2):S218–S223.

238. Paradise JL, Bluestone CD, Bachman RZ, et al: Efficacy of tonsillectomy for recurrent throat infection in severely affected children. Results of parallel randomized and nonrandomized clinical trials. N Engl J Med 1984; 310(11):674–683.

239. Han BK, Dunbar JS, Striker TW: Membranous laryngotracheobronchitis (membranous croup). AJR Am J Roentgenol 1979;133(1):53–58.

240. Jones R, Santos JI, Overall JC, Jr: Bacterial tracheitis. JAMA 1979;242(8):721–726.

241. Gallagher PG, Myer CM III: An approach to the diagnosis and treatment of membranous laryngotracheobronchitis in infants and children. Pediatr Emerg Care 1991;7(6):337–342.

242. Mahajan A, Alvear D, Chang C, et al: Bacterial tracheitis, diagnosis and treatment. Int J Pediatr Otorhinolaryngol 1985;10(3):271–277.

243. Liston SL, Gehrz RC, Siegel LG, Tilelli J: Bacterial tracheitis. Am J Dis Child 1983;137(8):764–767.

244. Donnelly BW, McMillan JA, Weiner LB: Bacterial tracheitis: Report of eight new cases and review. Rev Infect Dis 1990;12(5):729–735.

245. Bernstein T, Brilli R, Jacobs B: Is bacterial tracheitis changing? A 14-month experience in a pediatric intensive care unit. Clin Infect Dis 1998;27(3):458–462.

246. Brook I: Aerobic and anaerobic microbiology of bacterial tracheitis in children. Pediatr Emerg Care 1997;13(1):16–18.

247. Liston SL, Gehrz RC, Jarvis CW: Bacterial tracheitis. Arch Otolaryngol 1981;107(9):561–564.

248. Sofer S, Duncan P, Chernick V: Bacterial tracheitis—an old disease rediscovered. Clin Pediatr (Phila) 1983;22(6):407–411.

249. Dudin AA, Thalji A, Rambaud-Cousson A: Bacterial tracheitis among children hospitalized for severe obstructive dyspnea. Pediatr Infect Dis J 1990;9(4):293–295.

250. Feigin R, Stechenberg B: Diphitheria. In Feigin R, Cherry J (eds): Textbook of Pediatric Infectious Diseases. Philadelphia, WB Saunders, 1987, pp 1134–1140.

251. Briggs WH, Altenau MM: Acute epiglottitis in children. Otolaryngol Head Neck Surg 1980;88(6):665–669.

252. Faden HS: Treatment of *Haemophilus influenzae* type B epiglottitis. Pediatrics 1979;63(3):402–407.

253. Losek JD, Dewitz-Zink BA, Melzer-Lange M, Havens PL: Epiglottitis: Comparison of signs and symptoms in children less than 2 years old and older. Ann Emerg Med 1990;19(1):55–58.

254. Breivik H, Klaastad O: Acute epiglottitis in children. Review of 27 patients. Br J Anaesth 1978;50(5):505–510.

255. Lacroix J, Gauthier M, Lapointe N, et al: *Pseudomonas aeruginosa* supraglottitis in a six-month-old child with severe combined immunodeficiency syndrome. Pediatr Infect Dis J 1988;7(10):739–741.

256. Battaglia JD, Lockhart CH: Management of acute epiglottitis by nasotracheal intubation. Am J Dis Child 1975; 129(3):334–336.

257. Coker SB, Scherz RG: Safe alternative to tracheostomy in acute epiglottitis [letter]. Am J Dis Child 1975;129(1):136.

258. Heldtander P, Lee P: Treatment of acute epiglottitis in children by long-term intubation. Acta Otolaryngol 1973;75(4):379–381.

259. Lacroix J, Blanc V, Weber M, et al: Etude de 100 cas consecutifs d'epiglottite aigue. L'Union Medicale du Canada 1982;111:774–779.
260. Oh TH, Motoyama EK: Comparison of nasotracheal intubation and tracheostomy in management of acute epiglottitis. Anesthesiology 1977;46(3):214–216.
261. Kissoon N, Mitchell I: Adverse effects of racemic epinephrine in epiglottitis. Pediatr Emerg Care 1985;1(3):143–144.
262. Granoff DM, Daum RS: Spread of *Haemophilus influenzae* type b: Recent epidemiologic and therapeutic considerations. J Pediatr 1980;97(5):854–860.
263. American Academy of Pediatrics Red Book, Report of the Committee on Infectious Diseases 25th ed. *Haemophilus influenzae* infections 262–272.
264. Denny FW, Murphy TF, Clyde WA, Jr, et al: Croup: An 11-year study in a pediatric practice. Pediatrics 1983;71(6):871–876.
265. Lenny W, Milner AD: Treatment of acute viral croup. Arch Dis Child 1978;53(9):704–706.
266. Bourchier D, Dawson KP, Fergusson DM: Humidification in viral croup: A controlled trial. Aust Paediatr J 1984;20(4):289–291.
267. Kristjansson S, Berg-Kelly K, Winso E: Inhalation of racemic adrenaline in the treatment of mild and moderately severe croup. Clinical symptom score and oxygen saturation measurements for evaluation of treatment effects. Acta Paediatr 1994;83(11):1156–1160.
268. Henry R: Moist air in the treatment of laryngotracheitis. Arch Dis Child 1983;58(8):577.
269. Sasaki CT, Suzuki M: The respiratory mechanism of aerosol inhalation in the treatment of partial airway obstruction. Pediatrics 1977;59(5):689–694.
270. Adair JC, Ring WH, Jordan WS, Elwyn RA: Ten-year experience with IPPB in the treatment of acute laryngotracheobronchitis. Anesth Analg 1971;50(4):649–655.
271. Baugh R, Gilmore BB Jr: Infectious croup: A critical review. Otolaryngol Head Neck Surg 1986;95(1):40–46.
272. Waisman Y, Klein BL, Boenning DA, et al: Prospective randomized double-blind study comparing l-epinephrine and racemic epinephrine aerosols in the treatment of laryngotracheitis (croup). Pediatrics 1992;89(2):302–306.
273. Hinton W, Goss IJ: Croup, nebulised adrenaline and preservatives [letter]. Anaesthesia 1987;42(4):436–437.
274. Taussig LM, Castro O, Beaudry PH, et al: Treatment of laryngotracheobronchitis (croup). Use of intermittent positive-pressure breathing and racemic epinephrine. Am J Dis Child 1975;129(7):790–793.
275. Fogel JM, Berg IJ, Gerber MA, Sherter CB: Racemic epinephrine in the treatment of croup: Nebulization alone versus nebulization with intermittent positive pressure breathing. J Pediatr 1982;101(6):1028–1031.
276. Corneli HM, Bolte RG: Outpatient use of racemic epinephrine in croup [editorial; comment]. Am Fam Physician 1992;46(3):683–684.
277. Prendergast M, Jones JS, Hartman D: Racemic epinephrine in the treatment of laryngotracheitis: Can we identify children for outpatient therapy? Am J Emerg Med 1994;12(6):613–616.
278. Ledwith CA, Shea LM, Mauro RD: Safety and efficacy of nebulized racemic epinephrine in conjunction with oral dexamethasone and mist in the outpatient treatment of croup. Ann Emerg Med 1995;25(3):331–337.
279. Kunkel NC, Baker MD: Use of racemic epinephrine, dexamethasone, and mist in the outpatient management of croup. Pediatr Emerg Care 1996;12(3):156–159.
280. Kuusela AL, Vesikari T: A randomized double-blind, placebo-controlled trial of dexamethasone and racemic epinephrine in the treatment of croup. Acta Paediatr Scand 1988;77(1):99–104.
281. Schimmer B, Parker K: Adrenocorticotropic hormone: Adrenocortical steroids and their synthetic analogs; inhibitors of the synthesis and actions of adrenocortical hormones. In Hardman J, Limbird L (eds): The Pharmacological Basis of Therapeutics, 9th ed. New York, McGraw-Hill, 1996, pp. 1459–1485.
282. Kairys SW, Olmstead EM, O'Connor GT: Steroid treatment of laryngotracheitis: A meta-analysis of the evidence from randomized trials [see comments]. Pediatrics 1989;83(5):683–693.
283. Super DM, Cartelli NA, Brooks LJ, et al: A prospective randomized double-blind study to evaluate the effect of dexamethasone in acute laryngotracheitis [see comments]. J Pediatr 1989;115(2):323–329.
284. Cruz MN, Stewart G, Rosenberg N: Use of dexamethasone in the outpatient management of acute laryngotracheitis. Pediatrics 1995;96(2 Pt 1):220–223.
285. Geelhoed GC: Sixteen years of croup in a Western Australian teaching hospital: Effects of routine steroid treatment. Ann Emerg Med 1996;28(6):621–626.
286. Geelhoed GC, Macdonald WB: Oral dexamethasone in the treatment of croup: 0.15 mg/kg versus 0.3 mg/kg versus 0.6 mg/kg. Pediatr Pulmonol 1995;20(6):362–368.
287. Rittichier KK, Ledwith CA: Outpatient treatment of moderate croup with dexamethasone: Intramuscular versus oral dosing [in process citation]. Pediatrics 2000;106(6):1344–1348.
288. Burton DM, Seid AB, Kearns DB, Pransky SM: *Candida* laryngotracheitis: A complication of combined steroid and antibiotic usage in croup. Int J Pediatr Otorhinolaryngol 1992;23(2):171–175.
289. Johansson SA, Andersson KE, Brattsand R, et al: Topical and systemic glucocorticoid potencies of budesonide, beclomethasone dipropionate and prednisolone in man. Eur J Respir Dis Suppl 1982;122:74–82.
290. Newhouse MT, Dolovich MB: Control of asthma by aerosols [see comments]. N Engl J Med 1986;315(14):870–874.
291. Husby S, Agertoft L, Mortensen S, Pedersen S: Treatment of croup with nebulised steroid (budesonide): A double blind, placebo controlled study. Arch Dis Child 1993;68(3):352–355.
292. Klassen TP, Watters LK, Feldman ME, et al: The efficacy of nebulized budesonide in dexamethasone-treated outpatients with croup. Pediatrics 1996;97(4):463–466.
293. Klassen TP, Feldman ME, Watters LK, et al: Nebulized budesonide for children with mild-to-moderate croup [see comments]. N Engl J Med 1994;331(5):285–289.
294. Mitchell DP, Thomas RL: Secondary airway support in the management of croup. J Otolaryngol 1980;9(5):419–422.
295. Tibballs J, Shann FA, Landau LI: Placebo-controlled trial of prednisolone in children intubated for croup. Lancet 1992;340(8822):745–748.
296. Duncan PG: Efficacy of helium-oxygen mixtures in the management of severe viral and post-intubation croup. Can Anaesth Soc J 1979;26(3):206–212.
297. Nelson DS, McClellan L: Helium-oxygen mixtures as adjunctive support for refractory viral croup. Ohio State Med J 1982;78(10):729–730.
298. Breese BB, Disney FA, Talpey WB: β-hemolytic streptococcal illness. A comparison of the effectiveness of penicillin G, triacetyloleandomycin, and erythromycin estolate. Am J Dis Child 1966;111(2):128–132.
299. Jackson H, Cooper J, Mellinger WJ, Olsen AR: Group A beta-hemolytic streptococcal pharyngitis—results of treatment with lincomycin. JAMA 1965;194(11):1189–1192.
300. Breese BB, Disney FA, Talpey WB, Green J: Beta-hemolytic streptococcal infection. Comparison of penicillin and lincomycin in the treatment of recurrent infections or the carrier state. Am J Dis Child 1969;117(2):147–152.

301. Randolph MF, DeHaan RM: A comparison of lincomycin and penicillin in the treatment of group A streptococcal infections: Speculation on the "L" form as a mechanism of recurrence. Del Med J 1969;41(2):51–62.

302. Randolph MF, Redys JJ, Hibbard EW: Streptococcal pharyngitis. 3. Streptococcal recurrence rates following therapy with penicillin or with clindamycin(7-chlorolincomycin). Del Med J 1970;42(4):87–92.

303. Randolph MF, Redys JJ, Cope J, Morris KE: Streptococcal pharyngitis: Posttreatment carrier prevalence and clinical relapse in children treated with clindamycin palmitate or phenoxymethyl penicillin. Clin Pediatr (Phila) 1975;14(2):119–122.

304. Raz R, Hamburger S, Flatau E: Clindamycin in the treatment of an outbreak of streptococcal pharyngitis in a kibbutz due to beta-lactamase producing organisms. J Chemother 1990;2(3):182–184.

305. Mehra S, van Moerkerke M, Welck J, et al: Short course therapy with cefuroxime axetil for group A streptococcal tonsillopharyngitis in children. Pediatr Infect Dis J 1998;17(6):452–457.

306. Adam D, Scholz H, Helmerking M: Comparison of short-course (5 day) cefuroxime axetil with a standard 10 day oral penicillin V regimen in the treatment of tonsillopharyngitis. J Antimicrob Chemother 2000;45(Suppl):23–30.

307. Gardner HG, Powell KR, Roden VJ, Cherry JD: The evaluation of racemic epinephrine in the treatment of infectious croup. Pediatrics 1973;52(1):52–55.

308. Westley CR, Cotton EK, Brooks JG: Nebulized racemic epinephrine by IPPB for the treatment of croup: A double-blind study. Am J Dis Child 1978;132(5):484–487.

309. Massicotte P, Tetreault L. [Evaluation of methyl-prednisolone in the treatment of acute laryngitis in children.] Union Med Can 1973;102(10):2064–2072.

310. Eden A, Larkin V: Corticosteroid treatment of croup. Pediatrics 1964;33:768–769.

311. Eden A, Kaufman A, Yu R: Corticosteroids and croup: Controlled double-blind study. JAMA 1967;200:403–404.

312. James J: Dexamethasone in croup: A controlled study. Am J Dis Child 1969;117:511–516.

313. Leipzig B, Oski FA, Cummings CW, et al: A prospective randomized study to determine the efficacy of steroids in treatment of croup. J Pediatr 1979;94(2):194–196.

314. Martinez F, Sanchez G, Rica E: Randomized double-blind study of treatment of croup with adrenaline and/or dexamethasone in children. An Esp Pediatr 1993;38:29–32.

315. Skowron P. The use of corticosteroid (dexamethasone) in the treatment of acute laryngotracheitis. CMAJ 1966;94:528–531.

316. Geelhoed GC, Turner J, Macdonald WB. Efficacy of a small single dose of oral dexamethasone for outpatient croup: A double blind placebo controlled clinical trial [see comments]. BMJ 1996;313(7050):140–142.

317. Muhlendahl K, Kahn D, Spohr H: Steroid treatment in pseudo-croup. Helv Pediatri Acta 1982;37:431–436.

318. Fitzgerald D, Mellis C, Johnson M, et al: Nebulized budesonide is as effective as nebulized adrenaline in moderately severe croup. Pediatrics 1996;97(5):722–725.

319. Geelhoed GC, Macdonald WB: Oral and inhaled steroids in croup: A randomized, placebo-controlled trial. Pediatr Pulmonol 1995;20(6):355–361.

320. Johnson DW, Schuh S, Koren G, Jaffee DM: Outpatient treatment of croup with nebulized dexamethasone [see comments]. Arch Pediatr Adolesc Med 1996;150(4):349–355.

321. Godden CW, Campbell MJ, Hussey M, Cogswell JJ: Double blind placebo controlled trial of nebulised budesonide for croup. Arch Dis Child 1997;76(2):155–158.

322. Johnson DW, Jacobson S, Edney PC, et al: A comparison of nebulized budesonide, intramuscular dexamethasone, and placebo for moderately severe croup [see comments]. N Engl J Med 1998;339(8):498–503.

323. Klassen TP, Craig WR, Moher D, et al: Nebulized budesonide and oral dexamethasone for treatment of croup: A randomized controlled trial. JAMA 1998;279(20):1629–1632.

section

3

Lower Respiratory Tract Infections

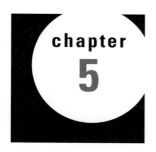

LIONEL A. MANDELL, MD, FRCP(C)

chapter 5

Bronchitis and Pneumonia

Lower respiratory tract infections involve the trachea, bronchi, terminal airways, and pulmonary parenchyma and manifest as bronchitis and pneumonia, respectively. The former is typically divided into acute and chronic bronchitis, and pneumonia is usually subdivided into community-acquired and hospital-acquired infections.

Together these diseases are significant causes of morbidity and mortality, and pneumonia continues to be the most common cause of death from infectious diseases worldwide. Despite advances in our understanding of the various etiologic agents and pathogenic mechanisms, we are often unable to accurately determine the etiologic agent in time to have an impact upon the initial treatment decision.

This chapter is divided into sections dealing with airway infection (acute bronchitis, acute exacerbation of chronic bronchitis) and pneumonia (community-acquired, hospital-acquired).

ACUTE BRONCHITIS

Etiology and Epidemiology

Acute bronchitis typically refers to an acute inflammation of the airways in patients who may have no underlying lung disease. The inflammation may be due to infection or environmental pollutants such as ammonia and sulfur dioxide. Although it is usually not a serious condition, it has considerable economic impact because of the frequency of physician visits and because physicians who diagnose acute bronchitis prescribe antibiotics for 66% of such patients despite the lack of any compelling evidence supporting antimicrobial therapy.[1] In the United States it is estimated that acute bronchitis results in approximately 12 million physician visits per year at a cost of 200 to 300 million dollars.[2]

Of the infecting agents, those typically associated with acute bronchitis are rhinovirus, coronavirus, adenovirus, and, of course, influenza virus, particularly during influenza outbreaks. A number of other viral agents have been reported as well including respiratory syncytial virus (RSV) and parainfluenza virus.

Other pathogens that have been associated with acute bronchitis include *Bordetella pertussis*, the etiologic agent of whooping cough, and *Mycoplasma pneumoniae* and *Chlamydia pneumoniae*.[3,4]

As one would expect with most respiratory infections, acute bronchitis is typically seen during the winter months. In the United Kingdom, weekly attack rates will reach 171/100,000 in winter and will fall to a low of 26/100,000 in summer.[5]

It is possible that respiratory bacterial pathogens such as *Streptococcus pneumoniae* and *Haemophilus influenzae* may cause secondary infections, possibly as a result of the mucosal changes and impaired ciliary function.

Diagnosis

Like the diagnosis of any medical condition, the diagnosis of infection relies on information from a carefully obtained history, a detailed physical examination, and appropriate laboratory tests or procedures. Depending on the type of infection and the circumstances of a particular case, laboratory and ancillary tests may be done to varying degrees. The diagnosis of acute bronchitis in an otherwise well adult is usually not difficult. The clinical presentation of an acute respiratory illness with cough as the predominant symptom and the absence of physical findings other than rales and rhonchi is usually sufficient to make the diagnosis. If there is any question of pneumonia, a chest radiograph should be done to rule out the presence of a pulmonary infiltrate.

For the average case of bronchitis it is not worth obtaining blood samples for serology or sputum for Gram stain and culture.

Treatment

Acute bronchitis typically is treated in the outpatient setting; few patients are hospitalized. Usually management is symptomatic and consists of maintenance of hydration and cough suppression when necessary. If the cough is unusually severe or keeps the patient from sleeping, a narcotic-based cough suppressant may be given as well as a nonsteroidal anti-inflammatory agent.[6] Currently, there is insufficient evidence for the routine use of oral or inhaled steroids for patients with persistent or troublesome cough.

If bronchospasm is a problem, inhaled β_2-adrenergic bronchodilators have been used, but this practice is not based on firm evidence.[7]

Patients with underlying cardiopulmonary disease may experience clinical deterioration following an attack of acute bronchitis and on occasion have required admission to the hospital and ventilatory and cardiac support. More specific treatment in the form of antimicrobial therapy generally is not recommended. Several placebo-controlled trials have evaluated the role of antibiotics in acute bronchitis, and benefit is minimal at best.

Specific antiviral agents are not used, however, given the possible etiologic agents (e.g., *M. pneumoniae* and *C. pneumoniae*) or secondary infecting pathogens (e.g., *S. pneumoniae* and *H. influenzae*). Drugs such as macrolides (azithromycin or clarithromycin) or doxycycline could be considered in the following situations:

1. A patient with a particularly severe attack on initial presentation
2. A patient whose symptoms have persisted for longer than 1 week and that show no evidence of resolving or whose symptoms are worsening

3. A patient with known cardiopulmonary disease whose underlying condition is known to be worsened by an attack of acute bronchitis

If acute bronchitis happens in the setting of an influenza outbreak, a number of agents may be used. Amantadine and rimantadine are available for treatment of influenza A infection only, Zanamivir and oseltamivir are two newer neuraminidase inhibitors with activity against both influenza A and B viruses. Both these agents are approved for treatment of uncomplicated influenza and if given within 48 hours of onset of symptoms may decrease the severity and duration of symptoms[8,9] (see Acute Exacerbations of Chronic Bronchitis, Prevention).

Prevention

There is little that one can do specifically to avoid infective causes of acute bronchitis. Patients who wish to protect themselves against influenza, however, should be vaccinated yearly with influenza vaccine. This is particularly recommended for older patients and those of any age with known pulmonary or cardiac disease.[10] Children should be vaccinated to protect them against whooping cough.

Obviously cigarette smoking should be avoided as should exposure to any chemicals or toxins known to cause episodes of acute bronchitis.

ACUTE EXACERBATIONS OF CHRONIC BRONCHITIS

To understand and appreciate acute exacerbations of chronic bronchitis (AECB) one must first understand the associated clinical conditions and the corresponding terminology. Chronic bronchitis is a clinical diagnosis for a condition defined by the presence of a productive cough occurring on most days during at least 3 months in each of 2 successive years.[11] If the situation is compounded by airflow obstruction, the term chronic obstructive pulmonary disease (COPD) is used. The prognosis for COPD correlates best with the forced expiratory volume in 1 second (FEV_1) and worsens considerably when it falls below 50% of predicted value.

Etiology and Epidemiology

Chronic bronchitis is common. It is estimated that up to one-quarter of the adult population may be affected.[11] Chronic bronchitis is the result of a variety of insults to the lung over time including cigarette smoke, infection, and environmental pollutants and irritants. Once chronic bronchitis is established, the episodic worsening is referred to as an acute exacerbation of chronic bronchitis, which can be triggered by similar causes. For the purposes of this chapter, however, we will focus on infective triggers.

Although there is general consensus that infection will initiate episodes of AECB, there is some debate over the role of viruses vs. bacterial pathogens. In support of bacteria as etiologic agents are studies that have shown increases in the number of bacteria in the mucus of patients during an exacerbation as well as acute antibody responses to such pathogens during the exacerbation.

It is estimated that viruses account for up to 50% of acute exacerbations, and those most frequently implicated are RSV, rhinovirus, influenza virus, and parainfluenza virus. The remaining 50% of acute exacerbations are thought to be due to bacteria, which include *H. influenzae, S. pneumoniae,* and *Moraxella catarrhalis.* The role of atypical pathogens such as *M. pneumoniae* and *C. pneumoniae* is unclear, but it is thought that they may account for a small percentage of infections in this population.

Infection results in the release of inflammatory mediators and further impairment of mucociliary clearance. This in turn alters the local milieu, making it easier for pathogens to further colonize the airways. Progressive airway damage is thought to be the result of injury caused by the pathogens themselves or by the host's response to the various infecting agents.

Diagnosis

One problem in diagnosis is that there is no single agreed upon definition of an acute exacerbation, nor is there a common cause or uniform therapy. Through common usage an acute exacerbation of chronic bronchitis has come to be defined by any one of or any combination of the following: an increase in cough and volume of sputum, an increase in purulence of sputum, and an increase in shortness of breath. The Anthonisen classification refers to patients with one of these findings as type 3, two of the findings as type 2, and three of the findings as type 1.[12]

A diagnosis typically is made clinically, and it is often the patient who makes it.

A sputum Gram stain may not be of much help, since many if not most persons with chronic bronchitis normally have bacteria in their respiratory secretions. These bacteria colonize the airways and during an exacerbation are present in higher numbers. Typically, pathogens such as *H. influenzae, S. pneumoniae,* and *M. catarrhalis* are present. In those with more severe exacerbations, however, these pathogens are present less often, and organisms such as *Haemophilus parainfluenzae* and *Pseudomonas aeruginosa* are more frequently found.[13,14] It appears that as the severity of the illness increases, as indicated by markers such as illness lasting longer than 10 years, more than four exacerbations per year, steroid therapy, recent antibiotics, and severe airway obstruction (FEV$_1$ < 35% predicted), the microbiology becomes more complex.[15,16] Despite problems with sensitivity and specificity of sputum culture, it may still be worth

obtaining samples from patients experiencing an exacerbation, particularly if it is serious, in the chance that a resistant pathogen may be found.

Because AECB represents an airway rather than a pulmonary parenchymal infection, a chest radiograph will not show any infiltrate. Depending upon the patient and the circumstances it may be worth doing a chest radiograph to rule out pneumonia or other possible disease entities that may be confounding the clinical picture.

Treatment

The treatment of AECB has evolved over the past 15 years. Although it would seem quite straightforward that patients experiencing an exacerbation should be given an antibiotic, data demonstrate that such routine treatment fails in one in seven to one in four patients.[17] Such failures are associated with considerable economic impact, since additional costs are generated related to return physician visits, alternate drug treatments, and work absence. The concept of risk stratification slowly developed and took shape with the idea that if higher risk populations could be identified and treated more aggressively, treatment failure rates might be reduced.

One of the first studies to assess response to treatment based upon stratification of patients according to their symptoms was by Anthonisen et al.[12] In this study it was shown that patients with at least two of the three findings—increased shortness of breath, increased sputum volume, and increased sputum purulence—who were treated with relatively broad-spectrum agents such as amoxicillin, TMP-SMZ, or doxycycline had better outcomes and faster recovery of lung function than patients given placebo. This trial was among the first to demonstrate that a response to treatment could be linked to stratification.

A recent meta-analysis of nine randomized placebo controlled trials of patients treated for AECB demonstrated a statistically significant improvement in outcome in those given an antibiotic.[18]

Treatment failure has been associated with a number of risk factors including cardiopulmonary disease and increased frequency of pulmonary infections during the previous year (more than 4).[17] A subgroup of patients is at risk not only for treatment failure but also for respiratory failure. Mortality rates during hospitalization of 10% to 30% have been reported, usually in patients older than 65 years, those with comorbid respiratory and extrapulmonary organ dysfunction, and those residing in hospital before transfer to the intensive care unit (ICU).[19,20]

It has been suggested that stratification of patients according to risk factors will allow physicians to treat more appropriately. No single stratification scheme has been agreed upon, but those schemes that do exist attempt to rank patients according to increased risk of treatment failure and hospitalization. Three schemes have been published to date: Lode[21] in Germany in 1991,

TABLE 5–1 ■ Stratification and Treatment—United Kingdom

Category	Characteristics	Suggested treatment
Group 1	Postviral tracheobronchitis; previously healthy person	None
Group 2	Simple chronic bronchitis; young person; mild-to-moderate impairment of lung function (FEV$_1$ > 50% predicted); <4 exacerbations per year	β-lactam antibodies
Group 3	Chronic bronchitis plus older person; FEV$_1$ 50% predicted or FEV$_1$ 50%–60% predicted but concurrent medical illnesses; congestive heart failure, diabetes mellitus, chronic renal disease, chronic liver disease, >4 exacerbations per year	Fluoroquinolones Amoxicillin-clavulanic acid Second- or third-generation cephalosporins Second-generation macrolides
Group 4	Chronic bronchial sepsis, bronchiectasis, chronic airway colonization	Tailor antimicrobial treatment to airway pathogens

FEV$_1$, forced expiratory volume 1 second.
From Wilson R: Outcome predictors in bronchitis. Chest 1995;108(suppl):53–57.

Balter et al[22] in Canada in 1994, and Wilson[23] in the United Kingdom in 1995. The British approach is summarized in Table 5–1.

In the discussions dealing with etiology and epidemiology and diagnosis, it is clear that a variety of microorganisms ranging from viruses to *P. aeruginosa* may be pathogens depending upon the circumstances associated with any given patient. The potential advantage of a hierarchical approach implicit in a stratification scheme is that it may identify patients at increased risk of treatment failure so that treatment may be initiated with an antibiotic regimen most likely to be effective against the potential etiologic agent(s) in that patient.

The patients at risk of infection with *P. aeruginosa* are the most difficult to manage. Typically they have severe structural lung damage such as bronchiectasis or cystic fibrosis. Other risk factors for infection with *P. aeruginosa* include steroid therapy and recent courses of antibiotics. The most effective agent for oral management is ciprofloxacin, as it is the only fluoroquinolone with consistently reliable antipseudomonal activity.

The optimal duration of treatment for AECB is unknown, although standard therapy is currently approximately 10 days. The newer "respiratory fluoroquinolones" may be given for only 5 days and are still effective.[24,25] This shorter course of treatment is of significant benefit, since it improves patient compliance and reduces antibiotic selection pressure with the attendant risk of antimicrobial resistance.

A variety of adjunctive or supportive measures including the use of bronchodilators, steroids (oral or inhaled or both), and oxygen therapy may be necessary as well.

Prevention

A number of steps can be taken to prevent episodes of AECB. These include cessation of smoking, avoidance of exposure to known environmental pollutants or chemicals, annual influenza vaccination, and administration of the pneumococcal vaccine. Annual prophylaxis using the influenza vaccine offers protection against the strains included in the vaccine (see Community-Acquired Pneumonia, Prevention). Four drugs are currently available for use in the prevention or treatment of influenza. Amantadine and rimantadine may be used for chemoprophylaxis and treatment of influenza A infection only. Zanamivir and oseltamivir are active against influenza A and B. Zanamivir is given intranasaly, and oseltamivir is administered orally. Both are effective in reducing febrile illness during the influenza season.[26,27] Both agents are also approved for treatment of uncomplicated influenza and if given within 48 hours of onset of symptoms may decrease their severity and duration.[9,28]

The pneumococcal vaccine is discussed under Community-Acquired Pneumonia, Prevention.

COMMUNITY-ACQUIRED PNEUMONIA

Community-acquired pneumonia (CAP) is a potentially lethal infection that has been the subject of considerable discussion and controversy in recent years. Although medical societies in North America and western Europe have published guidelines dealing with CAP management, it is clear that we still have much to learn about this disease.[10,29–32] CAP has a significant impact on individual patients and on society. It currently is the sixth leading cause of death in the United States, with an estimated 3 to 4 million cases occurring annually, resulting in 64 million days of restricted activity, 600,000 hospitalizations, and 45,000 deaths.[33]

Etiology and Epidemiology

As with many other infections, the incidence rates of pneumonia are greatest at the extremes of age. The overall annual rate of pneumonia in the United States is 12/1000 persons, and the incidence of CAP requiring hospitalization in adult patients is 2.6/1000.[34,35] Risk factors for pneumonia include alcoholism, asthma, immunosuppression, institutionalization, and age 70 years or older vs. age 60 to 69 years.[36] Specific risk factors for infection with *S. pneumoniae* include dementia, seizure disorders, congestive heart failure, cerebrovascular disease, COPD, human immunodeficiency virus (HIV) infection, and African-American race.[37,38]

The etiology of CAP is somewhat complicated, since it is not a single homogeneous entity and must be considered according to the site of acquisition of infection, that is, the community at large vs. a nursing home, the site of patient care (e.g., outpatient vs. inpatient), and the presence of any comorbid illnesses (e.g., congestive heart failure, COPD). The issue is further complicated by the fact that more than one pathogen may be responsible for disease in any given patient. Such mixed infections are well known in hospital-acquired pneumonia, in which it has been shown that multiple pathogens are present in more than half of the patients.[39] In CAP, the incidence of mixed infections is less, ranging from 2.7% to 10% in three studies of hospitalized CAP patients.[40–42]

Undoubtedly, the most important etiologic agent is *S. pneumoniae*. In a meta-analysis covering a 30-year period and 7000 cases of pneumonia in which an etiologic diagnosis was made, *S. pneumoniae* accounted for two-thirds of all cases and for two-thirds of fatalities.[43]

The "atypical" pathogens include a number of agents; however, those most commonly included in this category are *M. pneumoniae, C. pneumoniae,* and *Legionella* spp. A recent study of more than 2700 patients hospitalized with CAP ranked these three pathogens second, third, and fourth of all etiologic agents meeting the criteria for a "definite" diagnosis.[44] A Canadian study described three outbreaks of *C. pneumoniae* in nursing homes in which the attack rates and mortality were high.[45] These two studies have helped to dispel earlier misconceptions that the atypicals usually caused only mild disease and did not affect the elderly.

Gram-negative rods such as *Escherichia coli* and *Klebsiella* spp are not particularly common causes of CAP but are nevertheless important to consider, particularly in the elderly or in those with comorbid illness, especially if they are ill enough to require hospitalization. There has also been considerable debate about whether *P. aeruginosa* is a significant pathogen requiring treatment. The consensus is that although it is certainly not common, it can occur in selected patients if risk factors such as a recent course of antibiotics or a prolonged stay in hospital are present.

Diagnosis

The diagnosis of CAP has generated considerable debate among physicians involved in the care and management of patients with pneumonia. There are essentially two steps involved in assessing such patients. The first is to determine whether the patient in fact has pneumonia as opposed to some other infective or noninfective process. If a diagnosis of pneumonia is made, the next step is to determine the etiologic agent if possible. Depending upon the circumstances, we are reasonably good at making the clinical determination of pneumonia but we are quite poor when it comes to determining the etiologic agent. Despite extensive testing in university medical centers, a specific etiologic agent may not be found in up to one-half of CAP cases.[40,46] Knowledge of the etiologic agent has several advantages including identification of microorganisms with potential epidemiologic significance and the opportunity to use directed as opposed to empiric antimicrobial treatment. This is associated with a reduction in antibiotic costs, reduced adverse effects, and a reduction in antibiotic selection pressure resulting in less antimicrobial resistance.

Unfortunately, however, a study in the United Kingdom demonstrated that in routine clinical practice the etiologic agent is determined in only approximately 25% of cases but that this determination results in a change in antimicrobial therapy in less than 10% of cases.[47]

Diagnostic testing generally falls into two categories: clinical and invasive-quantitative. Clinical testing relies upon information obtained from a patient history, physical examination, and selected tests or procedures such as a chest radiograph, sputum Gram stain, and blood and sputum cultures. Invasive-quantitative methods include bronchoscopic techniques, pleural fluid aspiration, and in selected cases lung biopsy. As a rule the clinical method is too sensitive and lacks specificity, whereas the invasive-quantitative method requires special expertise and laboratory support and is more costly.

Clinical Evaluation

It is now generally accepted that it is not possible to accurately identify the etiologic agent based upon clinical findings, routine laboratory data, or the chest radiographic appearance.[40] There is significant interobserver variation in the ability to elicit abnormal physical findings, and the sensitivity and specificity of the history and physical examination are currently undetermined.[48,49]

Chest Radiograph

An infiltrate on the chest radiograph can help to establish the diagnosis of pneumonia but does not determine the causative pathogen. The radiograph is important, however, not only in defining the presence of an infiltrate but also in assessing the severity of illness and the prognosis. For example, if extensive or multilobar infiltrates are noted, consideration should be given to treatment of the patient in the ICU setting.

Ideally, posteroanterior and lateral chest radiographs should be obtained in all patients in whom pneumonia is suspected. This may not always be possible, however. In such situations a trial of empiric therapy without radiographic confirmation of the diagnosis may be a reasonable approach to initial patient management.

Laboratory Assessment

Routine laboratory assessment is unnecessary for ambulatory patients with CAP who are likely to be managed as outpatients. For those ill enough to require admission to the hospital (or for those even considered for admission) the following routine laboratory tests should be performed: a complete blood count (CBC) and differential, serum electrolytes, liver function tests, serum creatinine, and an oxygen saturation assessment. Significant abnormalities have been identified as risk factors for a complicated course or increased mortality. These are also used as the basis for assigning points to patients based upon Fine's rule to assess mortality risk and to help in the site-of-care decision.[50]

Microbiologic Assessment

Sputum Gram Stain and Culture

A meta-analysis of the sputum Gram stain in CAP shows that the test is neither sensitive nor specific.[51] At least a third of patients are unable to even produce a sputum sample, and of those samples obtained, at best only 40% are ranked as being of good quality. If patients have recently taken antibiotics, this may well affect the culture results, and although it is now estimated that 20% to 25% of all CAP cases are caused by atypicals, these organisms are not detectable by either of these tests.

Blood Cultures

The incidence of positive blood cultures in ambulatory patients is unknown, but in hospitalized patients it ranges from 6.6% to 17.6% and can reach 27% in ICU patients.[52] The most common pathogen is *S. pneumoniae*.

Serology

Routine serologic testing is not recommended for the management of CAP patients.

Legionella Urinary Antigen

This test is relatively easy to perform and rapidly provides results with a sensitivity and specificity of 70% and 100%, respectively. Its main limitation is that it can only identify *Legionella pneumophila* serogroup 1; however, serogroup 1 accounts for over 90% of *Legionella* infections.

DNA Probes and Amplification

Rapid diagnostic techniques are generally not available, and even if they were, identifying the presence of a particular microorganism does not allow one to say with certainty whether it is simply colonizing the patient or is an active invader causing disease. There are, however, a few microorganisms whose mere presence indicates infection. These include *Mycobacterium tuberculosis*, *Coxiella burnetii*, and *Pneumocystis carinii*.

Invasive Procedures

For most CAP patients, invasive procedures such as bronchoscopy, bronchoalveolar lavage, and percutaneous lung needle aspiration are not necessary. In selected circumstances such as patients with fulminant pneumonia or those unresponsive to a standard course of broad-spectrum antimicrobials, an invasive procedure may help to identify a resistant or fastidious pathogen or to rule out a noninfectious cause. Thoracentesis should be considered in CAP patients with significant pleural effusions as defined by a collection greater than 10 mm thick on the lateral decubitus view.[53]

Treatment

Before the actual therapeutic regimens that are used in the management of CAP are discussed, two important issues deserve attention: the site-of-care decision and antimicrobial resistance. The former refers to the decision regarding whether management should be outpatient or in hospital, and the latter deals with the issues of in vitro resistance and their relevance to clinical management.

The site-of-care decision has considerable economic implications. The cost of inpatient management exceeds that of outpatient care by a factor of 15 to 20 and accounts for most of the estimated 4 billion dollars spent annually on CAP in the United States.[54,55]

In some cases it is immediately obvious that outpatient management is appropriate, whereas in other cases it is just as apparent that hospitalization and possibly admission to an ICU is required. Because of the marked variability among physicians in dealing with such issues, it became clear that effective scoring and outcome-assessment tools were necessary to help physicians to make the site-of-care decision. Such assessment tools provide physicians with objective methods of assessing the risk of adverse outcomes, including death.

A number of prognostic tools are available to help physicians in identifying patients at risk of poor outcomes:

1. The Appropriateness Evaluation Protocol 1981
2. The British Thoracic Society Statement on CAP in Adults in British Hospitals 1987
3. The American Thoracic Society Guidelines for Community-acquired Pneumonia 1993
4. The Modified Appropriateness Evaluation Protocol 1996[56–58]

In addition to this, several studies by Fine et al outline evaluation tools to identify at risk patients.[59,60] These and a number of other studies have attempted to identify CAP patients at increased risk for adverse outcomes and to define independent predictors of mortality or poor outcome. Unfortunately many of these have weaknesses or design flaws, but the best and most widely used is the one by Fine et al published in the *New England Journal of Medicine*.[50] Although not originally developed as a triage rule, the Fine et al paper provides a two-step prediction rule designed to identify CAP patients at low risk for death. This may help to minimize unnecessary hospital admissions and to identify patients who will benefit from care and intervention in a hospital setting. Points are assigned on the basis of age, coexisting disease, and abnormal physical and laboratory findings, and the patient is assigned to one of five classes depending upon the number of points. The mortality for the classes are class 1 = 0.1%, class 2 = 0.6%, class 3 = 2.8%, class 4 = 8.2%, and class 5 = 29.2%. On the basis of these rates it has been suggested that patients in classes 1 and 2 be managed outside the hospital, whereas those in classes 4 and 5 be admitted to hospital. Patients in class 3 should be admitted for observation and treatment for a day or two if hospital facilities are available. This rule has been adopted by the Infectious Diseases Society of America (IDSA) and by the joint guidelines prepared by the Canadian Infectious Disease Society and the Canadian Thoracic Society.

This rule does not deal with severe CAP and does not help physicians decide whether to admit a patient to the ICU. Criteria for severe CAP were developed and presented in the original American Thoracic Society (ATS) guidelines.[30]

Antimicrobial resistance has become increasingly common, and it is important that clinicians understand and appreciate the general mechanisms and implications of this phenomenon. The emergence of resistance to penicillin among strains of *S. pneumoniae* represents a gradual reduction of in vitro susceptibility. The National Committee on Clinical Laboratory Standards defines strains with minimum inhibitory concentrations (MIC) to penicillin of less than 0.06 µg/ml as sensitive, 0.1 to 1 µg/ml as intermediate, and 2 µg/ml or higher as resistant.[61] With *S. pneumoniae* the DNA that is incorporated and remodeled is from closely related oral commensal bacteria, and this process takes place in our mouths. By such a process, our own colonizing microflora can develop resistance when we are treated with antibiotics, and pathogens such as *S. pneumoniae* can acquire resistance coding DNA from our colonizing microflora.[62] Pneumococcal resistance to β-lactams primarily is due to the presence of low-affinity penicillin binding proteins. Macrolide resistance, on the other hand, can occur either by target-site modification or by an efflux pump. A change in 23 Sr RNA mediated by the *erm* gene can result in resistance to macrolides, lincosamides, and streptogramin-B type antibiotics (MLS_B phenotype).[63] The efflux mechanism is controlled by the *mef* gene and results in an M phenotype. Efflux accounts for low-level macrolide resistance with MICs in the range of 1 to 32 µg/ml, and target-site changes are characterized by high-level resistance with MICs of 64 µg/ml or higher. These two mechanisms account for approximately 55% and 45%, respectively, of resistant isolates in North America. Recent reports of breakthrough pneumococcal bacteremia in patients treated with macrolides have highlighted concerns about resistance to this class of drugs.[64] In North America the macrolides continue to be effective in most cases because of excellent concentrations achieved in the alveolar macrophage. The 14-hydroxy metabolite of clarithromycin achieves concentrations of 480 µg/ml, and azithromycin achieves concentrations of 464 µg/ml in these phagocytes.[65]

A report of resistance to ciprofloxacin and to newer fluoroquinolones among pneumococcal isolates has generated considerable interest world wide.[66] Pneumococcal resistance to fluoroquinolones may be mediated by changes in one or both target sites (topoisomerase II and IV), usually resulting from mutations in the *gyrA* and *parC* genes, respectively, and possibly by an efflux pump as well.[67] Of greatest concern, however, are the multidrug-resistant isolates: those resistant to two or more antibiotics having different mechanisms of action. Recent data on more than 1500 pneumococcal isolates from across the United States indicate that 10% are macrolide resistant and 9.1% are multidrug resistant.[68]

Pathogens such as *H. influenzae* and the Enterobacteriaceae are important as well. *H. influenzae* is the third most common cause of CAP requiring admission to the hospital in some series, and although the Enterobacteriaceae are not particularly common, they are important because of the high mortality associated with them. Among such pathogens, resistance is usually mediated by β-lactamases, and the highest prevalence of β-lactamase genes is found on plasmids rather than an chromosomes. Members of the TEM and SHV families are the most successful of the plasmid-encoded β-lactamases, and the TEM_1 β-lactamase accounts for almost 80% of all such plasmid-encoded enzymes.[69] The extended spectrum β-lactamases include oxyimino enzymes that are TEM and SHV mutants and cephalosporinases unrelated to TEM and SHV enzymes.

Chromosomal β-lactamases are produced in either an inducible or a constitutive manner by genes located on the chromosome. Unfortunate sequelae may result because certain antibiotics are potent inducers of chromosomal β-lactamases and because bacteria mutate with reasonable regularity. When a spontaneous mutation occurs in the bacterial genome of a pathogen during treatment with an antibiotic that is an inducer of β-lactamase, the result may be the overgrowth of a stable derepressed mutant that is a hyperproducer of such enzymes. Recently a novel class of TEM_1-derived β-lactamases resistant to β-lactamase inhibitors has been described.[70] They are called inhibitor-resistant TEM–derived β-lactamases.

Therapeutic Regimens

The correct regimen for the initial treatment of the CAP patient has generated considerable discussion and controversy among respirologists, infectious disease specialists, internists, and emergency room physicians, and a number of societies have produced guidelines to help physicians with this task.[10,29–32,71–74] One of the guidelines is from the United Kingdom, but most are from North America. The fact that there are four distinct sets of North American guidelines highlights the controversy associated with this topic.

Some have argued that physicians should not rely upon guidelines and that each physician should make his or her own decision based on the circumstances of a particular case. An interesting paper discussing the use of antibiotics for CAP at several prominent U.S. medical centers before the development of the guidelines revealed a disturbing trend in the number and type of antibiotics used.[75] It demonstrated quite clearly that before the advent of the guidelines the treatment of CAP was far from ideal. Over 20 different types of antibiotics were used for outpatients, and over 23 types were used for inpatients, with many patients being given three or more drugs.

The guidelines serve a number of useful functions. They have codified our management of patients with CAP and have helped to highlight the gaps in our knowledge and to direct future studies and research. The guidelines also result in less money spent on antibiotics, lower mortality, and less time in hospital.[76,77]

The original guidelines published in North America in 1993 by the Canadian Infectious Disease Society and subsequently by the American Thoracic Society suggested that macrolides be used for the management of outpatients.[29,30] This had nothing to do with concerns about pneumococcal resistance to penicillin but was an attempt to deal with the atypical pathogen issue. If penicillin was used, it would be the agent of choice for *S. pneumoniae*, but it would be ineffective against any of the atypicals; however, a macrolide would provide good-to-excellent coverage for all the likely pathogens.

Recently, the fluoroquinolones have assumed a more important role in the management of CAP. This coincides with concerns about resistance to β-lactams and macrolides, the appreciation of the potential importance of gram-negative rods in selected CAP patients, and the recent appearance of the "respiratory fluoroquinolones." For patients admitted to a hospital, the fluoroquinolones offer logistic and financial benefits, since a single drug is given once daily compared to the multiple dosing required if a β-lactam plus macrolide regimen is used.

One of the fundamental differences between the Centers for Disease Control (CDC) document and the other current North American guidelines is that the CDC assumes that the physician knows that he or she is dealing with a pneumococcal infection.[10,72–74] The CDC believes there are no treatment failures for infection with *S. pneumoniae* with penicillin MICs of up to 1 μg/ml. For strains with penicillin MICs of 2 to 4 μg/ml, some data suggest that there is no increase in treatment failure, whereas other data suggest increased mortality or complications.[78–81]

Many experts believe that penicillin still has a role to play in the treatment of pneumoccocal pneumonia and that it is an effective agent for infections caused by susceptible organisms. For strains of *S. pneumoniae* with intermediate levels of resistance to penicillin, higher doses may be used. Unfortunately the question of penicillin efficacy is often moot, since in most cases our current diagnostic methods do not allow us to determine the identity or susceptibility of the etiologic agent at the time the decision is made regarding initial antibiotic treatment.

The efflux mechanism of macrolide resistance results in low-level resistance, and the target-change mechanism results in high-level resistance. The efflux mechanism is predominant in North America, and the target-change mechanism is more common in Europe. In the United States and Canada, therefore, macrolides are still seen as having a role to play in the management of many CAP patients. It should be emphasized, however, that the issue of both penicillin and macrolide resistance is one that is in a constant state of flux, and the usefulness of β-lactams and macrolides must be reassessed on a regular basis.

Approaches to the initial empiric treatment of patients with CAP based upon the Canadian guidelines are given in Table 5–2.

The IDSA, ATS, and Canadian documents are remarkably similar.[10,72,74] Although the IDSA statement lists outpatients as a single group, specific considerations are provided in their main treatment table and are addressed in the body of the IDSA document.[10] For example, the IDSA indicates that some clinicians may prefer to use macrolides or doxycycline for patients less than 50 years of age without comorbidity and fluoroquinolones for those older than 50 years of age or with comorbidity. In the Canadian guidelines, outpatients are divided into those without modifying factors in whom a macrolide may be used and those with modifying factors such as COPD who have or have not received antibiotics or steroids within 3 months.[72] A final grouping is patients with suspected gross aspiration. Fluoroquinolones are reserved for patients with COPD who recently have taken antibiotics, that is, those at increased risk of infection with penicillin-resistant *S. pneumoniae* or possibly infection with gram-negative rods. The ATS guidelines are similar to the Canadian ones in terms of how the outpatient groups are stratified and the suggested regimens.[74]

For patients treated in hospital, all three guidelines divide cases into (1) those treated on a medical ward and (2) those treated in the ICU, and they all use the risk of infection with *P. aeruginosa* as a means of further subdividing ICU patients. In previous guidelines the first choice for ward patients was a β-lactam with or without a macrolide.[29,30] In the most recent guidelines the Canadian document recommends monotherapy with a respiratory fluoroquinolone as first choice and a β-lactam plus a macrolide as second choice for ward patients. The IDSA suggests that either regimen may be used. For those treated in the ICU, a fluoroquinolone or macrolide in combination with a β-lactam is suggested if *P. aeruginosa* is not a concern. If it is a concern, an antipseudomonal β-lactam plus ciprofloxacin is recommended.

The ATS differs from the IDSA and Canadian guidelines in the management of ward patients in one

TABLE 5–2 ■ Empirical Antimicrobial Selection for Adults with Community-Acquired Pneumonia

Type of patient, factor(s) involved	Treatment regimen	
	First choice	Second choice
Outpatient without modifying factors	Macrolide*	Doxycycline
Outpatient with modifying factors		
COPD (no recent antibiotics or oral steroids within past 3 mo)	Newer macrolide†	Doxycycline
COPD (recent antibiotics or oral steroids within past 3 mo)	Respiratory fluoroquinolone‡	Amoxicillin-clavulanate + macrolide or 2G cephalosporin + macrolide
Suspected macroaspiration	Amoxicillin-clavulanate ± macrolide	Respiratory fluoroquinolone, e.g., levofloxacin + clindamycin or metronidazole
Nursing home acquired		
Treat in nursing home	Respiratory fluoroquinolone alone *or* amoxicillin-clavulanate + macrolide	2G cephalosporin + macrolide
Treat in hospital	Identical to treatment for other hospitalized patients (see below)	
Hospitalized patient on medical ward	Respiratory fluoroquinolone	2G, 3G, or 4G cephalosporin + macrolide
Hospitalized patient in intensive care unit		
Pseudomonas aeruginosa not suspected	IV respiratory fluoroquinolone + cefotaxime, ceftriaxone, *or* β-lactam–β-lactamase inhibitor	IV macrolide + cefotaxime, ceftriaxone, or β-lactam–β-lactamase inhibitor
P. aeruginosa suspected	Antipseudomonal fluoroquinolone (e.g., ciprofloxacin) + antipseudomonal β-lactam or aminoglycoside	Triple therapy with antipseudomonal β-lactam (e.g., ceftazidime, piperacillin-tazobactam, imipenem, or meropenem) + aminoglycoside (e.g., gentamicin, tobramycin, or amikacin) + macrolide

COPD, chronic obstructive pulmonary disease; 2G, second-generation; 3G, third-generation; 4G, fourth-generation.

*Erythromycin, azithromycin, or clarithromycin.

†Azithromycin or clarithromycin.

‡Levofloxacin, gatifloxacin, or moxifloxacin; use of trovafloxacin is restricted because of its association with severe hepatotoxicity.

important aspect.[10,72,74] It suggests that azithromycin alone may be used for patients without cardiopulmonary disease and with no modifying factors. Neither the IDSA nor the Canadian guidelines have such a category, and neither group suggests monotherapy with azithromycin as an option.

Of the four North American guidelines the only one that is not evidence based is the CDC document.[73] Interestingly, it is the only guideline that offers a regimen without atypical coverage as an option for outpatients with CAP, that is, macrolide, doxycycline, or a β-lactam.

Institution of antimicrobial therapy should not be delayed, particularly when dealing with patients older than 65 years. A study of elderly subjects presenting to emergency departments with CAP showed that those who received antibiotics within 8 hours of presentation had a significantly lower 30-day mortality than those who waited longer for initiation of their treatment.[82]

Intravenous-to-oral sequential treatment is strongly recommended, since it reduces costs, encourages patient mobility, and allows earlier discharge from the hospital. Ancillary measures such as supplemental oxygen, drainage of significant pleural effusions, and hydration are important as well.

The patient should be followed and objective parameters monitored: cough, shortness of breath, and elevated temperature should resolve and for those in hospital, the oxygen saturation and white blood cell count should improve.

Prevention

The two major steps that can be taken to reduce the impact of CAP are (1) influenza vaccine and (2) pneumococcal vaccine.

Influenza Vaccine

The incidence of influenza is variable, but when an outbreak occurs, it can have an effect on CAP in one of two ways. The first is by primary influenza pneumonia, and the second is by a secondary bacterial infection following the initial viral insult. Influenza is an acute febrile illness caused by infection with influenza virus A or B. It usually occurs in outbreaks of varying degrees of severity and may on occasion result in pandemics with devastating consequences. Antigenic variants in the external glycoproteins HA and NA give rise to minor (drift) or major (shift) antigenic changes, and scientists attempt to determine the viral antigenic variances likely to cause disease in the upcoming season. On the basis of such assessments the components of the inactivated trivalent vaccine are determined.

TABLE 5–3 ■ Target Groups for Influenza Immunization

GROUPS AT INCREASED RISK FOR INFLUENZA-RELATED COMPLICATIONS
Persons 65 years of age and older
Residents of nursing homes and other long-term care facilities that house persons of any age who have chronic conditions
Adults and children who have chronic disorders of the pulmonary or cardiovascular system, including children with asthma
Children and teenagers (ages 6 months to 18 years) who are receiving long-term aspirin therapy
Women who will be in the second or third trimester of pregnancy during the influenza season.

OCCUPATIONAL GROUPS WITH INCREASED POTENTIAL FOR TRANSMISSION OF INFLUENZA TO PERSONS AT HIGH RISK
Physicians, nurses, and other health care professionals
Employees of nursing homes and other long-term care facilities who have patient contact
Providers of home care and household contacts of persons at high risk

The vaccine ideally should be administered in the early fall to allow sufficient time for development of a protective antibody response. A meta-analysis showed that the vaccine reduced pneumonia by 53%, hospitalization by 50%, and mortality by 68%.[83]

The target groups for whom the vaccine is indicated are given in Table 5–3.

Immunoprophylaxis through the use of a vaccine is the optimal way to prevent influenza infection. Should an outbreak occur, however, particularly among an unprotected population living in a closed environment (e.g., unvaccinated elderly in a nursing home), other means of protection must be used. Chemoprophylaxis provides immediate protection but only while the drug is taken. The optimal approach in such a situation is to immediately vaccinate those who have not been immunized and to begin a 2-week regimen with an appropriate chemoprophylactic agent. The 2-week period should be sufficient time for an immune response to the vaccine to develop.

Pneumococcal Vaccine

Currently there are two types of pneumococcal vaccine: one is recommended for use in adults and older children, and the other is recommended for children ages 2 to 3 months and 24 to 59 months at increased risk for pneumococcal disease. The former is a 23-valent polysaccharide vaccine, and the latter is a 7-valent pneumococcal polysaccharide–protein conjugate vaccine.

The pneumococcal polysaccharide vaccine is effective in preventing invasive pneumococcal disease; effectiveness varies from 65% to 84%, depending upon the patient subgroup.[84]

Immunization is recommended for the following groups:

1. Persons age 65 years or older
2. Persons 2 to 64 years of age who have chronic illnesses, such as cardiovascular disease (congestive heart failure or cardiomyopathies), chronic pulmonary disease (COPD or emphysema, but not asthma), diabetes mellitus, alcoholism, chronic liver disease (cirrhosis), or cerebrospinal fluid leaks
3. Persons 2 to 64 years of age who have functional or anatomic asplenia

4. Persons 2 to 64 years of age who are living in special environments or social settings (Alaskan natives, certain Native American populations, residents of long-term care facilities).

The following immunocompromised persons over 2 years of age should also be immunized: persons with HIV infection, leukemia, lymphoma, Hodgkin's disease, multiple myeloma, generalized malignancy, chronic renal failure, nephrotic syndrome, or other conditions associated with immunosuppression and persons receiving immunosuppressant chemotherapy including long-term corticosteroids.[85]

HOSPITAL-ACQUIRED PNEUMONIA

Nosocomial or hospital-acquired pneumonia (HAP) is defined as pneumonia that occurs 48 hours or more after admission to the hospital. Although it is the second most common nosocomial infection in the United States, accounting for 13% to 18% of all hospital-acquired infections, it is the one most frequently associated with a fatal outcome.[86,87] It is associated not only with significant morbidity and mortality but also with a substantial economic burden, since it prolongs length of hospital stay by an average of 8 days.[86]

It is estimated that the rate of occurrence varies from four to eight episodes per 1000 hospitalizations in nonteaching and teaching hospitals, respectively.[88,89] In patients who are intubated the rate increases dramatically, in some cases being 20-fold higher than in nonintubated patients. Rates of ventilator-associated pneumonia (VAP) are reported to be approximately 15/1000 ventilator days.[87]

Mortality among patients with nosocomial pneumonia remains high; however, it is important to distinguish between crude and attributable mortality. Crude mortality is simply the percentage of patients with pneumonia who die. Rates in the order of 30% to 50% have been described[90]; however, since many of these patients often have significant underlying disease, the true importance of the crude mortality is difficult to determine.[87,90] Attributable mortality on the other hand represents death caused directly by pneumonia, and figures ranging from 10% to 20% have been reported.[91,92]

Etiology and Epidemiology

The most common pathogens encountered in nosocomial pneumonia are the gram-negative bacilli, which have been reported in up to 60% of cases, and *Staphylococcus aureus*, which has been reported in up to 40% of patients.[93–96] For infections occurring during the first 4 days of hospital stay, bacteria that typically are associated with CAP such as *S. pneumoniae* and *H. influenzae* have been reported as well.[97,98]

The Enterobacteriaceae are gram-negative facultative anaerobes widely distributed in nature, and those of interest in nosocomial pneumonia are *Escherichia coli*, *Klebsiella* spp, *Enterobacter* spp, *Proteus* spp, and *Serratia marcescens*. *E. coli* is the third most common coliform isolated from patients with HAP and appears to affect predisposed hosts such as the critically ill.[99] Of the *Klebsiella* spp, *K. pneumoniae* is most commonly isolated and may cause severe necrotizing lobar pneumonia in the elderly and in alcoholics and diabetics.[100] *K. pneumoniae* and *E. coli* are the bacteria that most commonly carry the extended spectrum β-lactamase enzymes, rendering them resistant to oxyimino-β-lactams such as cefotaxime, ceftazidime, and aztreonam.[101]

Enterobacter spp are among the most common of the Enterobacteriaceae implicated as causes of HAP, with *E. cloacae* and *E. aerogenes* being chiefly responsible. These bacteria are relatively opportunistic pathogens and frequently colonize patients who have received a course of antibiotics. Resistance to third-generation cephalosporins by these pathogens may develop within days of treatment.

Proteus mirabilis and *Proteus vulgaris* can act as opportunistic respiratory pathogens in a manner similar to that of the *Enterobacter* species. Indole-positive species such as *P. vulgaris* may also undergo single-step mutation to become constitutive high-level producers of β-lactamase enzymes, which is manifested as resistance to third-generation cephalosporins. *S. marcescens* preferentially colonizes the respiratory and urinary tracts and has been associated with common source outbreaks of pneumonia in the setting of inhalation therapy and contaminated bronchoscopes.[102,103] Like all Enterobacteriaceae, this organism may be spread to patients by hand transfer from health care personnel.

The nonfermentative gram-negative bacilli of importance are *P. aeruginosa* and *Acinetobacter* spp. *P. aeruginosa* is one of the leading gram-negative causes of pneumonia.[99,104] The most common mechanism of infection is direct contact with environmental reservoirs including respiratory devices such as contaminated nebulizers or humidifiers. *Acinetobacter* spp can also result in serious nosocomial infection and has been shown to be an important cause of VAP.[105]

H. influenzae frequently colonizes the upper respiratory tract of persons with predisposing conditions such as chronic obstructive lung disease. Most adult infections are caused by nontypeable strains, and *H. influenzae*

along with *S. pneumoniae* can often be isolated from tracheal secretions following intubation.[106] *S. pneumoniae* is an encapsulated gram-positive diplococcus that, like *H. influenzae*, colonizes the oropharynx. Although it is predominantly a pathogen associated with CAP, *S. pneumoniae* is being recognized with increasing frequency in cases of hospital-acquired infection.[97,105]

S. aureus is a gram-positive coccus that resides primarily in the anterior nares. From there, it may colonize the skin, groin, axillae, and perineal regions. It is spread through the hospital primarily by the hands of health care personnel. Adhesion of the organism to endothelial structures is an important mechanism for colonization.

Anaerobes may be found as pathogens in patients predisposed to aspiration[39] but are infrequently isolated from patients with VAP. The anaerobes that have been implicated in nosocomial pneumonia are those that colonize the oropharynx such as anaerobic gram-positive cocci and gram-negative bacilli, for example, *Fusobacterium* spp, *Prevotella melaninogenica*, and *Bacteroides ureolyticus*.[107]

Legionella pneumophila serogroup 1 is the most common of the *Legionella* species to be associated with both community-acquired and hospital-acquired pneumonia. The exact mode of transmission is controversial, and there is evidence for both aspiration and aerosolization.[108,109] Contaminated potable water and contaminated aerosols have been reported as sources of infection in hospitals.[110]

It is important to realize that nosocomial pneumonia may be caused by multiple pathogens in any one patient, emphasizing the need for broad coverage when empiric treatment is initiated. It has been demonstrated that more than one pathogen could be documented in almost half of HAP cases.[39]

Diagnosis

The diagnosis of HAP is similar in many ways to the diagnosis of CAP. The major difference is that for those with VAP, it is considerably easier to obtain bronchoscopic or deep suction samples for culture and Gram stain.

In taking the history, the physician must seek details that might help to suggest pneumonia as opposed to some other disease entity. For example, a history of a nonproductive cough and weight loss in a heavy smoker suggests carcinoma of the lung, whereas fever, chills, and a cough productive of purulent sputum might suggest pneumonia. Inquiries should also be made about risk factors for HAP and for specific pathogens (Tables 5–4 and 5–5).[111,112]

On physical examination, evidence should be sought not only of pulmonary involvement (e.g., findings suggestive of consolidation or pleural effusion) but also of extrapulmonary infection. As part of the general assessment of the patient, evidence of a systemic response to infection, such as elevated temperature and tachycardia,

TABLE 5–4 ■ Risk Factors for Nosocomial Pneumonia

Risk factor	Odds ratio (range)
Age	2.1–4.6
Chronic obstructive pulmonary disease	1.9–3.7
Low albumin	12.4–15.6
Neuromuscular disease	3.9–18
Decreased consciousness	1.9–5.8
Impaired reflexes	2.9–3.5
Trauma	2.6–3
Severity of illness	2.9–6.4
Aspiration	5–10.6
Intracranial pressure monitor	4.2
Endotracheal intubation	3–12.9
Emergent intubation	2.7
Prolonged mechanical ventilation	1.2–3.1
Thoracic or upper abdominal surgery	4.3–6
Nasogastric intubation	6.5

is also important. Signs suggestive of respiratory distress, such as a markedly elevated respiratory rate, cyanosis, and use of accessory muscles of respiration, are important to document as well.

The chest radiograph is not specific for pneumonia; however, the appearance of a new pulmonary infiltrate in the absence of any other obvious causes in conjunction with a clinical constellation of signs and symptoms, such as fever and purulent sputum, is suggestive of the diagnosis of pneumonia. None of these findings, however, enable the physician to determine the etiologic pathogen.[40] Chest radiography is also useful in helping to determine the extent of the pneumonia. Multilobe involvement, cavitation, or rapid radiographic progression indicates a severe infection. The chest film can also be used to determine whether a pleural effusion is present.

Routine blood counts and chemistry may indicate evidence of end organ dysfunction (rising liver function test results or serum creatinine) and are helpful in adjusting dosage regimens of antibiotics. Blood cultures may be useful in identifying the etiologic pathogen in up to 20% of patients with nosocomial pneumonia.[86]

The presence of a pathogen in blood not only indicates that it is the etiologic agent but also that the patient is at increased risk of a complicated course.[86,113] When blood cultures do yield a pathogen, it is important to exclude other sites of infection. In patients in whom carbon dioxide retention is possible, arterial blood gases should be measured, but if this is not possible, oximetry will suffice. There is also a role for oximetry in defining the severity of illness and determining whether supplemental oxygen is necessary.

Serology normally is not useful in the management of individual patients with nosocomial pneumonia. Serologic testing may be helpful for epidemiologic purposes, although this is more likely to be the case in patients with CAP.

The value of sputum Gram stain and culture is controversial, as there are significant problems with both the sensitivity and specificity of these tests. Most studies have been carried out in patients with CAP; however, the results can be extrapolated to patients with nosocomial pneumonia. For the results to be useful in the management of patients with pneumonia, a proper sample of respiratory secretions is necessary, the patient should not be receiving any antimicrobials, and the

TABLE 5–5 ■ Risk Factors for Specific Pathogens

Pathogens	Risk factors
Enterobacteriaceae	Oropharyngeal colonization (increased with underlying disease)
	Gastric colonization (antacids, H_2 antagonists)
Haemophilus influenzae	No prior antibiotics
	Smoking
Penicillin-resistant	β-lactam antibiotics or hospitalization during previous 3 months
Streptococcus pneumoniae	Nosocomial pneumonia
	Pneumonia during previous year
	Critical condition on presentation
	Immunosuppressive illness
Staphylococcus aureus	Head injury
	Coma > 24 h
	Intravenous drug use
	Diabetes mellitus
	Renal failure
Pseudomonas aeruginosa	Prior antibiotics
	Malnutrition
	Structural lung disease
	Steroid treatment
	Mechanical ventilation
	Contaminated water reservoirs
Acinetobacter spp	Prior antibiotics
Anaerobes	Recent abdominal surgery
	Witnessed aspiration event
Legionella spp	Contaminated water supply

sputum Gram stain should be assessed by someone with expertise in this area. Generally these tests are most helpful if they identify a pathogen that was unexpected or a pathogen with an unexpected in vitro susceptibility pattern. In selected cases, however, direct staining of sputum samples for fungi or mycobacteria or direct fluorescent antibody staining for *Legionella* may help in selecting therapy.

Invasive techniques are not performed routinely in patients with HAP. For patients with mild-to-moderate illness a diagnosis based on the clinical presentation is standard. Invasive techniques should be considered in selected cases, such as:

- Patients receiving appropriate empiric antimicrobial coverage but who are failing to respond
- Certain immunocompromised patients
- Patients in whom an alternative diagnosis (e.g., carcinoma) is suspected

A number of methods have been developed in an attempt to obtain samples of lower respiratory tract secretions that are not contaminated by oropharyngeal microorganisms. These vary from noninvasive techniques, such as endotracheal aspiration, to methods employing fiberoptic bronchoscopy. Essentially four methods are used to obtain secretions: endotracheal aspirate, protected catheter aspirate, protected specimen brush, and bronchoalveolar lavage. The studies that claim to support these techniques suffer from a lack of standardization, which makes comparison difficult at best. The discordant findings among the investigators studying these techniques make it difficult for practitioners to determine the best method. Most physicians would usually not rely on tests with such unstable properties to rule in or rule out a specific disease entity.

Other invasive tests include transthoracic needle aspiration, transbronchial biopsy, thoracoscopy, and open lung biopsy. There are no data to show that the use of invasive diagnostic testing alters mortality in patients in general and in VAP patients in particular.

Treatment

Before I go on to discuss the actual treatment regimen, a few brief comments about antimicrobial resistance are in order. In the section dealing with CAP, pneumococcal resistance to penicillins and macrolides was discussed and the extended spectrum β-lactamases were touched upon as well. *S. aureus*, however, although not particularly important in CAP, is the most common pathogen in HAP. Resistance of *S. aureus* to methicillin and to almost all β-lactam drugs is mediated by an acquired chromosomal gene (*mecA*) that encodes for the drug-resistant target *PBP2A*.[114] The presence of methicillin-resistant strains of *S. aureus* precludes the use of penicillinase-resistant semisynthetic penicillins (oxacillin, cloxacillin, nafcillin, methicillin) in many centers until the susceptibility patterns have been determined.

In the selection of an antimicrobial regimen for the management of HAP, the interactive triad of the patient, the pathogen, and the drug should be considered.

Patient-Related Factors

The physician must be aware of any previous history of adverse reaction and, in particular, of anything that suggests type I hypersensitivity to any antimicrobial. Age is also important, since adverse drug effects appear to be more common in the elderly, and with increasing age, impairment of renal and hepatic function is more likely. The macrolides, lincosamides, chloramphenicol, and metronidazole are eliminated via the liver, whereas most other antibiotics are eliminated by the kidney.

In the treatment of women in their child-bearing years, it is important to determine if the patient is pregnant, since teratogenicity has been associated with some agents, and risk of toxicity to the fetus is a concern when any drug is being used. The site of infection is important as well. A number of drugs, such as the aminoglycosides and many of the β-lactams, do not cross the blood-brain barrier easily. It is often not appreciated that barriers to certain antimicrobials exist in the lung as well. Aminoglycosides do not generally achieve high levels in lung tissue, and this problem is compounded by the fact that they are also relatively inactivated by the acidic pH present at the site of infection.[115,116]

It is also important to determine what other drugs the patient is taking. Drug interactions are always a concern, since they may be associated with adverse and occasionally fatal outcomes.

Pathogen-Related Factors

The identity of the pathogen(s) causing the infection is often not known. If this information is available, specific therapy directed against the pathogen can be used. Ideally, the narrowest spectrum agent with the least toxicity and the lowest price should be administered. Unfortunately, empiric therapy is usually the norm, and one must consider the likely pathogens on the basis of the local epidemiology, the risk factors for pneumonia and for specific pathogens, and the severity of the illness. The prevalence of resistance of certain pathogens to various antimicrobials must also be considered.

In many cases, monotherapy may be used; however, combination treatment should be employed for pathogens such as enterococci and *P. aeruginosa*.[117] As a general rule, combinations of antibiotics are used to broaden the antimicrobial spectrum, to provide additive or synergistic activity against certain pathogens, and to prevent the emergence of resistance.

Drug-Related Factors

In the selection of any antibiotic regimen the first step is to select an agent to which the pathogen is known or likely to be susceptible. There are, however, other features to be considered, including pharmacokinetic and pharmacodynamic properties, toxicity, drug interactions, and cost. Pharmacokinetics refers to the absorption, distribution, and elimination of drugs; pharmacodynamics is the relationship between the concentration of the drug in serum and its pharmacologic and toxicologic effects. Depending upon the class of antibiotic used, different pharmacokinetic and pharmacodynamic parameters correlate more or less closely with clinical or therapeutic efficacy. For β-lactam drugs, macrolides, and clindamycin, the time that the antibiotic concentration at the site of action in the tissues is above the MIC of the organism correlates best with efficacy. However, for aminoglycosides, fluoroquinolones, and vancomycin, the 24-hour area-under-the-curve (AUC)/MIC ratio correlates best. Higher ratios of peak serum concentrations to MIC have been shown to prevent the emergence of resistance during treatment with fluoroquinolones and aminoglycosides.

As a general rule, doses sufficient to achieve levels above the MIC of a particular pathogen at the site of infection should be administered. In immunocompetent patients, however, even subinhibitory concentrations of an antibiotic may be effective. Although the drug may not be able to kill or even inhibit the microorganism, it may alter it sufficiently so that it is more readily disposed of by intact host defenses such as opsonins and phagocytes.

Issues such as the significance of protein binding of antibiotics have not yet been fully resolved. It is known that only the unbound form of the drug is active in vitro, and presumably the same is true in vivo. It should be appreciated that the protein binding process itself is rapidly reversible, however, and even highly protein bound antibiotics are known to be clinically effective.

Toxicity and adverse drug reactions are important considerations in choosing an antibiotic. These reactions may range from mild gastrointestinal upset to fatal reactions. In all cases, physicians must try to select the drug that is the most efficacious and that is associated with the fewest side effects. Physicians should also be aware that certain drugs exhibit synergistic toxicity when administered in combination. Examples include aminoglycosides and loop diuretics, and aminoglycosides in combination with vancomycin or platinum derivatives.

Specific Issues

Given the shortcomings of the diagnostic methods available, the physician is usually faced with having to initiate therapy empirically. In effect, an educated guess is made regarding the most likely causative pathogens in a given situation. Two sets of guidelines have been developed that provide a structured approach to this problem.[86,118] The U.S. and Canadian guidelines are similar and are based upon the same premises and assumptions. Their approach takes into account risk factors, severity of illness, and time of onset of the illness in relation to hospitalization. The risk factors are for infection with specific pathogens; severity of illness is either mild to moderate or severe; and time of onset refers to early versus late, with these being less than 5 or 5 or more days, respectively.

Based upon these variables, 3 tables were developed that represent a hierarchical approach to the patient with nosocomial pneumonia. Although it is recognized that a large number of bacteria are potential pathogens, there is a "core" group of organisms that must be considered in each case and for which antimicrobial coverage must be provided. This core group consists of gram-negative bacilli such as *Enterobacter* spp, *E. coli*, *Klebsiella* spp, *Proteus* spp, *S. marcescens*, and *H. influenzae* and gram-positive cocci such as *S. aureus* and *S. pneumoniae*. Depending upon the risk factors present and the severity of illness, anaerobes, methicillin-resistant *S. aureus*, and *Legionella*, *Pseudomonas*, and *Acinetobacter* spp should be considered as well.

The ATS regimens are presented in Tables 5–6 to 5–8.[86] The treatments listed are not meant to represent priority of administration. The decision to pick any one agent should be made on the basis of the host, pathogen,

TABLE 5–6 ■ Initial Empiric Treatment of Patients with Mild-to-Moderate Hospital-Acquired Pneumonia, No Unusual Risk Factors, and Onset at Any Time or with Severe, Early-Onset Hospital-Acquired Pneumonia

Core organisms	Core antibiotics
Enteric gram-negative bacilli (nonpseudomonal), *Enterobacter* spp *Escherichia coli* *Klebsiella* spp	Cephalosporin Second-generation or nonpseudomonal Third-generation β-lactam–β-lactamase inhibitor combination, e.g., piperacillin-tazobactam
Proteus spp *Serratia marcescens* *Haemophilus influenzae* Methicillin-sensitive *Staphylococcus aureus* *Streptococcus pneumoniae*	If allergic to penicillin Fluoroquinolone or Clindamycin + aztreonam

Adapted from American Thoracic Society: Hospital-acquired pneumonia in adults: Diagnosis, assessment of severity, initial antimicrobial therapy, and preventive strategies: a consensus statement. Am J Respir Crit Care Med 1995;153:1711–1725.

TABLE 5–7 ■ **Initial Empiric Treatment of Patients with Mild-to-Moderate Hospital-Acquired Pneumonia with Risk Factors, Onset at Any Time**

Core organisms	Core antibiotics plus
Anaerobes (recent abdominal surgery, witnessed aspiration)	Clindamycin or β-lactam–β-lactamase inhibitor (alone) e.g., piperacillin-tazobactam
Staphylococcus aureus (coma, head trauma, diabetes mellitus, renal failure)	+/- Vancomycin (until methicillin-resistant S. aureus is ruled out)
Legionella (high-dose steroids)	Erythromycin +/- rifampin
Pseudomonas aeruginosa (prolonged ICU stay, steroids, antibiotics, structural lung disease)	Treat as severe hospital-acquired pneumonia

Adapted from American Thoracic Society: Hospital-acquired pneumonia in adults: Diagnosis, assessment of severity, initial antimicrobial therapy, and preventive strategies: a consensus statement. Am J Respir Crit Care Med 1995;153:1711–1725.

TABLE 5–8 ■ **Initial Empiric Treatment of Patients with Severe, Early-Onset Hospital-Acquired Pneumonia with Risk Factors or with Severe, Late-Onset Hospital-Acquired Pneumonia**

Core organisms plus	Therapy		
Pseudomonas aeruginosa	Antipseudomonal penicillin or		
Acinetobacter spp	Piperacillin-tazobactam or Ceftazidime or Carbapenem*	+	Aminoglycoside or Ciprofloxacin

*Imipenem or meropenem.
Adapted from American Thoracic Society: Hospital-acquired pneumonia in adults: Diagnosis, assessment of severity, initial antimicrobial therapy, and preventive strategies: a consensus statement. Am J Respir Crit Care Med 1995;153:1711–1725.

and drug-related issues outlined earlier. A few specific issues, however, deserve comment. As can be seen from the tables, single-agent therapy is recommended in many situations. Combinations of antibiotics are used to extend antimicrobial coverage, provide synergy, or prevent the emergence of resistance. The issue of broader coverage was a concern a decade ago before the introduction of broader spectrum agents such as some of the third-generation cephalosporins, the carbapenems, and more recently, the β-lactam–β-lactamase inhibitor combinations. Now, however, agents such as piperacillin-tazobactam provide coverage for most of the aerobic and anaerobic pathogens of concern. The issue of synergistic or additive activity is important for bacteria such as Enterococcus spp or P. aeruginosa, but there are no data to support the routine use of combination therapy for other bacterial pathogens in nonneutropenic patients.

Enterobacter is the most common genus of Enterobacteriaceae implicated as a cause of HAP.[99] One of the major concerns with infection caused by this organism is that in the presence of a third-generation cephalosporin, a mutation in the bacterial genome may occur, resulting in a pathogen that becomes a hyperproducer of β-lactamase.[119,120]

In patients who are severely ill with risk factors and early onset or severely ill without risk factors but with late onset, aggressive combination therapy should be instituted. If the patient had not received any antibiotics and deep suction aspirates or bronchoscopy samples fail to yield P. aeruginosa or other often resistant pathogens such as Acinetobacter spp, treatment may be modified to a single-drug regimen.

The Canadian guidelines go a step further and suggest that in patients with mild-to-moderate pneumonia without risk factors, an oral regimen alone may suffice.[118] This, of course, assumes that an agent with appropriate in vitro and pharmacokinetic-pharmacodynamic properties is selected.

The final issue is that of duration of therapy. Unfortunately there are no appropriately designed randomized controlled trials that specifically address this issue. The general consensus, however, is that patients with severe infection caused by pathogens such as P. aeruginosa or Acinetobacter spp should be treated for a minimum of 14 days, whereas patients with less severe infection may only require 7 to 10 days of treatment.

Prevention

Prevention of pneumonia in the hospital setting is somewhat more complicated than prevention of CAP. It includes prophylactic measures directed at patients on a medical or surgical ward as well as prevention of VAP, which complicates the process considerably. Recently a review of risk factors for nosocomial pneumonia with particular emphasis on prophylaxis was published, and

TABLE 5–9 ■ Centers for Disease Control and Hospital Infection Control Practices Advisory Committee (CDC–HICPAC) Guidelines for Prevention of Hospital-Acquired Pneumonia and Kollef's Guidelines for Prevention of Ventilator-Associated Pneumonia (VAP)

Risk factor	Preventive measure	CDC–HICPAC category[*]	Kollef category[†] (VAP)
Age	Primary prevention, health care maintenance	NS	NS
Underlying disease	Treat COPD, incentive spirometry	II	NS
	Influenza, pneumococcal vaccination	IA	D
Immunosuppression	Minimize duration of neutropenia ± G-CSF	NS	D
Depressed consciousness	Cautious use of CNS depressants	IB	NS
	Position patient upright at 30°–45°	IB/IA	B
Oral hygiene	Use chlorhexidine gluconate (0.12%) oral rinse (cardiac patients)	NS	B
Cross-infection	Educate and train personnel	IA	NS
	Appropriate handwashing, use of gloves and gowns	IA	B
	Feedback of surveillance data to staff	IA	NS
	Identification of MDR pathogens	NS	NS
Enteral feeding	Verify tube placement	IB	U
	Use sterile water	NS	NS
	Use orogastric tube, if possible	NS	D
	Acidification of gastric feedings	NR	U
	Use of intermittent versus continuous feedings	NR	NS
Avoid reflux	Position patient upright at 30°–45°	IB/IA	B
Antibiotic administration	Antibiotic prophylaxis for nosocomial pneumonia not recommended	IA	U
	Judicious administration of appropriate antibiotics	IA	C
	Rotation of empiric antibiotic regimens	NS	C

G-CSF, granulocyte colony stimulating factor.

[*]Key to CDC-HICPAC categories:

IA, measure strongly recommended for all hospitals, and well-designed studies are available to support recommendation.

IB, measure strongly recommended for all hospitals, although definitive studies may not exist, but there is a consensus of opinion among experts on the value of the measure.

II, measure is suggested for use in many hospitals on the basis of suggestive clinical studies.

NR, no recommendation can be given because of insufficient data or a lack of consensus.

NS, measure not specified.

[†]Key to Kollef categories:

A, data supported by at least two randomized controlled trials.

B, data supported by at least one randomized controlled trial.

C, data supported by nonrandomized concurrent-cohort investigations, historical-cohort investigations, or a case series.

D, data supported by randomized controlled investigations of other nosocomial infections.

NS, measure not specified.

U, undetermined or not yet studied measures.

the interested reader is referred to this paper.[121] The majority of the recommendations are based upon the Centers for Disease Control–Hospital Infection Control Practices Advisory Committee (CDC–HICPAC) guidelines for prevention of HAP and prevention of VAP as outlined in a paper by Kollef.[93,122]

Preventive measures are aimed at a number of host-related factors and infection control practices as well as medication and device-associated risk factors. Many of these preventive measures are listed in Tables 5–9 and 5–10 together with the status of the recommendations as given in the CDC–HICPAC statement and the paper by Kollef.[93,122] In the CDC–HICPAC document a number of categories are used. IA and IB imply that the preventive measure is strongly recommended for all hospitals and that in the first case, data from well-designed studies are available, in IB,

definitive studies may not exist, but there is a consensus of opinion among experts on the value of the measure. Category II means that the measure is suggested for use in many hospitals based upon suggestive clinical studies. NR means that no recommendation can be given as the issue is unresolved because of insufficient data or a lack of consensus, NS means that the preventive measure is not specified by the CDC–HICPAC guidelines. The Kollef criteria are somewhat different. Categories A and B refer to data supported by at least two or one randomized controlled trial, respectively. Category C refers to data supported by nonrandomized concurrent-cohort investigations, historical-cohort investigations, or a case series; category D refers to data supported by randomized controlled investigations of other nosocomial infections; U refers to measures that are undetermined or not yet studied.

TABLE 5–10 ■ Centers for Disease Control and Hospital Infection Control Practices Advisory Committee (CDC–HICPAC) Guidelines for Prevention of Nosocomial Pneumonia and Kollef's Guidelines for Prevention of Ventilator-Associated Pneumonia (VAP)

Risk factor	Preventive measure	CDC–HICPAC category*	Kollef category[†] (VAP)
DEVICE-RELATED			
Invasive devices	Appropriate cleaning and sterilization	IB	NS
	Expeditious removal	IB	NS
Spirometer–O$_2$ sensor	Clean, sterilize/disinfect between patients	IA	NS
Resuscitation bag	Clean, sterilize/disinfect between patients	IA	NS
Nasogastric tube	Refer to enteral feeding (above)	IA	
	Remove tube as soon as is feasible	IA	C
Endotracheal intubation	Continuous aspiration of subglottic secretions	NR	A
	Adequate cuff pressure at all times	IB	C
	Oral intubation	NR	D
Ventilator circuits	Do not change more often than every 48 hours	IA	A
	Use heat-moisture exchanger	NR	A
	Schedule drainage condensate away from patients	IA	C
In-line nebulizer	Disinfect between treatments	IB	NS
	Sterilize between patients	IB	NS
Suction catheter	Aseptic technique	IA	NS
	Sterile single-use catheter for open system	II	NS
	Closed-circuit tracheal suction catheter	NR	NS
Tracheostomy care	Use aseptic technique when changing tracheostomy tubes	IB	NS
Immobility	Lateral rotational bed	NR	NS
	Semirecumbent positioning	NS	B
Cross-infection	Handwashing, glove and gown	IA	B
	Infection control program	IA	C
PHARMACOLOGIC			
Orogastric colonization	Selective digestive decontamination not recommended	NR	A
Stress bleeding prophylaxis	Use nonalkalinizing cytoprotective agents	II	B
Bacterial resistance	Antibiotic class rotation	NS	C

G-CSF, granulocyte colony stimulating factor.

*Key to CDC-HICPAC categories:

IA, measure strongly recommended for all hospitals, and well-designed studies are available to support recommendation.

IB, measure strongly recommended for all hospitals, although definitive studies may not exist, but there is a consensus of opinion among experts on the value of the measure.

II, measure is suggested for use in many hospitals on the basis of suggestive clinical studies.

NR, no recommendation can be given because of insufficient data or a lack of consensus.

NS, measure not specified.

[†]Key to Kollef categories:

A, data supported by at least two randomized controlled trials.

B, data supported by at least one randomized controlled trial.

C, data supported by nonrandomized concurrent-cohort investigations, historical-cohort investigations, or a case series.

D, data supported by randomized controlled investigations of other nosocomial infections.

NS, measure not specified.

U, undetermined or not yet studied measures.

REFERENCES

1. Gonzales R, Steiner JF, Sande MA: Antibiotic prescribing for adults with colds, upper respiratory tract infections, and bronchitis by ambulatory care physicians. JAMA 1997;278:901–904.

2. Rodnick JE, Gude JK: The use of antibiotics in acute bronchitis and acute exacerbations of chronic bronchitis. West J Med 1988;149:347–351.

3. Smith CB, Golden CA, Kanner RE, et al: Association of viral and *Mycoplasma pneumoniae* infections with acute respiratory illness in patients with chronic obstructive pulmonary diseases. Am Rev Respir Dis 1980;121:225–232.

4. Niroumand M, Grossman RF: Airway infection. Infect Dis Clin North Am 1998;12(3):671–687.

5. Ayres JG: Seasonal patterns of acute bronchitis in general practice in the United Kingdom. Thorax 1986;41:106–110.

6. Gwaltney J Jr: Clinical and mechanistic perspectives on acute self-limited cough. Symposium Report from the World Congress of Pharmacy and Pharmaceutical Sciences. Int Pharm J 1997;11:5–7.

7. Littenberg B, Wheeler M, Smith DS: A randomized controlled trial of oral albuterol in acute cough. J Fam Pract 1996;42:49–53.

8. Read RC: Treating influenza with zanamivir. Lancet 1998;352:1872–1873.

9. Hayden FG, Treanor JJ, Fritz RS, et al: Use of the oral neuraminidase inhibitor oseltamivir in experimental human influenza. JAMA 1999;282:1240–1248.

10. Bartlett JG, Dowell SF, Mandell LA, et al: Practice guidelines for the management of community-acquired pneumonia in adults. Guidelines from the Infectious Diseases Society of America. Clin Infect Dis 2000;31:347–382.

11. Celli BR, Snider GL, Heffner J, et al: American Thoracic Society Statement—Standards for the diagnosis and care of patients with chronic obstructive pulmonary disease. Am J Respir Crit Care Med 1995;152:S77–S120.

12. Anthonisen NR, Manfreda J, Warren CPW, et al: Antibiotic therapy in exacerbations of chronic obstructive lung disease. Ann Intern Med 1987;106:196–204.

13. Monso E, Ruiz J, Rosell A, et al: Bacterial infection in chronic obstructive pulmonary disease: A study of stable and exacerbated outpatients using the protected specimen brush. Am J Respir Crit Care Med 1995;152:1316–1320.

14. Soler N, Torres A, Ewig S, et al: Bronchial microbial patterns in severe exacerbations of chronic obstructive pulmonary disease (COPD) requiring mechanical ventilation. Am J Respir Crit Care Med 1998;157:1498–1505.

15. Eller J, Ede A, Schaberg T, et al: Infective exacerbations of chronic bronchitis: Relation between bacteriologic etiology and lung function. Chest 1998;113:1542–1548.

16. Miravitlles M, Espinosa C, Fernandez-Laso E, et al: Relationship between bacterial flora in sputum and functional impairment in patients with acute exacerbations of COPD. Chest 1999;116:40–46.

17. Ball P, Harris JM, Lowson D, et al: Acute infective exacerbations of chronic bronchitis. Q J Med 1995;88:61–68.

18. Saint S, Vittinghoff E, Grady D: Antibiotics in chronic obstructive pulmonary disease exacerbations. A meta-analysis. JAMA 1995;273:957–960.

19. Derenne JP, Fleury B, Parienta R: Acute respiratory failure of chronic obstructive lung disease. Am Rev Respir Dis 1988;138:1006–1033.

20. Seneff MG, Wagner DP, Wagner RP, et al: Hospital and 1-year survival of patients admitted to intensive care units with acute exacerbation of chronic obstructive lung disease. JAMA 1999;274:1852–1857.

21. Lode H: Respiratory tract infections: When is antibiotic therapy indicated? Clin Ther 1991;13:149–156.

22. Balter NS, Hyland RH, Low DE, et al: Recommendations on the managements of chronic bronchitis. CMAJ 1994;151(Suppl):7–23.

23. Wilson R: Outcome predictors in bronchitis. Chest 1995;108(Suppl):53–57.

24. Wilson R, Kubin R, Ballin I, et al: Five day moxifloxacin therapy compared with 7 day clarithromycin therapy for the treatment of acute exacerbations of chronic bronchitis. J Antimicrob Chemother 1999;44:501–513.

25. Wilson R, Ball P, Mandell LA, et al: Efficacy of once daily gemifloxacin for 5 days compared with twice daily clarithromycin for 7 days for the treatment of AECB. Intercontinental Conference on Antimicrobial Agents and Chemotherapy, San Francisco, September 1999.

26. Hayden FG, Atmar RI, Schilling M, et al: Safety and efficacy of oral GS4104 in long-term prophylaxis of natural influenza [abstract LB-6]. Final Program, Abstracts and Exhibits Addendum: 38th Annual Intercontinental Conference on Antimicrobial Agents and Chemotherapy, San Diego, 1998;22(abstract LB-7).

27. Monto AS, Robinson DP, Herlocher L, et al: Efficacy and safety of zanamivir in prevention of influenza among healthy adults. Final Program, Abstracts and Exhibits Addendum: 38th Annual Intercontinental Conference on Antimicrobial Agents and Chemotherapy, San Diego, 1998.

28. Hayden FG, Osterhaus ADME, Treanor JJ, et al: Efficacy and safety of the neuraminidase inhibitor zanamivir in the treatment of influenza virus infections. N Engl J Med 1997;337:874–879.

29. Mandell LA, Niederman MS: Antimicrobial treatment of community-acquired pneumonia in adults: A conference report. The Canadian Community-Acquired Pneumonia Consensus Group. Can J Infect Dis 1993;4:25–28.

30. Niederman MS, Bass JB Jr, Campbell GD, et al: Guidelines for the initial management of adults with community-acquired pneumonia: Diagnosis, assessment of severity, and initial antimicrobial therapy. American Thoracic Society, Medical Section of the American Lung Association. Am Rev Respir Dis 1993;148:1418–1426.

31. British Thoracic Society: Guidelines for the management of community-acquired pneumonia in adults admitted to hospital. Br J Hosp Med 1993;49:346–350.

32. European Respiratory Society Task Force Report: Guidelines for management of adult community-acquired lower respiratory tract infections. Eur Respir J 1998;11:986–991.

33. National Center for Health Statistics National Hospital Discharge Survey: Annual summary 1990. Vital Health Stat 1998;13:1–225.

34. Foy HM, Cooney MK, Allan I, et al: Rates of pneumonia during influenza epidemics in Seattle, 1964 to 1975. JAMA 1979;241:253–258.

35. Koivula I, Sten M, Makela PH: Risk factors for pneumonia in the elderly. Am J Med 1994;96:313–320.

36. Sankilampi U, Herva E, Haikala R, et al: Epidemiology of invasive *Streptococcus pneumoniae* infections in adults in Finland. Epidemiol Infect 1997;118:7–15.

37. Nielsen SV, Henrichsen J: Incidence of invasive pneumococcal disease and distribution of capsular types of pneumococci in Denmark, 1989–94. Epidemiol Infect 1996;117:411–416.

38. Zangwill KM, Vadheim CM, Vannier AM, et al: Epidemiology of invasive pneumococcal disease in southern California: Implications for the design and conduct of a pneumococcal conjugate vaccine efficacy trial. J Infect Dis 1996;174:752–759.

39. Bartlett JG, O'Keefe P, Tally FP, et al: Bacteriology of hospital-acquired pneumonia. Arch Intern Med 1986;146(5):868–871.

40. Fang GD, Fine M, Orloff J, et al: New and emerging etiologies for community-acquired pneumonia with implications for therapy: A prospective multicenter study of 359 cases. Medicine 1990;69(5):307–316.

41. Marrie TJ: Community-acquired pneumonia. Clin Infect Dis 1994;18:501–515.

42. Moine P, Vercken J-B, Chevret S, et al: Severe community-acquired pneumonia: Etiology, epidemiology and prognostic factors. Chest 1994;105:1487–1495.

43. Fine MJ, Smith MA, Carson CA, et al: Prognosis and outcomes of patients with community-acquired pneumonia. JAMA 1996;275:134–141.

44. Marston BJ, Plouffe JF, File TM Jr, et al: Incidence of community-acquired pneumonia requiring hospitalization. Results of a population based surveillance study in Ohio. The Community-Based Pneumonia Incidence Study Group. Arch Intern Med 1997;157:1709–1718.

45. Troy CJ, Peeling RW, Ellis AG, et al: *Chlamydia pneumoniae* as a new source of infectious outbreaks in nursing homes. JAMA 1997;277:1217–1218.

46. Bates JH, Campbell GD, Barron AL, et al: Microbial etiology of acute pneumonia in hospitalized patients. Chest 1992;101:1005–1012.

47. Woodhead MA, Arrowsmith J, Chamberlain-Webber R, et al: The value of routine microbial investigation in community-acquired pneumonia. Respir Med 1991;85:313–317.

48. Spiteri MA, Cook DG, Clark SW: Reliability of eliciting physical signs in examination of the chest. Lancet 1988;1:873–875.

49. Schilling RSF, Hughes JPW, Dingwall-Fordyce I: Disagreement between observers in an epidemiological study of respiratory disease. BMJ 1955;230:55–68.

50. Fine MJ, Auble TE, Yealy DM, et al: A prediction rule to identify low-risk patients with community-acquired pneumonia. N Engl J Med 1997;336:243–250.

51. Reed WW, Byrd GS, Gates RH Jr, et al: Sputum Gram's stain in community-acquired pneumococcal pneumonia. A meta-analysis. West J Med 1996;165:197–204.

52. Moine P, Vercken JB, Chevret S, et al: Severe community-acquired pneumococcal pneumonia. The French Study Group of Community-Acquired Pneumonia in ICU. Scand J Infect Dis 1995;27:201–206.

53. Light RW, Girard WM, Jenkinson SG, et al: Parapneumonic effusions. Am J Med 1980;69:507–512.

54. Auble TE, Yealy DM, Fine MJ: Assessing prognosis and selecting an initial site of care for adults with community-acquired pneumonia. Infect Dis Clin North Am 1998;12:741–759.

55. Niederman MS, McCombs JS, Unger AN, et al: The cost of treating community-acquired pneumonia [abstract]. Am J Respir Crit Care 1998;157:A292.

56. German PM, Restuccia JD: The appropriateness evaluation protocol: A technique for assessing unnecessary days of hospital care. Med Care 1981;19:855–871.

57. British Thoracic Society and Public Health Laboratory Service: Community-acquired pneumonia in adults in British hospitals in 1982–1983: A survey of aetiology, mortality, prognostic factors, and outcome. Q J Med 1987;62:195–222.

58. Porath A, Schlaeffer F, Lieberman D: Appropriateness of hospitalization of patients with community-acquired pneumonia. Ann Emerg Med 1996;27:176–183.

59. Fine MJ, Smith MA, Carson CA, et al: Prognosis and outcomes of patients with community-acquired pneumonia. A meta-analysis. JAMA 1996;275:134–141.

60. Fine MJ, Hanusa BH, Lave JR, et al: Comparison of a disease-specific and a generic severity of illness measure for patients with community-acquired pneumonia. J Gen Intern Med 1995;10:359–368.

61. National Committee for Clinical Laboratory Standards: Performance Standards for Antimicrobial Susceptibility Testing. Villanova, Pa, National Committee for Clinical Laboratory Standards, 1994. NCCLS document M100-S5 supplement, vol 24, no 16.

62. Ferrandiz MJ, Fernoll A, Linares J, de la Campa AG: Horizontal transfer of parC and parA in fluoroquinolone-resistant clinical isolates of Streptococcus pneumoniae. Antimicrob Agents Chemother 2000;44:840–847.

63. Johnston NJ, deAzavedo JC, Kellner JD, et al: Prevalence and characterization of the mechanisms of macrolide, lincosamide, and streptogramin resistance in Streptococcus pneumoniae from across Canada. Abstracts from the 37th Intercontinental Conference on Antimicrobial Agents and Chemotherapy, Toronto, Ontario, Canada, Sept 28–Oct 1, 1997. Abstract C-77a.

64. Kelley MA, Weber DJ, Gilligan P, et al: Breakthrough pneumococcal bacteremia in patients being treated with azithromycin and clarithromycin. Clin Infect Dis 2000;31:1008–1011.

65. Nix DE: Intrapulmonary concentrations of antimicrobial agents. Infect Dis Clin North Am 1998;12(3):631–646.

66. Wise R, Brenwald N, Gill M, et al: Streptococcus pneumoniae resistance to fluoroquinolones [letter]. Lancet 1996;348:1660.

67. Kohler T, Pechere JC: Bacterial resistance to quinolones. In Andriole VT (ed): The Quinolones. San Diego, Academic Press, 1998, pp 117–142.

68. Doern GV, Brueggemann A, Holley HP Jr, et al: Antimicrobial resistance of Streptococcus pneumoniae recovered from outpatients in the United States during the winter months of 1994 to 1995: Results of a 30-center national surveillance study. Antimicrob Agents Chemother 1996;40:1208–1213.

69. Livermore DM: Beta-lactamases in laboratory and clinical resistance. Clin Microbiol Rev 1995;8:557–584.

70. Henquell C, Chanal C, Sirot D, et al: Molecular characterization of nine different types of mutants among 107 inhibitor-resistant TEM beta-lactamases from clinical isolates of Escherichia coli. Antimicrob Agents Chemother 1995;39:427–430.

71. Bartlett JG, Breiman RF, Mandell LA, et al: Community-acquired pneumonia in adults: Guidelines for management. Clin Infect Dis 1998;26:811–838.

72. Mandell LA, Marrie TH, Grossman RF, et al and the Canadian Community-Acquired Pneumonia Working Group: Canadian guidelines for the initial management of community-acquired pneumonia: An evidence-based update by the Canadian Infectious Disease Society and the Canadian Thoracic Society. Clin Infect Dis 2000;31:383–421.

73. Heffelfinger JD, Dowell SF, Jorgensen JH, et al: Management of community-acquired pneumonia in the era of pneumococcal resistance: A report from the Drug-Resistant Streptococcus pneumoniae Therapeutic Working Group. Arch Intern Med 2000;160(10):1399–1408.

74. American Thoracic Society: Guidelines for the management of adults with community-acquired pneumonia: Diagnosis, assessment of severity, antimicrobial therapy and prevention. Am J Respir Crit Care Med 2001;163:1730–1754.

75. Gilbert K, Gleason PP, Singer DE, et al: Variations in antimicrobial use and cost in more than 2,000 patients with community-acquired pneumonia. Am J Med 1998;104:17–27.

76. Gleason PP, Meehan TP, Fine JM, et al: Associations between initial antimicrobial therapy and medical outcomes for elderly patients with pneumonia. Arch Intern Med 1999;159(21):2562–2572.

77. Stahl JE, Barza M, DesJardin J, et al: Effect of macrolides as part of initial empiric therapy on length of stay in patients with community-acquired pneumonia. Arch Intern Med 1999;159(21):2576–2580.

78. Choi E, Lee H: Clinical outcome of invasive infections by penicillin-resistant Streptococcus pneumoniae in Korean children. Clin Infect Dis 1998;26:1346–1354.

79. Deeks SL, Palacio R, Ruinsky R, et al: Risk factors and course of illness among children with invasive penicillin-resistant Streptococcus pneumoniae. Pediatrics 1999;103:409–413.

80. Feikin D, Schuchat A, Kolczak M, et al: Mortality from invasive pneumococcal pneumonia in the era of antibiotic resistance, 1995–1997. Am J Public Health 2000;90:223–229.

81. Dowell SF, Smith T, Leversedge K, et al: Pneumonia treatment failure associated with highly resistant pneumococci. Clin Infect Dis 1999;29:462–463.

82. Meehan TP, Fine MJ, Krumholz HM, et al: Quality of care, process and outcomes in elderly patients with pneumonia. JAMA 1997;278(23):2080–2084.

83. Fedson DS, Harward MP, Reid RA, et al: Hospital-based pneumococcal immunization: Epidemiologic rationale from the Shenandoah Study. JAMA 1990;264:1117–1122.

84. Gross PA: Vaccines for pneumonia and new antiviral therapies. Med Clin North Am 2001;85(6):1531–1544.

85. CDC: Prevention of pneumococcal disease: Recommendations of the advisory committee on immunization practices (ACIP). MMWR Morb Mortal Wkly Rep 1997;46(RR-8):1–24.

86. American Thoracic Society: Hospital-acquired pneumonia in adults: Diagnosis, assessment of severity, initial antimicrobial therapy, and preventative strategies: A consensus statement. Am J Respir Crit Care Med 1995;153:1711–1725.

87. Craven DE, Steger KA: Hospital-acquired pneumonia: Perspectives for the healthcare epidemiologist. Infect Control Hosp Epidemiol 1997;18:783–795.

88. Craven DE, Steger KA, LaForce FM: Pneumonia. In Bennett JV, Brachman PS (eds): Hospital Infections, 4th ed. Philadelphia, Lippincott-Raven Press, 1998.

89. Gross PA: Epidemiology of hospital-acquired pneumonia. Semin Respir Infect 1987;2:2–7.

90. Celis R, Torres A, Gatell JM, et al: Nosocomial pneumonia: A multivariate analysis of risk and prognosis. Chest 1988;93:318–324.

91. Leu H-S, Kaiser DL, Mori M, et al: Hospital-acquired pneumonia: Attributable mortality and morbidity. Am J Epidemiol 1989;129:1258–1267.

92. Fagon J-Y, Chastre J, Hance AJ, et al: Nosocomial pneumonia in ventilated patients: A cohort study evaluating attributable mortality and hospital stay. Am J Med 1993;94:281–288.

93. Tablan OC, Anderson LJ, Arden NH, et al: Guidelines for prevention of nosocomial pneumonia. Infect Control Hosp Epidemiol 1994;15:587–627.

94. Craven DE, Steger KA, Barber TW: Preventing nosocomial pneumonia: State of the art and perspectives for the 1990s. Am J Med 1991;91(Suppl 3B):44S–53S.

95. Craven DE, Steger KA: Nosocomial pneumonia in mechanically ventilated adult patients: Epidemiology and prevention in 1996. Semin Respir Infect 1996;11:32–53.

96. Johanson WG Jr, Pierce AK, Sanford JP, et al: Nosocomial respiratory infections with gram-negative bacilli: The significance of colonization of the respiratory tract. Ann Intern Med 1972;77:701–706.

97. Schleupner CJ, Cobb DK: A study of the etiologies and treatment of nosocomial pneumonia in a community-based teaching hospital. Infect Control Hosp Epidemiol 1992;13:515–525.

98. Rello JM, Ricart M, Ausina V, et al: Pneumonia due to *Haemophilus influenzae* among mechanically ventilated patients: Incidence, outcome, and risk factors. Chest 1992;102:1562–1565.

99. Hospital Infections Program, National Center for Infectious Disease, Centers for Disease Control and Prevention, US Department of Health and Human Services, National Nosocomial Infections Surveillance (NNIS) report, data summary from October 1986–April 1996, issued May 1996. Am J Infect Control 1996;24:380–388.

100. Verghese A, Berk SL: Bacterial pneumonia in the elderly. Medicine (Baltimore) 1983;62:271–285.

101. Jacoby GA, Medeiros AA: More extended-spectrum beta-lactamases. Antimicrob Agents Chemother 1991;35:1697–1704.

102. Sanders CV, Luby JP, Johanson WG Jr, et al: *Serratia marcescens* infections from inhalation therapy medications: Nosocomial outbreak. Ann Intern Med 1970;73:15–21.

103. Webb SF, Vall-Spinosa A: Outbreak of *Serratia marcescens* associated with the flexible fiberbronchoscope. Chest 1975;68:703–708.

104. Rello J, Quintana E, Ausina V, et al: Incidence, etiology, and outcome of nosocomial pneumonia in mechanically ventilated patients. Chest 1991;100:439–444.

105. Fagon J-Y, Chastre J, Domart Y, et al: Nosocomial pneumonia in patients receiving continuous mechanical ventilation: Prospective analysis of 52 episodes with use of a protected specimen brush and quantitative culture techniques. Am Rev Respir Dis 1989;139:877–884.

106. Sanderson PJ: The sources of pneumonia in ITU patients. Infect Control 1986;7:104–106.

107. Lorber B: Bacteroides, Prevotella, and Fusobacterium species (and other medically important anaerobic gram-negative bacilli). In Mandell GL, Bennett JE, Dolin R (eds): Principles and Practice of Infectious Disease, 4th ed. New York, Churchill Livingstone, 1995, pp 2195–2204.

108. Keller DW, Hajjeh R, DeMaria A Jr, et al: Community outbreak of legionnaires' disease: An investigation confirming the potential for cooling towers to transmit *Legionella* species. Clin Infect Dis 1996;22:257–261.

109. Blatt SP, Parkinson MD, Pace E, et al: Nosocomial legionnaires' disease: Aspiration as a primary model of disease acquisition. Am J Med 1993;95:16–22.

110. Mermel LA, Josephson SL, Giorgio CH, et al: Association of legionnaires' disease with construction: Contamination of potable water? Infect Control Hosp Epidemiol 1995;16:76–81.

111. Wiblin RT, Wenzel RP: Hospital-acquired pneumonia. Curr Clin Top Infect Dis 1996;16:194–214.

112. Loeb M, Mandell LA: Microbiology of hospital-acquired pneumonia. Semin Respir Crit Care Med 1997;18(2):111–120.

113. Bryan CS, Reynolds KL: Bacteremic nosocomial pneumonia: Analysis of 172 episodes from a single metropolitan area. Am Rev Respir Dis 1984;129:668–671.

114. Jacoby GA, Archer GL: New mechanisms of bacterial resistance to antimicrobial agents. N Engl J Med 1991;324:601–612.

115. Pennington JE: Penetration of antibiotics into respiratory secretions. Rev Infect Dis 1981;3:67–73.

116. Bodem CR, Lampton LM, Miller DP, et al: Endobronchial pH: Relevance to aminoglycoside activity in gram-negative bacillary pneumonia. Am Rev Respir Dis 1983;127:39–41.

117. Hilf M, Yu VL, Sharp J, et al: Antibiotic therapy for *Pseudomonas aeruginosa* bacteremia: Outcome correlations in a prospective study of 200 patients. Am J Med 1989;87:540–546.

118. Mandell LA, Marrie TJ, Niederman MS, et al: Initial antimicrobial treatment of hospital-acquired pneumonia in adults: A conference report. Can J Infect Dis 1993;4(6):317–321.

119. Sanders CC, Sander WE Jr: Clinical importance of inducible beta-lactamases in gram-negative bacteria. Eur J Clin Microbiol 1987;6:435–438.

120. Chow JW, Fine MJ, Shlaes DM, et al: *Enterobacter* bacteremia: Clinical features and emergence of antibiotic resistance during therapy. Ann Intern Med 1991;115:585–590.

121. Fleming CA, Balaguera HU, Craven DE: Risk factors for nosocomial pneumonia: Focus on prophylaxis. Med Clin North Am 2001;85(6):1545–1563.

122. Kollef MH: The prevention of ventilator-associated pneumonia. N Engl J Med 1999;340:627–634.

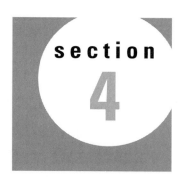

Cardiovascular Infections

Infections Associated with Intravascular Catheters

MARK E. RUPP, MD

The ability to routinely gain access to the vascular system, via intravascular (IV) catheters, to sample blood and instill fluids, blood products, and medications was a major advance in medical practice. Unfortunately, infection associated with IV catheters is a significant medical problem resulting in thousands of deaths and millions of dollars of excess medical cost in the United States each year. Despite the importance of these infections there is little controlled, comparative data regarding their most effective treatment. This chapter provides a brief summary of the epidemiology and pathogenesis of IV catheter infections and seeks to offer the clinician advice on therapy based on the limited data available. Controversies and questions regarding therapy are delineated.

EPIDEMIOLOGY AND SIGNIFICANCE

IV catheters are one of the most frequently used devices in the practice of modern medicine. Of the more than 150 million IV catheters used in the United States yearly, over 5 million are inserted in the central venous system (CVC)[1]. The risk of infection varies with the type of device used and the patient population. For instance, according to the Division of Healthcare Quality Promotion of the Centers for Disease Control and Prevention, the rate of CVC-associated bloodstream infection (BSI) in patients cared for in cardiothoracic intensive care units (ICU) is 2.8/1000 CVC days, and in patients cared for in burn ICUs the rate is 10/1000 CVC days.[2] The rate of infection for subcutaneously tunneled CVCs, such as Hickman or Broviac catheters, is lower than for nontunneled CVCs and is approximately 2.6 BSI/1000 CVC days.[3] The rate of infection with totally implanted catheters that are accessed via a subcutaneous port are quite low and are approximately 0.8 BSI/1000 CVC days.[3] It is estimated that as many as 250,000 patients experience IV catheter–associated BSI per year in the United States.[4] The attributable mortality of these infections has been observed to be as high as 25%.[5] Owing to the preponderance of infections due to relatively less virulent coagulase-negative staphylococci, however, a meta-analysis examining over 3000 episodes of IV catheter–associated BSI found the mean attributable mortality to be 2%.[6] The attributable cost of IV catheter–associated BSI ranges from $3700 to over $40,000.[7,8]

PATHOGENESIS

The pathogenesis of IV catheter-associated infections involves complex interactions between the host, the microbes, and the catheter. Host factors include such items as the site of insertion and underlying conditions, microbial factors include the presence or absence of various adhesins, and catheter factors include such items as biomaterial composition and design.[9] Microbes most frequently causing IV catheter–associated infection include coagulase-negative staphylococci and *Staphylococcus aureus*, *Enterococcus* spp. aerobic gram-negative bacilli, and *Candida* spp. The prevalence of infection due to Enterococci and *Candida* spp. appears to be increasing.

The route by which organisms gain access to the IV catheter is shown in Figure 6–1. It appears that in short-term nontunneled catheters the main route of colonization and infection is via transcutaneous migration down the external surface of the catheter. Conversely, in catheters that remain in place for longer periods and in tunneled catheters the main route of infection is via hub contamination and migration via the luminal surface of the catheter.

DIAGNOSIS

The diagnosis of IV catheter–associated infection depends on clinical signs and symptoms as well as microbiologic cultures of the blood and catheter. A full description of the clinical presentation and diagnosis of IV catheter–associated infection is beyond the scope of this chapter, and interested readers are referred to recent reviews.[10–15]

MANAGEMENT OF IV CATHETER INFECTION

The treatment of patients with IV catheter–associated infection depends on a number of variables including the type of catheter involved (e.g., peripheral vs. CVC), the site of infection (e.g., exit site vs. tunnel tract, with or without associated bacteremia), the causative pathogen (e.g., *S. aureus* vs. coagulase-negative staphylococci), host factors (e.g., ease of alternative vascular access, neutropenia), and clinical presentation (e.g., severity of systemic inflammatory response). Therefore, simple "one size fits all" recommendations are not possible. To further confound matters, there is little controlled data on which to base recommendations. Therefore, the following discussion is intended to help guide therapy but does not substitute for clinical experience and judgment.

Generally, the most pressing questions clinicians have when treating patients with IV catheter–associated infections are

1. Does the catheter need to be removed?
2. What antimicrobial agent should be given and by what route?
3. How long should the antimicrobial agent be administered?
4. What complications are possible and how are they evaluated and treated?

These practical questions will be stressed.

Peripheral IV Catheters

Because short-term peripheral IV catheters are generally easily removed and re-established, management issues are minimized. Peripheral IV catheters suspected to be infected should be promptly removed, the tip sent for culture (semi-quantitative or quantitative), and blood cultures obtained. In addition, any purulent exudate at the insertion site should be taken for Gram stain and culture. Empiric antibiotics should be initiated, and the regimen adjusted depending on culture results. The length of therapy depends on the causative organism and the clinical scenario (see Specific Pathogens).

Patients with septic thrombophlebitis of a peripheral vein usually have local signs of venous inflammation

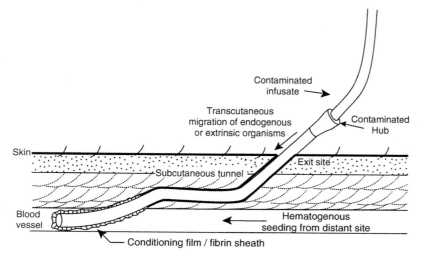

FIGURE 6–1. Potential sources for bacterial contamination of intravascular catheters. Bacteria gain access to the catheter by the following routes: contamination of the catheter hub, contamination of the infusate, transcutaneous migration, or hematogenous seeding. (From Rupp ME: Infections of intravascular catheters. In Crossley KB, Archer GL [eds]: The Staphylococci in Human Disease. New York, Churchill Livingstone, 1997, p 381.)

such as a palpable cord, abscess, tenderness, erythema, or purulent drainage.[16,17] Generally, because of its peripheral location, the involved vessel is excised or ligated.

Peripheral Arterial Catheters

Data suggest that peripheral arterial catheters are associated with a lower risk of infection per day of use than peripheral venous catheters are. As is the case with peripheral venous catheters, if a peripheral arterial catheter is suspected of being infected, it should be removed and its tip as well as any insertion site exudate should be cultured. Also, blood cultures should be obtained, and empiric antibiotics should be given. Infective arteritis of peripheral arteries, similar to infectious venous thrombophlebitis of peripheral veins, is usually manifest by local signs of inflammation. A pseudoaneurysm may form or embolic lesions may be noted.[18–20] Surgical excision and repair are often indicated.

Nontunneled Central Venous Catheters

In patients with clinically obvious nontunneled CVC-associated infection, manifested by purulence or evidence of inflammation at the site of insertion and systemic signs of infection (e.g., fever, hypotension), the CVC should be promptly removed, tip cultured, and empiric antimicrobials initiated. Unfortunately, CVC-associated infections rarely present with such overtly obvious signs, and most CVCs associated with bacteremia do not have significant local signs of infection.[21] Mild erythema at the CVC insertion site is usually a sign of localized foreign body–associated inflammation and does not necessarily indicate catheter-associated infection. To add to the complexity, many patients with CVCs are acutely ill because of a number of conditions and often have a variety of potential sources for fever. Eighty to ninety percent of febrile episodes in intensive care unit patients are not due to IV catheters, and most CVCs removed for presumed catheter-associated infection are removed unnecessarily.[13,22–24] Therefore, CVCs should not be removed routinely from patients with fever and limited severity of illness. CVCs should be removed from patients with obvious signs of CVC-associated infection (febrile patient with purulent drainage from CVC site) or patients with severe signs of infection and no other obvious source. Many clinicians choose to exchange CVCs via guidewires in subjects with ambiguous clinical situations. This allows the clinician to thoroughly evaluate the patient for a CVC-associated infection but protects the patient from some of the mechanical complications (e.g., pneumothorax, arterial puncture) associated with de novo CVC insertion. If cultures of the CVC confirm significant colonization of the catheter, the guidewire-exchanged catheter should be removed and a new CVC inserted at another site.[25]

There are limited data to support treatment of infected nontunneled CVCs without removal of the CVC. This

has been tried most successfully in subjects infected with less virulent organisms such as *Staphylococcus epidermidis*. In a retrospective survey, Raad and colleagues found that in 70 subjects with nontunneled CVC–associated coagulase-negative staphylococcal bacteremia, the mortality rate was similar whether the CVC was removed or treated in situ.[26] However, 29% of the 34 subjects in whom the catheters were treated in situ had the CVC exchanged over a guidewire, and the recurrence rate of bacteremia 6/30 (20%) was significantly higher than in those subjects in whom the CVC was removed 1/32 (3%).[26] All subjects with recurrent bacteremia were successfully treated with CVC removal and antibiotic therapy. Therefore, if it is elected to treat patients with a nontunneled CVC–associated infection without removal of the CVC they should be monitored closely. Continued fever or persistent bacteremia is a strong indication for CVC removal. It should also be noted that a significant number of persons with CVC-associated *S. aureus* bacteremia develop endocarditis. Fowler and colleagues found in a series of 59 subjects with *S. aureus* endocarditis that 45.8% were due to an infected intravascular device.[27] Therefore, some investigators suggest that transesophageal echocardiography (TEE) should be performed to assess for endocarditis in persons with *S. aureus* IV catheter–associated bacteremia.[28]

On occasion, the clinician will be faced with a febrile patient who in the course of the evaluation is found to have CVC cultures that indicate significant colonization (greater than or equal to 15 CFU) while blood cultures are sterile. There are no studies to guide the practitioner in how to proceed in this situation. If the CVC cultures reveal *S. aureus* or *Candida* spp. and the patient has underlying valvular heart disease or a significant immunosuppressive disorder, some authorities would recommend a short course (5 to 7 days) of antimicrobial therapy.[15] In all cases, these patients should be monitored closely, and appropriate cultures and treatment initiated if clinical signs or symptoms of significant infection develop. At other times a catheter culture may reveal significant colonization, but blood cultures were not obtained or were not obtained before empiric antibiotics were initiated. In these situations clinicians must rely on their clinical acumen, and if bacteremia is suspected, the patient must be appropriately treated. Recently the suggestion was made for clinical laboratories to reject catheter tip cultures if they were not accompanied by recently obtained blood cultures.[29] A general clinical approach to the patient with a suspected CVC-associated infection is outlined in Figure 6–2.

Tunneled CVCs and Subcutaneously Implanted CVCs

Surgically implanted CVCs consist of either subcutaneously tunneled devices such as Hickman, Broviac, or Groshong catheters or totally implanted devices such as

General Approach to the Patient with a Suspected Central Venous Catheter-Associated Infection

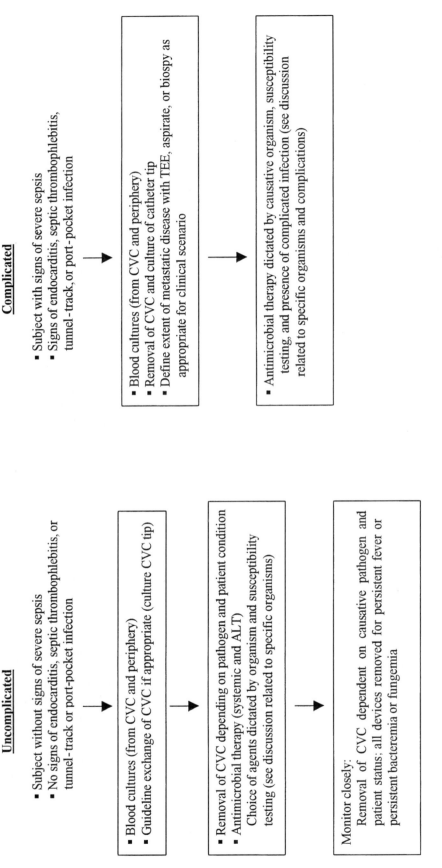

Uncomplicated

- Subject without signs of severe sepsis
- No signs of endocarditis, septic thrombophlebitis, or tunnel-track or port-pocket infection

↓

- Blood cultures (from CVC and periphery)
- Guideline exchange of CVC if appropriate (culture CVC tip)

↓

- Removal of CVC depending on pathogen and patient condition
- Antimicrobial therapy (systemic and ALT) Choice of agents dictated by organism and susceptibility testing (see discussion related to specific organisms)

↓

Monitor closely:
  Removal of CVC dependent on causative pathogen and patient status; all devices removed for persistent fever or persistent bacteremia or fungemia

Complicated

- Subject with signs of severe sepsis
- Signs of endocarditis, septic thrombophlebitis, tunnel-track, or port-pocket infection

↓

- Blood cultures (from CVC and periphery)
- Removal of CVC and culture of catheter tip
- Define extent of metastatic disease with TEE, aspirate, or biospy as appropriate for clinical scenario

↓

- Antimicrobial therapy dictated by causative organism, susceptibility testing, and presence of complicated infection (see discussion related to specific organisms and complications)

CVC — central venous catheter, TEE — transesophageal echocardiogram; ALT — antibiotic lock technique.

FIGURE 6-2. General approach to the patient with a suspected central venous catheter infection.

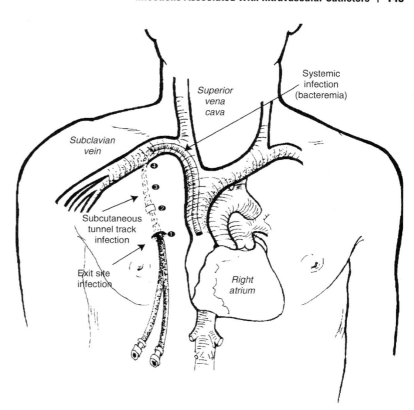

FIGURE 6–3. Anatomic landmarks and potential sites of infection for subcutaneously tunneled central venous catheters. 1, Cutaneous exit site; 2, Dacron cuff; 3, subcutaneous tunnel; 4, venous entrance site.

Port-a-Caths or Infuse-a-Ports. Figure 6–3 illustrates anatomic landmarks and potential sites of infection for subcutaneously tunneled CVCs. Because these devices are implanted in persons who require prolonged and repeated venous access, their removal often results in significant management issues, and particular care should thus be exercised in documenting the CVC as the source of infection.

Unfortunately, there are no randomized prospective studies to guide the clinician in management issues. A large prospective observational study was conducted by Groeger and colleagues at the Memorial Sloan-Kettering Cancer Center. In it 1630 surgically implanted, subcutaneously tunneled devices were studied for 443,563 device days.[30] During the 2-year study period, 341 (43%) catheters and 57 (8%) ports became infected. Of the catheters associated with bacteremia or fungemia, 72% were successfully treated with the catheters in situ.[30] However, 43% of the catheters were associated with repeated infection.[30] Unfortunately, the authors did not state which organisms were associated with recurrence and did not offer specific predictors of treatment success. A similar success rate was related by Mermel and colleagues, who reviewed 14 open trials of standard parenteral therapy for CVC-associated BSI and found that 342 (66.5%) of 514 episodes were treated successfully with the CVC in situ.[15] Lastly, it was observed that tunnel tract infections (Fig. 6–4) and port pocket infections required device removal, whereas exit site infections usually were treated successfully without device removal.[15,30]

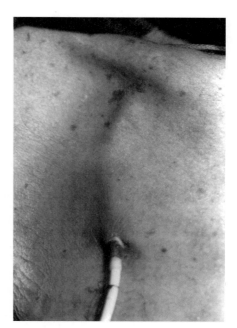

FIGURE 6–4. Typical appearance of a tunnel and exit site infection of a surgically implanted long-term central venous catheter exhibiting erythema, induration, and purulence. *Staphylococcus aureus* was recovered from purulent material expressed at the exit site, from blood cultures obtained from the catheter and peripheral blood, and from the catheter tip at time of removal. (From Rupp ME: Infections of intravascular catheters. In Crossley KB, Archer GL [eds]: The Staphylococci in Human Disease. New York, Churchill Livingstone, 1997, Plate 15–1.)

In general, many clinicians feel comfortable treating patients with a surgically implanted CVC-associated infection due to coagulase-negative staphylococci or other less virulent organisms with the CVC in situ. Infections due to *S. aureus*, gram-negative aerobic bacilli, and *Candida* spp. are associated with greater morbidity, and mortality, and many clinicians opt to remove the CVC rather than attempt in situ treatment (see Specific Pathogens). In all cases, if there is evidence of septic emboli, hypotension-sepsis, or persistently positive blood cultures, the CVC should be removed.

Hemodialysis Catheters

In 1999 approximately 200,000 patients were maintained on hemodialysis (HD) in the United States.[31] HD is dependent on prolonged vascular access either via surgically constructed fistulas and grafts or indwelling vascular catheters, and thus patients are at high risk for vascular catheter–associated infection. In a 1996 survey, 31.8% of patients undergoing HD did so via a CVC.[32] Recently the Centers for Disease Control and Prevention released guidelines on prevention of infection in HD patients.[33,34]

CVCs used for HD frequently become colonized with bacteria and often result in BSI.[35,36] In a study of French HD centers, 33% of infections involved the vascular access site.[37] Staphylococci are the organisms most frequently incriminated as a cause of HD catheter–associated BSI.[35,36,38] HD patients are often nasal carriers of *S. aureus*,[39,40] and efforts to reduce nasal carriage have successfully decreased rates of staphylococcal bacteremia.[39,41] Oliver and Schwab outlined a strategy for management of HD catheter–associated BSI that depended on the clinical severity of infection and the site of infection (presence of exit site or tunnel track infection).[42] Their review of the literature indicated success rates in treating HD catheter–associated bacteremia using their plan ranging from 32% to 100%.[42] As with other types of CVCs however, there are no randomized, prospective trials to document optimal methods of treating HD catheter–associated infections. The management of HD catheter– associated infection is similar to the management of other types of CVC-associated infection as previously discussed.

PERSISTENCE OF BIOMATERIAL-BASED INFECTION AND ANTIBIOTIC LOCK THERAPY

Biomaterial-associated infections are notoriously difficult to eradicate without removal of the device. A partial explanation for this problem is that organisms growing in a mature biofilm-associated environment are quite resistant to the effects of antimicrobial agents. Vaudaux and colleagues have demonstrated this effect in several studies using tissue cages experimentally infected with *S. aureus*.[43] In addition, there is a marked defect in host defense in the vicinity of a foreign body. Many studies have shown that in the presence of a foreign body, inocula of bacteria that would otherwise be subinfective result in clinical infection. For instance, in the presence of suture, inoculation of as few as 100 CFU of *S. aureus* results in an infection, whereas without the foreign body present, 10^7 organisms are noninfective.[44] Similar observations have been made in IV catheter models of infection.[45] Phagocytic and bactericidal activity of neutrophils is decreased when they are incubated with biomaterials.[46,47] Increased hexose-monophophate shunt activity and exocytosis of secondary granules result in cells with decreased bactericidal activity, the so-called frustrated phagocyte.[46,47] Also there may be local defects in cytokine levels in the vicinity of foreign bodies leading to decreased phogocyte activity.[48] The persistence of staphylococci in biomaterial-based infections despite treatment with appropriate antibiotics may be due to the presence of metabolically inactive small colony variants.[49,50]

To overcome the increased resistance of biomaterial-associated organisms to antibiotics, some investigators have supported the use of the antibiotic lock technique (ALT). The ALT consists of simply filling the lumen of a catheter with a solution containing a high concentration of antibiotic and then leaving the solution in place for a period of hours or days. The antibiotic solution is removed before the next use of the catheter. For example, vancomycin is often used at a concentration of 1 to 5 mg/ml. Generally, 2 to 3 ml are instilled into the catheter to fill the lumen, resulting in a local concentration of 1000 to 5000 µg/ml (well above the usual MIC of staphylococci and other susceptible organisms). This technique is most useful in situations in which the catheter can remain idle (antibiotic solution is indwelling) for at least several hours. In fact the ALT has been used most frequently in CVCs used for long-term total parenteral nutrition (TPN) administration in which TPN is infused overnight and the CVC is idle during the day. Studies have demonstrated the stability of various antibiotics when used under these conditions,[50,51] and in-vitro studies support the improved efficacy of ALT.[52,53] Mermel et al. reviewed 11 open trials of ALT involving 167 episodes of catheter-associated bacteremia and noted a success rate of 82.6%.[15] The duration of therapy varied, but most often was approximately 2 weeks.

It should be emphasized that these studies are not randomized comparative trials. Also, most clinicians using the ALT combine it with conventional systemic therapy, particularly in subjects with bacteremia or underlying neutropenia. Some pathogens may be difficult to eradicate, and indeed 7 of 10 attempts to treat fungal infections with the ALT failed.[54]

SPECIFIC PATHOGENS

There have been no prospective randomized trials with adequate sample size to indicate optimal therapy for IV catheter–associated infection due to any specific pathogen. The following recommendations are based on limited data and expert opinion:

Coagulase-Negative Staphylococci

Coagulase-negative staphylococci, such as *S. epidermidis*, are uniquely suited to cause IV catheter infections. *S. epidermidis* is the most prominent organism colonizing human skin[55] and it possesses a number of adhesins, allowing it to adhere and proliferate on IV catheter materials.[9,56] Indeed, coagulase-negative staphylococci are the most common cause of IV catheter–associated infection.[57–59] Fortunately, coagulase-negative staphylococci are relatively avirulent and although they are responsible for significant morbidity, they rarely cause severe sepsis or death.[6,15,60,61]

Although IV catheter–associated infections due to coagulase-negative staphylococci often resolve with the removal of the offending device, most authorities recommend antimicrobial therapy. Methicillin-resistant strains are responsible for 85% to 90% of nosocomially acquired coagulase-negative staphylococci infections.[2] Therefore, until susceptibility data are available, vancomycin is generally the drug of choice. Patients intolerant to vancomycin may be treated with one of the newer antistaphylococcal antibiotics such as quinupristin-dalfopristin or linezolid.

Available data suggest that CVCs infected with coagulase-negative staphylococci, particularly tunneled or totally implanted catheters, can be retained.[26, 29, 58, 62] If the catheter is retained, systemic therapy and ALT should be used for 10 to 14 days. If the catheter is removed, a shorter course of therapy (5 to 7 days) is appropriate.[63] It should be kept in mind that if the catheter is retained, a significant proportion may relapse. In one study, 20% of subjects experienced recurrent infection within the 12-week observation period.[26] Also, in patients who experience persistent fever or persistent bacteremia the catheter should be promptly removed.

Staphylococcus aureus

Because *S. aureus* is intrinsically a more virulent pathogen than coagulase-negative staphylococci and has a high propensity for metastatic seeding of heart valves, bones, joints, and other tissues, many clinicians favor prompt removal of all IV catheters infected with *S. aureus*. Several small observational studies associate removal of infected catheters with a more rapid clearance of bacteremia and higher cure rate.[64–66] Other studies, however, have not documented adverse outcomes associated with delayed removal of catheters infected with *S. aureus*, and thus the recommendation for removal should be made in the context of the clinical situation.[7,67,68] Clearly, easily removable, nontunneled IV catheters should be promptly removed, and all patients experiencing severe sepsis should have their catheters removed regardless of type. Patients with surgically implanted catheters who are not exhibiting signs of sepsis and in whom removal of the catheter presents a major hardship, may be treated expectantly with a combination of systemic and ALT treatment. In patients who remain febrile or bacteremic, the CVC should be removed.

A major controversy surrounding the treatment of *S. aureus* catheter-related bacteremia is the optimal duration of antibiotic therapy. In a study performed during the 1940's and 1950's by Wilson and Hamburger[69] a high prevalence of endocarditis (64%) was noted among patients with *S. aureus* bacteremia. This observation led to the practice of treating all patients with *S. aureus* bacteremia with 4 to 6 weeks of antibiotics. More recently this practice has been challenged, and a shorter course of therapy has been advocated. As was pointed out in a review by Jernigan and Farr,[70] however, most of the existing studies on this topic are flawed. A small randomized trial testing 2 weeks of therapy vs. 4 weeks of therapy revealed a higher relapse rate in the short-course therapy group (29% vs. 0).[71] The sample size was too small, however, and statistical significance was not demonstrated. Therefore, if short-course therapy is used, it must be done cautiously. One group of investigators recommended differentiating patients who could be treated with short-course therapy from those requiring longer courses of treatment by monitoring fever and bacteremia. The conditions of patients who remain febrile or bacteremic for more than 3 days following antibiotic initiation were considered complicated and these patients required at least 4 weeks of therapy.[67] An alternate method of triaging patients to short- or long-course therapy utilizes transesophageal echocardiography (TEE). Using the Duke endocarditis diagnostic criteria, Fowler and colleagues found that 23% of 69 patients with catheter-associated bacteremia had endocarditis.[72] The authors suggested that use of TEE to determine the length of therapy would be a cost-effective alternative to routine administration of 4 weeks of antibiotics to all patients with *S. aureus* IV catheter–associated bacteremia.[28] It should be noted that transthoracic echocardiography (TTE) should not be used in place of TEE, as the sensitivity of TTE in this study was only 27%.[28] Last, patients with AIDS who experience IV catheter–associated *S. aureus* bacteremia have been reported to have increased rates of adverse outcome.[74] Therefore, many clinicians caring for HIV-infected patients treat them with longer courses of therapy when they present with *S. aureus* IV catheter–associated infection.

The choice of antimicrobial agent to be used in the treatment of IV catheter–associated infection is complicated by the rising rate of antibiotic resistance observed in *S. aureus* strains. Over 50% of *S. aureus* isolates associated with nosocomial infection in ICU patients are resistant to methicillin.[2] Therefore in many institutions vancomycin is empirically used until data from susceptibility studies are known. Lastly some investigators advocate 2 weeks of oral therapy after completion of IV treatment.[71] Clearly this is an area in which there is a need for well-formulated, prospective, randomized treatment protocols.

Gram-Negative Aerobic Bacilli

A variety of gram-negative aerobic bacilli have been described to cause IV catheter–associated infections. In general, infections caused by *Pseudomonas aeruginosa*, *Burkholderia cepacia*, *Acinetobacter baumannii*, and *Stenotrophomomas* spp. require removal of the offending catheter.[15] Infections due to gram-negative aerobic bacilli, other than those noted above, in subjects with surgically implanted CVCs and without evidence of severe sepsis, can be treated expectantly with the CVC in situ. Systemic treatment and ALT should be employed for 14 days. The choice of antimicrobial agent should be governed by susceptibility studies and many clinicians would employ double coverage. For example, an anti-pseudomonal β-lactam, such as ceftazidime or cefepime, in combination with an aminoglycoside, such as gentamicin, or fluorquinoline, such as ciprofloxacin.

Candida Species

In the past, many clinicians thought that IV catheter infections due to *Candida* spp. could be treated by removal of the offending device. Because of increasingly recognized deep-seated or disseminated candidiasis, however, essentially all patients experiencing IV catheter–associated candidemia require systemic antifungal therapy. For instance, Rose described a 15% incidence of Candida endophthalmitis in 26 subjects with candidemia who were treated with catheter removal alone.[74] Several studies have shown that failure to promptly remove IV catheters associated with candidemia increases morbidity and mortality.[75–77] Therefore, all IV catheters infected with *Candida* spp. should be promptly removed. The evidence for this recommendation is strongest in non-neutropenic patients.[75,76] In neutropenic subjects the gut can also serve as a source for candidemia. In individual patients, however, it is often difficult to differentiate between possible sources for candidemia. Features that strongly suggest the IV catheter as the source in patients with candidemia include the following: isolation of *Candida parapsilosis*, non-neutropenic host, host receiving hyperalimentation, quantitative blood cultures revealing greater than 5 fold increase in burden of *Candida* in catheter-drawn blood compared to peripheral blood and greater than 2-hour differential time to positivity in peripheral and catheter-drawn blood cultures.

A number of studies suggest that fluconazole and amphotericin B are similarly effective in the treatment of IV catheter–associated fungemia.[78–81] However, the clinician should note that infections due to non-albicans candida are becoming more prevalent[82,83] and that *Candida krusei* and *Candida glabrata* are often resistant to fluconazole, whereas *Candida lusitaniae* is often resistant to amphotericin B.[82] Therapy should be continued for 2 weeks after the last positive blood culture is observed and after resolution of signs and symptoms of infection.[82]

Miscellaneous Organisms

Various other microorganisms have been described to occasionally cause IV catheter infections. In most cases experience is limited and specific recommendations based on scientifically rigorous data are impossible. It has been noted, however, that infections due to *Bacillus* spp., *Corynebacterium* spp., or *Mycobacterium* spp., generally require removal of the offending device.[15,84,85] The choice of antimicrobial agent should be guided by susceptibility studies and the duration of treatment is dictated by clinical response but generally is at least 2 weeks.

COMPLICATIONS

IV catheter–associated infections can be complicated by severe sepsis and death depending on the intrinsic virulence of the pathogen and underlying medical status of the patient. Septic thrombophlebitis and arteritis associated with peripheral vascular catheters were described in the discussions on peripheral IV catheters and peripheral arterial catheters. Infections of CVCs can also lead to septic thrombosis.

Patients with septic thrombophlebitis involving the central venous system often do not have clinical signs at the site of catheterization. However, examination often reveals signs of venous obstruction with swelling of the arm and shoulder or even superior vena cava syndrome.[9,86] Septic thrombophlebitis should be considered in any patient with persistent bacteremia or fungemia despite appropriate antimicrobial treatment and removal of the CVC. Definitive diagnosis generally is made by venography, venous Doppler studies, computed tomography, or magnetic resonance imaging with contrast.

S. aureus is the pathogen most commonly associated with septic thrombophlebitis, and up to 12% of cases of CVC-associated bacteremia may be associated with this complication.[87] However, *Candida* spp. and other organisms can also occasionally cause septic thrombophlebitis.[15,88] When septic thrombophlebitis is suspected, the CVC should be promptly removed and appropriate antibiotics initiated. Many clinicians favor the use of anticoagulant therapy with heparin,[89,90] although there are no randomized trials demonstrating optimal practice. Use of thrombolytic agents has been discouraged in the treatment of septic thrombophlebitis,[91] but has proven useful in the treatment of noninfected thrombi.[92]

As previously mentioned, a significant number of persons with *S. aureus* CVC-associated bacteremia develop endocarditis. In addition, metastatic seeding resulting in osteomyelitis, septic arthritis, epidural abscess, endophthalmitis, or abscesses in other organs occurs in 7% to 25% of cases.[7,25,93] Other organsims such as *Candida* spp. and gram-negative aerobic bacilli less commonly cause metastatic seeding of other sites. Treatment of these conditions depends on the site of involvement and causative pathogen, but in general terms, usually requires longer courses of antibiotics (4 to 6 weeks) and surgical resection or drainage.

CONCLUSION

Although in recent years our understanding of the pathogenesis of IV catheter infections has improved and some progress has been realized in optimizing techniques for the diagnosis of IV catheter–associated infection, there remains a great need for additional studies regarding optimal management of these infections. For instance, there is little data to guide clinicians as to when catheters infected with *S. aureus* or *Candida* spp. can be treated with the catheter in situ. Likewise, optimal duration of therapy is not clear. How should subjects with significant microbial colonization of catheters but without evidence of systemic infection be treated? What is the role of anticoagulants or thrombolytic agents? Clearly, there is great need for studies addressing optimal methods of treatment of IV catheter–associated infection. Until studies addressing these questions are completed, the reader should find the preceding discussion of value in managing these infections. Clinicians should understand that in the local environment of a prosthetic device, such as an IV catheter, the host defense is altered, and organisms are often relatively resistant to antimicrobial agents. Therefore, when in doubt, infected IV catheters should be removed. Also, some microbes (such as *S. aureus*) have a greater propensity for metastatic disease, and when the clinical situation is ambiguous, subjects infected with these species of bacteria should be treated with longer courses of antimicrobial therapy.

ACKNOWLEDGMENTS: This work was supported in part by a Grant-in-Aid from the American Heart Association, #9951167Z.

REFERENCES

1. Maki DG, Mermel LA: Infections due to infusion therapy. In Bennett JV, Bachman PS (eds): Hospital Infections. Philadelphia, Lippincott-Raven, 1998, pp 689–724.
2. National Nosocomial Infections Surveillance (NNIS) System Report, Data Summary from January 1992–April 2000, Issued June 2000: Am J Infect Control 2000;28:429–448.
3. Henderson DK: Infections due to percutaneous intravascular devices. In Mandell GL, Bennett JE, Dolin R (eds): Principles and Practice of Infectious Diseases. vol 1, Philadelphia, Churchill Livingstone, 2000, pp 3005–3020.
4. Maki DG, Stolz SM, Wheeler S, et al: Prevention of central venous catheter–related bloodstream infection by use of an antiseptic-impregnated catheter: A randomized, controlled trial. Ann Intern Med 1997;127:257–266.
5. Pittet D, Tamara D, Wenzel RP: Nosocomial bloodstream infection in critically ill patients: Excess length of stay, extra costs, and attributable mortality. JAMA 1994;271:1598–1601.
6. Byers K, Adal K, Anglim A, et al: Case fatality rate for catheter-related bloodstream infections (CRSBI): a meta-analysis (abstract 43). Infect Control Hosp Epidemiol 1995;16:23.
7. Arnow PM, Quimosing EM, Beach M: Consequences of intravascular catheter sepsis. Clin Infect Dis 1993; 16:778–784.
8. Veenstra DL, Saint S, Sullivan SD: Cost-effectiveness of antiseptic-impregnated central venous catheters for the prevention of catheter-related bloodstream infection. JAMA 1999;282:554–560.
9. Rupp ME: Infections of intravascular catheters and vascular devices. In Crossley KB, Archer GL (eds): The Staphylococci in Human Disease. New York, Churchill Livingstone, 1997, pp 379–399.
10. Mayhall CG: Diagnosis and management of infections of implantable devices used for prolonged venous access. In Remington JS, Swartz MN (eds): Current Clinical Topics in Infectious Diseases. Boston, Blackwell Scientific Publications, 1992, pp 83–110.
11. Raad I, Hanna H: Nosocomial infections related to use of intravascular devices inserted for long-term vascular access. In Mayhall CG (ed): Hospital Epidemiology and Infect Control, 2nd ed. Philadelphia, Lippincott Williams & Wilkins, 1999, pp 165–172.
12. Farr BM: Nosocomial infections related to use of intravascular devices inserted for short-term vascular access. In Mayhall CG (ed), Hospital Epidemiology and Infect Control, 2nd ed. Philadelphia, Lippincott Williams & Wilkins, 1999, pp 157–164.
13. Siegman-Igra Y, Anglim AM, Shapiro DE, et al: Diagnosis of vascular catheter–related bloodstream infection: A meta-analysis. J Clin Microbiol 1997;35(4):928–936.
14. Sherertz RJ, Raad II, Belani A, et al: Three-year experience with sonicated vascular catheter cultures in a clinical microbiology laboratory. J Clin Microbiol 1990;28:76–82.
15. Mermel LA, Farr BM, Sherertz RJ, et al: Guidelines for the management of intravascular catheter–related infections. Clin Infect Dis 2001;32:1249–1272.
16. Baker CC, Petersen SR, Sheldon GF: Septic phlebitis: a neglected disease. Am J Surg 1979;138:97–103.
17. Berkowitz FE, Argent AC, Faise T: Suppurative thrombophlebitis: A serious nosocomial infection. Pediatr Infect Dis J 1987;6:64–67.
18. Maki DG, McCormick RD, Uman SJ, et al: Septic endarteritis due to intra-arterial catheters for cancer chemotherapy. I. Evaluation of an outbreak. II. Risk factors, clinical features and management. III. Guidelines for prevention. Cancer 1979;44:1228–1240.
19. Cohen A, Reyes R, Kirk M, et al: Osler's nodes, pseudoaneurysm formation and sepsis complicating percutaneous radial artery cannulation. Crit Care Med 1984;12:1078–1079.
20. Falk PS, Scuderi PE, Sherertz RJ, et al: Infected radial artery pseudoaneurysms occurring after percutaneous cannulation. Chest 1992;101:490–495.
21. Pittet D, Chuard C, Rae AC, et al: Clinical diagnosis of central venous catheter line infections: a difficult job. In Programs and abstracts of the 31st Interscience Conference of Antimicrobial Agents and Chemotherapy, Chicago, IL Sept 29–Oct 2, 1991 (abstract 453) p 174.

22. Cercenado E, Ena J, Rodriguez-Creixems M, et al: A conservation procedure for the diagnosis of catheter-related infections. Arch Intern Med 1990;150:1417–1420.

23. Brun-Bruisson C, Abrouk F, Legrand P, et al: Diagnosis of central venous catheter-related sepsis: Critical level of quantitative tip cultures. Arch Intern Med 1987;147:873–877.

24. Ryan JA, Abel RM, Abbott WM, et al: Catheter complications in total parenteral nutrition: A prospective study of 200 consecutive patients. N Engl J Med 1974;290:757–761.

25. Pettigrew RA, Land SDR, Haydock DA, et al: Catheter-related sepsis in patients on intravenous nutrition: A prospective study of quantitative catheter cultures and guide wire changes for suspected sepsis. Br J Surg 1985;72:52–55.

26. Raad I, Davis S, Khan A, et al: Impact of central venous catheter removal on the recurrence of catheter-related coagulase-negative staphylococcal bacteremia. Infect Control Hosp Epidemiol 1992;13:215–221.

27. Fowler VG, Sanders LL, Kong LK, et al: Infective endocarditis due to *Staphylococcus aureus:* 59 prospectively identified cases with follow-up. Clin Infect Dis 1999;28:106–114.

28. Rosen AB, Fowler VG, Corey GR, et al: Cost-effectiveness of transesophageal echocardiography to determine the duration of therapy for intravascular catheter-associated to *Staphylococcus aureus* bacteremia. Ann Intern Med 1999;130:810–820.

29. Schreckenberger PC. Questioning dogmas: Proposed new rules and guidelines for the clinical microbiology laboratory. ASM News 2001;67:388–389.

30. Groeger JS, Lucas AB, Thaler HT, et al: Infectious morbidity associated with long-term use of venous access devices in patients with cancer. Ann Intern Med 1993;119:1168–1174.

31. National Institutes of Health: 1999 annual data report. US Renal Data System. Bethesda, MD: US Department of Health and Human Services, National Institute of Health, National Institute of Diabetes and Digestive and Kidney Diseases, April 1999.

32. United States Renal Data System: The USRDS dialysis morbidity and mortality study: Am J Kidney Dis 1997;30:S67–S85.

33. CDC MMWR Recommendations and Reports: Recommendations for preventing transmission of infections among chronic hemodialysis patients. April 27, 2001;50(RR05):1–43.

34. Pearson ML, HICPAC: Special report: Guideline for prevention of intravascular-device-related infections. Infect Control Hosp Epidemiol 1996;17(7):438–473.

35. Dahlberg PJ, Yutuc WR, Newcomer KL: Subclavian hemodialysis catheter infections. Am J Kidney Dis 1986;7:421–427.

36. Cheeseborough JS, Finch RG, Burden RP: A prospective study of the mechanism of infection associated with hemodialysis catheters. J Infect Dis 1986;154:579–589.

37. Kessler M, Hoen B, Mayeux D, et al: Bacteremia in patients on chronic hemodialysis: a multicenter prospective survey. Nephron 1993;64:95–100.

38. Almirall J, Gonzalez J, Rello J, et al: Infection of hemodialysis catheters: incidence and mechanisms. Am J Nephrol 1989;9:454–459.

39. Yu VL, Goetz A, Wagener M, et al: *Staphylococcus aureus* nasal carriage and infection in patients of hemodialysis: efficacy of antibiotic prophylaxis. N Engl J Med 1986;315:91–96.

40. Goldblum SE, Ulrich JA, Reed WP: Nasal and cutaneous flora among hemodialysis patients and personnel: quantitative characterization and pattern of staphylococcal carriage. Am J Kidney Dis 1982;2:281–286.

41. Boelaert JR, Van Landyt HW, Godard CA, et al: Nasal mupirocin ointment decreases the incidence of *Staphylococcus aureus* bacteremia in hemodialysis patients. Nephrol Dial Transplant 1993;8:235–239.

42. Oliver MJ, Schwab SJ: Infections related to hemodialysis and peritoneal dialysis. In Waldvogel FA, Bisno AL (eds): Infections Associated with Indwelling Medical Devices, 3rd ed. Washington, DC, ASM Press, 2000, pp 345–372.

43. Vaudaux P, Francois P, Lew DP, et al: Host factors predisposing to and influencing therapy of foreign body infections. In Waldvogel FA, Bisno AL (eds): Infections Associated with Indwelling Medical Devices, 3rd ed. Washington, DC, ASM Press, 2000, pp 1–26.

44. Noble WC: The production of subcutaneous staphylococcal skin lesions in mice. Br J Exp Pathol 1965;46:254.

45. Ulphani JS, Rupp ME: Novel rat model of *Staphylococcus aureus* central venous catheter-associated infection. Laboratory Animal Science 1999;49:283–287.

46. Yanai M, Quie PG: Chemiluminescence by polymorphonuclear leukocytes adhering to surfaces. Infect Immun 1981;123:285–289.

47. Zimmerli W, Lew DP, Waldvogel FA: Pathogenesis of foreign body infection: Evidence for a local granulocyte defect. J Clin Invest 1984;73:1191–1198.

48. Proctor RA, Peters G: Small colony variants in staphylococcal infections; Diagnostic and therapeutic implications. Clin Infect dis 1998;27:419–423.

49. Von Eiff C, Vaudaux P, Kahl BC, et al: Bloodstream infections caused by small-colony variants of coagulase-negative staphylococci following pacemaker implantation. Clin Infect Dis 1999;29:932–934.

50. Vaudaux P, Grau GE, Huggler E, et al: Contribution of tumor necrosis factor to host defense against staphylococci in a guinea pig model of foreign body infections. J Infect Dis 1992;166:58.

51. Anthony TU, Rubin LG: Stability of antibiotics used for antibiotic-lock treatment of infections of implantable venous devices (ports). Antimicrob Agents Chemother 1999;43(8):2074–2076.

52. Yao JDC, Arkin CF, Karchmer AW: Vancomycin stability in heparin and total parenteral nutrition solutions: novel approach to therapy of central venous catheter–related infections. J Parenter Interal Nutr 1992;16:268–274.

53. Gaillard JL, Merlino R, Pajot N, et al: Conventional and nonconventional modes of vancomycin administration to decontaminate the internal surface of catheters colonized with coagulase-negative staphylococci. J Parenter Interal Nutr 1990;14:593–597.

54. Andris DA, Krzywda EA, Edmiston CE, et al: Elimination of intraluminal colonization by antibiotic lock in silicone vascular catheters. Nutrition 1998;14:427–432.

55. Kloos WE: Ecology of human skin. In Mardh PA, Schleifer KH (eds): Coagulase-Negative Staphylococci. Stockholm, Bohuslaningens Boktryckeri AV, Uddevalla, 1986, pp 37–50.

56. Gotz F, Peters G: Colonization of medical devices by coagulase-negative staphylococci. In Waldvogel FA, Bisno AL (eds): Infections Associated with Indwelling Medical Devices, 3rd ed. Washington DC, ASM Press, 2000, pp 55–88.

57. Rupp ME, Archer GL: Coagulase-negative staphylococci: pathogens associated with medical progress. Clin Infect Dis 1994;19:231–245.

58. Winston DJ, Dudnick DV, Chapin M, et al: Coagulase-negative staphylococcal bacteremia in patients receiving immunosuppresive therapy. Arch Intern Med 1983;143:32–36.

59. Christensen GD, Bisno AL, Parisi JT, et al: Nosocomial septicemia due to multiple antibiotic-resistant *Staphylococcus epidermidis*. Ann Intern Med 1982;96:1–10.

60. Kirchhoff LV, Sheagren JN: Epidemiology and clinical significance of blood cultures positive for coagulase-negative staphylococcus. Infect Control 1985;6(12):479–486.

61. Thylefors JD, Harbarth S, Pittet D: Increasing bacteremia due to coagulase-negative staphylococci: fiction or reality? Infect Control Hosp Epidemiol 1998;19:581–589.

62. Rupp MR: Coagulase-negative staphylococcal infections: an update regarding recognition and management. Curr Clin Top in Infect Dis 1997;17:51–87.

63. Herrmann M, Peters G: Catheter-associated infections caused by coagulase-negative staphylococci: clinical and biological aspects. In Seifert H, Jansen B, Farr BM (eds): Catheter-Related Infections. New York, Marcel Dekker, 1997, pp 79–109.

64. Dugdale DC, Ramsey P: *Staphylococcus aureus* bacteremia in patients with Hickman catheters. Am J Med 1990;89:137–141.

65. Malanoski G, Samore M, Pefanis A, et al: *Staphylococcus aureus* bacteremia: minimal effective therapy and unusual infectious complications associated with arterial sheath catheters. Arch Intern Med 1995;155:1161–1166.

66. Fowler VG, Sander LL, Sexton DJ, et al: Outcome of *Staphylococcus aureus* bacteremia according to compliance with recommendations of infectious diseases specialists: Experience with 244 patients. Clin Infect Dis 1998;27:478–486.

67. Raad II, Sabbagh MF: Optimal duration of therapy for catheter-related *Staphylococcus aureus* bacteremia: a study of 55 cases and review. Clin Infect Dis 1992;14:75–82.

68. Marr KA, Sexton DJ, Conlon PJ, et al: Catheter-related bacteremia and outcomes of attempted catheter salvage in patients undergoing hemodialysis. Ann Intern Med 1997;127:275–280.

69. Wilson R, Hamburger M: Fifteen years' experience with *Staphylococcus* septicemia in a large city hospital: analysis of fifty-five cases in the Cincinnati General Hospital 1940 to 1954. Am J Med 1957;22:437–457.

70. Jernigan JA, Farr BM: Short-course therapy of catheter-related *Staphylococcus aureus* bacteremia: A meta-analysis. Ann Intern Med 1993;119:304–311.

71. Rahal JJ: Preventing second-generation complications due to *Staphylococcus aureus*. Arch Intern Med 1989;149:503–507.

72. Fowler VG, Li J, Corey GR, et al: Role of echocardiography in evaluation of patients with *Staphylococcus aureus* bacteremia: Experience in 103 patients. J Am Coll Cardiol 1997;30:1072–1078.

73. Jacobson M, Gellermann H, Chambers H: *Staphylococcus aureus* bacteremia and recurrent staphylococcal infection in patients with acquired immunodeficiency syndrome and AIDS related complex. Am J Med 1988;85:172–176.

74. Rose HD: Venous catheter-associated candidemia. Am J Med Sci 1978;275:265–269.

75. Nguyen MH, Peacock JE Jr, Tanner DC, et al: Therapeutic approaches in patients with candidemia: evaluation in a multicenter prospective observational study. Arch Intern Med 1995;155:2429–2435.

76. Rex JH, Bennett JE, Sugar AM, et al: Intravascular catheter exchange and duration of candidemia. Clin Infect Dis 1995;21:994–996.

77. Anaissie E, Rex JH, Uzun O, et al: Prognosis and outcome of candidemia in cancer patients. Am J Med 1998;104:238–245.

78. Rello J, Gatell JM, Almirall J, et al: Evaluation of culture techniques for identification of catheter-related infection in hemodialysis patients. Eur J Clin Microbiol Infect Dis 1989;8:620–622.

79. Saltissi D, Macfarlane DJ: Successful treatment of *Pseudomonas paucimobilis* haemodialysis catheter-related sepsis without catheter removal. Postgrad Med 1994;70:47–48.

80. Kairraitis LK, Gottlieb T: Outcome and complications of temporary haemodialysis catheters. Nephrol Dial Transplant 1999;14:1710–1714.

81. Carlisle EJ, Blake P, McCarthy F, et al: Septicemia in long-term jugular hemodialysis catheters: eradicating infection by changing the catheter over a guide wire. Int J Artif Organs 1991;14:150–153.

82. Rex JH, Walsh TJ, Sobel JD, et al: Practice guidelines for the treatment of candidiasis. Clin Infect Dis 2000;30:662–678.

83. Pfaller MA, Jones RN, Doern GV, et al: Bloodstream infections due to *Candida* species: SENTRY antimicrobial surveillance program in North America and Latin America, 1997–1998. Antimicrob Agents Chemother 2000;44(3):747–751.

84. Voss A: Miscellaneous organisms. In Seifert H, Jansen B, Farr BM (eds): Catheter-Related Infections. New York, Marcel Dekker, 1997, pp 157–182.

85. Gill MV, Klein NC, Cunhna BA: Unusual organisms causing intravenous line infections in compromised hosts. 1. Bacterial and algal infections. Infect Dis Clin Pract 1996;5:244–255.

86. Kaufman J, Demas C, Stark K, et al: Catheter-related septic central venous thrombosis: Current therapeutic options. West J Med 1986;145:200–203.

87. Shapiro ED, Wald ER, Nelson KA, et al: Broviac catheter-related bacteremia in oncology patients. Am J Dis Child 1982;136:679–683.

88. Benoit D, Decruyenaere J, Vandewoude K, et al: Management of candidal thrombophlebitis of the central veins: case report and review. Clin Infect Dis 1998;26:393–397.

89. Verghese A, Widrich WC, Arbeit RD: Central venous septic thrombophlebitis: the role of medical therapy. Medicine (Baltimore) 1985;64:394–400.

90. Topiel MS, Bryan RT, Kessler CM, et al: Case report: treatment of Silastic catheter-induced central vein septic thrombophlebitis. Am J Med Sci 1986;291:425–428.

91. Atkinson JB, Chamberlin K, Boody BA: A prospective randomized trial of urokinase as an adjuvant in the treatment of proven Hickman catheter–sepsis. J Pediatr Surg 1998;33:714–716.

92. Ponec D, Irwin D, Haire WD, et al. Recombinant tissue plasminogen activator (alteplase) for restoration of flow in occluded central venous access devices: A double-blind placebo-controlled trial—the cardiovascular thrombolytic to open occluded lines (COOL) efficacy trial. J Vasc Intervent Radiol 2001;12:951–955.

93. Libman H, Arbeit RD: Complications associated with *Staphylococcus aureus* bacteremia. Arch Intern Med 1984;144:541.

Endocarditis

LARRY M. BADDOUR, MD

Infective endocarditis is an uncommon illness. Nevertheless the disease is frequently considered in the differential diagnosis of several more commonly seen febrile syndromes, particularly those associated with bacteremia or fungemia. Thus the clinical evaluation for the presence of infective endocarditis occurs much more often than does the need to choose a specific regimen for the treatment of infective endocarditis. In other words, only a small minority of patients in whom the diagnosis of infective endocarditis is initially considered will ultimately complete antimicrobial therapy for it. It is therefore appropriate to devote a portion of this treatment chapter to the initial evaluation of patients in whom infective endocarditis is a possible diagnosis.

Although not a common illness, infective endocarditis is a financially expensive one. In one survey[1] that included a mean follow-up of 8 years, 20 patients with infective endocarditis accounted for almost $1 million (1990 dollars) in hospitalization and ambulatory care costs. Over 50% of health care charges were accrued after the initial hospitalization for infective endocarditis complicating mitral valve prolapse.

CASE DEFINITIONS

Specific clinical criteria that have been recognized for over a century are used to secure an endocarditis diagnosis. These include bacteremia or fungemia, embolic phenomena, active valvular involvement, and immunologic peripheral vascular events. When all of these features are present, the diagnosis of infective endocarditis is obvious. Most patients, however, do not manifest all four clinical criteria, and securing a correct diagnosis in this setting is often difficult.

Specific case definitions have been devised to assist in the diagnosis of infective endocarditis. The use of case definitions are not only helpful to epidemiologists and clinical trials investigators to ensure the appropriate inclusion of endocarditis patients in studies but also to clinicians who manage the care of individual patients. In the latter scenario, case definitions provide a tool that assists the clinician in making critical diagnostic and treatment decisions. The use of case definitions should represent the best possible compromise between sensitivity and specificity in disease diagnosis so that the most appropriate treatment will be administered. Nevertheless case definitions should complement clinical judgment and should not replace it.

Several case definitions have been used since the time of Osler. Most recently, two sets of criteria have received wide acceptance.[2,3] The Beth Israel scheme[2] has been used for almost 2 decades. According to its criteria, only cases with pathologic confirmation can be included as "definite" endocarditis cases. Most patients with infective endocarditis, however, do not require surgical intervention for valve replacement or embolectomy, and most patients survive the illness so that postmortem examination is not performed. Also, the Beth Israel definition does not include echocardiographic findings as part of the case definition.

In 1994, the Duke criteria[3] were presented and have quickly gained acceptance for use in a variety of patient populations. These criteria, unlike the Beth Israel case definitions, list specific clinical features (Tables 7–1 and 7–2) that can be used to satisfy a "definite" diagnosis of infective endocarditis. These include echocardiographic findings defined as (1) an oscillating intracardiac mass on a valve or supporting structures, in the path of regurgitant jets, or on implanted material in the absence of an alternative anatomic explanation or (2) myocardial abscess, or (3) new partial dehiscence of a prosthetic valve. More recent proposed modifications[4] to the Duke criteria should enhance both the sensitivity and specificity of the case definitions.

TABLE 7–1 ■ Proposed New Criteria for Diagnosis of Infective Endocarditis

DEFINITE INFECTIVE ENDOCARDITIS
PATHOLOGIC CRITERIA
Microorganisms, demonstrated by culture or histology in a vegetation, or in a vegetation that has embolized, or in an intracardiac abscess, or
Pathologic lesions: vegetation or intracardiac abscess present, confirmed by histology showing active endocarditis

CLINICAL CRITERIA (USING SPECIFIC DEFINITIONS LISTED IN TABLE 7–2)
2 major criteria, or
1 major and 3 minor criteria, or
5 minor criteria

POSSIBLE INFECTIVE ENDOCARDITIS
Findings consistent with infective endocarditis that fall short of "definite" but not rejected

REJECTED
Firm alternate diagnosis for manifestations of endocarditis, or
Resolution of manifestations of endocarditis, with antibiotic therapy for ≤4d, or
No pathologic evidence of infective endocarditis at surgery or autopsy after antibiotic therapy for ≤4d

Reprinted from Durack DT, Lukes AS, Bright DK: New criteria for diagnosis of infective endocarditis: Utilization of specific echocardiographic findings: Duke Endocarditis Service. Am J Med 1994;96:200–209. Copyright 1994 with permission from Excerpta Medica Inc.

TABLE 7–2 ■ Definitions of Terminology Used in the Proposed New Criteria

MAJOR CRITERIA
1. Positive blood culture for infective endocarditis
   a. Typical microorganism for infective endocarditis from two separate blood cultures
      (1) Viridans streptococci, *Streptococcus bovis,* HACEK group, or
      (2) Community-acquired *Staphylococcus aureus* or enterococci, in the absence of a primary focus, or
   b. Persistently positive blood culture, defined as recovery of a microorganism consistent with infective endocarditis from
      (1) Blood cultures drawn more than 12 h apart, or
      (2) All of three or a majority of four or more separate blood cultures, with first and last drawn at least 1 h apart
2. Evidence of endocardial involvement
   a. Positive echocardiogram for infective endocarditis
      (1) Oscillating intracardiac mass, on valve or supporting structures, or in the path of regurgitant jets, or on implanted material, in the absence of an alternative anatomic explanation, or
      (2) Abscess, or
      (3) New partial dehiscence of prosthetic valve, or
   b. New valvular regurgitation (increase or change in preexisting murmur not sufficient)

MINOR CRITERIA
1. Predisposing: predisposing heart condition or intravenous drug use
2. Fever: ≥38°C (100.4°F)
3. Vascular phenomena: major arterial emboli, septic pulmonary infarcts, mycotic aneurysm, intracranial hemorrhage, conjunctival hemorrhages, Janeway lesions
4. Immunologic phenomena: glomerulonephritis, Osler's nodes, Roth spots, rheumatoid factor
5. Microbiologic evidence: positive blood culture but not meeting major criterion as noted previously[†] or serologic evidence of active infection with organisms consistent with infective endocarditis
6. Echocardiogram: consistent with infective endocarditis but not meeting major criterion as noted previously

HACEK, *Haemophilus* spp, *Actinobacillus actinomycetemcomitans, Cardiobacterium hominis, Eikenella* spp, and *Kingella kingae.*
[*]Including nutritional variant strains.
[†]Excluding single positive cultures for coagulase-negative staphylococci and organisms that do not cause endocarditis.
Reprinted from Durack DT, Lukes AS, Bright DK: New criteria for diagnosis of infective endocarditis: Utilization of specific echocardiographic findings: Duke Endocarditis Service. Am J Med 1994;96:200–209. Copyright 1994 with permission from Excerpa Medica Inc.

LABORATORY PROCEDURES

With some infectious disease syndromes such as community-acquired pneumonia, empiric therapy is initiated with the expectation that the offending pathogen will not be defined in most settings. The selection of empiric antibiotic therapy therefore is based on the more common bacteriologic causes of pneumonia.

Because of the duration, cost, and potential toxicity of many endocarditis treatment regimens, every effort is made to define the microbiologic cause of infective endocarditis rather than to administer empiric therapy. Both the identification of the pathogen and its antimicrobial drug susceptibility testing results are crucial in choosing therapy for infective endocarditis. Susceptibility testing should include a broad array of antibiotic classes, and the causative bacterium should not be discarded for several months in case additional susceptibility testing is required. This is because unpredictable events can occur that mandate treatment changes. For example, new onset of allergic manifestations or other drug-related toxicities during treatment can necessitate revisions in the initial treatment regimen.

Blood cultures are paramount for several reasons in infective endocarditis. First, positive blood cultures are the key to the diagnosis of infective endocarditis and may be one of a few early clinical clues that endocardial infection is present. Second, blood cultures are the only specimen that is sampled in most patients that yields the causative organism. Third, serial blood cultures can be obtained to evaluate response to therapy.

Serum bactericidal titers, often referred to as "Schlichter testing," are mentioned here largely for historical reasons. Such testing is labor intense, and the methodology varies with the laboratory performing the procedure. Currently recommended antibiotics achieve good cure rates. The impact of serum bactericidal titers on treatment and outcome is limited, and currently they are not performed in many centers.

Antibiotic therapy should be bactericidal. We learned years ago that bacteristatic therapy with agents such as chloramphenicol and tetracycline could improve symptoms but were associated with high relapse rates once therapy was discontinued.

PATHOGENESIS

Gram-positive cocci account for most cases of endocarditis; these include *Staphylococcus aureus*, viridans group streptococci, and enterococci. They harbor unique virulence factors[5,6] that allow them to bind either to endothelial cells or to wounds of the endothelial layer that are covered with fibrin and platelets. In the latter case the nidus is referred to as nonbacterial thrombotic endocarditis, or NBTE. An expanding appreciation of pathogenesis has led to potentially new therapeutic and preventive modalities. For example, antiplatelet drugs including aspirin and ticlopidine[7] have been used in animal models of endocarditis to reduce the size of infected vegetations. Platelet-derived peptides[8] that have antimicrobial properties may also be useful as adjunctive therapies in the future. It is expected that novel therapeutics will be available in the future in the treatment of human endocardial disease.

The presence of metabolically inactive bacterial cells theoretically can diminish endocarditis cure rates. Cell-wall active agents including penicillins may not be bactericidal for organisms that are not actively involved in cell-wall synthesis. These metabolically inactive cells have been demonstrated in vegetations and are thought to give rise to small colony variant forms. In one animal endocarditis model,[9] there was a selection for small colony forms among isolates recovered from infected vegetations as compared to colony populations in inocula of *Staphylococcus epidermidis* used for animal challenge.

TREATMENT

Before specific treatment recommendations are addressed, the following comments should be noted. First, treatment decisions can vary from day-to-day for patients with infective endocarditis. This is particularly true for patients with left-sided infections. The sudden onset of infection- or drug-related complications can dictate immediate treatment strategy changes. Second, some of the treatment and prevention regimens that are commonly recommended have not been critically examined in appropriate trials because of the infrequency of endocarditis, which makes it difficult to accrue enough patients for such trials. Also, ethical issues have prohibited placebo-controlled trials of prophylaxis. Third, guidelines for the treatment and prevention of infective endocarditis may differ, depending on the recommending body and the country of origin of the recommendations.

Treatment will be discussed according to type of pathogens, site of infection, and whether infection involves native or prosthetic valves. Antimicrobial susceptibility testing results and prior history of drug allergies are additional factors that have to be considered in formulating treatment guidelines. Because there is a legion of microorganisms that has been reported to cause infective endocarditis, a review of therapy for each potential pathogen is not feasible. Therefore, treatment for the more common and better recognized microorganisms will be addressed.

The viridans group of streptococci cause most cases of infective endocarditis involving native valves in nonintravenous drug users. The taxonomic names of species of the viridans group of streptocci have varied, which has led to some confusion. The current nomenclature includes at least 18 species. Three other groups of gram-positive cocci are discussed with the viridans group of streptococci regarding treatment considerations and include *Streptococcus bovis*, *Abiotrophia* spp, and *Gemella morbillorum*. *Abiotrophia* spp and *G. morbillorum* were formally known as "nutritionally variant" streptococci and *Streptococcus morbillorum*, respectively.

Treatment of viridans group streptococci, *S. bovis*, and *G. morbillorum* (VBG) organisms is divided into two groups based on in vitro susceptibility testing to penicillin G.[10] The two groups include organisms that are highly susceptible to penicillin G (defined as a minimum inhibitory concentration (MIC) of 0.1 µg/ml or less) and those that are relatively resistant to penicillin G (defined as a MIC greater than 0.1 µg/ml). For VBG bacteria that are highly sensitive to penicillin, 4 weeks of aqueous crystalline penicillin G administered intravenously have been used for over 20 years with microbiologic cure rates exceeding 95% (Table 7–3). Penicillin, 12 to 18 million units is given every 24 hours as either a continuous infusion or as six equally divided doses. Ceftriaxone sodium, 2 g daily, represents a second regimen that can be administered for 4 weeks by either intravenous or intramuscular injection with cure rates comparable to those of aqueous crystalline penicillin G. Ceftriaxone has gained acceptance because of its relative ease of administration and can be used as outpatient therapy in appropriately selected patients. In addition the surgical placement of a permanent central venous catheter (CVC) can be avoided in patients who tolerate intramuscular injections of ceftriaxone.

Vancomycin is recommended in patients with a history of immediate-type hypersensitivity reaction to penicillin or other β-lactam antibiotics including ceftriaxone. The drug must be given per intravenous route, and dosage is based on obtainable serum concentrations. Therapy is administered for 4 weeks.

Regardless of whether aqueous crystalline penicillin G, ceftriaxone, or vancomycin is selected for use, patients should be monitored for certain drug adverse events associated with the high dosages of prolonged therapy required in the treatment of endocarditis. Drug-induced neutropenia has been described with all three agents,[11] and peripheral white blood cell counts should be serially monitored. Although uncommon, renal toxicity can be seen with vancomycin, and serial assays of serum creatinine should be performed. Patients receiving prolonged ceftriaxone should be monitored for the formation of biliary sludge; patients may develop signs or symptoms of biliary tract disease.

Two combination regimens have been used in selected patients as 2-week treatment courses of endocarditis due to penicillin-susceptible VBG bacteria. The same dose of aqueous crystalline penicillin G as in the 4-week course is combined with gentamicin, 1 mg/kg

TABLE 7–3 ■ Suggested Regimens for Therapy of Native Valve Endocarditis Due to Penicillin-Susceptible Viridans Streptococci and *Streptococcus bovis* (Minimum Inhibitory Concentration ≤ 0.1 µg/ml)*

Antibiotic	Dosage and route	Duration (wk)	Comments
Aqueous crystalline penicillin G sodium *Or*	12–18 MU/24 h IV either continuously or in six equally divided doses	4	Preferred in most patients older than 65 y and in those with impairment of N VIII or renal function
Ceftriaxone sodium	2 g once daily IV or IM[†]	4	
Aqueous crystalline penicillin G sodium	12–18 MU/24 h IV either continuously or in six equally divided doses	2	When serum is obtained 1 h after a 20–30 min IV infusion or IM injection, serum concentration of gentamicin of approximately 3 µg/ml is desirable; trough concentration should be <1 µg/ml
With gentamicin sulfate[‡]	1 mg/kg IM or IV q8h	2	
Vancomycin hydrochloride[§]	30 mg/kg/24 h IV in two equally divided doses, not to exceed 2 g/24 h unless serum levels are monitored	4	Vancomycin therapy is recommended for patients allergic to β-lactams; peak serum concentrations of vancomycin should be obtained 1 h after completion of the infusion and should be in the range of 30–45 µg/ml for twice-daily dosing

*Dosages recommended are for patients with normal renal function. For nutritionally variant streptococci, see Table 7–6.

[†]Patients should be informed that IM injection of ceftriaxone is painful.

[‡]Dosing of gentamicin on a mg/kg basis will produce higher serum concentrations in obese patients than in lean patients. Therefore, in obese patients, dosing should be based on ideal body weight. (Ideal body weight for men is 50 kg + 2.3 kg per inch over 5 feet, and ideal body weight for women is 45.5 kg + 2.3 kg per inch over 5 feet). Relative contraindications to the use of gentamicin are age >65 y, renal impairment, or impairment of N VIII. Other potentially nephrotoxic agents (e.g., nonsteroidal anti-inflammatory drugs) should be used cautiously in patients receiving gentamicin.

[§]Vancomycin dosage should be reduced in patients with impaired renal function. Vancomycin given on a mg/kg basis will produce higher serum concentrations in obese patients than in lean patients. Therefore, in obese patients, dosing should be based on ideal body weight. Each dose should be infused over at least 1 h to reduce the risk of the histamine-release "red man" syndrome.

From Wilson WR, Karchmer AW, Dajani AS, et al: Antibiotic treatment of adults with infective endocarditis due to streptococci, enterococci, staphylococci, and HACEK microorganisms. JAMA 1995;274:1706–1713. Copyright 1995, American Medical Association.

administered every 8 hours by either intramuscular or intravenous injections (Table 7–3). Because synergistic killing of bacteria with penicillin G is the goal, lower peak (~3 μg/ml) and trough (less than 1 μg/ml) levels of gentamicin are desired.

The other regimen includes ceftriaxone, 2 g daily in combination with netilmicin or gentamicin. It should be emphasized that neither of the 2-week combination treatment regimens for highly penicillin-susceptible VBG bacteria should be used in all patients. Exclusions include those with underlying renal or cranial nerve VIII dysfunction, myocardial abscess, extracardiac foci of infection, prolonged (longer than 3 months) symptoms before initiation of therapy, or congestive heart failure, or in shock.

Patients who are infected with VBG bacteria that are highly susceptible to penicillin and that cause prosthetic valve endocarditis or infection of other intracardiac prosthetic materials should be treated more aggressively. Six weeks of penicillin G should be administered. In addition, dual therapy with gentamicin added to the first 2 weeks of penicillin treatment is recommended.

Patients with native valve endocarditis due to VBG bacteria with penicillin MICs greater than 0.1 μg/ml require more aggressive antibiotic therapy (Table 7–4). Combination therapy with penicillin and gentamicin is recommended; the duration of gentamicin administration depends on the level of penicillin resistance. When the penicillin MIC is <0.5 μg/ml, gentamicin is given for the first 2 of 4 weeks of penicillin G. Also, higher-dose (18 million units per 24 hours) penicillin G is recommended. When the penicillin MIC is 0.5 μg/ml or higher, combination therapy should be continued for 4 to 6 weeks. In addition, the dosage of penicillin G should be increased to 30 million units per 24 hours. Alternative therapies to be used in patients with penicillin allergy include cefazolin or other first-generation cephalosporins when the penicillin allergy is not an immediate type of reaction. For those with immediate-type penicillin reactions, vancomycin should be employed. In the latter case, gentamicin is not required. As recommended for infections due to highly penicillin-susceptible VBG bacteria, patients with prosthesis infections caused by more resistant VBG organisms should be given extended (6 weeks) treatment.

Enterococci are another group of gram-positive cocci that commonly produce infective endocarditis. This group of bacteria has garnered a tremendous amount of attention over the past decade because of the development of multidrug resistance—including resistance to vancomycin—particularly for the *faecium* species. For this reason, in vitro susceptibility testing is now more important than ever in selecting a treatment regimen. For endocarditis due to enterococci that are susceptible to penicillin and gentamicin, combination therapy with both antibiotics should be given for 4 to 6 weeks (Table 7–5). Six weeks of treatment is favored if symptoms have been present for longer than 3 months before initiation of antibacterial therapy or if prosthetic valve endocarditis is present. Ampicillin, 12 g IV per 24 hours divided into every 6-hour dosing or by continuous infusion can be used as an alternative to penicillin G. Vancomycin should be combined with gentamicin if the isolate's MIC to penicillin G is greater than 16 μg/ml. If the enterococcal isolate is high-level resistant to both gentamicin and streptomycin, then more prolonged therapy (8 to 12 weeks) with high-dose penicillin or ampicillin can be used.

Currently there is no recommended therapy for vancomycin-resistant enterococcal endocarditis.[12] There are case reports that include the use of a variety of agents. Whether newer drugs that include streptogramins (quinupristin-dalfopristin), glycopeptides (teicoplanin),

TABLE 7–4 ■ Therapy for Native Valve Endocarditis Due to Strains of Viridans Streptococci and *Streptococcus bovis* Relatively Resistant to Penicillin G (Minimum inhibitory Concentration > 0.1 μg/ml and <0.5 μg/ml)*

Antibiotic	Dosage and route	Duration (wk)	Comments
Aqueous crystalline penicillin G sodium	18 MU/24 h IV either continuously or in six equally divided doses	4	Cefazolin or other first-generation cephalosporins may be substituted for penicillin in patients whose penicillin hypersensitivity is not of the immediate type
With gentamicin sulfate†	1 mg/kg IM or IV q8h	2	
Vancomycin hydrochloride‡	30 mg/kg/24 h IV in two equally divided doses, not to exceed 2 g/24 h unless serum levels are monitored	4	Vancomycin therapy is recommended for patients allergic to β-lactams

*Dosages recommended are for patients with normal renal function.
†For specific dosing adjustment and issues concerning gentamicin (obese patients, relative contraindications), see Table 7–3 footnotes.
‡For specific dosing adjustment and issues concering vancomycin (obese patients, length of infusion), see Table 7–3 footnotes.
From Wilson WR, Karchmer AW, Dajani AS, et al: Antibiotic treatment of adults with infective endocarditis due to streptococci, enterococci, staphylococci, and HACEK microorganisms. JAMA 1995;274:1706–1713. Copyright 1995, American Medical Association.

TABLE 7–5 ■ Standard Therapy for Endocarditis due to Enterococci*

Antibiotic	Dosage and route	Duration (wk)	Comments
Aqueous crystalline penicillin G sodium	18–30 MU/24 h IV either continuously or in six equally divided doses	4–6	4-wk therapy recommended for patients with symptoms <3 mo in duration; 6-wk therapy recommended for patients with symptoms >3 mo in duration
With gentamicin sulfate[†]	1 mg/kg IM or IV q8h	4–6	
Ampicillin sodium	12 g/24 h IV either continuously or in six equally divided doses	4–6	
With gentamicin sulfate[†]	1 mg/kg IM or IV q8h		
Vancomycin hydrochloride[†‡]	30 mg/kg/24 h IV in two equally divided doses, not to exceed 2 g/24 h unless serum levels are monitored	4–6	Vancomycin therapy is recommended for patients allergic to β-lactams; cephalosporins are not acceptable alternatives for patients allergic to penicillin
With gentamicin sulfate[†]	1 mg/kg IM or IV q8h	4–6	

*All enterococci causing endocarditis must be tested for antimicrobial susceptibility in order to select optimal therapy. This table is for endocarditis due to gentamicin- or vancomycin-susceptible enterococci, viridans streptococci with a minimum inhibitory concentration of >0.5 μg/ml, nutritionally variant viridans streptococci, or prosthetic valve endocarditis caused by viridans streptococci or *Streptococcus bovis*. Antibiotic dosages are for patients with normal renal function.

[†]For specific dosing adjustment and issues concerning gentamicin (obese patients, relative contraindications), see Table 7–3 footnotes.

[‡]For specific dosing adjustment and issues concerning vancomycin (obese patients, length of infusion), see Table 7–3 footnotes.

From Wilson WR, Karchmer AW, Dajani AS, et al: Antibiotic treatment of adults with infective endocarditis due to streptococci, enterococci, staphylococci, and HACEK microorganisms. JAMA 1995;274:1706–1713. Copyright 1995, American Medical Association.

cyclic lipopeptides (daptomycin), and oxazolidinones (linezolid) will prove efficacious is yet to be determined.

Endocardial infections due to *Abiotrophia* spp characteristically present problems in in vitro antibiotic susceptibility testing because of their fastidious nature and clincially have been associated with difficulties in eradication of endocardial infections. Therefore, treatment of *Abiotrophia* endocarditis should follow the regimens outlined for enterococcal infection.

Staphylococci are important causes of native valve infective endocarditis. Although most infections are due to the species *aureus*, there have been increasing numbers of cases due to coagulase-negative staphylococci. The coagulase-negative isolates are often methicillin susceptible and due to a variety of species. This is in contrast to coagulase-negative staphylococci that cause early prosthetic valve infections, which are usually methicillin resistant and are identified as the species *epidermidis*. The species *lugdunensis* has received considerable attention recently as a cause of native valve endocarditis. In many respects its virulence is more akin to that of coagulase-positive staphylococci (*S. aureus*), and infection complications, including death, have been reported frequently.

Treatment of native valve infective endocarditis due to *S. aureus* will be addressed according to site of involvement. Right-sided infection is most often seen in intravenous drug users, is due to methicillin-susceptible strains, and is associated with a high cure rate. Data from three series[13–15] of patients treated with a short course (2 weeks) of combined antibiotics for selected patients showed that cure rates exceeded 95% among patients completing treatment. Recognizing that treatment compliance and frequent patient refusal of prolonged hospitalization among the intravenous drug using population are concerns, short-course combination therapy seems reasonable to consider in the selected patient. Nafcillin or cloxacillin given every 4 hours is combined with an aminoglycoside for 14 days. Patients treated with a 2-week regimen should be hemodynamically stable and have had no systemic embolic event or metastatic infection. In the only comparative trial,[16] intravenous drug users with right-sided *S. aureus* endocarditis were given either cloxacillin (2 g IV every 4 hours) alone or cloxacillin plus gentamicin. Cure rates (92% vs. 94%) were comparable in the two groups for those who completed 2 weeks of monotherapy vs. dual therapy, respectively. If the patient has responded quickly to treatment and has suffered no systemic complications, combination therapy for two weeks can be considered. Monotherapy with cloxacillin for 14 days is currently not recommended but deserves further study. Whether two-week treatment is appropriate for populations other than intravenous drug users has not investigated.

Three additional points deserve comment regarding therapy of right-sided native valve endocarditis in intravenous drug users. First, a 2-week regimen with vancomycin in the penicillin-allergic (immediate-type) patient or the patient infected with a methicillin-resistant strain is not recommended. Therapy with vancomycin for 4 to 6 weeks should be given; the addition of an aminoglycoside is not routinely recommended, and the combination with vancomycin can increase the risks of ototoxicity and nephrotoxicity. Second, vancomycin should not be used to treat methicillin-susceptible

S. aureus infection in patients who are not allergic to penicillin. Intravenous drug users who have been treated with vancomycin for endocardial infection due to methicillin-susceptible *S. aureus* appeared to do less well than patients given semisynthetic penicillins did.[17] Third, infection with human immunodeficiency virus (HIV), a well-known complication of intravenous drug use, does not directly impact response to endocarditis therapy.[18] Rather the resultant immunosuppression seen in patients with later stage HIV disease has been associated with increased mortality due to infective endocarditis.

One other combination regimen that has been used in intravenous drug users includes ciprofloxacin and rifampin.[19,20] In one prospective, randomized, nonblinded trial,[20] a regimen of 28 days of oral therapy consisting of ciprofloxacin (750 mg) and rifampin (300 mg), both given twice daily, was compared with oxacillin (or vancomycin in penicillin-allergic patients) administered intravenously for 28 days with gentamicin given for the first 5 days of treatment. Although efficacy was comparable in the two groups, more drug toxicity (3% vs. 62%, *P* < .0001) was seen with the parenteral regimen. Although oral therapy would be attractive for use in selected intravenous drug users, recommendations for the routine use of oral therapy cannot be made at this time. Further evaluation, however, is warranted.

Left-sided native valve infective endocarditis due to methicillin-susceptible staphylococci requires more prolonged treatment than right-sided disease and is associated with a much higher mortality. Nafcillin should be administered for 4 to 6 weeks (Table 7–6). Some advocate the addition of gentamicin in a low dose (1 mg/kg every 8 hours) for the first 3 to 5 days of nafcillin to more quickly reduce the duration of systemic toxicity and bacteremia. By limiting the number of days of gentamicin therapy, it is thought that the benefit of drug synergy can be gained with a low likelihood of drug toxicity due to the aminoglycoside. The addition of gentamicin, however, has not been shown to improve the cure rates or mortality of monotherapy with nafcillin.

Cefazolin should be used in patients who are allergic to penicillin but who have not had an immediate-type hypersensitivity reaction (Table 7–6). For those with immediate-type hypersensitivity reactions, vancomycin should be given, and cefazolin and other first-generation cephalosporins should be avoided. Vancomycin is the

TABLE 7–6 ■ Therapy for Endocarditis Due to Staphylococcus in the Absence of Prosthetic Material*

Antibiotic	Dosage and route	Duration	Comments
METHICILLIN-SUSCEPTIBLE STAPHYLOCOCCI			
Regimen for non-β-lactam-allergic patients			Benefit of additional aminoglycosides has not been established
Nafcillin sodium or oxacillin sodium	2 g IV q4h	4–6 wk	
With optional addition of gentamicin sulfate†	1 mg/kg IM or IV q8h	3–5 d	
Regimens for β-lactam-allergic patients			Cephalosporins should be avoided in patients with immediate-type hypersensitivity to penicillin
Cefazolin (or other first-generation cephalosporins in equivalent dosages)	2 g IV q8h	4–6 wk	
With optional addition of gentamicin†	1 mg/kg IM or IV q8h	3–5 d	
Vancomycin hydrochloride‡	30 mg/kg/24 h IV in two equally divided doses, not to exceed 2 g/24 h unless serum levels are monitored	4–6 wk	Recommended for patients allergic to penicillin
METHICILLIN-RESISTANT STAPHYLOCOCCI			
Vancomycin hydrochloride‡	30 mg/kg/24 h IV in two equally divided doses, not to exceed 2 g/24 h unless serum levels are monitored	4–6 wk	

*For treatment of endocarditis due to penicillin-susceptible staphylococci (minimum inhibitory concentration ≤ 0.1 µg/ml) aqueous crystalline penicillin G sodium (Table 7–4, first regimen) can be used for 4 to 6 wk instead of nafcillin or oxacillin. Shorter antibiotic courses have been effective in some drug addicts with right-sided endocarditis due to *Staphylococcus aureus*.

†For specific dosing adjustment and issues concerning gentamicin (obese patients, relative contraindications), see Table 7–3 footnotes.

‡For specific dosing adjustment and issues concerning vancomycin (obese patients, length of infusion), see Table 7–3 footnotes.

From Wilson WR, Karchmer AW, Dajani AS, et al: Antibiotic treatment of adults with infective endocarditis due to streptococci, enterococci, staphylococci, and HACEK microorganisms. JAMA 1995;274:1706–1713. Copyright 1995, American Medical Association.

drug of choice for endocarditis due to methicillin-resistant strains of *S. aureus*.

Prosthetic valve endocarditis due to staphylococci should be treated with combination antibiotic therapy, and treatment should be for at least 6 weeks (Table 7–7). Methicillin resistance among infecting strains is frequently isolated, particularly for coagulase-negative staphylococci producing infection within 1 year of prosthetic valve placement.[21] Thus vancomycin is often the central drug of a triple-drug regimen. Rifampin, 300 mg PO every 8 hours, is also administered for 6 weeks in patients infected with staphylococcal strains susceptible to this agent. Gentamicin, 1 mg/kg IV or IM every 8 hours, is given for the first 2 weeks of combination therapy. If the infecting staphylococcal strain is gentamicin resistant, then another aminoglycoside should be examined in susceptibility testing. If the infecting strain is resistant to all aminoglycosides, susceptibility to a newer fluoroquinolone should be tested. If the isolate is fluoroquinolone susceptible, a new fluoroquinolone should be used to replace aminoglycoside therapy and should be given over the initial 2 weeks of combination therapy. High-dose nafcillin (12 g/d) can be used in place of vancomycin for infections due to methicillin-susceptible strains. A first-generation cephalosporin can be given instead of nafcillin in patients who are allergic to penicillin but who have not manifested signs and symptoms of immediate-type hypersensitivity reactions to penicillin in the past. For those with immediate-type hypersensitivity reactions, vancomycin should be administered, and all β-lactam antibiotics should be avoided.

Additional comments are in order regarding the syndrome of prosthetic valve endocarditis due to *S. aureus*. An enlarging body of evidence[22–24] indicates that a combined medical-surgical approach that includes prosthetic valve replacement improves survival. Some now advocate early surgical intervention once the diagnosis of prosthetic valve infection due to *S. aureus* is established. There is general agreement that patients with this illness should be managed only in medical centers with cardiothoracic surgery services.

Other gram-positive cocci also produce native valve infective endocarditis. *Streptococcus pneumoniae* was a common cause of infective endocarditis in the preantibiotic era and continues to cause endocarditis but much less often. Endocarditis can be associated with pneumonia and meningitis, so-called Osler's triad. Even without meningitis and pneumonia, native valve endocarditis due to *S. pneumoniae* is frequently a complicated illness that necessitates surgical intervention for valve replacement.[25–27] The mortality is sizeable.

Therapy for pneumococcal native valve endocarditis is largely undefined because the rarity of the syndrome largely precludes therapeutic trial investigations. Adding

TABLE 7–7 ■ **Treatment of Staphylococcal Endocarditis in the Presence of a Prosthetic Valve or Other Prosthetic Material***

Antibiotic	Dosage and route	Duration (wk)	Comments
REGIMEN FOR METHICILLIN-RESISTANT STAPHYLOCOCCAL			
Vancomycin hydrochloride[†]	30 mg/kg/24 h IV in two or four equally divided doses, not to exceed 2 g/24 h unless serum levels are monitored	≥6	
With rifampin[‡]	300 mg PO q8h	≥6	Rifampin increases the amount of warfarin sodium required for antithrombotic therapy
And with gentamicin sulfate[§//]	1 mg/kg IM or IV q8h	2	
REGIMEN FOR METHICILLIN-SUSCEPTIBLE STAPHYLOCOCCI			
Nafcillin sodium or oxacillin sodium	2 g IV q4h	≥6	First-generation cephalosporins or vancomycin should be used in patients allergic to β-lactam; cephalosporins should be avoided in patients with immediate-type hypersensitivity to penicillin or with methicillin-resistant staphylococci
With rifampin[‡]	300 mg PO q8h	≥6	
And with gentamicin sulfate[§//]	1 mg/kg IM or IV q8h	2	

*Dosages recommended are for patients with normal renal function.

[†]For specific dosing adjustment and issues concerning vancomycin (obese patients, length of infusion), see Table 7–3 footnotes.

[‡]Rifampin plays a unique role in the eradication of staphylococcal infection involving prosthetic material; combination therapy is essential to prevent emergence of rifampin resistance.

[§]For specific dosing adjustment and issues concerning gentamicin (obese patients, relative contraindications), see Table 7–3 footnotes.

[//]Use during initial 2 weeks.

From Wilson WR, Karchmer AW, Dajani AS, et al: Antibiotic treatment of adults with infective endocarditis due to streptococci, enterococci, staphylococci, and HACEK microorganisms. JAMA 1995;274:1706–1713. Copyright 1995, American Medical Association.

uity of preferred therapy is the recognition s been a recent worldwide increase in multidrug resistance among pneumococcal isolates. It seems reasonable to use high-dose (18 million units every 24 hours) intravenous aqueous crystalline penicillin G for endocarditis due to strains with an MIC less than 0.1 μg/ml. For infections due to intermediately resistant (MIC = 0.1 to 1 μg/ml) and highly resistant (MIC 2 μg/ml and higher) strains of *S. pneumoniae*, the optimum therapy is unknown. Some have advocated that treatment of pneumococcal endocarditis parallel that recommended for pneumococcal meningitis due to nonsensitive strains. If this approach were taken, vancomycin would be recommended for endocarditis treatment. An alternative treatment option might include ceftriaxone, 2 g daily, provided that the isolate is susceptible to it. Duration of therapy should be 4 to 6 weeks.

There have been suggestions that early valve replacement combined with parenteral antibiotic therapy might improve the mortality due to *S. pneumoniae* native valve endocarditis. The data analyzed that led to this opinion were retrospectively reviewed,[25–27] and on multivariate analysis in one study,[27] valve replacement appeared to have a protective effect as far as mortality goes. Nevertheless, no firm recommendations for early valve replacement can be made.

β-Hemolytic streptococci represent another group of gram-positive cocci that uncommonly produce native valve endocarditis. Generally the infection is aggressive, destructive, and associated with frequent complications, particularly embolic phenomena. Despite the increased complication rate, the mortality is low according to one recently published series of cases.[28] In that series of 31 cases, group B streptococcus was most commonly identified as a pathogen and accounted for over two-thirds (67.7%) of endocarditis cases due to β-hemolytic streptococci.

Aqueous crystalline penicillin G should be administered for β-hemolytic streptococcal endocarditis. The rec-

ommended dosage and duration of therapy is largely undefined, but 18 millions units per 24 hours for 4 to 6 weeks seems reasonable. There are limited data to suggest that the addition of gentamicin to the first 14 days of penicillin may decrease the mortality as compared with that associated with penicillin monotherapy. A first-generation cephalosporin can be used as alternative therapy in patients who are allergic to penicillin provided the allergy is not manifested by an immediate-type hypersensitivity reaction. If the latter is present, cephalosporins should not be administered, and vancomycin should be given. If vancomycin is used in combination with gentamicin, monitoring for ototoxicity and nephrotoxicity is required. As in the case of pneumococcal native valve endocarditis, there is a clinical impression that a combined medical-surgical approach reduces mortality, but that impression is not based on controlled data and is yet to be confirmed.

Some gram-negative bacilli that make up the HACEK (*Haemophilus* spp., *Actinobacillus actinomycetemcomitans, Cardiobacterium hominis, Eikenella* spp., and *Kingella kingae*) group are well recognized[10] as causes of endocarditis; they account for a small portion of native valve infections. The organisms are fastidious and can be slow growing and include *Haemophilus parainfluenzae, Haemophilus aphrophilus, A. actinomycetemcomitans, C. hominis, Eikenella corrodens*, and *K. kingae*. Treatment choice ideally is based, in part, on in vitro susceptibility test results. Unfortunately, because of the growth characteristics of this group of bacilli, in vitro susceptibility testing is difficult to secure. This limitation coupled with the demonstration that some HACEK isolates produce β-lactamase have prompted a recent change in recommended therapy. Ceftriaxone or other third-generation cephalosporin should be administered for 4 weeks (Table 7–8). If it can be determined that the HACEK organism is β-lactamase negative, one set of guidelines has included the combination of ampicillin, 12 g every 24 hours either given continuously by intravenous infusion or administered in six divided doses, with gentamicin,

TABLE 7–8 ■ Therapy for Endocarditis Due to HACEK Microorganisms*

Antibiotic	Dosage and route	Duration (wk)	Comments
Ceftriaxone sodium[†]	2 g once daily IV or IM[†]	4	Cefotaxime sodium or other third-generation cephalosporins may be substituted
Ampicillin sodium[‡]	12 g/24 h IV either continuously or in six equally divided doses	4	
With gentamicin sulfate[§]	1 mg/kg IM or IV q8h	4	

HACEK, *Haemophilus parainfluenzae, Haemophilus aphrophilus, Actinobacillus actinomycetemcomitans, Cardiobacterium hominis, Eikenella corrodens*, and *Kingella kingae*

*Antibiotic dosages are for patients with normal renal function.

[†]Patients should be informed that IM injection of ceftriaxone is painful. For patients unable to tolerate β-lactam therapy, consult text.

[‡]Ampicillin should not be used if laboratory tests show β-lactamase production.

[§]For specific dosing adjustment and issues concerning gentamicin (obese patients, relative contraindications), see Table 7–3 footnotes.

From Wilson WR, Karchmer AW, Dajani AS, et al: Antibiotic treatment of adults with infective endocarditis due to streptococci, enterococci, staphylococci, and HACEK microorganisms. JAMA 1995;274:1706–1713. Copyright 1995, American Medical Association.

1 mg/kg every 8 hours. I have difficulty in recommending 4 weeks of aminoglycoside therapy because of my personal bias due to ototoxicity and nephrotoxicity risks. No mention was made regarding the use of β-lactam–β-lactamase inhibitor agents including ampicillin-sulbactam, and studies examining its use in this setting have not been performed. Nevertheless, it seems intuitive that such an agent should be efficacious in the treatment of HACEK native valve endocarditis.

In vitro susceptibility test results indicate that there are several non-β-lactam antibiotics that have activity against HACEK bacteria and that should be useful in patients who are not candidates for cephalosporin or ampicillin therapy. These include fluoroquinolones and TMP-SMX; aztreonam is a monobactam type of antibiotic with activity against HACEK microorganisms and has been used safely in penicillin-allergic patients. Nevertheless concern remains about its use in patients with immediate-type hypersensitivity reactions, and a decision to use this agent should be carefully scrutinized.

Endocarditis due to *Pseudomonas aeruginosa* usually occurs in two settings: native valve involvement in intravenous drug users and prosthetic valve infection in patients who are within both the early and late postoperative periods. The illness has been associated with the use of pentazocine and tripelennamine among drug users in at least two cities[29,30] in the United States. *Pseudomonas* endocarditis can be right sided, left sided, or mixed in intravenous drug users; it is usually left sided in prosthetic valve recipients who develop infection.

Medical therapy of right-sided endocarditis with a combination of third-generation cephalosporin such as ceftazidime, cefepime, or ureidopenicillin (piperacillin) combined with tobramycin, the aminoglycoside with the most activity against *P. aeruginosa*, is often successful. A high dose (8 mg/kg/d) of aminoglycoside has been advocated by some in more refractory cases.[31] In addition, tricuspid valve removal (without replacement) or vegectomy or annuloplasty may be required for control of infection. The duration of medical therapy should be a minimum of 4 weeks.

Because of the poor outcome with medical therapy of left-sided native valve *Pseudomonas* endocarditis, early valve replacement with at least 6 weeks of combined antibiotic treatment is recommended.

Fungal endocarditis is largely a disease of medical progress.[32–34] Patients who require complex medical care are at risk. This includes patients with central venous catheters and those with prosthetic cardiac valves. Intravenous drug users represent another "at risk" population. The clinical course is frequently complicated, and despite combined medical-surgical treatment the mortality rate is alarming. In one recent literature review[35] the mortality for yeast-related (predominately *Candida* species) endocarditis was 40%; that for mold-induced endocarditis exceeded 80%.

No prospective clinical trial has been conducted to attempt to define the most appropriate therapy for patients with fungal endocarditis. Surgical removal of the infected valve, particularly if it is a prosthetic valve, is advocated. Amphotericin B is used because it is the only fungicidal agent available to date in this country. Patients are given 0.5 mg/kg/d or higher for yeast-related infections and ≥ 1 mg/kg/d or higher for mold-related endocarditis. Of course, nephrotoxicity risks are increased with the higher and more prolonged dosing required for endocarditis treatment. Lipid-based preparations of amphotericin B have been used in patients with nephrotoxicity due to amphotericin B, and stabilization or improvement in renal function has been documented in many patients. Nevertheless the lipid-based products harbor some nephrotoxicity risks, and renal function must be monitored with their use. Currently there are three lipid-based products available for use in this country. Amphotericin B lipid complex (ABLC) is dosed 5 mg/kg/d; amphotericin B colloidal dispersion (ABLD) is dosed 3 to 4 mg/kg/d, and the liposomal amphotericin B (LAB) dose is 3 to 5 mg/kg/d. Some recommend the addition of flucytosine to amphotericin B for susceptible yeast infections. If flucytosine is used with amphotericin B, close monitoring of renal function must be done because flucytosine is renally eliminated. Toxicity risks increase if clearance of flucytosine is delayed because of amphotericin B–induced renal dysfunction. This could result in potentially life-threatening bone marrow suppression due to flucytosine.

A novel form of antifungal therapy has been used for patients who are not candidates for valve replacement for potential cure. Once acute treatment was completed and a clinical response was achieved, long-term suppression therapy has been used with success in some cases.[34] This is largely due to the availability of oral azole drugs including fluconazole and itraconazole for long-term suppression. Some have also advocated long-term suppressive therapy for patients who have undergone valve replacement for fungal endocarditis because the relapse rate following acute medical and surgical treatment is high. This new form of endocarditis therapy has raised many unanswered questions: (1) What is the appropriate dose of oral azole? (2) Is this form of treatment cost effective? (3) What is the safety of long-term suppressive therapy? and (4) Will suppressive therapy result in selection of azole resistance among endocarditis isolates?

The recovery of a pathogen from blood cultures is critical in the diagnosis and treatment of infective endocarditis. Multiple positive blood cultures, particularly with certain pathogens such as viridans group streptococci, can be the sentinel clue that leads to the diagnosis of infective endocarditis. In addition, key treatment decisions are based on the identification and susceptibility testing of blood culture isolates. Unfortunately, for either iatrogenic or microbiologic reasons, blood cultures can be culture negative, which has led to a syndrome designation of "culture-negative endocarditis."

Culture-negative endocarditis presents a treatment conundrum. The choice of therapy is empiric and is associated with several concerns that linger throughout the treatment course. These include whether the regimen will be efficacious, whether it is appropriate in regard to exposing a patient to unnecessary drug(s) and potential drug adverse events, and whether the empiric choice of therapy will only hamper the ability to discern the cause of the infection by interfering with subsequent blood and tissue cultures.

Empiricism begets empiricism. It is the empiric administration of antibiotics for reasons other than the treatment of endocarditis that is the most common cause of culture-negative endocarditis. Typically, patients present with nonspecific febrile syndromes that are ascribed to illnesses other than infective endocarditis and are given antibiotics without prior blood cultures being secured. Subsequent microbiologic evaluation is compromised when the diagnosis of endocarditis is entertained.

If antibiotics were recently given before blood cultures are obtained and the cultures are negative, a treatment regimen to "cover" the most likely pathogens should be selected. In the case of native valve infection, antibiotic therapy for community-acquired endocarditis is based on the clinical presentation. If the illness is acute, a regimen that includes high-dose (12 g/d) nafcillin or other penicillinase-resistant penicillins should be used. For subacute presentations, coverage for S. aureus, viridans group streptococci, and enterococci should be provided. In addition, therapy for the HACEK group of organisms should be considered. Ampicillin-sulbactam (3 g IV every 6 hours) combined with gentamicin (1 mg/kg/ IV or IM every 8 hours) is one appropriate option.

Vancomycin should be given with rifampin for prosthetic valve infections that are culture negative and occur within 1 year of valve placement to cover methicillin-resistant strains of coagulase-negative staphylococci. Coverage of aerobic gram-negative bacilli with ceftazidime, 2 g IV every 8 hours, should probably be included. If the prosthetic valve infection occurs after the first postoperative year, coverage for methicillin-susceptible staphylococci, enterococci, and viridans group streptococci should be included. Duration of therapy for prosthetic valve infection should be at least 6 weeks.

The other major cause of culture-negative endocarditis (that has an infectious cause) is microbiologic related.[36-38] Some microorganisms do not grow in routine blood culture media or grow slowly. These include the nutritionally deficient streptococci, the HACEK group of organisms, and fungi, all of which have been addressed. Numerous bacterial and fungal organisms that produce culture-negative endocarditis have been identified by other laboratory-based methods. Selected pathogens discussed here include Coxiella burnetii, Chlamydia psittaci, and the species of Legionella, Bartonella, and Brucella. At least three of the organisms, C. burnetii,

C. psittaci, and Brucella spp, represent zoonotic infections. Bartonella is probably a fourth group of bacteria that is transmitted from animals to humans. Legionella spp have caused prosthetic valve infections.

Before listing specific treatment regimens, several additional comments are noteworthy. First, delays in treatment are characteristic in culture-negative endocarditis and account for, in part, the poorer outcomes frequently seen. Second, there are no clinical trial data to define the most appropriate treatment regimen or its duration. Third, the modeling of a treatment regimen must take into account epidemiologic features, the clinical course of the illness, and whether prior antibiotic exposure was administered or not.

Combination therapy for C. burnetii is recommended. A tetracycline, usually doxycycline, is combined with rifampin, a fluoroquinolone, or TMP-SMZ. Therapy is administered for years, and both IgG and IgA antibodies should be monitored to judge both the response to therapy and duration of treatment. Some advocate indefinite or life-long therapy. In addition, surgical intervention with valve removal is recommended by some. Valve replacement is needed if a prosthetic valve is infected.

Similar combination regimens have been recommended in the cases of C. psittaci and Brucella spp endocardial infections. The most appropriate duration of therapy for both syndromes is undefined. Treatment is usually measured in months rather than weeks.

Macrolides plus rifampin have been used for endocarditis treatment due to Legionella spp and Bartonella spp. Again, the most appropriate duration of therapy is unknown. In one report, 6 months of antibiotic treatment was given for Legionella endocarditis.

Most persons who develop infective endocarditis do not require surgical intervention. There is, however, a subpopulation of patients who harbors or develops clinical features that serve as indicators for valve replacement to improve patient outcome.[39-41] The technical approaches of surgical intervention and the variety of materials used to replace or repair intracardiac structures will not be addressed in this review.

Uncontrolled or persistent infection despite optimal antimicrobial therapy is the most common reason for surgical intervention. This can be manifested in two clinical syndromes that are not mutually exclusive. In one case, continued or worsening sepsis prompts operative intervention. In the other case, progressive cardiac tissue destruction or enlarging vegetations serve as indicators for surgery.

Recurrent systemic emboli to major organs are another indication for valve replacement. Also, the embolic event may prompt a second surgical procedure, embolectomy, when limb viability is in question or if there is concern that the embolus could serve as an intravascular nidus of continued bloodstream seeding in the setting of a newly placed prosthetic valve or other intracardiac device.

Congestive heart failure due to valvular insufficiency that is refractory to medical management is another indication for surgery. Timing of surgery is crucial and should be done before severe hemodynamic instability occurs. It is also important to remember that valvular insufficiency leading to congestive heart failure can occur not only acutely but also weeks to months after microbiologic cure of infection. This phenomenon is due to the daily "wear-and-tear" of an abnormal valvular structure caused by prior infection. In addition, preexisting valvular abnormalities that predisposed to infective endocarditis can contribute to valvular dysfunction and subsequent congestive heart failure.

There are microbiologic features that serve as relative indications for surgery. Some advocate valve replacement if fungal endocarditis (native valve or prosthetic valve related) is present or if *S. aureus* is causing prosthetic valve infection. Recent investigations indicate that the mortality is lower in patients with prosthetic valve endocarditis due to *S. aureus* who undergo prosthetic valve replacement as compared with those given medical therapy alone.

Relapsing endocardial infection is another indication for valve replacement. Unlike the syndrome of uncontrolled infection discussed earlier in this section, some patients may respond to medical therapy with resolution of systemic toxicity and bacteremia or fungemia. It is only when antimicrobial therapy is completed that a return of clinical signs and symptoms of endocarditis is seen. Valve replacement should be considered in these patients, particularly if relapsing infection occurs despite appropriate antimicrobial treatment.

OUTPATIENT MANAGEMENT

The outpatient management of certain infectious disease syndromes including infective endocarditis was not considered an appropriate treatment option not too long ago. Because endocarditis is a potentially life-threatening illness, treatment was confined to the inpatient setting. Medical advances on two fronts now allow us to consider outpatient therapy for infective endocarditis as a treatment option for selected patients. Routine availability of echocardiography has allowed us to stratify patients into risk groups for complications. For example, patients with enlarging vegetations demonstrated on echocardiography despite appropriate therapy should not be considered for home care. Also, patients with mobile vegetations on the anterior leaflet of the mitral valve are at high risk for embolization and would not be good candidates for outpatient management. Advances in therapy and in medical devices used for intravenous infusions have also allowed clinicians to consider outpatient therapy as a useful and safe treatment option.

As detailed elsewhere,[42] most of our early published experience in outpatient therapy has included cases of endocarditis due to viridans group streptococci. Both the more traditional regimens of penicillin with or without aminoglycoside and the newer regimens of ceftriaxone with or without aminoglycoside[43,44] or with amoxicillin[45] have been employed.

Much less published data are available for the outpatient treatment of endocarditis caused by other types of microorganisms. Nevertheless, selected patients in this category can be considered for outpatient treatment if they are deemed low risk for complications.

It cannot be emphasized enough that patient selection is key when outpatient treatment of infective endocarditis is considered. Patients who are at the lowest risk for complications, who are hemodynamically stable, who have access to knowledgable health care professionals with state-of-the-art infusion-related devices, and who have dedicated and involved family members represent the best population for home therapy. Even in the ideal situations, complications—particularly embolic phenomena—occur, and all professional and family members who are providing care should be educated about the clinical manifestations of these potential complications and have plans for immediate transfer of patients to appropriately staffed medical facilities.

PREVENTION

Although many physicians are not involved in the medical management of patients with infective endocarditis, a wide variety of them in numerous specialties, dentists, and oral surgeons routinely participate in endocarditis prophylaxis decisions. Unfortunately, recommended guidelines for the use of antibiotic prophylaxis in patients considered at risk for the development of infective endocarditis are often not followed despite recent attempts to simplify the recommendations. Therefore, current guidelines[46] from the American Heart Association are reviewed in this chapter. Also addressed is the expectation of vaccine availability as a novel preventive tool in infective endocarditis.

Several qualifying remarks are in order as we evaluate the administration of antibiotic prophylaxis for the prevention of infective endocarditis. First, many clinicians have the misconception that dental and surgical procedures account for most cases of infective endocarditis. The percentage of cases of endocarditis linked to invasive procedures is thought to be in the single digits. Thus, even with the best prophylactic regimens employed, the number of endocarditis cases that can be prevented is small. Recently published data from the Philadelphia area support the notion that the contribution of dental procedures to the number of cases of infective endocarditis is limited. Second, antibiotic regimens were derived from work using animal models of experimental endocarditis and are not based on clinical trials data in humans. Third, questions linger requiring the efficacy of antibiotic prophylaxis, since no placebo-controlled trials have been or are likely to be conducted to examine this issue. Fourth, failures have been recorded even when appropriate antibiotic regimens are used. Fifth, medicolegal concerns in this country make it difficult for clinicians to recommend discontinuance of the use of prophylaxis among patients who have previously been administered prophylaxis for reasons not recognized as appropriate in published guidelines.

Cardiac conditions predisposing to the development of infective endocarditis have been stratified into moderate and highest risk categories (Table 7–9). Some of the more common conditions that increase the risk of endocarditis include prosthetic cardiac valves, prior episode of endocarditis, bicuspid aortic valve, acquired valvular dysfunction, and mitral valve prolapse with valvular regurgitation. Patients with mitral valve prolapse who have leaflet thickening and redundancy demonstrated on echocardiography should receive prophylaxis regardless of whether regurgitation is demonstrated. This latter subset of mitral valve prolapse patients is often older and is male.

There are several other conditions or settings in which the risk of endocarditis is no greater than that of the general population. Congenital lesions including secundum atrial septal defect and atrial or ventricular septal defect or patent ductus arteriosus more than 6 months after repair fall into this low-risk category. Also in this group is the adult patient with an innocent or physiologic murmur defined by echocardiography.

Once it is determined that a patient is at increased risk of developing infective endocarditis because of underly-ing structural abnormalities, the type of invasive procedure is examined to decide whether prophylaxis is warranted. The procedure usually involves one of four mucosal sites: oral, respiratory, gastrointestinal, and genitourinary. Although the resultant bacteremia may be polymicrobial, prophylaxis is selected to treat bacteremia due to either viridans group streptococci or enterococci. These organisms along with S. aureus have virulence features that make them uniquely qualified to produce endocarditis. In contrast, other types of bacteria such as anaerobes are commonly present in the bloodstream following some invasive dental procedures but rarely produce endocardial infection.

It is impossible to list the myriad invasive procedures at all mucosal sites that can result in bacteremia. The American Heart Association has addressed some of the more common procedures in tabular form (Tables 7–10 and 7–11) and indicated whether antibiotic prophylaxis should be considered. Unlike some invasive procedures at mucosal sites, procedures involving the puncture or incision of skin are not associated with significant bacteremia and do not warrant antibiotic prophylaxis.

A single dose of amoxicillin, 2 g, is recommended as the prophylactic agent of choice for dental, oral, respiratory, and esophageal procedures in adults (Table 7–12). The dose is taken orally 1 hour before the procedure to prevent endocarditis due to viridans group streptococci. No subsequent dosing of amoxicillin is recommended. For patients who cannot take oral drugs, ampicillin is recommended and is given as a 2-g dose 30 minutes before the procedure by intravenous or intramuscular route. For

TABLE 7–9 ■ Cardiac Conditions Associated with Endocarditis

ENDOCARDITIS PROPHYLAXIS RECOMMENDED
HIGH-RISK CATEGORY
Prosthetic cardiac valves, including bioprosthetic and homograft valves
Previous bacterial endocarditis
Complex cyanotic congenital heart disease (e.g., single ventricle states, transposition of the great arteries, tetralogy of Fallot)
Surgically constructed systemic pulmonary shunts or conduits

MODERATE-RISK CATEGORY
Most other congenital cardiac malformations (other than above and below)
Acquired valvular dysfunction (e.g., rheumatic heart disease)
Hypertrophic cardiomyopathy
Mitral valve prolapse with valvular regurgitation or thickened leaflets or both

ENDOCARDITIS PROPHYLAXIS NOT RECOMMENDED
NEGLIGIBLE-RISK CATEGORY (NO GREATER RISK THAN THE GENERAL POPULATION HAS)
Isolated secundum atrial septal defect
Surgical repair of atrial septal defect, ventricular septal defect, or patent ductus arteriosus (without residua beyond 6 mo)
Previous coronary artery bypass graft surgery
Mitral valve prolapse without valvular regurgitation
Physiologic, functional, or innocent heart murmurs
Previous Kawasaki disease without valvular dysfunction
Previous rheumatic fever without valvular dysfunction
Cardiac pacemakers (intravascular and epicardial) and implanted defibrillators

From Dajani AS, Taubert KA, Wilson W, et al: Prevention of bacterial endocarditis. Recommendations by the American Heart Association. JAMA 1997;227:1794–1801. Copyright 1997, American Medical Association.

TABLE 7–10 ■ Dental Procedures and Endocarditis Prophylaxis

ENDOCARDITIS PROPHYLAXIS RECOMMENDED*
Dental extractions
Periodontal procedures including surgery, scaling and root planning, probing, and recall maintenance
Dental implant placement and reimplantation of avulsed teeth
Endodontic (root canal) instrumentation or surgery only beyond the apex
Subgingival placement of antibiotic fibers or strips
Initial placement of orthodontic bands but not brackets
Intraligamentary local anesthetic injections
Prophylactic cleaning of teeth or implants where bleeding is anticipated

ENDOCARDITIS PROPHYLAXIS NOT RECOMMENDED
Restorative dentistry[†] (operative and prosthodontic) with or without retraction cord[‡]
Local anesthetic injections (nonintraligamentary)
Intracanal endodontic treatment; following placement and buildup
Placement of rubber dams
Postoperative suture removal
Placement of removable prosthodontic or orthodontic appliances
Taking of oral impressions
Fluoride treatments
Taking of oral radiographs
Orthodontic appliance adjustment
Shedding of primary teeth

*Prophylaxis is recommended for patients with high- and moderate-risk cardiac conditions.
[†]This includes restoration of decayed teeth (filling cavities) and replacement of missing teeth.
[‡]Clinical judgment may indicate antibiotic use in selected circumstances that may create significant bleeding.
From Dajani AS, Taubert KA, Wilson W, et al: Prevention of bacterial endocarditis. Recommendations by the American Heart Association. JAMA 1997;227:1794–1801. Copyright 1997, American Medical Association.

TABLE 7–11 ■ Other Procedures and Endocarditis Prophylaxis

ENDOCARDITIS PROPHYLAXIS RECOMMENDED
RESPIRATORY TRACT
Tonsillectomy or adenoidectomy
Surgical operations that involve respiratory mucosa
Bronchoscopy with rigid bronchoscope

*GASTROINTESTINAL TRACT**
Sclerotherapy for esophageal varices
Esophageal stricture dilation
Endoscopic retrograde cholangiography with biliary obstruction
Biliary tract surgery
Surgical operations that involve intestinal mucosa

GENITOURINARY TRACT
Prostatic surgery
Cytoscopy
Urethral dilation

ENDOCARDITIS PROPHYLAXIS NOT RECOMMENDED
RESPIRATORY TRACT
Endotracheal intubation
Bronchoscopy with flexible bronchoscope, with or without biopsy[†]

Tympanostomy tube insertion
GASTROINTESTINAL TRACT
Transesophageal echocardiography[†]
Endoscopy with or without gastrointestinal biopsy[†]

GENITOURINARY TRACT
Vaginal hysterectomy[†]
Vaginal delivery[†]
Cesarean section
In uninfected tissue:
  Urethral catheterization
  Uterine dilatation and curettage
  Therapeutic abortion
  Sterilization procedures
  Insertion or removal of intrauterine devices

OTHER
Cardiac catheterization, including balloon angioplasty
Implanted cardiac pacemakers, implanted defibrillators, and coronary stents
Incision or biopsy of surgically scrubbed skin
Circumcision

*Prophylaxis is recommended for high-risk patients; it is optional for medium-risk patients.
[†]Prophylaxis is optional for high-risk patients.
From Dajani AS, Taubert KA, Wilson W, et al: Prevention of bacterial endocarditis. Recommendations by the American Heart Association. JAMA 1997;227:1794–1801. Copyright 1997, American Medical Association.

patients with a history of immediate-type hypersensitivity reactions, clindamycin (600 mg), azithromycin (500 mg), or clarithromycin (500 mg) can be given orally 1 hour before the procedure. Oral cephalexin (2 g) or cefadroxil (2 g) can be used in patients who are penicillin-allergic but who have not had immediate-type reactions to penicillin.

Clindamycin, 600 mg IV, or cefazolin, 1 g IV, can be given 30 minutes before the procedure in patients who cannot take oral medications and who are allergic to penicillin. As with the case of cephalexin and cefadroxil, cefazolin should not be used in patients with a history of immediate-type hypersensitivity reactions to penicillin.

TABLE 7–12 ■ Prophylactic Regimens for Dental, Oral, Respiratory Tract, or Esophageal Procedures

Situation	Agent	Regimen
Standard general prophylaxis	Amoxicillin	**Adults:** 2 g; children*: 50 mg/kg PO 1 h before procedure
Unable to take oral medications	Ampicillin	**Adults:** 2 g IM or IV; children*: 50 mg/kg IM or IV within 30 min before procedure
Allergic to penicillin	Clindamycin or	**Adults:** 600 mg; children*: 20 mg/kg PO 1 h before procedure
	Cephalexin† or Cefadroxil† or	**Adults:** 2 g; children*: 50 mg/kg PO 1 h before procedure
	Azithromycin or Clarithromycin	**Adults:** 500 mg; children*: 15 mg/kg PO 1 h before procedure
Allergic to penicillin and unable to take oral medications	Clindamycin or	**Adults:** 600 mg; children*: 20 mg/kg IV within 30 min before procedure
	Cefazolin†	**Adults:** 1 g; children*: 25 mg/kg IM or IV within 30 min before procedure

*Total children's dose should not exceed adult dose.

†Cephalosporins should not be used for persons with immediate-type hypersensitivity reaction (urticaria, angioedema, or anaphylaxis) to penicillins.

From Dajani AS, Taubert KA, Wilson W, et al: Prevention of bacterial endocarditis. Recommendations by the American Heart Association. JAMA 1997;227:1794–1801. Copyright 1997, American Medical Association.

TABLE 7–13 ■ Prophylactic Regimens for Genitourinary or Gastrointestinal (Excluding Esophageal) Procedures

Situation	Agent	Regimen*
High-risk patients	Ampicillin plus gentamicin	**Adults:** ampicillin 2 g IM or IV plus gentamicin 1.5 mg/kg (not to exceed 120 mg) within 30 min of starting procedure; 6 h later, ampicillin 1 g IM or IV or amoxicillin 1 g PO **Children†:** ampicillin 50 mg/kg IM or IV plus gentamicin 1.5 mg/kg within 30 min of starting the procedure; 6 h later, ampicillin 25 mg/kg IM or IV or amoxicillin 25 mg/kg PO
High-risk patients allergic to ampicillin and amoxicillin	Vancomycin plus gentamicin	**Adults:** vancomycin 1 g IV over 1–2 h plus gentamicin 1.5 mg/kg IV or IM (not to exceed 120 mg); complete injection or infusion within 30 min of starting procedure **Children†:** vancomycin 20 mg/kg IV over 1–2 h plus gentamicin 1.5 mg/kg IV or IM; complete injection or infusion within 30 min of starting procedure
Moderate-risk patients	Amoxicillin or Ampicillin	**Adults:** amoxicillin 2 g PO 1 h before procedure, or ampicillin 2 g IM or IV within 30 min of starting procedure **Children†:** amoxicillin 50 mg/kg PO 1 h before procedure, or ampicillin 50 mg/kg IM or IV within 30 min of starting procedure
Moderate-risk patients allergic to ampicillin and amoxicillin	Vancomycin	**Adults:** vancomycin 1 g IV over 1–2 h; complete infusion within 30 min of starting procedure **Children†:** vancomycin 20 mg/kg IV over 1–2 h; complete infusion within 30 min of starting procedure

*No second dose of vancomycin or gentamicin is recommended.

†Total children's dose should not exceed adult dose.

From Dajani AS, Taubert KA, Wilson W, et al: Prevention of bacterial endocarditis. Recommendations by the American Heart Association. JAMA 1997;227:1794–1801. Copyright 1997, American Medical Association.

Enterococcal bacteremia is a concern with certain genitourinary and gastrointestinal procedures (Table 7–13). Amoxicillin, 2 g PO, can be used in patients at moderate risk of the development of endocarditis. Ampicillin, 2 g IV or IM, can be used in patients who cannot take oral antibiotic dosing. Patients who are deemed moderate risk and who are allergic to penicillin should be given vancomycin, 1 g IV over 1 to 2 hours, and the infusion should be completed within 30 minutes of the procedure initiation.

High-risk patients should receive more aggressive prophylaxis. A combination of ampicillin and gentamicin is administered intravenously before the procedure and is followed with a subsequent dose of parenteral ampicillin or oral amoxicillin 6 hours later. Vancomycin is combined with gentamicin in penicillin-allergic patients.

The recognition that only a small portion of endocardial infections occur as a result of identifiable invasive procedures has made us appreciate that antibiotic prophylaxis is of limited value in reducing the number of endocarditis cases. Because at-risk patients can be identified, there has been an interest in other forms of prophylaxis, including immunization. Currently, there is active investigation in the development of efficacious and safe vaccines for use in the prevention of systemic infections due to gram-positive cocci. Although no vaccine is currently available for use, several potential candidate vaccines against both staphylococci and streptococci are being examined. Immunization experiments using animal models of experimental endocarditis indicate that certain surface components of viridans group streptococci,[47] *S. aureus*,[48] and coagulase-negative staphylococci[49] serve both as critical virulence factors and potent immunogens. Whether these or other vaccines will be useful in infection prevention in humans awaits further study. We are encouraged by these preliminary animal investigations and firmly believe that immunization in patients with recognized risk factors for the development of endocarditis will be an integral part of the disease prevention strategy in these patients.

REFERENCES

1. Frary CJ, Devereux RB, Kramer-Fox R, et al: Clinical and health care cost consequences of infective endocarditis in mitral valve prolapse. Am J Cardiol 1994;73:263–267.
2. Von Reyn CF, Levy BS, Arbeit RD, et al: Infective endocarditis: An analysis based on strict case definitions. Ann Intern Med 1981;94:505–518.
3. Durack DT, Lukes AS, Bright DK: New criteria for diagnosis of infective endocarditis: Utilization of specific echocardiographic findings: Duke Endocarditis Service. Am J Med 1994;96:200–209.
4. Li JS, Sexton DJ, Mick N, et al: Proposed modifications to the Duke criteria for the diagnosis of infective endocarditis. Clin Infect Dis 2000;30:633–638.
5. Baddour LM: Virulence factors among gram-positive bacteria in experimental endocarditis. Infect Immun 1994;62:2143–2148.
6. Baddour LM, Sullam PM, Bayer AS: Pathogenesis of infective endocarditis. In Sussman M (ed): Molecular Medical Microbiology. London, Academic Press, 2001, pp. 999–1020.
7. Nicolau DP, Tessier PR, Nightingale CH: Beneficial effect of combination antiplatelet therapy on the development of experimental *Staphylococcus aureus* endocarditis. Int J Antimicrob Agents 1999;11:159–161.
8. Yeaman MR, Bayer AS: Antimicrobial peptides from platelets. Drug Resist Updat 1999;2:116–126.
9. Baddour LM, Simpson WA, Weems JJ Jr, et al: Phenotypic selection of small-colony variant forms of *Staphylococcus epidermidis* in the rat model of endocarditis. J Infect Dis 1988;157:757–763.
10. Wilson WR, Karchmer AW, Dajani AS, et al: Antibiotic treatment of adults with infective endocarditis due to streptococci, enterococci, staphylococci, and HACEK microorganisms. J Am Med Assoc 1995;274:1706–1713.
11. Himelright IM, Keerasuntonpong A, McReynolds JA, et al: Gender predilection of antibiotic-induced granulocytopenia in outpatients with septic arthritis or osteomyelitis. Infect Dis Clin Pract 1997;6:183–187.
12. Rybak MJ, Coyle EA: Vancomycin-resistant *Enterococcus*: Infectious endocarditis treatment. Curr Infect Dis Rep 1999;1:148–152.
13. Chambers HF, Miller RT, Newman MD: Right-sided *Staphylococcus aureus* endocarditis in intravenous drug abusers: Two-week combination therapy. Ann Intern Med 1988;109:619–624.
14. Torres-Tortosa M, de Cueto M, Vergara A, et al: Prospective evaluation of a two-week course of intravenous antibiotics in intravenous drug addicts with infective endocarditis. Grupo de Estudio de Engermedades Infecciosas de la Provincia de Cadiz. Eur J Clin Microbiol Infect Dis 1994;13:559–564.
15. Espinosa FJ, Valdes M, Martin-Luengo F, et al: [Right endocarditis caused by *Staphylococcus aureus* in parenteral drug addicts: Evaluation of a combined therapeutic scheme for 2 weeks versus conventional treatment]. Enferm Infecc Microbiol Clin 1993;11:235–240.
16. Ribera E, Gómez-Jiménez J, Cortés E, et al: Effectiveness of cloxacillin with and without gentamicin in short-term therapy for right-sided *Staphylococcus aureus* endocarditis: A randomized, controlled trial. Ann Intern Med 1996;125:969–974.
17. Small PM, Chambers HF: Vancomycin for *Staphylococcus aureus* endocarditis in intravenous drug users. Antimicrob Agents Chemother 1990;34:1227–1231.
18. Ribera E, Miro JM, Cortés E, et al: Influence of human immunodeficiency virus 1 infection and degree of immunosuppression in the clinical characteristics and outcome of infective endocarditis in intravenous drug users. Arch Intern Med 1998;158:2043–2050.
19. Dworkin RJ, Lee BL, Sande MA, Chambers HF: Treatment of right-sided *Staphylococcus aureus* endocarditis in intravenous drug users with ciprofloxacin and rifampicin. Lancet 1989;2(8671):1071–1073.
20. Heldman AW, Hartert TV, Ray SC et al: Oral antibiotic treatment of right-sided staphylococcal endocarditis in injection drug users: Prospective randomized comparison with parenteral therapy. Am J Med 1996;101:68–76.
21. Karchmer AW, Archer GL, Dismukes WE: *Staphylococcus epidermidis* prosthetic valve endocarditis: Microbiological and clinical observations as guide to therapy. Ann Intern Med 1983;98:447–455.
22. Yu VL, Fang GD, Keys TF et al: Prosthetic valve endocarditis: Superiority of surgical valve replacement versus medical therapy only. Ann Thorac Surg 1994;58:1073–1077.
23. Wolff M, Witchitz S, Chastang C, et al: Prosthetic valve endocarditis in the ICU. Prognostic factors of overall survival in a series of 122 cases and consequences for treatment decision. Chest 1995;108:688–694.
24. John MDV, Hibberd PL, Karchmer AW, et al: *Staphylococcal aureus* prosthetic valve endocarditis: Optimal management and risk factors for death. Clin Infect Dis 1998;26:1302–1309.
25. Lindberg J, Prag J, Schønheyder C: Pneumococcal endocarditis is not just a disease of the past: An analysis of 15 cases diagnosed in Denmark 1986–1997. Scand J Infect Dis 1998;30:469–472.
26. Aronin SI, Mukherjee SK, West JC, Cooney EL: Review of pneumococcal endocarditis in adults in the penicillin era. Clin Infect Dis 1998;26:165–171.
27. Lefort A, Mainardi JL, Selton-Suty C, et al: *Streptococcus pneumoniae* endocarditis in adults. A multicenter study in France in the era of penicillin resistance (1991–1998). The Pneumococcal Endocarditis Study Group. Medicine (Baltimore) 2000;79:327–337.
28. Baddour LM and the Infectious Diseases Society of America's Emerging Infections Network: Infective endocarditis caused by ß-hemolytic streptococci. Clin Infect Dis 1998;26:66–71.
29. Shekar R, Rice TW, Zierdt CH, Kallick CA: Outbreak of endocarditis caused by *Pseudomonas aeruginosa* serotype 011 among pentazocine and tripelennamine abusers in Chicago. J Infect Dis 1985;151:203–208.
30. Komshian SV, Tablan DC, Palutke W, Reyes MP: Characteristics of left-sided endocarditis due to *Pseudomonas aeruginosa* in the Detroit Medical Center. Rev Infect Dis 1990;12:693–702.

31. Bayer AS, Bolger AF, Taubert KA, et al: Diagnosis and management of infective endocarditis and its complications. Circulation 1998;98:2936–2948.

32. Nasser RM, Melger GR, Longworth DL, Gordon SM: Incidence and risk of developing fungal prosthetic valve endocarditis after nosocomial candidemia. Am J Med 1997;103:25–32.

33. Nguyer MH, Nguyer ML, Yu VL, et al: *Candida* prosthetic valve endocarditis: Prospective study of six cases and review of the literature. Clin Infect Dis 1996;22:262–267.

34. Baddour LM: Long-term suppressive therapy for fungal endocarditis. Clin Infect Dis 1996;23:1338–1339.

35. Pierrotti L, Baddour LM. Fungal endocarditis, 1995–2000. Chest 2002;122:302–310.

36. Berbari EF, Cockerill FR III, Steckelberg JM: Infective endocarditis due to unusual or fastidious microorganisms. Mayo Clin Proc 1997;72:532–542.

37. Barnes PD, Crook DWM: Culture negative endocarditis. J Infect 1997;35:209–213.

38. Fournier P-E, Raoult D: Nonculture laboratory methods for the diagnosis of infective endocarditis. Curr Infect Dis Rep 1999;1:136–141.

39. Jamieson SW: Surgical therapy for infective endocarditis. Mayo Clin Proc 1995;70:598–600.

40. Drinkwater DC Jr, Laks H, Child JS: Diagnosis and management of infective endocarditis. Issues in surgical treatment of endocarditis including intraoperative and postoperative management. Cardiol Clin 1996;14:451–464.

41. Mullany CJ, Chua YL, Schaff HV, et al: Early and late survival after surgical treatment of culture-positive active endocarditis. Mayo Clin Proc 1995;70:517–525.

42. Rehn SJ: Outpatient intravenous antibiotic therapy for endocarditis. Infect Dis Clin North Am 1998;12:879–901.

43. Francioli P, Etienne J, Hoigne R, et al: Treatment of streptococcal endocarditis with a single daily dose of ceftriaxone sodium for 4 weeks: Efficacy and outpatient treatment feasibility. JAMA 1992;267:264–267.

44. Sexton DJ, Tenenbaun MJ, Wilson WR, et al: Ceftriaxone once daily for four weeks compared with ceftriaxone plus gentamicin once daily for two weeks for treatment of endocarditis due to penicillin-susceptible streptococci. Clin Infect Dis 1998;27:1470–1474.

45. Stamboulian D, Bonvehi P, Arevalo C, et al: Antibiotic management of outpatients with endocarditis due to penicillin-susceptible streptococci. Rev Infect Dis 1991;13(suppl 2):S160–S163.

46. Dajani AS, Taubert KA, Wilson W, et al: Prevention of bacterial endocarditis. Recommendations by the American Heart Association. JAMA 1997;227:1794–1801.

47. Viscount HB, Munro CL, Burnette-Curley D, et al: Immunization with FimA protects against *Streptococcus parasanguis* endocarditis in rats. Infect Immun 1997;65:994–1002.

48. Lee JC, Park J-S, Shepherd SE, et al: Protective efficacy of antibodies to the *Staphylococcus aureus* type 5 capsular polysaccharide in a modified model of endocarditis in rats. Infect Immun 1997;65:4146–4151.

49. Takeda S, Pier GB, Kojima Y, et al: Protection against endocarditis due to *Staphylococcus epidermidis* by immunization with capsular polysaccharide/adhesin. Circulation 1991;11:452–463.

chapter 8

Pericarditis and Myocarditis

CATHERINE DIAMOND, MD, MPH

JEREMIAH G. TILLES, MD

Because the management and outcome of pericarditis and myocarditis may vary with the etiology, pathogenesis, or clinical presentation, it will be useful to first review the essential aspects of each of these topics. We refer the reader to Chapter 70 in *Infectious Diseases* for a detailed discussion of these topics.

PERICARDITIS

Etiology

Noninfectious causes of pericarditis include systemic disorders such as collagen vascular disease, uremia, and neoplasia, insults to the thoracic cavity such as chest trauma, radiation, or surgery, myocardial infarction, and drug reactions to hydralazine or procainamide. Many cases of idiopathic pericarditis are believed to be due to undiagnosed viral infections. Enteroviruses, particularly coxsackievirus group B, are the most frequently implicated viral etiology of myocarditis, although other viruses such as influenza and cytomegalovirus (CMV) are also common causes.[1–4] Small, asymptomatic pericardial effusions are common in AIDS patients, whereas tuberculosis, opportunistic infections, malignancies, and bacterial infection are included in the differential diagnosis when the effusion becomes large and symptomatic.[5,6]

In the past, bacterial pericarditis was most common in youths with pneumonia. Bacterial pericarditis has become less common with the advent of antibiotics and typically occurs in debilitated adults as a result of pulmonary infection, endocarditis, chest wall injury, or bacteremia.[7] *Streptococcus pneumoniae* used to be the most common agent and is still an important pathogen.[8] *Staphylococcus aureus*, streptococci other than the pneumococcus, gram-negative rods, and anaerobes have been prominent causes in more recent reports.[9–12] Both *Haemophilus influenzae* and meningococcus have been notable causes of pericarditis in children. In recent years, however, the conjugated *H. influenzae* vaccine has become less prominent as a cause of childhood infection, but the meningococcus still affects both adults and children.[13,14] Tuberculosis is an important cause of pericarditis in underdeveloped countries and in patients with AIDS. Fungal pericarditis is uncommon but can occur following cardiothoracic surgery or with disseminated infection.[15,16]

Pathogenesis

Normally there is about 30 ml of pericardial fluid between the visceral and parietal pericardium that drains into the thoracic and the right lymphatic ducts. The inflammatory infiltrate of pericarditis may disturb lymphatic drainage and cause accumulation of pericardial fluid. When the volume of the fluid is sufficient to restrict ventricular filling, cardiac tamponade can occur. Recurrent pericarditis is thought to be due to an autoimmune mechanism.[17] Constrictive pericarditis is characterized by a fibrotic pericardium that impairs the motion of the heart.

Clinical Diagnosis

The most common symptom of acute pericarditis is chest pain, and a friction rub is the most noteworthy physical sign.[18] Since the rub is not present in every case and may be evanescent, the lack of a rub should not exclude the diagnosis of pericarditis.[19,20] Elevations in simple laboratory test results such as the erythrocyte sedimentation rate (ESR), white blood cell count (WBC), and cardiac isoenzymes may support the diagnosis of pericarditis. The most sensitive electrocardiographic feature is widespread elevation of the ST segments.[21] Although a chest radiograph may show cardiac enlargement if a sizeable effusion is present, echocardiography is the best way to evaluate for pericardial effusion.[22,23] Computed tomography or magnetic resonance imaging (MRI) may show pericardial thickening or masses in cases when echocardiography does not provide sufficient information.[24–26]

When a patient also has a condition such as uremia or myocardial infarction that is a frequent cause of pericarditis, the etiologic diagnosis of the pericarditis is straightforward.[27] Microbiologic evidence of systemic infection or infection in the chest near the pericardium similarly allows a presumptive diagnosis. In the workup of suspected viral pericarditis, human immunodeficiency virus (HIV) serology, viral cultures from sites such as blood, throat, or rectum, acute and convalescent serologies for Coxsackievirus B or other suspected viral pathogens and viral immunoglobulin M antibodies are recommended. Because of the number of viruses that cause pericarditis and their ubiquity, the results of these cultures and serologic tests, whether negative or positive, may be difficult to interpret and only provide a presumptive diagnosis at best.

In a study of over 250 patients with clinically diagnosed pericarditis that required a workup to determine etiology, 86% were idiopathic, 5% neoplastic, and 2% due to collagen vascular disease. For only 7% of the patients was an infectious etiology identified (4% tuberculous, 1% viral, 1% toxoplasmal, and 1% bacterial pericarditis).[28] When patients in the study received pericardiocentesis for the treatment of tamponade, the diagnostic yield was 28% as opposed to a diagnostic yield of 5% when the procedure was undertaken for diagnosis only. The diagnostic yield was 54% when the patients received a pericardial biopsy or pericardiectomy for tamponade, which allowed examination of pericardial tissue as well as fluid. These figures indicate that pericardiocentesis with tissue examination is more likely to result in a diagnosis than drainage of pericardial fluid without biopsy. Diagnostic

pericardiocentesis is necessary only in patients with possible purulent effusion, immunocompromised status, cardiac tamponade, or a disease duration longer than 3 weeks.[29] When pericardial fluid (with or without biopsy) is obtained, the following studies are recommended: cultures and stains for bacteria, mycobacteria, and fungi; culture and polymerase chain reaction (PCR) for suspected viral pathogens; and histology studies.[30] Cell count, protein, glucose, amylase, and cholesterol levels, and cytology may be helpful in the workup for cases of noninfectious and infectious origins.

Treatment and Prognosis

Viral or Idiopathic Pericarditis

Nonsteroidal anti-inflammatory agents such as indomethacin (25 to 75 mg four times a day), ibuprofen (400 mg four times a day), or aspirin (650 mg four to six times a day) are first-line medical therapy for viral or idiopathic pericarditis.[31,32] Nonsteroidal anti-inflammatory agents, however, are deleterious in mouse models of myocarditis and thus should not be used in patients with either myocarditis or pericarditis with a myocarditis component. Patients with acute idiopathic pericarditis unresponsive to nonsteroidal anti-inflammatory agents may respond to prednisone 60 mg daily for 3 days followed by a rapid taper. Because of the side effects of corticosteroids and suspicions that they may prolong disease or promote recurrence, this therapy is reserved for patients who do not respond to nonsteroidal anti-inflammatory agents within 2 to 3 days.[31] Like nonsteroidal anti-inflammatory agents, corticosteroids have been shown to be harmful in mouse myocarditis models and thus should be avoided in patients with viral myocarditis or pericarditis with a myocarditis component. There are no prospective clinical trials of nonsteroidal anti-inflammatory agents or corticosteroids in human viral pericarditis.

If a patient with viral pericarditis is infected with a virus sensitive to antiviral agents, the patient may benefit from antiviral therapy administered for up to 4 weeks (see Myocarditis, Treatment discussion for information on individual drugs). Anticoagulants increase the risk of hemorrhage and tamponade in pericarditis and should not be used. A patient with tamponade must receive emergent pericardiocentesis or surgical drainage for the purposes of diagnosis and therapy.

Although acute viral or idiopathic pericarditis is usually self-limited, lasting 1 to 3 weeks, the course may be complicated by associated myocarditis, recurrent pericarditis, cardiac tamponade, or the late development of constrictive pericarditis. About 15% to 30% of patients with idiopathic acute pericarditis have at least one recurrent episode.[33,34] Although the timing and number of recurrences vary, recurrent episodes are generally less severe than the first episode. Deaths, cardiac tamponade, or constrictive pericarditis are uncommon. Most patients respond to intermittent treatment with nonsteroidal anti-inflammatory agents, although a few require prolonged therapy. Colchicine at an initial dose of 3 mg followed by 1 mg daily for 6 months to 1 year is useful in cases of relapsing pericarditis to prevent recurrence.[35–37] The response rate is about 75%.[36] The most common side effect is diarrhea, which occurs in about 15% of recipients but typically does not require suspension of therapy.[38] Colchicine has been used in acute pericarditis as well as recurrent pericarditis, but there are no controlled trials in either setting.[39]

Corticosteroid therapy should only be considered for cases of recurrent pericarditis unresponsive to nonsteroidal anti-inflammatory agents and colchicine. Most patients will respond to 60 mg per day of prednisone within a few days. This dose may be continued for 1 to 3 weeks and then gradually tapered. When the dose is reduced to less than 10 to 15 mg per day, however, symptoms may recur, and patients with recalcitrant disease frequently require continued prednisone at 2 to 5 mg per day for months or years.[17,36] This long-term corticosteroid therapy may result in a Cushingoid appearance, myopathy, aseptic necrosis of the bone, and immunosuppression.[17] Although clinicians have used other drugs such as azathioprine, chlorambucil, and interferon to treat recurrent pericarditis, experience with these therapies is minimal.[36,40] One retrospective case series showed benefit from pericardiectomy in the setting of recurrent pericarditis, but the procedure is rarely necessary and then only in the few patients with severe or frequent episodes unresponsive to or intolerant of medical therapy or who have with constrictive pericarditis.[17,40,41]

Tuberculous Pericarditis

The antibiotic regimens recommended for tuberculous pericarditis are the same as those recommended for pulmonary tuberculosis. A systematic review of previous randomized trials of therapy in tuberculous pericarditis concluded that corticosteroids potentially have a large impact on survival but that published trials are too small to measure this and that future placebo-controlled trials are needed.[42] Despite the lack of conclusive data, most experts recommend corticosteroids in the setting of tuberculous pericarditis. In a South African study with 143 subjects, corticosteroids decreased mortality from 11% in controls to 4% in treated cases. Pericardiectomies were required in 30% of controls vs. 21% of steroid-treated cases.[43] In another study from the same group, corticosteroid-treated patients had significantly improved survival and were less likely to require pericardiectomy or repeat pericardiocentesis than controls were.[44] Adult doses used in these studies were prednisolone 60 mg for weeks 1 to 4, 30 mg for weeks 5 to 8, 15 mg for weeks 9 and 10, and 5 mg for week 11 of antituberculous therapy. In a randomized trial of HIV-associated tuberculous pericarditis in Zimbabwe, all patients received a standard short course of antituberculous chemotherapy; 29 patients received adjunctive prednisolone, and 29 received placebo. Mortality was significantly lower in the corticosteroid-treated group.[45] Corticosteroids are not indicated for the treatment of constrictive pericarditis.

Pericardial infection in patients with pulmonary tuberculosis may remain undiagnosed until the hemodynamic signs of constrictive pericarditis develop late in the course of the disease. Even with correct therapy, constrictive pericarditis develops in 30% to 50% of cases of tuberculous pericarditis, and the risk is greater in patients with tamponade.[46,47] In a controlled clinical trial conducted in Africa, open surgical drainage of tuberculous pericardial effusion permitted diagnosis and abolished the need for recurrent pericardiocentesis, but a pericardial window did not decrease mortality or need for pericardiectomy. In addition, the mortality directly attributed to the procedure was 2%. Since open surgical drainage adds expense and morbidity without any mortality benefit, it should not be performed routinely.[42,44]

About one-third to one-half of patients with tuberculous pericarditis will require pericardiectomy.[48] There are no clinical trial data from which to draw recommendations regarding indications for, and timing of, pericardiectomy.[42] Some authors recommend pericardiectomy for all patients with tuberculous pericarditis, whereas others recommend waiting for up to 3 months after starting therapy to determine if constriction will resolve without surgery.[46,49] Pericardiectomy is clearly required for patients with recurrent or life-threatening tamponade. Since tuberculous pericarditis that has progressed to calcification has a poor prognosis, it is better to perform pericardiectomy earlier in cases where it is indicated.[48,49] Although pericardiectomy usually improves hemodynamics; it may take months for venous congestion to resolve, and there may be residual damage to myocardial function if the procedure has been excessively delayed.[49]

Bacterial Pericarditis

A patient with bacterial pericarditis requires a prolonged course of high-dosage intravenous antibiotics. For example, pericarditis due to methicillin-sensitive *S. aureus* would be treated for 4 to 6 weeks with intravenous nafcillin at 2 g every 4 hours. Since intravenous antibiotics achieve sufficiently high levels in the inflamed pericardium, it is not necessary to irrigate with topical antibiotics. Surgical drainage in combination with appropriate antibiotics is usually necessary to treat bacterial pericarditis.[50] Although pericardiocentesis or a pigtail catheter may be able to drain thin fluid, thicker fluid requires a more definitive drainage procedure. A pericardiostomy tube drain, although effective, increases the risk of constrictive pericarditis. Although a pericardial window permits resorption of fluid from the left pleural space and recovers tissue for histologic and microbiologic testing, it increases the risk that wound infection, pneumonia, or a chronic sinus tract will develop.[50,51] Although there is an anecdotal report of the use of streptokinase as an intervention for purulent pericarditis, this procedure carries the risk of local irritation and recurrent tamponade.[50,52] When there is a thick effusion with loculations, pericardiectomy is needed for drainage and to prevent constriction. Pericardiectomy is usually indicated in patients with candidal or nocardial infections or continued sepsis. It is also indicated in patients with hemodynamic compromise from recurrent effusion or progressive pericardial thickening.

Reflecting the severity of the predisposing conditions in most contemporary patients with purulent pericarditis, the mortality from bacterial pericarditis was 16% to 44% in patients diagnosed antemortem and treated with combined medical and surgical therapy.[9,10,53] Poor prognostic indicators include intracardiac or postoperative source of infection, gram-negative rod infection, and absence of combined surgical and medical therapy. Mortality is highest in older and debilitated patients and when the diagnosis is delayed.[9,10]

MYOCARDITIS

Etiology

Myocarditis may have a wide variety of infectious causes (viral, bacterial, fungal, or parasitic) or noninfectious causes (idiopathic, drug, toxin, autoimmune, radiation, endocrine, or metastatic tumors). Most infectious causes are viral, with the most frequent in immunocompetent persons being enteroviruses (especially coxsackievirus B), adenovirus, and influenza A and B viruses (particularly during a recognized outbreak).[2,3,54–56] In immunocompromised persons the most common viral causes are CMV and HIV.[57] In parts of Central and South America the most common infectious cause is the parasite *Trypanosoma cruzi*.[58] Alcoholism, sarcoidosis, scleroderma, and systemic lupus erythematosus are among the relatively more frequent noninfectious causes.

Pathogenesis

Pathogenesis may vary with the variety and dose of the causal agent as well as with the immune status, genetics, age, and sex of the host. Little is known about the pathogenesis of myocarditis in general, or viral myocarditis in particular, for humans. On the other hand, viral myocarditis has been extensively studied in murine models. One can speculate from the murine models that damage in enteroviral myocarditis in humans usually is minimal because of low dose or low virulence of the virus strain or the robust response of the host. It may lead to rapid cardiac decompensation and death, however, if the viral dose is large, the strain is particularly virulent, or the host resistance is significantly reduced. When lysis of myocytes is acute, it may be due to infection by the virus or cytokines released from the inflammatory infiltrate. The inflammatory infiltrate is usually transient but can be persistent with a change in profile from polymorphonuclear leukocytes to mononuclear cells. When it persists, it may be accompanied by viral nucleic acid detectable by PCR, which implies persistent infection, or it may be accompanied by antimyosin antibodies, which implies an autoimmune component. It is believed that a small percent of patients with acute viral myocarditis go on to a state of chronic dilated cardiomyopathy. The myocardial biopsies of patients with dilated cardiomyopathy may or may not have an inflammatory infiltrate or enterovirus RNA by PCR.[59] The blood serum of these patients may contain antimyosin antibody.[60,61]

Clinical Diagnosis

It is well established that most cases of myocarditis are asymptomatic and would go undiagnosed unless the opportunity for histologic diagnosis is provided by autopsy, performed routinely or for sudden and unexpected natural death, or unless transient changes are detected on serial electrocardiogram or myocardial serum enzyme studies possibly drawn for routine or other reasons.[62–64] When symptomatic disease is due to virus, it may occur one to several weeks following a febrile episode with constitutional or acute respiratory symptoms. The most prominent symptom of acute myocarditis itself is chest pain that may be accompanied by palpitations, shortness of breath, or cough.[65] On physical examination the patient usually has tachycardia and may have a third heart sound, muffled first heart sound, pericardial friction rub, or signs of congestive heart failure. Troponin or creatine phosphokinase, C-reactive protein, ESR, and WBC count are frequently elevated.[66,67] The chest radiograph frequently shows cardiac enlargement, and is usually some ST segment elevation and T wave inversions are shown on serial electrocardiograms. Echocardiograms can be helpful in assessing ejection fraction and left ventricular wall motion abnormality.

Treatment and Prognosis

The modalities of treatment to consider for myocarditis depend on the degree of confidence one has in the identification of the specific etiologic agent, the stage of the disease that is being addressed, and state of the cardiovascular system. When one has a high level of confidence in the diagnosis of a specific agent, there may be specific treatment available that can be initiated along with supportive measures. For all other situations, management is necessarily confined to supportive measures alone.

Supportive Measures
General

Supportive care must be considered regardless of the causal agent but will vary with the stage of evolution of the disease and the degree of severity. Since the causal organism of viral myocarditis is usually unknown, the foundation of therapy often is limited to the supportive care that would be required regardless of the etiologic agent. Bed rest is recommended, since exercise worsens the outcome of coxsackievirus myocarditis in mice and exacerbates wall motion abnormalities in humans (Table 8–1).[68,69] Hospitalization, oxygen, and continuous cardiac monitoring are standard for all patients with myocarditis.

Although there is no evidence to determine how long to continue these supportive measures, it would be prudent for the patient to avoid strenuous exercise during the convalescent period until heart size and function have returned to normal and electrocardiogram changes have resolved. Given that excessive alcohol alone can cause cardiomyopathy, the patient should avoid alcohol intake. Anemia and fever should be treated urgently to decrease the demand on the heart. If a life-threatening arrhythmia occurs, electrophysiologic evaluation, antiarrhythmics, a pacemaker, or an implantable defibrillator may be necessary. Because the clinical manifestations of myocarditis typically resolve with conservative therapy and the treatment of myocarditis is usually supportive, endomyocardial biopsy is generally not indicated. If there is progressive clinical deterioration or a cause of myocarditis requiring specific therapy is a diagnostic consideration, the risk of biopsy may be justifiable.

Cardiovascular Agents

Patients with symptomatic heart failure or an ejection fraction under 40% require afterload reduction with an angiotensin-converting enzyme (ACE) inhibitor. ACE inhibitors may alter postinjury remodeling or decrease pathologic damage by scavenging oxygen free radicals.[70] In a mouse model, early administration of captopril improved histologic appearance and reduced heart weight.[71] Angiotensin II is elevated in mice with myocarditis, and a newly developed angiotensin II receptor antagonist (TCV-116) decreased myocardial cell necrosis, cellular infiltration, and calcification in a mouse model.[72] In mice infected with an encephalomyocarditis virus, captopril reduced myocardial necrosis and inflammation; enalapril improved only necrosis and not inflammation; and losartan, an FDA-approved angiotensin II receptor antagonist, did not influence myocardial necrosis or inflammation.[73] Because the animal data are strongest with captopril, captopril is recommended unless the patient develops related side effects such as renal failure, angioedema, or cough. Hydralazine and isosorbide dinitrate are recommended for afterload reduction if the patient cannot tolerate an ACE inhibitor. In addition to afterload reduction, patients with congestive heart failure should receive diuretics, and their salt intake should be restricted. Although spironolactone has not been studied specifically in mouse myocarditis models or human myocarditis, at a dose of 25 mg daily it reduced morbidity and mortality in patients with severe heart failure when given with ACE inhibitors.[74]

Although clinicians often employ digoxin in the treatment of myocarditis, digoxin increases proinflammatory cytokines, myocardial necrosis, cellular infiltration, and

TABLE 8–1 ■ Treatment for Myocarditis

	Animal data	Human data	Recommendation	Note
SUPPORTIVE MEASURES				
Bedrest	+	+	+	
CARDIOVASCULAR AGENTS				
Beta-blocker	–	No data	+/–	Carvedilol beneficial in humans with heart failure who are receiving concurrent therapy with digoxin, diuretics, and ACE inhibitors but not tested in humans with myocarditis
Calcium channel blocker	+	No data	+/–	Amlodipine reduced mortality in humans with nonischemic dilated cardiomyopathy but not in myocarditis specifically
Digoxin	–	No data	+/–	Use cautiously at low doses
Angiotensin converting enzyme (ACE) inhibitor	+	No data	+	Captopril preferable; there is human data on benefits of captopril in heart failure but not myocarditis
ANTIVIRALS				
Ribavirin	+	Minimal data	–	Ribavirin prevented viral shedding in humans, but adverse effects outweigh potential benefits
Pleconaril	+	Minimal data	+/–	Reported use in four patients with minimal adverse effects
IMMUNOSUPPRESSANTS AND IMMUNOMODULATORS				
Prednisone	–	No benefit	–	Many adverse events associated with therapy
Intravenous immunoglobulin	+	No benefit	–	Few adverse events associated with therapy
Interferon	+	Minimal data	–	Many adverse effects associated with therapy

+, Positive study results or recommended therapy; –, adverse study results or not recommended therapy.

mortality in a mouse model, suggesting that the drug should be used cautiously and only at low doses.[75] Dobutamine and dopamine may also be part of myocarditis treatment and are preferable to epinephrine, norepinephrine, or isoproterenol.[76] Vesnarinone, a quinolone-derived positive inotropic agent and also an immunomodulator, improved survival and reduced myocardial damage in a mouse model of myocarditis due to encephalomyocarditis virus, perhaps through inhibition of natural killer cell activity.[77] Vesnarinone, however, is not available in the United States because the drug has been associated with a dose-dependent increase in mortality in patients with severe heart failure.[78]

While beta-blockers may have a place in the armamentarium, they should be used with caution, particularly in acute severe disease. In a mouse model of coxsackievirus B3 myocarditis, metoprolol increased mortality.[79] Carvedilol, however, reduces the risk of death and hospitalization for cardiovascular causes in humans with heart failure who are receiving concurrent therapy with digoxin, diuretics, and ACE inhibitors.[80] Furthermore, in a recent study of immunoglobulin in acute dilated cardiomyopathy, an incidental finding was an improved natural history compared to historical data. The authors attributed this improvement in natural history to the use of beta-blockers in the management of systolic dysfunction. They noted that 18% of subjects received beta-blockers at baseline, but 45% were receiving these agents by their 1-year follow-up visit.[81]

In a mouse model of viral myocarditis, verapamil-treated mice had reduced microvascular changes and myocardial necrosis, suggesting calcium channel blockers may reduce microvascular spasm in viral myocarditis.[82] In a study comparing the effects of amlodipine vs. diltiazem or placebo in mice infected with an encephalomyocarditis virus, 70% of the amlodipine-treated mice survived compared with 50% in the diltiazem group and 33% in the control group; this therapeutic effect may be a result of inhibition of nitric oxide production.[83] In humans, amlodipine reduced mortality in patients with nonischemic dilated cardiomyopathy but not in myocarditis specifically.[84] Although anticoagulation is contraindicated in acute viral myopericarditis because of the risk of inducing cardiac tamponade, anticoagulation is indicated with atrial fibrillation or intracardiac thrombi and should be considered if the patient is in sinus rhythm but has a low ejection fraction.

Mechanical Support and Cardiac Transplant

In acute fulminant myocarditis with cardiogenic shock, aggressive circulatory supportive therapies such as intra-aortic balloon pumps, ventricular assist devices, or extracorporeal membrane oxygenation (ECMO) may be necessary. These devices support the circulation while the heart recovers or until cardiac transplant. Publications describing the use of these circulatory support techniques in myocarditis tend to report small numbers of patients with no controls. In a report of 11 myocarditis patients treated with an external ventricular assist device, nine patients survived to explantation or transplant.[85] Among four children treated with biventricular support devices, three improved and one underwent successful transplantation.[86] In two reports from Asia about the use of ECMO in myocarditis, one reports survival of four of five Taiwanese patients and the other survival of five of six Japanese patients.[87,88]

The medical team should select a treatment plan based on the characteristics of the particular patient and the expertise of the treating facility. During ventricular support there is a risk of thrombosis with inadequate anticoagulation or bleeding with excessive anticoagulation. ECMO also requires heparinization. ECMO has the advantage of providing oxygen support in the setting of pulmonary insufficiency. ECMO also allows gradual reduction of circulatory support for weaning. Inadequate decompression of the left ventricle with ECMO, however, can result in elevated left ventricular end diastolic pressure and pulmonary edema.[87,88]

The clinician generally should not consider cardiac transplant in the acute phase, because patients with fulminant myocarditis can recover completely. In the setting of persistent heart failure, however, the clinician should consider obtaining an endomyocardial biopsy and possibly cardiac transplant. Although there was a report of 12 patients undergoing transplantation for myocarditis who had shorter survival than controls undergoing cardiac transplant for other diagnoses, a much larger study did not confirm this finding.[89,90]

Pathogen-Specific Treatment
Viral and Autoimmune Myocarditis

ANTIVIRAL AGENTS. Although most cases of idiopathic myocarditis are presumed to be viral in origin, there are little data on the treatment of myocarditis with antiviral agents and no controlled studies of efficacy. Since the causative agent is usually not diagnosed, there has been little opportunity to study antivirals in humans with myocarditis. If the infection is acute and the specific organism is diagnosed, the clinician could prescribe antiviral agents such as ganciclovir or foscarnet for CMV, M2 (amantadine, rimantidine) or oral neuraminidase inhibitors (oseltamivir) for influenza, antiretrovirals for HIV, or pleconaril for enterovirus. Clearly the clinician must weigh the potential toxicity of the specific antiviral drug against the potential benefit of therapy, considering the severity and stage of the patient's illness.

Antiviral therapy with ganciclovir and hyperimmune globulin for severe CMV myocarditis is one of the therapies under investigation in the European Study of Epidemiology and Treatment of Cardiac Inflammatory Disease (ESET-CID). There is also a single case report of ganciclovir treatment of CMV myocarditis.[91] Although zidovudine has been linked to cardiomyopathy in patients with AIDS, antiretroviral therapy will prevent opportunistic infections and likely prolong life in AIDS patients with cardiomyopathy.

Ribavirin has shown activity against coxsackievirus B3 in vitro and in mice.[92,93] In a study of three patients with influenza myocarditis, viral shedding ceased with administration of intravenous ribavirin, but all three patients eventually died of myocarditis.[94] Given this scant and conflicting data, ribavirin currently does not have a role in the treatment of human myocarditis.

No drugs to treat enteroviruses are currently on the market. In March 2002, the FDA's Antiviral Drugs Advisory Committee voted against approval of pleconaril for treatment of acute picornaviral viral respiratory infection in adults, requesting more safety data and studies on more diverse patient populations.[95] Oral pleconaril (VP63843 or Picovir), however, is available for compassionate use through ViroPharma for serious enteroviral infection. Pleconaril inhibits enteroviral replication by preventing viral uncoating and attachment to host cell receptors. A precursor agent, WIN 54954, reduced coxsackievirus replication and mortality in murine myocarditis models, but adverse effects prevented its development for therapy of human myocarditis.[96,97] Pleconaril decreased symptoms and disease duration in a phase II study of enteroviral meningitis, and the drug appeared to have a clinical and virologic response in compassionate use.[95,98] Thus far there are only four published reports of patients with myocarditis who received pleconaril through compassionate use, and three had clinical responses temporally related to pleconaril administration. Myocarditis has a variable natural history, however, and there is the possibility of a postinfectious autoimmune component in these cases. Clinical efficacy could only be demonstrated by a properly designed and placebo-controlled phase III study.

Although there is no vaccine available to prevent enteroviral infection, there is an attenuated vaccine under development in a mouse model using a group B coxsackievirus–poliovirus 5′ nontranslated region chimera.[99] There is also a formalin-inactivated coxsackievirus B vaccine that has been protective in mouse models against infection with all six types of group B coxsackievirus.[100] It is also possible that avoiding strenuous exercise during viral infection may decrease the risk of myocarditis.

IMMUNOSUPPRESSANTS. It is difficult to conduct treatment trials of myocarditis. The incidence of recognized symptomatic myocarditis is low, limiting human studies. Myocarditis varies in presentation, ranging from inapparent infection to acute congestive heart failure to chronic dilated cardiomyopathy, making it difficult to generalize treatment. Myocarditis generally improves with conservative treatment; thus it is difficult to interpret the effectiveness of therapy in studies that did not include a control group.

The Myocarditis Treatment Trial, a randomized controlled trial that enrolled patients with a histopathologic diagnosis of myocarditis and a left ventricular ejection fraction of less than 0.45, is the best designed study to date (Table 8–2).[101,102] The study's results indicated that immunosuppressive therapy did not improve left ventricular ejection fraction or survival. Since the trial was

TABLE 8–2 ■ Studies of Myocarditis Treatment

Treatment category	Author	Study name	Setting	Number of subjects	Entry criteria	Intervention	Results
Immuno-suppressant	Mason et al[101]	Myocarditis Treatment Trial (MTT)	31 centers in North America and Japan	111 adults	Histologic evidence of myocarditis, LVEF <0.45, < 2 years of symptoms	Prednisone and either azathioprine or cyclosporine	No difference in 1 y mortality or LVEF at 28 wk
Immuno-modulator	McNamara et al[81]	Intervention in Myocarditis and Acute Cardiomyopathy (IMAC)	6 centers in United States	62 adults	LVEF <0.40, < 6 months of symptoms	Intravenous immuno-globulin	No difference in LVEF at 6 mo or 1 y follow-up
Immuno-suppressant and immuno-modulator	Maisch et al[111]	European Study of Epidemiology and Treatment of Cardiac Inflammatory Disease (ESETCID)	14 centers in Europe	250 anticipated	Histologic evidence of myocarditis, LVEF <0.45	Hyper-immune globulin +/– ganciclovir for cytomegalovirus Interferon-α for enterovirus Prednisolone and azathioprine for presumed autoimmune disease	Pending

LVEF, left ventricular ejection fraction.

conducted in adults with a duration of illness of up to 2 years, it is unknown whether the results apply to children or more acutely ill patients. It is also possible the duration, dosage, or choice of immunosuppressive treatment was not sufficient to produce an ameliorative effect.

There are multiple uncontrolled case series of myocarditis patients treated with immunosuppressive agents with apparent benefit, but controlled trials of therapy other than the Myocarditis Treatment Trial have not provided strong evidence to support immunosuppressive therapy.[103,104] A matched-cohort study demonstrated clinical, hemodynamic, and histologic improvement with prednisone combined with azathioprine or cyclosporine in children with active myocarditis and severe hemodynamic dysfunction.[105] This unblinded study, however, had a small number of patients and questionable histologic criteria. Another study found an initial marginal improvement in ventricular function in adults with dilated cardiomyopathy who received prednisone compared with control subjects who received conventional therapy.[106] At 3 months, improvement was observed in 53% of prednisone-treated patients vs. 27% of controls ($P < .05$). Patients with "reactive disease" (defined as lymphocytic infiltration, a positive gallium scan, or an elevated ESR) were more likely to improve with corticosteroids. By 9 months, however, there was no difference between treated and control groups, and the authors concluded that prednisone should not be administered as standard therapy.[106] A matched-cohort trial conducted in Germany found a significant improvement in left ventricular ejection fraction at 3 months but no difference with respect to prognosis.[107]

A potential reason for the conflicting results described above is the diagnostic limitations of light microscopy. Immunosuppressive treatment may only be beneficial if an active inflammatory process exists at treatment initiation. The diagnosis of an inflammatory process of the myocardium, however, is difficult to establish by routine light microscopy. Because cellular infiltrates are often sparse or focal, they are easily missed by sampling error or the misinterpretation of interstitial cells, resulting in high interobserver variability. In one study, only 7/130 (5%) had lymphocytic infiltrates on routine histologic examination vs. 48/130 (37%) using immunohistologic methods that allow better identification and quantification of infiltrating lymphocytes.[108]

In a murine model of coxsackievirus B infection, administration of cortisone during the viral replication phase increases myocardial necrosis.[109] Serious side effects associated with corticosteroids in humans include gastrointestinal bleeding, aseptic necrosis of the femoral head, psychosis, glucose intolerance, adrenal insufficiency, and increased susceptibility to infections. Cyclosporine may cause renal insufficiency and hypertension. Azathioprine can cause leukopenia and thrombocytopenia.

Since steroids cause serious adverse effects and are harmful in mouse models and since the best designed human trial did not show benefit, the use of immunosuppressive therapies outside of clinical trials cannot be recommended. In a meta-analysis of methodologically sound trials of biopsy-proven myocarditis the authors concluded that immunosuppressive therapy is ineffective in lymphocytic myocarditis.[110] The ESETCID will test the use of prednisolone with azathioprine for autoimmune myocarditis.[111] Various investigators report the use of immunosuppressive agents other than corticosteroids or aziothioprine, such as muromonab-CD3 (Orthoclone OKT3), cyclosporine, cyclophosphamide, and tacrolimus.[112] However, there is currently no evidence to support the use of these agents outside of a research setting.

IMMUNOMODULATORS. The effectiveness of high-dose intravenous immune globulin (IVIG) in Kawasaki disease, a coronary vasculitis of children, suggested its use as a therapy for myocarditis.[81,113] High-dose IVIG improves survival when given at the onset of viral infection in mice. When used later in the postviremic phase, IVIG-treated mice had less myocardial necrosis and inflammatory cell infiltration than control animals had.[114] IVIG could provide specific antibodies to viruses and thus a more rapid clearing of myocardial viral infection. Alternatively, IVIG may modulate immune response, resulting in decreased cardiac inflammation or down regulation of proinflammatory cytokines that have direct negative inotropic effects. The most common side effects of IVIG are mild flulike symptoms or headaches in 5% to 10% of patients. However, there are case reports of worsening renal function in patients treated with immune globulin.[115]

In a retrospective study of IVIG treatment of presumed acute myocarditis in 21 children, high-dose IVIG was associated with superior recovery of left ventricular function compared with historical controls; there was a trend toward improved survival 1 year after presentation.[116] In a case series of 10 adults with new-onset dilated cardiomyopathy treated with high-dose IVIG, left ventricular ejection fraction improved 17 EF units at 1-year follow-up.[117] In a retrospective study of women with peripartum cardiomyopathy, six patients treated with immune globulin had a greater improvement in ejection fraction during early follow-up than 11 control patients treated conventionally.[118]

In contrast to the smaller studies that were either uncontrolled or that used historical controls a recent randomized placebo-controlled study of the use of IVIG in myocarditis failed to demonstrate any benefit.[81] The Intervention in Myocarditis and Acute Cardiomyopathy Trial (IMAC) enrolled 62 subjects, half of whom received 2 mg/kg IVIG divided over 2 consecutive days. The controlled design and larger size of this study indicates that IVIG does not improve outcomes in adult myocarditis, despite its positive effect in a mouse model. Although the IMAC study results do not rule out a benefit of IVIG in children with myocarditis or with a more prolonged dosing schedule, there have been no prospective randomized studies to test these variations.

In mouse models of myocarditis, interferon inhibits virus replication, inflammation, and myocardial damage.[119–121] The ESETCID uses interferon vs. placebo in myocarditis with enterovirus detected in myocardial tissue by PCR, but results of the study are not yet available.[111] In 40 patients with idiopathic myocarditis or dilated cardiomyopathy randomized to receive either interferon or thymic hormones or conventional therapy, left ventricular reserve was significantly higher at 2-year follow-up in subjects treated with immunomodulators.[122] In four patients with myocarditis with enterovirus detectable by PCR in cardiac tissue, hemodynamic parameters improved with treatment with interferon, and in two of the four, enterovirus was no longer detectable.[123] Adverse effects of interferon therapy include neurologic symptoms, hematologic abnormalities, thyroid dysfunction, depression, myalgia, fever, headache, and fatigue. At this time the use of interferon for human myocarditis should be confined to research protocols.

NONSTEROIDAL ANTI-INFLAMMATORY DRUGS. The use of nonsteroidal anti-inflammatory agents in acute myocarditis in mouse models increased mortality and viral titers and worsened cardiac inflammation and necrosis.[124,125] Although there are no human studies, it is wise to avoid treatment with nonsteroidal anti-inflammatory drugs during the acute phase of myocarditis.

PROGNOSIS AND FOLLOW-UP. Since most myocarditis is asymptomatic and mild, it is likely that most patients recover completely within a few weeks without sequelae. Regarding seriously ill patients with acute myocarditis requiring mechanical support, long-term outcome is unpredictable.[126] Biopsy results generally have little prognostic value.[127] It should be noted that fulminant myocarditis is a specific clinical entity with a good long-term prognosis, and thus aggressive hemodynamic support is suggested for patients with this condition.[128] In the Myocarditis Treatment Trial, a higher left ventricular ejection fraction, less intensive conventional therapy, and shorter disease duration at baseline predicted a higher left ventricular ejection fraction at week 28 of the study.[101] The mortality was 20% at 1 year and 56% at approximately 4 years. In a meta-analysis, the left ventricular ejection fraction improved 10% over 6 months in survivors of lymphocytic myocarditis who did not receive immunosuppressive therapy.[110] In the IMAC study the mean improvement in left ventricular function at 1 year was approximately 16 EF units in both the placebo and IVIG arms, greater than the investigators expected based on previous studies.[81] IMAC, however, had different inclusion criteria than previous studies; patients with and without inflammation on biopsy were eligible for enrollment, and subjects were required to have no more than 6 months of symptoms. In addition, the subjects were more likely to have taken beta-blockers as part of their conventional therapy than subjects enrolled in previous studies, were.

Infectious Myocarditis Caused by Nonviral Agents

DIPHTHERITIC MYOCARDITIS. Clinical myocarditis occurs in 10% to 25% of cases of nasopharyngeal diphtheria but is responsible for 50% of diphtheritic mortality, which is particularly associated with atrioventricular and left bundle branch blocks. Myocarditis is more likely to occur with more severe pharyngitis and usually develops during the initial 2 weeks of disease. Even though diphtheria is now a rare cause of myocarditis in the United States, it should be immediately treated with antitoxin and either penicillin or erythromycin for 14 days along with bedrest and cardiac and airway monitoring.[129,130] Antitoxin is available through the Centers for Disease Control and Prevention, and the dose and route of antitoxin is dependent on the severity of disease. There is a risk of serum sickness with antitoxin administration, so skin testing for hypersensitivity is necessary before administration. In one study from Vietnam, penicillin was more effective than erythromycin, although there was no evidence of QT prolongation with erythromycin and erythromycin previously has been shown to be slightly better than penicillin in eradicating the carrier state.[130] Steroids do not prevent or ameliorate diphtheritic myocarditis.[131] The patient should remain in isolation during treatment, receive follow-up cultures 2 weeks after completing therapy, and be vaccinated during convalescence because natural disease does not always provide immunity. Chemoprophylaxis of contacts is necessary to prevent the spread of disease.

LYME MYOCARDITIS. Myocarditis occurs in up to 10% of adults in the disseminated phase of Lyme borreliosis, usually about 4 weeks after the appearance of erythema migrans.[132] The most typical manifestation is atrioventricular block with about half having third-degree block. Rhythm disturbances, pericarditis, and heart failure are less common.[133,134] Although it is unclear if antibiotics alter the outcome of heart block in Lyme myocarditis, most clinicians would treat this diagnosis with antibiotics because of the beneficial effect of antibiotics in other manifestations of Lyme disease. Mild Lyme carditis with a PR interval of less than or equal to 0.3 second may be treated with oral doxycycline or amoxicillin, similar to the treatment for early infection. If there is high-degree AV block or a PR interval of greater than 0.3 second, the patient should receive intravenous ceftriaxone or penicillin. Patients usually receive antibiotics for 2 to 4 weeks. Cardiac monitoring is required for patients with second-degree or complete atrioventricular block and for first-degree block if the PR interval is greater than 0.3 second. If the patient has improved, he or she can change to oral antibiotics. Heart block rarely persists more than 1 week in Lyme myocarditis, so a permanent pacemaker is not necessary, although temporary pacing may be required.[132] Anecdotally, prednisone at a dose of 40 to 60 mg per day tapered 5 to 10 mg per week may be helpful in Lyme myocarditis with complete heart block or congestive heart failure if the patient does not improve with antibiotics within 24 hours.[133] (There was a vaccine available to prevent Lyme disease but the manufacturer withdrew if from the market in February 2002, citing poor sales.) The risk of acquiring Lyme myocarditis would decrease with avoidance of endemic areas and the use of insecticides and protective clothing.

CHAGAS' MYOCARDITIS. While Chagas' myocarditis is much less common in North America than in endemic areas in Central and South America, infection with *Trypanosoma cruzi* is an important cause of cardiac disease that occurs in up to 30% of chronically infected individuals. Chagas' myocarditis requires supportive measures such as serial electrocardiograms, antiarrhythmics such as amiodarone, and therapy for congestive heart failure. Nifurtimox or benznidazole are both available through the Centers for Disease Control and Prevention for the treatment of Chagas' disease. These drugs have side effects, and their efficacy in advanced disease is debatable.[135,136] Interferon, itraconazole, fluconazole, and allopurinol have all been studied in mouse models for use in acute Chagas' disease, but these drugs currently are not standard therapy for Chagasic cardiomyopathy. An interferon inducer, poly inosine–poly cytosine, has been shown to aggravate Chagas' disease in a mouse model.[137,138] Patients with the greatest risk of death have left ventricular enlargement and dysfunction.[139] Although infection may recur following heart transplantation, studies indicate that survival is better for Chagas' than for other diagnoses requiring transplantation, and rejection is less common.[140,141] In endemic areas the likelihood of acquiring Chagas' myocarditis would decrease with use of insecticides and protective clothing or netting and avoidance of poorly constructed dwellings.

TOXOPLASMOSIS. Myocarditis due to toxoplasmosis in AIDS or cardiac transplant patients should be treated with conventional drugs for toxoplasmosis (e.g., pyrimethamine and sulfadiazine, using clindamycin as a second-line drug in patients intolerant of sulfadiazine).[142,143] Prophylaxis with TMP-SMZ would prevent this complication in the seropositive immunocompromised patient. The seronegative individual could prevent acquisition of toxoplasmosis through avoidance of raw meat and cat feces.

ACKNOWLEDGMENT: This work was sponsored in part by the California Collaborative Treatment Group (CC99-SD-003).

REFERENCES

1. Brodie HR, Marchessault V: Acute benign pericarditis caused by coxsackie group B. N Engl J Med 1960;262:1278.
2. Hirschman SZ, Hammer GS: Coxsackievirus myopericarditis. Am J Cardiol 1974;34:224.
3. Grist NR, Bell EJ: Coxsackie viruses and the heart. Am Heart J 1969;77:295–300.
4. Campbell PT, Li JS, Wall TC, et al: Cytomegalovirus pericarditis: A case series and review of the literature. Am J Med Sci 1995;309:229.
5. Rerkpattanapipat P, Wongpraparut N, Jacobs LE, et al: Cardiac manifestations of acquired immunodeficiency syndrome. Arch Intern Med 2000;160:602.
6. Chen Y, Brennessel D, Walters J, et al: Human immunodeficiency virus–associated pericardial effusion: Report of 40 cases and review of the literature. Am Heart J 1999;137:516.
7. Klacsmann PG, Bulkley BH, Hutchins GM: The changed spectrum of purulent pericarditis. An 86 year autopsy experience in 200 patients. Am J Med 1977;63:666.
8. Kauffman CA, Watanakumnakorn C, Phair JP: Purulent pneumococcal pericarditis. Am J Med 1973;54:743.
9. Rubin RH, Moellering RC: Clinical, microbiologic and therapeutic aspects of purulent pericarditis. Am J Med 1975;59:68.
10. Gould K, Barnett JA, Sanford JP: Purulent pericarditis in the antibiotic era. Arch Intern Med 1974;134:923.
11. Brook I, Frazier EH: Microbiology of acute purulent pericarditis. A 12 year experience in a military hospital. Arch Intern Med 1996;156:1857.
12. Skiest DJ, Steiner D, Werner M, et al: Anaerobic pericarditis: Case report and review. Clin Infect Dis 1994;19:435.
13. Fyfe DA, Hagler DJ, Puga FJ, et al: Clinical and therapeutic aspects of *Haemophilus influenzae* pericarditis in pediatric patients. Mayo Clin Proc 1984;59:415.
14. Blaser MJ, Reingold AL, Alsever RN, et al: Primary meningococcal pericarditis: A disease of adults associated with serogroup C *Neisseria meningitidis*. Rev Infect Dis 1984;6:625.
15. Schrank JH, Dooley DP: Purulent pericarditis caused by *Candida* species: Case report and review. Clin Infect Dis 1995;21:182.
16. Walsh TJ, Bulkley BH: *Aspergillus* pericarditis: Clinical and pathological features in the immunocompromised patient. Cancer 1982;49:48.
17. Fowler NO: Recurrent pericarditis. Cardiol Clin 1990;8:621.
18. Smith WG: Coxsackie B myopericarditis in adults. Am Heart J 1970;80:34.
19. Spodick DH: Acoustic phenomena in pericardial disease. Am Heart J 1971;81:114.
20. Spodick DH: Pericardial rub: Prospective multiple observer investigation of pericardial friction rub in 100 patients. Am J Cardiol 1975;35:357.
21. Spodick DH: Electrocardiogram in acute pericarditis. Distributions of morphologic and axial changes by stages. Am J Cardiol 1974;33:470.
22. Engel PJ, Hon H, Fowler NO, et al: Echocardiographic study of right ventricular wall motion in cardiac tamponade. Am J Cardiol 1982;50:1018.
23. Horowitz MS, Schultz CS, Stinson EB, et al: Sensitivity and specificity of echocardiographic diagnosis of pericardial effusion. Circulation 1974;50:239.
24. Isner JM, Carter BL, Bankoff MS, et al: Computed tomography in the diagnosis of pericardial heart disease. Ann Intern Med 1982;97:473.
25. Sechtem U, Tscholakoff D, Higgins CB: MRI of the abnormal pericardium. Am J Roentgenol AJR 1986;147:245.
26. Stark DD, Higgins CB, Lanzer P, et al: Magnetic resonance imaging of the pericardium: Normal and pathologic findings. Radiology 1984;150:469.
27. Spodick DH: Pericarditis in systemic diseases. Cardiol Clin 1990;8:709.
28. Soler-Soler J, Permanyer-Miralda G, Sagrista-Sauleda J: A systematic diagnostic approach to primary acute pericardial disease. The Barcelona experience. Cardiol Clin 1990;8:609.

29. Permanyer-Miralda G, Sagrista-Sauleda J, Soler-Soler J: Primary acute pericardial disease: A prospective series of 231 consecutive patients. Am J Cardiol 1985;56:623.
30. Maisch B: Pericardial diseases, with a focus on etiology, pathogenesis, pathophysiology, new diagnostic imaging methods, and treatment. Curr Opin Cardiol 1994;9:379.
31. Houghton JL: Pericarditis and myocarditis. Postgrad Med 1992;91:273.
32. Shabetai R: Acute pericarditis. Cardiol Clin 1990;8:639.
33. Connolly DC, Burchell HB: Pericarditis: A ten year survey. Am J Cardiol 1961;7:7.
34. Carmichael DB, Sprague HB, Wyman SM, et al: Acute nonspecific pericarditis. Circulation 1951;3:321.
35. Adler Y, Finkelstein Y, Guindo J, et al: Colchicine treatment for recurrent pericarditis a decade of experience. Circulation 1998;97:2183.
36. Millaire A, de Groote P, Decoulx E, et al: Treatment of recurrent pericarditis with colchicine. Eur Heart J 1994;15:120.
37. Brucato A, Cimaz R, Balla E: Prevention of recurrences of corticosteroid-dependent idiopathic pericarditis by colchicine in an adolescent patient. Pediatr Cardiol 2000;21:395.
38. Guindo J, Adler Y, Spodick DH, et al: Colchicine for recurrent pericarditis: 51 patients followed up for 10 years (abstract 157). Circulation 1997;96(Suppl I):I–29.
39. Millaire A, Ducloux G: Treatment of acute or recurrent pericarditis with colchicine [letter]. Circulation 1991;83:1458.
40. Fowler NO, Harbin AD: Recurrent acute pericarditis: Follow-up study of 31 patients. J Am Coll Cardiol 1986;7:300.
41. Hatcher CR, Logue RB, Logan WD, et al: Pericardiectomy for recurrent pericarditis. J Thorac Cardiovasc Surg 1971;62:371.
42. Mayosi BM, Volmink JA, Commerford PJ: Interventions for treating tuberculous pericarditis (Cochrane Review). In The Cochrane Library Issue 4, 2001. Oxford: Update Software.
43. Strang JIG, Kakaza HHS, Gibson DG, et al: Controlled trial of prednisolone as adjuvant in the treatment of tuberculous constrictive pericarditis in Transkei. Lancet 1987;2:1418.
44. Strang JIG, Kakaza HHS, Gibson DG, et al: Controlled clinical trial of complete open surgical drainage and of prednisone in treatment of tuberculous pericardial effusion in Transkei. Lancet 1988;2:759.
45. Hakim JG, Ternouth I, Mushangi E, et al: Double blind randomized placebo controlled trial of adjunctive prednisolone in the treatment of effusive tuberculosis in HIV seropositive patients. Heart 2000;84:183.
46. Carson TJ, Murray GF, Wilcox BR, et al: The role of surgery in tuberculous pericarditis. Ann Thorac Surg 1974;17:163.
47. Suwan PK, Potjalongsilp S: Predictors of constrictive pericarditis after tuberculous pericarditis. Br Heart J 1995;73:187.
48. Fowler NO: Tuberculous pericarditis. JAMA 1991;266:99.
49. Fennell WMP: Surgical treatment of constrictive pericarditis. S Afr Med J 1982;62:353.
50. Park S, Bayer AS: Purulent pericarditis. Curr Clin Top Infect Dis 1992;12:56.
51. Piehler JM, Pluth JR, Schaff HV, et al: Surgical management of effusive pericardial disease. J Thorac Cardiovasc Surg 1985;90:506.
52. Defouilloy C, Meyer G, Slama M, et al: Intrapericardial fibrinolysis: A useful treatment in the management of purulent pericarditis. Intensive Care Med 1997;23:117.
53. Sagrista-Sauleda J, Barrabes JA, Permanyer-Miralda G, et al: Purulent pericarditis: Review of a 20-year experience in a general hospital. J Am Coll Cardiol 1993;22:1661.
54. Pauschinger M, Bowles NE, Fuentes-Garcia FJ, et al: Detection of adenoviral genome in the myocardium of adult patients with idiopathic left ventricular dysfunction. Circulation 1999;99:1348.
55. Karjalainen J, Nieminen MS, Heikkila J: Influenza A1 myocarditis in conscripts. Acta Med Scand 1980;207:27.
56. Verel D, Warrack AJN, Potter CW, et al: Observations on the A2 England influenza epidemic. Am Heart J 1976;92:290.
57. Cheitlin MD: Cardiovascular complications of HIV infection. In Sande MA, Volberding PA (eds): The Medical Management of AIDS, 6th ed. Philadelphia, W.B. Saunders, 1999, p 275.
58. Rosenbaum MB: Chagasic myocardiopathy. Progr Cardiovasc Dis 1964;7:199.
59. Jin O, Sole MJ, Butany JW, et al: Detection of enterovirus RNA in myocardial biopsies from patients with myocarditis and cardiomyopathy using gene amplification by polymerase chain reaction. Circulation 1990;82:8.
60. Caforio ALP, Grazzini M, Mann JM, et al: Identification of alpha- and beta-cardiac myosin heavy chain isoforms as major autoantigens in dilated cardiomyopathy. Circulation 1992;85:1734.
61. Lauer B, Schannwell M, Kuhl U, et al: Antimyosin autoantibodies are associated with deterioration of systolic and diastolic left ventricular function in patients with chronic myocarditis. J Am Coll Cardiol 2000;35:11.
62. Gravanis MG, Sternby NH: Incidence of myocarditis. Arch Pathol Lab Med. 1991;115:390.
63. Neuspiel DR, Kuller LH: Sudden and unexpected natural death in childhood and adolescence. JAMA 1985;254:1321.
64. Wentworth PL, Jentz LA, Croal AE: Analysis of sudden unexpected death in Southern Ontario with emphasis on myocarditis. CMAJ 1979;120:676.
65. Karjalainen J: Clinical diagnosis of myocarditis and dilated cardiomyopathy. Scand J Infect Dis 1993;S88:33.
66. Lauer B, Niederau C, Kuhl U, et al: Cardiac troponin T in patients with clinically suspected myocarditis. J Am Coll Cardiol 1997;30:1354.
67. Smith SC, Ladenson JH, Mason JW, et al: Elevations of cardiac troponin I associated with myocarditis. Circulation 1997;95:163.
68. Tilles JG, Elson SH, Shaka JA, et al: Effects of exercise on coxsackie A9 myocarditis in adult mice. Proc Soc Exp Biol Med 1964;117:777.
69. Damm S, Andersson LG, Henriksen E, et al: Wall motion abnormalities in male elite orienteers are aggravated by exercise. Clin Physiol 1999;19:121.
70. Rezkalla SH, Raikar S, Kloner RA: Treatment of viral myocarditis with focus on captopril. Am J Cardiol 1996;77:634.
71. Rezkalla S, Kloner RA, Khatib G, et al: Beneficial effects of captopril in acute coxsackievirus B3 murine myocarditis. Circulation 1990;82:1039.
72. Tanaka A, Matsumori A, Wang W, et al: An angiotensin II receptor antagonist reduces myocardial damage in an animal model of myocarditis. Circulation 1994;90:2051.
73. Araki M, Kanda T, Imai S, et al: Comparative effects of losartan, captopril, and enalapril on murine acute myocarditis due to encephalomyocarditis virus. J Cardiovasc Pharm 1995;26:61.
74. Pitt B, Zammad F, Remme J, et al: The effect of spironolactone on morbidity and mortality in patients with severe heart failure. N Engl J Med 1999;341:709.
75. Matsumori A, Igata H, Ono K, et al: High doses of digitalis increase the myocardial production of proinflammatory cytokines and worsen myocardial injury in viral myocarditis: A possible mechanism of digitalis toxicity. Jpn Circ J 1999;63:934.
76. Drucker NA, Newburger JW: Viral myocarditis: Diagnosis and management. Adv Pediatr 1997;44:141.
77. Matsui S, Matsumori A, Matoba Y, et al: Treatment of virus-induced myocardial injury with a novel immunomodulating agent, vesnarinone: Suppression of natural killer cell activity and tumor necrosis factor-alpha production. J Clin Invest 1994;94:1212.
78. Cohn JN, Goldstein SO, Greenberg BH, et al: A dose-dependent increase in mortality with vesnarinone among patients with severe heart failure. N Engl J Med 1998;339:1810.

79. Rezkalla S, Kloner RA, Khatib G, et al: Effect of metoprolol in acute coxsackie B3 murine myocarditis. J Am Coll Cardiol 1988;12:412.

80. Packer M, Bristow MR, Cohn JN, et al: The effect of carvedilol on morbidity and mortality in patients with chronic heart failure. N Engl J Med. 1996;334:1349.

81. McNamara DM, Holubkov R, Starling RC, et al: Controlled trial of intravenous immune globulin in recent-onset dilated cardiomyopathy. Circulation 2001;103:2254.

82. Dong R, Liu P, Wee L, et al: Verapamil ameliorates the clinical and pathological course of murine myocarditis. J Clin Invest 1992;90:2022.

83. Wang WZ, Matsumori A, Yamada T, et al: Beneficial effects of amlodipine in a murine model of congestive heart failure induced by viral myocarditis. Circulation 1997;95:245.

84. Packer M, O'Connor CM, Ghali JK, et al: Effect of amlodipine on morbidity and mortality in severe chronic heart failure. Prospective Randomized Amlodipine Survival Evaluation Study Group. N Engl J Med. 1996;335:1107.

85. Chen JM, Spanier TB, Gonzalez JJ, et al: Improved survival in patients with acute myocarditis using external pulsatile mechanical ventricular assistance. J Heart Lung Transplant 1999;18:351.

86. Stiller B, Dahnert I, Weng YG, et al: Children may survive severe myocarditis with prolonged use of biventricular assist devices. Heart 1999;82:237.

87. Kawahito K, Murata S-I, Yasu T, et al: Usefulness of extracorporeal membrane oxygenation for treatment of fulminant myocarditis and circulatory collapse. Am J Cardiol 1998;82:910.

88. Chen Y-S, Wang M-J, Chou N-K, et al: Rescue for acute myocarditis with shock by extracorporeal membrane oxygenation. Ann Thorac Surg 1999;68:2220.

89. O'Connell JB, Dec GW, Goldenberg IF, et al: Results of heart transplantation for active lymphocytic myocarditis. J Heart Transplant 1990;9:351.

90. O'Connell JB, Breen TJ, Hosenpud JD: Heart transplantation in dilated heart muscle disease and myocarditis. Eur Heart J 1995;16(Suppl O):137

91. McCormack JG, Bowler SD, Donnelly JE, et al: Successful treatment of severe cytomegalovirus infection with ganciclovir in an immunocompetent host. Clin Infect Dis 1998;26:1007.

92. Kishimoto C, Crumpacker CS, Abelmann WH: Ribavirin treatment of murine coxsackievirus B3 myocarditis with analyses of lymphocyte subsets. J Am Coll Cardiol 12:1334–1341.

93. Heim A, Grumbach I, Pring-Akerblom P, et al: Inhibition of coxsackievirus B3 carrier state infection of cultured human myocardial fibroblasts by ribavirin and human natural interferon-alpha. Antiviral Res 1997;34:101.

94. Ray CG, Icenogle TB, Minnich LL, et al: The use of intravenous ribavirin to treat influenza virus–associated acute myocarditis. J Infect Dis 1989;159:829.

95. Rotbart HA, Webster AD for the Pleconaril Treatment Group: Treatment of potentially life-threatening enterovirus infections with pleconaril. Clin Infect Dis 2001;32:228.

96. Fohlman J, Pauksen K, Hyypia T, et al: Antiviral treatment with WIN 54954 reduces mortality in murine coxsackievirus B3 myocarditis. Circulation 1996;94:2254.

97. See DM, Tilles JG: Treatment of coxsackievirus A9 myocarditis in mice with WIN 54954. Antimicrob Agents Chemother 1992;36:425.

98. Rotbart HA, O'Connell JF, McKinlay MA: Treatment of human enterovirus infection. Antiviral Res. 1998;38:1.

99. Chapman NM, Ragland A, Leser JS, et al: A group B coxsackievirus/poliovirus 5′ nontranslated region chimera can act as an attenuated vaccine strain in mice. J Virol. 2000;74:4047.

100. See DM, Tilles JG: Efficacy of a polyvalent inactivated-virus vaccine in protecting mice from infection with clinical strains of group B coxsackieviruses. Scand J Infect Dis 1994;26:739.

101. Mason JW, O'Connell JB, Herskowitz A, et al: A clinical trial of immunosuppressive therapy for myocarditis. N Engl J Med 1995;333:269.

102. Hahn EA, Hartz VL, Moon TE, et al: The Myocarditis Treatment Trial: Design, methods and patient enrollment. Eur Heart J 1995;16(Suppl O):162.

103. Lee KJ, McCrindle BW, Bohn DJ, et al: Clinical outcomes of acute myocarditis in childhood. Heart 1999;82:226.

104. Kleinert S, Weintraub RG, Wilkinson JL, et al: Myocarditis in children with dilated cardiomyopathy: Incidence and outcome after dual therapy with immunosuppression. J Heart Lung Transplant 1997;16:1248.

105. Camargo PR, Snitcowsky R, da Luz PL, et al: Favorable effects of immunosuppressive therapy in children with dilated cardiomyopathy and active myocarditis. Pediatr Cardiol 1995;16:61.

106. Parrillo JE, Cunnion RE, Epstein SE, et al: A prospective, randomized, controlled trial of prednisone for dilated cardiomyopathy. N Engl J Med 1989;321:1061.

107. Maisch B, Schonian U, Hengstenberg C, et al: Immunosuppressive treatment in autoreactive myocarditis—results from a controlled trial. Postgrad Med J 1994;70(Suppl 1):S29–S34.

108. Kuhl U, Schultheiss H-P: Treatment of chronic myocarditis with corticosteroids. Eur Heart J 1995;16 (Suppl O):168.

109. Kilbourne ED, Wilson CB, Perrier D: The induction of gross myocardial lesions by a coxsackie (pleurodynia) virus and cortisone. J Clin Invest 1956;35:362.

110. Garg A, Shiau J, Guyatt G: The ineffectiveness of immunosuppressive therapy in lymphocytic myocarditis: An overview. Ann Intern Med 1998;128:317.

111. Maisch B, Hufnagel G, Schonian U, et al: The European study of epidemiology and treatment of cardiac inflammatory disease. Eur Heart J 1995;16 (Suppl O):173.

112. Ahdoot J, Galindo A, Alejos JC, et al: Use of OKT3 for acute myocarditis in infants in children. J Heart Lung Transplant 2000;19:1118.

113. Newburger JW, Takahashi M, Burns JC, et al: The treatment of Kawasaki syndrome with intravenous gamma globulin. N Engl J Med 1986;315:341.

114. Takada H, Kishimoto C, Hiraoka Y: Therapy with immunoglobulin suppresses myocarditis in a murine coxsackie B3 model. Circulation 1995;92:1604.

115. MMWR: Renal insufficiency and failure associated with immune globulin intravenous therapy—United States, 1985–1998. Morb Mortal Wkly Rep 1999;48:518.

116. Drucker NA, Colan SD, Lewis AB, et al: Gamma globulin treatment of acute myocarditis in the pediatric population. Circulation 1994;89:252.

117. McNamara DM, Rosenblum WD, Janosko KM, et al: Intravenous immune globulin in the therapy of myocarditis and acute cardiomyopathy. Circulation 1997;95:2476.

118. Bozkurt B, Villaneuva FS, Holubkov R, et al: Intravenous immune globulin in the therapy of peripartum cardiomyopathy. J Am Coll Cardiol 1999;34:177.

119. Matsumori A, Crumpacker CS, Abelmann WH: Prevention of viral myocarditis with recombinant human leukocyte interferon-alpha A/D in a murine model. J Am Coll Cardiol 1987;9(6):1320.

120. Lutton CW, Guantt CJ: Ameliorating effects of interferon beta and anti-interferon beta on coxsackievirus B3-induced myocarditis in mice. Interferon Res 1985;5:137.

121. Matsumori A, Tomioka N, Kawai C: Protective effect of recombinant alpha interferon on coxsackievirus B3 myocarditis in mice. Am Heart J 1988;115:1229.

122. Miric M, Miskovic A, Vasiljevic JD, et al: Interferon and thymic hormones in the therapy of human myocarditis and idiopathic dilated cardiomyopathy. Eur Heart J 1995;16(Suppl O):150.

123. Stille-Siegener M, Heim A, Figulla HR: Subclassification of dilated cardiomyopathy and interferon treatment. Eur Heart J 1995;16(Suppl O):147.

124. Khatib R, Reyes MP, Smith F, et al: Enhancement of coxsackievirus B4 virulence by indomethacin. J Lab Clin Med 1990;116:116.

125. Costanzo-Nordin MR, Reap EA, O'Connell JB, et al: A nonsteroid anti-inflammatory drug exacerbates coxsackie B3 murine myocarditis. J Am Coll Cardiol 1985;6:1078.

126. Houel R, Vermes E, Tixier DB, et al: Myocardial recovery after mechanical recovery for acute myocarditis: Is sustained recovery predictable? Ann Thorac Surg 1999;68:2177.

127. Grogan M, Redfield MM, Bailey KR, et al: Long-term outcome of patients with biopsy-proven myocarditis: Comparison with idiopathic dilated cardiomyopathy. J Am Coll Cardiol 1995;26:80.

128. McCarthy RE, Boehmer JP, Hruban RH, et al: Long-term outcome of fulminant myocarditis as compared with acute (nonfulminant) myocarditis. N Engl J Med 2000;342:690.

129. Kadirova R, Kartoglu HU, Strebel PM: Clinical characteristics and management of 676 hospitalized diphtheria cases, Kyrgz Republic, 1995. J Infect Dis 2000;181 (Suppl 1):S110.

130. Kneen R, Giao PN, Solomon T, et al: Penicillin vs. erythromycin in the treatment of diphtheria. Clin Infect Dis 1998;27:845.

131. Thisyakorn U, Wongvanich J, Kumpeng V: Failure of corticosteroid therapy to prevent diphtheric myocarditis or neuritis. Pediatr Infect Dis 1984;3:126.

132. McAlister HF, Klementowicz PT, Andrews C, et al: Lyme carditis: An important cause of reversible heart block. Ann Intern Med 1989;110:339.

133. Steere AC, Batsford WP, Weinberg M, et al: Lyme carditis: Carditis abnormalities of Lyme disease. Ann Intern Med 1980;93:8.

134. Van Der Linde MR: Lyme carditis: Clinical characteristics of 105 cases. Scand J Infect Dis 1991;Suppl 77:81.

135. Viotti R, Vigliano C, Armenti H, et al: Treatment of chronic Chagas' disease with benznidazole: Clinical and serologic evolution of patients with long-term follow-up. Am Heart J 1994;127:151.

136. Sgambatti de Andrade ALS, Zicker F, de Oliveira RM, et al: Randomised trial of efficacy of benznidazole in treatment of early *Trypanosoma cruzi* infection. Lancet 1996;348:1407.

137. Martinez-Silva R, Lopez VA, Chiriboga J: Effects of poly I-C on the course of infection with *Trypanosoma cruzi*. Proc Soc Exp Biol Med 1970;134:885.

138. Kumar R, Worthington M, Tilles JG, et al: Effect of the interferon stimulator polyinosinic-polycytidylic acid on experimental Trypanosoma cruzi infection. Proc Soc Exp Biol Med 1971;137:884.

139. Hagar JM, Rahimtoola SH: Chagas' heart disease in the United States. N Engl J Med 1991;325:763.

140. de Carvalho VB, Sousa EFL, Vila JHA, et al: Heart transplantation in Chagas' disease 10 years after the initial experience. Circulation 1996;94:1815.

141. Bocchi EA, Fiorelli A: The paradox of survival results after heart transplantation for cardiomyopathy caused by *Trypanosoma cruzi*. Ann Thorac Surg 2001;71:1833.

142. Hofman P, Drici M-D, Gibelin P, et al: Prevalence of toxoplasma myocarditis in patients with the acquired immunodeficiency syndrome. Br Heart J 1993;70:376.

143. St Georgiev V: Management of toxoplasmosis. Drugs 1994;48:179.

section

5

Intra-abdominal Infections

ATUL KUMAR MADAN, MD
RONALD LEE NICHOLS, MD

chapter 9
Peritonitis, Abscess, Liver Abscess, Biliary Tract Infections

Intra-abdominal infections continue to cause significant patient morbidity and mortality. Peritonitis, intra-abdominal abscesses, liver abscesses, and biliary tract infections account for most of these infections. Early diagnosis and treatment are essential to decrease the morbidity and mortality. Prevention and treatment of these life-threatening infections are emphasized in the following discussion.

PERITONITIS

By definition, peritonitis refers to inflammation of the entire peritoneum (generalized) or a part of it (local). Although the peritoneum is only a single layer of mesothelial cells with underlying loose connective tissue, it comprises an area of 1.8 m^2. Thus only 1-mm thickening of the peritoneum due to edema requires up to 8 liters of third space fluid.[1] When this shift of fluid occurs, it can create significant hypovolemia and multiple systemic events.

Infectious peritonitis frequently has been categorized as primary, secondary, or tertiary. Intra-abdominal abscess often is defined as a form of localized secondary peritonitis. Although prevention of intra-abdominal abscess often entails the same measures required to prevent secondary peritonitis, treatment can vary significantly and thus will be discussed separately.

Primary Peritonitis

Primary peritonitis is defined as an infection of the peritoneum not related to other intra-abdominal organ pathology. Since most primary peritonitis is secondary to bacterial infections, it is also referred to as spontaneous bacterial peritonitis. The usual underlying predisposing factor is ascites. In fact, primary peritonitis develops in up to 25% of patients with alcoholic cirrhosis.[2] Since the incidence of peritonitis is not as high in other causes of ascites, it is felt that intrahepatic shunting may be an important factor in the development of primary peritonitis, especially since the hepatic reticuloendothelial system is a major site for the removal of bacteria from the blood. Infection due to primary peritonitis is thought to be spread by hematogenous or lymphatogenous seeding, by translocation through the intact intestinal wall, or from the vagina through the fallopian tubes.

Diagnosis usually is made by paracentesis. Fluid should be analyzed for cell and differential count, protein, Gram stain, pH, and culture. Peritoneal biopsy obtained at laparotomy or by a laparoscope may be necessary to differentiate primary from secondary peritonitis. Polymicrobial infections are more common with secondary peritonitis than

ml), compared to 3 to 4 liters of the polyethylene glycol, generally is well tolerated by most of our patients. Although it is generally agreed that the antibiotics prescribed should be able to suppress both aerobes and anaerobes, there is less agreement about which agents are ideal and what route of administration is preferred.

Advocates of the oral administration of antibiotics typically emphasize the importance of reducing the number of microorganisms in the colonic lumen before opening the colon, whereas advocates of parenteral administration emphasize the importance of adequate tissue levels of antibiotics. Two regimens of oral antibiotics are most commonly used: (1) neomycin with erythromycin base

Although the literature lacks a multitude of randomized prospective studies that demonstrate that bowel preparation with mechanical cleansing and antibiotics decreases intra-abdominal infections after elective surgery, most experts agree that proper mechanical and antibiotic bowel preparation is a necessary adjunct to decrease secondary peritonitis and intra-abdominal abscesses in addition to decreasing the incidence of surgical site infections. We believe that this practice is the standard of care to be used in all elective colorectal operations.

Meticulous surgical technique, proper preoperative skin preparation, careful tissue handling, and thorough hemostasis are all requirements that appear to help with primary peritonitis which usually is associated with monomicrobial infection. Patients with primary peritonitis most often have predisposing factors and lack evidence of intra-abdominal disease. If the diagnosis is not obvious, operative exploration usually is required to differentiate primary from secondary peritonitis.

Prevention of Primary Peritonitis

Prevention of primary peritonitis has been suggested despite lack of any proven survival advantage.[3] Oral norfloxacin (400 mg daily) does reduce the incidence of spontaneous bacterial peritonitis.[4] The obvious disadvantage is the potential for superinfection with gram-positive

TABLE 9–1 ■ Suggested Empiric Therapies for Peritonitis

Organisms involved	Suggested antibiotic regimens
PRIMARY PERITONITIS	
Enterobacteriaceae	Cefotaxime
Streptococcus pneumoniae	Ciprofloxacin
	Levofloxacin
Enterococci	Piperacillin-tazobactam
	Ticarcillin-clavulanate
SECONDARY PERITONITIS	
AEROBIC: ENTEROBACTERIACEAE	**AEROBIC COVERAGE (PLUS ANAEROBIC)**

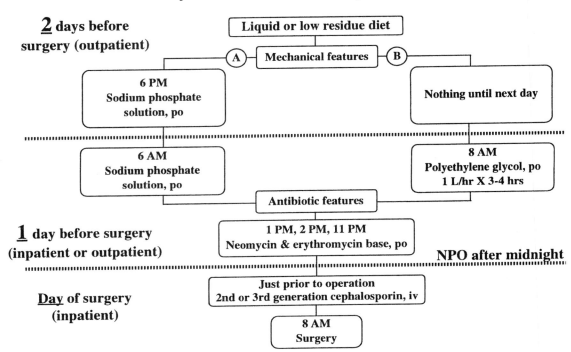

FIGURE 9–1. Bowel preparation. Our recommendation concerning the mechanical and antibiotic features of preoperative intestinal antisepsis before colorectal surgery.

prevent intra-abdominal infections after any intra-abdominal operation. Painstaking care must be taken to minimize spillage of any intraluminal contents into the peritoneal cavity. If an ostomy is required during an operation, closure and isolation of the initial primary incision needs to be performed before maturation of the ostomy. Drains should be kept to a minimum and used only for treatment and not "prophylactically." When drains are used, closed-suction drains usually are chosen and brought out of the skin in areas away from the primary surgical incision. Operatively placed drains carry the risk that erosion into the visceral organs or vascular structure will cause fistulization or bleeding. Also, drains acting as a foreign body may potentiate infection or anastomotic dehiscence. Bacterial adherence and biofilm formation on the drains are the mechanism that may encourage the development of infection.[11] Bacteria may also enter sterile tissues with the retrograde spread via drains.[12] In fact, the use of drains has lengthened the hospital stay of patients with perforated appendicitis.[13]

Supportive Management in Secondary Peritonitis and Intra-abominal Abscess

Patients with secondary peritonitis require a significant amount of supportive care. Although many patients may appear hemodynamically stable, it is imperative that a careful assessment be made frequently, especially in regard to their fluid and electrolyte status.[3] A urinary catheter is used to evaluate whether urine output is adequate, since many of these patients will have some element of hypovolemia. The source of this hypovolemia may be twofold. First, third-space loss is considerable with diffuse peritonitis. There is not only thickening of the peritoneum, which increases fluid requirements, but also bowel edema and luminal fluid retention. Additionally, capillary leak syndrome results in severe total-body third space losses. Many of these patients will also have septicemia, which will cause a vasodilation and a subsequent relative hypovolemia.

The treatment of secondary peritonitis includes surgery with antibiotics, which takes place after the initial management, which centers around proper rapid resuscitation. Although tachycardia due to pain or fever may be present, hypovolemia should always be a strong consideration as the true underlying cause of tachycardia in the patient with acute abdominal findings. Urinary output needs to be maintained, and hypotension should be avoided. Crystalloid solutions and blood products should be given intravenously through a large-bore access. Often central venous catheters are necessary for proper monitoring and the delivery of the large volumes of fluid required. In patients who have underlying cardiac and renal pathology a pulmonary artery catheter may be useful in assessing adequate volume status, although its use, in general, has recently come into question.[14] Pressor support is sometimes required but should not be initiated until adequate volume resuscitation has been achieved. Proper resuscitation to achieve adequate fluid volume should not delay operative treatment, but general anesthesia in a severely hypovolemic patient can have dire consequences.

Postoperatively, care must be taken diligently to continue to avoid hypotension and hypovolemia. Additionally, resuscitation with crystalloid and blood products can forestall renal failure. Mechanical ventilation may be needed until the patient is hemodynamically stable and adequate tissue perfusion is obvious. Nutrition via parenteral alimentation or enteral feedings should be initiated early in the severely septic patient or in a patient with evidence of preoperative malnutrition. Fluid resuscitation in a patient with a history of congestive heart failure or renal insufficiency can often provide a challenge to even a critical care intensivist. It is imperative to maximize tissue perfusion, however, to prevent the dreaded complication of multiple system organ failure.

Recent research has indicated that patients with severe sepsis may also benefit from new drug therapies such as recombinant human activated protein C.[15] A recent prospective, double-blinded, placebo-controlled trial, which was carefully designed and carried out at 164 centers in 11 countries, demonstrated that recombinant human activated protein C reduced by more than 19% the relative risk of 28-day mortality in patients with systemic inflammation and organ failure due to acute infection.[15] This study also analyzed subgroups divided by APACHE II score, number of dysfunctional organs or systems, other indicators of the severity of disease, sex, age, the site of infection, the type of infection, and the presence or absence of protein C deficiency. These subgroup analyses demonstrated consistent reduction of mortality with the use of recombinant human activated protein C. This drug appears to represent a new avenue in the treatment options for the severely septic patient.

Surgical Treatment of Secondary Peritonitis

The surgical treatment of secondary peritonitis has three underlying goals: (1) control of the infection source, (2) removal of microbial contamination of the abdominal cavity, and (3) prevention of further infection. The source of the infection is identified and controlled during surgical exploration. When secondary peritonitis is suspected, most often a midline abdominal incision is used, which can be extended with ease according to the site of the pathology. In the laparoscopic era, exploration may be done via a laparoscope even though frank peritonitis is generally considered a relative contraindication to laparoscopic surgery.[16] For certain suspected disease processes such as appendicitis and cholecystitis, simple removal of the diseased organ through a small local incision is the best treatment. In perforation or frank gangrene of the small bowel, resection with primary anastomosis is recommended. Perforated gastric or duodenal ulcers can be resected or covered with an omental patch, depending on their location. In the absence of peritonitis, localized large-bowel ischemia can be resected and primary anastomosis performed. In cases in which ischemia is not localized or when it is associated with generalized peritonitis, resection with colostomy is recommended. Traumatic colon perforations most often call for primary closure or resection with primary anastomosis.[17] Depending on surgeon preference, patient condition, and degree of initial peritoneal infection, surgery options are a resection with primary anastomosis (single stage), resection with end-colostomy and mucous fistula (double stage), or resection with end-colostomy and closure of the distal end (double stage). If secondary peritonitis occurs after an elective gastrointestinal operation, anastomotic leakage from disruption should be suspected. If the integrity of the anastomosis is in question, an ostomy at the anastomotic site may be the only option. At the conclusion of the operation the large and small bowel should be manually and visually explored for any inadvertent enterotomies, and any found should be primarily repaired. Rarely a colostomy may be required if a colonic hole is associated with generalized fecal contamination.

During surgical exploration most surgeons recommend removal of all bacterial contamination. Adequate identification and control of the primary source of infection is imperative to the prevention of further infection. Intraoperatively all debris and particulate matter should be removed. Hudspeth in 1975 advocated radical peritoneal débridement,[18] but Polk and Fry in 1980 reported a randomized trial that demonstrated no advantage to this technique compared with standard cleansing methods.[19] Intraoperative peritoneal irrigation with antibiotics or antiseptics is less commonly used today.[20,21] The usual irrigant is 2 to 3 liters of warm saline, which should be removed from the peritoneal cavity before closure.[22]

Other techniques have been described to prevent the recurrence or persistence of infection. Major techniques to reduce infection include proper drainage, continuous postoperative peritoneal lavage, planned relaparotomy, and the open peritoneal cavity.

Drains should not be used indiscriminately. Their purpose is to evacuate a well-defined abscess cavity or to establish a controlled fistula. Drains also have been used to provide continuous postoperative peritoneal lavage.

Closed peritoneal lavage was a technique performed in the postoperative period that used intraoperatively placed drains. The catheter drains were lavaged with a large volume of solution, usually more than 2 liters over a 3-hour period. This lavage was continued for 2 to 3 days or until the effluent became clear. The addition of antibiotics and low-dose heparin theoretically reduced the risk of infection and adhesions. In a critical review of 39 studies describing closed postoperative catheter peritoneal lavage for generalized peritonitis, the authors concluded that the therapeutic value of this procedure remains unknown.[23] Since continuous peritoneal lavage can be labor intense, requiring intensive care unit admission, and can be complicated by the development of fistulas, we have never used this technique in our treatment plan.

Teichmann and colleagues in 1986 reported a prospective study of a new concept of scheduled multiple laparotomies with abdominal lavage for the treatment of diffuse secondary peritonitis.[24] This process, referred to as *Etappenlavage* in the German literature, involved scheduled reoperations to ensure exclusion of the infection source, promote maximal elimination of necrotic material, and allow prompt recognition of complications to effect immediate repair. In 1990 Wittmann and colleagues used this technique and compared retention sutures, simple zippers, slide fasteners, and a Velcro analog (artificial blur).[25] Their patients with diffuse peritonitis required over six reoperations, but mortality was substantially lower in this group than in historical controls in whom this approach was not used. The Velcro analog was the most practical method of closure, with retention sutures having the highest complication rate. Also, decompression of the abdomen was not allowed by retention sutures or the zipper. Some have suggested that reoperation should be based on clinical findings or laboratory tests indicating continued intra-abdominal infection.[26,27] In fact, planned relaparotomy still has not been shown to improve results compared to relaparotomy on demand.[28]

Because continued reoperations can make closure of the abdomen difficult, leaving the abdomen open (laparotomy) is sometimes the only option. In 1979, Steinberg used this technique successfully in 12 of 14 patients.[29] Laparotomy involves leaving the fascia open and packing the abdominal defect with saline gauze. The benefit of this technique included the conceptual advantage of treating the entire peritoneal cavity as one large collection with open exposure allowing for excellent drainage and improved ventilation, improved renal perfusion, and ultimately the prevention of abdominal compartment syndrome. Complications included evisceration, massive fluid losses, spontaneous fistulas, and contamination of the open wound. This technique may require other major operations because the fascial defect is often too large to close primarily. We reserve leaving the abdomen open to cases of proved or suspected abdominal compartment syndrome, although a recent report has suggested that the Velcro analog (artificial bur) may prove to be an effective treatment for abdominal compartment syndrome.[30]

Antimicrobial Treatment of Secondary Peritonitis and Intra-abdominal Abscess

The antibiotic therapy of secondary peritonitis is based on the most likely source of bacterial contamination. In most cases the source of this contamination is the endogenous flora of the digestive tract. Although the biliary tract or the genitourinary system usually is sterile, injury or disease can permit contamination of these fluids with normal bowel flora.[31] In normal states the stomach has a sparse bacterial flora, primarily because of the acid environment, hence the use of H_2 blockers or proton pump inhibitors as well as certain disease states such as gastric outlet obstruction and small bowel obstruction may encourage bacterial growth in the stomach.[31] The small bowel, which normally has significant bacterial flora only in the distal ileum, can also have bacterial overgrowth due to long-standing partial or total bowel obstructions. In normal states the bacterial concentrations of the colon can exceed 10^{12} bacteria per gram of feces. Endogenous colonic flora include both facultative gram-negative aerobes such as *E. coli* and anaerobic organisms such as *Bacteroides fragilis* and species of *Fusobacterium*, *Clostridium*, and *Peptostreptococcus*, which represent the majority of bacteria in the colonic microflora. Obviously spillage of any of these enteric contents can result in a secondary peritonitis.

It is clear that antimicrobial therapy alone is not an effective treatment for patients with secondary peritonitis. Antibiotics cannot replace surgical management. Timely surgical intervention is a requirement in the treatment of secondary peritonitis. Antibiotics along with appropriate surgical management should be used to help stop or prevent early septicemia, wound infection, and intra-abdominal abscess.

The actual antimicrobial agent(s) to use, as well as the length of their use, is under much debate. No definite single superior choice can be found in the literature. There is little disagreement that the spectrum of activity of the antibiotics should include both the colonic aerobes and anaerobes based on experimental studies reported over 20 years ago.[32–34] Two decades of clinical studies have confirmed these experimental observations. Overall *E. coli* and *B. fragilis* are the most frequently isolated pathogens and the ones most associated with bacteremia in the patient with intra-abdominal sepsis.[35]

A traditional 1970s choice of treatment for severe intra-abdominal infections was "triple drug therapy," usually ampicillin, gentamicin, and clindamycin. In the last two decades, many intravenous antibiotics, either as part of a combination regimen or as monotherapy, have been investigated for patients with intra-abdominal infections. In Table 9–1 we list the agents most commonly used in the treatment of secondary peritonitis. Many factors influence antibiotic selection, such as patient hypersensitivity status, tolerability, toxicity, local hospital microbial sensitivity patterns, frequency of dosing, and cost, but often physician preference and hospital formularies guide antibiotic therapy choices.

In patients with penetrating abdominal wounds there is a trend to reduce the duration of antibiotic therapy in preventative clinical situations. We showed that risk factor analysis can be used to identify low-risk patients who require only short-term antibiotic therapy.[36] High-risk patients were those who were older, had colon injuries in which colostomy was done, suffered significant blood loss, and experienced multiple organ damage.[37] We found no difference in results between 2 and 5 days of antibiotic therapy in the high-risk patients who suffered penetrating abdominal trauma with intestinal leakage.[36] Only leaving their abdominal incision open with packing decreased the incidence of subsequent wound infection. Low-risk patients in whom the gastrointestinal tract had not been penetrated were given only one preoperative dose of antibiotics with low subsequent infection rates. Intraoperative peritoneal cultures collected at the time of the initial laparotomy for penetrating abdominal trauma had no value for predicting subsequent infections or the pathogen identified from such infections when they did occur.[37]

The duration of antibiotic treatment for intra-abdominal infections has been addressed by a guideline of the Surgical Infection Society, which was published in a policy statement.[38] Antibiotic treatment for generalized peritonitis or localized abdominal abscess is recommended for 5 to 7 days. Some investigators, however, have advised against such fixed treatment courses and have found that if fever or leukocytosis was still present, the recurrent infection rate approaches 55%.[39] Previous investigations have found that the risk of recurrent infection was negligible if antibiotics were discontinued when the patient had no fever or leukocytosis and had a differential blood count that showed less than 73% granulocytes and less than 3% immature granulocytes.[40] We believe that antibiotics can be terminated when the patient is becoming close to afebrile (< 37.7°C [100°F]) for 24 hours and appears to be clinically improving. If the patient continues to have febrile episodes or leukocytosis after 7 days of antibiotic therapy, antibiotics should be discontinued and the patient should be recultured while being observed. Often this "antibiotic vacation" is successful, but if fever continues, the workup for a source of infection should continue under the safety net of a new antibiotic choice. A few of the clinical settings of intra-abdominal infection in which antibiotics are rarely needed for more than 1 to 3 days are listed in Table 9–2.

Intravenous drug administration is the ideal choice for initial drug therapy for intra-abdominal infection. However, completion therapy with oral antibiotic regimens may be effective.[41] The long-term continued use of oral antibiotic agents should be discouraged. In our experience it is rarely necessary to use them for more than a few days, if at all, if initial parenteral antibiotic therapy was adequate.

TABLE 9–2 ■ Disease Processes in Which Preventive Antibiotics Are Not Needed for More Than 3 Days

Early acute appendicitis
Acute suppurative appendicitis
Acute cholecystitis
Localized ischemic bowel
Perforated Gastric or Duodenal Ulcer within 24 Hours of Perforation
Penetrating abdominal trauma with associated enteric perforations within 12 Hours of trauma

Tertiary Peritonitis

Tertiary peritonitis has been well described by Rotstein and Meakins.[42] This term is synonymous with "recurrent peritonitis" and also has been defined as a later stage of peritonitis when clinical peritonitis and sepsis persist after treatment of secondary peritonitis. The infection cannot be contained because of inadequate host defense mechanisms, inadequate source control, or inadequate antibiotic therapy. Occasionally no organisms are isolated from the cultures of peritoneal exudate, but more often low-virulence pathogens such as enterococci and fungi are found. It has been hypothesized that these organisms gain access to the peritoneal cavity by contamination during operative interventions, by selection from the initial polymicrobial antibiotic interventions, or by translocation of bowel flora.[6] Translocation may be promoted by intestinal ischemia, endotoxemia, malnutrition, or proliferation of resistant bowel flora due to antibiotic choices. Risk factors include malnutrition, elevated APACHE (acute physiological assessment and chronic health evaluation) II scores, and the presence of colonizing or infecting resistant organisms.

These patients have a clinical picture of occult or obvious sepsis with hyperdynamic cardiovascular findings, low-grade fevers, and a hypermetabolic state. Operative treatment is similar to that for secondary peritonitis; however, antimicrobial choices differ as seen in Table 9–1. Fungal therapy is needed if evidence of fungal infection exists or is highly suspect. Many patients with this infection die with multiple organ system failure, and the mortality from tertiary peritonitis ranges from 30% to 64%.[27,43]

Special Clinical Situations—Peritonitis

Barium Peritonitis

A diagnostic barium enema may perforate a diseased or normal bowel segment, with subsequent spillage of the colonic contents mixed with barium sulfate. In experimental studies the combination of barium and intestinal contents produces a more virulent peritonitis than either alone.[44,45] Water-insoluble barium is thought to tenaciously bind to the bacteria, and this lethal mixture is difficult, if not impossible, to remove mechanically from the peritoneal cavity. The end result is multiple foci of intra-abdominal infection that continue despite antibiotics and operative intervention! If the barium spillage is localized, survival is increased; however, the best treatment is prevention by avoidance of the use of barium in patients with gastrointestinal disease that may lead to rupture. A water-soluble contrast medium should be used when radiologic studies are indicated. The patient who has had barium peritonitis and survived will usually require many antibiotic courses and multiple surgical procedures with the goal to divert, débride, and drain the affected areas.

Peritonitis Associated with Intraperitoneal Devices

Patients with indwelling synthetic catheters for peritoneal dialysis, peritoneal venous shunts, or ventriculoperitoneal shunts may develop peritonitis that deserves special attention. Although this complication is common in patients with continuous ambulatory peritoneal dialysis (CAPD), the frequency is decreasing with improvement in catheter design.[46] Any break in aseptic technique during the daily connecting and disconnecting of the administration sets can be associated with CAPD peritonitis. The average rate of peritonitis is reported to be 1.3 to 1.4 episodes per patient per year.[47] The skin flora is often the source of the contamination, with coagulase-negative staphylococci responsible for 30% to 45% of the infections.[48,49] The remaining infections are most often caused by Staphylococcus aureus (10% to 20%), streptococci (10% to 15%), and gram-negative organisms (20% to 35%).

Diagnosis is usually suggested when a cloudy peritoneal effluent is observed. Clinical signs and symptoms including abdominal pain or tenderness, fever, nausea, vomiting, and chills may or may not be present. In uncomplicated cases, outpatient treatment with intraperitoneal antibiotic administration will suffice. Various antibiotics including cephalosporins, aminoglycosides, and penicillins have been used to treat CAPD peritonitis. Vancomycin delivered either intravenously or intraperitoneally is most commonly used for gram-positive infections, and similarly delivered aminoglycosides are most commonly used for gram-negative infections. Success with oral quinolones has been reported for CAPD peritonitis, although their efficacy has not been proved conclusively.[50,51] Successful treatment usually mandates only large doses of specific systemic antimicrobials, but it may be necessary to remove and subsequently replace the affected catheter if no response is seen. Also when there is associated infection of the subcutaneous tunnel, the catheter, which acts as a foreign body, needs to be removed. In patients with tuberculous peritonitis complicating CAPD, one report has outlined treatment plans not calling for removal of the dialysis catheter.[52]

Fungal peritonitis associated with peritoneal dialysis only accounts for 10% of the cases, but nevertheless it necessitates a special discussion. The mortality of fungal peritonitis ranges from 5% to 25%, and peritoneal dialysis cannot be resumed in up to 40% of the patients.[53–55] The International Society of Peritoneal Dialysis currently recommends antifungal treatment for 4 to 6 weeks with catheter removal if there is no clinical improvement after 4 to 7 days,[56] but more recent reports suggest that removal of the catheter early (within 24 hours of diagnosis) may reduce mortality.[57] Our clinical practice calls for immediate removal of the catheter and treatment with oral fluconazole (200 mg per day) or with intravenous amphotericin B (0.5 mg/kg daily) if the fungal culture revealed an organism other than Candida albicans.

Tuberculous Peritonitis

Although tuberculous peritonitis is rare the increase in the number of reported cases of tuberculosis demands special attention be given to this disease process.[58] The source of the Mycobacterium tuberculosis is usually a primary pulmonary focus that is spread hematogenously to the peritoneal cavity. The peritoneal cavity is the sixth most common site of extrapulmonary tuberculosis in the United States.[59] The onset is insidious, frequently lasting several weeks to months.[60] Nonspecific signs and symptoms include abdominal pain or tenderness, progressively increasing abdominal girth, fever, weight loss, night sweats, diarrhea, and ascites. Paracentesis usually is performed but rarely is helpful. The measurement of the adenosine deaminase activity of the ascitic fluid (>33 U/L) has been used to diagnose tuberculous peritonitis.[61–64] Diagnosis frequently requires laparoscopy or laparotomy, which discloses multiple tubercles scattered throughout the peritoneal cavity (Fig. 9–2). Blind percutaneous peritoneal biopsy is not recommended, as death has been reported as a complication.[60] Triple drug therapy may be necessary, especially with the emergence of multidrug-resistant tuberculosis. Susceptibilities should be checked to determine the correct antibiotic therapy. Isoniazid, rifampin, ethambutol, pyrazinamide, and streptomycin are some first-line drugs used in the treatment of extrapulmonary tuberculosis.

Diverticulitis

Patients with acute diverticulitis commonly present with the classic triad of left lower quadrant pain, fever, and leukocytosis. Since perforation and the subsequent development of barium peritonitis is a serious complication of barium enema, it is never indicated in the acute setting of diverticulitis. Computed tomography (CT) scans have a high degree of sensitivity (90% to 95%), a specificity of 72%, and a false-negative rate of 7% to 21%.[65,66] Initial treatment for acute diverticulitis consists of bowel rest and antibiotics. Those persons with mild cases of

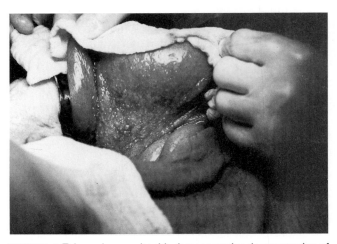

FIGURE 9–2. Tuberculous peritonitis. Intraoperative demonstration of intraperitoneal tubercles on the small bowel mesentery.

diverticulitis can be treated as outpatients with oral antibiotics. Antibiotics chosen should cover bowel flora and are the same ones used to treat other intra-abdominal infections (Table 9–1). Complications develop in about 20% of patients during their first episode of diverticulitis,[67] although complications develop in about 60% of patients with recurrent episodes.[68] For these reasons, surgical resection is recommended after two documented episodes of simple acute diverticulitis. Acute diverticulitis in younger patients (less than 50 years of age) is not common and comprises only about 2% to 5% of all cases of diverticulitis.[69,70] In younger patients, the higher rates of recurrence and complications justify operation after only one episode of diverticulitis.[71] Surgery should be performed 6 to 8 weeks after resolution of acute diverticulitis. Surgical resection classically has been performed with open laparotomy; however, the use of the laparoscope is becoming more common.[72,73] As expertise in laparoscopic technique grows, laparoscopic surgery may replace open laparotomy as the treatment of choice for surgical resection after acute diverticulitis.

Complications of diverticulitis require surgical resection after one episode or at the time of initial surgery. Abscess, fistula, perforation, and obstruction are common complications of acute diverticulitis. Surgical resection after percutaneous drainage of a diverticulitis-associated abscess is the recommended treatment. Percutaneous drainage has been used effectively to drain abscesses secondary to acute diverticulitis.[74] If percutaneous drainage is unsuccessful, operative treatment will depend on the size and nature of the abscess. Small abscesses can sometimes be treated with antibiotic treatment without percutaneous drainage (Fig. 9–3). Colovesical and colovaginal fistulas require preoperative workup to rule out malignancy. If there is any question of a malignant colonic fistula, *en bloc* resection should be performed. Even though these operations previously have been recommended as staged procedures, they frequently can be done in one stage.[75]

Perforation with generalized peritoneal contamination is a complication of diverticulitis that requires emergent operation. Although resection and primary anastomosis with intraoperative colonic lavage can be done,[76–78] extensive peritoneal contamination usually requires the formation of a diverting colostomy. Obstruction as a result of diverticular disease, due either to mass effect or diverticular mass or stricture, will require an operation (Fig. 9–4). Again primary anastomosis with intraoperative colonic lavage can be considered, but in the presence of proximal unprepped dilated bowel a colostomy is usually required. Intraoperatively a proper oncologic resection is often carried out, since it may be difficult to discern whether the obstruction is due to malignancy or diverticulitis.

Appendicitis

Appendectomy is the primary treatment of acute appendicitis. It can be achieved via the laparoscopic approach or via the open approach. Although the benefit in thin male patients is probably marginal, laparoscopic appendectomy is our choice. Simple or suppurative acute appendicitis does not require prolonged antibiotic therapy

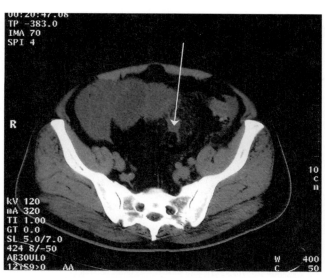

FIGURE 9–3. Acute diverticulitis with associated intra-abdominal abscess. Computed tomography scan demonstrating haziness and fat stranding along the sigmoid colon as well as an associated 2 cm area of low attenuation (*arrow*) consistent with a diverticulitis-associated abscess. The patient was successfully treated with intravenous antibiotics and elective resection and primary anastomosis.

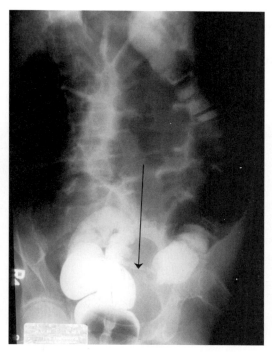

FIGURE 9–4. Diverticular stricture. Barium enema demonstrating a diverticular stricture (*arrow*) confirmed during operation and by pathology. Preoperatively carcinoma must be considered in the differential diagnosis, although this is unlikely since the mucosal folds of the colon are present.

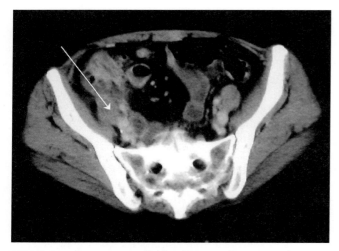

FIGURE 9–5. Acute appendicitis. Computed tomography scan demonstrating an inflammatory process (*arrow*) seen in the right lower quadrant at the base of the cecum. Although the appendix is not seen, this is preoperatively consistent with acute appendicitis, which was confirmed at operation. The patient was treated with appendectomy and short-term antibiotics.

(Fig. 9–5).[38,79] Appendicitis with established peritonitis, diffuse peritonitis, or intra-abdominal abscess requires a longer duration of antibiotic therapy (5 to 7 days). Intraoperative cultures are not useful in the treatment of acute appendicitis with or without perforation.[79–81]

Intra-abdominal abscesses due to acute perforative appendicitis can frequently be treated with percutaneous drainage in stable patients (Fig. 9–6).[82,83] After successful drainage an appendectomy frequently can be done on an elective basis (interval appendectomy). Antibiotic treatment is similar to that for other secondary intra-abdominal infections (Table 9–1).

INTRA-ABDOMINAL ABSCESS

Intra-abdominal abscesses are collections of purulent material often secondary to organ perforation with localized peritonitis that are separated from the remainder of the peritoneal cavity by inflammatory adhesions, loops of intestine, the mesentery, the greater omentum, or other viscera. The formation of an abscess reflects the localization of disseminated infection by the local host defense mechanisms. Complete resolution of the infection is halted by the inability of immune cells to function within the abscess cavity. The microenvironment of the abscess cavity may render the usual local host defense mechanism useless. Hypoxia, low pH, hyperosmolarity, and hypercapnia effect neutrophil activity and phagocyte function, which may hinder the normal defense mechanism.[84–89]

One large review of the causes for intra-abdominal abscesses conducted from 1961 to 1972 found that appendicitis was the underlying pathologic process in 50% of the patients.[90] Also, it has been demonstrated that more that 30% of abscesses are associated with an anastomotic leak.[91]

The diagnosis of intra-abdominal abscess depends on clinical signs and radiologic tests. Unlike patients with diffuse generalized peritonitis, diagnosis can be elusive. The signs and symptoms of infections, such as fever, leukocytosis, anorexia, general malaise, and weakness, are not specific only to the abdominal cavity or the abscess within! Palpation of masses or localized tenderness on examination may seem to be a worthwhile effort, but in a clinical setting this often proves to be futile. Clinical signs such as hiccups, cough, tachypnea, and jaundice may suggest a subphrenic abscess.[92] Psoas

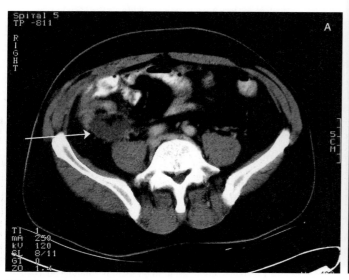

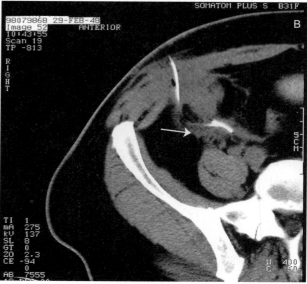

FIGURE 9–6. Periappendiceal abscess. *A,* Computed tomography (CT) scan demonstrating an intra-abdominal abscess (*arrow*) from acute appendicitis. *B,* CT guided catheter was placed percutaneously and successfully used to drain the abscess (*arrow*) in the patient in *A.*

abscess may present with hip and back pain along with a flexion deformity of the hip and quadriceps femoris wasting.[93] Retroperitoneal abscess can produce lumbar or ileopsoas spasm or referred pain to the hip, groin, or knee.[94] Diarrhea is the presenting symptom in 20% of the patients with a pelvic abscess because of the associated irritation of the sigmoid colon.[95] In a postoperative patient a deep mass palpated on rectal examination along with a decrease in sphincter tone can be diagnostic of a pelvic abscess similar to a deep ischiorectal abscess.

Multiple radiologic techniques have been used in the diagnosis of intra-abdominal abscess. Abdominal roentgenograms are taken routinely but rarely are helpful. A displacement of gastric air shadow, an extraluminal air-fluid level, or retroperitoneal air is helpful in making the diagnosis. Loss of the psoas shadow is a subtle finding that suggests an intra-abdominal abscess. Fry and coworkers demonstrated, in a series of 143 patients with abdominal abscess, that physical examination and a three-view abdominal roentgenographic series were not very useful in making the diagnosis.[96] They showed that abdominal roentgenography was of value in only about 15% of patients. Fry has suggested with the availability of other noninvasive radiologic techniques that abdominal roentgenography alone generally is not worthwhile.[97]

Upper and lower gastrointestinal contrast studies have been used in the past to identify intra-abdominal abscesses. In Figure 9–7 displacement of the stomach by a lesser sac abscess is seen. Because of the widespread availability of more sophisticated radiologic tests, contrast studies have little use in the diagnosis of intra-abdominal abscesses in today's medicine.

In the 1970s, ultrasonography seemed to gain popularity in the diagnosis of intra-abdominal abscess (Fig. 9–8)[98–101]; in experienced hands the accuracy rate can exceed 90%.[99,102] Its relatively low cost and the small size of the equipment and its ease of transport would seem to make ultrasound an attractive choice for diagnosing postoperative intra-abdominal abscesses. However, ultrasonography has some serious shortcomings: Postoperative ileus may make differentiating extraluminal air-fluid levels from intraluminal contents difficult. Obese patients, open wounds, ostomies, and bulky abdominal dressings may also make ultrasongraphy problematic.

In our practice, CT scan is the radiologic test most often used to identify intra-abdominal abscess. In fact the CT scan has become the gold standard imaging method for the diagnosis of intra-abdominal abscess.[103,104] A greater than 95% accuracy in the diagnosis of abdominal abscess has been reported with CT scan.[105] Examples of abscesses diagnosed by CT scan are demonstrated in Figure 9–9. Another advantage of CT scan is that it enables percutaneous catheter drainage of the abscess to be performed with guidance.

Management of intra-abdominal abscess is analogous to that for secondary peritonitis. Supportive management and antibiotic administration also are similar to those for secondary peritonitis. Without the necessity for open operative management, as is frequently the case in secondary peritonitis, percutaneous drainage may be used.

Drainage of Intra-abdominal Abscess

Today percutaneous abscess drainage has replaced open operative drainage as the first line of therapy (Fig. 9–10). At first it was suggested that percutaneous drainage be

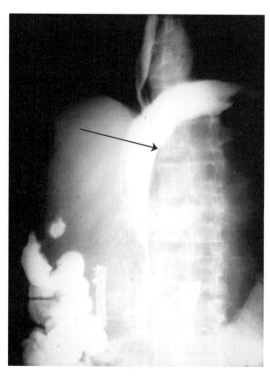

FIGURE 9–7. Lesser sac abscess. Upper gastrointestinal study demonstrating a lesser sac abscess (*arrow*) displacing the stomach.

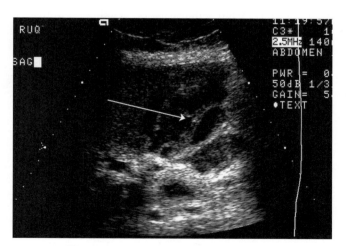

FIGURE 9–8. Ultrasonography of intra-abdominal abscess. Septated fluid-filled mass in the right upper quadrant (*arrow*) consistent with an intra-abdominal abscess seen by ultrasonography. The patient had an intra-abdominal abscess from a perforated gallbladder.

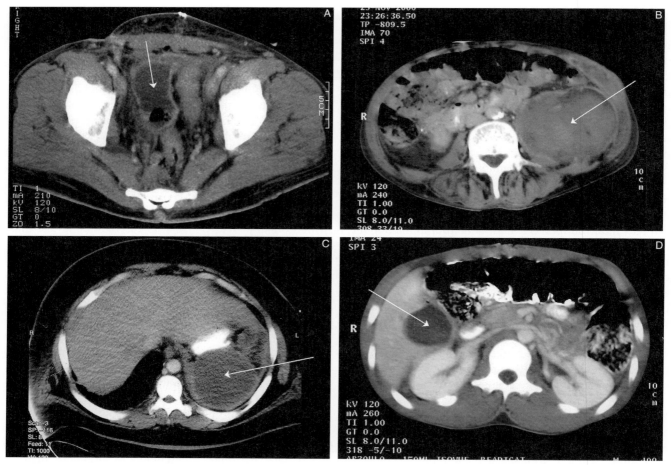

FIGURE 9–9. Intra-abdominal abscesses. *A*, Computed tomography (CT) scan of the pelvis demonstrating a low attenuation area (*arrow*) compressing the rectum. This pelvic abscess was treated with CT-guided drainage and intravenous antibiotics. *B*, CT scan demonstrating an extensive mixed attenuation fluid collection (*arrow*) arising near the left psoas muscle. Intraoperatively, this was found to be a large infected hematoma. The patient did well after operative placement of drains and intravenous antibiotics. *C*, CT scan demonstrating a large left-upper-quadrant intra-abdominal abscess (*arrow*) after a splenectomy. During drainage, care must be taken to enter below the pleural margin to avoid seeding the pleural space, hemothorax, and pneumothorax. *D*, CT scan demonstrating a subhepatic intra-abdominal abscess (*arrow*) after a cholecystectomy for acute cholecystitis.

limited to simple abscesses only. Now percutaneous drainage has been successfully used for complex abscesses. However, successful drainage is extremely operator dependent. Although CT often is used as the imaging test to help place the percutaneous catheter in localized fluid collection, ultrasonography is especially useful in the critically ill patient when safe transport to the CT suite is impossible.

After the abscess is visualized by either technique, a modified Seldinger technique is used in percutaneous drainage. A fine needle (20 or 22 gauge) is guided into the abscess for localization and aspiration of a sample of the fluid so it can be sent for laboratory analysis. A guidewire placed through the needle into the cavity is used to introduce a catheter (8 to 14 French) into the cavity. Although a large-bore tube does not necessarily result in more effective drainage, a drain with multiple side holes is imperative to prevent catheter occlusion. The catheter should be placed on gravity or low-suction drainage. Irrigation with 10 to 15 ml of normal saline two

or three times a day helps assure continued catheter patency, although some suggest this is unnecessary.[106] Also the catheter must be secured with suture along with tape reinforcement so that its position is maintained.

Repeat radiologic examination with ultrasound, CT, or sinogram helps to ensure abscess cavity size has been reduced and to determine if any enteral communication exists. The percutaneous catheter can be removed when certain criteria are met: clinical resolution of septic parameters signaled by normal temperature, normal leukocyte count, minimal serous drainage from the catheter, and radiologic evidence of abscess resolution as judged by sinogram or other abdominal imaging. Some authors recommend catheter removal be based simply on normal temperature, normal leukocyte count, and daily drainage of less than 10 ml.[106] The duration of drainage varies widely from 7 to 47 days.[107] Complications of percutaneous drainage are low but include hemorrhage, intestinal perforation, enteric fistulas, and empyemas due to inadvertent transpleural passage of the catheter.[108]

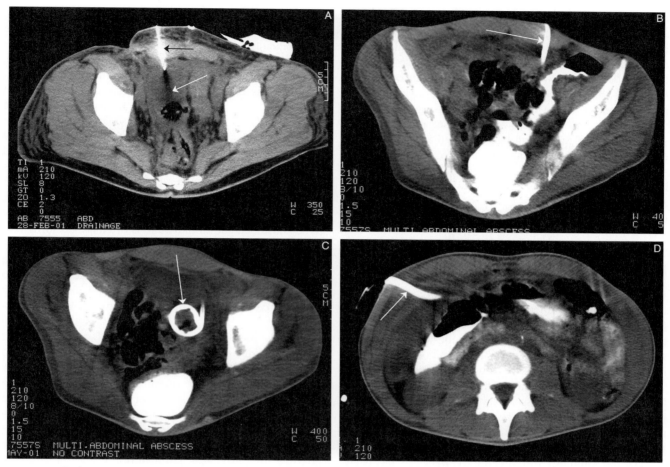

FIGURE 9–10. Drainage catheters. *A*, Computed tomography (CT) scan demonstrating a pelvic abscess (*white arrow*) being drained by a percutaneous catheter (*black arrow*). *B*, CT scan demonstrating a percutaneous drainage catheter (*arrow*) entering the pelvis. *C*, CT scan demonstrating the pigtail portion (*arrow*) of the catheter in *B* in the pelvis after an intra-abdominal abscess has been successfully drained through it. *D*, CT scan demonstrating a drainage catheter (*arrow*) that also has successfully drained an intra-abdominal abscess.

Improved clinical response usually is seen 48 to 72 hours after drainage ceases; persistent fever or leukocytosis after this time requires reevaluation.[109] Ineffective drainage may be due to inadequate catheter size, poor catheter position, undrained area of contiguous abscess, large enteric communication, or a second abscess. A formal laparotomy may be needed if effective drainage cannot be achieved.

Subphrenic, subhepatic, or pelvic abscesses usually can be easily accessed percutaneously. Abscesses located in the lesser sac or the presence of multiple abscesses, however, usually requires an open laparotomy for effective drainage. Also, fluid collections developing within the first 72 hours after an operation usually are not localized and therefore are not amenable to percutaneous drainage. These early collections usually are due to an anastomotic dehiscence and require a laparotomy with resection, ostomy, and drainage.

When operative drainage of subphrenic abscesses is necessary, a flank or subcostal incision may afford an extraserosal approach to drain the abscess. The twelfth rib sometimes may be resected to provide dependent drainage of the subphrenic abscess. Also, a limited lateral abdominal incision can be used to provide access to a pericolic gutter abscess or pelvic collections via an extraserosal route of drainage that avoids contamination of the remaining peritoneal cavity.

Multiple studies have demonstrated that percutaneous drainage is equal to operative drainage in rates of complications, rates of inadequate drainage, duration of drainage, and success rates.[106,110,111] As stated by Ochsner and Debakey in 1938, ideal drainage is "characterized by directness, simplicity, and above all, avoidance of unnecessary contamination of uninvolved areas."[112] Whether this is accomplished with operative drainage or percutaneous drainage should depend on each unique patient situation.

LIVER ABSCESS

In 1938, Ochsner and colleagues published a classic review of 575 cases of liver abscesses.[113] In this review, 35% were amebic and 34% occurred in association with appendicitis and had a mortality of 80%. Today more sophisticated imaging techniques, refinements in microbiology, the availability of many antimicrobial agents, and percutaneous drainage have helped decrease the mortality to 10% to 20%. Hepatic abscesses can be single, multiple, amebic, or pyogenic. Pyogenic abscesses are more common in the United States and are associated with a higher mortality than amebic abscesses are. In the southern United States and in areas with a large number of immigrants from Central and South America, the incidence of amebic abscess may actually equal or exceed that of pyogenic abscess.[114,115] In the immunocomprised host, fungi, cytomegaloviruses, and other organisms also cause liver abscess but are less common and are associated with more diffuse hepatic disease.

Pyogenic Liver Abscess

Penetrating trauma, spread of virulent organisms from the gastrointestinal tract via the portal system, infection from the biliary tract, direct extension of infection from a contiguous disease process, and blood-borne infection via the hepatic artery are possible mechanisms involved in the development of pyogenic liver abscesses. "Cryptogenic" abscesses account for approximately 15% to 30% of all liver abscesses. Although ascending cholangitis only accounted for 14% of hepatic abscesses in the review by Ochsner,[113] it now accounts for about 30% of hepatic abscesses.[116]

The microbiology of pyogenic liver abscess has been shown to have anaerobes and aerobes including *E. coli* and species of *Streptococcus*, *Staphylococcus*, *Proteus*, *Klebsiella*, *Enterobacter*, *Bacteroides*, *Clostridium*, and *Actinomyces*. Today CT scan is considered the most sensitive imaging technique and specific method of detecting pyogenic liver abscesses. Lesions are usually sharply demarcated, low-density masses (20 to 30 Hounsfield units). In up to 30% of abscesses, gas is detected

(Fig. 9–11*A*). As with other intra-abdominal abscesses, CT scan and ultrasound have the potential for assisting in percutaneous aspiration and drainage (Fig. 9–11*B*).

The primary treatment of pyogenic liver abscess includes drainage and antibiotics. Although some pyogenic abscesses can respond to antimicrobial treatment alone,[117,118] most often drainage is necessary in effective treatment. Thus treatment options for pyogenic liver abscess are (1) broad-spectrum antibiotics only (rarely used), (2) needle aspiration with antibiotics (sometimes used), (3) percutaneous catheter drainage with antibiotics (most commonly used), and (4) surgical drainage with antibiotics (commonly used). The underlying condition that promoted the development of the liver abscess needs to be addressed additionally and is often the deciding factor on what therapy is given.

The empiric antibiotics chosen are similar to those used to treat other intra-abdominal infections (Table 9–1). Often Gram stain or culture from the abscess cavity helps guide the choice of the definitive antibiotic regimen.

As in intra-abdominal abscesses, pyogenic liver abscesses can be drained percutaneously via a modified Seldinger technique. Multiple drains may be used for multiple abscesses. The literature has demonstrated the morbidity and mortality with percutaneous drainage to be better than or at least equal to the morbidity and mortality with open surgical drainage.[119]

Sometimes percutaneous drainage is not successful or possible. In these cases, surgical options are undertaken. Pyogenic liver abscesses can be approached operatively via extraserous drainage or transperitoneal drainage. With the extraserous approach, contamination of the peritoneum can be avoided, but full exploration of the peritoneum is impossible. Thus the transperitoneal approach often is recommended to thoroughly examine the liver and to look for other possible abscesses and any possible underlying lesions.

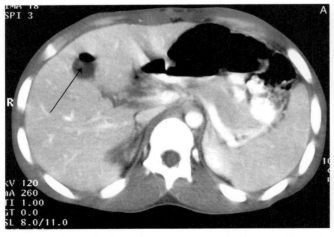 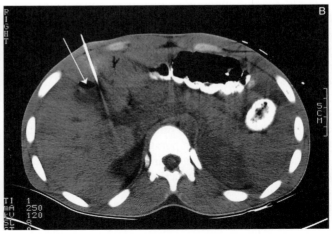

FIGURE 9–11. Pyogenic liver abscess. *A,* Computed tomography (CT) scan of the abdomen displaying a pyogenic liver abscess (*arrow*) that developed after a gunshot wound to the liver. Air is seen in the abscess cavity. *B,* CT-guided percutaneous drainage of the pyogenic liver abscess in the patient in *A* (*arrow*) is noted.

Amebic Liver Abscess

The difference between amebic and pyogenic liver abscess is not always obvious, although patients with amebic abscesses are less febrile and have lower absolute neutrophil counts. The indirect hemagglutinin and gel diffusion tests to detect the amebas are the best methods for distinguishing between the two entities. Unluckily, clinical distinctions and laboratory tests are no true substitute for the serologic tests that are definitive in establishing the presence or absence of an amebic liver abscess.[120] Often while waiting for the results of the tests, metronidazole is started empirically, since it is the treatment of choice for amebic liver abscess and because it is a valid treatment of the anaerobic component in pyogenic liver abscess. Prompt resolution of symptoms after initiation of metronidazole supports the diagnosis of amebic abscess. The distinction between amebic and pyogenic liver abscess is essential, since amebic liver abscesses are usually treated with antibiotic therapy only.

Metronidazole is the mainstay treatment for amebic liver abscess. The dosage is 750 mg three times a day for 10 days orally. If oral medication is not tolerated, a loading dose of 15 mg/kg intravenously is followed by 7.5 mg/kg every 6 hours. Chloroquine (600 mg of the base daily for 2 days, then 300 mg of base daily for 2 to 3 weeks) or emetine (1 mg/kg daily for no more than 10 days) can be added if the patient is critically ill and if the fever does not fall or no clinical improvement is seen in 72 hours.

Usually aspiration of amebic liver abscess is not necessary for resolution of symptoms or therapy.[114,115,121] Aspiration of an amebic liver abscess should be limited to those situations in which (1) a pyogenic abscess cannot be ruled out, (2) a secondary infection is suspected, (3) the abscess enlarges, or (4) treatment with metronidazole fails.[114,115]

Prevention of amebic liver abscess requires the prevention of amebic infection. No immunization exists, so that prevention requires efforts to decrease fecal contamination of food and water. Low doses of chlorine and iodine do not effectively kill the amebas; only boiling is effective. Effective waste disposal and water purification are necessary to decrease amebic infections. Prevention of contact with feces during sexual acts can help prevent infections also.

BILIARY TRACT INFECTIONS

The three classic biliary tract infections encountered are acute cholecystitis, pancreatitis, and cholangitis. Acute cholecystitis can be divided into either calculous or acalculous cholecystitis. Advanced acute cholecystitis may result in empyema, "pus bag," of the gallbladder. Acute cholangitis also can be divided into acute cholangitis, acute suppurative cholangitis, and recurrent pyogenic cholangitis. Acute cholecystitis and cholangitis due to choledocholithiasis can be prevented by removal of the gallbladder. Thus patients who have symptomatic cholelithiasis should be offered a cholecystectomy to prevent these serious complications of gallstones.

Acute Cholecystitis

The treatment of acute cholecystitis entails patient admission, hydration, bowel rest, intravenous antibiotics, and cholecystectomy. Antibiotic treatment for acute cholecystitis should cover both gram-negative and gram-positive organisms. Before the advent of laparoscopic surgery, morbidity, mortality, and length of hospital stay were significantly greater for acute cholecystitis than for open cholecystectomy for chronic disease processes.[122] Also the exact timing of surgical intervention has been debated, with some of the literature suggesting early surgical intervention,[123,124] although studies have demonstrated no difference in mortality and morbidity for early versus delayed surgical procedures.[125,126] During the early laparoscopic years, acute cholecystitis was considered a contraindication for laparoscopic cholecystectomy.[127] As the technique of the laparoscopic approach became more refined, laparoscopic cholecystectomy was performed successfully for acute cholecystitis.[128,129] The debate about the timing of surgical intervention was thus renewed. Although surgeons often try to "cool down" the gallbladder, the literature suggests that waiting for the inflammation to decrease may actually increase the adhesions and scar tissue, making the subsequent cholecystectomy more difficult. Thus laparoscopic surgery should be undertaken within 48 to 72 hours of the onset of symptoms.[130,131] Sometimes delayed patient presentation can make operation in this window impossible. If this is the case, the patient should be given bowel rest, hydration, and intravenous antibiotics until symptoms subside. Diet should be restarted slowly and advanced to a low-fat diet in hope of decreasing gallbladder contraction. If this is successful, surgery can be undertaken in 4 to 6 weeks after the resolution of the inflammatory process. Although much of the literature has focused on the timing of surgery, one investigation demonstrated that the "who" and "where" determine outcomes as much as the "when" in patients undergoing laparoscopic cholecystectomy for acute cholecystitis.[132] Proper facilities with the appropriate equipment and technically savvy surgeons well versed in laparoscopic skills are requirements in utilizing the laparoscopic technique in patients with acute cholecystitis.

In high-risk patients, conservative management should be undertaken and cholecystectomy performed when the patient is in medically optimal condition. If symptoms do not resolve, a percutaneous cholecystostomy should be placed, and a formal cholecystectomy (laparoscopic or open) can be performed later. In cases of empyema of the gallbladder, cholecystectomy is performed either by open or laparoscopic technique with appropriate antibiotic treatment.

Emphysematous cholecystitis generally occurs in diabetic patients with acute cholecystitis. Diagnosis is made when air is noted in the gallbladder wall or lumen on radiologic studies. Stones may or may not be present in acute emphysematous cholecystitis. Appropriate and timely surgical and antimicrobial treatment is needed in this disease process that often develops rapidly and generally has a relatively high morbidity and mortality.

In acalculous cholecystitis the management depends on the situation and condition of the patient. In patients who can tolerate an operation, a laparoscopic or an open cholecystectomy should be performed immediately because of the high risk of gangrenous changes with ultimate perforation. Percutaneous cholecystostomy with radiologic guidance can be performed with local anesthesia in those high-risk critically ill patients who cannot tolerate general anesthesia (Fig. 9–12A). When the patient has recovered, 6 to 8 weeks after surgery, the catheter can be removed after radiologic imaging via the catheter demonstrates no obstruction of the gallbladder (Fig. 9–12B). In those patients who have gallstones, elective laparoscopic cholecystectomy is the procedure of choice after their condition is stabilized and they are in medically optimal condition.

Acute Pancreatitis

Treatment of mild pancreatitis usually requires bowel rest, intravenous fluids, and often hyperalimentation. The treatment of severe hemorrhagic pancreatitis, on the other hand, is still controversial. Although bowel rest and intravenous fluids are the mainstay treatment of severe pancreatitis without necrosis or infection, preventative antibiotics appear to have a role in the treatment plan. CT scanning with thin cuts through the pancreas is helpful in determining the extent of pancreatitis (Fig. 9–13) and the presence of necrosis (Fig. 9–14). Percutaneous aspiration can be used to identify the presence of infection (Fig. 9–15).[133] If the Gram stain or culture is positive, proper antibiotic treatment should be initiated. Lumsden and Bradley reviewed over 1100 cases of secondary pancreatic infections and demonstrated the infecting organisms to be *E. coli* (35%), *K. pneumoniae* (24%), *Enterococcus* spp (24%), *Staphylococcus* spp (14%), *Pseudomonas* spp (11%), *Proteus* spp (8%), aerobic *Streptococcus* spp (7%), other Enterobacteriaceae (7%), *Bacteroides* spp (6%), and a wide variety of other organisms.[134] Fungal infections recently have been implicated in acute necrotizing infections.[135]

The use of preventative antibiotics in patients with pancreatitis without evidence of associated infection is still a subject of much debate. Early reported studies using ampicillin failed to demonstrate a benefit.[136,137] Failure of efficacy in these studies may be due to poor secretion of ampicillin into the pancreas. Recent studies have demonstrated a benefit for antibiotics in pancreatitis,[138–142] and a critical review of the subject recommends antibiotic use.[143] Kramer and Levy recommended the routine use of antibiotics in pancreatitis in patients with a Ranson score of 3 or greater, necrosis involving one-third of the pancreas, or 2 or more acute fluid collections.[144] Since infection usually becomes apparent within 14 to 22 days after the initial attack, antibiotic use is recommended for at least 14 days. Two intravenous antibiotic therapy strategies used for prophylaxis in severe pancreatitis include (1) imipenem 0.5 g every 8 hours combined with fluconazole 400 mg daily and (2) ciprofloxacin 400

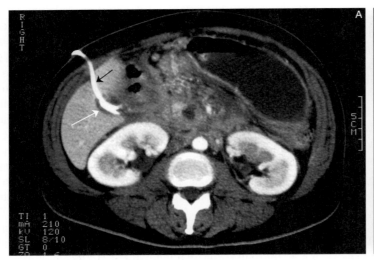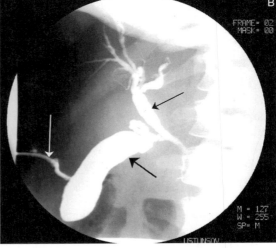

FIGURE 9–12. Cholecystostomy catheter. *A*, Computed tomography (CT) demonstrating a cholecystostomy tube (*black arrow*) in the gallbladder (*white arrow*) in a patient who had developed acute acalculus cholecystitis during a prolonged intensive care unit stay. *B*, Dye placed via the cholecystostomy tube (*white arrow*) from the patient in *A* demonstrating no gallstones in the gallbladder (*large black arrow*) and a patent cystic duct that drains into the common bile duct (*small black arrow*). Because of the patient's overall poor surgical risk factors, the catheter was removed without cholecystectomy. The patient has had no right-upper-quadrant complaints to date.

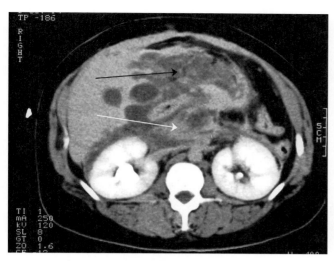

FIGURE 9–13. Acute pancreatitis. Computed tomography scan demonstrating extensive mesenteric fat plane changes (*black arrow*). Inflammatory changes with associated edema and peripancreatic fluid are also seen. Normal pancreatic architecture is lost (*white arrow*). These findings are consistent with severe acute pancreatitis.

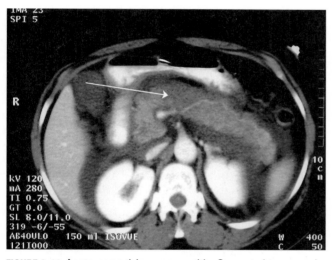

FIGURE 9–14. Acute necrotizing pancreatitis. Computed tomography scan of the abdomen demonstrating an edematous pancreas. Some areas of necrosis (*arrow*) are suspected because of the loss of enhancement.

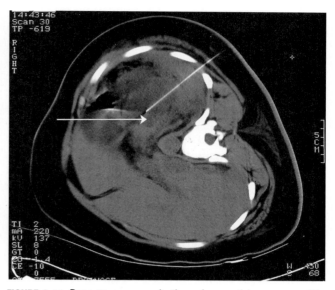

FIGURE 9–15. Percutaneous aspiration of necrotizing pancreatitis. Computed tomography–guided needle aspiration of suspected necrotizing pancreatitis (*arrow*) is performed while the patient is in the decubitus position. Five milliliters of aspirate were obtained and sent for Gram stain and culture.

débridement can be taken. Proper pancreatic débridement can require more than one operative procedure. Drains may or may not be used. Often when multiple operations are required, the abdomen is left open, marsupialized, and closed with a sterile intravenous bag or cassette cover or a sterile zipper.[145] Operative choice is usually determined by the responsible surgeon's experience.

Treatment of Acute Cholangitis

In 1877, Charcot described a triad of fever, jaundice, and right-upper-quadrant pain associated with acute cholangitis.[147] Almost 75 years later, Reynolds and Dargon described a more severe form of cholangitis with Charcot's triad plus septic shock and mental obtundation.[148] The two factors involved in acute cholangitis are (1) biliary stasis and obstruction and (2) significant bacterial concentrations in the bile. Although complete biliary obstruction causes complete stasis, it is not associated with bacteria in the bile as often as partial obstruction is. Thus partial obstruction due to benign strictures, choledocholithiasis, chronic pancreatitis, pancreatic pseudocyst compression, an obstructed biliary anastomosis, or an obstructed endoprosthesis is more likely to be associated with clinical acute cholangitis.

Two decades ago, common duct stones were the most common cause of obstructive cholangitis.[149] Today, with the various nonoperative and surgical biliary interventions, manipulation of the biliary tract has become the most common cause of cholangitis.[150] The aerobic microbiology of acute cholangitis is similar to that of pancreatitis. *B. fragilis* is the anaerobic organism most commonly isolated in acute cholangitis, followed by

mg every 12 hours with metronidazole 500 mg every 6 hours and fluconazole 400 mg daily.[145] A recent randomized study demonstrated a reduced need for operative intervention in patients with severe pancreatitis when early treatment with imipenem is employed.[146] The investigators used the higher dose of imipenem (1 g). Again, although use of antibiotics is still controversial, evidence seems to be mounting for their efficacy in all patients with severe pancreatitis. No one antibiotic regimen has been proven superior.

Once established pancreatic abscess is diagnosed, operative intervention is most frequently added to the antibiotic therapy. A variety of operative approaches to

Clostridium spp. Diagnosis can be made via ultrasonography or CT scan. Jaundice, spiking fever, and abdominal pain are most commonly found in acute cholangitis. With the appropriate clinical symptoms and signs along the dilated ductal system on imaging studies, the diagnosis of acute cholangitis can be made with certainty. Rarely, air in the biliary ductal system on CT scan can be seen in acute cholangitis.

All patients who present with acute cholangitis or acute suppurative cholangitis require proper resuscitation with intravenous fluid and electrolytes. Patients with clinical signs of sepsis require more aggressive intensive care monitoring, often including pressor support. Appropriate intravenous antimicrobial therapy is initiated empirically. Classically, an aminoglycoside combined with a penicillin and metronidazole have been used for acute cholangitis. Second- and third-generation cephalosporins provide broad coverage, but they do not cover *Enterococcus*, which frequently is the reported pathogen. Newer antibiotics (single or combined) such as imipenem or meropenem are useful for the treatment of acute cholangitis, as are β-lactamase inhibitors including ampicillin-sulbactam, ticarcillin-clavulanate, and piperacillin-tazobactam.

Patients with external biliary drains presenting with acute cholangitis should have the drains opened to gravity. The bile should be gram stained and cultured, and antibiotic therapy should be initiated based on those results as well as on knowledge of the usual infecting flora. Radiologic studies can be used to confirm patency and appropriate location of the biliary drains.

Patients with acute cholangitis who fail to respond to appropriate resuscitation and antibiotic therapy require a prompt drainage intervention. Biliary duct decompression is best performed nonoperatively, either via a percutaneous transhepatic or endoscopic approach. The choice of approach is determined by the cause of the obstruction and local hospital expertise. If only intrahepatic ductal dilation is seen, percutaneous transhepatic cholangiography with drainage is recommended. If the patient's clinical status is stable and extrahepatic choledocholithiasis is noted, endoscopic retrograde cholangiography and papillotomy with basket retrieval of stones may be needed. Nasobiliary catheters or biliary stents can be used as well to help relieve the obstruction. If endoscopic attempts are not successful, percutaneous decompression should be undertaken immediately. Nonoperative intervention can be performed with relatively lower rates of morbidity (less than 40%) and mortality (less than 10%).[151]

Since emergent open surgical decompression is associated with a mortality of greater than 30%,[151] it should be undertaken only when nonoperative procedures are not successful or available. Operative intervention should decompress the biliary system with a choledochotomy with placement of a T-tube. Although some surgeons have developed laparoscopic experience that allows the exploration of the common bile duct, this approach is not recommended when there is a need for urgent common duct decompression as is required in acute cholangitis. However, laparoscopic surgery does have a role in the treatment of choledocholithiasis after resolution of the acute cholangitis episode.

Recurrent pyogenic cholangitis, also known as Oriental infestational cholangitis,[152] intrahepatic stone disease,[153] or simply hepatolithiasis,[154,155] is characterized by recurrent episodes of cholangitis. Its pathogenesis is unknown, although infection with parasites such as *Clonorchis*, *Ascaris*, or *Fasciola* has been suggested to be the principal cause.[152,156–158] The parasites may cause ductal injury and strictures leading to bile stasis, stone formation, and obstruction. The damaged biliary system appears to be more susceptible to secondary infection by bacteria. Acute episodes of cholangitis may respond to antibiotics or may require immediate biliary duct decompression. Surgical interventions are needed to correct the underlying biliary disease. Procedures include sphincteroplasty, choledochotomy, lithotomy, bilioenteric bypass, cholecystectomy, and liver resection.[159–163] Unfortunately the disease often recurs after surgery, since complete correction of strictures and complete removal of all hepatic stones is usually impossible.[160,161,163–165] Thus treatment is seen as long-term management with establishment of access to the biliary system via a dilated T-tube tract[166–168] or a hepaticocutaneous jejunostomy.[163,169] Stricture dilation, stone removal, or lithotripsy additionally can be performed via this access.[155,162,163,165,170,171]

REFERENCES

1. Condon RE, Wittmann DH: Intraabdominal Infections. In Gorbach SL, Bartlett JG, Blacklow NR (eds): Infectious Diseases. Philadelphia, WB Saunders, 1998, pp 793–800.
2. Conn HO, Fessel JM: Spontaneous bacterial peritonitis in cirrhosis: Variations on a theme. Medicine 1971;50:161–197.
3. Such J, Runyon BA: Spontaneous bacterial peritonitis. Clin Infect Dis 1998;27:669–674.
4. Gines P, Rimola A, Planas R, et al: Norfloxacin prevents spontaneous bacterial peritonitis recurrence in cirrhosis: Results of a double-blind, placebo-controlled trial. Hepatology 1990; 12:716–724.
5. Singh N, Gayowski T, Yu VL, et al: Trimethoprim-sulfamethoxazole for the prevention of spontaneous bacterial peritonitis in cirrhosis: A randomized trial. Ann Intern Med 1995;122:595–598.
6. Johnson CC, Baldessarre J, Levison ME: Peritonitis: Update on pathophysiology, clinical manifestations, and management. Clin Infect Dis 1997;24:1035–1045.
7. Nichols RL, Smith JW, Garcia RY, et al: Current practices of preoperative bowel preparation among North American colorectal surgeons. Clin Infect Dis 1997;24:609–619.
8. Nichols RL: Bowel Preparation. In Wilmore DW, Cheung LY, Harken AH, et al (eds): Scientific American: Surgery. New York, Scientific American, 1995, pp 1–11.
9. Nichols RL, Condon RE, Gorbach SL, et al: Efficacy of preoperative antimicrobial preparation of the bowel. Ann Surg 1972;176:227–232.
10. Coppa GF, Eng K: Factors involved in antibiotic selection in elective colon and rectal surgery. Surgery 1988;104:853–858.
11. Costerton JW, Irwin RT, Cheung KJ: The bacterial glycocalyx in nature and disease. Annu Rev Microbiol 1981;35:299–324.

12. Cerise EJ, Pierce WA, Diamond DL: Abdominal drains: Their role as a source of infection following splenectomy. Ann Surg 1970;171:764–769.

13. Haller JD, Shaker IJ, Donahoo JS: Peritoneal drainage versus non-drainage for generalized peritonitis from ruptured appendicitis in children. Ann Surg 1973;177:595–600.

14. Connors AF, Speroff T, Dawson NV, et al: The effectiveness of right heart catheterization in the initial care of critically ill patients. SUPPORT Investigators. JAMA 1996;18:889–897.

15. Bernard GR, Vincet JL, Laterre PF, et al: Efficacy and safety of recombinant human activated protein C for severe sepsis. N Engl J Med 2001;344:699–709.

16. Olson JA, Moley JF: Patient selection and preparation. In Jones DB, Wu JS, Soper NJ (eds): Laparoscopic surgery: Principles and procedures. St. Louis, Quality Medical Publishing, 1997.

17. Chappuis CW, Frey DJ, Dietzen CD: Management of penetrating colon injuries. A prospective trial. Ann Surg 1991;213:492–497.

18. Hudspeth AS: Radical surgical débridement in the treatment for established peritonitis. Arch Surg, 1975;110:1233–1236.

19. Polk HC, Fry DE: Radical peritoneal débridement for established peritonitis. The results of a prospective randomized clinical trial. Ann Surg 1980;192:350–355.

20. Roth RM, Gleckman RA, Gantz NM, et al: Antibiotic irrigations—A plea for controlled clinical trials. Pharmacotherapy 1985;5:222–227.

21. Pissiotis CA, Nichols RL, Condon RE: Absorption and excretion of intraperitoneally administrated kanamycin sulfate. Surg Gynecol Obstet 1972;134:995–998.

22. Nathens AB, Rotstein OD: Therapeutic options in peritonitis. Surg Clin North Am 1994;74:677–692.

23. Leiboff AR, Soroff HS: The treatment of generalized peritonitis by closed postoperative peritoneal lavage: A critical review of the literature. Arch Surg 1987;122:1005–1010.

24. Teichmann W, Wittmann DH, Andreone PA: Scheduled reoperations (*Etappenlavage*) for diffuse peritonitis. Arch Surg 1986;121:147–152.

25. Wittmann DH, Aprahamian C, Bergstein JM: *Etappenlavage*: Advanced diffuse peritonitis managed by planned multiple laparotomies utilizing zippers, slide fastener, and Velcro analogue for temporary abdominal closure. World J Surg 1990;14:218–226.

26. Andrus C, Doering M, Herrmann VM, et al: Planned reoperation for generalized intraabdominal infection. Am J Surg 1986;152:682–686.

27. Butler JA, Huang J, Wilson SE: Repeated laparotomy for postoperative intraabdominal sepsis. Arch Surg 1987;122:702–706.

28. Hau T, Ohmann C, Wolmershauser A, et al: Planned relaparotomy vs. relaparotomy on demand in the treatment of intraabdominal infections. Arch Surg 1995;130:1193–1196.

29. Steinberg D: On leaving the peritoneal cavity open in acute generalized suppurative peritonitis. Am J Surg 1979;137:216–220.

30. Wittmann DH, Iskander GA: The compartment syndrome of the abdominal cavity: A state of the art review. J Intensive Care Med 2000;15:201–206.

31. Condon RE: Microbiology of intra-abdominal infection and contamination. Eur J Surg 1996;576S:9–12.

32. Weinstein WM, Onderdonk AB, Bartlett JG, et al: Antimicrobial therapy of experimental intraabdominal sepsis. J Infect Dis 1975;132:282–286.

33. Nichols RL, Smith JW, Fossedal EN, et al: Efficacy of parenteral antibiotics in the treatment of experimentally induced intraabdominal sepsis. Rev Infect Dis 1979;1:302–312.

34. Weinstein WN, Onderdonk AB, Bartlett JG, et al: Experimental intra-abdominal abscesses in rats: Development of an experimental model. Infect Immun 1974;10:1250–1255.

35. Lorber B, Swenson RM: The bacteriology of intraabdominal infections. Surg Clin North Am 1975;55:1349–1354.

36. Nichols RL, Smith JW, Robertson GD, et al: Prospective alterations in therapy for penetrating abdominal trauma. Arch Surg 1993;128:55–63.

37. Nichols RL, Smith JW, Klein DB: Risk of infection after penetrating abdominal trauma. N Engl J Med 1984;311:1065–1070.

38. Bohen JMA, Solomkin JS, Dellinger EP, et al: Guidelines for clinical care: Anti-infective agents for intra-abdominal infection. A Surgical Infection Society policy statement. Arch Surg 1992;127:83–89.

39. Lennard ES, Dellinger EP, Wertz MJ, et al: Implications of leukocytosis and fever at conclusion of antibiotic therapy for intra-abdominal sepsis. Ann Surg 1982;195:19–24.

40. Stone HH, Bourneuf AA, Stinson LD: Reliability of criteria for predicting persistent or recurrent sepsis. Arch Surg 1985;120:17–20.

41. Solomkin JS, Reinhart HH, Dellinger EP, et al: Results of a randomized trial comparing sequential intravenous/oral treatment with ciprofloxacin plus metronidazole to imipenem/cilastatin for intra-abdominal infections. The Intra-Abdominal Infection Study Group. Ann Surg 1996;223:303–315.

42. Rotstein OD, Meakins JL: Diagnostic and therapeutic challenges of intra-abdominal infections. World J Surg 1990;14:159–166.

43. Nathens AB, Rotstein OD, Marshall JC: Tertiary peritonitis: Clinical features of a complex nosocomial infection. World J Surg 1998;22:158–163.

44. Bartlett JG, Onderdonk AB, Louie T, et al: A review: Lessons from an animal model of intraabdominal sepsis. Arch Surg 1978;113:853–857.

45. Nichols RL, Smith JW, Balthazar ER: Peritonitis and intraabdominal abscess: An experimental model for the evaluation of human disease. J Surg Res 1978;25:129–134.

46. Rubin J, Ray R, Barnes T, et al: Peritonitis in continuous ambulatory peritoneal dialysis patients. Am J Kidney Dis 1983;2:602–609.

47. Bailie GR, Eisele G: Continuous ambulatory peritoneal dialysis: A review of its mechanics, advantages, complications, and areas of controversy. Ann Pharmacother 1992;26:1409–1420.

48. von Graevenitz A, Amsterdam D: Microbiological aspects of peritonitis associated with continuous ambulatory peritoneal dialysis. Clin Microbiol Rev 1992;5:36–48.

49. Saklayen MB: CAPD peritonitis. Incidence, pathogens, diagnosis and management. Med Clin North Am 1990;74:997–1010.

50. Smith JA: Treatment of intra-abdominal infections with quinolones. Eur J Clin Microbiol Infect Dis 1991;10:330–333.

51. Janknegt R: CAPD peritonitis and fluoroquinolones: A review. Perit Dial Int 1991;11:53–58.

52. Lui SL, Lo CY, Choy BY, et al: Optimal treatment and long-term outcome of tuberculous peritonitis complicating continuous ambulatory peritoneal dialysis. Am J Kidney Dis 1996;28:747–751.

53. Nagappan R, Collins JF, Lee WT. Fungal peritonitis in continuous ambulatory peritoneal dialysis. Am J Kidney Dis 1992;20:492–496.

54. Chan TM, Chan CY, Cheng SW, et al: Treatment of fungal peritonitis complicating continuous ambulatory peritoneal dialysis with oral fluconazole: A series of 21 patients. Nephrol Dial Transplant 1994;9:539–542.

55. Michel C, Courdavault L, al Khayat R, et al: Fungal peritonitis in patients on peritoneal dialysis. Am J Nephrol 1994;14:113–120.

56. Keane WF, Alexander SR, Bailie GR: Peritoneal dialysis–related peritonitis treatment recommendations. Perit Dial Int 1996;16:557–573.

57. Wang AY, Yu AW, Li PK, et al: Factors predicting outcome of fungal peritonitis in peritoneal dialysis: Analysis of a 9-year experience of fungal peritonitis in a single center. Am J Kidney Dis 2000;36:1183–1192.

58. Dineen P, Homan WP, Grage WR: Tuberculous peritonitis: 43 years' experience in diagnosis and treatment. Ann Surg 1976;184:717–721.

59. Mehta JB, Dutt A, Harvill L, et al: Epidemiology of extra-pulmonary tuberculosis: A comparative analysis with pre-AIDS era. Chest 1991;99:1134–1138.

60. Marshall JB: Tuberculosis of the gastrointestinal tract and peritoneum. Am J Gastroenterol 1993;88:989–999.

61. Dwivedi M, Misra SP, Misra V, et al: Value of adenosine deaminase estimation in the diagnosis of tuberculous ascites. Am J Gastroenterol 1990;85:1123–1125.

62. Martinez-Vazquez JM, Ocana I, Ribera E, et al: Adenosine deaminase activity in the diagnosis of tuberculous peritonitis. Gut 1986;27:1049–1053.

63. Voigt MD, Kalvaria I, Trey C, et al: Diagnostic value of ascites adenosine deaminase in tuberculous peritonitis. Lancet 1989;1:751–754.

64. Fernandez-Rodriguez CM, Perez-Arguelles BS, Ledo L, et al: Ascites adenosine deaminase activity is decreased in tuberculous ascites with low protein content. Am J Gastroenterol 1991;86:1500–1503.

65. Smith TR, Cho KC, Morehouse HT, et al: Comparison of computed tomography and contrast enema evaluation of diverticulitis. Dis Colon Rectum 1990;33:1–6.

66. Doringer E: Computed tomography of colonic diverticulitis. Crit Rev Diagn Imaging 1992;33:421–435.

67. Kohler L, Sauerland S, Neugebauer E: Diagnosis and treatment of diverticular disease: Results of a consensus development conference. Surg Endosc 1999;13:430–436.

68. Farmakis N, Tudor RG, Keighley MR: The 5-year natural history of complicated diverticular disease. Br J Surg 1997;81:733–735.

69. Freischlag J, Bennion RS, Thompson JE: Complications of diverticular disease of the colon in young people. Dis Colon Rectum 1986;29:639–643.

70. Spivak H, Weinrauch S, Harvey JC, et al: Acute colonic diverticulitis in the young. Dis Colon Rectum 1997;40:570–574.

71. Wolff BG, Devine RM: Surgical management of diverticulitis. Am Surg 2000;66:153–156.

72. Bruce CJ, Coller JA, Murray JJ, et al: Laparoscopic resection for diverticular disease. Dis Colon Rectum 1996;39:S1–S6.

73. Franklin ME, Dorman JP, Jacobs M, et al: Is laparoscopic surgery applicable to complicated colonic diverticular disease? Surg Endosc 1997;11:1021–1025.

74. Saini S, Mueller PR, Wittenberg J, et al: Percutaneous drainage of diverticular abscess. Arch Surg 1986;121:475–478.

75. Vasilevsky CA, Belliveau P, Trudel JL, et al: Fistulas in complicating diverticulitis. Int J Colorect Dis 1998;13:57–60.

76. Lee EC, Murray JJ, Coller JA, et al: Intraoperative colonic lavage in nonelective surgery for diverticular disease. Dis Colon Rectum 1997;40:669–674.

77. Belmonte C, Klas JV, Perez JJ, et al: The Hartmann procedure: First choice or last resort in diverticular disease? Arch Surg 1996;131:612–615.

78. Wedell J, Banzhaf G, Chaoui R, et al: Surgical management of complicated colonic diverticulitis. Br J Surg 1997;84:380–383.

79. Browder W, Smith JW, Vivoda LM, et al: Nonperforative appendicitis: A continuing surgical dilemma. J Infect Dis 1989;159:1088–1094.

80. McNamara MJ, Pasquale MD, Evans SR: Acute appendicitis and the use of intraperitoneal cultures. Surg Gynecol Obstet 1993;177:393–397.

81. Mosdell DM, Morris DM, Fry DE: Peritoneal cultures and antibiotic therapy in pediatric perforated appendicitis. Am J Surg 1994;167:313–316.

82. Gerzof SG, Johnson WC, Robbins AH, et al: Expanded criteria for percutaneous abscess drainage. Arch Surg 1985;120:227–232.

83. Nunez D, Huber JS, Yrizarry JM, et al: Nonsurgical drainage of appendiceal abscesses. AJR Am J Roentgenol 1986;146:587–589.

84. Mandell GL: Bactericidal activity of aerobic and anaerobic polymorphonuclear neutrophils. Infect Immun 1974;9:337–341.

85. Knighton DR, Halliday B, Hunt TK: Oxygen as an antibiotic. The effect of inspired oxygen on infection. Arch Surg 1984;119:191–195.

86. Simchowitz L, Cragoe EJ: Regulation of human neutrophil chemotaxis by intracellular pH. J Biol Chem 1986;261:6492–6500.

87. Rotstein OD, Feigel VD, Simmons RL, et al: The deleterious effect of reduced pH and hypoxia on neutrophil migration in vitro. J Surg Res 1988;45:298–303.

88. Kazilek CJ, Merkle CJ, Chandler DE: Hyperosmotic inhibition of calcium signals and exocytosis in rabbit neutrophils. Am J Physiol 1988;23:C709–C718.

89. Hampton MB, Chambers ST, Vissers MC, et al: Bacterial killing by neutrophils in hypertonic environments. J Infect Dis 1994;169:839–846.

90. Altemeier WA, Culbertson WR, Fullen WD, et al: Intra-abdominal abscesses. Am J Surg 1973;125:70–79.

91. Olson MM, Allen MO: Results of an eight-year prospective study of 32,284 operations. Arch Surg 1989;124:356–361.

92. Sherman NJ, Davis JR, Jesseph JE: Subphrenic abscess. A continuing hazard. Am J Surg 1969;117:117–123.

93. During P, Schofield PF: Diagnosis and management of psoas abscess in Crohn's disease. J R Soc Med 1984;77:33–34.

94. Crepps JT, Welch JP, Orlando R: Management and outcome of retroperitoneal abscesses. Ann Surg 1987;205:276–281.

95. Longo WE, Milsom JW, Lavery IC, et al: Pelvic abscess after colon and rectal surgery—What is optimal management? Dis Colon Rectum 1993;36:936–941.

96. Fry DE, Garrison RN, Heitch RC, et al: Determinants of death in patients with intraabdominal abscess. Surgery 1980;88:517–523.

97. Fry DE: Noninvasive imaging tests in the diagnosis and treatment of intra-abdominal abscesses in the postoperative patient. Surg Clin North Am 1994;74:693–709.

98. Bergnan AB, Neiman HL, Kraut B: Ultrasonographic evaluation of pericholecystic abscesses. AJR Am J Roentgenol 1979;132:201–203.

99. Doust BD, Quiroz F, Stewart JM: Ultrasonic distinction of abscesses from other intra-abdominal fluid collections. Radiology 1977;125:213–218.

100. Doust BD, Thompson R: Ultrasonography of abdominal fluid collections. Gastrointest Radiol 1978;3:273–279.

101. Maklad NF, Doust BD, Baum JK: Ultrasonic diagnosis of postoperative intra-abdominal abscess. Radiology 1974;113:417–422.

102. Taylor KJW, Wasson JF, De Graff C, et al: Accuracy of grey-scale ultrasound diagnosis of abdominal and pelvic abscesses in 220 patients. Lancet 1978;1:83–84.

103. Koehler PR, Moss AA: Diagnosis of intra-abdominal and pelvic abscesses by computerized tomography. JAMA 1980;244:49–52.

104. Robison JG, Pollack TW: Computed tomography and localization in the diagnosis of intra-abdominal abscesses. Am J Surg 1980;140:783–786.

105. Mueller PR, Simeone JF: Intra-abdominal abscesses: Diagnosis by songraphy and computed tomography. Radiol Clin North Am 1983;21:425–443.

106. Gerzof SG, Johnson WC: Radiologic aspects of diagnosis and treatment of abdominal abscesses. Surg Clin North Am 1984;64:53–65.

107. Stabile BE, Puccio E, van Sonnenberg E, et al: Preoperative percutaneous drainage of diverticular abscesses. Am J Surg 1990;159:99–104.

108. Samuelson SL, Ferguson MK: Empyema following percutaneous drainage of upper abdominal abscesses. Chest 1992;102:1612–1614.

109. Brolin RE, Flancbaum L, Ercoli FR, et al: Limitations of percutaneous catheter drainage of abdominal abscesses. Surg Gynecol Obstet 1991;173:203–210.

110. Malangoni MA, Shumate CR, Thomas HA: Factors influencing the treatment of intra-abdominal abscesses. Am J Surg 1990;159:167–171.

111. Johnson WC, Gerzof SG, Robbins AH, et al: Treatment of abdominal abscesses: Comparative evaluation of operative drainage versus percutaneous catheter drainage guided by computed tomography or ultrasound. Ann Surg 1981;194:510–520.

112. Ochsner A, Debakey M: Subphrenic abscess: A collective review and an analysis of 3608 collected and personal cases. Int Abstr Surg 1938;66:426.

113. Ochsner A, Debakey M, Murray S: Pyogenic abscesses of the liver. II. An analysis of forty-seven cases with review of the literature. Am J Surg 1938;49:292.

114. Barnes PF, DeCock KM, Reynolds TN, et al: A comparison of amebic and pyogenic abscess of the liver. Medicine 1987;66:472–483.

115. Conter RL, Pitt HA, Thompkins RK, et al: Differentiation of pyogenic from amebic hepatic abscesses. Surg Gynecol Obstet 1986;162:114–120.

116. Frey CF, Zhu Y, Suzuki M, et al: Liver abscesses. Surg Clin North Am 1989;69:259–271.

117. Maher JA, Reynolds TB, Yellin AE: Successful medical treatment of pyogenic liver abscess. Gastroenterology 1979;77:618–622.

118. Reynolds TB: Medical treatment of pyogenic liver abscess. Ann Intern Med 1982;96:373–374.

119. Bertel CK, van Heerden JA, Sheedy PF: Treatment of pyogenic hepatic abscesses. Surgical vs. percutaneous drainage. Arch Surg 1986;121:554–558.

120. Goh KL, Wong NW, Paramosothy M, et al: Liver abscess in the tropic: Experience in the University Hospital, Kuala Lumpur. Postgrad Med J 1987;63:551–554.

121. Ralls PW, Barnes PF, Johnson MB, et al: Medical treatment of hepatic amebic abscess. Rare need for percutaneous drainage. Radiology 1987;165:805–807.

122. Roslyn JJ, Binns GS, Hughes EFX: Open cholecystectomy: A contemporary analysis of 42,274 patients. Ann Surg 1993;218:129–137.

123. van der Linden W, Edlund G: Early versus delayed cholecystectomy: The effect of a change in management. Br J Surg 1981;68:753–757.

124. Reiss R, Nudelman I, Gutman C, et al: Changing trends in surgery for acute cholecystitis. World J Surg 1990;14:567–570.

125. Norrby S, Herlin P, Holmin T, et al: Early or delayed cholecystectomy in acute cholecystitis? A clinical trial. Br J Surg 1983;70:163–165.

126. Jarvinen HJ, Hastbacka J: Early cholecystectomy for acute cholecystitis: A prospective randomized study. Ann Surg 1980;191:501–505.

127. Cameron JC, Gadacz TR: Laparoscopic cholecystectomy. Ann Surg 1991;213:1–2.

128. Eldar S, Sabo E, Nash E, et al: Laparoscopic cholecystectomy for acute cholecystitis: Prospective trial. World J Surg 1997;21:540–545.

129. Wiesen SM, Unger SW, Barkin JS, et al: Laparoscopic cholecystectomy: The procedure of choice for acute cholecystitis. Am J Gastroenterol 1993;88:334–337.

130. Pessaux P, Tuech JJ, Rouge C, et al: Laparoscopic cholecystectomy in acute cholecystitis: A prospective comparative study in patients with acute vs. chronic cholecystitis. Surg Endosc 2000;14:358–361.

131. Lo CM, Liu CL, Fan ST, et al: Prospective randomized study of early versus delayed laparoscopic cholecystectomy for acute cholecystitis. Ann Surg 1998;227:461–467.

132. Greenwald JA, McMullen HF, Coppa GF, et al: Standardization of surgeon-controlled variables: Impact on outcome in patients with acute cholecystitis. Ann Surg 2000;231:339–344.

133. Gerzof SG, Banks PA, Robbins AH, et al: Early diagnosis of pancreatic infection by computed tomography–guided aspiration. Gastroenterology 1987;93:1315–1320.

134. Lumsden A, Bradley EL: Secondary pancreatic infections. Surg Gynecol Obstet 1990;170:459–467.

135. Grewe M, Tsiotos GG, de-Leon EL: Fungal infection in acute necrotizing pancreatitis. J Am Coll Surg 1999;188:408–414.

136. Howes R, Zuidema GD, Cameron JL: Evaluation of prophylactic antibiotics in acute pancreatitis. J Surg Res 1975;18:197–200.

137. Finch WT, Sawyers JL, Schenker S: A prospective study to determine the efficacy of antibiotics in acute pancreatitis. Ann Surg 1976;183:667–671.

138. Pederzoli P, Bassi C, Vesentini S, et al: A randomized multicenter clinical trial of antibiotic prophylaxis of septic complications in acute necrotizing pancreatitis with imipenem. Surg Gynecol Obstet 1993;176:480–483.

139. Sainio V, Kemppainen E, Puolakkainen P, et al: Early antibiotic treatment in acute necrotising pancreatitis. Lancet 1995;346:663–667.

140. Delcenserie R, Yzet T, Ducroix JP: Prophylactic antibiotics in treatment of severe acute alcoholic pancreatitis. Pancreas 1996;13:198–201.

141. Schwarz M, Isenmann R, Meyer H, et al: Antibiotic use in necrotizing pancreatitis: Results of a controlled study. Dtsch Med Wochenschr 1997;122:356–361.

142. Ho HS, Frey CF. The role of antibiotic prophylaxis in severe acute pancreatitis. Arch Surg 1997;132:487–492.

143. Barie PS: A critical review of antibiotic prophylaxis in severe acute pancreatitis. Am J Surg 1996;172(Suppl6A):38S–43S.

144. Kramer KM, Levy H: Prophylactic antibiotics for severe acute pancreatitis: The beginning of an era. Pharmacotherapy 1999;19:592–602.

145. Laws HL, Kent RB III: Acute pancreatitis: Management of complicating infection. Am Surg 2000;66:145–152.

146. Nordback I, Sand J, Saaristo R, et al: Early treatment with antibiotics reduces the need for surgery in acute necrotizing pancreatitis—A single-center randomized study. J Gastrointest Surg 2001;5:113–118.

147. Charcot JM: Lecons sur les maladies du fore des voices biliares et des veins. In Bourneville et Severstre; Faculte de Medicine de Paris, Paris, 1877.

148. Reynolds BM, Dargan EL: Acute obstructive cholangitis: A distinct clinical syndrome. Ann Surg 1959;150:299.

149. Pitt HA, Longmire WPJ: Suppurative cholangitis. In Hardy JM (ed): Critical Surgical Illness, 2nd ed. Philadelphia, WB Saunders, 1980.

150. Lillemoe KD: Surgical treatment of biliary tract infections. Am Surg 2000;66:138–144.

151. Lai ECS, Mok FPT, Tan ESY, et al: Endoscopic biliary drainage for severe acute cholangitis. N Engl J Med 1992;326:1582–1586.

152. Seel DJ, Park YK: Oriental infestational cholangitis. Am J Surg 1983;146:366–370.

153. Lim JH, Ko YT, Lee DH, et al: Oriental cholangiohepatitis: Sonographic findings in 48 cases. AJR Am J Roentgenol 1990;155:511–514.

154. Chan FL, Chan JKF, Leong LLY: Modern imaging in the evaluation of hepatolithiasis. Hepatogastroenterology 1997;44:358–369.

155. Jan YY, Chen MF: Percutaneous trans-hepatic cholangioscopic lithotomy for hepatolithiasis. Gastrointest Endosc 1995;42:1–5.

156. Lim JH: Oriental cholangiohepatitis: Pathologic, clinical, and radiologic features. AJR Am J Roentgenol 1991;157:1–8.

157. Turner WW, Cramer CR: Recurrent oriental cholangiohepatitis. Surgery 1983;93:397–401.

158. Yellin AE, Donovan AJ: Biliary lithiasis and helminthiasis. Am J Surg 1981;142:128–136.

159. Fan ST, Lai ECS, Wong J: Hepatic resection for hepatolithiasis. Arch Surg 1993;128:1070–1074.

160. Gott PE, Tieva MH, Barcia PJ, et al: Biliary access procedure in the management of oriental cholangiohepatitis. Am Surg 1996;62:930–934.

161. Harris HW, Kumwenda ZL, Sheen-Cheen SM, et al: Recurrent pyogenic cholangitis. Am J Surg 1998;176:34–37.

162. Pitt HA, Venbrux AC, Coleman J: Intrahepatic stones: The transhepatic team approach. Ann Surg 1994;219:527–535.

163. Stain SC, Incarbone R, Guthrie CR, et al: Surgical treatment of recurrent pyogenic cholangitis. Arch Surg 1995;130:527–532.

164. Sperling RM, Koch J, Sandhu JS, et al: Recurrent pyogenic cholangitis in Asian immigrants to the United States: Natural history and role of therapeutic ERCP. Dig Dis Sci 1997;42:865–871.

165. Yeh YH, Huang MH, Yang JC, et al: Percutaneous transhepatic cholangioscopy and lithotripsy in the treatment of intrahepatic stones: A study with 5 year follow-up. Gastrointest Endosc 1995;42:13–18.

166. Jeng KS, Yang FS, Chiang HJ, et al: Bile duct stents in the management of hepatolithiasis with long-segment intrahepatic biliary strictures. Br J Surg 1992;79:663–666.

167. Sheen-Cheen SM, Cheng YF, Chou FF, et al: Ductal dilatation and stenting making routine hepatectomy unnecessary for left hepatolithiasis with intrahepatic biliary stricture. Surgery 1995;117:32–36.

168. Yoon HK, Sung KB, Song HY, et al: Benign biliary strictures associated with recurrent pyogenic cholangitis: Treatment with expandable metallic stents. AJR Am J Roentgenol 1997;169:1523–1527.

169. Fan ST, Mok F, Zheng SS, et al: Appraisal of hepaticocutaneous jejunostomy in the management of hepatolithiasis. Am J Surg 1993;165:332–335.

170. Choi BI, Han JK, Park YH, et al: Retained intrahepatic stones: Treatment with piezoelectric lithotripsy combined with stone extraction. Radiology 1991;178:105–108.

171. Sheen-Cheen SM, Chou FF, Lee CM, et al: The management of complicated hepatolithiasis with intrahepatic biliary stricture by the combination of T-tube tract dilation and endoscopic electrohydraulic lithotripsy. Gastrointest Endosc 1993;39:168–171.

chapter
10

Viral Hepatitis

RAYMOND S. KOFF, MD

Hepatic involvement may complicate a number of infectious diseases, but the various forms of viral hepatitis are the predominant and most important infectious diseases of the liver. In fact, infections by the five well-described and serologically distinct hepatitis viruses have been among the most common infections in the world and are likely to remain so for many years. The generally self-limited, enterically transmitted hepatitis viruses—hepatitis A virus (HAV) and hepatitis E virus (HEV)—are prevalent in many parts of the developing world. In many of the same countries, as well as in many parts of the developed world, the bloodborne hepatitis viruses—hepatitis B virus (HBV)—hepatitis D virus (HDV), and hepatitis C virus (HCV)—are endemic and responsible for extensive morbidity and mortality resulting from HBV-, HBV-HDV-, and HCV-induced chronic liver disease.

HBV infection is now recognized as the most common bloodborne infection in the world. More than 2 billion people have been infected by HBV, and of these, 350 million are chronically infected. Without treatment, as many as 25% of those chronically infected will die from cirrhosis and hepatocellular carcinoma. Globally, HBV-related deaths occur at a rate of over 1 million per year. Concurrent HBV-HDV infection is responsible for a small proportion of these deaths, but HDV infection appears to be declining.[1] Although the global prevalence of HCV infection appears to be lower than that of HBV, in excess of 175 million people may be chronically infected by HCV. In most countries HCV prevalence rates vary from 1% to 3%. In some regions, rates may exceed 10%. In the United States, with a seroprevalence of 1.8%, nearly 4 million people have been infected; of these, 2.7 million are actively infected, and HCV is the major cause of death from liver disease. Mortality for HCV sequelae—end-stage liver disease and hepatocellular carcinoma—is rising, and because mortality increases with duration of infection, it will continue to rise as the number of persons infected for more than 20 years increases during the next 15 years.[2]

Despite intensive study the immunologically mediated or virus-dependent mechanisms underlying the development of chronic liver disease in HBV, HDV, and HCV infections remain ill-defined. It seems likely that an appropriate early response by CD8+ cytotoxic T lymphocytes together with the induction of neutralizing antibodies usually results in viral clearance. The presence and role of viral genes that interact with host cells to evade immune clearance require further study. Impaired, unbalanced, and evaded immune responses, which favor the development of persistent infection, are thought to lead to chronic liver disease.

In the United States the incidence of acute viral hepatitis is decreasing. The decline in HAV infections appears to have begun decades ago, whereas the reduction in new HBV and HCV infections has been recognized only during the past decade. Changes in risk factor exposure, rather than vaccine immunoprophylaxis, are responsible, since the declines in HAV and HCV incidence began well before the introduction of the inactivated HAV vaccines and in the absence of a vaccine for HCV. The decline in HBV incidence has been seen in both sexes, all racial groups, and in those age groups with the highest infection rates, namely the 20- to 39-year-old age group. The decline began after the introduction of HBV vaccines but before widespread implementation of a national vaccination program. Therefore changes in risk-taking behavior among injection drug users and among high-risk heterosexuals may be responsible for the decline in HBV and HCV infection rates. Among health care workers, the disappearance of hepatitis B can be attributed to widespread HBV vaccine use. Although available data are limited at present, the prevalence of HDV infection is also rapidly declining.

Despite the falling incidence of acute viral hepatitis, viral hepatitis continues to be among the leading notifiable infectious diseases in the United States, and correcting for underreporting, between 200,000 to 300,000 annual new infections can be expected for the next few years. The use of HAV and HBV vaccines is the key strategy for the control of these infections in the United States.

HEPATITIS A

Prevention of HAV Infection

Immune Globulin

Administration of human immune globulin containing IgG anti-HAV has been the major form of immunoprophylaxis of HAV for more than 5 decades. Its effectiveness in pre- and postexposure settings was established before HAV infection could be serologically identified and before anti-HAV could be measured. Intramuscular injection results in low levels of circulating anti-HAV and protects against clinical disease in a large proportion (75% to 90%) of recipients for a finite period of no more than 2 to 6 months. The intramuscular immune globulin preparations produced in the United States have had a superb safety record, but in recent years shortages have limited availability. Fortunately the need for this product is diminishing with the increases in HAV vaccine use. Nonetheless, in the United States immune globulin continues to be recommended for HAV immunoprophylaxis for children less than 2 years of age and for postexposure prophylaxis of household contacts of infected persons.

Absence of a recommendation for use of HAV vaccine in infants results from early data suggesting that passively acquired, maternal anti-HAV in the infant may interfere with vaccine immunogenicity (see below for further discussion). In infants of mothers who are seronegative, HAV vaccine elicits excellent seroconversion rates and high titers of antibody.[3] Immune globulin is still recommended for postexposure prophylaxis because data on vaccine efficacy in this setting remains sparse (see below). Current recommendations call for administration of immune globulin to all susceptible household members or intimate contacts of persons with hepatitis A as soon as possible after identification of the index case. If given more than 2 weeks after exposure, efficacy is reduced. The duration of protection is dose dependent and relatively short. Immune globulin has not been shown to be effective in the control of community-wide or common-source outbreaks.

Hepatitis A Vaccines

Two highly immunogenic, formaldehyde-inactivated, alum-adjuvanted, safe and effective whole-virus HAV vaccines are approved for use in the United States.[4,5] Both are given in a two-dose schedule with intervals between the first and second doses of 6 to 12 months, and both are well tolerated. Both Havrix (manufactured by SmithKline Beecham) and Vaqta (manufactured by Merck) provide protection by inducing neutralizing antibodies and specific memory B cells. Both vaccines are available in adult and pediatric dose forms. The pediatric vaccines are approved for use in children ages 2 through 18 years. In addition to the two licensed HAV vaccines available in the United States, a live attenuated vaccine has been used in China but is unlikely to receive approval for use in the United States. In Europe a formaldehyde-inactivated vaccine also is in use in which the HAV antigen is bound to immunopotentiating, reconstituted influenza virosome membranes.[6] For those HAV vaccines produced from inactivated virus, vaccination during pregnancy probably carries no additional risks for the developing fetus.

The protective efficacy of the two United States–approved vaccines is likely to be similar. Head-to-head field trials comparing protective efficacy, however, are not currently available. Nonetheless the vaccines appear to have similar immunogenicity when evaluated by identical immunoassays for induced HAV-antibody.[7] Following a single dose of either vaccine, seroconversion rates of 100% were observed at 4 to 8 weeks; by the end of the second week seroconversion had occurred in nearly 90% of recipients. Levels of anti-HAV sufficient to provide protection for at least 1 year have been observed in about 95% of vaccinees following a single dose.[8]

Whether a single vaccine dose would provide more durable immunoprophylaxis is uncertain, although in one study a single dose of HAV vaccine in children appeared to provide protection for those at risk who were exposed before the second dose.[9] Even assuming that anti-HAV levels may decline or disappear following a single vaccine dose, memory B cells capable of the rapid production of neutralizing antibodies upon re-exposure to HAV are likely to extend protection. Because studies of the effectiveness of a single dose of HAV vaccine are still limited, the conventional two-dose regimen is recommended.

With concurrent administration of HAV vaccine and immune globulin peak, anti-HAV levels are lower than levels seen when vaccine alone is given.[10] Although lower during the first 24 weeks after immunization, the levels are sufficiently high to provide protection against infection, and after the second vaccine dose, given at 24 weeks, concentrations of anti-HAV are not significantly different in the two groups. Concurrent HAV and immune globulin prophylaxis is used predominantly for the traveler who is leaving for an endemic area shortly (within 2 weeks of the office encounter).

Pre-exposure vaccination is recommended by the Advisory Committee on Immunization Practices (ACIP) for individuals at high risk for HAV infection[11] (Table 10–1). Vaccination has been recommended for children 2 years of age or older residing in those communities (e.g., states, counties, and localities) in which HAV attack rates are twice the U.S. national average of 10/100,000 population. Vaccination of children also should be considered by local health authorities when HAV infection rates are above the national average but below the twofold threshold level of 20/100,000.

Patients with chronic liver diseases and those who have received liver transplants who are susceptible to HAV infection should be vaccinated, since HAV superinfection may result in acute liver failure.[12] In patients with chronic liver disease, particularly those with chronic hepatitis C, HAV vaccines may be slightly less immunogenic than in healthy subjects, but the two-dose regimen induced anti-HAV in nearly 95% of vaccines[13] (Table 10–2), and vaccination appears to be cost effective, although conflicting assumptions have made the question controversial.[14] Early immunization after diagnosis of chronic liver disease is reasonable, since patients with decompensated liver disease and patients with a liver transplant may respond less well than those with milder disease.[15]

Food handlers are not necessarily at increased risk because of their occupation, but if infected, they are capable of amplifying infection by contaminating foods served to hundreds of customers. Vaccination of food handlers should be considered whenever local conditions suggest that it would be cost effective to do so. Sewage and waste water treatment workers and workers in day

TABLE 10–1 ■ Candidates for Pre-exposure Hepatitis A Virus (HAV) Vaccine

Children in communities with HAV attack rates twice the national average
International travelers to endemic regions (tourists)
Persons working in HAV endemic countries
  Business visitors
  Peace-keeping or military forces
Homosexual and bisexual men
Recipients of solvent-detergent-treated clotting factor concentrates
Persons who work with HAV or HAV-infected nonhuman primates
Injecting and noninjecting illicit drug users
Persons with chronic liver disease or liver transplants
Food handlers, depending on local conditions

TABLE 10–2 ■ Immunogenicity of Hepatitis A Virus (HAV) Vaccine in Healthy Adults and Patients with Chronic Liver Diseases

Vaccinated subjects	Seroconversion rate 1 month after second vaccine dose (%)	Geometric mean anti-HAV titer (mIU/ml)
Healthy adults	98.2	1315
Chronic hepatitis B	97.7	749
Chronic hepatitis C	94.3	467
Other liver diseases	95.2	562

Adapted from Keeffe EB, Iwarson S, McMahon BJ, et al: Safety and immunogenicity of hepatitis A vaccine in patients with chronic liver disease. Hepatology 1998;27:881–886.

care centers may also be appropriate candidates for HAV vaccine, but national recommendations are lacking.

The general failure of immune globulin in controlling community-wide outbreaks and its limited availability have turned attention to the use of HAV vaccine as a public health measure. Early experiences in Alaska suggested that transmission could be interrupted if a large proportion, approximately 80%, of the at-risk population could be immunized.[16] In the absence of controlled studies, however, firm conclusions about the effectiveness of HAV vaccine cannot be drawn.[17] High vaccine costs and the uncertainty about the feasibility of rapidly identifying and delivering vaccine to groups at risk are obstacles, but general acceptance of vaccine as a control measure seems likely in the future.

HAV vaccine has yet to be incorporated into routine infant immunization programs, in part because early studies suggested that passively acquired maternal anti-HAV in the infant would reduce vaccine immunogenicity. More recent data however, indicate that a 100% seroconversion rate can be achieved in infants despite the presence of maternal anti-HAV when vaccine is given at 5 and 11 months of age. The geometric mean titer of anti-HAV was lower than in vaccinated infants without maternal antibodies, raising concerns about the duration of protection in these infants.[18] Further studies are needed before infant immunization can be recommended.

Whether HAV vaccine administered in the post-HAV exposure setting is effective remains uncertain. The vaccine appeared to reduce the postexposure infection rate in one study.[5] If vaccine is effective in the control of community-wide outbreaks, perhaps part of its effectiveness is also due to prevention of infection after exposure. In one trial, household contacts of hospitalized index cases of hepatitis A were randomized to receive HAV vaccine within 8 days of onset of symptoms in the index case or were not vaccinated.[19] Although a protective efficacy rate of 82% was reported in vaccinated contacts, the 95% confidence intervals were quite large (20% to 96%). These data require confirmation in additional controlled clinical trials before HAV vaccine can be generally recommended for postexposure prophylaxis.

A highly immunogenic bivalent hepatitis A and B vaccine (Twinrix, manufactured by SmithKline Beecham), is available in the United States and elsewhere for individuals susceptible to both infections.[20] A three-dose regimen simplifies immunization schedules and should reduce administration costs and improve compliance.

Treatment of HAV Infection

Specific drug treatment is unavailable. Most patients are treated at home unless persistent vomiting or severe anorexia cannot be controlled by home care. No specific diet, with the exception of a prohibition on alcohol during the acute phase, can be recommended. Prolonged or highly strenuous physical activity is proscribed. The extent of rest is best determined by the severity of fatigue and malaise as assessed by the patient. Clinical and biochemical recovery is anticipated to be complete within a few months of the onset of illness in most cases. For the rare patient with acute liver failure due to HAV infection, survival rates of about 65% or greater may be achieved by early referral for liver transplantation. Effective antiviral treatment in this setting is unavailable. In cholestatic forms of hepatitis A with prolonged jaundice the prognosis is excellent with or without a short course of corticosteroid treatment. Similarly, despite occasional relapses following apparent recovery or near-recovery in hepatitis A, complete recovery is anticipated without intervention.

HEPATITIS E

Prevention of HEV Infection

Immune Globulin

Immune globulin manufactured in the United States is not effective in the prophylaxis of HEV infection. Immune globulin produced in HEV endemic regions also is probably ineffective, but one study suggested possible benefit in reducing infection rates in pregnant women.[21] The key to prevention of HEV infection lies in increasing the availability of clean water supplies in endemic areas. Currently the best advice for the traveler to endemic regions is to avoid drinking water or ice of uncertain origin, uncooked bivalve mollusks, and uncooked fruits and vegetables.

HEV Vaccine

Commercial HEV vaccines are not yet available. If they were, the principal candidates for vaccination would be susceptible pregnant women, in whom the risk of fatal acute liver failure due to HEV is high. Women living in endemic regions or traveling to such regions would be the first targeted. An inexpensive, safe HEV vaccine, however, would be of considerable general value in endemic regions to reduce HEV-associated morbidity. Because replication of HEV in cell culture has been relatively inefficient, resulting in low virus yields, an inactivated vaccine seems unlikely at this time. Similarly, although a vaccine prepared from one HEV isolate would presumably provide protection against all isolates, a live, attenuated vaccine is not currently on the drawing boards, and reversion to wild-type would be a concern if such a vaccine were developed. A subunit HEV vaccine would obviate this concern.

Much interest has focused on the protein expressed from the second open reading frame (ORF-2) of HEV as a promising immunogen for vaccine development. Inoculation of a purified recombinant plasmid vector containing the ORF-2 elicited a long-term humoral immune response in mice, and the elicited antibodies have been shown to recognize native HEV.[22] In other studies using DNA immunization with a plasmid expressing the ORF-2 structural protein the antibody response was enhanced with the use of plasmids expressing interleukin-2 and granulocyte-macrophage colony-stimulating factor (GM-CSF) or with viruslike particles expressed through a baculovirus expression system.[23]

A prototype recombinant ORF-2 protein vaccine reduced the duration and extent of viremia and fecal shedding of HEV following challenge with live HEV in rhesus monkeys. Pre-exposure vaccination did not reduce the frequency of infection after intravenous challenge with homologous or heterologous strains. It did provide protection from hepatitis as defined by serum alanine aminotransferase (ALT) levels and histopathology.[24]

Gene gun delivery to cynomolgus macaques of a plasmid DNA construct encoding and expressing ORF-2 protected the animals from challenge with a heterologous HEV strain.[25] Intradermal inoculation of this DNA vaccine was ineffective.

Treatment of HEV Infection

As in the case of HAV infection no specific drug therapy is available. Treatment is symptomatic and supportive. Whether early delivery of the pregnant woman with acute hepatitis E will reduce fetal mortality remains to be determined.

HEPATITIS B

On the basis of nucleotide divergence, HBV has been genotypically classified into seven groups, termed genotypes A to G, which vary in global distribution. Their impact on natural history, clinical outcome, and treatment are poorly understood, but they do not appear to influence immunoprophylaxis.[26]

Prevention of HBV Infection

Hepatitis B Immune Globulin

Antibody against the hepatitis B surface antigen (anti-HBs) is the protective, HBV-neutralizing antibody. Immune globulin preparations containing high levels of this antibody are termed hepatitis B immune globulin (HBIG) and have been available for the immunoprophylaxis of HBV infection for over 2 decades. They are relatively expensive, less effective than HBV vaccine for pre-exposure immunoprophylaxis, and now have limited utility: they are more-or-less reserved for coadministration with HBV vaccines in a few specific settings such as for neonates of HBsAg-positive mothers, for susceptible nonvaccinated victims of HBV-contaminated needlesticks, and for sexual partners of acutely infected persons. The principal use of HBIG is in the control of post-liver-transplantation HBV infection, where it has been shown to delay or prevent HBV reinfection of the graft.

Hepatitis B Vaccines

The first HBV vaccines were plasma derived. Although no longer available in the United States, at one time these vaccines comprised about 80% of worldwide HBV vaccine production. Recombinant, subunit HBV vaccines, produced by cloning the gene encoding HBsAg through use of a plasmid vector inserted into common baker's yeast, have been commercially available since the mid-1980s. The HBsAg particles, which comprise the immunogen in the vaccine, induce immunity by eliciting anti-HBs. Anti-HBs levels of 10 mIU/ml or higher are thought to be seroprotective. Antibody to the hepatitis B core antigen (anti-HBc) is not induced by the recombinant HBV vaccines. Transiently positive tests for HBsAg in serum may be found within 24 hours following vaccine administration and rarely may remain detectable for days to weeks after vaccine administration.[27]

The recombinant HBV vaccines are highly immunogenic, safe, and well tolerated. They no longer contain thimerosal as a preservative. No causal association with autoimmune or neurologic disorders such as multiple sclerosis or Guillain-Barré syndrome has been established.[28] Because the HBV vaccines are subunit vaccines, vaccination during pregnancy should carry no additional risks for the developing fetus. The vaccines are usually given intramuscularly in a three-dose schedule at a deltoid injection site or, in infants, the anterolateral muscle of the thigh. Recombivax HB (Merck) is formulated to contain a 10-μg adult dose of HBsAg protein given in a three-dose schedule at 0, 1, and 6 months. It can be given in a 5-μg three-dose schedule to children up to age 19 years. For children ages 11 to 15 years a 10-μg, two-dose schedule (0 and 4 to 6 months) is an option. Engerix-B (SmithKline Beecham), the second recombinant HBV vaccine approved in the United States, contains a 20-μg dose of HBsAg protein for older children and adults, given in a three-dose schedule. For children between ages 5 to 16 years the 10-μg dose of Engerix-B is also approved for a three-dose regimen in which the injections are spaced 1 year apart (0, 12, and 24 months). It should be noted that dose scheduling is now less rigid than in the past. For example, vaccination of infants at 2, 4, and

12 to 15 months of life provides immunogenicity comparable to the standard schedule of 0, 1, and 6 months. A two-dose vaccine regimen may also be shown to be effective in adults but is not yet approved in the United States.[29]

Both HBV vaccines are close to 95% effective in preventing HBV infection or clinical hepatitis B. Vaccine-induced immunity appears to be prolonged, despite the fact that anti-HBs concentrations may fall below the seroprotective threshold of 10 mIU/ml and become undetectable after several years. Immunologic memory cells that participate in anamnestic boosts in anti-HBs levels on exposure to HBV are believed to be responsible for this persistence of immunity. Immunologic memory may be retained for a few years even after a single vaccine dose. The precise duration of protection remains uncertain but is more than 10 years in healthy young people who receive all three doses. It has been reported to be as long as 15 years in children vaccinated at 16 months of age[30] and may be lifelong. Booster doses are recommended only for immunocompromised persons in whom anti-HBs levels fall below 10 mIU/ml on annual testing.

A number of factors appear to reduce the response to vaccination (Table 10–3). Use of higher doses of vaccine may augment antibody response in some of these patient groups, for example, those on hemodialysis. Novel HBV vaccines containing the pre-S (middle and large surface) proteins in addition to HBsAg have been developed. None are currently approved for use in the United States. Their principal role may be in the revaccination of nonresponders to the conventional HBsAg-containing vaccines.[31,32] This genetically based vaccine non-responsiveness is seen in no more than 5% of people. The absence of a dominant immune response gene capable of mediating anti-HBs production appears to be associated with a T lymphocyte defect and an impaired or absent cytokine response to HBsAg but not to a defect in antigen presenting cells.[33] Nonresponders should probably be revaccinated with three additional doses of the same or the other recombinant vaccine if they are at high risk. Seroprotective levels are reached in few of the genetically determined nonresponders but in as many as one-half of other nonresponders. Another potential approach to enhancing the response to HBV vaccines may be the

TABLE 10–3 ■ Populations with a Reduced Response to Hepatitis B Virus Vaccine

Persons over 40 years of age
Obese persons
Smokers
Patients with chronic cardiac, pulmonary, or renal disease
Hemodialysis patients
Organ transplant recipients
Human immunodeficiency virus–positive patients with low CD4+ counts
Genetically determined nonresponsiveness

use of oligonucleotide adjuvants.[34] Studies in human subjects are awaited.

Another innovative concept is the use of genetic (DNA) HBV vaccines encoding the structural genes of HBV. These have been shown to both induce and boost anti-HBs levels in mice[35] and to protect chimpanzees against challenge with live HBV.[36] Studies in human volunteers utilizing low doses of a DNA vaccine encoding HBsAg delivered into the skin have been initiated.[37]

Over 110 countries have incorporated HBV vaccine into national immunization programs. The effectiveness of these programs has been demonstrated most dramatically in formerly high prevalence regions, for example, Taiwan[38] and Alaska.[39] In Taiwan, the HBsAg carrier rate among young children has fallen by more than 85% in just under 10 years after introduction of infant immunization in 1984. Alaskan natives have participated in an immunization program begun in 1983. Persons born before the initiation of routine infant HBV vaccination had a 16% rate of chronic HBV infection, while no chronic infections were identified in children born since the introduction of that program, indicating that elimination of new chronic HBV infection is a feasible goal.

Current vaccination strategies in the United States are focused on the screening of pregnant women for HBsAg, followed by early immunization of the neonates of HBsAg-positive women, and vaccination of infants of HBsAg-negative women, children and adolescents through 18 years of age, and high-risk adult groups. Each year, about 20,000 women with persistent HBV infection give birth in the United States. Approximately one-third of HBV-infected children have acquired their infections from their HBsAg-positive mothers. In the remaining two-thirds, close contact with other HBsAg-positive household contacts is responsible. Hence early vaccination in the newborn period should protect against both infant and early childhood infection. Furthermore, infants receiving the vaccine during the first 7 days of life are more likely to complete the full series than are infants who received the first dose later.[40]

For infants born to HBsAg-positive mothers, administration of HBIG and HBV within 12 hours of birth is recommended in the United States. HBV vaccine alone, however, may have comparable efficacy to coadminstration of HBV vaccine and HBIG. In a 10-year follow-up of high-risk infants immunized at birth, HBIG administration was not correlated with long-term efficacy.[41] In many countries HBIG is no longer used in the prevention of maternal-neonatal HBV transmission.

For infants born to HBsAg-negative mothers, HBV vaccine preferably should be given during the newborn period. For infants who are at high risk of early childhood infection because their mothers belong to populations with a high or moderate prevalence of HBV infection the first dose of vaccine should be given before nursery discharge. For infants with a low risk of early childhood

TABLE 10–4 ■ Hepatitis B Virus (HBV) Vaccination Strategies in the United States

Antenatal screening of pregnant women for HBsAg
  Hepatitis B immune globulin plus HBV vaccine for neonates of HBsAg-positive mothers
  Routine immunization with HBV vaccine of infants of HBsAg-negative mothers
Catch-up vaccination of previously unvaccinated children through age 19 years
Routine immunization of household and intimate contacts of HBsAg carriers, Alaskan natives, Pacific Islanders, children of immigrants from HBV-hyperendemic regions
Vaccination of high-risk adolescents and adults
First-responders
Health care workers
Users of illicit injection drugs
Patients with bleeding disorders
Persons with more than one sexual partner in a 6-month period
Homosexual and bisexual males
Attendees at sexually transmitted disease clinics
Adolescents living in areas with high rates of teenage pregnancy
Patients with chronic renal failure
Patients with non-HBV chronic liver disease
Persons in correctional institutions
Persons residing in institutions for the mentally retarded
Travelers to hyperendemic regions (when visits are prolonged)
Hepatitis B immune globulin plus HBV vaccine for susceptible contaminated needlestick victims and for sexual partners of acutely infected persons

infection the first dose can be given before discharge from the nursery or later, but before 2 months of age.

When the HBsAg status of the mother is unknown, the vaccine should be given to the newborn within 12 hours of birth. If the mother then tests positive, the infant should receive HBIG as soon as possible but no later than 7 days after birth.

Infant, high-risk, and other groups targeted for HBV vaccination are listed in Table 10–4. Unfortunately a small proportion, generally under 5%, of infants born to infected mothers acquire infection despite immunization. The precise mechanisms responsible for these "breakthrough" infections in the HBIG and HBV vaccine-immunized infants of HBV-infected mothers are poorly understood (Table 10–5). Considerable attention has been directed to the role of HBV escape mutant viruses, which are widely distributed globally but generally in low prevalence. Whether it will become necessary to incorporate the HBsAg antigens from the mutant strains into

TABLE 10–5 ■ Potential Mechanisms of Breakthrough Hepatitis B Virus (HBV) Infections in Immunized Infants

Infection in utero before immunization
Genetic vaccine nonresponsiveness
HBV escape mutant transmission from mother to infant
Appearance of HBV escape mutant de novo

future HBV vaccines remains uncertain. Some comfort has been derived from studies showing that the currently licensed recombinant HBV vaccines can protect chimpanzees against infection with the prototype HBsAg escape mutant virus.[42] Of course, other mutant strains may subsequently emerge.

Treatment of Acute HBV Infection

Antiviral treatment of acute hepatitis B would be welcome, particularly for infants and young children in whom the risk of developing persistent infection is high, for that 1% of patients who develop acute liver failure, and for patients with acute HBV infection after liver transplantation. Unfortunately, few studies of the efficacy of treatment with lamivudine or interferon are available.[43,44] Because less than 5% of HBV-infected adults develop chronic HBV infection and because it is impossible to identify those who would develop persistent infection, many would need to be treated to prevent progression in the few.

Treatment of Chronic HBV Infection

A large body of data support the notion that sustained suppression of HBV replication is associated with reduction of hepatic inflammation and necrosis, recovery of structural damage, and interruption of progression to advanced liver disease. The goals of treatment are shown in Table 10–6. End-points of treatment include loss of HBV DNA by non–polymerase chain reaction (PCR) assays, loss of HBeAg and development of anti-HBe, loss of HBsAg and development of anti-HBs, and normalization of serum ALT levels.

Candidates for treatment include HBsAg-positive patients who are HBV DNA–positive and who have elevated serum ALT levels. Patients with the HBV precore mutant, in whom HBeAg is not synthesized but in whom circulating HBsAg and HBV DNA are present, are also candidates. Patients with signs and symptoms of hepatic decompensation may be treated with the oral antiviral lamivudine, but referral for liver transplantation is essential. No therapy is currently available for healthy HBsAg carriers with normal serum ALT levels and minimal histologic findings on liver biopsy.

Interferon

Subcutaneous injections of interferon alfa-2b in doses of 5 MU (daily) or 10 MU (three times weekly) for periods of 4 to 6 months achieve HBV clearance by non-PCR assays, loss of HBeAg, biochemical resolution, and histologic improvement in 30% to 40% of cases. After completion of therapy about 10% of patients may experience relapse. A short course of prednisone before initiation of interferon has been used in some centers, but its benefits remain uncertain, and it carries the risk of precipitating hepatic failure. It cannot be recommended. Factors linked with a favorable response to initial therapy are shown in Table 10–7.

The appearance of anti-HBe and clearance of HBV DNA by PCR assay may be delayed for several months after the treatment period. Loss of HBsAg and the appearance of anti-HBs may be delayed for years. Flares in serum ALT levels occur in most responders during treatment and are usually well tolerated except in patients with pre-existing hepatic decompensation. Interferon-associated adverse events require dose reductions in about 25% of treated patients. Cirrhosis does not affect response rates. Among patients who respond, life expectancy and survival free of complications return to normal,[45,46] and as might be expected, treatment is cost saving.[47]

Lamivudine

Lamivudine, a well-tolerated, orally administered deoxycytosine analogue, given in a dose of 100 mg daily, results in premature chain termination during reverse transcription of HBV DNA, thereby inhibiting HBV replication. It also may reverse T cell hyporesponsiveness to HBV antigens.[48] In over 50% of treated patients histologic improvement in hepatocyte necrosis and inflammation is seen, and fibrosis appears to be slowed. Serum ALT levels return to normal in nearly 75% of patients, but loss of HBV DNA and HBeAg seroconversion may occur in no more than 20% of patients after 1 year of lamivudine treatment. Lamivudine has been administered for periods exceeding 1 year; the optimal length of treatment remains unknown.[49] Discontinuation may be attempted after 1 year of treatment if the patient is HBeAg-negative and anti-HBe-positive and if HBV DNA has cleared.[50] Lamivudine infrequently induces biochemical flares. As many as 30% of patients will develop a lamivudine-resistant HBV mutant—the

TABLE 10–6 ■ Goals of Treatment in Chronic Hepatitis B

Sustained inhibition of hepatitis B virus replication
Biochemical remission
Histologic remission
Reduction in risk of cirrhosis
Reduction in risk of hepatic decompensation
Reduction in risk of hepatocellular carcinoma
Return to normal life expectancy

TABLE 10–7 ■ Positive Pretreatment Predictors of Virologic Response to Interferon Therapy in Chronic Hepatitis B

High serum alanine aminotransferase levels
Low circulating hepatitis B virus DNA levels
Short duration of chronic infection
Active necroinflammatory histologic lesions
Absence of hepatitis D virus coinfection
Absence of human immunodeficiency virus coinfection

YMDD mutation within the HBV DNA polymerase gene—within 1 to 2 years of treatment, which may result in breakthrough infection with reappearance of HBV. These mutants appear to be less replication competent and possibly less virulent. The management of lamivudine-associated breakthrough infections is uncertain; continuation of lamivudine resulting in suppression of wild-type HBV may be appropriate, but further study is needed.

For patients with end-stage liver disease due to chronic hepatitis B, limited experience suggests that lamivudine treatment increases pretransplantation survival, reduces the risk of reinfection of the graft in those patients with a liver transplant, and may be effective in managing posttransplantation HBV recurrence.

Lamivudine and alpha interferon combination treatment has been reported to be more effective than monotherapy with either agent,[51] but confirmation is not yet available. For patients with HBeAg-negative chronic hepatitis B, lamivudine appears to induce high early biochemical and virologic response rates, but breakthroughs with the YMDD mutant increase during extended treatment beyond the first year.[52]

Future Treatment

Approaches currently under study include novel nucleoside analogues (adefovir, entecavir, emtricitabine), therapeutic vaccines incorporating a cytotoxic T lymphocyte epitope derived from the hepatitis B core protein, DNA-based vaccines, and pre-S-containing vaccines with newer adjuvants, thymosin, antisense oligonucleotides, and ribozymes. It seems likely that combination therapies will prove more useful than monotherapy with any agent.

HEPATITIS D

Prevention of HDV Infection

Although pre-exposure administration of HBV vaccines will protect against HBV-HDV coinfections, neither passive immunoprophylaxis with immune globulin nor active immunization with an HDV vaccine is available for the prevention of HDV superinfection. Candidates for immunoprophylaxis would be HBsAg-positive hemodialysis patients, injection drug users, recipients of multiple blood products, and persons with multiple sexual contacts. DNA vaccines comprising plasmids encoding the large hepatitis D antigen or coexpressing this antigen and HBsAg have induced both humoral and cellular immune responses in mice.[53] This approach holds promise, but clinical studies are years away.

Treatment of HDV Infection

Satisfactory treatment of acute HDV infection is not available. Short-term interferon therapy for chronic HDV infection has been generally disappointing with high recurrence rates after discontinuance of treatment. Virologic, biochemical, and histologic resolution of chronic HDV infection after high-dose interferon therapy given daily for 12 years has been reported[54] in a single patient. In an early study of five patients with chronic hepatitis D, 1 year of treatment with lamivudine in a dose of 100 mg daily was ineffective in improving liver histology or serum ALT levels, and all patients remained HDV RNA–positive.[55] Novel antiviral agents, for example, drugs that inhibit prenylation of the large HDV antigen, are under development.[56]

HEPATITIS C

Prevention of HCV Infection

Immune Globulin

Conventional immune globulin is not recommended for HCV prophylaxis. A number of studies have indicated the existence of HCV-neutralizing antibodies. Unfortunately these appear to be isolate specific and may lose effectiveness as a result of the emergence of escape HCV mutants. As a consequence of screening donors for anti-HCV it is likely that immune globulins prepared in the United States have little or no HCV-neutralizing antibodies. Current preparations of immune globulin are therefore unlikely to have any efficacy in HCV immunoprophylaxis. Repeated injections of high doses of immune globulins made in Switzerland in 1991 from unscreened plasma appeared to be effective in preventing sexual transmission in a single Italian study.[57] This preparation is no longer available.

Hepatitis C Immune Globulin

HCV immune globulins are experimental, and none are commercially available. In a small number of studies using chimpanzees, human plasma from an HCV-infected patient and antibodies induced by inoculation of a synthetic HCV peptide have been reported to neutralize HCV when mixed with HCV in vitro.[58,59] In another study, HCV hyperimmune globulin prepared from anti-HCV-positive human plasma containing antibodies to HCV core NS3 and NS4 proteins but negative for HCV RNA did not induce sterilizing immunity but may have restricted the extent of intrahepatic replication in chimpanzees.[60] Further study of these preparations is needed.

Hepatitis C Vaccine

Failure to propagate HCV in tissue culture, the absence of susceptible small animals, and HCV's remarkable heterogeneity and high mutation rate have been obstacles in vaccine development. Although no HCV vaccine is currently available, novel approaches to vaccine development are promising.

A vaccine consisting of recombinant HCV envelope glycoproteins (gpE1/E2) has been shown to induce antibodies to these antigens in mice and chimpanzees[61] but failed, in general, to induce sterilizing immunity in chimpanzees challenged with infectious virus.[62] Nonetheless, immunization may have reduced the severity of infection and the likelihood of chronic infection. The immunogenicity, safety, and protective efficacy of this candidate has not been reported in human volunteers. Phase 1 trials have been initiated.

Immunization with plasmid DNA has been another innovative approach. A plasmid DNA derived from an HCV genomic clone has induced humoral immunity to HCV proteins and cytotoxic T lymphocytes against HCV epitopes,[63] and the elongation factor 1-alpha promoter may be useful in the induction of T cell immunity.[64]

Immunization of chimpanzees with a plasmid DNA encoding the cell-surface E2 envelope protein of HCV[65] has been reported to produce variable levels of anti-E2 and cytotoxic T lymphocyte responses to E2.[66] Challenged with homologous monoclonal HCV, animals developed evidence of infection, but liver injury appeared earlier in the course of infection, and infection resolved completely in the vaccinated animals. In contrast, infection in the unvaccinated challenged chimpanzee became chronic. Although the small number of animals studied is a limitation of this work, this DNA vaccine appeared to modify infection.

Once an HCV vaccine is available, populations at risk will be studied. Potential candidates for effective HCV immunoprophylaxis are listed in Table 10–8.

Treatment of Acute Hepatitis C

A number of small studies indicate that interferon monotherapy during the acute phase of HCV infection reduces the risk of progression to chronic infection.[67] The role of combination therapy (interferon and ribavirin) in acute hepatitis C has yet to be established. Initiation of interferon or combination therapy shortly after the appearance of HCV RNA in the serum when serum ALT levels are still normal, during the incubation period, might be even more effective in reducing the risk of chronic infection, but data to support this notion are not available.

TABLE 10–8 ■ Potential Candidates for Hepatitis C Virus (HCV) Vaccine Immunoprophylaxis

Persons who inject illicit drugs or snort cocaine
Renal failure patients likely to receive long-term hemodialysis
Patients with blood-clotting disorders
Sexual partners of patients with HCV infection
Patients with non-HCV chronic liver diseases
Persons residing in or likely to return to prison or juvenile detention centers
Persons considering receipt of tattoos or bodypiercing
Health care workers regularly exposed to blood
Newborn of HCV-infected mothers

Treatment of Chronic Hepatitis C

Patients with elevated serum ALT levels and circulating HCV RNA are candidates for treatment. Treatment of patients with persistently normal ALT levels remains controversial. Pretreatment liver biopsy has been routine in clinical trials and has been widely recommended, but it increases costs without improving health outcomes.[68] It may be reasonable to reserve liver biopsy to aid management decisions in nonresponders to current treatment. HCV viral load measurement and HCV genotyping do not generally influence treatment decisions but have prognostic value regarding optimal length of treatment and the probability of a sustained virologic response. Among patients with sustained virologic responses, defined as being HCV RNA negative (undetectable) 6 months after completion of therapy, health-related quality of life improves, and the virologic, biochemical, and histologic responses are maintained in more than 95% of patients on prolonged follow-up (approaching 12 years).

Combination therapy consisting of interferon alfa-2b in its conventional dose of 3 MU given by subcutaneous injection three times weekly and the guanosine analogue, ribavirin, in an oral divided (twice daily) total dose of 1000 to 1200 mg, has resulted in sustained virologic response rates of about 40%.[69] Ribavirin has weak antiviral activity. Its efficacy when given with interferon may be a result of an anti-inflammatory or immunomodulatory action coupled with a mild inhibition of HCV polymerase. Among previously untreated patients, combination therapy given for 12 months has a sustained virologic response in just 28% of genotype 1 patients, who are most resistant to therapy. Sustained response rates for patients with HCV genotype 2 or 3 are about 60% to 70% when combination therapy is given for 6 months. Higher response rates are seen in women, in persons under 40 years of age, and in those with low viral loads.

Relapsing patients in whom HCV RNA reappears after discontinuing treatment will have about a 50% sustained virologic response rate following re-treatment with combination therapy for 6 months or treatment with interferon alfacon-1 in a dose of 15 µg three times weekly for 12 months. Re-treatment of nonresponders to interferon monotherapy remains unsatisfactory: sustained response rates are generally less than 15%.

The ubiquitous development of hemolytic anemia in ribavirin-treated patients and concerns about the drug's teratogenicity and mutagenicity, persisting for months after completion of therapy, suggest a cautious approach to the selection of patients. Discontinuation of therapy for adverse events occurs in 20% of treated patients compared with about 5% of patients receiving interferon monotherapy. Interruption of combination therapy for less than 2 weeks, however, does not decrease the response rate.

Antivirals in development include HCV serine protease inhibitors, helicase inhibitors, polymerase inhibitors, inhibitors of inosine monophosphate dehydrogenase, ribozymes, and oligonucleotides. Pegylated interferons, with delayed clearance from the circulation, and given in a once-a-week subcutaneous injection, appear to be nearly as effective as the combination of alpha interferon three times a week plus daily oral ribavirin. It is likely that pegylated interferons will replace current combination therapy, and that the combination of pegylated interferon plus ribavirin is the treatment of choice, with a sustained response rate of 40% to 55% in genotype 1 when given for 12 months and 75% to 85% in genotypes 2 and 3 when treatment is given for 6 months.

The use of histamine hydrochloride as an adjuvant to interferon appears promising,[70] but the results of prospective, randomized, and sufficiently powered controlled trials are not yet available. Combining interferon with amantidine does not improve virologic or biochemical response rates in previously untreated patients.[71]

It should be noted that histologic improvement and slowing of the progression of fibrosis may occur in the absence of complete HCV eradication in interferon-treated patients. Hence, continuing interferon monotherapy in patients who are virologic nonresponders may be beneficial. Proof of such an effect is not yet available, but trials of maintenance therapy with long-acting pegylated interferons have been initiated.

Although end-stage liver disease due to HCV infection is the single most common indication for liver transplantation in the United States, HCV infection recurs in nearly all surviving patients. Unfortunately the liver injury seen in this setting appears to be both aggressive and accelerated, increasing the occurrence of graft failure and death. Reinfection of second allografts can be expected. The combination of interferon and ribavirin given early in the posttransplant period as prophylaxis may reduce the likelihood of infection, but large-scale, long-term studies of efficacy and safety in this setting are not yet available, and studies with pegylated interferons with or without ribavirin are ongoing.[72]

REFERENCES

1. Gaeta GB, Stroffolini T, Charamonte M, et al: Chronic hepatitis D: A vanishing disease? An Italian multicenter study. Hepatology 2000;32:824–827.
2. Armstrong GL, Alter MJ, McQuillan GM, Margolis HS: The past incidence of hepatitis C virus infection: Implications for the future burden of chronic liver disease in the United States. Hepatology 2000;31:777–782.
3. Troisi CL, Hollinger FB, Krause DS, Pickering LK: Immunization of seronegative infant with hepatitis A vaccine (HAVRIX;SKB): A comparative study of two dosing schedules. Vaccine 1997;15:1613–1617.
4. Innis BL, Snitbhan R, Kunasol P, et al: Protection against hepatitis A by an inactivated vaccine. JAMA 1994;271:1328–1334.
5. Werzberger A, Mensch B, Kuter B, et al: A controlled trial of a formalin-inactivated hepatitis A vaccine in healthy children. N Engl J Med 1992;327:453–457.
6. Zurbriggen R, Novak-Hofer I, Seelig A, Gluck R: IRIV-adjuvanted hepatitis A vaccine: In vivo absorption and biophysical characterization. Prog Lipid Res 2000;39:3–18.
7. Ashur Y, Adler R, Rowe M, et al: Comparison of immunogenicity of two hepatitis A vaccines—VAQTA and HAVRIX—in young adults. Vaccine 1999;17:2290–2296.
8. Clemens R, Safary A, Hepburn A: Clinical experience with an inactivated hepatitis A vaccine. J Infect Dis 1995;171:S44–S49.
9. Werzberger A, Kuter B, Nalin D: Six years' follow-up after hepatitis A vaccination. N Engl J Med 1998;338:1160.
10. Walter EB, Hornick RB, Poland GA, et al: Concurrent administration of inactivated hepatitis A vaccine with immune globulin in healthy adults. Vaccine 1999;17:1468–1473.
11. Centers for Disease Control and Prevention: Prevention of hepatitis A through active or passive immunization: Recommendations of the Advisory Committee on Immunization Practices (ACIP). MMWR Recomm Rep 1996;45(RR-15):1–30.
12. Vento S, Garofano T, Renzini C, et al: Fulminant hepatitis associated with hepatitis A virus superinfection in patients with chronic hepatitis C. N Engl J Med 1998;338:286–290.
13. Keeffe EB, Iwarson S, McMahon BJ, et al: Safety and immunogenicity of hepatitis A vaccine in patients with chronic liver disease. Hepatology 1998;27:881–886.
14. Jacobs RJ, Koff RS: Cost-effectiveness of hepatitis A vaccination in patients with chronic hepatitis C. Hepatology 2000;32:873–874.
15. Dumot JA, Barnes DS, Younossi Z, et al: Immunogenicity of hepatitis A vaccine in decompensated liver disease. Am J Gastroenterol 1999;94:1601–1604.
16. McMahon BJ, Beller M, Williams J, et al: A program to control an outbreak of hepatitis A in Alaska by using an inactivated hepatitis A vaccine. Arch Pediatr Adolesc Med 1996;150:733–739.
17. Craig AS, Sockwell DC, Schaffner W, et al: Use of hepatitis A vaccine in a community-wide outbreak of hepatitis A. Clin Infect Dis 1998;27:531–535.
18. Piazza M, Safary A, Vegnente A, et al: Safety and immunogenicity of hepatitis A vaccine in infants: A candidate for inclusion in the childhood vaccination programme. Vaccine 1999;17:585–588.
19. Sagliocca L, Amoroso P, Stroffolini T, et al: Efficacy of hepatitis A vaccine in prevention of secondary hepatitis A infection: A randomised trial. Lancet 1999;353:1136–1139.
20. Thoelen S, Van Damme P, Leentvaar-Kuypers A, et al: The first combined vaccine against hepatitis A and B: An overview. Vaccine 1999;17:1657–1662.
21. Arankalle VA, Chadha MS, Dama BM, et al: Role of immune serum globulin in pregnant women during an epidemic of hepatitis E. J Viral Hepat 1998;5:199–214.
22. He J, Binn LN, Caudill JD, et al: Antiserum generated by a DNA vaccine binds to hepatitis E virus (HEV) as determined by PCR and immune electron microscopy (IEM): Application for HEV detection by affinity-capture RT-PCR. Virus Res 1999;62:59–65.
23. Tuteja R, Li TC, Takeda N, Jameel S: Augmentation of immune responses to hepatitis E virus ORF2 DNA vaccination by codelivery of cytokine genes. Viral Immunol 2000;13:169–178.
24. Tsarev SA, Tsareva TS, Emerson SU, et al: Recombinant vaccine against hepatitis E: Dose response and protection against heterologous challenge. Vaccine 1997;15:1834–1838.
25. Kamili S, Spelbring J, Krawczynski K: DNA vaccination protects nonhuman primates against hepatitis E virus. Hepatology 2000;32:380a.

26. Stuyver L, De Gendt S, Van Geyt C, et al: A new genotype of hepatitis B virus: Complete genome and phylogenetic relatedness. J Gen Virol 2000;81:67–74.

27. Lunn ER, Hoggarth BJ, Cook WJ: Prolonged hepatitis B surface antigenemia after vaccination. Pediatrics 2000;105:E81.

28. Monteyne P, Andre FE: Is there a causal link between hepatitis B vaccination and multiple sclerosis? Vaccine 2000;18:1994–2001.

29. Gellin BG, Greenberg RN, Hart RH, et al: Immunogenicity of two doses of yeast recombinant hepatitis B vaccine in healthy older adults. J Infect Dis 1997;175:1494–1497.

30. Liao S-S, Li R-C, Li H, et al: Long-term efficacy of plasma-derived hepatitis B vaccine: A 15-year follow-up study among Chinese children. Vaccine 1999;17:2661–2666.

31. McDermott AB, Cohen SB, Zuckerman JN, et al: Human leukocyte antigens influence the immune response to a pre-S/S hepatitis B vaccine. Vaccine 1999;17:330–339.

32. Zuckerman J: Hepatitis B third-generation vaccines: Improved response and conventional vaccine non-response—third generation preS/S vaccines overcome nonresponse. J Viral Hepat 1998;5(Suppl 2):13–15.

33. Larsen CE, Xu J, Lee S, et al: Complex cytokine responses to hepatitis B surface antigen and tetanus toxoid in responders, nonresponders and subject naïve to hepatitis B surface antigen. Vaccine 2000;18:3021–3030.

34. Davis HL, Suparto I, Weeratna R, et al: CpG DNA overcomes hyporesponsiveness to hepatitis B vaccine in orangutans. Vaccine 2000;18:1920–1924.

35. Geissler M, Tokushige K, Chante CC, et al: Cellular and humoral immune response to hepatitis B virus structural proteins in mice after DNA-based immunization. Gastroenterology 1997;112:1307–1320.

36. Prince AM, Whalen R, Brotman B: Successful nucleic acid based immunization of newborn chimpanzees against hepatitis B virus. Vaccine 1997;15:916–919.

37. Tacket CO, Roy MJ, Widera G, et al: Phase 1 safety and immune response studies of a DNA vaccine encoding hepatitis B surface antigen delivered by a gene delivery device. Vaccine 1999;17:2826–2829.

38. Chen H-L, Chang M-H, Ni Y-H, et al: Seroepidemiology of hepatitis B virus infection in children. Ten years of mass vaccination in Taiwan. JAMA 1996;276:906–908.

39. Harpaz R, McMahon BJ, Margolis HS, et al: Elimination of new chronic hepatitis B virus infections: Results of the Alaska immunization program. J Infect Dis 2000;181:413–418.

40. Yusuf HR, Daniels D, Smith P, et al: Association between administration of hepatitis B vaccine at birth and completion of the hepatitis B and 4:3:1:3 vaccine series. JAMA 2000;284:978–983.

41. Wu JS, Hwang L-Y, Goodman KJ, et al: Hepatitis B vaccination in high-risk infants: 10-year follow-up. J Infect Dis 1999;179:1319–1325.

42. Ogata N, Cote PJ, Zanetti AR, et al: Licensed recombinant hepatitis B vaccines protect chimpanzees against infection with the prototype surface gene mutant of hepatitis B virus. Hepatology 1999;30:779–786.

43. Andreone P, Caraceni P, Grazi GL, et al: Lamivudine treatment for acute hepatitis B after liver transplantation. J Hepatol 1998;29:985–989.

44. Reshef R, Sbeit W, Kaspa RT: Lamivudine in the treatment of acute hepatitis B. N Engl J Med 2000;343:1123–1124.

45. Niederau C, Heintges T, Lange S, et al: Long-term follow-up of HBeAg-positive patients treated with interferon alfa for chronic hepatitis B. N Engl J Med 1996;334:1422–1427.

46. Lin SM, Sheen IS, Chien RN, et al: Long-term beneficial effect of interferon therapy in patients with chronic hepatitis B virus infection. Hepatology 1999;29:971–975.

47. Wong JB, Koff RS, Tine F, Pauker, SG: Cost-effectiveness of interferon alfa-2b treatment for hepatitis B e antigen–positive chronic hepatitis B. Ann Intern Med 1995;122:664–675.

48. Boni C, Bertoletti A, Penna A, et al: Lamivudine treatment can restore T-cell responsiveness in chronic hepatitis B. J Clin Invest 1998;102(5):968–975.

49. Dienstag JL, Schiff ER, Wright TL, et al: Lamivudine as initial treatment for chronic hepatitis B in the United States. N Engl J Med 1999;341(17):1256–1263.

50. Dienstag JL, Schiff ER, Mitchell M, et al: Extended lamivudine retreatment for chronic hepatitis B: Maintenance of viral suppression after discontinuation of therapy. Hepatology 1999;30:1082–1087.

51. Schalm SW, Heathcote J, Cianciara J, et al: Lamivudine and alpha interferon combination treatment of patients with chronic hepatitis B infection: A randomized trial. Gut 2000;46:562–568.

52. Hadziyannis SJ, Papatheodoridis GV, Dimou E, et al: Efficacy of long-term lamivudine monotherapy in patients with hepatitis B e antigen–negative chronic hepatitis B. Hepatology 2000;32:847–851.

53. Huang YH, Wu JC, Tao MH, et al: DNA-based immunization produces Th1 immune responses to hepatitis delta virus in a mouse model. Hepatology 2000;32:104–110.

54. Lau DT, Kleiner DE, Park Y, et al: Resolution of chronic delta hepatitis after 12 years of interferon alfa therapy. Gastroenterology 1999;117:1229–1233.

55. Lau DT, Doo E, Park Y, et al: Lamivudine for chronic delta hepatitis. Hepatology 1999;30:546–549.

56. Glenn JS, Marsters JC Jr, Greenberg HB: Use of a prenylation inhibitor as a novel antiviral agent. J Virol 1998;72:9303–9306.

57. Piazza M, Sagliocca L, Tosone G, et al: Sexual transmission of the hepatitis C virus and efficacy of prophylaxis with intramuscular immune serum globulin. A randomized controlled trial. Arch Intern Med 1997;157:1537–1544.

58. Farci P, Alter HJ, Wong DC, et al: Prevention of hepatitis C virus infection in chimpanzees after antibody-mediated in vitro neutralization. Proc Natl Acad Sci USA 1994;91:7792–7796.

59. Farci P, Shimoda A, Wong D, et al: Prevention of HCV infection in chimpanzees by hyperimmune serum against the hypervariable region I (HVRI): Emergence of neutralization escape mutants in vivo. Hepatology 1995;22:220A.

60. Krawczynski K, Alter MJ, Tankersley DL, et al: Effect of immune globulin on the prevention of experimental hepatitis C virus infection. J Infect Dis 1996;173:822–828.

61. Choo QL, Kuo G, Ralston R, et al: Vaccination of chimpanzees against infection by the hepatitis C virus. Proc Natl Acad Sci USA 1994;91:1294–1298.

62. Houghton M, Choo QL, Kuo G, et al: HCV vaccine: Interim report. IX Triennial International Symposium on Viral Hepatitis and Liver Disease, Rome, April, 1996.

63. Gordon EJ, Bhat R, Liu Q, et al: Immune responses to hepatitis C virus structural and nonstructural proteins induced by plasmid DNA immunizations. J Infect Dis 2000;181:42–50.

64. Nishimura Y, Kamei A, Uno-Furuta S, et al: A single immunization with a plasmid encoding hepatitis C virus (HCV) structural proteins under the elongation factor 1-alpha promoter elicits HCV-specific cytotoxic T-lymphocytes (CTL). Vaccine 2000;18:675–680.

65. Forns X, Allander T, Rohwer-Nutterr P, Bukh J: Characterization of modified hepatitis C virus E2 proteins expressed on the cell surface. Virology 2000;274:75–85.

66. Forns X, Payette PJ, Ma X, et al: Vaccination of chimpanzees with plasmid DNA encoding the hepatitis C virus (HCV) envelope E2 protein modified the infection after challenge with homologous monoclonal HCV. Hepatology 2000;32:618–625.

67. Poynard T, Leroy V, Cohard M, et al: Meta-analysis of interferon randomized trials in the treatment of viral hepatitis C: Effects of dose and duration. Hepatology 1996;24:778–789.

68. Wong JB, Bennett WG, Koff RS, Pauker SG: Pretreatment evaluation of chronic hepatitis C. Risks, benefits, and costs. JAMA 1998;280:2088–2093.

69. McHutchison JG, Gordon SC, Schiff ER, et al: Interferon alfa–2b alone or in combination with ribavirin as initial treatment for chronic hepatitis C. N Engl J Med 1998;339:1485–1492.

70. Lurie Y, Nevens F, Hyle S, Gehlsen K: A phase II dose-ranging study of histamine dihydrochloride (Maxamine) and interferon -2b in naïve chronic hepatitis C patients:12- and 24-week analysis. Antiviral Ther 2000;5:61.

71. Zeuzem S,Teuber G, Naumann U, et al: Randomized, double-blind, placebo-controlled trial of interferon alfa2a with and without amantidine as initial treatment for chronic hepatitis C. Hepatology 2000;32:835–841.

72. Szabo G, Katz E, Bonkovsky HL: Management of recurrent hepatitis C after liver transplantation: A concise review. Am J Gastroenterol 2000;95:2164–2170.

section

6

Central Nervous System Infections

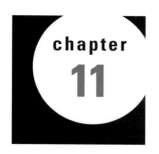

Therapy of Acute Bacterial Meningitis and Focal Intracranial Bacterial Infections

chapter 11

JOHN SEGRETI, MD
ALAN A. HARRIS, MD

Acute bacterial meningitis remains a significant cause of morbidity and mortality in the United States. The annual incidence is approximately three cases per 100,000 persons per year.[1] The most common etiologic agents vary according to the age of the patient and the presence of comorbidities. Until recently, *Haemophilus influenzae* type b was the most common cause of bacterial meningitis in childhood followed by *Neisseria meningitidis* and *Streptococcus pneumoniae*. Following the introduction of effective vaccines for *H. influenzae* type b, there has been a dramatic decline in the incidence of invasive disease due to this organism.[2] In fact many states now have no reported cases of meningitis, bacteremia, or epiglottitis due to *H. influenzae* type b. *S. pneumoniae* and *N. meningitidis* now are more common than *H. influenzae* type b in children.[3] Over the past few years there has been an alarming rise in multidrug resistance among pneumococci, requiring a modification of recommendations for the empiric and definitive therapy of pneumococcal meningitis.[4] In adults, *S. pneumoniae*, *N. meningitidis*, and *Listeria monocytogenes* are the most common organisms associated with community-acquired meningitis.[3] Group B streptococcus, *L. monocytogenes*, and gram-negative bacilli are common causes of meningitis in neonates.[3,5] In elderly, debilitated, or immunosuppressed patients, *S. pneumoniae*, *L. monocytogenes*, and gram-negative bacilli are important causes of meningitis.[3,5,6] Hospital-acquired bacterial meningitis remains unusual but now accounts for an increasing number of cases, especially in centers with active neurosurgical programs. The organisms most commonly associated with hospital-acquired meningitis are gram-negative bacilli, *Staphylococcus aureus*, coagulase-negative staphylococci, and streptococci.[7]

PHARMACOKINETICS AND PHARMACODYNAMICS OF ANTIBACTERIAL AGENTS FOR INFECTIONS OF THE CENTRAL NERVOUS SYSTEM

Much of our understanding of the use of antibiotics in the treatment of meningitis has been derived from animal models. These models allow us to distinguish in vivo activity from in vitro susceptibility. Successful eradication of bacteria from the cerebrospinal fluid (CSF) is determined by several factors including CSF penetration, antibacterial activity in the CSF, and the bactericidal activity of the drug.[8,9]

It is well known that drug kinetics in the CSF differs from that in other physiologic compartments.[8,9] The presence of the blood brain barrier is crucial in determining which antibiotics will penetrate into the CSF. The cited percentages of antibiotic CSF penetration are sometimes inconsistent. This is because of the methodologic differences between investigations.[8,9] For example, if the CSF is sampled at the same time as the serum, the CSF penetration may be underestimated, as the time to peak concentration in the CSF may be delayed. Following penetration into the CSF, the half-life in the CSF may be significantly longer than that in the serum.[8,9] Table 11–1 shows the CSF penetration of antibiotics commonly used to treat meningitis.

Lipid solubility, molecular size, and protein binding are important determinants of the ability to penetrate into the CSF.[8,9] The more lipophilic the compound, the better the CSF penetration. In general, smaller compounds penetrate better than larger more complicated compounds. Drugs with a high degree of protein binding do not penetrate as well as drugs that have a low degree of protein binding. In the presence of CSF inflammation or meningeal damage, even drugs with poor penetration may achieve concentrations adequate to treat meningitis.[8,9] The tight junctions between cerebral capillary endothelial cells are damaged in the presence of CSF inflammation, thus increasing the permeability of the blood brain barrier. As CSF inflammation resolves with appropriate therapy, the tight junctions are repaired, and CSF levels of the antibiotic will decline.[8,9]

β-Lactam antibiotics penetrate the uninflamed CSF poorly.[10–12] Their penetration into the CSF is greatly enhanced by meningeal inflammation.[10–21] Many types of penicillin achieve CSF concentrations of 5% to 55% of serum levels in the setting of meningitis.[20] Such levels are usually adequate for the treatment of meningitis due to susceptible gram-positive bacteria. Gram-negative rods (GNRs), however, with the exception of ampicillin-susceptible *H. influenzae*, are usually not adequately treated. First- and second-generation cephalosporins, except for cefuroxime, do not penetrate well into the CSF and should not be used to treat meningitis.[12] The third-generation cephalosporins, especially cefotaxime,

ceftriaxone, ceftazidime, and cefepime, achieve levels in the CSF adequate to treat susceptible *S. pneumoniae*, *H. influenzae*, and aerobic GNRs.[10–12,16,19,20] The carbapenems reach CSF levels in the range of 10% to 40% of serum values.[8,9] These concentrations are adequate for the above bacteria with the possible exception of some GNRs, such as *Pseudomonas*.

Aztreonam, a monobactam, has been shown to achieve CSF penetration adequate for treating susceptible GNRs, including *H. influenzae*, Enterobacteriaceae, and *Pseudomonas aeruginosa*.[13–15] Aztreonam has no microbiologic or pharmacologic advantage over third- or fourth-generation cephalosporins. In fact, it has no activity against the pneumococcus and other gram-positive cocci. It is especially useful, however, for empiric treatment of the patient with possible GNR meningitis and a history suggestive of IgE-mediated immediate hypersensitivity reactions to penicillin.[22]

Like the β-lactams, vancomycin does not penetrate well through uninflamed meninges.[23–26] However, adequate levels are achieved in the presence of meningeal irritation. Until recently there was little call for the routine use of vancomycin to treat bacterial meningitis. The emergence of penicillin- and cephalosporin-resistant pneumococci has given new prominence to vancomycin. The report of therapeutic failure in 4 of 11 patients with pneumococcal meningitis raised concerns about the adequacy of vancomycin in treating meningitis.[27] Recent studies in rabbits and humans showing adequate CSF levels of vancomycin have been reassuring.[23–26]

Fluoroquinolones penetrate well into the CSF, including uninflamed meninges.[8,9,28] Levels in the CSF approach 20% to 60% of serum levels. They would be expected to treat a variety of GNRs such as *H. influenzae* and *Escherichia coli*. Effectiveness in the therapy of pseudomonal, streptococcal, and staphylococcal meningitis, however, requires further study.

Metronidazole, a drug with a low molecular weight and simple chemical structure, penetrates well into the CSF.[8,9] Chloramphenicol, rifampin, sulfonamides, and trimethoprim are all highly lipid soluble and penetrate well into the CSF.[8,9] With the exception of TMP-SMX, these drugs have limited utility in the treatment of meningitis. TMP-SMX may be an appropriate drug for meningitis due to *Listeria* and susceptible GNRs, especially in the setting of penicillin allergy.[29,30] Rifampin is occasionally added to ceftriaxone and vancomycin to treat recalcitrant penicillin-resistant *S. pneumoniae* (PRSP) or staphylococcal meningitis.

Once an antibiotic penetrates the blood brain barrier into the CSF, it confronts the acidic pH that typically occurs with bacterial meningitis. Aminoglycosides are not active at low pH and thus tend to perform poorly in meningitis. Protein concentration is increased in purulent CSF, and drugs that have a high degree of protein binding are expected to perform poorly. Bacteria do not divide as rapidly in CSF, and so antibiotics that are primarily effective against dividing organisms have diminished activity.

TABLE 11–1 ■ Percent Penetration of Selected Antibiotics into the Cerebrospinal Fluid in Humans with Meningitis

Antibiotic	Penetration (%)
Penicillin G	7.8
Ampicillin	35
Nafcillin	5–27
Cefotaxime	27
Ceftazidime	20–40
Cefepime	10
Aztreonam	5
Imipenem	8.5
Meropenem	21
Aminoglycosides	<1
Ciprofloxacin	6–37
Trovafloxacin	23
Vancomycin	1–53
TMP-SMZ	24–35

Bactericidal antibiotics are preferred to bacteriostatic drugs.[31] Meningitis is an infection in an area of impaired host resistance. Low CSF concentrations of immunoglobulin and complement further add to the impaired bacterial killing, and purulent CSF adversely affects white blood cell activity. It has been estimated that the optimal killing of bacteria in the CSF is accomplished when drugs attain CSF concentrations at least ten times the minimum bactericidal concentration (MBC).[8,9]

The bactericidal activity of antibiotics can be characterized as either concentration dependent or time dependent. Aminoglycosides and fluoroquinolones demonstrate concentration-dependent killing.[8,9] In the serum, optimal killing of bacteria is achieved when the peak serum level exceeds the MIC of the organism by a factor of 10 or greater. Bacterial killing has also been associated with the area under the inhibitory curve (AUC). Killing of bacteria is optimal when the AUC exceeds the MIC of gram-positive bacteria by at least 30 times and of gram-negative bacteria by at least 125 times. Time above the MIC does not appear to be important for these antibiotics.[8,9]

Although data are few on the optimal dosing of aminoglycosides in the treatment of meningitis, animal data suggest that aminoglycosides exhibit concentration-dependent killing in the CSF as well as in the serum. One study of experimental *E. coli* meningitis showed that once-daily dosing was more effective than traditional dosing.[32] The optimal AUC/MIC ratio was ≥50. Given the poor penetration of these drugs into the CSF, intrathecal or intraventricular administration of aminoglycosides should improve outcomes. Studies of intraventricular and intrathecal lumbar injection of aminoglycosides, however, have been inconsistent.[33–37] Therefore the routine use of intrathecal or intraventricular aminoglycosides remains controversial. We suggest that intrathecal and intraventricular aminoglycosides be reserved for the patient who fails to respond to conventional therapy and for meningitis due to organisms resistant to conventional therapy.

The pharmacodynamic characteristics of fluoroquinolones are similar to those of aminoglycosides.[8,9] Higher CSF concentrations of fluoroquinolones are associated with improved bacterial killing in experimental meningitis. The AUC/MBC and peak/MBC ratios appear to be good predictors of bactericidal activity. As in nonmeningeal infections, a CSF peak/MBC ratio ≥10 appears to be predictive of bacterial eradication.[38–40]

Almost all other antibiotics, including penicillins, cephalosporins, and vancomycin demonstrate time-dependent killing. With these antibiotics, time above the MIC is critical. Optimal activity is achieved when the antibiotic maintains levels above the MIC for at least 40% of the dosing interval. Given the differences between serum and CSF pharmacokinetics, however, data obtained from serum concentration studies may not extrapolate well to the CSF. In most animal studies, optimal killing is seen when the CSF concentration of a time-dependent drug is above the MBC for more than 50% of the dosing interval. Therefore β-lactams and vancomycin should either be given as a constant infusion or dosed at frequent intervals. The duration of antibiotic therapy may also be important. Tauber et al were able to show that survival of rabbits with experimental pneumococcal meningitis improved when four doses of ampicillin were given over a 72-hour interval compared with the same amount of drug administered over 12- or 36-hour intervals.[41]

EMPIRICAL THERAPY

Once a diagnosis of bacterial meningitis is considered, a spinal tap should be performed and blood cultures obtained. The contraindications to lumbar puncture, the CSF studies required, and the differential diagnosis of the cellular, biochemical, and microbiologic studies are beyond the scope of this chapter. Administration of appropriate antibiotics should not be delayed while a brain CT or MRI scan is awaited. For the rare patient with focal neurologic findings who requires a CT scan prior to spinal tap, empiric antibiotic therapy should be given pending the scan. A short course of antibiotics will reduce the microbiologic yield to some degree. It is unlikely, however, that the white blood cell count, white blood cell differential, or the glucose or protein in the CSF will be significantly affected.[42]

When the clinical scenario or CSF findings suggest bacterial meningitis, appropriate antibiotics should be started that will have activity against the most likely organisms. *S. pneumoniae, N. meningitidis,* and *H. influenzae* are the organisms most commonly associated with community-acquired meningitis. Therefore, a third-generation cephalosporin such as ceftriaxone or cefotaxime is usually indicated.[43] In communities where high-level PRSP is common, it is recommended that vancomycin be added pending culture and antibiotic susceptibility results.[43] Once the organism has been identified, antibiotics can be adjusted on the basis of susceptibility patterns.

In elderly and immunosuppressed patients, *L. monocytogenes* should also be treated empirically. This requires the addition of high-dose ampicillin or penicillin in addition to the cephalosporin and vancomycin.[44–46] Vancomycin has in vitro activity against *L. monocytogenes*; however, clinical results have been mixed. Both treatment failures and successes have been reported.[44–46] With the declining incidence of *H. influenzae* as a cause of meningitis, we expect that *L. monocytogenes* will account for a larger proportion of cases of bacterial meningitis.

Enteric GNRs are also more common in elderly and immunosuppressed patients. Ceftriaxone and cefotaxime are usually adequate for most enteric GNRs. Aztreonam is an alternative in the penicillin-allergic patient.[22] Its CSF penetration has been found to be adequate to treat a susceptible GNR.[13–15] Of the carbapenems, imipenem is generally not recommended because of its epileptogenic potential.[47,48] Meropenem is less likely to trigger seizures and should be as effective as imipenem.[49] Carbapenem resistance in *P. aeruginosa*, however, is an issue of increasing importance. Quinolones may be alternatives in selected cases. A growing number of GNRs, however, especially *P. aeruginosa*, are becoming resistant to quinolones.

P. aeruginosa and *S. aureus* should be suspected in the postneurosurgical patient. Ceftazidime, cefepime, meropenem, or aztreonam along with vancomycin are appropriate in this setting.[50] Meningitis following neurosurgery can be exceedingly difficult to treat. Generally an antipseudomonal cephalosporin such as ceftazidime or cefepime is used. Concomitant intrathecal or intraventricular aminoglycoside should be considered for patients not responding to conventional therapy.

Suggestions for empiric antibiotic therapy based on the patient population are listed in Table 11–2.

SPECIFIC ANTIBIOTIC THERAPY (TABLE 11–3)

Haemophilus influenzae

Approximately one-third of *H. influenzae* B strains in the United States are β-lactamase producers and therefore resistant to ampicillin. Most β-lactamase-producing

H. influenzae B strains are susceptible to cefuroxime, but a recent clinical trial found lower rates of clearing of *H. influenzae* from the CSF with this drug than with ceftriaxone.[51] Therefore it is recommended that cefuroxime not be used for definitive therapy of *H. influenzae* meningitis. If *H. influenzae* B is not a β-lactamase producer, then ampicillin at a dose of 2 g IV every 4 hours is adequate. If the organism is a β-lactamase producer, then either ceftriaxone at a dose of 2 g IV every 12 hours or cefotaxime at 2 g IV every 4 to 6 hours is usually recommended. In general, ceftazidime does not offer any advantages over either cefotaxime or ceftriaxone.[52] A new fourth-generation cephalosporin, cefepime, is equivalent to cefotaxime for the treatment of bacterial meningitis in infants and children.[53] Meropenem is another alternative, but because of its cost is not considered first-line therapy.

Streptococcus pneumoniae

Over the last few years the incidence of resistance to penicillin among *S. pneumoniae* strains has increased[4] worldwide. Organisms that have a penicillin MIC of ≤ 0.06 μg/ml are considered susceptible. Organisms with an MIC of greater than 0.06 μg/ml but less than 1 μg/ml are called intermediately susceptible. *S. pneumoniae* strains with an

TABLE 11–2 ■ Recommended Empiric Antibiotic Therapy in Patients with Suspected Bacterial Meningitis

Age	Likely pathogen	Antibiotics	Alternatives
Neonate–3 mo	Group B streptococci, *Escherichia coli*, *Listeria monocytogenes*	Ampicillin and cefotaxime or ceftriaxone	Aztreonam and vancomycin
3 mo–5 y	*Neisseria meningitidis*, *Haemophilus influenzae*, *Streptococcus pneumoniae*	Cefotaxime or ceftriaxone and vancomycin if penicillin-resistant *S. pneumoniae* suspected	Aztreonam and vancomycin
5–50 y	*N. meningitidis*, *S. pneumoniae*	Cefotaxime or ceftriaxone and vancomycin	Aztreonam and vancomycin
Over 50 y	*S. pneumoniae*, Enterobacteriaceae, *L. monocytogenes*	Cefotaxime or ceftriaxone, vancomycin, and ampicillin	Aztreonam or TMP-SMX and vancomycin
Postneurosurgery	*Staphylococcus aureus*, *Pseudomonas aeruginosa*	Vancomycin and ceftazidime, cefepime, or meropenem	Aztreonam and vancomycin +/– an aminoglycoside

TABLE 11–3 ■ Pathogen-Specific Therapy for Bacterial Meningitis

Organism	Antibiotic	Alternative in patient with allergy
Streptococcus pneumoniae		
Penicillin susceptible	Penicillin G	
Penicillin intermediately susceptible	Cefotaxime or ceftriaxone	Vancomycin
Penicillin resistant	Cefotaxime or ceftriaxone and vancomycin	Vancomycin and rifampin
Haemophilus influenzae		
β-lactamase negative	Ampicillin	Aztreonam
β-lactamase positive	Cefotaxime or ceftriaxone	Aztreonam
Neisseria meningitidis	Ampicillin or penicillin G	Aztreonam
Listeria monocytogenes	Ampicillin +/– gentamicin	TMP-SMX
Staphylococcus aureus	Nafcillin or oxacillin	Vancomycin
Enterobacteriaceae	Ceftazidime, cefepime, or meropenem	Aztreonam or TMP-SMX
Pseudomonas aeruginosa	Ceftazidime, cefepime, or meropenem +/– intrathecal aminoglycoside	Aztreonam +/– aminoglycoside

MIC of ≥ 2 µg/ml are considered highly resistant (PRSP). Although the significance of PRSP in the treatment of non-meningeal infections continues to be debated, it is accepted that PRSP affects the management of bacterial meningitis. The optimal management of PRSP bacterial meningitis is still evolving, but it is clear that penicillin- and cephalosporin-resistant isolates have failed therapy with penicillin, cephalosporins, and chloramphenicol.[54] PRSP remains universally susceptible to vancomycin, and it is currently recommended that vancomycin be added to whatever regimen is initially started. A third-generation cephalosporin, such as ceftriaxone or cefotaxime, is usually given along with vancomycin.[54] This combination is synergistic in vitro against PRSP.[35] Some experts recommend continuation of both drugs in the setting of PRSP meningitis regardless of cephalosporin susceptibility.[54–56] Imipenem and meropenem have some activity against PRSP, but resistance is increasing. In a recent survey, 16% of all *S. pneumoniae* strains and 52% of PRSP strains were resistant to carbapenems.[4] Therefore it is recommended that vancomycin also be added when therapy consists of imipenem or meropenem. The recent reports of vancomycin-tolerant pneumococci are worrisome.[57–59] Although the clinical significance of this laboratory phenomenon is unknown, continued surveillance is necessary.

Traditionally, patients with bacterial meningitis who are clinically improving do not require repeat lumbar puncture. Many experts, however, recommend that patients with PRSP meningitis have a repeat spinal tap performed within 24 to 48 hours to determine that the infection is clearing.[54–56] If cultures remain positive on the repeat tap, rifampin should be added to the treatment regimen.

A number of new agents recently have been released that have activity against PRSP. Synercid is a member of the streptogramin family of antibiotics. It is a combination of two streptogramins, quinupristin and dalfopristin. Quinupristin-dalfopristin appears to inhibit bacterial growth by interfering with protein synthesis. Most PRSP and macrolide-resistant *S. pneumoniae* strains remain susceptible.[60] An intriguing finding has been that dalfopristin-quinupristin does not increase CSF concentrations of teichoic acid, lipoteichoic acid, and tumor necrosis factor.[61] Theoretically this should attenuate the inflammatory response in the CSF and thereby improve clinical outcomes. However, there are few clinical data on the effects of this drug combination for the treatment of pneumococcal meningitis. In a rabbit model of experimental pneumococcal meningitis, quinupristin-dalfopristin was less bactericidal than ceftriaxone.[60]

Another new drug with in vitro activity against PRSP is linezolid, a member of a new class of antibiotics known as oxazolidinones. In an animal meningitis model, linezolid penetrated well into the CSF.[62] Linezolid, however, was slightly inferior to ceftriaxone plus vancomycin in the treatment of a strain of PRSP. Linezolid was also less effective than ceftriaxone against a penicillin-susceptible pneumococcal strain.[62] It is unlikely that linezolid will be a primary therapy for the treatment of pneumococcal meningitis.

Quinolone antibiotics are not routinely considered in the treatment of pneumococcal meningitis. However, most PRSP strains remain susceptible to fluoroquinolones. Trovafloxacin and gatifloxacin have demonstrated bactericidal activity against PRSP in an animal model of meningitis.[39–41,63] Given the lack of clinical data and the potential for emergence of quinolone-resistant pneumococcal isolates, these drugs are currently not recommended for routine treatment of pneumococcal meningitis.

Neisseria meningitidis

N. meningitidis continues to be an important cause of community-acquired meningitis. Most isolates are β-lactamase negative and penicillin susceptible. Therefore, penicillin G or ampicillin are the drugs of choice for menigococcal meningitis. In the United States only about 3% of menigococci exhibit reduced susceptibility to penicillin.[64] High-level penicillin resistance has been described as a result of β-lactamase production, but to date such isolates are rare.[65] Third-generation cephalosporins are reasonable alternative therapies of menigococcal meningitis and are preferred if the organisms are β-lactamase producers.[66]

Listeria monocytogenes

L. monocytogenes meningitis is usually treated with ampicillin or penicillin G.[44–46] Consideration for the addition of an aminoglycocide reflects the demonstrated in vitro synergy and enhanced in vivo killing of *Listeria* with combination therapy in animal models.[67] Proof that combination therapy in humans is superior to ampicillin or penicillin alone is not available. Cephalosporins should not be used because of their lack of activity. In the penicillin-allergic patient, TMP-SMX has been found to be effective against *L. monocytogenes* and should be strongly considered.[44–46,68] Despite in vitro activity against *Listeria*, erythromycin and vancomycin have been associated with failure rates and are not recommended for definitive therapy. Meropenem is active in vitro, but there are no clinical data.[44–46]

Staphylococcus aureus

While *S. aureus* is often seen as a pathogen in the setting of recent neurosurgery, it is an unusual cause of community-acquired bacterial meningitis.[69–72] *S. aureus* accounted for 2.4% of community-acquired adult bacterial meningitis in Denmark.[70] The mortality was high— 43%. *S. aureus* meningitis could not be clinically distinguished from meningitis due to other pathogens. It was often associated with endocarditis and pneumonia.[70]

TABLE 11–6 ■ Empiric Antibiotic Therapy for Suspected Focal Intracranial Infection

Predisposing condition	Antibiotic	Alternative
Otitis media, mastoiditis, or sinusitis	Metronidazole and cefotaxime or ceftriaxone	Aztreonam, vancomycin, and Flagyl or aztreonam and clindamycin
Dental abscess	Penicillin G and metronidazole	Aztreonam, vancomycin, and Flagyl or aztreonam and clindamycin
Trauma or neurosurgery	Ceftriaxone or cefotaxime with vancomycin	Aztreonam, vancomycin, and Flagyl or aztreonam and clindamycin
Infective endocarditis	Vancomycin and gentamicin	Aztreonam, vancomycin, and Flagyl or aztreonam and clindamycin
Congenital heart disease	Cefotaxime or ceftriaxone	Aztreonam, vancomycin, and Flagyl or aztreonam and clindamycin
Unknown	Cefotaxime or ceftriaxone, vancomycin, and metronidazole	Aztreonam, vancomycin, and Flagyl or aztreonam and clindamycin

at 2, 4, and 6 months of age followed by a booster at 12 to 15 months.[108] The effectiveness of the protein-conjugate HiB vaccines is related to their excellent immunogenicity as well as their ability to reduce nasopharyngeal colonization.[2] Thus unimmunized children benefit from the lower rates of nasopharyngeal colonization in the community. An unresolved issue is the effect of simultaneous inoculation with multiple protein-conjugate vaccines.

Over 90% of the invasive meningococcal infections are due to serotypes A, B, and C.[109] The only meningococcal vaccine currently available in the United States is a quadrivalent vaccine that consists of the purified bacterial capsular polysaccharide of serotypes A, C, Y, and W-135. Unfortunately, serogroup B polysaccharide vaccine is poorly immunogenic.[109] Attempts to improve immune response by conjugating the polysaccharide antigen to a protein such as tetanus or diphtheria toxin are in progress.[110,111] The patient population that would most benefit from menigococcal vaccination is not known. Endemic, sporadic meningococcal disease is sufficiently uncommon that routine meningococcal vaccination is not justified.[100] The vaccine is relatively ineffective in children under 2 years of age. Protection in the absence of repeat exposure or a booster is for a relatively short duration.[100] Vaccination has proven to be effective in terminating outbreaks, however, especially those due to serotype C.[112,113] The use of meningococcal vaccine in populations potentially at risk, such as entering freshman college students living in dormitories or residence halls, is justified if the potential infection rate surpasses the endemic rate.[100] The Centers for Disease Control and Prevention and the Advisory Committee on Immunization Practices recently have issued guidelines for the use of meningococcal vaccine in college students. Routine vaccination is also recommended for persons at high risk of meningococcal disease.[100] These include persons with deficiency of the terminal components of complement and those who have functional or anatomic asplenia. The vaccine may also be useful in travelers to countries in which *N. meningitidis* is hyperendemic or epidemic.[100]

Close contacts of patients with meningococcal meningitis are at increased short-term risk of meningococcal disease; they may also have increased long-term risk. Therefore we recommend that close contacts of a patient with a vaccine-preventable strain receive vaccine in addition to chemoprophylaxis. Whether this will decrease the long-term risk of meningococcal disease is unknown at present.

The recent availability of a heptavalent pneumococcal protein-conjugate vaccine hopefully will result in a decline in invasive pneumococcal disease in children comparable to that seen for invasive HiB infection following vaccination.[114] Protein-conjugate vaccines have been developed because the polysaccharide vaccines are ineffective in children under 2 years of age. Although polysaccharide vaccines have been effective in preventing invasive pneumococcal disease in immunocompetent adults, results have not been as good in asplenic, immunosuppressed, or elderly persons.[115–121] The usual recommendation is to give the first dose at 2 to 6 months of age.[100] Two more doses are given at 2-month intervals and are followed by an additional dose at 12 to 15 months of age.[100] This schedule is identical to that of HiB vaccine, and concomitant inoculation with both vaccines has been shown to be safe and effective. Healthy children 24 to 59 months of age require a single injection.[100] Children of this age who have sickle cell disease, human immunodeficiency virus (HIV), asplenia, or other immunocompromising condition should receive two doses 2 months apart.[100] Protein-conjugate pneumococcal vaccine has been shown to be highly effective in preventing pneumococcal pneumonia and otitis media in children.[122] An ongoing study is evaluating the efficacy of protein-conjugate vaccines in preventing pneumococcal meningitis. It is also hoped that this vaccine will decrease nasopharyngeal colonization with *S. pneumoniae*. This should reduce horizontal transmission of pneumococci, including PRSP.

FOCAL INTRACRANIAL INFECTIONS

Cerebritis, brain abscesses, subdural empyema, epidural empyema, and suppurative thrombosis of the intracranial sinuses are focal intracranial processes associated with high morbidity and mortality. Timely diagnosis and therapy are imperative. It is necessary to maintain a high degree of suspicion for these entities as patients may present in a subtle or insidious manner.

Of the focal intracranial infections, brain abscesses are the most frequently seen. Nonetheless they are uncommon.[123] They are estimated to occur 50 times less often than brain malignancies. The annual incidence in the United States is about 1 in 10,000 hospital admissions.[123] Brain abscesses may arise from hematogenous spread, contiguous infection, or penetrating injury.[124–128] Hematogenous sources are more likely to result in multiple lesions—usually in the distribution of the middle cerebral artery. Infective endocarditis is the most common infection associated with hematogenous brain abscesses. Congenital heart disease (especially conditions with a right-to-left shunt with hypoxemia and cyanosis) and structural lung diseases (e.g., lung abscess, empyema, and bronchiectasis) may also result in hematogenous brain abscesses.[123–128] Brain abscesses related to a contiguous focus of infection are more likely to be solitary lesions. The location of the lesion suggests but does not prove the source of the infection. Temporal lobe abscesses are more likely to be associated with otitis media or mastoiditis. Frontal lobe abscesses are more likely to be seen in patients with sinusitis or a dental infection as the source. Approximately one-third of cases have no identifiable underlying source.[123]

Anaerobic bacteria or microaerophilic streptococci are present in about 70% of brain abscesses.[127,129] Most of these streptococci can be classified as *Streptococcus milleri*.[127,129] Other streptococci, including *S. pneumoniae* or β-hemolytic streptococci, are seen much less frequently. *S. aureus* and GNRs are also infrequent causes. Patient characteristics also affect the cause of brain abscess. Patients with abnormal cell-mediated immunity (e.g., HIV, high-dose steroids, cancer chemotherapy) are at greater risk for infection with organisms such as *L. monocytogenes*, *Toxoplasma gondii*, *Nocardia asteroides*, *Cryptococcus neoformans*, and mycobacteria.[123] Patients with neutropenia or severe neutrophil defects are more prone to infection with aerobic gram-negative bacteria and fungi.[123] Penetrating injuries put patients at risk for anaerobes, staphylococci, GNRs, soil mycobacteria, and fungi.[123] Brain abscess following a neurosurgical procedure more likely is due to staphylococci and GNRs.[123] Treatment of cerebral toxoplasmosis, fungi, and mycobacterial infections are detailed in other chapters.

Brain abscess remains a difficult diagnosis. Fewer than 50% of patients present with the classic triad of headache, fever, and focal neurologic defect.[123–128] Most patients present within 2 weeks of the onset of symptoms. However, the time course from onset of symptoms to establishment of the diagnosis ranges from a few hours to over a month. Once the diagnosis is entertained, a computed tomography (CT) scan with infusion of contrast or magnetic resonance imaging (MRI) with gadolinium should be obtained. The MRI is more sensitive than the CT and is preferred.[123] In fact, MRI may show a lesion even in the setting of a negative CT scan. Infections due to *Toxoplasma*, mycobacteria, and *Cryptococcus* often present as a homogeneous tissue mass on CT or MRI rather than as an abscess. If the CT or MRI shows a ring-enhancing lesion, neurosurgical consultation should be obtained to aspirate or remove the lesion. This is both a diagnostic and therapeutic procedure. Histopathology and culture of the biopsy or aspirate of the lesion reveals the identity of the infectious agent in 80% to 95% of cases.[123] Studies such as the peripheral leukocyte count, sedimentation rate, and C-reactive protein are not reliable in establishing or excluding a diagnosis of brain abscess. The yield from blood cultures is only about 10%.[130] Nonetheless blood cultures should be routinely obtained given their low cost, low morbidity, and ready availability. A positive blood culture should heighten consideration of underlying endocarditis. Performing a lumbar puncture in the setting of a brain abscess has been associated with increased morbidity and mortality and is usually contraindicated. Even when a lumbar puncture can be safely performed, the CSF findings are usually nonspecific and rarely help in establishing a diagnosis.[128]

The presence of a focal intracranial lesion, regardless of causes, may be associated with increased intracranial pressure.[98] Treatment of elevated intracranial pressure is detailed above and may consist of hyperventilation, hyperosmolar agents, or corticosteroids. Steroids have been most effective in the setting of severe cerebral edema and midline shift associated with intracranial malignancy.[127,131] These measures are usually of little benefit in the setting of brain abscess. A good outcome for patients with brain abscesses is dependent on definitive treatment with surgical intervention and antibiotics.

No study has yet to demonstrate that excision of the abscess is superior to aspiration. Therefore the timing and type of procedure should be individualized for each patient. Occasional patients may be considered for medical treatment alone. These are patients who are poor surgical candidates and whose mental status is unlikely to improve with surgery. The location of some abscesses, such as in the brain stem, may preclude a surgical procedure. The presence of multiple lesions may also make complete excision or drainage impractical but should not prohibit a diagnostic aspiration.

Anti-infective therapy should be initiated as soon as the diagnosis of brain abscess is strongly suspected and a diagnostic plan is defined. Although it is reasonable to withhold therapy in a clinically stable patient, it is unlikely that a few doses of antibiotics will adversely affect the microbiologic yield of a biopsy or aspirate. Viable bacteria have been obtained from patients treated with appropriate antibiotics for up to 10 days before aspiration.[127] Appropriate empiric therapy depends on the location of the abscess, the presence of single or multiple abscesses, and the immune status of the patient. In a patient with a single temporal lobe lesion, contiguous otitis media or mastoiditis should be suspected. For patients with a frontal lobe abscess, sinusitis or a dental source should be suspected. The most likely bacteria are streptococci, anaerobes, and Enterobacteriaceae. Empiric antibiotics should consist of a third-generation cephalosporin along with metronidazole with or without penicillin. *S. aureus* may be involved in frontal lobe abscesses. Brain abscess following a neurosurgical procedure is most likely due to staphylococci and gram-negative bacilli, including *Pseudomonas*. Empiric therapy should consist of vancomycin and an antipseudomonal β-lactam such as ceftazidime, cefepime, aztreonam, or meropenem. *Nocardia* should be considered in immunosuppressed persons and in patients with a lung abscess. TMP-SMX usually is suggested if *Nocardia* is suspected. Third-generation cephalosporins and meropenem, however, also have in vitro activity and should provide adequate coverage pending culture results. In patients with multiple abscesses, infective endocarditis, noncardiac sources of bacteremia, and toxoplasmosis should be considered as the source.[127] Vancomycin and gentamicin are appropriate if endocarditis is suspected. TMP-SMX is active against both *Nocardia* and *Toxoplasma*.

Once the cultures identify the organisms and susceptibility data are available, therapy should be adjusted. The optimal duration and route of antibiotic therapy are unknown. Many authorities suggest 2 to 6 weeks of IV antibiotics followed by 2 to 4 months of oral therapy if available.[123–127] We prefer 6 weeks of intravenous antibacterial therapy. This duration of therapy is usually adequate, and no further oral therapy is needed. Therapy needs to be individualized, however, based on follow-up clinical examination and CT or MRI scan. A scan may continue to appear abnormal at the completion of a course of therapy.[131] This does not necessarily call for prolonging the therapy. In fact, CT and MRI scans continue to improve with time even after antibiotics are discontinued.

Therapy recommendations will likely change as antibiotics with enhanced oral bioavailability become available. For example, there is no reason for metronidazole to be given intravenously if the patient has a functional gastrointestinal tract and is able to tolerate oral medications. Serum drug levels should be obtained if there is concern about adequate gastrointestinal absorption. There is never an indication for direct instillation of antibiotic into the brain.

Intracranial subdural empyema is a true medical emergency.[130] It is a collection of pus between the dura and the subarachnoid space and is seen primarily in post-neurosurgery patients, after trauma, or in the setting of sinusitis, mastoiditis, and otitis. Subdural empyema accounts for about 15% to 25% of focal intracranial infections.[130] MRI with gadolinium usually establishes the diagnosis. Neurosurgical intervention should occur as soon as possible. Pending culture and susceptibility data,

empiric antibiotic therapy should consist of vancomycin, metronidazole, and a third-generation cephalosporin. An antipseudomonal antibiotic should be used in the post-neurosurgery patient.

An intracranial epidural abscess consists of a collection of pus between the dura mater and the overlying skull.[130] The clinical settings and bacteriology of intracranial epidural abscesses are identical to those of intracranial subdural abscesses. Virtually all cases are associated with frontal sinusitis, mastoiditis, trauma, or a neurosurgical procedure.[130] As with other focal intracranial infections, therapy consists of drainage along with antibiotics that cover *S. aureus*, microaerophilic streptococci, GNRs, and anaerobes. This usually consists of a third-generation cephalosporin along with vancomycin and metronidazole. Antibiotics are adjusted on the basis of the antibiotic susceptibilities of the identified bacteria.

Thrombosis of the intracranial venous sinuses may complicate bacterial meningitis but is more likely to follow otitis media or mastoiditis.[132–134] This is uncommon today compared with the preantibiotic era. Suppurative thrombosis most commonly affects the cavernous sinus, lateral sinus, and the superior sagittal sinus. Severe headache, confusion, vomiting, and seizures should arouse suspicion of a venous sinus thrombosis. CT scan or MRI of the head usually suggests the diagnosis. Treatment includes appropriate antibiotics and measures to decrease the elevated intracranial pressure. The role of anticoagulation is unclear. Some authors suggest anticoagulation because of the potentially severe outcomes.[132–134] Controlled studies are needed but are unlikely given the rarity of this complication.

REFERENCES

1. Segreti J, Harris AA: Acute bacterial meningitis. Infect Dis Clin North Am 1996;10:797–809.
2. Adams WG, Deaver KA, Cochi SL, et al: Decline of childhood *Haemophilus influenzae* type b (HiB) disease in the HiB vaccine era. JAMA 1993;269:221–226.
3. Schuchat A, Robinson K, Wenger JD, et al: Bacterial meningitis in the United States in 1995. N Engl J Med 1997;337:970–976.
4. Whitney CG, Farley MM, Hadler J, et al: Increasing prevalence of multidrug-resistant *Streptococcus pneumoniae* in the United States. N Engl J Med 2000;343:1917–1924.
5. Sigurdardottir B, Bjornsson OM, Jonsdottir KE, et al: Acute bacterial meningitis in adults: A 20-year overview. Arch Intern Med 1997;157:425–430.
6. Behrman RE, Meyers BR, Mendelson MH, et al: Central nervous system infections in the elderly. Arch Intern Med 1989;149:1596–1599.
7. Durand ML, Calderwood SB, Weber DJ, et al: Acute bacterial meningitis in adults. N Engl J Med 1993;328:21–28.
8. Andes DR, Craig WA: Pharmacokinetics and pharmacodynamics of antibiotics in meningitis. Infect Dis Clin North Am 1999;13:595–618.
9. Lutsar I, McCracken GH, Friedland IR: Antibiotic pharmacodynamics in cerebrospinal fluid. Clin Infect Dis 1998;27:1117–1129.
10. Fong IW, Tomkins KB: Penetration of ceftazidime into the cerebrospinal fluid of patients with and without evidence of meningeal inflammation. Antimicrob Agents Chemother 1984;26:115–116.

11. Nau R, Prange HW, Muth P, et al: Passage of cefotaxime and ceftriaxone into cerebrospinal fluid of patients with uninflamed meninges. Antimicrob Agents Chemother 1993;37:1518–1524.

12. Cherubin CE, Eng RHK, Norrby R, et al: Penetration of newer cephalosporins into cerebrospinal fluid. Rev Infect Dis 1989;11:526–548.

13. McCracken GH, Sakata Y, Olsen KD: Aztreonam therapy in experimental meningitis due to *Haemophilus influenzae* type b and *Escherichia coli* K1. Antimicrob Agents Chemother 1985;27:655–656.

14. Modai J, Vittecoq D, Decazes JM, et al: Penetration of aztreonam into cerebrospinal fluid of patients with bacterial meningitis. Antimicrob Agents Chemother 1986;29:281–283.

15. Strausbaugh LJ, Bodem CR, Laun PR: Penetration of aztreonam into cerebrospinal fluid and brain of noninfected rabbits and rabbits with experimental meningitis caused by *Pseudomonas aeruginosa*. Antimicrob Agents Chemother 1986;30:701–704.

16. Latif R, Dajani AS: Ceftriaxone diffusion into cerebrospinal fluid of children with meningitis. Antimicrob Agents Chemother 1983;23:46–48.

17. Jacobs RF, Kearns GL, Brown AL, et al: Cerebrospinal fluid penetration of imipenem and cilastatin (primaxin) in children with central nervous system infections. Antimicrob Agents Chemother 1986;29:670–674.

18. Hieber JP, Nelson JD: A pharmacologic evaluation of penicillin in children with purulent meningitis. N Engl J Med 1977;297:410–413.

19. Del Rio M, McCracken GH, Nelson JD, et al: Pharmacokinetics and cerebrospinal fluid bactericidal activity of ceftriaxone in the treatment of pediatric patients with bacterial meningitis. Antimicrob Agents Chemother 1982;22:622–627.

20. Barrett FF, Eardley WA, Yow MD, et al: Ampicillin in the treatment of acute suppurative meningitis. J Pediatr 1966;69:343–353.

21. Modai J, Vittecoq D, Decazes JM, et al: Penetration of ceftazidime into cerebrospinal fluid of patients with bacterial meningitis. Antimicrob Agents Chemother 1983;24:126–128.

22. Segreti J, Trenholme GM, Levin S: Antibiotic therapy in the allergic patient. Med Clin North Am 1995;79:935–942.

23. Ahmed A: A critical evaluation of vancomycin for treatment of bacterial meningitis. Pediatr Infect Dis J 1997;16:895–903.

24. Ahmed A, Jafri H, Lutsar I, et al: Pharmacodynamics of vancomycin for the treatment of experimental penicillin- and cephalosporin-resistant pneumococcal meningitis. Antimicrob Agents Chemother 1999;43:876–881.

25. Krontz DP, Strausbaugh LJ: Effect of meningitis and probenecid on the penetration of vancomycin into cerebrospinal fluid in rabbits. Antimicrob Agents Chemother 1980;18:882–886.

26. Albanese J, Leone M, Bruguerolle B, et al: Cerebrospinal fluid penetration and pharmacokinetics of vancomycin administered by continuous infusion to mechanically ventilated patients in an intensive care unit. Antimicrob Agents Chemother 2000;44:1356–1358.

27. Viladrich PF, Gudiol F, Linares J, et al: Evaluation of vancomycin for therapy of adult pneumococcal meningitis. Antimicrob Agents Chemother 1991;35:2467–2472.

28. Nau R, Schmidt T, Kaye K, et al: Quinolone antibiotics in therapy of experimental pneumococcal meningitis in rabbits. Antimicrob Agents Chemother 1995;39:593–597.

29. Levitz RE, Quintiliani R: Trimethoprim-sulfamethoxazole for bacterial meningitis. Ann Intern Med 1984;100:881–890.

30. McConville JH, Manzella JP: Parenteral trimethoprim/sulfamethoxazole for gram negative bacillary meningitis. Am J Med Sci 1984;287:43–45.

31. Scheld WM, Sande MA: Bactericidal versus bacteriostatic antibiotic therapy of experimental pneumococcal meningitis in rabbits. J Clin Invest 1983;71:411–419.

32. Ahmed A, Paris MM, Trujillo M, et al: Once-daily gentamicin therapy for experimental *Escherichia coli* meningitis. Antimicrob Agents Chemother 1997;41:49–53.

33. Kaiser AB, McGee ZA: Aminoglycoside therapy of gram-negative bacillary meningitis. N Engl J Med 1975;293:1215–1220.

34. McCracken GH, Mize SG, Threlkeld N: Intraventricular gentamicin therapy in gram-negative bacillary meningitis of infancy: Report of the second neonatal meningitis cooperative study group. Lancet April 12, 1980, pp. 787–791.

35. Rahal JJ, Hyams PH, Simberkoff MS, et al: Combined intrathecal and intramuscular gentamicin for gram-negative meningitis: Pharmacologic study of 21 patients. N Engl J Med 1974;290:1394–1398.

36. McCracken GH, Mize SG: A controlled study of intrathecal antibiotic therapy in gram-negative enteric meningitis of infancy. J Pediatr 1976;89:66–72.

37. Swartz MN: Intraventricular use of aminoglycosides in the treatment of gram-negative bacillary meningitis: Conflicting views. J Infect Dis 1981;143:293–296.

38. Perrig M, Acosta F, Cottagnoud M, et al: Efficacy of gatifloxacin alone and in combination with cefepime against penicillin-resistant *Streptococcus pneumoniae* in a rabbit meningitis model and *in vitro*. J Antimicrob Chemother 2001;47:701–704.

39. Ostergaard C, Sorensen TK, Knudsen JD, et al: Evaluation of moxifloxacin, a new 8-methoxyquinolone, for the treatment of meningitis caused by penicillin-resistant *Pneumococcus* in rabbits. Antimicrob Agents Chemother 1998;42:1706–1712.

40. McCracken GH: Pharmacodynamics of gatifloxacin in experimental models of pneumococcal meningitis. Clin Infect Dis 2000;31:S45–S50.

41. Tauber MG, Kunz S, Zak O, et al: Influence of antibiotic dose, dosing interval, and duration of therapy on outcome in experimental pneumococcal meningitis in rabbits. Antimicrob Agents Chemother 1989;33:418–423.

42. Talan DA, Hoffman JR, Yoshikawa TT, et al: Role of empiric parenteral antibiotics prior to lumbar puncture in suspected bacterial meningitis: State of the art. Rev Infect Dis 1988;10:365–376.

43. Quagliarello VJ, Scheld WM: Treatment of bacterial meningitis. N Engl J Med 1997;336:708–716.

44. Blanot S, Boumaila C, Berche P: Intracerebral activity of antibiotics against *Listeria monocytogenes* during experimental rhombencephalitis. J Antimicrob Chemother 1999;44:565–568.

45. Bartt R: *Listeria* and atypical presentations of *Listeria* in the central nervous system. Semin in Neurol 2000;20:361–373.

46. Mylonakis E, Hohmann EL, Calderwood SB: Central nervous system infection with *Listeria monocytogenes*: 33 years' experience at a general hospital and review of 776 episodes from the literature. Medicine 1998;77:313–336.

47. Eng RHK, Munsif AN, Yangco BG, et al: Seizure propensity with imipenem. Arch Intern Med 1989;149:1881–1883.

48. Wong VK, Wright HT, Ross LA, et al: Imipenem/cilastatin treatment of bacterial meningitis in children. Pediatr Infect Dis J 1991;10:122–125.

49. Odio CM, Puig JR, Feris JM, et al: Prospective, randomized, investigator-blinded study of the efficacy and safety of meropenem vs. cefotaxime therapy in bacterial meningitis in children. Pediatr Infect Dis J 1999;18:581–590.

50. Morris A, Low DE: Nosocomial bacterial meningitis, including central nervous system shunt infections. Infect Dis Clin North Am 1999;13:735–750.

51. Schaad UB, Suter S, Gianella-Borradori A, et al: A comparison of ceftriaxone and cefuroxime for the treatment of bacterial meningitis in children. N Engl J Med 1990;322:141–147.

52. Norrby SR: Role of cephalosporins in the treatment of bacterial meningitis in adults: Overview with special emphasis on ceftazidime. Am J Med 1985;79:56–61.

53. Saez-Llorens X, Castano E, Garcia R, et al: Prospective, randomized, comparison of cefepime and cefotaxime for treatment of bacterial meningitis in infants and children. Antimicrob Agents Chemother 1995;39:937–940.

54. Friedland IR, McCracken GH: Management of infections caused by antibiotic-resistant *Streptococcus pneumoniae*. N Engl J Med 1994;331:377–382.

55. Klugman KP, Friedland IR, Bradley JS: Bactericidal activity against cephalosporin-resistant *Streptococcus pneumoniae* in cerebrospinal fluid of children with acute bacterial meningitis. Antimicrob Agents Chemother 1995;39:1988–1992.

56. Paris MM, Ramilo O, McCracken GH: Management of meningitis caused by penicillin-resistant *Streptococcus pneumoniae*. Antimicrob Agents Chemother 1995;39:2171–2175.

57. Novak R, Henriques B, Charpentier E, et al: Emergence of vancomycin tolerance in *Streptococcus pneumoniae*. Nature 1999;399:590–593.

58. McCullers JA, English BK, Novak R: Isolation and characterization of vancomycin-tolerant *Streptococcus pneumoniae* from the cerebrospinal fluid of a patient who developed recrudescent meningitis. J Infect Dis 2000;181:369–373.

59. Henriques Normark B, Novak R, Ortqvist A, et al: Clinical isolates of *Streptococcus pneumoniae* that exhibit tolerance of vancomycin. Clin Infect Dis 2001;32:552–558.

60. Tarasi A, Dever LL, Tomasz A: Activity of quinupristin/dalfopristin against *Streptococcus pneumoniae* in vitro and in vivo in the rabbit model of experimental meningitis. J Antimicrob Chemother 1997;39:121–127.

61. Heer C, Stuertz K, Reinert RR, et al: Release of teichoic and lipoteichoic acids from 30 different strains of *Streptococcus pneumoniae* during exposure to ceftriaxone, meropenem, quinupristin/dalfopristin, rifampicin and trovafloxacin. Infection 2000;28:13–20.

62. Cottagnoud P, Gerber CM, Acosta F, et al: Linezolid against penicillin-sensitive and -resistant pneumococci in the rabbit meningitis model. J Antimicrob Chemother 2000;46:981–985.

63. Paris MM, Hickey SM, Trujillo M, et al: Evaluation of CP-99,219, a new fluoroquinolone, for treatment of experimental penicillin- and cephalosporin-resistant pneumococcal meningitis. Antimicrob Agents Chemother 1995;39:1243–1246.

64. Brunen A, Peetermans W, Verhaegen J, et al: Meningitis due to *Neisseria meningitidis* with intermediate susceptibility to penicillin. Eur J Clin Microbiol Infect Dis 1993;12:969–970.

65. Campos J, Fuste MC, Trujillo G: Genetic diversity of penicillin-resistant *Neisseria meningitidis*. J Infect Dis 1992;166:173–177.

66. Tuncher AM, Ertem U, Ece A, et al: Once daily ceftriaxone for meningococcemia and meningococcal meningitis. Pediatr Infect Dis J 1988;7:711–713.

67. Scheld WM, Fletcher DD, Fink FN, et al: Response to therapy in an experimental rabbit model of meningitis due to *Listeria monocytogenes*. J Infect Dis 1979;140:287–294.

68. Winslow DL, Pankey GA: In vitro activities of trimethoprim and sulfamethoxazole against *Listeria monocytogenes*. Antimicrob Agents Chemother 1982;22:51–54.

69. Lu CH, Chang WN: Adults with meningitis caused by oxacillin-resistant *Staphylococcus aureus*. Clin Infect Dis 2000;31:723–727.

70. Lerche A, Rasmussen N, Wandall JH, et al: *Staphylococcus aureus* meningitis: A review of 28 consecutive community-acquired cases. Scand J Infect Dis 1995;27:569–573.

71. Jensen AG, Espersen F, Skinhoj P, et al: *Staphylococcus aureus* meningitis: A review of 104 nationwide, consecutive cases. Arch Intern Med 1993;153:1902–1908.

72. Kim JH, van der Horst C, Mulrow CD, et al: *Staphylococcus aureus* meningitis: Review of 28 cases. Rev Infect Dis 1989;11:698–706.

73. Wasson Dunne D, Quagliarello V: Group B streptococcal meningitis in adults. Medicine 1993;72:1–10.

74. Sepkowitz KA, Kasemsri T, Brown A, et al: Meningitis due to beta-hemolytic non-A, non-D streptococci among adults at a cancer hospital: Report of four cases and review. Clin Infect Dis 1992;14:92–97.

75. Radetsky M: Duration of treatment in bacterial meningitis: A historical inquiry. Pediatr Infect Dis J 1990;9:2–9.

76. Viladrich PF, Pallares R, Ariza J, et al: Four days of penicillin therapy for meningococcal meningitis. Arch Intern Med 1986;146:2380–2382.

77. Roine I, Ledermann W, Foncea LM, et al: Randomized trial of four vs. seven days of ceftriaxone treatment for bacterial meningitis in children with rapid initial recovery. Pediatr Infect Dis J 2000;19:219–222.

78. Bradley JS, Farhat C, Stamboulian D, et al: Ceftriaxone therapy of bacterial meningitis: Cerebrospinal fluid concentrations and bactericidal activity after intramuscular injection in children treated with dexamethasone. Pediatr Infect Dis J 1994;13:724–728.

79. Kilpi T, Anttila M, Kallio MJT, et al: Length of prediagnostic history related to the course and sequelae of childhood bacterial meningitis. Pediatr Infect Dis J 1993;12:184–188.

80. Radetsky M: Duration of symptoms and outcome in bacterial meningitis: An analysis of causation and the implications of a delay in diagnosis. Pediatr Infect Dis J 1992;11:694–698.

81. Talan DA, Zibulewsky J: Relationship of clinical presentation to time to antibiotics for the emergency department management of suspected bacterial meningitis. Ann Emerg Med 1993;22:1733–1738.

82. Kallio MJT, Kilpi T, Anttila M, et al: The effect of a recent previous visit to a physician on outcome after childhood bacterial meningitis. JAMA 1994;272:787–791.

83. Aronin SI, Peduzzi P, Quagliarello VJ: Community-acquired bacterial meningitis: Risk stratification for adverse clinical outcome and effect of antibiotic timing. Ann Intern Med 1998;129:862–869.

84. Lebel MH, Freij BJ, Syrogiannopoulos GA, et al: Dexamethasone therapy for bacterial meningitis: Results of two double-blind, placebo-controlled trials. N Engl J Med 1988;319:964–971.

85. Schaad UB, Lips U, Gnehm HE, et al: Dexamethasone therapy for bacterial meningitis in children. Lancet 1993;342:457–461.

86. Tauber MG, Sande MA: Dexamethasone in bacterial meningitis: Increasing evidence for a beneficial effect. Pediatr Infect Dis J 1989;8:842–845.

87. Girgis NI, Farid Z, Mikhail IA, et al: Dexamethasone treatment for bacterial meningitis in children and adults. Pediatr Infect Dis J 1989;8:848–851.

88. Kanra GY, Ozen H, Secmeer G, et al: Beneficial effects of dexamethasone in children with pneumococcal meningitis. Pediatr Infect Dis J 1995;14:490–494.

89. McIntyre PB, Berkey CS, King SM, et al: Dexamethasone as adjunctive therapy in bacterial meningitis: A meta-analysis of randomized clinical trials since 1988. JAMA 1997;278:925–931.

90. Wald ER, Kaplan SL, Mason EO Jr, et al: Dexamethasone therapy for children with bacterial meningitis: Meningitis Study Group. Pediatrics 1995;95:21–28.

91. Arditi M, Mason EO Jr, Bradley JS, et al: Three-year multicenter surveillance of pneumococcal meningitis in children: Clinical characteristics and outcome related to penicillin susceptibility and dexamethasone use. Pediatrics 1998;102:1087–1097.

92. Gupta A, Singh NK: Dexamethasone in adults with bacterial meningitis. J Assoc Physicians India 1996;44:90–92.

93. Qazi SA, Khan MA, Mughal N, et al: Dexamethasone and bacterial meningitis in Pakistan. Arch Dis Child 1996;75:482–488.

94. Rintala E, Seppala OP, Kotilainen P, et al: Protein C in the treatment of coagulopathy in meningococcal disease. Crit Care Med 1999;27:2849–2850.

95. Smith OP, White B, Vaughan D, et al: Use of protein-C concentrate, heparin, and haemodiafiltration in meningococcus-induced purpura fulminans. Lancet 1997;350:1590–1593.

96. Sheridan RL, Briggs SE, Remensnyder JP, et al: Management strategy in purpura fulminans with multiple organ failure in children. Burns 1996;22:53–56.

97. Bernard GR, Vincent J-L, Laterre P-F, et al: Efficacy and safety of recombinant human activated protein C for severe sepsis. N Engl J Med 2001;344:699–709.

98. Rauf SJ, Roberts NJ Jr: Supportive management in bacterial meningitis. Infect Dis Clin North Am 1999;13:647–659.

99. Zangwill KM, Schuchat A, Riedo FX, et al: School-based clusters of meningococcal disease in the United States. JAMA 1997;277:389–395.

100. Centers for Disease Control and Prevention: Prevention and Control of Meningococcal Disease in College Students: Recommendations of the Advisory Committee on Immunization Practices (ACIP). MMWR – Recommendations and Reports, June 30, 2000, vol 49, No. RR-7.

101. Peltola H: Prophylaxis of bacterial meningitis. Infect Dis Clin North Am 1999;13:685–710.

102. De Wals P, Hertoghe L, Borlee-Grimee I, et al: Meningococcal disease in Belgium: Secondary attack rate among household, day-care nursery and pre-elementary school contacts. J Infect 1981;3:53–61.

103. Dworzack DL, Sanders CC, Horowitz EA, et al: Evaluation of single-dose ciprofloxacin in the eradication of *Neisseria meningitidis* from nasopharyngeal carriers. Antimicrob Agents Chemother 1988;32:1740–1741.

104. Schwartz B, Al-Ruwais A, A'ashi J, et al: Comparative efficacy of ceftriaxone and rifampin in eradicating pharyngeal carriage of group A *Neisseria meningitidis*. Lancet, June 4, 1988, pp. 1239–1242.

105. Renkonen O-V, Sivonen A, Visakorpi R: Effect of ciprofloxacin on carrier rate of *Neisseria meningitidis* in army recruits in Finland. Antimicrob Agents Chemother 1987;31:962–963.

106. Takala AK, Eskola J, Peltola H, et al: Epidemiology of invasive *Haemophilus influenzae* type b disease among children in Finland before vaccination with *Haemophilus influenzae* type b conjugate vaccine. Pediatr Infect Dis J 1989;8:297–302.

107. Booy R, Hodgson S, Carpenter L, et al: Efficacy of *Haemophilus influenzae* type b conjugate vaccine PRP-T. Lancet 1994;344:362–366.

108. Centers for Disease Control and Prevention: Recommended Childhood Immunization Schedule – United States, 2001. MMWR Weekly, January 12, 2001;50(01):7–10, 19.

109. Rosenstein NE, Perkins BA, Stephens DS, et al: Meningococcal disease. N Engl J Med 2001;344:1378–1388.

110. MacLennan JM, Shackley F, Heath PT, et al: Safety, immunogenicity, and induction of immunologic memory by serogroup C meningococcal conjugate vaccine in infants: A randomized controlled trial. JAMA 2000;283:2795–2801.

111. Tappero JW, Lagos R, Maldonado-Ballesteros A, et al: Immunogenicity of 2 serogroup B outer-membrane protein meningococcal vaccines: A randomized controlled trial in Chile. JAMA 1999;281:1520–1527.

112. Rosenstein N, Levine O, Taylor JP, et al: Efficacy of meningococcal vaccine and barriers to vaccination. JAMA 1998;279:435–439.

113. De Wals P, De Serres G, Niyonsenga T: Effectiveness of a mass immunization campaign against serogroup C meningococcal disease in Quebec. JAMA 2001;285:177–181.

114. Centers for Disease Control and Prevention: Preventing pneumococcal disease among infants and young children: Recommendations of the Advisory Committee on Immunization Practices (ACIP). MMWR, October 6, 2000;49 (No. RR-9).

115. Sims RV, Steinmann WC, McConville JH, et al: The clinical effectiveness of pneumococcal vaccine in the elderly. Ann Intern Med 1988;108:653–657.

116. Weaver M, Krieger J, Castorina J, et al: Cost-effectiveness of combined outreach for the pneumococcal and influenza vaccines. Arch Intern Med 2001;161:111–120.

117. Shapiro ED, Berg AT, Austrian R, et al: The protective efficacy of polyvalent pneumococcal polysaccharide vaccine. N Engl J Med 1991;325:1453–1460.

118. Breiman RF, Keller DW, Phelan MA, et al: Evaluation of effectiveness of the 23-valent pneumococcal capsular polysaccharide vaccine for HIV-infected patients. Arch Intern Med 2000;160:2633–2638.

119. Simberkoff MS, Cross AP, Al-Ibrahim M, et al: Efficacy of pneumococcal vaccine in high-risk patients. N Engl J Med 1986;315:1318–1327.

120. Forrester HL, Jahnigen DW, LaForce FM: Inefficacy of pneumococcal vaccine in a high-risk population. Am J Med 1987;83:425–430.

121. Bolan G, Broome CV, Facklam RR, et al: Pneumococcal vaccine efficacy in selected populations in the United States. Ann Intern Med 1986;104:1–6.

122. Eskola J, Kilpi T, Palmu A, et al: Efficacy of a pneumococcal conjugate vaccine against acute otitis media. N Engl J Med 2001;344:403–409.

123. Fischer SA, Harris AA: Brain abscess. In: Gorbach SL, Bartlett JS, Blacklow NR (eds): Infectious Diseases, 2nd ed. Philadelphia, WB Saunders, 1998, pp 1431–1444.

124. Jadavji T, Humphreys RP, Prober CG: Brain abscesses in infants and children. Pediatr Infect Dis 1985;4:394–398.

125. Brewer NS, MacCarty CS, Wellman WE: Brain abscess: A review of recent experience. Ann Intern Med 1975;82:571–576.

126. Saez-Llorens XJ, Umana MA, Odio CM, et al: Brain abscess in infants and children. Pediatr Infect Dis J 1989;8:449–458.

127. Chun CH, Johnson JD, Hofstetter M, et al: Brain abscess: A study of 45 consecutive cases. Medicine 1986;65:415–431.

128. Gelfand MS, Stephens DS, Howell EI, et al: Brain abscess: Association with pulmonary arteriovenous fistula and hereditary hemorrhagic telangiectasia: Report of three cases. Am J Med 1988;85:718–720.

129. Ariza J, Casanova A, Fernandez Viladrich P, et al: Etiological agent and primary source of infection in 42 cases of focal intracranial suppuration. J Clin Microbiol 1986;24:899–902.

130. Heilpern KL, Lorber B: Focal intracranial infections. Infect Dis Clin North Am 1996;10:879–898.

131. Whelan MA, Hilal SK: Computed tomography as a guide in the diagnosis and follow-up of brain abscesses. Radiology 1980;135:663–671.

132. Pfister HW, Borasio GD, Dirnagl U, et al: Cerebrovascular complications of bacterial meningitis in adults. Neurology 1992;42:1497–1504.

133. DiNubile MJ, Boom WH, Southwick FS: Septic cortical thrombophlebitis. J Infect Dis 1990;161:1216–1220.

134. Southwick FS, Richardson EP Jr, Swartz MN: Septic thrombosis of the dural venous sinuses. Medicine 1986;65:82–106.

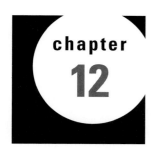

chapter

12

Viral Infections of the Central Nervous System

KEVIN CASSADY, MD
JOHN W. GNANN, MD
RICHARD J. WHITLEY, MD

Encephalitis is an unusual manifestation of, for the most part, common human viral infections. Although many people develop systemic viral infections, only a few develop symptomatic infection of the central nervous system (CNS). Viruses vary widely in their potential to produce significant CNS infection. For some viruses (e.g., mumps), CNS infection is a common but a relatively benign component of the clinical syndrome. For others (e.g., Japanese encephalitis), neurologic disease is the most prominent clinical feature of the systemic infection. A third group of viruses are those that commonly cause infection, but only rarely cause encephalitis (e.g., herpes simplex virus [HSV]). Lastly there are viruses for which human infection inevitably and exclusively results in CNS disease (e.g., rabies). In addition to acute pathology, other viruses (e.g., measles or influenza) can cause syndromes of postinfectious encephalopathy.

CNS symptoms usually include headache, lethargy, and impaired psychomotor performance. The infections that cause these symptoms have tremendous importance because of the potential for death and neurologic damage. Neural tissues are exquisitely sensitive to metabolic derangements, and injured brain tissue recovers slowly and often incompletely.[1,2] Clinical presentation and patient history, although frequently suggestive of a diagnosis, remain unreliable methods for determining the specific cause of CNS disease.[3,4] Tumors, infections, and autoimmune processes in the CNS often produce similar signs and symptoms.[4]

DEFINITIONS

The definitions of viral CNS disease are often based on both virus tropism and disease duration. Inflammation can occur at multiple sites within the CNS and accounts for the myriad clinical descriptors of viral neurologic disease. Inflammation of the spinal cord, leptomeninges, dorsal nerve roots, or nerves results in myelitis, meningitis, radiculitis, and neuritis, respectively. Aseptic meningitis is a misnomer frequently used to refer to a benign, self-limited, viral infection causing inflammation of the leptomeninges.[5,6] The term hinders epidemiologic studies, as the definition fails to differentiate between infectious (fungal, tuberculous, viral, or other infectious organisms) and noninfectious causes of meningitis. Encephalitis refers to inflammation of

Studies performed by the authors and herein reported were initiated and supported under a contract (NO1-AI-62554) with the Development and Applications Branch of the National Institute of Allergy and Infectious Diseases (NIAID), a Program Project Grant (PO1 AI 24009), by grants from the General Clinical Research Center Program (RR-032), and the State of Alabama.

parenchymal brain tissue and is usually accompanied by an altered level of consciousness, altered cognition, and frequently focal neurologic signs. Acute encephalitis occurs over a relatively short time (days), whereas chronic encephalitis presents over weeks to months. The temporal course of slow infections of the CNS (kuru, visna, variant Creutzfeldt-Jacob disease) overlaps with the chronic encephalitides. Slow infections of the CNS are distinguished by their long incubation period and eventually result in death or extreme neurologic disability.[7]

Viral disease in the CNS can also be classified by pathogenesis. Neurologic disease is frequently categorized as either primary or postinfectious. Primary encephalitis results from direct viral entry into the CNS that produces clinically evident cortical or brainstem dysfunction.[8] Subsequent damage results from a combination of virus-induced cytopathic effects and the host immune response. Viral invasion, however, remains the initiating event.[8] The parenchyma exhibits neuronophagia and the presence of viral antigens or nucleic acids.[8] A

postinfectious encephalitis produces signs and symptoms of encephalitis, temporally associated with a systemic viral infection, without evidence of direct viral invasion in the CNS. Pathologic specimens demonstrate demyelination, perivascular aggregation of immune cells, but no evidence of virus or viral antigen, leading some to hypothesize an autoimmune etiology.[8]

Meningitis and encephalitis represent separate clinical entities; however, there is a continuum between these distinct forms of disease. With the exception of rabies, any other neurotropic virus can cause meningitis, encephalitis, or a combination of the two (meningoencephalitis). A change in a patient's clinical condition can reflect disease progression with involvement of different regions of the brain. Therefore in many cases it is difficult to accurately and prospectively predict the cause and extent of CNS infection. Epidemiologic data in many cases provide clues to the cause of the illness. An overview is difficult, as each pathogen fills a different ecologic niche with unique seasonal, host, and vector properties. (Tables 12–1 to 12–3).[9] Instead it is useful to

TABLE 12–1 ■ DNA VIRUSES: Type of Disease, Epidemiologic Data, and Pathogenesis of Viral Infections of the CNS

Viral agent	CNS disease	Temporal course	Transmission	Pathway to CNS	Relative frequency	Laboratory confirmation
HERPESVIRIDAE						
Herpes simplex virus type 1 (HSV-1)	Encephalitis Meningo-encephalitis	Acute Congenital Sporadic reactivation	Human	Neuronal Blood	+++	CSF PCR Cell culture: brain biopsy sample
HSV-2	Meningitis	Primary or recurrent			++	Cell culture: genital, rectal, skin CSF PCR
Varicella zoster virus (VZV)	Cerebellitis Encepahlitis Meningitis Myelitis	Postinfectious Acute and latent reactivation (zoster)		Blood Neuronal	++	Clinical findings Cell culture from a lesion Brain biopsy Necroscopy rarely
Human herpes virus 6 (HHV-6)	Encephalitis Febrile seizures	Acute		Blood	?	Culture, PCR (high frequency of detection) Unknown significance
B Virus	Latent form? Encephalitis	Acute	Animal bite and human	Neuronal	+	Culture
Cytomegalovirus (CMV)	Encephalitis (immuno-suppressed and neonate)	Acute Subacute		Blood	++	PCR Cell culture: brain biopsy or CSF
Epstein-Barr virus (EBV)	Encephalitis Meningitis Myelitis Guillain-Barré	Acute			+	PCR
ADENOVIRIDAE						
Adenovirus	Meningitis Encephalitis	Acute	Human	Blood	+	Cell culture of CSF or brain
POXVIRIDAE						
Vaccinia virus	Encephalo-myelitis	Postinfectious	Vaccine	Blood	Extinct	Recent vaccination

Frequency: +++, frequent; ++, infrequent; +, rare; ?, unknown.
CSF, cerebrospinal fluid; PCR, polymerase chain reaction.

TABLE 12–2 ■ RNA Viruses: Type of Disease, Epidemiologic Data, and Pathogenesis of Viral Infections of the CNS

Viral taxonomy	CNS disease	Case fatality rate	Vector	Geographic distribution
TOGAVIRIDAE: ALPHAVIRUS (ARBOVIRUS)				
Western equine encephalitis virus	Meningitis Encephalitis	3%–10%	Mosquito Birds	United States west of Mississippi river
Eastern equine encephalitis virus		>30%		United States in Atlantic and Gulf Coast states
Venezuelan equine encephalitis virus		<1%	Mosquito Horses	Central and South America Southwestern United States and Florida
FLAVIVIRIDAE: FLAVIVIRUS (ARBOVIRUS)				
Japanese encephalitis virus	Meningitis Encephalitis	25%	Mosquito Swine Birds	Japan, China, Korea, Taiwan, Southeast Asia, India, Nepal
St. Louis encephalitis virus		7%		United States
West Nile fever virus		Higher attack rate in elderly 11%–33%		Africa, Middle East, India, Eastern Europe; imported into United States, in 1999
Murray Valley virus	Encephalitis	20%–60%		Australia
Tick-borne encephalitis virus (TBE complex)		20%	Tick Unpasteurized milk	Eastern Russia and Central Europe
BUNYAVIRIDAE (ARBOVIRUS)				
California (La Cross) encephalitis virus	Meningitis Encephalitis	<1%	Mosquito Rodents	Northern Midwest and Northeastern United States
REOVIRIDAE: COLTIVIRUS (ARBOVIRUS)				
Colorado tick fever virus	Meningitis Encephalitis	<1%	Tick Rodents	Rocky Mountains and Pacific Coast states in United States
PICORNAVIRIDAE (ENTEROVIRUS)				
Poliovirus	Meningitis Myelitis	4.5%–50%*	Fecal oral	Worldwide
Coxsackievirus	Meningitis	Rarely†		
Echovirus	Meningo- encephalitis Myelitis			
PARAMYXOVIRIDAE (EXANTHEMATOUS VIRUS)				
Measles virus	Encephalitis Subacute selerosing panen- cephalitis	15%	Postinfectious Blood	Worldwide
Mumps virus	Meningitis Encephalitis Myelitis	<1%	Blood	
ORTHOMYXOVIRIDAE (UPPER RESPIRATORY TRACT VIRUS)				
Influenza viruses	Encephalitis	<1%	Postinfectious	Worldwide
RHABDOVIRIDAE				
Rabies	Encephalitis Encephalo- myelitis	~100%	Mammal	Worldwide
RETROVIRIDAE				
Human immunodeficiency virus type 1 (HIV-1)	Encephalopathy Encephalitis Leukoen- cephalopathy	Majority	Human	Worldwide
ARENAVIRIDAE				
Lymphocytic choriomenigitis virus	Meningitis Encephalitis	<2.5%	Rodent	Worldwide

*The case fatality rate from poliomyelitis is increased in sporadic cases. With vaccination the epidemic forms of polio have decreased, as has morbidity. In turn the calculated case fatality rate in the United States has increased as sporadic and vaccine-associated disease has increased relative to the number of cases of disease.

†Rarely fatal except in nenonates and agammaglobulinemic patients in whom case fatality rates can approach 50% even with treatment.

TABLE 12–3 ■ RNA Viruses: Type of Disease, Epidemiologic Data, and Pathogenesis of Viral Infections of the CNS

Viral taxonomy	Disease pattern	Pathway to CNS	Frequency	Laboratory confirmation
TOGAVIRIDAE: ALPHAVIRUS (ARBOVIRUS)				
Western equine encephalitis virus	Epidemic	Blood	++	Serologic titers (HI, CF, NA, IFA) Viral antigen detection in brain Rarely culture
Eastern equine encephalitis virus	Sporadic		+	Viral culture or antigen detection in brain Serologic titers (HI, CF, NA, IFA) CSF IgM ELISA
Venezuelan equine encephalitis virus	Sporadic Epidemic		+	Serologic titers (HI, CF, NA, IFA) CSF IgM ELISA
FLAVIVIRIDAE: FLAVIVIRUS (ARBOVIRUS)				
Japanese encephalitis virus	Epidemic Endemic	Blood	+++	Peripheral blood ELISA Serologic titers (HI, CF, NA, IFA) CSF antigen tests or PCR
St. Louis encephalitis virus			+++	CSF IgM ELISA Serologic titers (HI, CF, NA, IFA) PCR Rarely culture
West Nile fever virus			+	Rarely culture Serology (HI, IFA), PCR
Murray Valley virus			++	Viral culture Serologic titer (HI, CF, NA)
Tick-born encephalitis virus (TBE complex)	Epidemic Sporadic		++	Serologic titer (HI, CF, NA) IgM ELISA PCR
BUNYAVIRIDAE (ARBOVIRUS)				
California (La Crosse virus [LCV]) encephalitis virus (CEV)	Endemic	Blood	+++ (LCV) + (CEV)	Viral culture CSF IgM ELISA Serologic titers (HI, CF, NA, IFA, CIE) PCR
REOVIRIDAE: COLTIVIRUS (ARBOVIRUS)				
Colorado tick fever virus	Endemic	Blood	+	Antigen detection on RBC membrane Viral culture Serologic titers (HI, CF, NA, IFA)
PICORNAVIRIDAE: ENTEROVIRUS				
Poliovirus	Endemic	Blood and neuronal	++	Viral culture CSF or Brain Viral culture from other site Serologic testing for some serotypes PCR
Coxsackievirus		Blood	+++	
Echovirus			+++	
PARAMYXOVIRIDAE (EXANTHEMATOUS VIRUS)				
Measles virus	Sporadic	Blood	++	Serology ELISA Clinical examination
Mumps virus			+++	CSF viral culture
ORTHOMYXOVIRIDAE (UPPER RESPIRATORY TRACT VIRUS)				
Influenza viruses	Sporadic	Blood	+	Viral culture from another site
RHABDOVIRIDAE				
Rabies	Sporadic	Neuronal	+++	Antigen detection in brain Serologic tests (IFA, CF, HA, CIE) Viral culture
RETROVIRIDAE				
Human immunodeficiency virus type 1 (HIV-1)	?Progressive	Blood	++	CSF PCR Autopsy samples MRI findings Isolation in situ Antigen detection

Continued

TABLE 12–3 ■ RNA Viruses: Type of Disease, Epidemiologic Data, and Pathogenesis of Viral Infections of the CNS (*Continued*)

Viral taxonomy	Disease pattern	Pathway to CNS	Frequency	Laboratory confirmation
ARENAVIRIDAE				
Lymphocytic choriomenigitis virus	Sporadic	Blood	+	CSF and blood culture Urine culture Serology

CF, complement fixation; CIE, counter-immunoelectrophoresis; CSF, cerebrospinal fluid; ELISA, enzyme-linked immunosorbent assay; HI, hemagglutination inhibition; IFA, immunofluorescent antibody; IgM, immunoglobulin M; MRI, magnetic resonance imaging; NA, neutralizing antibody titer; PCR, polymerase chain reaction.)
Frequency: +++, frequent; ++, infrequent; +, Rare; ?, unknown.

analyze the prototypes of viral CNS infection, meningitis, and encephalitis and the approach to patients with presumed viral infections of the CNS.

VIRAL MENINGITIS

Epidemiology

Acute viral meningitis and meningoencephalitis represent most viral CNS infections and frequently occur in epidemics or in seasonal distribution.[9,10] Enteroviruses cause an estimated 90% of cases (in countries that immunize against mumps), whereas arboviruses constitute most of the remaining reported cases in the United States.[5,11–13] Mumps is also an important cause of viral CNS disease in countries that do not immunize against this virus. In a recent study performed in Japan, mumps infection was the second leading cause of aseptic meningitis, accounting for approximately 30% of the cases.[14] Viral meningitis is no longer a reportable disease to the Centers for Disease Control and Prevention (CDC). There are more than 74,000 cases a year in the United States.[13,15] Most cases occur from the late spring to autumn months, reflecting the increased incidence of enteroviral and arboviral infections during these seasons.[13,16] A retrospective survey performed in the 1980s found that the annual incidence of "aseptic meningitis" was approximately 10.9/100,000 persons or at least four times the incidence passively reported to the CDC during the period.[10] A viral cause was identified in only 11% of patients in this study. This low viral isolation rate likely reflects the technologic limits of the period, the infrequency with which viral cultures were performed, and the decreased incidence of viral CNS disease resulting from widespread vaccination against mumps and polioviruses.[10] With the advent of more rapid molecular diagnostic techniques the rate of identification of etiologic agents now approaches 50% to 86% for some syndromes and will provide more reliable epidemiologic estimates.[12,14]

Pathogenesis

The pathogenesis of viral meningitis is incompletely understood. Inferences regarding the pathogenesis of viral meningitis are largely derived from data on encephalitis, experimental animal models of meningitis, and clinical observations.[5,9] Viruses use two basic pathways to gain access to the CNS: hematogenous and neuronal spread. Most cases of viral meningitis occur following secondary viremia. Host and viral factors combined with seasonal, geographic, and epidemiologic events determine the probability of the development of viral CNS infection. For example, arboviral infections occur more frequently in epidemics and show a seasonal variation, reflecting the prevalence of the transmitting vector.[16] Enteroviral meningitis occurs with greater frequency during the summer and early autumn months, reflecting the seasonal increase in enteroviral infections. Enteroviral infections also exemplify the difference host physiology plays in determining the extent of viral disease. In children less than 2 weeks of age, enterovirus infections can produce a severe systemic infection, including meningitis or meningoencephalitis.[13] Approximately 50% of neonates with systemic enteroviral infections die, and 76% of the survivors are left with permanent sequelae. In children over 2 weeks of age, however, enteroviral infections are rarely associated with severe disease or significant morbidity.[13]

The sequence of viral hematogenous spread to the CNS is illustrated in Figure 12–1.[17] A virus must first enter host epithelial cells to produce infection. Virus then spreads and initially replicates in the regional lymph

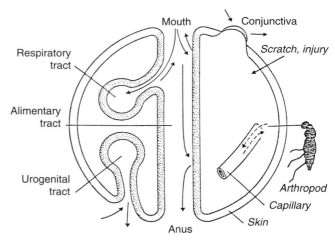

FIGURE 12–1. Body surfaces as sites of virus infection and shedding.

nodes (e.g., measles, influenza) or alternatively enters the circulatory system, where it seeds other tissues (e.g., arboviruses, enteroviruses, varicella).[9] This primary viremic phase allows virus to seed distant locations of the body and, frequently, marks the onset of clinical illness. In rare circumstances, such as disseminated neonatal herpes simplex virus (HSV) infection, viruses infect the CNS during primary viremia[18,19]; however, most viral infections involve an intermediate organ before reaching the CNS. The liver and spleen provide ideal locations for secondary viral replication because of their highly vascular structure and reticuloendothelial network. Secondary viremia generally results in high titers of virus in the bloodstream for prolonged periods, facilitating viral CNS spread. The pathophysiology of viral transport from blood to brain and viral endothelial cell tropism are poorly understood. Virus infects endothelial cells, leaks across damaged endothelium, passively channels through endothelium (pinocytosis or colloidal transport), or bridges the endothelium within migrating leukocytes.[9,20] This transendothelial passage occurs in vessels of the choroid plexus, meninges, or cerebrum, as depicted in Figure 12–2.

Numerous barriers and host defenses limit viral dissemination to the CNS. The skin and mucosal surfaces possess mechanical, chemical, and cellular defenses that protect the cells from viral infection.[9] Leukocytes and secretory factors (interleukins, interferons, antibodies) further augment these defenses and help eliminate viruses that bridge the epithelial layer. Local immune responses are crucial in limiting systemic viral infection. A swift inflammatory response can limit viremia and symptoms of infection. In the liver and spleen, the high degree of parenchymal contact and the large number of fixed mononuclear macrophage cells provide an excellent opportunity for host termination of viremia.[9] The

blood-brain or blood—cerebrospinal fluid (CSF) barrier, a network of tight endothelial junctions sheathed by glial cells that regulate molecular access to the CNS, further limits viral access to the CNS.[21–23]

Viral meningitis is a relatively benign self-limited illness, and pathologic specimens are rarely available for study.[13] The CSF, however, is frequently sampled and demonstrates a mononuclear immune cell response to most viral infection. Certain viral infections, most notably mumps and some enterovirus infections, elicit a polymorphonuclear cell infiltrate in the CSF early during disease. The initial CSF formula mimics bacterial meningitis and later shifts to a mononuclear predominance. Viral antigen presentation by mononuclear histiocytes stimulates the influx of immune cells. Recruited immune cells release soluble factors (interleukins, vasoactive amines) that mobilize other cells and change the permeability of the blood-brain barrier.[24,25] Physical and chemical changes in the blood-brain barrier allow the entry of serum proteins like immunoglobulins and interleukins, further augmenting the antiviral process. The cell-mediated immune response is important for eliminating virus from the CNS; however, immunoglobulin also has a role in protecting the host in some viral infections. This is best illustrated by the devastating clinical course of enteroviral meningitis in agammaglobulinemic patients as well as X-linked hyper-IgM syndrome.[13,26,27] Patients with impaired cell-mediated immunity have a higher incidence of CNS infections with certain viruses (varicella-goster virus [VZV], measles, cytomegalovirus [CMV]).[9]

Clinical Manifestations

The age and immune status of the patient and the particular virus involved influence the clinical manifestations of viral meningitis. Patients with enteroviral meningitis

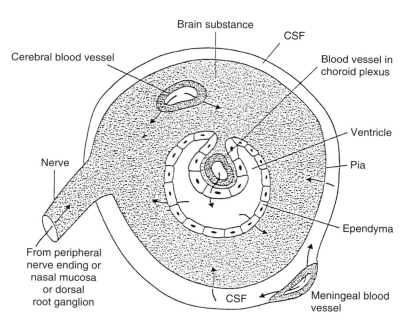

FIGURE 12–2. Routes of viral invasion of the central nervous system. CSF, cerebrospinal fluid.

often present with nonspecific symptoms such as fever (38°C to 40°C) of 3- to 5-day duration, malaise, and headache.[13,28] Approximately 50% of patients have nausea or vomiting.[28] Nuccal rigidity and photophobia are the hallmark sign and symptom for meningitis, but 33% of patients with viral meningitis have no evidence of meningismus.[28] Less than 10% of children younger than 2 years of age develop signs of meningeal irritation. Most of these children with meningitis present with fever and irritability.[29] Children may also present with seizures secondary to fever, electrolyte disturbances, or the infection itself. The clinician must have a high index of suspicion for meningitis, especially in younger patients. In the immunocompromised host, enteroviral infection is both a diagnostic quandary and a potentially life-threatening disease. Immunocompromised patients frequently do not mount a brisk immune cell response. Therefore CSF analysis does not reflect evidence of disease, namely, CNS involvement.

Symptoms of meningitis (stiff neck, headache, and photophobia) occur in approximately 11% of men and 36% of women with primary HSV-2 genital infection. In one study, 5% of patients with primary HSV genital infection had meningitis severe enough to require hospitalization. All the hospitalized patients had evidence of a lymphocytic pleocytosis on CSF analysis.[30] In another study, HSV-2 was cultured from the CSF of 78% of patients with meningitis symptoms during primary genital infection. These patients also exhibited a CSF leukocytosis and increases in CSF antibody titers.[31] Recurrent HSV-2 meningitis (with or without genital lesions) has been reported, although cases associated with primary infection are more common.[32] HSV meningitis may spread to the CSF by neuronal routes along the sacral nerves. Alternatively, the virus may reach the CSF by hematogenous spread, as the virus has been cultured from the blood buffy coat layer.[5] VZV, CMV, Epstein-Barr virus (EBV), and parainfluenza virus have all been cultured or detected by polymerase chain reaction (PCR) from the CSF of patients with meningitis.[5,14,33–35]

Laboratory Findings

Initial CSF samples, although frequently suggestive of a diagnosis, are not sensitive or specific enough predictors to differentiate viral from bacterial meningitis.[36] Instead, epidemiologic trends, patient history, and accompanying laboratory information are important adjuncts in predicting the cause of meningitis. CSF in patients with viral meningitis typically exhibits a pleocytosis with 10 to 500 leukocytes and a slightly elevated protein level (< 100 mg/dl). The glucose level in the CSF typically is 40% or more of that in a simultaneously drawn serum sample. There is tremendous variation in CSF formulas, with significant overlap between viral and bacterial CSF laboratory findings.[36] In a retrospective review of over 400 patients with acute viral or bacterial meningitis

performed before the existence of the *Haemophilus influenza* B conjugate vaccine, investigators found that approximately 20% of the CSF samples that grew bacteria exhibited a CSF pleocytosis of less than 250 white blood cells (WBC)/mm^3.[5] Of the patients with bacterial meningitis, 15% had a CSF lymphocytosis, whereas 40% of the patients with viral meningitis had a predominance of polymorphonuclear cells. Some investigators recommend repeating the lumbar puncture 6 to 12 hours later, as the CSF profile of patients with viral meningitis will shift from a polymorphonuclear neutrophil (PMN) to a lymphocytic pleocytosis over this period.[37] In one study performed during an echovirus epidemic, however, eight of nine children with presumed enteroviral meningitis had failed to develop CSF lymphocyte predominance when a lumbar puncture was repeated 5 to 8 hours later.[38] A recent retrospective study found that during an enterovirus outbreak, 51% of patients demonstrated PMN predominance in their CSF profile despite symptoms of longer than 24 hours duration. Of note, the investigators in this study were unable to confirm the cause of the meningitis in most cases, as this was a retrospective study.[36] Other investigators have confirmed that the change to a lymphocytic CSF profile occurs 18 to 36 hours into the illness.[39] Most clinicians do not send viral cultures on CSF, and furthermore certain enteroviruses are extremely difficult to culture. More recently PCR has been used to diagnose enteroviral meningitis in both normal and agammaglobulinemic patients and has demonstrated great sensitivity and specificity.[40,41] The PCR assay provides a rapid, reliable test for verifying the cause of certain types of meningitis. This technique provides results within 24 to 36 hours and therefore may limit the duration of hospitalization, antibiotic use, and excessive diagnostic procedures.[42]

Etiologic Diagnosis

Historically the techniques for identifying viral meningitis were insensitive and often impractical. Depending upon the study cited and diagnostic methods used, investigators identified an agent in only 25% to 67% of presumed CNS infections.[4,40] The diagnosis of viral meningitis relied on viral culture, and CSF viral culture rates differ based on etiology.[28] Some viruses can only be diagnosed presumptively by acute and convalescent serologic testing or isolation of virus from another location in the body.[5]

A synopsis of viral detection techniques for different viruses is presented in Tables 12–1 and 12–3.[9] The rapidity and sensitivity of enterovirus diagnosis has improved with the advent of molecular diagnostic techniques such as PCR. Demonstration of viral nucleic acid in the CSF of patients with symptoms of meningitis has replaced viral culture and serologic diagnosis. One of the advantageous features of viral culture is the ability to identify virus serotypes for epidemiologic studies; however, for clinical purposes, PCR has replaced culture because of the speed and sensitivity of the technique.[13,42] As with any PCR-based technique, nucleic acid contamination of the laboratory area is a concern, and results must always be interpreted within the clinical context.

In the past serologic testing confirmed the clinical suspicion of an arboviral infection. Although virus can be cultured from CSF during the early stages of the infection, this has little utility in the acute management of a patient with CNS disease.[43] Recently the use of PCR for the diagnosis of arbovirus infections in the CNS has met with mixed results. Because of the diverse viral causes of arboviral infection, the development of specific primers that can hybridize across multiple viral families (Alphaviridae, Flaviviridae, Bunyaviridae) has been difficult. Currently there is an emphasis on the development of improved "universal group primers" to perform an initial group screening followed by PCR using higher specificity primers as a second viral diagnostic test.[44] Such a technique would likely not be cost effective except for a reference laboratory. For other infections, molecular techniques are the standard for diagnosing viral meningitis.[12,15] Enterovirus is the cause of approximately 90% of aseptic meningitis cases for which a pathogen is detected.[13] The technique is invaluable in detecting low-titer infections or serotypes that fail to grow in conventional cell culture.[9,45]

Differential Diagnosis

Unusual but treatable infections should always be considered and investigated in patients with a CSF pleocytosis and negative conventional bacterial cultures. Spirochetes (*Treponema, Borrelia, Leptospira*), *Mycoplasma, Bartonella*, and *Mycobacterium* can produce a pleocytosis when both Gram stain and bacterial culture are negative. Fastidious bacteria (*Listeria*) may fail to grow in culture and occasionally produce a mononuclear pleocytosis similar to that of viral meningitis. This is of particular concern in infants, the elderly, and immunocompromised patients. Some bacteria, although not directly infecting the CNS, can release toxins that create a change in the level of consciousness, specifically *Staphylococcus aureus* and *Streptococcus pyogenes* exotoxin-mediated toxic shock syndrome. Frequently, children with streptococcal throat infections present with "neck stiffness" secondary to localized pharyngeal inflammation and tender anterior cervical lymphadenopathy. Parameningeal infections, especially from infected sinuses, produce a pleocytosis and CNS symptoms; however, these infections more frequently present as encephalitis with focal neurologic changes and altered mental status. Similarly, partially treated bacterial infections can have CSF findings resembling those of viral meningitis

Fungal and parasitic infections can produce CNS infections, although they uncommonly produce only meningitis. The exceptions to this rule are coccid-ioidomycosis and cryptococcosis. These pathogens characteristically produce meningitis rather than any focal CNS disease. *Cryptococcus*, for example, produces subacute meningitis in both normal and immunosuppressed patients and remains the leading cause of fungal meningitis.[6] Many of these infections are treatable and need to be investigated with a thorough history for possible exposures. Fungi such as *Candida, Aspergillus, Histoplasma*, and *Blastomyces* most frequently cause focal parenchymal disease when infecting the CNS. These fungi, although they are frequently in the differential diagnosis for an immunocompromised host, can also cause disease in the normal host. Parasites like *Naegleria fowleri* produce meningoencephalitis with purulent CSF findings. A history of recent summertime swimming in a stagnant pond should raise suspicion for this infection.

Noninfectious processes that can produce true aseptic meningitis include hematologic malignancies, medications (especially immunomodulatory, nonsteroidal anti-inflammatory, and TMP-SMZ medications), autoimmune diseases, and foreign material and proteins. Leukemia produces a CSF pleocytosis with cancerous cells and occurs most frequently with acute lymphocytic leukemia, although subarachnoid involvement can also occur in acute myelogenous leukemia. Immunomodulatory drugs such as intravenous immunoglobulin or antilymphocyte globulin (muromonab-CD3 [Orthoclone OKT3]) also cause aseptic meningitis. Of the medications associated with meningitis, nonsteroidal anti-inflammatory agents, sulfa-containing drugs, and cytosine arabinoside are the most common offenders. Drug-induced aseptic meningitis frequently occurs in patients with underlying connective tissue or rheumatologic diseases. A patient with drug-induced aseptic meningitis warrants investigation for a possible underlying autoimmune disease.[5,6] Epithelial or endothelial cysts can rupture and spill their contents (keratin, protein), producing a brisk inflammatory response, mimicking acute viral meningitis.

Treatment and Prognosis

The fundamental principle of therapy for viral meningitis lies in the identification of potentially treatable diseases. Until recently, no therapy existed for most cases of viral meningitis. Efforts instead focused on preventive strategies (largely through vaccination) as well as identification of treatable nonviral causes of meningitis. Antiviral therapies are emerging for the treatment of enteroviral meningitis.[46,47] Despite these recent chemotherapeutic and diagnostic advances in the diagnosis of enteroviral infection, patients with meningitis warrant careful assessment for treatable nonviral causes of meningitis. The clinician must also anticipate and treat the complications of viral CNS disease (seizures, inappropriate secretion of antidiuretic hormone hydrocephalus, raised intracranial pressure). Supportive therapy includes hydration and an antipyretic-analgesic.

In the normal host, viral meningitis is a relatively benign self-limited disease. A prospective study in children less than 2 years of age, for example, found that even in the 9% of children who develop evidence of acute neurologic disease (complex seizures, increased intracerebral pressure, or coma) their long-term prognosis is excellent. During long-term follow up (42 months), children with acute CNS complications performed neurodevelopmental tasks and achieved developmental milestones as well as children with an uncomplicated course.[29]

Currently antibody preparations and an antiviral agent, pleconaril, have shown activity against enterovirus infections, including those of the CNS, in case reports and animal studies. Randomized controlled trials, however, have not supported their use in routine treatment of enterovirus meningitis. In case reports immunoglobulin preparations, given systemically or intrathecally, retarded mortality and morbidity in agammaglobulinemic patients with chronic enteroviral meningitis. Despite the administration of immunoglobulin, the virus was not eliminated from the CSF, and these patients developed chronic enteroviral meningitis.[48,49] Enteroviral infections in neonates frequently produce overwhelming viremia and CNS disease. A blinded, randomized, controlled trial did not demonstrate clinical benefit from intravenous immunoglobulin for neonates with severe life-threatening enteroviral infection.[50]

A recently developed antiviral agent (3-[3,5-dimethyl-4-[[3-(3-methyl-5-isoxazolyl)propyl]oxy]phenyl]-5-trifluoromethyl-1,2,4-oxadiazole), pleconaril (ViroPharma Inc., Exton, PA), is a bioavailable small-molecule inhibitor of picornavirus replication that binds the capsid and prevents receptor uncoating of viral RNA. Because of homology between the picornaviruses, namely, enterovirus and rhinovirus capsid structure, the drug has activity against these human pathogens. Initial cell culture and animal studies of pleconaril demonstrated that the drug had potent antienteroviral activity.[46] Randomized, controlled, double-blind clinical trials, although demonstrating slight improvements in adults with enteroviral meningitis, have not demonstrated the dramatic efficacy initially anticipated and have not been published in peer-reviewed literature. In the 32 adults with aseptic meningitis studied, shortening the duration of headache was the most dramatic improvement, with the pleconaril group experiencing on average 6.5 days of headache vs. 18.3 days of headache for the placebo control population.[47] The duration of headache in the placebo control group is much longer than previously published for enteroviral meningitis. Similarly, if one uses an objective measurement, such as the duration of analgesic use (historical average control is 5 days) vs. that reported in the pleconaril study (placebo group is 11.5 days), the statistically significant 5.3 days of analgesic use by the pleconaril group is less dramatic.[47,51] Although pleconaril does not have the dramatic effect previously predicted in cases of uncomplicated enterovirus meningitis, it may

still prove beneficial in the treatment of severe life-threatening disease (neonatal sepsis, disease in the immunocompromised patient, encephalomyelitis). A multicenter randomized, controlled trial is ongoing, evaluating pleconaril in severe neonatal infection, but preliminary information is unavailable at this time (David Kimberlin, personal communication, 2002).

Specific antiviral agents are available for several other viral causes of meningitis. Although no definitive clinical trials have been conducted, most authors recommend the use of intravenous acyclovir for HSV meningitis, as it decreases the duration of primary herpes disease and may limit meningeal involvement.[52] Recurrent HSV-2 meningitis is rare, and recently a single case of meningitis associated with HSV-1 reactivation was reported. At this time there are no data on the benefit of antiviral treatment or on suppressive therapy for recurrent HSV CNS disease.[32,53] VZV, CMV, EBV, and parainfluenza virus have all been cultured from the CSF of patients with meningitis. Effective antiviral therapy exists for VZV infections of the CNS and should be instituted in these patients.[54–56] The issue of therapy for CMV CNS infection in the immunocompromised host is more problematic, and therapy should be tailored to the clinical likelihood of infection.

VIRAL ENCEPHALITIS

Epidemiology and Prevalence

As is the case with viral meningitis, passive reporting systems underestimate the incidence of viral encephalitis.[10] An estimated 20,000 cases of encephalitis occur each year in the United States; however, the CDC received only 740 (0.3/100,000) to 1340 (0.54/100,000) annual reports of persons with encephalitis from 1990 to 1994.[8,57] A review of the cases in Olmsted county, Minnesota, from 1950 to 1980 found the incidence of viral encephalitis was at least twice the incidence reported by the CDC.[10] A recent prospective multicenter study in Finland demonstrated results similar to those of the Olmstead study and demonstrated the incidence of encephalitis to be 10.5/100,000.[58] HSV CNS infections occur without seasonal variation, affect all ages, and cause most of the fatal cases of endemic encephalitis in the United States.[9] Arboviruses, a group of over 500 arthropod-transmitted RNA viruses, are the leading cause of encephalitis worldwide and in the United States.[59] Arboviral infections occur in epidemics and have a seasonal predilection, reflecting the prevalence of the transmitting vector.[60] Asymptomatic infections vastly outnumber symptomatic infections. Patients with disease may develop a mild systemic febrile illness or viral meningitis.[43] Encephalitis occurs in a minority of persons with arboviral infections, but the case fatality rate varies extremely from 5% to 70%, depending upon the responsible virus and age of the patient. La Crosse encephalitis is the most commonly reported arboviral disease in the United States, whereas St. Louis encephalitis is the most common cause of epidemic encephalitis.[60] Interestingly a case of eastern equine encephalitis (EEE) in the coastal region of Alabama was reported in January 1996 (the first case since 1964). Characteristically EEE and most arboviral infections occur in the late summer following amplification of the virus and peak mosquito activity.[60] This case report demonstrates that in warm climates the clinician must have a high index of suspicion for insect-born diseases. More recently, as will be described, West Nile virus (WNV) has caused disease in the United States as well as significant outbreaks in the Mideast.

Japanese B encephalitis and rabies constitute most cases of encephalitis outside of North America. Japanese encephalitis virus (JEV), a member of the Flavivirus genus, occurs throughout Asia and causes epidemics in China despite routine immunization.[9] In warmer locations, the virus occurs endemically.[61] The disease typically affects children, although adults with no history of exposure to the virus are also susceptible.[8] As with the other arboviral infections, asymptomatic infections occur more frequently than symptomatic infections do. Japanese encephalitis, however, has a high case fatality rate and leaves half of the survivors with a significant degree of neurologic morbidity.[9] Rabies virus remains endemic around much of the world. Human infections in the United States decreased over the last decades to 1 to 3 cases per year because of the immunization of domesticated animals. Bat exposure is increasingly recognized as the source of infection. Fifteen percent (685 of 4470) of bats tested carried the rabies virus in one study analyzing the risk of bat exposure and rabies.[62] Since 1990, bat-associated variants of the virus have accounted for 24 of the 32 reported cases. In most cases (22 of 24) there was no evidence of bite; however, in half of the cases, direct contact (handling of the bats) was documented.[63] In areas outside the United States, human cases of rabies encephalitis number in the thousands and are caused by unvaccinated domestic animals following contact with infected wild animals.

Postinfectious encephalitis, an acute demyelinating process, has also been referred to as acute disseminated encephalomyelitis (ADEM) or autoimmune encephalitis and accounts for approximately 100 to 200 additional cases of encephalitis annually.[57] The disease historically produced approximately one-third of the encephalitis cases in the United States and was associated with measles, mumps, and other exanthematous viral infections.[9,64] Postinfectious encephalitis is now associated with antecedent upper respiratory tract virus (notably influenza virus) and varicella infections in the United States.[8,9] Measles continues to be the leading cause of postinfectious encephalitis worldwide and complicates 1 of every 1000 measles infections.[8]

The slow infections of the CNS, or transmissible spongiform encephalopathies (TSE), occur sporadically worldwide. The prototypical TSE, Creutzfeld-Jakob disease (CJD), occurs at high rates within families and has an estimated incidence of 0.5 to 1.5 cases per million population.[7] In 1986, cases of a TSE in cattle, bovine spongiform encephalopathy (BSE), were reported in the United Kingdom. In addition to affecting other livestock throughout Europe that were fed supplements containing meat and bone meal, cross-species transmission of BSE has been documented, leading to a ban in the use of bovine offal in fertilizers, pet food, or other animal feed.[7] A decrease in the number of recognized cases of BSE has occurred since the institution of these restrictions. Concomitant with the increased cases of BSE in Europe, an increase in cases of an atypical Creutzfeldt-Jakob disease also occurred, suggesting animal-to-human transmission. The report of atypical CJD (unique clinical and histopathologic findings) affecting young adults (an age at which CJD rarely has been diagnosed) led to the designation of a new disease, new variant Creutzfeldt-Jakob disease (nvCJD). As of this writing, 88 cases of nvCJD have been reported in the United Kingdom, 3 cases in France, and one in Ireland.*

Pathogenesis

The pathogenesis of encephalitis requires that viruses reach the CNS by hematogenous or neuronal spread. As in the case with meningitis, viruses most frequently access the CNS following secondary viremia and cell-free or cell-associated CNS entry.[5,19] Other than direct entry via cerebral vessels, virus initially can infect the meninges and CSF and then enter the parenchyma across either ependymal cells or the pial linings. Viruses exhibit differences in neurotropism and neurovirulence. For example, reovirus types 1 and 3 produce different CNS diseases in mice based on differences in receptor affinities. Viral hemagglutinin receptors on reovirus type 3 bind to neuronal receptors, enabling fatal encephalitis. Reovirus type 1 has a distinct hemagglutinin antigen and binds to ependymal cells and produces a hydrocephalus and an ependymitis.[65] Receptor difference is only one determinant of viral neurotropism. For example, enteroviruses with similar receptors produce very different diseases. Five serotypes of coxsackie virus B (B1 to B5) readily produce CNS infections, whereas type B6 rarely produces neurologic infection.[6] Viral genes have been discovered that influence the neurovirulence of HSV-1.[66] Mutant HSV-1 viruses with either γ_1 34.5 gene deletions or stop codons inserted into the gene have less ability to cause encephalitis and death following intracerebral inoculation in mice than wild type virus has.[66]

In addition to viral factors, host physiology is also important in determining the extent and location of viral CNS disease. Age, sex, and genetic differences between

---

*WHO Fact Sheet No. 180, 2001. Variant Creutzfeld-Jakob disease (VCJD).

hosts influence viral infections and clinical course.[13,32] Host age influences the clinical manifestations and sequelae of a viral infection. For example, Sindbis virus infection produces lethal encephalitis in newborn mice, whereas weanling mice experience persistent but nonfatal encephalitis. The reason for the difference in outcome is twofold: Mature neurons resist virus-induced apoptosis, and older mice have an improved antibody response, thus limiting viral replication.[67] Variations in macrophage function between persons can result in clinically distinct infections and disease. Moreover, macrophage-antigen response can change with age and is important in limiting spread of infection within a patient.[68,69] In addition to age, physical activity may be another important host factor that determines the severity of infection. Exercise has been associated with increased risk for paralytic poliomyelitis and may increase the incidence of enteroviral myocarditis and aseptic meningitis.[70,71] Increasingly host differences are recognized as equally important determinants of disease at the cellular and molecular level.

Historically the peripheral neural pathway was considered the only pathway of viral neurologic infection.[72] Contemporary data, however, demonstrate that the circulatory system provides the principal pathway for most CNS infections in humans.[9] HSV and rabies provide examples of viruses that infect the CNS by neuronal spread. Sensory and motor neurons contain transport systems that carry materials along the axon to (retrograde) and from (anterograde) the nucleus. Peripheral or cranial nerves provide access to the CNS and shield the virus from immune regulation.

Rabies classically infects by the myoneural route and provides a prototype for peripheral neuronal spread.[73] Rabies virus replicates locally in the soft tissue following a rabid animal bite. After primary replication the virus enters the peripheral nerve by acetylcholine receptor binding. Once in the muscle the virus buds from the plasma membrane, crosses myoneural spindles, or enters across the motor end plate.[73,74] The virus travels by anterograde and retrograde axonal transport to infect neurons in the brainstem and limbic system. Eventually the virus spreads from the diencephalic and hippocampal structure to the remainder of the brain, killing the animal.[73] Virus also infects the CNS through cranial nerves. Animal studies have shown that HSV can infect the brain through the olfactory system as well as the trigeminal nerve.[75,76] Early HSV encephalitis damages the inferomedial temporal lobe and contains direct connections with the olfactory bulb.[9] The route of human HSV infections, however, is less clear. Despite data supporting olfactory and trigeminal spread of virus to the CNS, definitive proof in humans is lacking. The association of viral latency in the trigeminal ganglia, the relative infrequency of herpes simples encephalitis (HSE), and the confusing data regarding encephalitis from HSV reactivation suggests that the pathogenesis is more complex than described above.[77]

In patients with acute encephalitis the parenchyma exhibits neuronophagia and cells containing viral nucleic acids or antigens. The pathologic findings are unique for different viruses and reflect differences in pathogenesis and virulence. In the case of typical HSV encephalitis a hemorrhagic necrosis[8] occurs in the inferomedial temporal lobe with evidence of perivascular cuffing, lymphocytic infiltration, and neuronophagia.[78] Pathologic specimens in animals with rabies encephalitis demonstrate microglial proliferation, perivascular infiltrates, and neuronal destruction. The location of the pathologic findings can be limited to the brainstem areas (dumb rabies) or the diencephalic, hippocampal, and hypothalamic areas (furious rabies) based on the immune response mounted against the infection.[73] Pathologic findings relate to the viral cause and are described in subsequent discussions.

Some viruses do not directly infect the CNS but produce immune system changes that damage the parenchyma. Patients with postinfectious encephalitis (ADEM) exhibit focal neurologic deficits and altered consciousness associated temporally with a recent (within 1 to 2 weeks) viral infection or immunization.[64] Pathologic specimens, although they show evidence of demyelination by histologic or radiographic analysis, do not demonstrate evidence of viral infection in the CNS by culture or antigen tests. Patients with postinfectious encephalitis have subtle differences in their immune system, and some authors have proposed an autoimmune reaction as the pathogenic mechanism of disease.[8] Postinfectious encephalitis occurs most commonly following measles, VZV, mumps, influenza, and parainfluenza infections. With immunization the incidence of postinfectious encephalitis has decreased in the United States; however, measles continues to be the leading cause of postinfectious encephalitis worldwide.[8]

The TSEs are noninflammatory CNS diseases involving the accumulation of an abnormal form of a normal glycoprotein, the prion protein (PrP).[79] These encephalopathies differ in mode of transmission. Although most of the TSEs are experimentally transmissible by direct inoculation in the CNS, this mode rarely occurs except for iatrogenic transmissions.[7] The scrapie agent spreads by contact and lateral transmission. There is no evidence for lateral transmission in the case of BSE or nvCJD, and all cases appear to have occurred following parenteral injection or ingestion of affected materials. The transmissible agents remain infectious after treatments that would normally inactivate viruses or nucleic acids (detergent formalin, ionizing radiation, nucleases).[79] Most of the experimental work on TSEs has involved analysis of the scrapie agent. The current working model is that posttranslational alteration of the normally α-helical form of the PrP protein creates a protease resistant β-pleated sheet structure that accumulates in neurons, leading to progressive dysfunction, cell death, and subsequent astrocytosis. In studies on the scrapie agent, gastrointestinal tract involvement with infection of abdominal lymph nodes occurs first, followed by brain involvement a year or more later.[7] Experimental subcutaneous inoculation in mice and goats also leads to local lymph node involvement followed by splenic spread and then CNS involvement. The mode of transmission to the CNS (direct vs. hematogenous) as well as the infectivity of body fluids at different stages of infection are not known at this time.

Clinical Manifestations

Clinical symptoms have a pathophysiologic basis. Patients with encephalitis have clinical and laboratory evidence of parenchymal disease; however, infection rarely involves only the brain parenchyma. Some viruses (rabies, B virus) produce encephalitis without significant meningeal involvement; however, most patients with encephalitis have a concomitant meningitis. Most patients also have a prodromal illness with myalgias, fever, and anorexia reflecting the systemic viremia. Neurologic symptoms can range from fever, headache, and subtle neurologic deficits or change in level of consciousness to severe disease with seizures, behavioral changes, focal neurologic deficits, and coma.[59] Clinical manifestations reflect the location and degree of parenchymal involvement and differ according to the viral cause. For example, HSE infects the inferomedial frontal area of the cortex, resulting in focal seizures, personality changes, and aphasia. These symptoms reflect the neuroanatomic location of infection with inflammation near the internal capsule, limbic, and broca's regions.[9] Paresthesias near the location of the animal bite and change in behavior correlate temporally with the axoplasmic transport of rabies and the viral infection of the brainstem and hippocampal region.[9,73] Rabies has a predilection for the limbic system, producing personality changes. The damage spares cortical regions during this phase, allowing humans to vacillate between periods of calm, normal activity and short episodes of rage and disorientation.[73] Alternatively, Japanese encephalitis virus (JEV) initially produces a systemic illness with fever, malaise, and anorexia, followed by photophobia, vomiting, headache, and changes in brainstem function. Most children die from respiratory failure and frequently have evidence of cardiac and respiratory instability, reflecting viremic spread via the vertebral vessels and infection of brainstem nuclei.[8] Other patients have evidence of multifocal CNS disease involving the basal ganglia, thalamus, and lower cortex and develop tremors, dystonia, and parkinsonian symptoms.[8]

Encephalitis, unlike meningitis, has higher mortality and complication rates. Case fatality rates differ based on the viral cause and host factors.[9] For example, within the arthropod-born viral encephalitides, St. Louis encephalitis virus has an overall case mortality of 10%. The mortality is only 2% in children but increases to 20% in the elderly.[59] Other viruses like western equine and eastern equine encephalitis produce higher mortality and morbidity in children than in adults.[59]

The TSEs are slowly progressing diseases with long incubation periods. Sporadic CJD occurs between the ages of 50 and 70 years of age and is characterized by dementia, tremors, and more rarely abnormal movements and ataxia. Unlike sporadic CJD, nvCJD disease affects young adults and adolescents and produces cerebellar ataxia and sensory involvement (dysesthesias), with florid amyloid plaques detected in the brain on autopsy. Neurologic deterioration progresses relentlessly, and most patients die less than a year after onset of their neurologic manifestations.

Laboratory Findings and Diagnosis

Establishing a diagnosis requires a meticulous history, knowledge of epidemiologic factors, and a systematic evaluation of possible treatable diseases. In the past, investigators failed 50% to 75% of the time to identify the virus responsible for the encephalitis depending on the study and diagnostic tests used.[59] Encephalitis can occur as a separate clinical entity, although meningitis usually coexists with it. A CSF pleocytosis usually occurs in encephalitis but is not necessary for the diagnosis. White blood cell counts typically number in the 10s to 100s in viral encephalitis, although higher counts occur.[59] Cerebrospinal glucose levels are usually normal, although some viruses (EEE) produce CSF studies consistent with acute bacterial meningitis.[9] Some viruses (HSV) produce a hemorrhagic necrosis, and the CSF exhibits this with moderately high protein levels and evidence of red blood cells. Supratentorial and cerebellar tumors can increase intracranial pressure and mimic encephalitis. A careful fundoscopic examination should be performed to rule out any evidence of papilledema and increased intracranial pressure before CSF is obtained.

Unlike meningitis, encephalitis often requires additional laboratory and radiologic tests to establish the diagnosis. The clinical circumstances of the patient and the likely causes dictate specific laboratory and radiologic evaluations. Historically the standard for diagnosis has been brain biopsy and viral culture. For some viruses (HSV, enterovirus, VZV, JC virus) PCR detection of viral nucleic acids from the CSF has replaced culture and brain biopsy as the standard for diagnosing encephalitis.[12,14,41,80–84] Radiographic studies that support the diagnosis of focal encephalitis are computed tomography (CT scan) and magnetic resonance imaging (MRI). The sensitivity of MRI to alterations in brain water content and the lack of bone artifacts make this the neuroradiologic modality of choice for CNS infections.[85] MRI detects parenchymal changes earlier than CT scan does and better defines the extent of a lesion.[85] Furthermore MRI is more sensitive for detecting evidence of demyelinating lesions in the periventricular and deep white matter, thus allowing the differentiation of parainfectious from acute viral encephalitis.[85] Patients with viral encephalitis frequently have diffuse or focal epileptiform discharges with background slowing.[3] These electroencephalogram (EEG) changes precede CT scan evidence of encephalitis and provide a sensitive, although nonspecific, diagnostic test. EEG changes in the temporal lobe area strongly support the diagnosis of HSE; however, the absence of these changes does not rule out HSE.

Historically, patients with viral encephalitis required a battery of different diagnostic tests. HSE, for example, could be diagnosed acutely by brain biopsy and viral culture, or retrospectively by CSF antibody and convalescent serologic tests, albeit not optimally.[78] The diagnosis of enterovirus meningitis previously required virus isolation from the throat or rectum acutely or serologic studies retrospectively. The advent of PCR has simplified and improved the diagnosis of many viral CNS infections. CSF PCR has been used for the diagnosis of enteroviral, human herpervirus (HHV)-6, EBV, and CMV parenchymal diseases.[86] Primers also exist for the detection of certain arboviral encephalitides (California encephalitis group, Japanese encephalitis virus, West Nile fever virus, St. Louis encephalitis, dengue fever virus serotypes 1 to 4, and yellow fever virus); however, the development of universal arboviral primers has been more difficult.[12,41,44,84] The successful detection of viral DNA in the CSF is influenced by the duration, extent, and cause of the disease. The laboratory test is relatively rapid, has high sensitivity, and provides a less invasive means to diagnose encephalitis. For example, only 4% of CSF cultures are positive in patients with sporadic HSE; however, 53 of 54 patients with biopsy proven HSE had evidence of HSV DNA in the CSF by PCR. CSF PCR has a greater than 95% sensitivity and a specificity approaching 100% in patients with HSE.[87] Interestingly, in the three cases in which the CSF PCR was positive but the brain biopsy negative, biopsy samples had been improperly prepared before viral culture or the biopsy site was suboptimal.[87] Recently efforts have focused on correlating viral nucleic acid copy as a reflection virus quantity to predict clinical outcome.[88]

The TSEs are currently only diagnosed by histologic examination, characteristic EEG and MRI changes, and the clinical context. Most laboratory tests are of little value in the diagnosis. CSF examination shows normal values or slightly elevated protein levels. The EEG in classic CJD reveals generalized slowing early in the disease, which late in the disease is punctuated by biphasic or triphasic peaks with the onset of myoclonus. MRI changes late in the illness reveal global atrophy with hyperintense signal from the basal ganglia.[7] Fluid attenuation inversion recovery (FLAIR) MRI provides greater sensitivity and demonstrates signal intensity changes in the cortex that T2-weighted spin-echo MRI cannot detect.[89] Histopathologic examination of the brain using a specific antibody to the PrP-res protein confirms the disease. In addition evidence of gliosis, neuronal loss, and spongiform changes support the diagnosis. In cases of nvCJD, characteristic amyloid plaques (so called florid

plaques) microscopically define the disease. The florid plaques are not seen in other TSEs and consist of flower-like amyloid deposits surrounded by vacuolar halos. The detection of PrP-res in the tonsillar tissue by immunohistochemical staining is also strongly supportive of nvCJD diagnosis.[7]

Differential Diagnosis

Identifying treatable disease expeditiously is a priority in patients presenting with neurologic changes. In patients with suspected HSE undergoing brain biopsy for confirmation of disease, alternate diagnoses are frequently found. Of 432 patients, only 45% had biopsy-confirmed HSE, and 22% had another cause established by brain biopsy. Of these, 40% had a treatable disease (9% of the biopsy group), including bacterial abscess, tuberculosis, fungal infection, tumor, subdural hematoma, or autoimmune disease. Viruses were the cause in most of the remaining 60% who had identifiable but nontreatable encephalitis. A third group of 142 patients (33%) went undiagnosed even after brain biopsy and the conventional diagnostic tests.[4]

Pathologic processes in the CNS have limited clinical expressions, and thus different diseases often produce similar signs and symptoms.[4] Diseases that may mimic viral encephalitis or meningitis are presented in Table 12–4. Mass lesions in the CNS (tumor, abscess, or blood) can cause focal neurologic changes, fever, and seizures, similar to those of encephalitis. Metabolic (hypoglycemia, uremia, inborn-errors of metabolism) and toxin-mediated disorders (ingestions, tick paralysis, or Reyes syndrome) can cause decreased consciousness, seizures, and evidence of background slowing on EEG. Limbic encephalitis can produce protracted encephalitis and is caused by paraneoplastic phenomena. Furthermore, treatable infectious causes of encephalitis must be vigorously investigated. *Mycoplasma* produces demyelinating brainstem encephalitis in approximately 0.1% of infections.

Prevention

Prevention remains the mainstay of therapy. Historically the most frequent cause of viral CNS disease, mumps, has largely been eliminated through vaccination. Live attenuated vaccines against measles, mumps, and rubella have dramatically decreased the incidence of encephalitis in industrialized countries. Measles continues to be the leading cause of postinfectious encephalitis in developing countries, however, and complicates 1 of every 1000 measles infections.[8] Vaccination has also changed the character of previously common viral CNS disease. In 1952, poliomyelitis affected 57,879 Americans. Widespread vaccination has eradicated the disease currently from the Western Hemisphere.[90] Vaccines exist for some arboviral infections. Vaccination against Japanese encephalitis virus (JEV) has reduced the incidence of

TABLE 12–4 ■ Diseases That Mimic Herpes Simplex Encephalitis

Diseases	Number of patients
TREATABLE (No. = 46)	
Infection	
Abscess or subdural empyema	
Bacterial	5
Listeria	1
Fungal	2
Mycoplasma	2
Tuberculosis	6
Cryptococcosis	3
Rickettsial fevers	2
Toxoplasmosis	1
Zygomycosis (mucormycosis)	1
Meningococcal meningitis	1
Other viruses	
Cytomegalovirus	1
Influenza A*	4
Echovirus*	3
Tumor	5
Subdural hematoma	2
Systemic lupus erythematosus	1
Adrenal leukodystrophy	6
NONTREATABLE (No. = 49)	
Vascular disease	11
Toxic encephalopathy	5
Reye's syndrome	1
Viral (no. = 40)	
Arbovirus infection	
St. Louis encephalitis	7
Western equine encephalitis	3
California encephalitis	4
Eastern equine encephalitis	2
Other herpesviruses	
Epstein-Barr virus	8
Other viruses	
Mumps virus	3
Adenovirus	1
Progressive multifocal leukoencephalopathy (JC virus)	1
Lymphocytic choriomeningitis virus	1
Subacute sclerosing panencephalitis (measles virus)	2

*Investigational drug therapy.

Adapted from Whitley RJ, Cobbs CG, Alford CA Jr, et al: Diseases that mimic herpes simply encephalitis. Diagnosis, presentation, and outcome. JAMA 1989;262:234–239. Copyright 1989, American Medical Association.

encephalitis in Asia; however, in China where 70 million children are immunized for JEV, 10,000 cases still occur annually.[91]

Vaccination is not cost effective for preventing all viral infections. For example, vector avoidance, mosquito deterrents, and mosquito abatement programs are less costly strategies for preventing arboviral encephalitides in the United States.[3,60] Ideally, chemoprophylaxis taken during outbreaks would provide the least costly and most effective prevention; however, at this time no such drug exists.[43]

Pre-exposure and immediate postexposure prophylaxis are the only ways known to prevent death in rabies-exposed persons.[73] There are case reports of patients

surviving symptomatic rabies, but all of these patients had some prior immunity or received postexposure prophylaxis before symptoms developed. Persons exposed to rabies require vigorous cleansing of the wound, postexposure vaccination, and direct administration of rabies hyperimmunoglobulin at the site of the animal bite. Persons with frequent contact with potentially rabid animals (veterinarians, animal control staff, workers in rabies laboratories, and travelers to rabies-endemic areas) should receive pre-exposure vaccination.

The United States Food and Drug administration (FDA), to reduce the potential exposure to TSE agents in the blood supply, has implemented guidelines eliminating whole blood or blood components prepared from individuals who later developed CJD or nvCJD. Changes in agricultural practices in Europe and bans on infected cattle have been associated with a decline in cases of nvCJD. In North America no cases of nvCJD have been reported, and the Department of Agriculture has programs in place to monitor for TSEs in livestock.

Treatment

Patients with encephalitis, depending on the cause and the extent of CNS involvement, require treatment tailored to their clinical situation. Currently few antiviral medications are available to treat CNS infections. Antiviral therapy exists for HSV-1, HSV-2, VZV, CMV, and HIV. Acyclovir and Vidarabine have sharp by reduced mortality and morbidity from herpes infections. Neonatal mortality from disseminated HSV disease and HSE has declined from 70% to 40% since the development of acyclovir and vidarabine.[9] Antiviral treatment decreases the incidence of morbidity from disseminated HSE from 90% of survivors to 50% of survivors and reduces the severity of their neurologic impairment.[9] Varicella immunoglobulin (VZIG) and acyclovir have reduced the complications from primary VZV infection and zoster in the neonate and immunocompromised patient. Although controlled trials have not evaluated the efficacy of acyclovir in VZV encephalitis, the medication is routinely used to treat this complication.[92,93] With the increase of HIV infection, diseases previously limited to the neonatal and postnatal period now occur with increasing frequency in the adult population. Ganciclovir and foscarnet are used for the treatment of CMV encephalitis, although controlled clinical trials have not confirmed the efficacy of treatment. Data also suggest that antiretroviral therapy decreases the frequency and severity of HIV CNS disease. Studies have not determined if this is because of a direct reduction in HIV viral activity in the CNS or of an indirect effect due to improved immune function and fewer opportunistic infections affecting the CNS.[94,95] In cases of postinfectious encephalitis or ADEM, no randomized controlled trial has confirmed the benefit of immunomodulatory drugs. In practice, clinicians often treat ADEM with different immunomodulators in an attempt to limit

T cell–mediated destruction of the CNS.[64,96,97] It must be emphasized, however, that no placebo-controlled studies have been performed, and immunomodulatory therapy is based simply on isolated case reports. As with most case reports, clinical failures and iatrogenic morbidity from a therapeutic modality are rarely reported.

SELECTED CLINICAL SYNDROMES

Herpes Simplex Encephalitis

Human infection caused by HSV is ubiquitous, but encephalitis caused by this virus fortunately is uncommon. Nonetheless HSE has played an important role in our understanding of viral infections of the CNS. HSE was one of the first human infections to be routinely diagnosed using methods of molecular biology (i.e., PCR for detection of HSV DNA in CSF).[87,98–101] Furthermore, HSE is one of the first viral infections to be successfully treated with antiviral chemotherapy.[102,103]

HSV is the most common cause of nonepidemic, acute focal encephalitis in the United States.[104] The estimated frequency of occurrence is one case per 250,000 to 500,000 population annually. Occurring throughout the year, approximately one-third of the cases of HSE develop in patients less than 20 years of age, and one-half develop in individuals over the age of 50 years. In the absence of effective antiviral therapy the mortality for HSE is >70%, with only 2.5% of persons returning to normal function.

Acyclovir is the treatment of choice for HSE, but morbidity and mortality remain high; mortality is 28% at 18 months after acyclovir treatment.[102,105] Age of the patient, level of consciousness at presentation, and duration of encephalitis all influence the outcome in patients receiving acyclovir therapy. If the level of consciousness as measured by the Glasgow Coma Score was 6 or less, a poor outcome was uniform, irrespective of the age of the patient. If disease was present for 4 days or less, the likelihood of survival increased from 65% to 100% among acyclovir recipients. At 2 years after treatment, 30% of acyclovir recipients were judged to be normal or mildly impaired, 9% had moderate sequelae, and 53% of the patients were dead or severely impaired. Relapse of HSV infection of the CNS following therapy has been demonstrated. From studies of neonatal HSE, approximately 8% of babies who received acyclovir had a documented virologic relapse if treated for 10 days at a dosage of 10 mg/kg every 8 hours. Relapse has not been documented when a higher dose of 20 mg/kg every 8 hours is administered for 21 days. The exact percentage of adults and older children who suffer relapse is unknown, but reports have suggested that relapse can occur following therapy, and rater may be as high as 5%.[106]

A distinction must be made between HSV infections of the CNS that occur during the neonatal period and infections in older children and adults. Beyond the neonatal period, most cases of HSV encephalitis are attributable to HSV-1. On the basis of serologic studies, approximately one-third of these cases are caused by primary HSV-1 infection, and two-thirds result from viral reactivation.[107] Studies in animal models have demonstrated reactivation of latent HSV from the trigeminal ganglia with transport of virus along nerves of the olfactory tract to the brain. The pathogenesis of HSV encephalitis in humans is not completely known. The possibility of reactivation of latent virus in brain tissue has not been excluded. In contrast, neonates most often acquire HSV infection from virus shed in the maternal genital tract at the time of vaginal delivery. HSV-2 infection of the brain in newborns with multiorgan disseminated infection is likely blood borne and associated with a diffuse encephalitic process, resulting in generalized encephalomalacia. When disease involves only the CNS of the newborn, however, neuronal transmission of virus to the CNS initially results in unitemporal involvement that extends to bitemporal disease, as occurs in older children and adults (Fig. 12–3). Babies with HSV-1 infection of the CNS have a significantly better neurologic outcome than those with HSV-2 infection. Recently, giving a higher dose of acyclovir (20 mg/kg every 8 hours) for 21 days has decreased mortality to 5% for newborns with HSV encephalitis; approximately 40% of survivors develop normally. The reasons for the differences in the pathogenesis and tropism of HSV-1 and HSV-2 CNS infections are not well understood.[108,109]

B Virus

B virus (cercopithecine herpesvirus 1) causes enzootic infection of macaque monkeys that usually causes little or no disease in the animal.[110] However, B virus can cause severe and fatal encephalitis in humans when transmitted by the bite or scratch of an infected macaque.[111,112] Human disease is characterized by a nonspecific prodrome of fever and malaise (possibly with herpetic blisters at the inoculation site), progressing to a rapidly ascending encephalomyelitis. The mortality for human encephalitis caused by B virus encephalitis is 50% to 70% in the absence of therapy. No evidence suggests that B virus can cause a subclinical infection in humans.[113] Persons who experience a bite, scratch, or mucosal exposure from a potentially infected macaque should thoroughly decontaminate the wound. Prophylactic antiviral therapy is recommended for persons who have a high-risk exposure.[114] Because of the high mortality associated with B virus encephalitis, patients should be treated with intravenous acyclovir or ganciclovir, although the therapeutic experience with this disease is limited.

Rabies

Rabies, a zoonotic disease caused by a rhabdovirus, remains one of the few human infections with a near

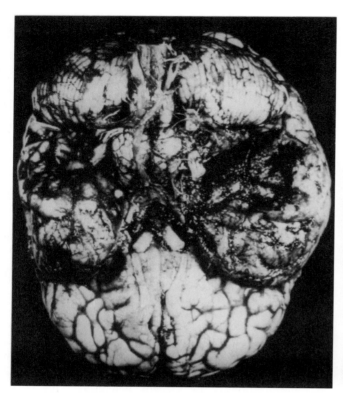
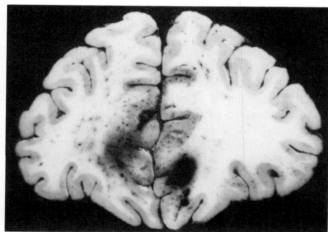

FIGURE 12–3. Coronal section of brain from patient with herpes simplex encephalitis.

100% mortality. Conversely, rabies can be readily prevented by judicious use of passive and active immunization, even after infection has occurred.[115] In the developing world, infected dogs remain the primary vector for human rabies.[116] In the United States and Western Europe, human infection is more likely due to exposure to bats or wild terrestrial mammals.[117] The incubation period for rabies in humans can range from 5 days to longer than 6 months, although the usual period is 20 to 60 days.[118] After a prodromal period of fever, malaise, anxiety, and pain or itching at the site of the bite wound, patients with rabies develop overt CNS findings, which may be predominantly encephalopathic or paralytic.[118] The patient progresses to coma, cardiorespiratory failure, and ultimately to death. Other than supportive care, no therapy for human rabies is available. The best diagnostic method for laboratory confirmation for rabies is detection of rabies virus RNA in saliva by reverse transcription (RT)-PCR, which has high sensitivity and specificity.[119,120] Alternative diagnostic methods include demonstration of rabies virus antigens in biopsies of brain, nuccal skin, or corneal impressions. Medical management of rabies is focused on prevention. Veterinarians and other individuals at high risk for exposure to rabies should receive preexposure vaccination. Unimmunized persons who have a risky exposure to a potentially rabid animal should receive postexposure vaccination with both rabies immune globulin (RIG, preferably human rather than equine) and rabies vaccine. Modern rabies vaccines produced in human tissue culture cell lines or avian embryo cultures are more efficacious and much better tolerated than older vaccines produced in animal nervous system tissues.[121]

Since 1996, several deaths have been reported in Queensland, Australia, from a rabies-like enzootic infection caused by Australia bat Lyssavirus (ABL), which is found in flying foxes and other bats.[122,123] Pre-exposure or postexposure administration of standard rabies vaccine appears to be protective against human infection with ABL.

Arthropod-Borne Encephalitis Viruses

Viruses transmitted to humans by the bites of arthropods (especially mosquitoes and ticks) are major causes of encephalitis worldwide, as illustrated in Tables 12–2 and 12–3.[124] These encephalitides are predominately caused by viruses from the Togaviridae (e.g., EEE), Flaviviridae (e.g., japanese encephalitis) and Bunyaviridae (e.g., La Crosse encephalitis) families. An antigenically related group of flaviviruses accounts for hundreds of thousands of cases of human infection around the globe each year. These include mosquito-borne diseases such as St. Louis encephalitis (North America), Murray Valley encephalitis (Australia), West Nile virus encephalitis (Africa and the Middle East), japanese encephalitis (Asia), far eastern tick-borne encephalitis (Russia), and western tick-borne encephalitis (Europe).[124]

JEV, transmitted by Culex mosquitoes, probably causes more cases of acute encephalitis than the other arthropod-borne viruses combined. Over the last 75 years, from its focus in China and Southeast Asia, JEV has expanded westward to India and Pakistan, northward to eastern Russia, eastward to the Philippines, and southward to Australia. In the northern range, epidemics of japanese encephalitis can occur during the warm summer months, and disease occurs throughout the year in the warmer southern areas.[125] In China alone at least 20,000 symptomatic cases of japanese encephalitis are reported annually.[126] The ratio of symptomatic to asymptomatic infections with JEV is estimated to be 1:25 to 1:1000.[125] In areas where japanese encephalitis is common, it is primarily a disease of children, and more cases are seen in adults when the virus moves into a previously unexposed population. After a few days of nonspecific symptoms, patients with japanese encephalitis present with headache, vomiting, and altered mentation; seizures are reported in 85% of children and 10% of adults. Other characteristic findings include coarse tremor, dystonia, rigidity, and a characteristic masklike facies. A variant of japanese encephalitis that presents with poliomyelitis-like acute flaccid paralysis has recently been reported.[127] MRI reveals a characteristic pattern of mixed intensity or hypodense lesions especially in the thalamus but also in the basal ganglia and midbrain.[128] Diagnosis is facilitated by detection of IgM in the CSF.[129] The mortality for patients hospitalized with japanese encephalitis is about 30%. Approximately 50% of survivors have severe neurologic sequelae, including motor weakness, intellectual impairment, and seizure disorders. Therapy for japanese encephalitis is limited to intensive supportive care. An effective formalin-inactivated vaccine against japanese encephalitis is available and is recommended for inhabitants of endemic areas as well as travelers entering rural endemic areas.[130] An attenuated live virus vaccine for japanese encephalitis has been developed in China but is less widely available than the inactivated vaccine.[131]

In the United States, most cases of arthropod-borne encephalitis in recent years have been attributed to La Crosse virus, EEE virus, and St. Louis encephalitis virus (Table 12–5). La Crosse virus, a Bunyavirus in the California encephalitis serogroup, causes aseptic meningitis and encephalitis, primarily in school-age children. Although the mortality associated with La Crosse encephalitis is low, 10% to 15% of survivors will have significant neurologic deficits.[132,133] EEE occurs during the summer months along the eastern and gulf coasts of the United States. In contrast to La Crosse encephalitis, EEE frequently occurs among older adults. Patients with EEE experience a short prodromal illness, then present with fever, headache, and generalized seizures which may progress to stupor or coma.[134] MRI reveals focal lesions in the basal ganglia, thalami, and brainstem. The mortality is 30% to 40%, and at least one-third of survivors have significant neurologic sequelae. High CSF white count ($>500/mm^3$) and low serum sodium (≤130 mmol/L) are associated with poor outcome.[134]

Beginning in August 1999 an epidemic of viral encephalitis occurred in and around New York City that ultimately resulted in 62 cases and 7 deaths. On the basis of positive serologic results the outbreak was initially attributed to St. Louis encephalitis. A simultaneous epidemic of deaths among wild and exotic captive birds, however, suggested that St. Louis encephalitis virus (which does not ordinarily kill the avian host) might not be the correct pathogen. Ultimately the etiologic agent was identified as WNV.[135–137] WNV encephalitis is a well-described disease in Africa and the Middle East but had not previously been encountered in the Western Hemisphere. As a harbinger of the appearance of WNV in North America, the first major WNV epidemic in Europe occurred in Romania in 1996 and was characterized by a high rate of neurologic complications.[138] On the

TABLE 12–5 ■ Characteristics of Selected Mosquito-Borne Arbovirus Encephalitides in the United States

Characteristic	Western equine	Eastern equine	Venezuelan	St. Louis	La Crosse	West Nile
Geographic distribution	West, Midwest United States	East, Gulf Coast, Southern United States	South America, Southern and Southwest United States	Central, West and Southern United States	Central and Eastern United States	East Coast United States
Age group affected	Infants and adults >50 y old	Children and adults	Adults	Adults >50 y old	Children	Adults
Mortality	5%–15%	30%–40%	1%	2%–20%	<1%	<5%
Sequelae	Moderate in infants; low in others	>30% of survivors	Rare	20% of survivors	10%–15%	Low
Symptoms	Headache, altered consciousness, seizures	Headache, altered consciousness, seizures	Headache, myalgia, pharyngitis	Headache, nausea, vomiting, disorientation, stupor, irritability	Seizures, paralysis, focal weakness	Seizures, myelitis, optic neuritis

Adapted from Whitley RJ: Viral encephalitis. *N Engl J Med* 1990;323:242–250 basis of hospital-based surveillance, 393 confirmed cases of WNV infection were identified in Romania, most of which involved meningoencephalitis. The mortality clearly increased with age; the overall fatality-to-case ratio was 4.3, with all deaths occurring in patients over 50 years of age. The number of mild cases occurring in the Romanian population could not be calculated, but the overall seroprevalence rate was 4.1%. Clinical findings were similar in the Romanian and New York outbreaks. Patients typically presented with abrupt onset of fever, headache, neck stiffness, and vomiting. Patients who progressed to encephalitis demonstrated depressed consciousness, disorientation, and generalized weakness. In both Romania and the United States, additional cases of WNV infection appeared during the following summer, with geographic expansion of human and animal infections proving successful over-wintering of WNV and establishment of an enzootic cycle of transmission involving birds and mosquitoes.[139,140] The pattern of recent epidemics of WNV in Europe and North America indicates that migratory birds contribute to dispersement of the virus, suggesting that WNV has the potential to cause new outbreaks.[141–143] In the summer of 2000 an unexpectedly large outbreak of WNV encephalitis occurred in Israel, with more than 250 confirmed cases and 19 deaths, all in patients over the age of 50 years.[144] There is currently no vaccine to prevent WNV infection. Preventive measures include vector avoidance and mosquito control programs.[145]

Enteroviral Infections

Enteroviruses (including polioviruses, coxsackieviruses, and echoviruses) cause a wide spectrum of human diseases, including myocarditis and pericarditis, exanthemas and enanthemas, conjunctivitis, and meningitis, most of which are mild and self-limited. Certain of the enteroviruses, however, have the potential to cause severe and even fatal neurologic disease, the best known of which is poliomyelitis. Other enteroviruses are frequent causes of seasonal aseptic meningitis and (less commonly) meningoencephalitis, especially in young infants. In 1998 a large outbreak of enteroviral infection (hand-foot-and-mouth disease and herpangina) occurred in Taiwan, with over 60% of the cases attributed to enterovirus 71.[146] What distinguished this enteroviral epidemic was the high rate of neurologic complications among children infected with enterovirus 71.[147] A total of 405 patients with serious enteroviral infection were identified. Most were under 5 years of age, and the mortality in this group was 19.3%. Among patients with positive viral cultures, enterovirus 71 was isolated from 75% of the hospitalized patients and from 92% of the patients who died.[146] The typical clinical presentation was rhombencephalitis, characterized by myoclonus, tremors, ataxia, and cranial nerve involvement.[147] The most severely affected children presented with evidence of brainstem involvement (including neurogenic shock and pulmonary edema), which indicated a poor prognosis.[148] MRI demonstrated distinctive high-intensity lesions localized to the midbrain, pons, and medulla.[148] Long-term neurologic sequelae were common in the children with rhombencephalitis who survived. Although other outbreaks of enterovirus 71 disease have been reported, none have had the level of serious neurologic involvement seen in the Taiwanese epidemic. There is currently no vaccine (other than for polio) or approved antiviral treatment of enteroviral infections, although the antiviral drug pleconaril shows promise and is currently undergoing clinical evaluation.[46]

New Paramyxoviruses: Nipah and Hendra Viruses

In 1997 an outbreak of encephalitis noted among pig farm workers in Malaysia was attributed to JEV. Encephalitis recurred in September 1998, and both clinical and epidemiologic characteristics made it clear that japanese encephalitis was not the correct diagnosis. A paramyxovirus isolated from a Malaysian patient with encephalitis demonstrated in vitro characteristics similar to those of Hendra virus, a new Morbillivirus isolated from horses and humans in Australia in 1995.[149] Subsequent virologic studies have shown that the Malaysian pathogen, now named Nipah virus, is closely related to but distinct from Hendra virus and that the two belong to a new genus within the family Paramyxoviridae.[150] Epidemiologic investigations demonstrated that Nipah virus is transmitted to humans by close contact with infected pigs, probably via the respiratory route.[151] The infection does not require an insect vector and is not readily transmitted from person to person. Patients with Nipah virus encephalitis present with fever, headache, dizziness, vomiting, and altered mental status.[151,152] Clinical features such as hypertension, tachycardia, areflexia, and hypotonia suggest brainstem involvement. MRI scanning shows a distinctive picture of discrete 2- to 7-mm lesions disseminated throughout the brain but occurring mainly in the subcortical and deep white matter of the cerebral hemispheres.[153] Pathologic correlation suggests that the lesions seen on MRI are due to widespread microinfarctions resulting from small-vessel vasculitis.[154] Among 94 patients hospitalized with Nipah virus encephalitis in Malaysia from February to June 1999, 32% died, 53% had full recovery, and 15% survived but had persistent neurologic deficits.[151] The epidemic was terminated by aggressive culling of all infected or exposed pigs. As with Hendra virus, the natural reservoir for Nipah virus appears to be pteropid bats, with pigs serving as hosts for viral amplification.[155]

APPROACH TO THE PATIENT WITH VIRAL CENTRAL NERVOUS SYSTEM DISEASE

The approach to a patient with a presumed CNS viral infection must be tailored to the severity and distribution of neurologic involvement. The degree of diagnostic as well as therapeutic intervention differs with the type of CNS disease. For example, a patient with photophobia and nuccal rigidity but a nonfocal neurologic examination result does not require invasive intracranial pressure monitoring like a patient with encephalitis and evidence of increased intracranial pressure needs. After establishing the degree of CNS disease by history and physical examination and stabilizing the patient (airway, breathing, circulation), the clinician next must ascertain a diagnosis. A simplified flow diagram reviewing the way to approach the patient with viral CNS disease is presented in Figure 12–4. The first step of any intervention hinges on establishing the correct diagnosis. A history and physical examination are logical first step. The thoroughness of the initial history and physical examination is tailored to the stability of the patient. A comatose person with apneustic respirations requires immediate intervention, whereas the person with nuccal rigidity and photophobia can be afforded a

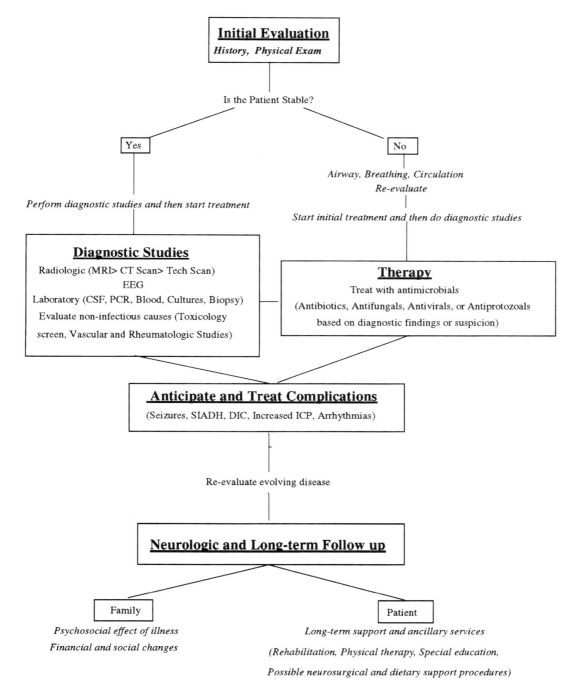

FIGURE 12–4. Approach to patient with presumed central nervous system viral infection. CSF, cerebrospinal fluid; CT, computed tomography; DIC, disseminated intravascular coagulation; EEG, electroencephalogram; ICP, intracranial pressure; MRI, magnetic resource imaging; PCR, polymerase chain reaction; SIADH, syndrome of inappropriate antidiurectic hormone.

more detailed investigation for the cause of the symptoms before any therapy is instituted.

Treatable causes of CNS dysfunction require rapid evaluation and intervention in an effort to prevent permanent or further CNS damage. Potentially treatable diseases (fungal CNS infections, partially treated bacterial meningitis, tuberculous meningitis, parameningeal infection, Mycoplasma infection, and fastidious bacterial infections) can mimic viral CNS disease and should be vigorously investigated before the illness is attributed to an untreatable viral cause. The same logic applies to treatable viral infections and noninfectious causes. The radiographic and laboratory studies available for establishing a diagnosis must be prioritized according to the likely cause and the stability of the patient.

After establishing a presumptive diagnosis and instituting therapy, the clinician must also vigilantly anticipate and treat complications associated with the viral CNS disease or the therapeutic interventions. Seizures secondary to direct viral CNS damage, inflammatory vasculitis, and electrolyte changes, require anticonvulsant therapy with benzodiazepines, phenytoin, and barbiturates.[3] Patients with cerebral edema may require intracranial pressure monitoring, hyperventilation, osmotic therapy, and CSF removal to maintain cerebral pressures at less than 15 mm Hg.[3] The ultimate goal of intracranial pressure monitoring is to maintain adequate cerebral perfusion. While a physician struggles to maintain an adequate intravascular blood volume, intracranial pressures can rise to dangerous levels as capillary leak complicates the patient's course. The risks of increased intracranial pressure from aggressive fluid resuscitation or SIADH release necessitate fastidious fluid management and frequent electrolyte monitoring. Cardiac arrhythmias can also develop secondary to electrolyte changes or brainstem damage in patients with encephalitis. Cardiac and respiratory arrest can occur early in disease; therefore equipment for intubation and cardioversion should be readily available for a patient with encephalitis. In addition to the direct damage the virus can cause in the CNS, certain viruses can also produce systemic damage that complicates the management of the CNS disease. Patients can develop overwhelming hepatitis, pneumonitis, disseminated intravascular coagulation, and shock. Patients in coma from encephalitis can recover after long periods of unconsciousness. The physician should limit the amount of iatrogenic damage and vigorously support the patient during the acute phase of the illness.

CONCLUSION

Numerous factors influence the clinical manifestations of viral CNS infections. A person's age, immune history, cultural practices, and genetic makeup can influence the clinical expression of viral infection as readily as the viral serotype, receptor preference, viral load, and cell tropism.[9] Changes in behavior and in cultural beliefs, increased travel, and modification of the environment alter disease patterns and expose people to new infectious agents. CNS infections therefore must be examined in a geographic, cultural, and environmental context as well as the cellular, molecular, and genetic levels.[136,142] Improvements in our ability to diagnose CNS infections will produce a better understanding of the pathogenesis and true extent of CNS viral disease.

REFERENCES

1. Moorthi S, Schneider WN, Dombovy ML: Rehabilitation outcomes in encephalitis—a retrospective study 1990–1997. Brain Inj 1999;13:139.
2. Schlitt M, Chronister RB, Whitley RJ: Pathogenesis and pathophysiology of viral infections of the central nervous system. In Scheld WM, Whitley RJ, Durack DT (eds): Infections of the Central Nervous System. New York, Raven Press, 1991, p 7.
3. Bale JF Jr: Viral encephalitis. Med Clin North Am 1993;77:25.
4. Whitley RJ, Cobbs CG, Alford CA Jr, et al: Diseases that mimic herpes simplex encephalitis: Diagnosis, presentation and outcome. JAMA 1989;262:234.
5. Hammer SM, Connolly KJ: Viral aseptic meningitis in the United States: Clinical features, viral etiologies, and differential diagnosis. Curr Clin Top Infect Dis 1992;12:1.
6. Rotbart HA: Viral meningitis and the aseptic meningitis syndrome. In Scheld WM, Whitley RJ, Durack DT (eds): Infections of the Central Nervous System. Philadelphia, Lippincott-Raven, 1997, p 23.
7. Whitley RJ, MacDonald N, Asher DM, et al: Technical report: Transmissible spongiform encephalopathies: A review for pediatricians. Pediatrics 2000;106:1160.
8. Johnson RT: The pathogenesis of acute viral encephalitis and postinfectious encephalitis. J Infect Dis 1987;155:359.
9. Cassady KA, Whitley RJ: Pathogenesis and pathophysiology of viral central nervous system infections. In Scheld WM, Whitley RJ, Durack DT (eds): Infections of the Central Nervous System. New York, Raven Press, 1997, p 7.
10. Nicolosi A, Hauser WA, Beghi E, et al: Epidemiology of central nervous system infections in Olmsted County, Minnesota, 1950–1981. J Infect Dis 1986;154:399.
11. Nigrovic LE, Chiang VW: Cost analysis of enteroviral polymerase chain reaction in infants with fever and cerebrospinal fluid pleocytosis. Arch Pediatr Adolesc Med 1986;154:817.
12. Pozo F, Casas I, Tenorio A, et al: Evaluation of a commercially available reverse transcription-PCR assay for diagnosis of enteroviral infection in archival and prospectively collected cerebrospinal fluid specimens. J Clin Microbiol 1998;36:1741.
13. Sawyer MH: Enterovirus infections: Diagnosis and treatment. Pediatr Infect Dis J 1999;18:1033.
14. Hosoya M, Honzumi K, Sato M, et al: Application of PCR for various neurotropic viruses on the diagnosis of viral meningitis. J Clin Virol 1998;11:117.
15. Rotbart HA: Enteroviral infections of the central nervous system. Clin Infect Dis 1995;20:971.
16. Summary of notifiable diseases, United States, 1994. MMWR Morb Mortal Wkly Rep 1994;43:1.
17. Cassady KA, Whitley RJ: Central nervous system infections. In Richman DD, Whitley RJ, Hayden FG (eds): Clinical Virology. New York, Churchill Livingstone, 1997, p 35.
18. Kimura H, Futamura M, Kito H, et al: Detection of viral DNA in neonatal herpes simplex virus infections: Frequent and prolonged presence in serum and cerebrospinal fluid. J Infect Dis 1991;164:289.

19. Stanberry LR, Floyd-Reising SA, Connelly BL, et al: Herpes simplex viremia: Report of eight pediatric cases and review of the literature. Clin Infect Dis 1994;18:401.

20. Wiestler OD, Leib SL, Brustle O: Neuropathology and pathogenesis of HIV encephalopathies. Acta Histochem Suppl 1992;42:107.

21. Bradbury MW: The blood-brain barrier. Exp Physiol 1993;78:453.

22. Edens HA, Parkos CA: Modulation of epithelial and endothelial paracellular permeability by leukocytes. Adv Drug Deliv Rev 2000;41:315.

23. Nagy Z, Martinez K: Astrocytic induction of endothelial tight junctions. Ann N Y Acad Sci 1991;633:395.

24. Abbott NJ: Inflammatory mediators and modulation of blood-brain barrier permeability. Cell Mol Neurobiol 2000;20:131.

25. Becher B, Prat A, Antel JP: Brain-immune connection: Immuno-regulatory properties of CNS-resident cells. Glia 2000;29:293.

26. Cunningham CK, Bonville CA, Ochs HD, et al: Enteroviral meningoencephalitis as a complication of X-linked hyper IgM syndrome. J Pediatr 1999;134:584.

27. Schmugge M, Lauener R, Seger RA, et al: Chronic enteroviral meningo-encephalitis in X-linked agammaglobulinaemia: Favorable response to anti-enteroviral treatment. Eur J Pediatr 1999;158:1010.

28. Wilfert CM, Lehrman SN, Katz SL: Enteroviruses and meningitis. Pediatr Infect Dis J 1983;2:333.

29. Rorabaugh ML, Berlin LE, Heldrich F, et al: Aseptic meningitis in infants younger than 2 years of age: Acute illness and neurologic complications. Pediatrics 1993;92:206.

30. Corey L, Adams HG, Brown ZA, et al: Genital herpes simplex virus infections: Clinical manifestations, course and complications. Ann Intern Med 1983;98:958.

31. Bergstrom T, Vahlne A, Alestig K, et al: Primary and recurrent herpes simplex virus type 2 induced meningitis. J Infect Dis 1990;162:322.

32. Jensenius M, Myrvang B, Storvold G, et al: Herpes simplex virus type 2 DNA detected in cerebrospinal fluid of 9 patients with Mollaret's meningitis. Acta Neurol Scand 1998;98:209.

33. Arisoy ES, Demmler GJ, Thaker S, et al: Meningitis due to parainfluenza virus type 3: Report of two cases and review. Clin Infect Dis 1993;17:995.

34. Echevarria JM, Casas I, Martinez-Martin P: Infections of the nervous system caused by varicella-zoster virus: A review. Intervirology 1997;40:72.

35. Echevarria JM, Casas I, Tenorio A, et al: Detection of varicella-zoster virus-specific DNA sequences in cerebrospinal fluid from patients with acute aseptic meningitis and no cutaneous lesions. J Med Virol 1994;43:331.

36. Negrini B, Kelleher KJ, Wald ER: Cerebrospinal fluid findings in aseptic versus bacterial meningitis. Pediatrics 2000;105:316.

37. Feigin RD, Shackelford PG: Value of repeat lumbar puncture in the differential diagnosis of meningitis. N Engl J Med 1973;289:571.

38. Harrison SA, Risser WL: Repeat lumbar puncture in the differential diagnosis of meningitis. Pediatr Infect Dis J 1988;7:143.

39. Varki B, Puthuran P: Value of second lumbar puncture in confirming the diagnosis of aseptic meningitis. Arch Neurol 1979;36:581.

40. Ahmed A, Brito F, Goto C, et al: Clinical utility of the polymerase chain reaction for diagnosis of enteroviral meningitis in infancy. J Pediatr 1997;131:393.

41. van Vliet KE, Glimaker M, Lebon P, et al: Multicenter evaluation of the Amplicor Enterovirus PCR test with cerebrospinal fluid from patients with aseptic meningitis. The European Union Concerted Action on Viral Meningitis and Encephalitis. J Clin Microbiol 1998;36:2652.

42. Ramers C, Billman G, Hartin M, et al: Impact of a diagnostic cerebrospinal fluid enterovirus polymerase chain reaction test on patient management. JAMA 2000;283:2680.

43. Tsai TF: Arboviral infections in the United States. Infect Dis Clin North Am 1991;5:73.

44. Kuno G: Universal diagnostic RT-PCR protocol for arboviruses. J Virol Meth 1998;72:27.

45. Webster AD, Rotbart HA, Warner T, et al: Diagnosis of enterovirus brain disease in hypogammaglobulinemic patients by polymerase chain reaction. Clin Infect Dis 1993;17:657.

46. Pevear DC, Tull TM, Seipel ME, et al: Activity of pleconaril against enteroviruses. Antimicrob Agents Chemother 1999;43:2109.

47. Rotbart HA: Antiviral therapy for enteroviral infections. Pediatr Infect Dis J 1999;18:632.

48. Dwyer JM, Erlendsson K: Intraventricular gamma-globulin for the management of enterovirus encephalitis. Pediatr Infect Dis J 1988;7(5 Suppl):S30.

49. McKinney RE, Katz SL: Chronic enteroviral meningoencephalitis in agammaglobulinemic patients. Rev Infect Dis 1987;9:334.

50. Abzug M, Keyserling HL, Lee ML, et al: Neonatal enterovirus infection: Virology, serology, and effects of intravenous immunoglubulin. Clin Infect Dis 1995;20:1201.

51. Rotbart HA, Brennan PJ, Fife KH, et al: Enterovirus meningitis in adults. Clin Infect Dis 1998;27:896.

52. Whitley RJ, Gnann J: Acyclovir: A decade later. N Engl J Med 1992;327:782.

53. Conway JH, Weinberg A, Ashley RL, et al: Viral meningitis in a preadolescent child caused by reactivation of latent herpes simplex (type 1). Pediatr Infect Dis J 1997;16:627.

54. De La Blanchardiere A, Rozenberg F, Caumes E, et al: Neurological complications of varicellazoster virus infection in adults with human immunodeficiency virus infection. Scand J Infect Dis 2000;32:263.

55. de Silva SM, Mark AS, Gilden DH, et al: Zoster myelitis: Improvement with antiviral therapy in two cases. Neurology 1996;47:929.

56. Gilden DH, Kleinschmidt-DeMasters BK, LaGuardia JJ, et al: Neurologic complications of the reactivation of varicella-zoster virus. N Engl J Med 2000;342:635.

57. Summary of notifiable diseases, United States, 1998. MMWR Morb Mortal Wkly Rep 1999;47:1.

58. Koskiniemi M, Korppi M, Mustonen K, et al: Epidemiology of encephalitis in children. A prospective multicenter study. Eur J Pediatr 1997;156:541.

59. Ho DD, Hirsch MS: Acute viral encephalitis. Med Clin North Am 1985;69:415.

60. Arboviral infections of the central nervous system—United States, 1996–1997. MMWR Morb Mortal Wkly Rep 1998;47:517.

61. Rantakallio P, Leskinen M, von Wendt L: Incidence and prognosis of central nervous system infections in a birth cohort of 12,000 children. Scand J Infect Dis 1986;18(4):287.

62. Pape WJ, Fitzsimmons TD, Hoffman RE: Risk for rabies transmission from encounters with bats, Colorado, 1977–1996. Emerg Infect Dis 1999;5:433.

63. Human rabies—California, Georgia, Minnesota, New York, and Wisconsin. MMWR Morb Mortal Wkly Rep 2000;49:1111.

64. Stuve O, Zamvil SS: Pathogenesis, diagnosis, and treatment of acute disseminated encephalomyelitis. Curr Opin Neurol 1999;12:395.

65. Sharpe AH, Fields BN: Pathogenesis of viral infections. Basic concepts derived from the reovirus model. N Engl J Med 1985;312(8):486.

66. Whitley RJ, Kern ER, Chatterjee S, et al: Replication, establishment of latency, and induced reactivation of herpes

simplex virus γ_1 34.5 deletion mutants in rodent models. J Clin Invest 1993;91:2837.

67. Griffin DE: A review of alphavirus replication in neurons. Neurosci Biobehav Rev 1998;22:721.

68. Goldsmith K, Chen W, Johnson DC, et al: Infected cell protein (ICP)47 enhances herpes simplex virus neurovirulence by blocking the CD8+ T cell response. J Exp Med 1998;187:341.

69. Johnson R: The pathogenesis of herpes virus encephalitis. II. A cellular basis for the development of resistance with age. J Exp Med 1964;120:359.

70. Gatmaitan BG, Chason JL, Lerner AM: Augmentation of the virulence of murine coxsackie-virus B-3 myocardiopathy by exercise. J Exp Med 1970;131(6):1121.

71. Russell WR: Poliomyelitis: Pre-paralytic stage and the effect of physical activity on the severity of paralysis. BMJ 1947;2(2):1023.

72. Friedemann U: Permeability of blood-brain barrier to neurotropic viruses. Arch Pathol 1943;35:912.

73. Mrak RE, Young L: Rabies encephalitis in humans: Pathology, pathogenesis and pathophysiology. J Neuropathol Exp Neurol 1994;53(1):1.

74. Lentz TL: The recognition event between virus and host cell receptor: A target for antiviral agents. J Gen Virol 1990;71(Pt 4):751.

75. Barnett EM, Cassell D, Perlman S: Two neurotropic viruses, herpes simplex virus type 1 and mouse hepatitis virus, spread along different neural pathways from the main olfactory bulb. Neuroscience 1993;57:1007.

76. Barnett EM, Jacobsen G, Evans G, et al: Herpes simplex encephalitis in the temporal cortex and limbic system after trigeminal nerve inoculation. J Infect Dis 1994;169:782.

77. Whitley RJ: Herpes simplex virus infections of the central nervous system: Encephalitis and neonatal herpes. In Sorkin EM (ed): Drugs. New Zealand, ADIS Press Limited, 1991, p 406.

78. Nahmias AJ, Whitley RJ, Visintine AN, et al: Herpes simplex encephalitis: Laboratory evaluations and their diagnostic significance. J Infect Dis 1982;145:829.

79. Pruisner SB: Novel proteinaceous infectious particles cause scrapie. Science 1982;216:136.

80. D'Arminio MA, Cinque P, Vago L, et al: A comparison of brain biopsy and CSF-PCR in the diagnosis of CNS lesions in AIDS patients. J Neurol 1997;244:35.

81. Fujimoto S, Kobayashi M, Uemura O, et al: PCR on cerebrospinal fluid to show influenza-associated acute encephalopathy or encephalitis. Lancet 1998;352:873.

82. Jeffery KJ, Read SJ, Peto TE, et al: Diagnosis of viral infections of the central nervous system: Clinical interpretation of PCR results. Lancet 1997;349:313.

83. Poggio GP, Rodriguez C, Cisterna D, et al: Nested PCR for rapid detection of mumps virus in cerebrospinal fluid from patients with neurological diseases. J Clin Microbiol 2000;38:274.

84. Read SJ, Kurtz JB: Laboratory diagnosis of common viral infections of the central nervous system by using a single multiplex PCR screening assay. J Clin Microbiol 1999;37:1352.

85. Smith RR: Neuroradiology of intracranial infection. Pediatr Neurosurg 1992;18(2):92.

86. Casas I, Pozo F, Trallero G, et al: Viral diagnosis of neurological infection by RT multiplex PCR: A search for entero- and herpesviruses in a prospective study. J Med Virol 1999;57:145.

87. Lakeman FD, Whitley RJ, the National Institute of Allergy and Infectious Diseases Collaborative Antiviral Study Group: Diagnosis of herpes simplex encephalitis: Application of polymerase chain reaction to cerebrospinal fluid from brain biopsied patients and correlation with disease. J Infect Dis 1995;172:857.

88. Domingues RB, Lakeman FD, Pannuti CS, et al: Advantage of polymerase chain reaction in the diagnosis of herpes simplex encephalitis: Presentation of 5 atypical cases. Scand J Infect Dis 1997;29:229.

89. Vrancken AF, Frijns CJ, Ramos LM: FLAIR MRI in sporadic Creutzfeldt-Jakob disease. Neurology 2000;55:147.

90. Expanded program on immunization. Certification of poliomyelitis eradication—the Americas. MMWR Morb Mortal Wkly Rep 1994;43:720.

91. Rosen L: The natural history of Japanese encephalitis virus. Annu Rev Microbiol 1986;40:395.

92. Balfour HH Jr: Current management of varicella zoster virus infections. J Med Virol 1993;Suppl 1:74.

93. Cinque P, Bossolasco S, Vago L, et al: Varicella-zoster virus (VZV) DNA in cerebrospinal fluid of patients infected with human immunodeficiency virus: VZV disease of the central nervous system or subclinical reactivation of VZV infection. Clin Infect Dis 1997;25:634.

94. Maschke M, Kastrup O, Esser S, et al: Incidence and prevalence of neurological disorders associated with HIV since the introduction of highly active antiretroviral therapy (HAART). Neurol Neurosurg Psychiatry 2000;69:376.

95. Soontornniyomkij V, Nieto-Rodriguez JA, Martinez AJ, et al: Brain HIV burden and length of survival after AIDS diagnosis. Clin Neuropathol 1998;17:95.

96. Balestri P, Grosso S, Acquaviva A, et al: Plasmapheresis in a child affectd by acute disseminated encephalomyelitis. Brain Dev 2000;22:123.

97. Pradhan S, Gupta RP, Shashank S, et al: Intravenous immunoglobulin therapy in acute disseminated encephalomyelitis. J Neurol Sci 1999;165:56.

98. Rowley A, Lakeman F, Whitley R, et al: Rapid detection of herpes simplex virus DNA in cerebrospinal fluid of patients with herpes simplex encephalitis. Lancet 1990;335:440.

99. Boerman RH, Arnoldus EP, Raap AK: Polymerase chain reaction and viral culture techniques to detect HSV in small volumes of cerebrospinal fluid: An experimental mouse encephalitis study. J Virol Methods 1989;25:189.

100. Puchhammer-Stockl E, Popow-Kraupp T, Heinz FX, et al: Establishment of PCR for the early diagnosis of herpes simplex encephalitis. J Med Virol 1990;32:77.

101. Powell KF, Anderson NE, Frith RW, et al: Non-invasive diagnosis of herpes simplex encephalitis. Lancet 1990;335:357.

102. Whitley RJ, Alford CA Jr, Hirsch MS, et al: Vidarabine versus acyclovir therapy in herpes simplex encephalitis. N Engl J Med 1986;314:144.

103. Longson M, Klapper PE, Cleator GM: The treatment of herpes encephalitis. J Infect 1983;6:15.

104. Whitely RJ, Lakeman F: Herpes simplex infections of the central nervous system: Therapeutic and diagnostic considerations. Clin Infect Dis 1995;20:414.

105. McGrath N, Anderson NE, Croxson MC, Powell KF: Herpes simplex encephalitis treated with acyclovir: Diagnosis and long term outcome. J Neurol Neurosurg Psychiatry 1997;63:321.

106. Ito Y, Kimura H, Yabuta Y, et al: Exacerbation of herpes simplex encephalitis after successful treatment with acyclovir. Clin Infect Dis 2000;30:185.

107. Whitley RJ: Herpes simplex virus. In Scheld WM, Whitley RJ, Durack DT (eds): Infections of the Central Nervous System. Philadelphia, Lippincott-Raven, 1996, p 73.

108. Vahlne A, Svennerholm B, Sandberg M, et al: Differences in attachment between herpes simplex type 1 and type 2 viruses to neurons and glial cells. Infect Immun 1980;28:675.

109. Gerber SI, Belval BJ, Herold BC: Differences in the role of glycoprotein C of HSV-1 and HSV-2 in viral binding may contribute to serotype differences in cell tropism. Virology 1995;214:29.

110. Jainkittivong A, Langlais RP: Herpes B virus infection. Oral Surg Oral Med Oral Pathol Oral Radiol Endod 1998;85:399.

111. Centers for Disease Control and Prevention: Fatal Cercopithecine herpesvirus 1 (B virus) infection following a mucocutaneous exposure and interim recommendations for worker protection. MMWR Morb Mortal Wkly Rep 1998;47:1073.

112. Ostrowski SR, Leslie MJ, Parrott T, et al: B virus from pet macaque monkeys: An emerging threat in the United States? Emerg Infect Dis 1998;4:117.

113. Freifeld AG, Hilliard J, Southers J, et al: A controlled seroprevalence survey of primate handlers for evidence of asymptomatic herpes B virus infection. J Infect Dis 1995;171:1031.

114. Holmes GP, Chapman LE, Stewart JE, et al: Guidelines for preventing and treating B virus infections in exposed persons. Clin Infect Dis 1995;20:421.

115. Moran GJ, Talan DA, Mower W, et al: Appropriateness of rabies postexposure prophylaxis treatment for animal exposures. Emergency ID Net Study Group. JAMA 2000;284:1001.

116. World survey of rabies, 1997. Wkly Epidemiol Rec 1997;74:381.

117. Krebs JW, Smith JS, Rupprecht CE, et al: Rabies surveillance in the United States during 1998. J Am Vet Med Assoc 2000;215:1786.

118. Plotkin SA: Rabies. Clin Infect Dis 2000;30:4.

119. Hanlon CA, Smith JS, Anderson GR: Recommendation of a national working group on prevention and control of rabies in the United States. Article II: Laboratory diagnosis of rabies. The National Working Group on Rabies Prevention and Control. J Am Vet Med Assoc 1999;215:1444.

120. Noah DL, Drenzek CL, Smith JS, et al: Epidemiology of human rabies in the United States, 1980 to 1996. Ann Intern Med 1998;128:922.

121. Centers for Disease Control and Prevention: Human rabies prevention–United States, 1999. MMWR Morb Mortal Wkly Rep 1999;48(Suppl RR-1):1.

122. Hanna JN, Carney IK, Smith GA, et al: Australian bat lyssavirus infection: A second human case with a long incubation period. Med J Aust 2000;172:597.

123. Samaratunga H, Searle JW, Hudson N: Non-rabies Lyssavirus human encephalitits from fruit bats: Australian bat Lyssavirus (pteropid Lyssavirus) infection. Neuropathol Appl Neurobiol 1998;24:331.

124. Whitley RJ: Viral encephalitis. N Engl J Med 1990;323:242.

125. Solomon T, Dung NM, Kneen R, et al: Japanese encephalitis. J Neurol Neurosurg Psychiatry 2000;68:405.

126. Vaughn DW, Hoke CH Jr: The epidemiology of Japanese encephalitis: Prospects for prevention. Epidemiol Rev 1992;14:197.

127. Solomon T, Kneen R, Dung NM, et al: Poliomyelitis-like illness due to Japanese encephalitis virus. Lancet 1998;351:1094.

128. Kalita J, Mista UK: Comparison of CT scan and MRI findings in the diagnosis of Japanese encephalitis. J Neurol Sci 2000;174:3.

129. Solomon T, Thao LT, Dung NM, et al: Rapid diagnosis of Japanese encephalitis by using an immunoglobulin M dot enzyme immunoassay. J Clin Microbiol 1998;36:2030.

130. Centers for Disease Control and Prevention: Inactivated Japanese encephalitis virus vaccine. Recommendations of the Advisory Committee on Immunization Practices (ACIP). MMWR Morb Mortal Wkly Rep 1993;42:1.

131. Tsai TF, Yu YX, Jia LL, et al: Immunogenicity of live attenuated SA 14-14-2 Japanese encephalitis vaccine—a comparison of 1- and 3-month immunization schedules. J Infect Dis 1998;177:221.

132. McJunkin JE, de los Reyes EC, Irazuzta JE, et al: La Crosse encephalitis in children. N Engl J Med 2001;344:801.

133. McJunkin JE, Khan RR, Tsai TF: California-LaCrosse encephalitis. Infect Dis Clin North Am 1998;12:83.

134. Deresiewicz RL, Thaler SJ, Hsu L, et al: Clinical and neuroradiographic manifestations of eastern equine encephalitis. N Engl J Med 1997;336:1867.

135. Centers for Disease Control and Prevention: Outbreak of West Nile–like viral encephalitis—New York, 1999. MMWR Morb Mortal Wkly Rep 1999;48:845.

136. Briese T, Jia XY, Huang C, et al: Identification of a Kunjin/West Nile–like flavivirus in brains of patients with New York encephalitis. Lancet 1999;354:1261.

137. Jia XY, Briese T, Jordan I, et al: Genetic analysis of West Nile New York 1999 encephalitis virus. Lancet 1999;354:1971.

138. Tsai TF, Popovici F, Cernescu C, et al: West Nile encephalitis epidemic in southeastern Romania. Lancet 1998;352:767.

139. Cernescu C, Nedelcu NI, Tardei G, et al: Continued transmission of West Nile virus to humans in southeastern Romania, 1997–1998. J Infect Dis 2000;181:710.

140. Centers for Disease Control and Prevention: Human West Nile virus surveillance—Connecticut, New Jersey, and New York, 2000. MMWR Morb Mortal Wkly Rep 2001;50:265.

141. Hubalek Z, Halouzka J: West Nile fever—A reemerging mosquito-borne viral disease in Europe. Emerg Infect Dis 1999;5:643.

142. Lanciotti RW, Roehrig JT, Deubel V, et al: Origin of West Nile virus responsible for an outbreak of encephalitis in the northeastern United States. Science 1999;286:2333.

143. Rappole JH, Derrickson SR, Hubalek Z: Migratory birds and spread of West Nile virus in the Western Hemisphere. Emerg Infect Dis 2000;6:319.

144. Siegel-Itzkovich J: Twelve die of West Nile virus in Israel. BMJ 2000;321:724.

145. Centers for Disease Control and Prevention: Guidelines for surveillance, prevention, and control of West Nile virus infection—United States. MMWR Morb Mortal Wkly Rep 2000;49:25.

146. Ho M, Chen ER, Hsu KH, et al: An epidemic of enterovirus 71 infection in Taiwan. Taiwan Enterovirus Epidemic Working Group. N Engl J Med 1999;341:929.

147. Huang CC, Liu CC, Chang YC, et al: Neurologic complications in children with enterovirus 71 infection. N Engl J Med 1999;341:936.

148. Wang SM, Liu CC, Tseng HW, et al: Clinical spectrum of enterovirus 71 infection in children in southern Taiwan, with an emphasis on neurological complications. Clin Infect Dis 1999;29:184.

149. Selvey LA, Wells RM, McCormack JG, et al: Infection of humans and horses by a newly described morbillivirus. Med J Aust 1995;162:642.

150. Chua KB, Bellini WJ, Rota PA, et al: Nipah virus: A recently emergent deadly paramyxovirus. Science 2000;288:1432.

151. Goh KJ, Tan CT, Chew NK, et al: Clinical features of Nipah virus encephalitis among pig farmers in Malaysia. N Engl J Med 2000;342:1229.

152. Paton NI, Leo YS, Zaki SR, et al: Outbreak of Nipah-virus infection among abattoir workers in Singapore. Lancet 1999;354:1253.

153. Sarji SA, Abdullah BJ, Goh KJ, et al: MR imaging features of Nipah encephalitis. A & R Am J Roentgenol 2000;175:437.

154. Chua KB, Goh KJ, Wong KT, et al: Fatal encephalitis due to Nipah virus among pig-farmers in Malaysia. Lancet 1999;354:1257.

155. Enserink M: Emerging diseases. Malaysian researchers trace Nipah virus outbreak to bats. Science 2000;289:518.

Cysticercosis

RAUL E. ISTURIZ, MD

Differences in larval characteristics (*Cysticercus cellulosae* vs. *Cysticercus racemosus*), parasite load, location, and viability, and distinct expressions of human defenses explain why cysticercosis is a disease of extreme clinical variability and prognosis.[1] Accordingly, no single treatment approach is possible, and strict individualization is pivotal for achieving a successful therapeutic outcome.

Many patients with cysticercosis do require some form of treatment, and for most the therapy of choice is pharmacologic. Nevertheless, surgical therapy, a combination of surgical and pharmacologic therapy, or no therapy at all are options for patients at different stages of cysticercosis, particularly in its most significant clinical picture, neurocysticercosis (NCC). Despite advances in therapy, cysticercosis of the central nervous system (CNS) remains a disease of guarded prognosis, considerable morbidity,[2] and still appreciable mortality.

ANTIPARASITIC DRUGS FOR THERAPY OF CYSTICERCOSIS

Praziquantel

Praziquantel is a pyrazinoisoquinolone with broad anthelmintic activity against adult trematodes and cestodes.[3] It is also active against cestodic larval forms. The (-) isomer is responsible for most of the drug's biologic properties. Although the molecular aspects of the mechanism of action of praziquantel in cysticercosis are unknown, it most likely produces tegumental damage affecting the membrane of intermediate cyst larvae. Its in vivo anticysticercal properties in humans were first demonstrated in the early 1980s.[4,5] Praziquantel is available as 600-mg film-coated tablets. Because of its bitter taste, it is advised that tablets be swallowed without chewing. After ingestion, it is rapidly and almost completely absorbed from the gastrointestinal tract, from which it undergoes first-pass hepatic metabolism. High levels of many inactive hydroxylated and conjugated compounds are produced that limit the bioavailability of the active drug. Peak serum levels of unchanged praziquantel of 1 µg/ml (0.2–2) are achieved 1 to 3 hours after oral administration of 50 mg/kg. Protein binding is 80%, and the half-life is 0.8–1.5 hours. Excretion is chiefly urinary. Approximately 80% is excreted in 4 days, and 90% of that amount in the first 24 hours. Fecal excretion of metabolites accounts for the difference. In cerebrospinal fluid (CSF), concentrations of praziquantel reach approximately 14% to 24% of the total plasma concentration.

Dexamethasone, a drug frequently used with praziquantel to prevent neural tissue inflammation and edema, decreases by about 50% the bioavailability of praziquantel[6,7] by mechanisms not clearly understood. Carbamazepine and phenobarbital may decrease levels of praziquantel by induction of the cytochrome P450 system.

Conversely, cimetidine,[8] ketaconazole, and other P450 inhibitors increase plasma levels of praziquantel by up to 100%. Under certain conditions, praziquantel may actually increase the bioavailability of albendazole, the other first-line anticysticercal drug, but the two are unlikely to be used together.

Praziquantel has been well tolerated by young adults and older children, but safety studies in patients younger that 4 years and in the elderly have not been properly conducted. Uncontrolled clinical use suggests that untoward effects are similar for all ages. Most adverse effects are directly related to the drug, are dose related, occur shortly after administration, and are short lived. They include gastrointestinal symptoms such as abdominal pain, nausea and vomiting, and neurologic complaints such as headache, drowsiness, and dizziness. Adverse reactions not due to intrinsic drug toxicity but to inflammation secondary to host responses to the dead parasites are common and may be severe, even lethal. Fever, urticaria, arthralgia, myalgia, and eosinophilia, uncommonly observed, may parallel the patient's level of parasitic burden. In NCC, inflammation of neural tissue surrounding the decaying larvae is common at 24 to 96 hours after initiation of therapy and may produce increased intracranial pressure, meningeal irritation, seizures, mental status changes, and CSF pleocytosis; therefore, outpatient therapy is seldom advisable. Patients should be instructed not to perform activities requiring mental alertness shortly after taking praziquantel, even for non-neural infections. In ocular cysticercosis, irreversible eye damage may ensue after therapy.[9]

Praziquantel is considered pregnancy category B. In rats and rabbits there has been no evidence of teratogenicity or impaired fertility. In the absence of well-controlled studies in pregnant women, however, the drug should be used during pregnancy only if clearly needed. Praziquantel is excreted in human milk at concentrations of one-fourth of that of maternal serum; therefore, women should not nurse while taking praziquantel and during the 72 to 96 hours following the last dose.

The current recommended dosage of praziquantel for therapy of NCC is 50 mg/kg daily for 15 to 30 days. Single day, 75 mg/kg total dose (25 mg/kg given every 2 hours for three doses)[10,11] or 100 mg/kg total dose (33 mg/kg given every 2 hours for three doses),[12] followed by three or more daily doses of dexamethasone or prednisone (avoiding cysticidal-steroidal drug interactions), can increase compliance as well as decrease length of therapy, cost, and adverse effects associated with longer regimens. Further evaluation of shorter regimens will be needed before widespread adoption.

Albendazole

Albendazole is a broad-spectrum benzimidazole carbamate that arrests assembly of helmintic cytoplasmic microtubules[13] by binding to β-tubulin and inhibiting its polymerization. Having proved useful in hydatidosis,

albendazole also exhibited cysticidal activity in vivo. This was initially demonstrated in humans in seven patients in whom an 86% reduction in the number of parenchymal cysts was documented after 30 days of treatment.[14] Albendazole is prepared for oral administration as 200-mg film-coated tablets. Because of its low water solubility the drug is poorly absorbed from the gastrointestinal tract, and plasma concentrations are nil after oral administration. Albendazole is rapidly converted to albendazole sulfoxide, the assumed cysticidal compound, by first-pass hepatic metabolism and by sulfoxidation in the gut.[15] When tablets are taken with a meal of high (approximately 40 g) fat content,[16] oral bioavailability is enhanced and higher albendazole sulfoxide serum levels are obtained. After a 400-mg dose, serum levels peak at 2 to 5 hours and range from 0.46 to 1.58 μg/ml (mean 1.31 μg/ml). Marked disparity in steady-state plasma levels among patients has been demonstrated. Elimination half-life ranges from 8 to 15 hours.[17] Protein binding is 70%, and distribution in body compartments is wide.

Albendazole sulfoxide undergoes extensive biliary elimination and enterohepatic recirculation as evidenced by concentrations in bile that are close to plasma levels. Urinary excretion of the parent drug and its principal metabolite is minimal. In the CNS, where it destroys living cysts, albendazole sulfoxide concentrations are roughly 40% of concentrations in serum[18] and in cyst fluid are approximately 50% of concentrations in serum. Penetration into the subarachnoid space allows killing of meningeal larvae. Dexamethasone increases steady-state trough serum levels of albendazole sulfoxide by approximately 50% to 60% when they are administered concomitantly.[7]

In young adults, tolerance of oral albendazole is generally good, but the drug has not been sufficiently studied in pediatric or geriatric patients. However, published studies of treatment in children as young as 1 year and in persons 65 years of age or older suggest no differences with results in young adults. The most commonly reported adverse event has been mild-to-moderate elevation of liver function test results, especially serum aminotransferase activity. Common symptoms include skin rash and to a lesser degree gastrointestinal complaints, such as abdominal pain and nausea and vomiting, headache, fever, fatigue, and reversible alopecia. Occasionally bone marrow suppression is manifested by leukopenia and thrombocytopenia. Rarely, a severe (even fatal) pancytopenia has been recorded.

There are no adequate studies of albendazole administration in pregnant or nursing women, but in rats and rabbits it has been shown to be highly teratogenic and embryotoxic even at oral doses below the human equivalent. It is labeled pregnancy category C. A negative pregnancy test should be required before it is prescribed for women. When pregnancy is known or suspected, the drug is contraindicated except in the extremely rare case in which the potential benefits outweigh the potential risks.

Caution should be exercised when the drug needs to be used in lactating women. Excretion in animal milk suggests that it may also be excreted in human milk.

Albendazole is administered at 10 to 15 mg/kg daily[19] for 8 to 30 days, given in two divided doses with meals. The maximum dose is 800 mg daily. For patients weighing 60 kg or more, 400 mg twice daily is a simple regimen.

Albendazole resistance in cysticercosis, although possible, has not been proven.

Flubendazole and mebendazole are not recommended for cysticercosis.

ANTIPARASITIC DRUGS FOR PREVENTING CYSTICERCOSIS BY ELIMINATING HUMAN TAENIASIS OR PORCINE CYSTICERCOSIS

Niclosamide

Niclosamide is effective in killing adult *Taenia solium* worms[20] but not cysticercus. In the United States, where the prevalence of tapeworm infections and undetected cerebral cysticercosis is low, niclosamide is no longer available and has been largely supplanted by praziquantel.[21] For patients from areas of high prevalence of asymptomatic NCC, niclosamide may be preferred to avoid the risk of CNS symptomatology. Although hard evidence is lacking, however, niclosamide treatment may possibly allow live ova to be liberated intraluminally in the human intestine and actually expose the patient to the risk of cysticercosis by autoinfection provoked by nausea and reverse peristalsis. Thus niclosamide, administered as a single chewed dose of 2 g (four 500-mg tablets) is usually followed by a laxative. In children, doses from 250 mg up to 2 g have been used. Absorption is minimal,[22] and for this reason its in vitro genotoxic effects in fungi[23] are unlikely to be observed in humans. The drug has few adverse effects[24] other than gastrointestinal symptoms, which usually are mild and self-limited.

Oxfendazole

As single-dose treatment of cysticercosis in pigs, oxfendazole has been advocated as an effective and inexpensive drug[25,26] for reservoir control. The drug is not approved, recommended, or used for humans.

CORTICOSTEROIDS

Clinical improvement from steroid treatment was demonstrated in the late 1950s and strongly suggested that allergic or inflammatory phenomena played an important role in the pathogenesis of NCC.

Corticosteroids are now firmly established as a therapeutic option for two main indications related to inflammation. They are the primary drugs for the therapy of cysticercotic encephalitis, arachnoiditis, and angiitis, and they are usually administered at the time of albendazole or praziquantel therapy to prevent or decrease neurologic symptoms related to the neural tissue damage caused by the rapid in situ death of parasites.

For the first indication, large doses are needed initially; up to 32 mg daily of dexamethasone, for example, with or without mannitol (2 g/kg/d) followed by 10 mg daily (or prednisone, 50 mg/d) until brain edema caused by encephalitis is clinically controlled or arachnoiditis subsides as evidenced clinically by improvement of the inflammatory reaction causing hydrocephalus and cranial nerve entrapment. In cysticercotic angiitis, similar doses may prevent occurrence and extension of cerebral infarcts. Monitoring CSF abnormalities during treatment aids in determining the length of therapy. For the second indication, steroids are mandatory before, during, and after cysticidal treatment[27] for the management of patients with large subarachnoid,[28] ventricular, spinal, and multiple parenchymal brain cysts and in the management of cysticercotic meningitis.[29,30] Steroids are advocated to reduce the risk of cerebral infarcts, acute hydrocephalus, and spinal cord and brain edema associated with those conditions. In patients with lower risk of complications (i.e., those with a few small intraparenchymal cysts), dexamethasone can be given preventively, or only if intracranial hypertension clinically expressed by headaches, vomiting, or seizures of focal neurologic symptoms develops during therapy. Symptoms appear typically from the second to the fifth day after the first dose and persist for 2 to 3 days.

Long-term prednisone may prevent the occurrence of CSF shunt dysfunction and blockage[31] and decrease the frequency of deleterious shunt revisions[32] in patients with ventricular derivations.

TREATMENT OF CLINICAL FORMS OF CYSTICERCOSIS

Larval Tissue Invasion Phase

After the eggs of *Taenia solium* are ingested, they liberate embryos that penetrate the intestinal mucosa and gain access to the circulation and thereby to numerous body sites and organs. This (still hypothetical) state of invasion is clinically silent or possibly accompanied by mild and nonspecific symptoms such as low-grade fever, fatigue, and myalgia, which usually go undiagnosed and untreated even when accompanied by eosinophilia. No therapy or only symptomatic analgesic or anti-inflammatory agents may be used.

Soft Tissue Localization

Most subcutaneous and musculoskeletal *T. solium* cysticerci mature slowly and are covered by a noninflammatory fibrous capsule until they enter a process of degeneration that culminates with the death of the larvae. A small, painless, often palpable nodular subcutaneous lesion results that may calcify with time. Although accompanied by some surrounding granulomatous inflammation, this slow involutional process is usually asymptomatic and requires no specific or nonspecific treatment. Rarely, painful lesions need to be treated with analgesics, nonsteroidal anti-inflammatory agents, or surgical excision. Nodules, apparently less common in America than in Asia or Africa,[33] sometimes serve as a clue to the diagnosis of neurologic disease.

Central Nervous System Localization (Neurocysticercosis)

The use of specific antiparasitic drugs, essentially albendazole and praziquantel, for therapy of infections by *Cysticercus cellulosae* continues to be a matter of controversy. Both drugs have demonstrated unequivocal cysticidal properties in vivo; both result in rapid improvement of certain computed tomography (CT) and magnetic resonance imaging (MRI) scans, and both have been shown to improve the prognosis of selected patients.[34] Their use may aid in making the differential diagnosis of single, enhancing, parenchymal cystic lesions in patients with seizures. If the causal association between NCC and human cancer[35–37] is established, the prevention of malignancies could constitute another reason to use antiparasitic drugs. Another potential benefit of cysticidal treatment is the sterilization of the intestinal tract, thereby eliminating the source of reinfection with ova. Albendazole and praziquantel, however, can exacerbate the local inflammatory reaction that occurs concomitantly with the rapid loss of cysticerci viability and may be responsible for the worsening of neurologic symptoms or the appearance of new ones. This fact limits their use. Moreover, certain clinical presentations such as encephalitis may worsen dramatically and even result in death with cysticidal therapy, rendering it contraindicated. In patients such as those who present with parenchymal cysts and hydrocephalus a ventricular shunt must be placed before initiation of treatment to prevent further elevation of intracranial pressure. In other persons, for example, those with large viable subarachnoid cysts, the administration of steroids is mandatory to prevent cerebral infarcts and death secondary to massive inflammatory response. Lesions that affect the basal or lateral cisternae and those caused by the racemous form do not respond well to antiparasitic agents and may have to be removed surgically. Calcified lesions represent dead parasites and require no specific therapy. Some studies suggest that antiparasitic therapy does not favorably affect the clinical prognosis of patients, even when dramatic reduction in cyst size and numbers is documented by neuroimaging studies. Therefore, cysticidal therapy for NCC has indications, contraindications, unresolved issues, and warnings. A precise evaluation of cyst

numbers, viability, and location and knowledge of the patterns of human inflammatory response to dying parasites are essential in deciding and planning specific drug therapy. No study has satisfactorily addressed all possible indications for anthelmintic treatment, and each case must be considered individually; frequently, therapeutic priorities must be set, especially in mixed forms of the disease.

Despite cysticidal drugs, a considerable number of patients continue to suffer from late neurologic sequelae such as seizure and headache.[38] Therefore, continuous attention and adjunctive therapy may be needed in most patients regardless of whether they receive cysticidal treatment.

TREATMENT OPTIONS FOR SPECIFIC CLINICAL SITUATIONS

Epilepsy Caused by Cysticercosis

Whether the prognosis of epilepsy, the most frequent sign of NCC, is improved by cysticidal therapy is a matter of sharp controversy. Observations suggesting that the course of cysticerci-induced seizures is positively influenced by anthelmintics[27,39–43] contrast with others that reach the opposite conclusion.[38,44–53] Some findings even suggest that treatment with praziquantel or albendazole may be associated with increased frequency of seizures during treatment and with long-term sequelae, possibly including seizures.[44] Pitfalls in research methods explain many of the differences.

First-line antiepileptic drugs frequently are used to control seizures in patients with NCC. Carbamazepine, phenobarbital, and phenytoin have stood the test of time and continue to be economically advantageous. Several new drugs[54,55] have not yet been formally tested for this indication. Standard doses are commonly required, and seizures do not recur so long as adequate levels are maintained. The possibility and timing of tapering or withdrawing antiepileptic drugs can be assessed only individually because data are conflicting as to the positive, indifferent, or even negative effects of specific treatment in the prognosis of seizures.[43,44,56,57] In cases in which neuroimaging studies normalize without cysticidal therapy and patients remain seizure free, anticonvulsants may be tapered and sometimes can be discontinued altogether, but the optimal timing has not been defined. Conversely, when cysticerci calcify, continued anticonvulsants are required to prevent convulsions. Seizure recurrence is more common in patients who develop parenchymal calcifications after albendazole therapy and in patients with a history of recurrent seizures and multiple brain cysts before initiation of antiparasitic treatment. Recent evidence suggests that patients with perilesional gliosis as identified by T1-weighted magnetization transfer MRI[58,59] or edema surrounding calcified lesions[48,49] need long-term antiepileptic drug administration. Because albendazole and praziquantel are toxic to the fetus, pregnant and lactating women should be given anticonvulsive medication before cysticidal drugs are considered. Antiparasitic drugs are delayed until birth has occurred and lactation has ended.

Solitary Cyst

Single CNS lesions are commonly found in children and young adults being studied for recent onset of focal or generalized seizures.[60] In patients with a single intraparenchymal cyst and a normal CSF analysis—especially those lacking a compatible epidemiologic history—the differential diagnosis of neurocysticercosis includes other infectious diseases, noninfectious granulomatous diseases, and tumors. The difficulty is compounded by the fact that with single cysts the sensitivity of serologic tests such as the electroimmunotransferblot assay (EITB) is low,[61–64] and making the differential diagnosis may require an invasive procedure, at times impossible or impractical. Early detection can be achieved with therapy.[65] Because spontaneous cyst resolution is slow, some authors consider the utilization of albendazole[53,66,67] and corticosteroids beneficial, but in many instances, patients may instead be treated with antiepileptics and carefully observed.[68] One randomized, placebo-controlled double-blind trial from India found that albendazole therapy resulted in significantly faster and complete resolution of solitary cysticercus lesions and appeared to reduce the risk of late seizure recurrence in children.[39] When a single parenchymal brain cysticercus causing epilepsy is recognized in the acute encephalitic phase, albendazole may improve the patient's prognosis for seizure-free status at 18 months.[42] Solitary cysticercus lesions located in the brainstem have been managed successfully with observation, albendazole, and surgery.[50,69] A growing cysticercus, even if single, usually constitutes an indication for cysticidal therapy, especially when eloquent areas of the CNS are affected. Surgical extirpation is still indicated for some cases of single cysticerci in parenchymal, intraventricular, spinal, and ocular locations and in patients with focal symptoms (i.e., cranial nerve entrapment).

Patients with a single lesion that exhibits imaging characteristics indicating that the cyst is either degenerating or already dead do not require cysticidal medication.

Multiple Active Parenchymal Cysts

No definitive study has established a clear benefit of antiparasitic drugs over symptomatic therapy in patients with three or more intraparenchymal lesions.[45] Therefore, both symptomatic therapy with adequate doses of anticonvulsants or albendazole or praziquantel therapy are options for selected clinical situations. Patients with growing cysts and those with focal neurologic deficits such as hemiparesis or hemiplegia, diminution of visual acuity, or involuntary movements may be better candidates for antiparasitic drugs because these symptoms cease after a trial of cysticidal agents.[34,70]

The indications for surgical treatment of patients with NCC who have parenchymal lesions have diminished since the advent of modern drugs and conservative management expertise, but a small subset of persons in whom medical therapy may fail requires surgical intervention.[71] Surgical strategies include catheter diversion into the subarachnoid space or peritoneal cavity, drainage of cyst fluid or removal of granulomatous tissue by craniotomy, and stereotactic aspiration of cyst contents with placement of an indwelling cyst catheter-reservoir for repeated aspiration as needed.[72–74]

Heavy Nonencephalitic Cerebral Cysticercosis in Tapeworm Carriers

A recently described presentation of NCC consists of massive brain infection with viable cysts and undetectable CNS inflammatory reaction. The disease is different from cysticercotic encephalitis and disseminated systemic cysticercosis[75] and may respond well to cysticidal drugs, but steroids and close imaging follow-up continue to be the preferred approach.

Intraventricular Cysticercosis

Invasive procedures play an important role in the management of cysticercal cysts migrating throughout the cerebrospinal fluid conduits where they move by gravity or bulk flow.[73] Intraventricular cysts tend to be solitary and are likely to be diagnosed in the absence of parenchymal involvement.[73] Viable cysticerci are most commonly found in the fourth ventricle.[77,78] During migration they can occlude vital communication pathways such as the cerebral aqueduct, resulting in sudden hydrocephalus, produce local mass effects and focal deficits, or, when decaying, generate ventriculitis,[79] ependymitis, and further occlusive symptoms.[71,73] Intraventricular cysts carry a guarded prognosis. They respond poorly to pharmacologic agents, which may lead to decompensated ependymitis; therefore, surgery is commonly indicated.[73,80] Craniotomy, stereotactic aspiration, and endoscopic management are possible[73,81–83] and, because of larval displacement,[84] should be guided by one of the latest imaging procedures.[85] Because cysts can be multiple and the hydrocephalus may be loculated, CSF shunting can be challenging at times requiring multiple origins.[72]

Subarachnoid and Basilar Cysticercosis

Basilar-subarachnoid cysticercosis frequently is due to *C. racemosus*, which forms large clusters of cysts, produces arachnoiditis vasculitis and hydrocephalus, and does not consistently respond to cysticidal therapy.[80] For patients with large lesions or who do not improve on medical therapy, neurologic surgery, essentially cyst excision by craniotomy and stereotactic drainage,[72] may be pursued. In the absence of arachnoiditis, cysts may be resected intact,[72] but when surrounding inflammation is present, successful resection is difficult, and marsupialization, while averting mass effects, may potentiate chemical meningitis.[72] Stereotactic aspiration is a suboptimal procedure because of the racemose nature of cysts in this location. Ventriculoperitoneal shunting or other form of CSF diversion is often necessary when hydrocephalus results from basilar arachnoiditis.[32,86] Because the inversion of CSF flow carries inflammatory cells and parasitic debris into the valve mechanism, shunt dysfunction is frequent, and the number of shunt exchanges negatively influences the already somber prognosis of these patients.[32] Long-term steroid administration improves useful shunt duration.[31] A new constant-flow system valve that impedes the back flow of cerebrospinal fluid into the ventricular system appears to be more effective.[87] Ventriculoperitoneal shunting to relieve hydrocephalus in patients with inactive NCC (scarring from previous subarachnoid or ventricular infection) is not associated with higher risk of shunt failure and requires no additional steroid therapy.[88]

Spinal Cysticercosis

Removal of individual cysts during surgical exploration for diagnosis or excision may improve the prognosis of this rare form of NCC.[89] Some cases of subarachnoid[90] and possibly intramedullary[91] disease may be treated with cysticidal agents.[92]

Ocular Cysticercosis

Surgical removal of individual intravitreal or subretinal lesions is the accepted approach for cysticercosis of the eye. Cysticercosis of the optic nerve has required a more invasive approach.[93] Albendazole plus long-term corticosteroid administration may be effective in a limited number of patients.

PREVENTION AND CONTROL OF CYSTICERCOSIS

Individual Prophylaxis

Avoiding the consumption of raw pork meat to prevent taeniasis is effective but not always possible. In endemic areas and occasionally in nonendemic situations,[91] infections may occur despite scrupulous eating habits and hygiene. Testing stools and possibly serology on return from a trip to suspect areas is reasonable but unproven.

Family Contacts of a Locally Acquired Case

In minimally endemic countries, investigation of family members, domestic employees coming from endemic regions,[94] and others possibly exposed to taenial eggs is easily undertaken by stool testing and immunoblot diagnostic serology.[95] Such tests may be rewarding in detecting not only the source of infection[96–98] in carriers but also asymptomatic patients for specific treatment, therefore preventing further cases.[99,100] Seropositivity in household family contacts with seizures strongly predicts a cysticercal cause for seizures.[60,101] By effectively decreasing reservoirs of infecting ova in the definitive host and consequently in the environment, early diagnosis and treatment of taeniasis with niclosamide or praziquantel in immigrants from endemic areas protects selected groups in developed countries.

Society

The magnitude of the disease burden from cysticercosis is great in developing societies,[102] and the disease is considered as emerging in developed countries.[70] Preventive health measures are the best way to manage global cysticercosis.[103] Global elimination is highly unlikely, however, because of the association with poverty of this feces-borne, food-borne, water-borne, and possibly air-borne disease. Interrupting the chain of transmission is possible. Actively searching for, treating, and reporting sources of contagion, identifying and treating exposed contacts, providing hygienic and sanitary infrastructure and education, and limiting the animal reservoir while enforcing meat inspection policies are necessary measures. A proposal has been made to declare NCC an international reportable disease,[104] the goal of which is to make possible the implementation of epidemiologic interventions.

T. solium has been successfully eradicated in industrialized countries by using strict porcine meat processing and inspection practices, hygienic measures and education, and by having a sanitary infrastructure that provides for the safe disposal of sewage. Large-scale anthelmintic treatment of populations[105] and community education have been tried with limited success in endemic areas,[70,106–108] but the efforts have not being sustained over time.[70] When praziquantel is used in mass treatment campaigns or when it is given for the treatment of taeniasis, treatment must be supervised by trained personnel to minimize the risk of CNS symptoms in asymptomatic NCC patients.[110]

Drugs used for veterinary purposes may improve control of human cysticercosis; oxfendazole, for example, is inexpensive and effective in the porcine host.

Despite these facts, in many developing countries the emergence, maintenance, and dissemination of cysticercosis continues to be a reality because poverty and disorganization have not permitted application of the preceding measures.

A vaccine against *T. solium* is theoretically possible,[111,112] but the absence of an animal model and possibly lack of economic incentives have delayed its advancement.

REFERENCES

1. Willms K: Cestodes (Tapeworms) In Gorbach SL, Bartlett JG, Blacklow NR: Infectious Diseases, 2nd ed. Philadelphia, WB Saunders, 1998.
2. White AC Jr: Neurocysticercosis: a major cause of neurological disease worldwide. Clin Infect Dis 1997;24:101.
3. King CH, Mahmoud AA: Drugs five years later: Praziquantel. Ann Intern Med 1989;110:290.
4. Sotelo J, Escobedo F, Rodriguez-Carbajal J, et al: Therapy of parenchymal brain cysticercosis with praziquantel. N Engl J Med 1984;301:1001.
5. Sotelo J, Torres B, Rubio-Donnadieu F, et al: Praziquantel in the treatment of neurocysticercosis: Long-term follow-up. Neurology 1985;35:752.
6. Vasquez ML, Jung H, Sotelo J: Plasma levels of praziquantel decrease when dexamethasone is given simultaneously. Neurology 1987;37:1561.
7. Jung H, Hurtado M, Medina MT, et al: Dexamethasone increases plasma levels of Albendazole. J Neurol 1990; 237:279.
8. Dachman WD, Adubofour KO, Bikin DS et al: Cimetidine-induced rise in praziquantel levels in a patient with neurocysticercosis being treated with anticonvulsants. J Infect Dis 1994;169:689.
9. Kestelyn P, Taelman H: Effect of praziquantel on intraocular cysticercosis: a case report. Br J Ophthalmol 1985;69:788.
10. Corona T, Lugo R, Medina R, et al: Single-day praziquantel therapy for neurocysticercosis. N Engl J Med 1996;334(2):125
11. Corona T, Lugo R, Medina R, et al: A short praziquantel regimen for the treatment of parenchymatous neurocysticercosis. Gac Med Mex 1999;35:369.
12. Del Brutto OH, Campos X, Sanchez J, et al: Single day praziquantel versus 1-week albendazole for neurocysticercosis. Neurology 1999;52:1079.
13. Ireland CM, Gull K, Gutteridge WE, et al: The interaction of benzimidazole carbamates with mammalian microtubule protein. Biochem Pharmacol 1979;28:2680.
14. Escobedo F, Penagos P, Rodriguez J, et al: Albendazole therapy for neurocysticercosis. Arch Intern Med 1987;147:738.
15. Lawrenz A, Eglit S, Kroker R: The metabolism of albendazole in the isolated perfused intestine of rats. DTW Dtsch Tierarztl Wochenschr 1992;99:416.
16. Eskazole: Clinical and Technical Review. SmithKline Beecham Pharmaceuticals 1990:A1-B28.
17. Jung H, Hurtado M, Sanchez M, et al: Clinical pharmacokinetics of albendazole in patients with brain cysticercosis. J Clin Pharmacol 1992;32:28.
18. Jung H, Hurtado M, Sanchez M, et al: Plasma and CSF levels of albendazole and praziquantel in patients with neurocysticercosis. Clin Neuropharmacol 1990;13:559.
19. Garcia HH, Gilman RH, Horton H: Albendazole therapy for neurocysticercosis: A prospective double-blind trial comparing 7 versus 14 days of treatment. Neurology 1997;48:1421.
20. Perera DR, Western KA, Schultz MG: Niclosamine treatment of cestodiasis: Clinical trials in the United States. Am J Trop Med Hyg 1970;19:610.
21. Rosenblatt JE: Antiparasitic agents. Mayo Clin Proc 1999;74:1161.
22. Pearson RD, Hewlett EL: Niclosamide therapy for tapeworm infections. Ann Intern Med 1985;102:550.
23. de la Torre RA, de la rua Barcelo R, Hernandez G, et al: Genotoxic effects of niclosamide in *Aspergillus nidulans*. Mutat Res 1989;222:337.
24. Gonnert R, Schraufstatter E: Experimentelle untersuchungen mit N-(2′-chlor-4′-nitrophenyl)-5-chlorsalicylamid, einen neuen bandwurmmitel. I Mitterlung: Chemotherapeutische Versuche Arzneimittlforschung 1960;10:881.
25. Gonzales AE, Garcia HH, Gilman RH, et al: Effective, single dose treatment of porcine cysticercosis with oxfendazole. Am J Trop Med Hyg 1996;54:391.
26. Gonzales AE, Falcon N, Gavidia C, et al: Treatment of swine cysticercosis with oxfendazole: A dose response trial. Vet Rec 1997;141:420.
27. Del Brutto OH: Cysticercosis and cerebrovascular disease: a review. J Neurol Neurosurg Psychiatry 1992;55:252.
28. Del Brutto OH, Sotelo J, Aguirre R, et al: Albendazole therapy for giant subarachnoid cysticerci. Arch Neurol 1992;49:535.
29. Barinagarrementeria F, Del Brutto OH: Lacunar syndrome due to neurocysticercosis. Arch Neurol 1989;46:415.
30. Ernest MP, Reller LB, Filley CM et al: Cysticercosis in the United States: 35 cases and a review. Rev Infect Dis 1987;9:961.
31. Suastegui RR, Soto J, Sotelo J: Effects of prednisone on ventriculoperitoneal shunt function in hydrocephalus secondary to cysticercosis: A preliminary study. J Neurosurg 1996;84:629.
32. Colli BO, Martelli N, Assirati JA et al: Results of surgical treatment of neurocysticercosis in 69 cases. J Neurosurg 1986;65:309.
33. Cruz I, Cruz ME, Teran W, et al: Human subcutaneous cysticercosis in an Andean population with neurocysticercosis. Am J Trop Med Hyg 1994;51:405.
34. Santoyo H, Corona R, Sotelo J: Total recovery of visual function after treatment for cerebral cysticercosis. N Engl J Med 1991;324:1137.
35. Del Brutto OH, Dolezal M, Castillo PR et al: Neurocysticercosis and oncogenesis. Arch Med Res 2000;31:151.
36. Herrera LA, Benita-Bordes A, Sotelo J et al: Possible relationship between neurocysticercosis and hematological malignancies. Arch Med Res 1999;30:154.
37. Del Brutto OH, Castillo PR, Mena IX et al: Neurocysticercosis among patients with cerebral gliomas. Arch Neurol 1997;54:1125.
38. Kim SK, Wang KC, Paek SH et al: Outcomes of medical treatment of neurocysticercosis: a study of 65 cases in Cheju Island, Korea. Surg Neurol 1999;52:563.
39. Baranwal AK, Singhi PD, Khandelwal MD et al: Albendazole therapy in children with focal seizures and single small enhancing computerized tomographic lesions: A randomized, placebo controlled, double blind trial. Pediat Infect Dis J 1998;17:696.
40. Caparros-Lefebvre D, Lannuzel A, Alexis C, et al: Cerebral cysticercosis: why it should be treated. Presse Med 1997;26:1574.
41. Rolfs A, Muhlschlegel F, Jansen-Rosseck R, et al: Clinical and immunologic follow up study of patients with neurocysticercosis after treatment with praziquantel. Neurology 1995;45:532.
42. Del Brutto OH: Single parenchymal brain cysticercus in the acute encephalitic phase: definition of a distinct form of neurocysticercosis with a benign prognosis. J Neurol Neurosurg Psychiatry 1995;58:247.
43. Vasquez N, Sotelo J: The course of seizures after treatment for cerebral cysticercosis. N Engl J Med 1992;327:696.
44. Carpio A, Santillan F, Leon P, et al: Is the course of neurocysticercosis modified by treatment with anthelmintic agents? Arch Intern Med 1995;155:1982.
45. Salinas R, Counsell C, Prasad K, et al: Treating neurocysticercosis medically: a systematic review of randomized, controlled trials. Trop Med and Internat Health 1999;4(11):713.
46. Salinas R, Prasad K: Drugs for treating neurocysticercosis (Cochrane Review). In The Cochrane Library. 1999 Issue 3. Updated Software, Oxford. *http://www.updateusa.com/cochrane.htm*
47. Cuellar R. Molinero M, Ramirez F, et al: Clinical findings in active cerebral neurocysticercosis in pediatrics. Rev Neurol 1999;29:334.
48. Nash TE, Patronas NJ: Edema associated with calcified lesions in neurocysticercosis. Neurology 1999;53:777.

49. Sheth TN, Lee C, Kucharczyk W, et al: Reactivation of neurocysticercosis: case report. Am J Trop Med Hy 1999;60:664.

50. Lath R, Rajshekhar V: Solitary cysticercus granuloma of the brainstem: report of four cases. J Neurosurg 1989;89:1047.

51. Del Brutto OH: Neurocysticercosis in children: clinical and radiological analysis and prognostic factors in 54 patients. Rev Neurol 1997;25:1681.

52. Padma MV, Behari M, Misra NK, et al: Albendazole in neurocysticercosis. Nat Med J India 1995;8:225.

53. Del Brutto OH: Prognostic factors for seizure recurrence after withdrawal of antiepileptic drugs in patients with neurocysticercosis. Neurology 1994;44:1706.

54. Anonymous: Two new drugs for epilepsy. Med Letter 2000;42:33.

55. Kwan P, Brodie MJ: Neuropsychological effects of epilepsy and antiepileptic drugs. Lancet 2001;357:216.

56. Medina MT, Genton P, Montoya MC et al: Effect of anticysticercal treatment in the prognosis of epilepsy in neurocysticercosis. A pilot trial. Epilepsy 1993;34:1024.

57. Del Brutto, Santibañez R, Noboa CA, et al: Epilepsy due to NCC analysis of 203 patients. Neurology 1992;42:389.

58. Gupta RK, Kathuria MK, Pradham S: Magnetization transfer magnetic resonance imaging demonstration of perilesional gliosis: Relationship with epilepsy in treated or healed neurocysticercosis. Lancet 1999;354:44.

59. Pradhan S, Kathuria MK, Gupta RK: Perilesional gliosis and seizure outcome: a study based on magnetization transfer magnetic resonance imaging in patients with neurocysticercosis. Ann Neurol 2000;48:181.

60. Singh G, Ram S, Kaushal V, et al: Risk of seizures and neurocysticercosis in household family contacts of children with single enhancing lesions. J Neurol Sci 2000;176:131.

61. Wilson M, Bryant RT, Fried JA, et al: Clinical evaluation of the cysticercosis enzyme-linked immunoelectrotransfer blot in patients with neurocysticercosis. J Infect Dis 1991;164:1007.

62. Feldman M, Plancarte A, Sandoval M, et al: Comparison of two assays (EIA and EITB) and two samples (saliva and serum) for the diagnosis of neurocysticercosis. Trans R Soc Trop Med Hyg 1990;84:559.

63. Diaz JF, Verastegua M, Gilman RH, et al: Immunodiagnosis of human cysticercosis (*Taenia solium*): a field comparison of an antibody-enzyme-linked immunosorbent assay (ELISA), an antigen-ELISA, and an enzyme-linked immunoelectrotransferblot (EITB) assay in Peru. Am J Trop Med Hyg 1992;46:610.

64. Mitchell WG, Crawford TO: Intraparenchymal cerebral cysticercosis in children: diagnosis and treatment. Pediatrics 1988;82:76.

65. Del Brutto OH: The use of albendazole in patients with single lesions enhanced on contrast CT. N Engl J Med 1993;328:356.

66. Padma MV, Behari M, Misra NK et al: Albendazole in single CT ring lesions in epilepsy. Neurology 1994;44:1334.

67. Rousseau MC, Guillotel B, Delmont J: Neurocysticercosis in the South-East of France 1988–1998. Presse Med 1999;28:2143.

68. Wadley JP, Shakir RA, Edwards JM: Experience with neurocysticercosis in the UK: correct diagnosis and neurosurgical management of the small enhancing brain lesion. Br J Neurosurg 2000;14:211.

69. Arruda WO, Ramina R, Pedrozo AA et al: Brainstem cysticercosis simulating cystic tumor lesion. A case report. Arq Neuropsiquiatr 1994;52:431.

70. Garcia HH, Del Brutto OH: Taenia solium cysticercosis. In Gotuzzo E, Isturiz R (eds): Emerging and re-emerging diseases in Latin America. Infect Dis Clin North Amer 2000;14(1):97.

71. Couldwell WT, Zee CS, Apuzzo MLJ: Definition of the role of contemporary surgical management in cisternal and parenchymatous cysticercosis cerebri. Neurosurgery 1991;28:231.

72. Amar AP, Ghosh S, Apuzzo MLJ: Treatment of central nervous system infections: A surgical perspective. Neuroimag Clin North Am 2000;10:445.

73. Couldwell WT, Apuzzo MLJ: Cysticercosis cerebri. In Haines SJ, Hall WJ (eds): Infections in Neurological Surgery. Neurosurg Clin North Am 1992;3:471.

74. Revuelta R, Juanbelz P, Balderrama J, et al: Contralateral trigeminal neuralgia: a new clinical manifestation of neurocysticercosis: Case report. Neurosurgery 1995;37:138.

75. Garcia HH and Del Brutto OH: Heavy nonencephalitic cerebral cysticercosis in tapeworm carriers. Neurology 1999;53:1582.

76. Apuzzo MLJ, Dobkin WR, Zee CS: Surgical considerations in treatment of intraventricular cysticercosis: an analysis of 45 cases. J Neurosurg 1984;60:400.

77. Cueter CA, Garcia Bobadilla J, Guerra LG, et al: Neurocysticercosis: Focus on intraventricular disease. Clin Infect Dis 1997;24:157.

78. Proaño JV, Madrazo I Garcia L, et al: Albendazole and praziquantel treatment in neurocysticercosis of the fourth ventricle. J Neurosurg 1997;87:29.

79. Salazar A, Sotelo J, Martinez H, et al: Differential diagnosis between ventriculitis and fourth ventricle cysts in neurocysticercosis. J Neurosurg 1983;59:660.

80. Sotelo J: Treatment of brain cysticercosis. Surg Neurol 1997;48:110.

81. Neal JH: An endoscopic approach to cysticercosis cysts of the posterior third ventricle. Neurosurgery 1995;36:1040.

82. Bergsneider M, Holly HT, Lee JH, et al: Endoscopic management of cysticercal cysts within the lateral and third ventricles. J Neurosurg 2000;92:14.

83. Cudlip SA, Wilkins PR, Marsh HT: Endoscopic removal of a third ventricular cysticercal cyst. Br J Neurosurg 1998;12:452.

84. Kramer J, Carrazana E, Crosgrove CR et al: Transaqueductal migration of a neurocysticercus cyst. J Neurosurg 1992;77:956.

85. Zee CS, Segall HD, Apuzzo MLJ et al: Intraventricular cysticercal cysts: Further neuroradiological observations and neurosurgical implications. Am J Neuroradiol 1984;5:727.

86. Sotelo J, Marin C: Hydrocephalus secondary to neurocysticercotic arachnoiditis: A long term follow up review of 92 cases. J Neurosurg 1987;66:686.

87. Sotelo J, Rubalcava MA, Gomez-Llata S: A new shunt for hydrocephalus that relies on CSF production rather than on ventricular pressure: Initial clinical experiences. Surg Neurol 1995;43:324.

88. White AC Jr: Neurocysticercosis: Updates in epidemiology, pathogenesis, diagnosis and management. Annu Rev Med 2000;50:187.

89. Mohanty A, Venkatrama SK, Das S et al: Spinal intramedullary cysticercosis. Neurology 1997;40:82.

90. Bandres J, White AC Jr, Samo T, et al: Extraparenchymal neurocysticercosis report of five cases and review of the literature on management. Clin Infect Dis 1992;5:799.

91. Garg RK, Nag D: Intramedullary spinal cysticercosis: response to albendazole: Case report. Spinal Cord 1998;36:67.

92. Corral I, Quereda C, Moreno A, et al: Intramedullary cysticercosis cured with drug treatment. A case report. Spine 1996;21:2284.

93. Bousquet CF, Dufour TF, Derome PC: Retrobulbar optic nerve cysticercosis. Case report. J Neurosurg 1996;84:293.

94. Schantz PM, Moore AC, Muñoz JL, et al: Neurocysticercosis in an Orthodox Jewish community in New York City. N Engl J Med 1992;327:692.

95. Moore AC, Lutwick LI, Schantz PM, et al: Seroprevalence of cysticercosis in an Orthodox Jewish community. Am J Trop Med Hyg 1995;53:439.

96. Anonymous: LA Public Health Lett. 1982;4:33.

97. Anonymous: LA Public Health Lett. 1987;10:1

98. Tsang VCW, Garcia HH: Immunoblot diagnostic test (EITB) for *Taenia solium* cysticercosis and its contribution to the definition of this under-recognized but serious health problem. In Garcia HH, Martinez SM (eds): *Taenia solium* Taeniasis/Cysticercosis, 2nd ed. Lima, Perú, Editorial Universo. 1999, p 245.

99. St. Geme III JW, Maldonado YA, Enzman D, et al: Consensus: diagnosis and management of neurocysticercosis in children. Pediatr Infect Dis J 1993;12:455.

100. Garcia-Noval J, Allan JC, Flates C, et al: Epidemiology of *Taenia solium* taeniasis and cysticercosis in two rural Guatemalan communities. Am J Trop Med Hyg 1996;55:282.

101. Goodman KA, Ballagh SA, Carpio A: Case-control study of seropositivity for cysticercosis in Cuenca, Ecuador. Am J Trop Med Hyg 1999;60:70.

102. Bern C, Garcia HH, Evans C, et al: Magnitude of the disease burden from neurocysticercosis in a developing country. Clin Infect Dis 1999;29:1203.

103. Garg RK: Neurocysticercosis. Postgrad Med J 1998;74:321.

104. Roman G, Sotelo J, Del Brutto O, et al: A proposal to declare neurocysticercosis an international reportable disease. Bull World Health Organ 2000;78:399.

105. Pawlowski ZS: Large-scale use of chemotherapy of taeniasis as a control measure for *Taenia solium* infections. In Geerts S, Kumar V, Brandt J (eds): Helminth Zoonoses. Dordrecht, Martius Nijhoff, 1987, pp 100–105.

106. Allan JC, Velasquez M, Fletes C, et al: Mass chemotherapy for intestinal *Taenia solium* infection: Effect on prevalence in humans and pigs. Trans R Soc Trop Med Hyg 1997;91:595.

107. Cruz M, Davis A, Dixon H, et al: Operational studies on the control of *Taenia solium* taeniasis/cysticercosis in Ecuador. Bull World Health Organ 1989;67:401.

108. Diaz-Camacho SP, Candil A, Suate V, et al: Epidemiologic study and control of *Taenia solium* infections with praziquantel in a rural village of Mexico. Am J Trop Med Hyg 1991;45:522.

109. Sarti E, Flisser A, Schantz PM, et al: Development and evaluation of a health education intervention against *Taenia solium* in a small community of Mexico. Am J Trop Med Hyg 1997;56:127.

110. Torres JR, Noya O, Noya BA, et al: Seizures and praziquantel. Rev Inst Med Trop Sao Paulo 1988;30:36.

111. Gauci CG, Flisser A, Lightowlers MW: *Taenia solium* oncosfere protein homologous to host-protective *Taenia ovis* and *Taenia saginata* 18 kDa antigens. Int J Parasitol 1998;28:757.

112. Johnson KS, Harrison GB, Lightowlers MW, et al: Vaccination against ovine cysticercosis using a defined recombinant antigen. Nature 1989;338:585.

Rabies

ROBERT V. GIBBONS, MD, MPH

It is even to be doubted whether any of the many diseases which afflict humanity, and are a source of dread, either because of their painfulness, their mortality, or the circumstances attending their advent and progress, can equal this [rabies] in the terror it inspires in the minds of those who are cognisant of its effects and who chance to be exposed to the risk of its attack, as well as the uniform fatality which terminates the distressing and hideous symptoms that characterise the disorder.

George Fleming, *Rabies and hydrophobia: their history, nature, causes, symptoms, and prevention (1872)*[1]

The rabies virus is one of seven neurotropic viruses of the genus Lyssavirus, family Rhabdoviridae.[2] The Rhabdoviridae are negative-stranded RNA, bullet (or rod)-shaped viruses. The Lyssavirus genus is composed of seven genotypes that share antigenic and nucleotide sequence homology (Table 14–1). All lyssaviruses likely cause a similar clinical disease, a rapidly progressive and usually fatal encephalomyelitis; however, only a handful of human cases have been documented to have been caused by lyssaviruses other than rabies.[2,3]

Rabies has been regarded with terror throughout recorded history, a reputation earned because of the apprehensive uncertainty of contracting rabies (worsened by a variable incubation period) and the inevitable and often excruciating death following the onset of symptoms. The word "rabies" is believed to derive from the Latin word *rabidus*, meaning "mad." *Rabidus* is probably related to the Sanskrit root *rabhas*, meaning "to do violence."[4] *Lyssa* is Greek, meaning "mad or frenzy," and the Greek word *rhabdos* means "rod."[5] Suggestions of the disease in man reportedly appear in the Eshnunna code written before 2300 BC. References are found in Chinese texts dating from the sixth century BC, and the disease is mentioned in literary works from ancient Greece. Democritus is believed to have made the first recorded description of canine rabies circa 500 BC.[6,7]

Rabies has been considered a possible explanation for the vampire legend in Europe, which dates back to the 1300s and reached maximum interest in the early 1700s.[8,9] In the mid-1700s, many French and other physicians believed in the spontaneous appearance of rabies, possibly because some cases were actually due to tetanus rather than rabies. By the late 1700s, it was recognized that rabies resulted only from the bites of rabid animals and that not all bites transmitted the disease. By 1884, Louis Pasteur was able to attenuate the virus in dried rabbit spinal cords. He found that injections with this material, unlike fresh central nervous system tissue, did not cause rabies but instead conferred protection. Human vaccinations began in 1885.[3,5,10]

TABLE 14–1 ■ Members of the Genus Lyssavirus of the Family Rhabdoviridae

Lyssavirus (genotype)	Range	Human infection?*	Rabies vaccine effective?
Rabies virus[1]	Worldwide, except for Australia, Antarctica, and a few island nations	Thousands each year	Effective
Lagos bat virus[2]	Africa	None reported	Probably ineffective
Mokola virus[3]	Africa	One fatal case and one nonfatal case	Probably ineffective
Duvenhage virus[4]	Africa	One case	Probably effective
European bat virus 1[5]	Europe	One confirmed case and one suspected case	Possibly effective
European bat virus 2[6]	Europe	One case	Possibly effective
Australian bat virus[7]	Australia	Two cases	Effective

*Because the Lagos bat, Mokola, and Duvenhage viruses occur where there is little surveillance and laboratory capability, deaths from these diseases could be reported as caused by the rabies virus.

Adapted from Smith GS: New aspects of rabies with emphasis on epidemiology, diagnosis, and prevention of the disease in the United States. Clin Microbial Rev 1996;9:166–176.

EPIDEMIOLOGY

Rabies is a zoonosis. All mammals are thought to be susceptible to infection, but reservoirs important to the maintenance and transmission of the virus are limited to Carnivora and Chiroptera (bats). Humans are dead-end hosts in that they do not contribute to the transmission cycle and human infection is not important to virus maintenance.[2,3]

In 1998 the World Health Organization (WHO) reported that there were 33,373 human deaths caused by rabies.[11] This reporting is incomplete, however, and it has been estimated that annually more than 50,000 rabies deaths occur worldwide.[12] According to the WHO, 112 nations reported the presence of rabies, and 49 reported its absence.[11]

Human rabies reflects the proximity and intimacy of dogs to humans. Dog bites are common, estimated to be between 200 and 800 per 100,000 persons in many countries.[13] In many developing countries, dogs account for more than 90% of rabies cases in animals. Most (95% to 98%) human rabies cases worldwide occur in areas of Africa, Asia, India, and Latin America, where canine rabies is endemic.[14] Rates range from 0.01 to 0.6 deaths per 100,000 population in Latin America to 2 to 18 deaths per 100,000 population in India and Ethiopia.[12]

In countries where canine rabies has been controlled (including the United States, Canada, and most European countries), most rabies cases in animals occur among specific wildlife species. In these countries, dogs account for less than 5% of cases in animals, and human cases are relatively rare. These countries account for less than 5% of human cases worldwide, and rates are typically less than 0.002 deaths per 100,000 population.[12]

Over the past century in the United States, domestic animal rabies has declined dramatically. The role of the dog in transmitting rabies to humans is illustrated by the declining incidence of human rabies closely following the declining prevalence of rabies in domestic dogs (Fig. 14–1). From 1946 to 1965 there were 236 human cases in the United States; 82% of these were attributable to dog

bites. This is an average of 12 cases per year, declining from 24 per year (90% due to dog bites) in 1946 to 1949 to 1.5 per year (67% due to dog bites) in 1962 to 1965.[15]

From 1960 through 1979 an average of two cases of rabies occurred annually in the United States.[16] From 1980 through 1989 there was an average of just one case of human rabies per year; seven were caused by a rabies variant associated with dogs outside the United States, two by a variant associated with indigenous bats, and one by a variant associated with indigenous skunks.[17-27] From 1990 through 2000 there were 32 human rabies cases (Table 14–2), of which 24 (75%) were caused by variants associated with bats, 6 (19%) were due to variants associated with foreign dogs, and 2 (6%) were due to a dog-coyote variant found in Texas.[17,28-46] Thus in the past decade 24 (92%) of 26 human deaths from domestically acquired rabies were due to bat variants of the rabies virus.

Rabies infections of terrestrial animals occur in geographically discrete areas. Transmission is primarily within

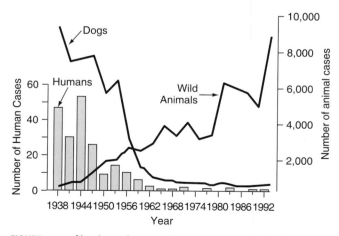

FIGURE 14–1. Number of reported human, dog, and wild animal rabies cases, United States, 1938–1992. (From Smith JS: New aspects of rabies with emphasis on epidemiology, diagnosis, and prevention of the disease in the United States. Clin Microbiol Rev 1996;9:166–176.)

TABLE 14–2 ■ Human Rabies Cases in the United States, 1990 through 2000 (MMWRs)

Mo/y state*	Time of diagnosis†	Onset of symptoms‡	Initial diagnosis(es)	Other diagnosis§	Variant‖	Exposure history¶
May90 Tex	PA	F, hand	Wound infection	Tetanus	Bat	Bite
Aug91 Tex	A	G	Panic disorder		Dog	Unknown
Aug91 Ark	PA	G	Pharyngitis	Drug intoxication, tetanus	Bat	Direct contact
Oct91 Ga	PA	G	Pharyngitis		Bat	Unknown
Apr92 Calif	A	G	Rabies		Dog#	Bite
Jul93 NY	P	F, hand	Musculoskeletal pain, otitis media	Pharyngitis	Bat	Bat indoors
Oct93 Tex	PA	G	Cerebrovascular accident	Upper respiratory tract infection, tetanus	Bat	Cow died 3 mo earlier
Nov93 Calif	A	G, jaw and shoulder	Myocardial ischemia	Anxiety disorder	Dog#	Bite
Jan94 Calif	P	F, arm	Cervical disc disease	Myelitis	Bat	Sick kitten 3 mo earlier
Jun94 Fla	P	G	Meningitis	Vasculitis	Dog#	Unknown
Oct94 WVa	A	G	Psychosis, drug intoxication	Tetanus, drug withdrawal	Bat	Direct contact
Nov94 Tex	A	G	Upper respiratory tract infection	Meningitis, brain abscess	Dog	Unknown
Nov94 Tenn	A	G, arm	Viral illness, herpes zoster	Anxiety, meningitis	Bat	Unknown
Oct94 Ala	P	G, arm	Musculoskeletal pain	Chest pain, seizures	Bat	Direct contact
Mar95 Wash	A	G	Upper respiratory tract infection	Drug intoxication, sepsis	Bat	Bat indoors
Mar95 Calif	A	G	Cephalgia	Pharyngitis, pneumonia	Bat	Direct contact
Sep95 Conn	A	F, arm	Cervical radiculopathy	Lyme	Bat	Bat indoors
Sep95 Calif	P	F, arm	Neuropathy	Cerebrovascular accident, pneumonia	Bat	Direct contact
Dec95 Fla	A	G	Constipation	Rabies, tetanus	Dog#	Bite
Aug96 NH	A	F, arm	Cervical radiculopathy	Rabies	Dog#	Bite
Sep96 Ky	A	G, arm	Pharyngitis	Sepsis	Bat	Unknown
Nov96 Mont	A	G	Sinusitis	Hyponatremia, pneumonia	Bat	Unknown
Dec96 Mont	P	G, arm	Temporary ischemic attack, worsening Parkinson's disease	Creutzfeldt-Jakob disease	Bat	Bat indoors
Dec96 Wash	P	F, arm	Myocardial infarction, cerebrovascular accident	Tetanus, Creutzfeldt-Jakob disease	Bat	Unknown
Oct97 Tex	A	F, face and ear	Sinusitis, alcohol withdrawal	Rabies	Bat	Direct contact
Oct97 NJ	A	F, shoulder and neck	Pharyngitis	Tetanus	Bat	Direct contact
Dec98 Va	A	G, wrist and arm	Anticholinergic poisoning, intoxication	Rabies	Bat	Unknown
Sep00 Calif	A	F, arm	Atypical neuropathy	Rabies	Bat	Bat indoors
Sep00 NY	A	G	Bowel obstruction	Rabies	Dog#	Bite
Oct00 Ga	PA	G	Encephalitis		Bat	Direct contact
Oct00 Minn	A	F, arm	Carpal tunnel syndrome	Epidural abscess, myelitis	Bat	Bite
Oct00 Wis	PA	G, arm	Myocardial ischemia	Sepsis	Bat	Direct contact

*Month, year, and state location when patient had the onset of symptoms.

†A, antemortem; P, postmortem; PA, postmortem but suspected antemortem.

‡F, focal; G, general.

§Encephalitis is invariably in the diagnosis late in the course of symptoms.

‖Animal species associated with the variant of the rabies virus.

¶Bite, history of an animal bite; direct contact, history of direct physical contact with the animal but not of a bite; bat indoors, history of a bat in the house but not of a bite or direct contact with a bat; unknown, no animal exposure history available.

#Foreign dog variant.

a species and involves a single, distinctive rabies variant that can be identified by monoclonal antibody techniques or genetic analysis. Spillover infection from one species to another does occur, but these cases are sporadic and rarely initiate sustained transmission in a new host. In the United States the reservoirs are raccoons along the eastern United States; the arctic and red fox in Alaska and intermittently in the New England states; gray foxes in Arizona and Texas; skunks in California, the north central states, and the south central states; and coyotes in Texas.[2]

Overlying the disease in terrestrial variants are multiple independent reservoirs for rabies in several species of bats. As in terrestrial species, distinct viral variants can be identified for different bat species; however, geographic boundaries cannot be easily defined.[2]

PATHOGENESIS

Rabies is transmitted by the introduction of the virus into the tissue of a susceptible host. This almost always involves the inoculation of virus-laden saliva via a bite. The risk of rabies infection (and hence, death) after a rabid animal bite ranges from 5% to 80% for untreated cases.[47] Factors that may increase the risk of transmission include a larger inoculum, an increased density of nerves in the exposed tissue, a shorter distance of the wound from the central nervous system (CNS), greater severity of the wound, the virus strain, and host factors.[13,14]

The virus may enter nervous tissue directly, or it may replicate in non-nervous tissue, particularly muscle, before entering the peripheral nerves.[14] Once in the peripheral nerves (sensory or motor), the virus can replicate and is transported by retrograde axoplasmic flow to the CNS.[6] Infection of the dorsal root ganglia in the spinal cord may result in local sensory prodromes. Infection can be disseminated widely in the CNS before the onset of clinical signs. The incubation period ranges from several days to several years but is usually 1 to 2 months.[48] The long incubation period is poorly understood; it might be due to a slow viral replication in muscle cells or latency in macrophages.[4,14,49] Once it reaches the CNS, the virus causes an acute nonsuppurative encephalomyelitis. After rapidly replicating and spreading throughout the CNS, the virus moves via anterograde axoplasmic flow down the peripheral nerves. Late in the infection, virus is released from axon terminals and may be taken up by a variety of non-nervous tissues.[6] Except for the salivary glands and other oral tissues, infection of non-nervous tissue is of little importance in transmission of the virus in nature.[2,4,14] Because the virus is not found in saliva, except immediately before and during the clinical manifestations, the host is generally noninfectious until that time.[2]

Exactly how the rabies virus causes such severe CNS dysfunction is unclear. As noted above, the virus can be widespread before the onset of symptoms; yet the amount of virus in the CNS does not appear to determine the severity of disease. In many cases the pathologic evidence of neuronal necrosis is absent or minimal.[4]

There is no evidence of viremia in naturally occurring infection and no evidence of an immune response until late in the clinical course after the development of encephalitis. It has been speculated that the lack of an immune response is due to insufficient antigenic load, viral replication at an immunologically privileged site, or the ability of the virus to evade or suppress the immune system.[4]

CLINICAL MANIFESTATIONS

The clinical history of rabies is often divided into stages: an incubation period, a prodrome, an acute neurologic phase, and coma followed by death. The incubation period has been documented to be as short as several days and as long as several years.[48] However, it is typically between a few weeks and a few months; 75% of patients become ill within 3 months and 95% within a year.[4]

Clinical symptoms of rabies may begin with a nonspecific prodrome of 2 to 10 days that includes symptoms common to many viral infections: fever, irritability, malaise, insomnia, anorexia, headache, upper respiratory tract symptoms, and nausea and vomiting. A local sensory prodrome, which may include pain, burning, pruritus, or numbness at the site of inoculation, may precede the general prodrome by a few days and is reported by 30% to 80% of patients. This stage is probably a manifestation of the virus reaching the dorsal root ganglia in the spinal cord.[14,50]

The acute neurologic manifestations last 2 to 10 days and are often categorized as either "furious" or "paralytic" rabies. It is not clear what determines whether a person develops furious or paralytic rabies. Both syndromes typically progress through paralysis and coma to death. Most (upwards of 80%) human cases are furious and have many features classically associated with rabies. These may include delirium and agitation, autonomic instability (hypersalivation, piloerection, anisocoria, nonreactive pupils, tachycardia, hypotension, temperature fluctuations, diaphoresis, lacrimation, and priapism), and pharyngeal, laryngeal, and diaphragmatic spasms (which may present as hydrophobia and aerophobia). Patients may develop generalized convulsions during a hydrophobic spasm.[14,50]

In paralytic rabies, lethargy and paralysis are the dominant features, and the clinical course may be days to weeks longer than in furious rabies. Paralysis often begins in the bitten extremity and progresses to paraplegia and involvement of the sphincter, laryngeal, pharyngeal, and facial and respiratory muscles. Inspiratory spasms occur preterminally. Because the paralysis may be of an ascending nature, this form of rabies may resemble Guillain-Barré syndrome (GBS). Although some classic symptoms of furious rabies may be present, they usually are mild and may appear only late in the course of the disease; consequently the paralytic form of rabies may be more often misdiagnosed.[14,50] Medical treatment, especially sedatives, may mask some of the classic symptoms of rabies.

Rabies is marked by a relentless progression to coma and death, often within a week of the onset of clinical symptoms. Death may be abrupt; however, with life support, survival has been reported for many weeks. The only four cases of documented human survival following rabies infection are in patients who had received at least some rabies vaccination prior to the onset of symptoms,[5,14] and most were left with neurologic sequelae. There are no well-documented cases of survival after the development of symptoms in patients who have not received prophylaxis before exposure or during the incubation period.[5,14]

Complications are common in both presentations of rabies and may contribute directly to the patient's death. The virus may affect the pituitary gland, causing diabetes insipidus or an inappropriate secretion of antidiuretic hormone. Diabetes inspidus may exacerbate volume depletion in patients already so predisposed because of their inability to swallow, and either condition can cause significant electrolyte abnormalities. Fluctuating body temperature may result from the effect of the virus on the thermoregulatory center in the hypothalamus. Paralysis of the respiratory muscles may result in respiratory collapse, pneumonia, hypoxia, and eventually death. Ventricular arrhythmias may be secondary to hypoxia or electrolyte disturbances or due to a primary rabies myocarditis. Increased intracranial pressure from cerebral hypoxia, edema, or hydrocephalus can lead to seizures and coma. Gastrointestinal bleeding has been described that resulted from esophageal tears caused by violent vomiting or from stress ulcers.[50]

Laboratory findings are nonspecific; they may reflect an infectious process and any underlying complications. The white blood cell count can be elevated, and chemistry results are often abnormal. The cerebrospinal fluid (CSF) is usually normal but may show a mild pleocytosis, an increase in protein, or an elevated opening pressure.[50] Likewise, CNS imaging with a computed tomography scan is usually normal and does not contribute to the diagnosis.

Management of the patient includes appropriate sedation and life support until the diagnosis is established. Nothing has been effective in preventing death once symptoms have begun. Ineffective therapies have included multisite intradermal vaccination with cell culture vaccine, alpha-interferon and rabies immune globulin (RIG) by intravenous and intrathecal routes, antithymocyte globulin, high-dose corticosteroids, vidarabine, inosine pranobex, ribavirin, and antibody-binding fragments of immunoglobulin G.[51]

DIAGNOSIS

Because rabies is rare in developed countries, it may not be readily considered in the differential diagnosis. Rabies should be considered in any patient who presents with an acute, progressive encephalopathy of unknown cause. The lack of an animal exposure history should not deter consideration of rabies. The patient (as well as family and friends) may not recall an exposure if there has been a long incubation period. Further the patient may be too sick or too young to provide an adequate history and may not have shared the history of a seemingly inconsequential animal bite with friends or family. Finally it is possible that some bat bites may not be recognized as a bat bite.

Worldwide most cases of human rabies occur in developing countries where laboratory facilities are largely unavailable or unaffordable; thus most patients are diagnosed clinically.[11] Where laboratory testing is available, antemortem tests may aid in the diagnosis. No studies are useful during the incubation period. The immune response to rabies does not occur until late in the disease; therefore it is important to examine a nuchal skin biopsy, saliva, and CSF for direct evidence of the virus. This testing is done with direct immunofluorescent-antibody (dIFA) or reverse transcription (Rt) of RNA and polymerase chain reaction (PCR). RT-PCR is also especially useful for determination of the virus variant by genetic sequencing. Although antibodies may not appear until late in the course of the disease, CSF and serum should be examined for antibodies against the virus. Any CSF antibody level is indicative of infection, even in patients who have received rabies vaccination. Serum antibodies must be interpreted in the light of such history. Virus isolation, through cell culture or mouse inoculation, is not routine but can be useful if other tests are inconclusive. Corneal impressions have been used but are not the sample of choice and are not as sensitive as nuchal skin biopsy specimens.[2,5]

The disease is most reliably confirmed after death. Since there is no effective treatment and rabies is rare in developed countries, antemortem brain biopsy is not indicated to diagnose rabies. However, biopsies done for other diseases (e.g., herpesvirus encephalitis), if negative, can be tested for evidence of rabies virus infection, usually using dIFA. Histologic staining for Negri bodies, classically associated with the disease, is positive in only 50% to 80% of cases and is not considered diagnostic in developed countries.[2] Postmortem examination is indicated in situations in which rabies is suspected but not confirmed.

PREVENTION

Because there is no effective treatment, the only way to limit human deaths from rabies is through prevention. This can be accomplished chiefly by avoiding human exposure to rabies through animal control, use of animal-vaccination programs, and education to prevent contact between humans and stray or wild animals. When exposure is unavoidable or likely to occur, pre-exposure prophylaxis is recommended. Finally, if exposure does occur, the administration of postexposure prophylaxis in a timely fashion can prevent rabies. As many as 7 million people receive rabies vaccine each year.[11] In the United States it is estimated that between 16,000 and 30,000 patients receive postexposure prophylaxis annually.[52]

Avoiding Exposure

Restriction of the movement of dogs, control of stray dogs, and vaccination have controlled canine rabies in the United States, Canada, and Europe. Efforts to control rabies in wildlife have been made by using oral rabies vaccines. This approach has been effective in controlling fox rabies in parts of Europe and Canada, and coyote rabies and raccoon rabies in the United States.[53–56] Oral vaccination programs appear to be most useful in the limited control of rabies in areas where natural barriers (e.g., bodies of water or mountains that prevent animal movement) to rabies already exist. Education about high-risk situations can potentially prevent exposures. Patients should be cautioned against handling wildlife and petting dogs and cats not known to be vaccinated. The importance of vaccinating domestic cats and dogs should be emphasized.

Pets or domestic animals exposed to a rabid animal need to be evaluated by a veterinarian and reported to the local health department immediately. Unvaccinated dogs, cats, and ferrets exposed to a rabid animal should be euthanized immediately. If the owner is unwilling to have this done, the animal should be placed in isolation for 6 months and vaccinated 1 month before release. Dogs, cats, and ferrets that have current vaccinations should be revaccinated immediately and observed for 45 days.

Those with an expired vaccination are evaluated on an individual basis.[57]

Livestock that have current vaccinations and are exposed to a rabid animal should be revaccinated immediately and observed for 45 days. Unvaccinated livestock should be euthanized immediately. Other animals exposed to a rabid animal should be euthanized immediately.[57]

Pre-exposure Prophylaxis

Pre-exposure prophylaxis is indicated for certain high-risk groups (Table 14–3).[58] The regimen consists of a dose of vaccine on day 0 (day of first dose), day 7, and day 21 or 28. Pre-exposure prophylaxis simplifies postexposure prophylaxis by eliminating the need for rabies immune globulin (RIG) and may provide a measure of protection in the event that a true exposure is not recognized. It does not eliminate the need for appropriate wound treatment and additional vaccinations in the case of a known exposure. Routine serologic testing to confirm seroconversion is not necessary except in the case of immunocompromised individuals and those with continuous or frequent exposure to the virus.

Exposure

Rabies is transmitted when the virus is introduced into bite wounds or breaks in the skin or onto mucous membranes. In determining whether exposure occurred and postexposure prophylaxis is indicated, three questions should be answered (Fig. 14–2):

TABLE 14–3 ■ Rabies Pre-exposure Prophylaxis Guide, United States (CDC, 1999)

Risk category	Nature of risk	Typical populations	Pre-exposure recommendations
Continuous	Virus present continuously, often in high concentrations; specific exposures likely to go unrecognized; bite, nonbite, or aerosol exposure	Rabies research laboratory workers*; rabies biologics production workers	Primary course; serologic testing every 6 mo; booster vaccination if antibody titer is below acceptable level†
Frequent	Exposure usually episodic, with source recognized, but exposure may also be unrecognized; bite, nonbite, or aerosol exposure	Rabies diagnostic laboratory workers*; spelunkers; veterinarians and staff; and animal-control and wildlife workers in rabies enzootic areas	Primary course; serologic testing every 2 y; booster vaccination if antibody titer is below acceptable level†
Infrequent (greater than the population at large)	Exposure nearly always episodic with source recognized; bite or nonbite exposure	Veterinarians and animal-control and wildlife workers in areas of low rabies rates; veterinary students; travelers visiting areas where rabies is enzootic and immediate access to appropriate medical care including biologics is limited	Primary course; no serologic testing or booster vaccination
Rare (population at large)	Exposures always episodic with source recognized; bite or nonbite exposure	U.S. population at large, including persons in rabies epizootic areas	No vaccination necessary

*Judgment of relative risk and extra monitoring of vaccination status of laboratory workers is the responsibility of the laboratory supervisor.
†Minimum acceptable antibody level is complete virus neutralization at a 1:5 serum dilution by rapid fluorescent focus inhibition test; a booster dose should be administered if the titer falls below this level.

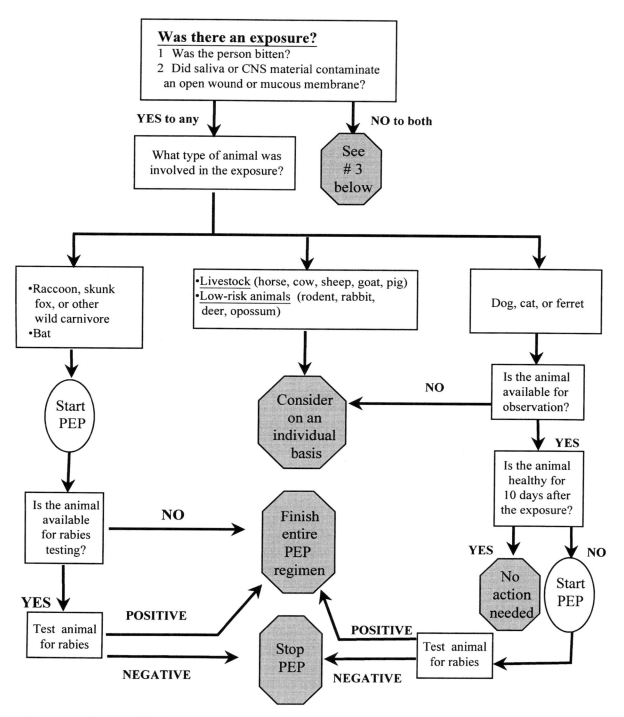

Was there an exposure?
1 Was the person bitten?
2 Did saliva or CNS material contaminate an open wound or mucous membrane?

YES to any

NO to both

What type of animal was involved in the exposure?

See # 3 below

•Raccoon, skunk fox, or other wild carnivore
•Bat

•Livestock (horse, cow, sheep, goat, pig)
•Low-risk animals (rodent, rabbit, deer, opossum)

Dog, cat, or ferret

Start PEP

Consider on an individual basis

Is the animal available for observation?

NO

Is the animal available for rabies testing?

Finish entire PEP regimen

Is the animal healthy for 10 days after the exposure?

YES

NO

YES

POSITIVE

YES

NO

Test animal for rabies

NEGATIVE

Stop PEP

POSITIVE

No action needed

Start PEP

Test animal for rabies

NEGATIVE

3 For assessing possible bat exposure: PEP should be considered when direct contact between a human and a bat has occurred unless the exposed person can be certain a bite, scratch, or mucous membrane exposure did not occur. PEP can be considered for persons who were in the same room as a bat who might be unaware that a bite or direct contact had occurred (e.g., a sleeping person awakens to find a bat in the room or an adult witnesses a bat in the room with a previously unattended child or incapacitated person).
IF POSSIBLE, TESTING THE BAT FOR RABIES SHOULD GUIDE THE NEED FOR PEP.

FIGURE 14–2. Algorithm to assist in determining the need for rabies postexposure prophylaxis (PEP).

1 Was the person bitten?

2 Did saliva or CNS material from a rabid animal contaminate an open wound or mucous membrane?

3 Was there a possibility of a bat bite (including finding a bat in a room with a young child or a sleeping or incapacitated person)?

If all can be answered no, then an exposure did not occur and postexposure prophylaxis is not required. Petting a rabid animal and contact with blood, urine, or feces of a rabid animal does not constitute an exposure and is not an indication for prophylaxis. If the answer to at least one of these questions is yes, then exposure to rabies is a possibility, and the likelihood that the animal has rabies must be considered (Table 14–4). Ideally, after an exposure occurs, an animal is captured and observed (for healthy dogs, cats, and ferrets) or euthanized (for all other animals) and tested for rabies. Obviously this is not always possible. The probability that any particular animal has rabies will vary according to the prevalence of rabies in species in particular geographic regions. Local public health departments can assist in determining whether postexposure prophylaxis is indicated.[58]

Nonbite exposures rarely result in transmission of rabies. Although the virus has been isolated from a variety of tissues and body fluids, only saliva and CNS tissue is considered to be infectious. Contamination of an open wound, scratch, abrasion, or mucous membrane by infected saliva or neural tissue may transmit the virus and is considered an exposure. In general, if the material containing the virus is dry, it can be considered noninfectious because the rabies virus is inactivated by thermal desiccation and ultraviolet light. Exposures to blood, feces, and unconcentrated urine are not a risk for transmission of the virus.[51,58]

Postexposure Prophylaxis

Wounds inflicted by a possibly rabid animal need immediate and thorough washing with soap and water. If available, a virucidal agent such as povidone-iodine can be used. Good wound care can reduce the risk of rabies by as much as 90%.[4] Tetanus vaccination and other measures to prevent bacterial infection may be indicated. Suturing may inoculate the virus deeper into the tissues and should be delayed or avoided.

When an exposure occurs, postexposure prophylaxis is required. All doses of vaccine are given intramuscularly in the deltoid area (anterolateral thigh is acceptable for small children). The gluteal area should not be used because administration in this area results in lower neutralizing titers. For those who have had prior vaccination with cell-culture vaccines (Table 14–5) or a documented history of antibody response to other vaccines, only two doses are required (one each on days 0 and 3), and RIG should not be used. Otherwise five doses are required (one each on days 0, 3, 7, 14, and 28), and RIG should be thoroughly infiltrated around the wound area. Any remaining RIG should be injected intramuscularly at a site distant from the vaccine administration. If RIG was not given when vaccination was begun, it can be administered through the seventh day after vaccination was started. Beyond the seventh day it is not indicated because an antibody response to the vaccine is presumed to have occurred (Table 14–6). Although no controlled trials have been performed, extensive experience from many parts of the world indicates that postexposure prophylaxis, consisting of local wound treatment, passive immunization (RIG), and vaccination, is effective if given in an appropriate and timely manner.[58] There have been no reported failures when the Advisory Committee on Immunization Practices (ACIP) recommendations have been followed. Failures with other accepted regimens of cell culture vaccines are rare and almost always involve deviations from the accepted vaccines or schedules.[59,60] Unfortunately many people are unaware of what constitutes an exposure and do not seek medical advice. Furthermore, because of the relatively rare need for postexposure prophylaxis, some medical providers

TABLE 14–4 ■ Rabies Postexposure Prophylaxis Guide, United States (CDC, 1999)

Animal type	Evaluation and disposition of animal	Postexposure prophylaxis recommendations
Dogs, cats, and ferrets	Healthy and available for 10 days observation	Should not begin prophylaxis unless animal develops clinical signs of rabies*
	Rabid or suspected rabid	Immediately vaccinate
	Unknown (e.g., escaped)	Consult public health officials
Skunks, raccoons, foxes, and most other carnivores; bats	Regard as rabid unless animal proven negative by laboratory tests†	Consider immediate vaccination
Livestock, small rodents, lagomorphs (rabbits and hares), large rodents (woodchucks and beavers), and other mammals	Consider individually	Consult public health officials; bites of squirrels, hamsters, guinea pigs, gerbils, chipmunks, rats, mice, other small rodents, rabbits, and hares almost never require antirabies postexposure prophylaxis

*During the 10-day observation period, begin postexposure prophylaxis at first sign of rabies in a dog, cat, or ferret that has bitten someone. If the animal exhibits clinical signs of rabies, it should be euthanized immediately and tested.

†The animal should be euthanized and tested as soon as possible. Holding for observation is not recommended. Discontinue vaccine if immunofluorescence test results of the animal are negative.

TABLE 14–5 ■ Cell-Culture Vaccines

Vaccine	Manufacturer
Immovax (HDCV)*	Aventis Pasteur
Immovax – Rabies vero (PVRV)	Aventis Pasteur
Lyssavac – HDC (HDCV)	Swiss Serum and Vaccine Institute (SSVI) Berna
Lyssavac N (PDEV)	Swiss Serum and Vaccine Institute (SSVI) Berna
Rabies Vaccine Adsorbed (RVA)*	Bioport
Rabipur/RabAvert (PCEC)*	Chiron Behring
Rabivac (HDCV)	Chiron Behring
Verorab (PVRV)	Aventis Pasteur

HDCV, human diploid cell vaccine; PCEC, purified chick embryo vaccine; PDEV, purified duck embryo vaccine; PVRV, purified vero cell vaccine
*Available in the United States.

may not understand what defines an exposure and the proper administration of rabies vaccine and RIG.

THE PREGNANT PATIENT

Pregnancy is not a contraindication to postexposure prophylaxis, and if the risk of exposure to rabies is substantial, pre-exposure prophylaxis might be indicated during pregnancy.[58] Additionally, if an expectant mother becomes ill with rabies, it is unlikely that the fetus will be infected. If mature enough for delivery, the fetus can be delivered. Postexposure prophylaxis should be considered as an additional preventive measure for the infant after delivery.

THE TRAVELER

The decision to give pre-exposure prophylaxis to travelers is complicated by the low incidence of rabies reported in travelers, the relatively high cost of pre-exposure rabies prophylaxis, and the need to begin the vaccination series at least 3 weeks before departure.[61] Nevertheless, pre-exposure prophylaxis should be considered for international travelers likely to come in contact with animals in areas where canine rabies is present and where immediate access to appropriate medical care, including safe and effective biologics, may be difficult. United States consulates may know whether or where cell culture vaccines for rabies can be obtained at a given destination.

If exposed, travelers should not accept a nerve tissue–derived vaccine, even if it delays start of treatment by 1 or 2 days. Most authorities feel that any of the cell culture–derived rabies vaccines (Table 14–5) can be used to complete a rabies vaccination series started with a different cell culture vaccine if it is not available. If a patient returns to the United States to complete a series and the type of vaccine used to initiate treatment cannot be verified, the series should be started from the beginning with one of the available cell culture vaccines. It is important for travelers and providers to remember that in many developing countries, testing of suspected rabid animals may be unreliable in determining whether rabies vaccination is needed.

TABLE 14–6 ■ Rabies Postexposure Prophylaxis Schedule, United States (CDC, 1999)

Vaccination status	Treatment	Regimen*
Not previously vaccinated	Wound cleansing	All postexposure treatment should begin with immediate thorough cleansing of all wounds with soap and water; if available, a virucidal agent such as povidone-iodine solution should be used to irrigate the wounds
	RIG	Administer 20 IU/kg body weight; if anatomically feasible, the full dose should be infiltrated around the wound(s), and any remaining volume should be administered IM at an anatomical site distant from vaccine administration; also, RIG should not be administered in the same syringe as vaccine; because RIG may partially suppress active production of antibody, no more than the recommended dose should be given
	Vaccine	HDCV, RVA, or PCEC 1 ml IM (deltoid area†), one each on days 0‡, 3, 7, 14, and 28.
Previously vaccinated§	Wound cleansing	All postexposure treatment should begin with immediate thorough cleansing of all wounds with soap and water; if available, a virucidal agent such as povidone-iodine solution should be used to irrigate the wounds
	RIG	RIG should NOT be administered
	Vaccine	HDCV, RVA, or PCEC 1 ml IM (deltoid area†), one each on days 0‡ and 3

HDCV, human diploid cell vaccine; PCEC, purified chick embryo cell vaccine; RIG = rabies immune globulin; RVA = rabies vaccine adsorbed.
*These regimens are applicable for all age groups, including children.
†The deltoid area is the only acceptable site of vaccination for adults and older children. For younger children the outer aspect of the thigh may be used. Vaccine should never be administered in the gluteal area.
‡Day 0 is the day the first dose of vaccine is administered.
§Any person with a history of pre-exposure vaccination with a cell culture vaccine (Table 14–5); prior postexposure prophylaxis with a cell culture vaccine (Table 14–5); or previous vaccination with another type of rabies vaccine *and* a documented antibody response to the vaccination.

BATS

The concern about bats is illustrated by the current situation in the United States. Excluding dog bites that occurred outside of the country, 24 (92%) of the 26 human cases of rabies in the United States since 1990 have been associated with bat rabies virus variants (Table 14–2). Although their histories sometimes have inconsistencies, only 2 of the 24 rabies patients reported a bat bite; at least another 9 patients reported direct contact with bats without being bitten; and another 5 patients had a history of bats in their place of residence. Several questions have been raised about the significance of this lack of bat bite history. Is it possible the bat variants have an altered pathophysiology (perhaps including the ability to infect via aerosol transmission)? Is it possible that "spillover" occurs in which the bat variants are acquired by other host animals, which then transmit the virus to humans? Or is it likely that bat bites are unreported or undetected.

In these cases without a reported bite, an unreported or undetected bat bite remains the most plausible hypothesis. There is some evidence that the variant of rabies virus associated with silver-haired bats might be more infectious than other variants associated with dogs and coyotes and that it may be better able to replicate at lower temperatures and in non-neural tissue.[62,63] However, this does not explain the means of initial transdermal transmission.

A review of the literature demonstrates few well-documented human cases that have been due to nonbite exposures. Ironically the data suggest that for nonbite transmission the greatest risk is iatrogenesis.[64–66] Eighteen cases of rabies in Brazil in 1960 were due to vaccine that had not been completely inactivated.[67] Eight cases have been linked to cornea transplants whose donors died of rabies.[68] Less well documented are cases due to saliva-contaminated scratches, open wounds, or mucous membranes.[65]

Accounts of rabies attributable to aerosol transmission are rare. Aerosol transmission of rabies has been reported as the only plausible mechanism of transmission in the laboratory in both animals and a human.[69–71] There is another purported aerosol case that occurred in a laboratory worker that is commonly attributed to aerosol, but other means of exposure seem likely and cannot be excluded.[72–74] Studies done on animals in captive situations in caves for several weeks or longer have supported the possibility of transmission of rabies via aerosol.[75] Two cases in humans from the 1950s are commonly attributed to aerosol exposure in caves,[13,49] but other means of transmission seem more probable and cannot be excluded.[75–77]

Possible transplacental transmission, perinatal transmission, and two possible cases of human-to-human transmission have been reported. These occurred in countries where human rabies is not uncommon, and ruling out more likely, verified modes of transmission was not possible.[66,78] In total there are only about 27 cases of well-documented and 17 poorly documented cases of nonbite transmission of human rabies. These rare cases must be considered in the perspective of the number of human rabies cases that have occurred annually worldwide; they are not indicative of the natural history of rabies.[79]

Studies have shown that bat variants rarely spillover to other host animals. A recent study of rabid cats and dogs showed that they were infected with the expected terrestrial rabies virus variant (e.g., raccoon variant in the eastern states, the coyote variant in Texas). Of 261 rabid cats and dogs, only one was infected with a variant associated with bats, a big brown bat variant.[80] Other animal studies have also shown that bat variants do not spillover into the terrestrial population in appreciable amounts.[81] In addition, histories of contact with other animals are diligently sought in investigations of human rabies, and such histories are not consistent with the possibility of spillover. If one consider the cases listed in Table 14–2, perhaps one patient who had contact with a sick kitten 6 to 9 months prior to his illness could fit this hypothesis. One other patient had contact with a sick cow that died 3 months earlier, but there is no history of a human rabies case resulting from an exposure to a rabid cow on record in the United States.

North American bats are small, and it is plausible that bat bites occur unrecognized. It may not be coincidental that the human cases attributable to bat variants are usually associated with the smallest of North American bats. The silver-haired and eastern pipistrelle bats weigh a third of an ounce or less. Their teeth are small, and evidence of a bite may be difficult to find.[82] In addition, these species generally do not form large colonies and can be found alone in trees, foliage, and crevices in wood and rock. Bites might occur outdoors and may not be recognized as such if the bat remains hidden in a tree or crevice (the bat bite may be considered a thorn prick, a spider bite, or an insect sting). Furthermore, small bites might go unrecognized if a person is asleep. If they do awaken, they may not do so quickly enough to recognize that they were bitten. A study from Colorado showed that 17 (50%) of 35 bats found by people upon awakening were rabid; 4 were not rabid, and 14 were not tested. Thus 17 (81%) of the 21 bats tested were rabid. The majority (23) of people had evidence of a bite, but the others did not.[83]

Perhaps an even more likely hypothesis is that people recognize when they are bitten by bats but minimize or do not appreciate the medical implications of a bat bite. In a recent survey, 15% of cavers (spelunkers) indicated that a bat bite was not a risk for rabies. This figure increased to 26% for those cavers with less education than a college degree.[84] In addition a bite by a dog, cat, or raccoon may warrant medical attention for the trauma alone and hence receive consideration for rabies prophylaxis. Regardless of whether a bat bite is recognized, it is unlikely to warrant medical attention for the minor trauma involved.

Indigenous rabid bats have been reported in every state except Hawaii, and human cases attributable to bat variants (Table 14-2) peak in September-October. This coincides with the peak of reported rabid bats in August plus a 4- to 8-week incubation period. In 1999, bats accounted for 14% of all reported rabid animals.[85] Of all bats submitted for testing, usually 4% to 15% are positive for rabies. This range reflects a sampling bias of sick bats, and the true prevalence is much lower, probably less than 1%.[81,86]

Postexposure prophylaxis should be considered when direct contact between a person and a bat might have occurred unless the person can be certain that a bite, scratch, or mucous membrane exposure did not occur. For example, consider the potential for exposure in situations in which a sleeping person wakes to find a bat in the room or an adult witnesses a bat in the room with a previously unattended child, mentally disabled person, or intoxicated person. Because of the minute size of bat teeth, examination for a bite wound alone is inadequate. If the bat in question is available for testing, and an exposure has not clearly occurred, initiation of postexposure prophylaxis may be delayed 24 to 48 hours for testing of the bat. If a bite or other clear exposure occurs, postexposure prophylaxis should begin immediately and may be stopped if laboratory testing shows that the bat is not rabid.[13,58]

On the basis of what is known about the pathogenesis of rabies and the studies available, bat bites remain the most plausible hypothesis for human cases of rabies associated with bat variants. People may minimize the importance of a bat bite, or bites from small solitary bats may not be recognized. Taken together, these two hypotheses probably explain most cases of cryptogenic rabies. The potential for the latter scenario is why the ACIP[58] recommends prophylaxis in the cases in which a bite cannot be reasonably excluded. Bat rabies spillover to other animals might explain a rare case, and nonbite transmission would be unlikely to explain many, if any, cryptogenic cases.

SUMMARY

It has been well over a century since Louis Pasteur performed the first rabies vaccination in 1885. Yet rabies remains an invariably fatal encephalitis and a significant cause of death worldwide. Human disease is rare in the United States and in other countries where canine rabies is well controlled. In the United States, bats rabies virus variants have emerged as the most common cause of human rabies. Rabies is almost always acquired through the bite from a rabid animal. Once symptoms of rabies develop, there is no effective medical treatment to prevent death. Avoiding exposure to stray and wild animals, however, and prophylaxis with wound care, RIG, and vaccination can prevent the development of rabies if given in an appropriate and timely manner.

ACKNOWLEDGMENTS: I would like to thank Chuck Rupprecht, Jean Smith, and Cathy Hanlon for their teaching and assistance with this manuscript and John O'Connor for his editorial work and Jennifer McQuiston for help with the Figures.

REFERENCES

1. Cited in Kaplan C: Rabies: The Facts, Oxford, Oxford University Press, 1977.
2. Smith JS: New aspects of rabies with emphasis on epidemiology, diagnosis, and prevention of the disease in the United States. Clin Microbiol Rev 1996;9:166–176.
3. Samaratunga H, Searle JW, Hudson N: Nonrabies Lyssavirus human encephalitis from fruit bats: Australian bat Lyssavirus (pteropid Lyssavirus) infection. Neuropathol Appl Neurobiol 1998;24:331–335.
4. Bleck TP, Rupprecht CE: Rhabdoviruses. In Richman DD, Whitley RJ, Hayden FG (eds): Clinical Virology. New York, Churchill Livingstone, 1997, pp 879–897.
5. Case records of the Massachusetts General Hospital (Case 21-1998). N Engl J Med 1998;339:105–112.
6. Dietzschold B, Rupprecht CE, Fu ZF, Koprowski H: Rhabdoviruses. In Fields BN, Knipe DM, Howley PM, et al (eds): Fields Virology, 3rd ed. Philadelphia, Lippincott-Raven, 1996, pp 1137–1159.
7. Steele JH, Fernandez PJ: History of rabies and global aspects. In Baer GM (ed): The Natural History of Rabies, 2nd ed. Boca Raton, Fla, CRC Press, 1991, pp 1–24.
8. Gomez-Alonso J: Rabies: A possible explanation for the vampire legend. Neurology 1998;51:856–859.
9. Heick A: Prince Dracula, rabies, and the vampire legend. Ann Intern Med 1992;117:172–173.
10. Patterson KD: Rabies. In Kiple KF (ed): The Cambridge World History of Human Disease, Cambridge, Cambridge University Press, 1993, pp 962–967.
11. World Health Organization (WHO): World survey of rabies no. 34 for the year 1998. Report no.: WHO/CDC/CSR/APH/99.6. Geneva, World Health Organization, 2000.
12. Haupt W: Rabies—risk of exposure and current trends in prevention of human cases. Vaccine 1999;17:1742–1749.
13. Fishbein DB, Robinson LE: Rabies. N Engl J Med 1993;329:1632–1638.
14. Hemachudha T, Phuapradit P: Rabies. Curr Opin Neurol 1997;10:260–267.
15. Held JR, Tierkel ES, Steele JH: Rabies in man and animals in the United States, 1946–65. Public Health Rep 1967;82:1009–1018.
16. Anderson LJ, Nicholson KG, Tauxe RV, Winkler WG: Human rabies in the United States, 1960 to 1979: Epidemiology, diagnosis, and prevention. Ann Intern Med 1984;100:728–735.
17. Noah DL, Drenzek CL, Smith JS, et al: Epidemiology of human rabies in the United States, 1980 to 1996. Ann Intern Med 1998;128:922–930.
18. Centers for Disease Control and Prevention: Human rabies—Oklahoma. MMWR Morb Mortal Wkly Rep 1981;30:343–349.
19. Centers for Disease Control and Prevention: Human rabies acquired outside the United States from a dog bite. MMWR Morb Mortal Wkly Rep 1981;30:537–540.
20. Centers for Disease Control and Prevention: Imported human rabies. MMWR Morb Mortal Wkly Rep 1983;32:78–80.

21. Centers for Disease Control and Prevention: Human rabies—Michigan. MMWR Morb Mortal Wkly Rep 1983; 32:159–160.

22. Centers for Disease Control and Prevention: Human rabies—Texas. MMWR Morb Mortal Wkly Rep 1984;33:469–470.

23. Centers for Disease Control and Prevention: Human rabies—Pennsylvania. MMWR Morb Mortal Wkly Rep 1984;33: 633–635.

24. Centers for Disease Control and Prevention: Human rabies acquired outside the United States. MMWR Morb Mortal Wkly Rep 1985;34:235–236.

25. Centers for Disease Control and Prevention: Human rabies diagnosed 2 months post-mortem—Texas. MMWR Morb Mortal Wkly Rep 1985;34:700, 705–707.

26. Centers for Disease Control and Prevention: Human rabies—California, 1987. MMWR Morb Mortal Wkly Rep 1988;37: 305–308.

27. Centers for Disease Control and Prevention: Human rabies—Oregon, 1989. MMWR Morb Mortal Wkly Rep 1989;38: 335–337.

28. Centers for Disease Control and Prevention: Human rabies—Texas, 1990. MMWR Morb Mortal Wkly Rep 1991;40:132–133.

29. Centers for Disease Control and Prevention: Human rabies—Texas, Arkansas, and Georgia, 1991. MMWR Morb Mortal Wkly Rep 1991;40:765–769.

30. Centers for Disease Control and Prevention: Human rabies—California, 1992. MMWR Morb Mortal Wkly Rep 1992;41: 461–463.

31. Centers for Disease Control and Prevention: Human rabies—New York, 1993. MMWR Morb Mortal Wkly Rep 1993; 42:799, 805–806.

32. Centers for Disease Control and Prevention: Human rabies—Texas and California, 1993. MMWR Morb Mortal Wkly Rep 1994;43:93–96.

33. Centers for Disease Control and Prevention: Human rabies—California, 1994. MMWR Morb Mortal Wkly Rep 1994; 43:455–457.

34. Centers for Disease Control and Prevention: Human rabies—Miami, 1994. MMWR Morb Mortal Wkly Rep 1994; 43:773–775.

35. Centers for Disease Control and Prevention: Human rabies—Alabama, Tennessee, and Texas, 1994. MMWR Morb Mortal Wkly Rep 1995;44:269–272.

36. Centers for Disease Control and Prevention: Human rabies—West Virginia, 1994. MMWR Morb Mortal Wkly Rep 1995;44:86–87, 93.

37. Centers for Disease Control and Prevention: Human rabies—Washington, 1995. MMWR Morb Mortal Wkly Rep 1995; 44:625–627.

38. Centers for Disease Control and Prevention: Human rabies—California, 1995. MMWR Morb Mortal Wkly Rep 1996; 45:353–356.

39. Centers for Disease Control and Prevention: Human rabies—Connecticut, 1995. MMWR Morb Mortal Wkly Rep 1996; 45:207–209.

40. Centers for Disease Control and Prevention: Human rabies—Florida, 1996. MMWR Morb Mortal Wkly Rep 1996; 45:719–720, 727.

41. Centers for Disease Control and Prevention: Human rabies—New Hampshire, 1996. MMWR Morb Mortal Wkly Rep 1997;46:267–270.

42. Centers for Disease Control and Prevention: Human rabies—Kentucky and Montana, 1996. MMWR Morb Mortal Wkly Rep 1997;46:397–400.

43. Centers for Disease Control and Prevention: Human rabies—Montana and Washington, 1997. MMWR Morb Mortal Wkly Rep 1997;46:770–774.

44. Centers for Disease Control and Prevention: Human rabies—Texas and New Jersey, 1997. MMWR Morb Mortal Wkly Rep 1998;47:1–5.

45. Centers for Disease Control and Prevention: Human rabies—Virginia. MMWR Morb Mortal Wkly Rep 1999; 48:95–97.

46. Centers for Disease Control and Prevention: Human rabies—California, Georgia, Minnesota, New York, and Wisconsin, 2000. MMWR Morb Mortal Wkly Rep 2000;49:1111–1115.

47. Hattwick MAW: Human rabies. Public Health Rev 1974;3:229–274.

48. Smith JS, Fishbein DB, Rupprecht CE, Clark K: Unexplained rabies in three immigrants in the United States. N Engl J Med 1991;324:205–211.

49. Plotkin SA: Rabies. Clin Infect Dis 2000;30:4–12.

50. Warrell DA: The clinical picture of rabies in man. Trans R Soc Trop Med Hyg 1976;70:188–195.

51. World Health Organization (WHO) Expert Committee on Rabies: Eighth report. WHO technical report series no. 824. Geneva, World Health Organization, 1992.

52. Krebs JW, Long-Marin SC, Childs JE: Causes, costs, and estimates of rabies postexposure prophylaxis treatments in the United States. J Public Health Management Practice 1998;4:56–62.

53. Schneider LG, Cox JH, Muller WW, Hohnsbeen KP: Current oral rabies vaccination in Europe: An interim balance. Rev Infect Dis 1988;10(Suppl):S654–S659.

54. Johnston DH, Voight DR, MacInnes CD, et al: An aerial baiting system for the distribution of attenuated or recombinant rabies vaccines for foxes, raccoons, and skunks. Rev Infect Dis 1988;10(Suppl):S660–S664.

55. Fearneyhough MG, Wilson PJ, Clark KA, et al: Results of an oral rabies vaccination program for coyotes. J Am Vet Med Assoc 1998;212:498–502.

56. Hanlon CA, Rupprecht CE: The reemergence of rabies. In Scheld IWM, Armstrong D, Hughes JM (eds): Emerging Infections. Washington, DC, ASM Press, 1998, pp 59–80.

57. National Association of State Public Health Veterinarians: Compendium of animal rabies control, 1999. MMWR Morb Mortal Wkly Rep 1999;48(RR-3):1–9.

58. Recommendations of the Advisory Committee on Immunization Practices (ACIP): Human rabies prevention—United States, 1999. MMWR Morb Mortal Wkly Rep 1999;48(RR-1):1–22.

59. Wilde H, Sirikawin S, Sabcharoen A, et al: Failure of postexposure treatment of rabies in children. Clin Infect Dis 1996;22:228–232.

60. Hemachudha T, Mitrabhakdi E, Wilde H, et al: Additional reports of failure to respond to treatment after rabies exposure in Thailand. Clin Infect Dis 1998;28:143–144.

61. Le Guerrier P, Pilon PA, Deshaies D, Allard R: Pre-exposure rabies prophylaxis for the international traveler: A decision analysis. Vaccine 1996;14:167–176.

62. Morimoto K, Patel M, Corisdeo S, et al: Characterization of a unique variant of bat rabies virus responsible for newly emerging human cases in North America. Proc Natl Acad Sci USA 1996;93:5653–5658.

63. Dietzschold B, Morimoto K, Hooper DC, et al: Genotypic and phenotypic diversity of rabies virus variants involved in human rabies: Implications for postexposure prophylaxis. J Hum Virol 2000;3:50–57.

64. Afshar A: A review of non-bite transmission of rabies virus infection. Br Vet J 1979;135:142–148.

65. Fishbein D: Rabies in humans. In Baer GM, (ed): The Natural History of Rabies, 2nd ed. Boca Raton, Fla, CRC Press, 1991, pp 519–550.

66. Feder HM, Nelson RS, Cartter ML, Sadre I: Rabies prophylaxis following the feeding of a rabid pony. Clin Pediatr 1998;37:477–482.

67. Para M: An outbreak of post-vaccinal rabies (rage de laboratoire) in Fortaleza, Brazil, in 1960. Bull World Health Organ 1965;33:177–182.

68. Javadi MA, Fayaz A, Mirdehghan SA, Ainollahi B: Transmission of rabies by corneal graft. Cornea 1996;15:431–433.

69. Centers for Disease Control and Prevention: Rabies in a laboratory worker—New York. MMWR Morb Mortal Wkly Rep 1977;26:183–184.

70. Centers for Disease Control and Prevention: Follow-up on rabies—New York. MMWR Morb Mortal Wkly Rep 1977;26:249–250.

71. Winkler WG, Baker EF JR, Hopkins CC: An outbreak of non-bite transmitted rabies in a laboratory animal colony. Am J Epidemiol 1972;95:267–277.

72. Centers for Disease Control and Prevention: Human rabies—Texas. MMWR Morb Mortal Wkly Rep 1972;21:113–114.

73. Conomy JP, Leibovitz A, McCombs W, Stinson, J: Airborne rabies encephalitis: Demonstration of rabies virus in the human central nervous system. Neurology 1977;27:67–69.

74. Winkler WG, Fashinell TR, Leffingwell L, et al: Airborne rabies transmission in a laboratory worker. JAMA 1973; 226:1219–1221.

75. Constantine DG: Rabies transmission by air in bat caves. Public Health Service Publication No. 1617. U.S. Department of Health, Education, and Welfare, Public Health Service, Atlanta, 1967.

76. Irons JV, Eads RB, Grimes JE, Conklin A: The public health importance of bats. Tex Rep Biol Med 1957;15:292–298.

77. Kent JR, Finegold SM: Human rabies transmitted by the bite of a bat. N Engl J Med 1960;263:1058–1065.

78. Fekadu M, Endeshaw T, Alemu W, et al: Possible human-to-human transmission of rabies in Ethiopia. Ethiop Med J 1996;34:123–127.

79. Gibbons RV, Cryptogenic rabies, bats, and the question of aerosol transmission. Ann Emerg Med 2002;39:528–536.

80. McQuiston JH, Yager PA, Smith JS, Rupprecht CE: Epidemiologic characteristics of rabies virus variants in dogs and cats in the United States, 1999. J Am Vet Med Assoc 2001;218:1939–1940.

81. Baer G, Smith JS: Rabies in nonhematophagous bats. In Baer GM (ed): The Natural History of Rabies, 2nd ed. Boca Raton, Fla, 1991, CRC Press, pp 341–366.

82. Feder HM, Nelson R, Reiher HW: Bat bite? Lancet 1997;350:1300.

83. Pape WJ, Fitzsimmons TD, Hoffman RE: Risk for rabies transmission from encounters with bats, Colorado, 1977–1996. Emerg Infect Dis 1999;5:433–438.

84. Gibbons RV, Holman RC, Mosberg SR, Rupprecht CE: Human rabies and exposure to bats: Implications of the knowledge among cavers in the United States. EID 2002;8:532–543

85. Krebs JW, Smith JS, Rupprecht CE, Childs JE: Rabies surveillance in the United States during 1999. J Am Vet Med Assoc 2000;216:1799–1811.

86. Brass DA: Prevalence and distribution of rabies in insectivorous bats. In Brass DA: Rabies in Bats, Natural History and Public Health Importance. Ridgefield, N.J., Livia Press, 1994, pp 131–150.

KENNETH C. GORSON, MD

JAYASHRI SRINIVASAN, MD, MRCP, PhD

Guillain-Barré Syndrome

Guillain-Barré syndrome (GBS) is one of the classic diseases in neurology with an easily appreciated clinical pattern of rapidly progressive, generalized weakness, limb paresthesias, and areflexia.[1] The recognition of unusual clinical and electrophysiologic patterns, so-called GBS variants, has warranted a reappraisal of the spectrum of the condition, which now includes acute inflammatory demyelinating polyneuropathy (AIDP, the most common pattern), acute motor sensory axonal neuropathy (AMSAN), acute motor axonal neuropathy (AMAN), and other regional variants, notably the Miller Fisher syndrome (acute ophthalmoplegia, ataxia, and areflexia, Table 15–1). As most patients with GBS have a preceding infectious illness, it is worthwhile to review various aspects of this condition in the context of a broader understanding of the evaluation and therapy of infectious diseases.

EPIDEMIOLOGY

GBS is the most common cause of acute paralysis in Western countries with an annual incidence of 1.8 cases per 100,000 population.[1] The incidence increases with age from 0.8 in those younger than 18 years to 3.2 for those over 60 years. There is a slight peak between 30 and 50 years, and the condition is less common at the extremes of age. GBS affects persons of all races but is slightly more common in whites. No genetic factors predispose to GBS, and there is no evidence that the disorder is communicable.

ETIOLOGY

The cause of GBS is not known. Approximately two-thirds of patients report a preceding immunologic trigger, most frequently an upper respiratory or gastrointestinal tract infection or an immunization 1 to 4 weeks prior to the onset of neurologic symptoms.[1,2] The infectious agent responsible for the prodromal illness frequently remains unidentified.[3] A number of anecdotal reports suggest a link between various bacterial and viral agents and GBS; however, a definite causal relationship has been established only with a few (Table 15–2).[1–5]

Bacterial Infections

The most common bacterial organism linked to GBS is *Campylobacter jejuni*.[5] Of patients with GBS who were studied prospectively, 26% had positive stool cultures or serology of *C. jejuni* infection, compared with 2% of controls.[5] Additional studies

TABLE 15–1 ■ Clinical Patterns of Guillain-Barré Syndrome

Acute inflammatory demyelinating polyneuropathy (AIDP, "typical GBS")
Acute motor-sensory axonal neuropathy (AMSAN)
Acute motor axonal neuropathy (AMAN)
Fisher syndrome (acute ophthalmoplegia, ataxia, areflexia)
Pure motor variant (demyelinating)
Pure sensory variant
Pure ataxic variant
Acute dysautonomia
Paraparetic variant
Cervico-pharyngeal-brachial variant
Acute lumbar polyradiculopathy with 6th nerve palsies

TABLE 15–2 ■ Infectious Agents Associated with Guillain-Barré Syndrome

BACTERIAL INFECTIONS
Campylobacter jejuni*
Mycoplasma pneumoniae*
Haemophilus influenzae
Salmonella
Listeria
Shigella
Legionella
Brucellosis
Yersinia enterocolitica
Pasturella tularensis

SPIROCHETAL INFECTIONS
Borrelia burgdorferi (Lyme disease)
Leptospira icterohaemorrhagiae

VIRAL INFECTIONS
Cytomegalovirus*
Epstein-Barr virus*
Herpes simplex virus I and II
Herpes zoster virus
Hepatitis A, B, C
HIV
Influenza A and B
Parainfluenza 1 and 2
Adenovirus
Echovirus
Cocksackievirus
Measles
Mumps
Rubella
Parvovirus B19
Respiratory syncytial virus
West Nile virus

*Epidemiological data support a statistical link between the agent and GBS.

have reported serologic evidence of recent C. jejuni infection in 17% to 39% of patients with GBS.[3,6–8] One study showed that the risk of developing GBS after confirmed C. jejuni infection was 30.4 cases per 100,000, substantially higher than the expected prevalence of 0.3 cases per 100,000 in the general population.[9] Patients with C. jejuni enteritis have fever, watery diarrhea, and abdominal cramping followed by the onset of GBS days or weeks later; however, approximately 30% of patients

have only serologic evidence of recent infection without enteritis.[5] The pathophysiology of GBS associated with C. jejuni infection is incompletely understood. Several studies have suggested a form of molecular mimicry in which acute infection stimulates the production of antibodies directed against C. jejuni lipopolysaccharides that inadvertently cross-react with ganglioside antigens on peripheral nerve myelin or axons.[8,10,11] Animal studies have shown that rabbits injected with lipopolysaccharides from certain strains of Campylobacter produced anti-GM_1, GA_1 and GQ_1 antibodies.[12] Patients with GBS associated with C. jejuni infection are more likely than those without infection to have severe axonal loss on electrodiagnostic studies, elevated anti-GM_1 antibodies, and a protracted recovery.[5,7] Another GBS pattern linked to the preceding C. jejuni infection predominantly involves distal weakness, spares cranial and sensory nerves, and has been associated with autoantibodies directed against the ganglioside N-acetylgalactosaminyl GD1a (anti-Ga1Nac-GD1a).[13,14]

Haemophilus influenzae infection has been related to an axonal form of GBS; a Japanese study showed 13% of patients with GBS had elevated anti–H. influenzae antibodies compared with controls.[15] Such cases are associated with prodromal respiratory infection, motor axon degeneration on electrophysiologic studies, elevated IgG anti-GM_1 antibodies, and less frequent cranial and sensory nerve involvement.[15]

Mycoplasma pneumoniae precedes GBS in approximately 5% of cases, and this agent should be considered when GBS develops after a prodromal illness characterized by fever, headache, and severe dry cough.[1,4] Infection with M. pneumoniae can be confirmed by complement-fixing antibody tests and is supported by the presence of cold agglutinin antibodies in the serum.[16] Infection due to Shigella, Salmonella, typhoid fever, brucellosis, and Yersinia enterocolitica also has been anecdotally reported to precede GBS, but an epidemiologic relationship is less convincing in these cases.[1,17–20]

The neurologic complications associated with Lyme disease include a chronic, axonal sensorimotor polyneuropathy (the most common pattern in the United States), painful polyradiculitis (Bannwarth's syndrome), and acute facial diplegia, which may resemble a regional variant of GBS.[21,22] The relationship between a GBS-like illness and antecedent infection with Lyme disease, however, remains unproven. A number of credible cases have been reported in Europe, but the association must be rare in North America.[23] A lymphocytic pleocytosis in the spinal fluid may distinguish these patients from typical forms of GBS.[1,23]

Viral Infections

Cytomegalovirus (CMV) is the most commonly identified viral infection that precedes GBS; as many as 15% of cases have serologic evidence of antecedent CMV infection.[3,4,24] In some instances the only indication that CMV is the preceding infectious agent may be elevated liver enzymes concomitant with the onset of GBS symptoms. In most patients the diagnosis can be confirmed by demonstrating elevated CMV IgM antibodies. GBS triggered by CMV infection occurs in younger persons and is associated with a more severe course with respiratory failure, prominent sensory loss, more frequent cranial nerve involvement, and raised antibodies directed against the peripheral nerve ganglioside GM_2.[24] CMV-infected fibroblasts express ganglioside-like epitopes that specifically recognize anti-GM_2 antibodies.[12] Anti-Ga1Nac-GD1a antibodies also have been elevated in patients with CMV infection, although in contrast to cases associated with *C. jejuni*, patients with GBS due to CMV and elevated anti-Ga1Nac-GD1a antibodies had a demyelinating polyneuropathy with slower progression, more frequent sensory deficits, and facial weakness.[25]

Epstein-Barr virus (EBV) infection precedes GBS in 2% to 10% of cases.[1–4] The infectious illness may be mononucleosis, pharyngitis, or hepatitis. Liver enzymes also may be elevated, and the diagnosis is supported by demonstrating a positive heterophile antibody or elevated EBV IgM antibodies.

GBS may be the initial manifestation of human immunodeficiency virus (HIV) infection or may occur soon after seroconversion.[26–28] Compared with seronegative patients, HIV-positive GBS patients were more likely to have generalized lymphadenopathy, cerebrospinal fluid (CSF), pleocytosis, and coexistent central nervous system deficits.[29]

Numerous anecdotal reports have linked GBS to infection with respiratory syncytial virus, parainfluenza virus, echovirus, coxsackievirus, measles, mumps, rubella, herpes zoster and simplex viruses, influenza, hepatitis A and B, and West Nile virus, but case reports preclude any conclusions about an epidemiologic relationship between these viruses and GBS.[1–4,30–32]

Vaccinations

Epidemiologic data have suggested a slight increase in cases of GBS following the 1976 swine influenza vaccine, although only a modest excess risk occurred with subsequent influenza vaccines.[33–35] One study concluded that there was no causal relationship between measles-mumps-rubella vaccination and GBS.[36] An increased incidence of GBS has been reported with other vaccines, notably tetanus and diphtheria toxoids, rabies, and oral poliomyelitis, but an epidemiologic relationship has not been demonstrated in large prospective studies.[37]

Other Factors Associated with GBS

Several systemic illnesses also have been tenuously linked to GBS, but most of these are implicated more often with chronic inflammatory demyelinating polyneuropathy.[38] GBS has been described in patients with Hodgkin's disease, lung cancer, thyroid disease, systemic lupus erythematosus, paraproteinemia, and sarcoidosis in single case reports or small series. It is difficult to be certain that the associations are anything more than chance.[1]

Several early series of GBS patients have contained a small proportion of cases that occurred after surgery.[1] Careful electrodiagnostic studies were performed inconsistently, however, and in retrospect these cases more likely represented critical illness polyneuropathy as a consequence of multiorgan failure or sepsis in the postoperative period.[39] Similarly, trauma rarely has been reported as a precipitant of GBS, but the association must remain uncertain.

Medications, drugs of abuse, bone marrow transplantation, and spinal epidural anesthesia have all been reported to precede GBS in a few cases, but these connections also remain unproven. GBS may occur at any time during pregnancy, the risk being greatest several months after delivery.[40]

CLINICAL FEATURES

GBS is principally a disorder that affects motor nerves, although distal limb paresthesias are frequently present at the onset of the condition (Table 15–3). The paresthesias are usually followed within hours or days by progressive leg weakness. Patients often complain of difficulty arising from a chair or climbing stairs because of involvement of the hip girdle muscles. The arms usually are affected as the condition advances, and the cranial nerves are involved in 30% to 50% of cases. Occasionally weakness remains restricted to the legs (paraparetic variant), or conversely the illness may begin with cranial nerves and arm weakness and involve the legs as the disorder

TABLE 15–3 ■ Clinical Features of Guillain-Barré Syndrome

Progressive weakness in the arms and legs
Generalized areflexia or hyporeflexia
Numbness and tingling in the limbs
Progression < 4 weeks

CRANIAL NERVE INVOLVEMENT
Facial diplegia
Ptosis
Ophthalmoplegia
Oropharyngeal weakness
Ventilatory failure (requiring mechanical ventilation)

DYSAUTONOMIA
Sinus tachycardia
Bradycardia (vagal spells)
Orthostatic hypotension
Hypertension
Ileus
Urinary retention

progresses.[41] Approximately one-third of patients have symmetrical, generalized arm and leg weakness at the onset of symptoms. The weakness is always bilateral, although some degree of asymmetry is common.

Another cardinal sign is reduced or absent deep tendon reflexes, presumably related to desynchronization of impulses carried by demyelinated fibers in the afferent loop of the reflex arc. Approximately 70% of patients have absent deep tendon reflexes at the time of presentation, and less than 5% of patients maintain reflexes throughout the course of the illness. Reflexes are almost always unobtainable in limbs that are too weak to move against gravity.

Approximately 50% of patients experience paresthesias of the hands and feet as the initial symptom. Most complain of "prickling" or "tingling" feelings, likened to an "asleep" feeling in an arm or leg after limb compression. The sensory symptoms are symmetrical and often precede weakness by a few days, ascending to the ankles and wrists as the illness worsens. Some describe a numb or dead sensation. Reduced vibration and joint position sensation in the distal limbs are common findings. Pain is also a common symptom and usually manifests as a deep aching sensation in large muscles of the back and legs, shooting pains radiating down the extremities, or as burning dysesthesias in the hands and feet.[42]

Cranial nerve involvement develops in approximately 50% of GBS patients, and the facial nerve is most commonly affected. As with limb weakness, facial paralysis is bilateral but may be asymmetrical. The ocular muscles are involved in 10% to 20% of patients, and in severe cases there may be complete ophthalmoplegia. Oropharyngeal weakness occurs in up to one-half of patients during the course of the illness and poses a substantial risk of aspiration.

Diaphragmatic weakness requiring assisted ventilation develops in approximately 30% of patients with GBS.[1,43,44] Most such patients have severe generalized weakness. Paralysis of the diaphragm reduces vital capacity and leads to atelectasis, arteriovenous shunting, and hypoxia. Patients also have difficulty clearing oral secretions, further aggravating ventilatory failure. Tachypnea develops, increasing the work of breathing, and eventually respiratory muscle fatigue with retention of carbon dioxide. These patients may rapidly deteriorate to a respiratory arrest. If diaphragmatic and respiratory muscle weakness have not occurred after 2 weeks from the onset of the condition, assisted ventilation is usually not required in the absence of other pulmonary or medical complications. Patients with GBS who require ventilator support have a less favorable prognosis for neurologic recovery, longer hospitalization, and higher mortality.[45]

Dysautonomia is a well-recognized feature in patients with fully developed GBS, occurring in up to 65% of cases.[46,47] The most common autonomic manifestation is sinus tachycardia, which usually does not require intervention unless the patient is hemodynamically unstable. Other features of autonomic instability include sinus bradycardia, sinus arrest, paroxysmal hypertension, and postural hypotension, ileus, and urinary retention.

GUILLAIN-BARRÉ SYNDROME VARIANTS

A number of restricted patterns are included within the limits of GBS because of similarities in the clinical and electromyographic (EMG) findings, temporal course, and prognosis (Table 15–1).

Axonal Forms of Guillain-Barré Syndrome (AMSAN and AMAN Variants)

A minority of patients with GBS develop an especially severe form of the illness, characterized by rapidly progressive paralysis, distal sensory loss, respiratory failure requiring prolonged ventilator support, and poor recovery.[48] The spinal fluid protein level is elevated, but in contrast to the demyelinating features of typical GBS, EMG studies show absent motor and sensory potentials and widespread active denervation, indicating an axonal process. Several studies have suggested that this syndrome, now called acute motor-sensory axonal neuropathy (AMSAN), represents a variant of GBS that is clinically indistinguishable from typical cases, but in which axons may be the target of the immune reaction.[49,50] In contrast to AMSAN, an acute motor axonal neuropathy (AMAN) afflicts primarily children in regions of northern China during the summer months.[51,52] The condition is characterized by acute symmetrical limb weakness, facial and oropharyngeal paralysis, and respiratory failure that progresses over several weeks. There are no sensory features and the extraocular muscles are spared. There is usually an antecedent gastrointestinal illness with abdominal pain and diarrhea, and most patients have elevated antibody titers of C. jejuni, anti-GM$_1$ and anti-GD$_{1a}$. The spinal fluid protein level is usually elevated. Electrophysiologic evaluation shows reduced or absent motor potential amplitudes without demyelinating features. Studies suggest that the pathogenesis of AMAN involves an antibody- and complement-mediated process directed primarily and selectively at the terminal aspects of motor axons.[53] Most patients have a favorable prognosis, similar to that of typical GBS, and in contrast to that of patients with AMSAN.[54]

Miller Fisher Variant

The triad of acute ophthalmoplegia, ataxia, and areflexia, described by C. Miller Fisher in 1956, has been accepted as a form of GBS on the basis of similar clinical and electrodiagnostic features.[55] Fisher syndrome accounts for approximately 5% of GBS cases, although in some patients the illness may evolve into a generalized form of the disorder.[56,57] Diplopia due to oculomotor or abducens nerve weakness is usually the first symptom, followed by limb or gait ataxia that appears within days. Large amplitude, discoordinated limb movements are indistinguishable from a cerebellar form of limb ataxia. Distal paresthesias, and bulbar and proximal limb weakness occur in as many as one-third of patients. Respiratory failure requiring ventilator support also develops in approximately one-third of patients, at which time the condition merges into typical GBS. The deep tendon reflexes are absent in all fully developed cases. Fisher syndrome rarely is confused with a form of brainstem encephalitis or infarction, but central nervous system findings (e.g., confusion, seizures, hemiparesis, Babinski signs) along with normal EMG studies suggest brainstem encephalitis or stroke. The CSF protein level may be elevated in Fisher syndrome but less frequently than in typical cases. The EMG shows absent sensory nerve action potentials and few or no motor conduction abnormalities. In virtually all cases there are elevated anti-ganglioside antibodies directed against the epitope GQ_{1b}.[58] The observation that paranodal regions of the oculomotor, trochlear, and abducens nerves are enriched with GQ_{1b} ganglioside supports a role of anti-GQ_{1b} antibodies in the pathogenesis of ophthalmoplegia.[59]

Other Guillain-Barré Syndrome Variants

A pure motor form of GBS has been reported to occur in 18% of cases in one large series.[60] These patients have rapidly progressive symmetrical limb paralysis and areflexia and lack any sensory symptoms or signs. This variant may be distinguished from typical GBS by a rapid onset of distally predominant weakness, sparing of cranial nerves, an early clinical nadir, higher than usual rates of elevated anti-GM_1 antibody titers, and a preceding *C. jejuni* infection.[60] These cases may be clinically similar to Chinese patients with the AMAN variant, but demyelinating changes detected by EMG studies are far more common in the pure motor form of GBS. There are rare cases of acute sensory polyneuropathy that may be appropriately classified as sensory variants of GBS on the basis of clinical, CSF, and EMG findings.[61–63] Sudden, rapidly progressive and severe large fiber sensory loss leads to limb and gait ataxia, Romberg sign, pseudoathetosis, and tremor. Other variants include acute pandysautonomia, a regional pattern of weakness restricted to the muscles of the arms, neck, and deglutition (cervical-oropharyngeal-brachial variant), and isolated leg weakness with areflexia (paraparetic variant).[1,41,57,64].

EVALUATION AND DIAGNOSIS

EMG studies confirm the diagnosis in virtually all patients.[65] Difficulty arises, however, when nerve conduction abnormalities are normal or show only modest changes, which may occur in a minority of cases early in the course of GBS; repeat studies are sometimes helpful when initial abnormalities are not specific.[66] The main finding is electrophysiologic evidence of multifocal nerve demyelination, demonstrated by slowing of motor nerve conduction velocities, conduction block, and prolonged distal motor latencies and F-responses (a measure of proximal nerve and nerve root conduction). Conduction block, defined as a progressive reduction (usually > 20%) in the amplitude of the motor potential following proximal nerve stimulation, is found in approximately one-third of patients with GBS. Seventy-five percent of patients have abnormal sensory conduction studies, usually reduced or absent sensory potentials. Patients with the severe "axonal" form of GBS have reduced or absent motor potentials, so-called inexcitable nerves, associated with widespread denervation on the needle electrode examination.[67] This is the typical pattern of AMSAN noted previously.

The CSF protein concentration is elevated in approximately 90% of patients at some time during the course of the illness. There are no inflammatory cells in the spinal fluid, and this "cyto-albuminologic dissociation" is a hallmark of GBS that distinguishes these patients from other febrile paralyses, notably poliomyelitis. A small number of patients, however, have a lymphocytic pleocytosis greater than 10 mm.[3] GBS associated with HIV or Lyme infection may involve inflammatory cells in the spinal fluid, presumably reflecting meningeal inflammation. Therefore, the presence of cells in the CSF does not exclude GBS. Patients with exceptionally high protein levels (for example, 1000 mg/dl) may develop papilledema and pseudotumor cerebri.[1,68] The protein concentration typically peaks within a few weeks and returns to normal after several months. The concentration of the spinal fluid protein and the clinical or EMG findings have no correlation with prognosis.

Most routine blood and urine studies are normal in patients with GBS (Table 15–4). The erythrocyte sedimentation rate and liver function study results are rarely abnormal, and abnormalities when found are most likely related to a preceding infectious illness. EBV and CMV antibody titers may be elevated and thus identify the triggering infectious agent in individual cases. Infection with *C. jejuni* can be demonstrated by finding increased serum IgM antibodies or culturing the bacteria from the stool. Approximately 25% of GBS patients have elevated anti-GM_1 antibodies, but the implications of this finding are not clear.[7,69] Anti-GQ_{1b} antibodies are found almost exclusively in patients with the Fisher variant.

DIFFERENTIAL DIAGNOSIS

GBS is easily recognized in typical cases, but unusual presentations expand the differential diagnosis to many other central nervous system and neuromuscular diseases (Table 15–5). These variant syndromes are

TABLE 15–4 ■ Evaluation of a Patient with Suspected Guillain-Barré Syndrome

LABORATORY STUDIES THAT MAY BE HELPFUL IN IDENTIFYING ANTECEDENT INFECTIOUS ILLNESS
HIV titer
Lyme titer
Campylobactor jejuni serum titer and stool culture
EBV and CMV titers
Mycoplasma pneumoniae titer

LABORATORY STUDIES THAT MAY BE HELPFUL IN EXCLUDING OTHER DISORDERS
Botulinum toxin titers and stool culture
Anti-acetylcholine receptor antibodies
Creatine kinase level
Acute and convalescent serum and spinal fluid poliovirus titers
Serum and urine heavy metal screen
Urine porphyrin screen

Anti-GM$_1$ antibody
Anti-GQ$_{1b}$ antibody (Fisher variant)

Cerebrospinal fluid protein and cell count

Electromyography

ADDITIONAL STUDIES IN SELECTED CASES
MRI of the cervical spinal cord (exclude acute transverse myelitis)
MRI of the lumbosacral spine (exclude compressive cauda equina syndrome)
Nerve biopsy

TABLE 15–5 ■ Differential Diagnosis of Guillain-Barré Syndrome

TOXIC NEUROPATHIES
Arsenic
Lead
Thallium
N-hexane (glue sniffing)
Organophosphates

OTHER ACUTE PERIPHERAL NERVE AND ROOT DISORDERS
Acute intermittent porphyria
Poliomyelitis
Diphtheria
Acute vasculitic neuropathy
Carcinomatous or lymphomatous polyradiculopathy
Cytomegalovirus-associated polyradiculopathy (with HIV infection)

NEUROMUSCULAR JUNCTION DISORDERS
Myasthenia gravis
Botulism

MUSCLE DISORDERS
Acute polymyositis
Rhabdomyolysis

METABOLIC DERANGEMENTS
Hypophosphatemia
Hypomagnesemia
Hypokalemia

encountered more frequently than are many of the rarer conditions that may simulate GBS. The initial task is to demonstrate that the condition is due to a disorder of the peripheral nerves.

There are numerous environmental, industrial (heavy metals), and occupational toxins that can cause demyelinating neuropathy resembling GBS. Thallium, arsenic, lead, N-hexane (glue-sniffers neuropathy), and organophosphate poisoning are common examples. In most cases, intoxication is manifested by gastrointestinal symptoms, and usually there is confusion, coma, seizures, alopecia (a finding specific for acute thallium intoxication), and involvement of other organ systems. Other instances include prescribed medications, and anecdotal cases of GBS have been linked to exposure to amiodarone, perhexiline, and gold therapy for rheumatoid arthritis.[1] An acute, rapidly progressive neuropathy, similar to GBS, also has been described in alcoholics.[70] These patients invariably have a long-standing history of alcohol abuse prior to onset of the acute neuropathy. Most develop progressive generalized weakness, severe distal sensory loss, and areflexia over days to weeks. The condition is differentiated from GBS by a normal CSF protein concentration and axonal features on EMG studies. Patients with acute intermittent porphyria may develop neuropathy that mimics GBS. Initial symptoms include vomiting, constipation, and abdominal pain. The weakness is symmetrical and begins in proximal muscles of the arms, but widespread weakness develops in most as the syndrome progresses. The EMG shows an axonopathy rather than demyelination, thus differentiating this condition from GBS. Increased urinary excretion of δ-aminolevulinic acid and porphobilinogen during an acute attack of acute intermittent porphyria establishes the diagnosis.

Poliomyelitis is now a rare illness except in underdeveloped countries. The condition is most commonly contracted by nonvaccinated persons after exposure to infants who recently have been vaccinated against the poliovirus. A number of other viruses, typically the enteroviruses, can produce an identical poliomyelitis syndrome simulating GBS.[71] Affected persons have a febrile illness, usually gastroenteritis, followed by a paralytic phase that develops within 2 weeks. Patients have fever, headache and neck stiffness, followed by muscle pain, asymmetrical flaccid limb paralysis, and fasciculations. Weakness progresses over days to weeks. Diaphragmatic and bulbar weakness is common, but the extraocular muscles and sensation are spared. The CSF shows a lymphocytic pleocytosis and a normal or mildly elevated protein level, in contrast to GBS. Similarly, nerve conduction studies in poliomyelitis show reduced or absent motor potentials without demyelinating features. Culture of the poliovirus from the pharynx or stool or detection of elevated antibodies directed against poliovirus with acute and convalescent sera establishes the diagnosis.

Diphtheria is also an unusual cause of acute polyneuropathy in developed countries because of effective vaccination programs. Infection with *Corynebacterium diphtheriae* produces a febrile syndrome with pharyngitis. The neurologic condition is manifested by weakness of the pharyngeal and limb muscles beginning weeks after the acute febrile illness. Cervical adenopathy and an exudate over the tonsils are present in most cases. Reflexes are absent but sensory findings are unusual, and there is no autonomic dysfunction. Progression is usually slower than with GBS, with maximal weakness occurring as long as 3 months after the onset of palatal involvement. The CSF is acellular with an elevated protein level, similar to GBS, and electrodiagnostic studies show an acute demyelinating neuropathy; accordingly, distinction from GBS can be difficult, but the low prevalence of diphtheria in developed countries makes GBS a far more common disorder.

Botulism is a rare disorder that often starts with diplopia and dysphagia and thus can be confused with certain regional variants of GBS. The illness occurs following ingestion of the neurotoxin produced by *Clostridium botulinum* types A, B, or E, usually after consumption of contaminated food. The toxin binds to the presynaptic terminal of the motor end plate and impairs the release of acetylcholine into the neuromuscular junction. The first symptoms are usually nausea and vomiting followed by constipation; the neurologic features develop hours to days later. Blurred vision is an early complaint and has been attributed to paralysis of accommodation with dilated pupils. Ptosis and oropharyngeal weakness are also common. The cranial nerve symptoms are followed by a variable degree of generalized limb and diaphragmatic weakness, leading to ventilatory failure in most cases. In contrast to GBS, the deep tendon reflexes are usually preserved. Electrodiagnostic studies show low motor amplitudes with marked increase of the amplitude (usually greater than 200% above baseline) after high-frequency repetitive nerve stimulation. This pattern confirms a presynaptic disorder of the neuromuscular junction; there are no demyelinating features distinquishing these cases from typical GBS. The CSF is normal. The detection of botulinum toxin in the serum, or culture of *C. botulinum* from the stool or contaminated food source confirms the diagnosis.

Other diseases that may simulate GBS include tick paralysis, fulminant forms of myasthenia gravis, acute vasculitic neuropathy, and central nervous system disorders such as acute occlusion of the basilar artery with brainstem stroke and cervical transverse myelitis.

PATHOGENESIS

A considerable body of evidence points to GBS as an immune disorder mediated by autoreactive T cells and humoral antibodies targeting peripheral nerve antigens.[72] The reader is referred to several excellent monographs that elucidate the pathogenesis in much greater detail.[1,72–74] An antibody response directed against an infectious agent targets certain epitopes on peripheral nerve. At the onset of disease, activated T cells disrupt the blood-nerve barrier and allow circulating antibodies access to peripheral nerve antigens. These T cells release proinflammatory cytokines (interleukin-6, interleukin-2, soluble interleukin-2 receptor, interferon-γ, tumor necrosis factor-α), which have been increased in the serum of some GBS patients.[72–75] These cytokines attract macrophages that are capable of inducing nerve demyelination and injury to Schwann cells and axons.[72–76] This complex immunologic process has been supported by observations in experimental allergic neuritis, an animal model of GBS.[76,77]

Several additional observations have indicated that humoral factors also participate in an immune attack targeted against peripheral nerve myelin: (1) pathologic studies have demonstrated deposits of immunoglobulin and complement on myelinated fibers of affected patients[78]; (2) intraneural injection of serum from patients with GBS into rat sciatic nerve has produced in vivo nerve demyelination[79]; (3) complement-fixing antiperipheral nerve antibodies have been detected in the serum of patients during the acute phase of GBS[80,81]; and (4) patients with GBS have improved following removal or neutralization of putative antibodies by plasma exchange or administration of intravenous immune globulin.[1,72,73,82–84]

Studies of typical GBS (cases of AIDP) have demonstrated endoneurial and perivascular mononuclear cell infiltration together with multifocal demyelination.[1,72–74,85,86] Inflammatory lesions may be widely distributed but are particularly prominent at the level of the spinal roots. Intense inflammation may lead to axonal degeneration as a consequence of a so-called bystander effect.[1,72–74] Ultrastructural studies have shown that macrophages strip myelin lamella from its axon, leading to demyelination.[85,86] The inflammatory infiltrates consist mainly of class II–positive monocytes, macrophages, and T lymphocytes. The expression of class II antigen is increased in Schwann cells, raising the possibility that Schwann cells present the antigen to autoreactive T cells and activate the destruction of myelin.[72,74]

In contrast, autopsy studies of early cases of AMAN have found deposition of activated complement components and immunoglobulins at nodal axolemma.[87] This was followed by disruption of the paranodal space, allowing the entry of complement and immunoglobulins along the axolemma, with subsequent recruitment of macrophages to affected nodes. Finally, macrophages have been shown to invade the periaxonal space, leading to wallerian degeneration of motor fibers.[88] These findings suggest that AMAN is caused by an antibody- and complement-mediated attack on axolemmal epitopes of motor fibers. The most attractive candidate targets are GM_1- and asialo-GM_1–like gangliosides, which are present in nodal and internodal membranes of motor fibers. Anti-GM_1 antibodies that cross-react to these lipopolysaccharide epitopes are found in a high proportion of AMAN and some GBS patients.[89,90] Axonal degeneration without significant inflammation or demyelination is the primary lesion in patients with AMSAN.[48,50]

PREVENTION

There are no methods to prevent the development of GBS.

TREATMENT

Supportive Care

Patients with mild limb weakness and no respiratory or oropharyngeal dysfunction can be managed on a ward, but most patients require close monitoring in an intensive care unit (ICU). The timely and skillful management of medical problems is as important as immune therapy in the outcome of patients with GBS (Table 15–6).

Ventilatory failure should be anticipated in any GBS patient with progressive limb or oropharyngeal weakness. Atelectasis develops early and leads to mild hypoxemia; hypercarbia is a late finding of neuromuscular, ventilatory failure. Therefore, arterial blood gases are not as sensitive as respiratory mechanics in monitoring

TABLE 15–6 ■ Guidelines for the Management of Guillain-Barré Syndrome

GENERAL SUPPORTIVE MEASURES

Admit to intensive care unit if:
  Rapidly progressive limb weakness
  Dysphagia with poor ability to handle secretions
  Cardiovascular instability (e.g., wide blood pressure and pulse fluctuations)
  Deteriorating respiratory function (vital capacity <18 ml/kg)

Routine monitoring of vital capacity and tidal volume every 4–6 h
  Intubation if vital capacity <12–15 ml/kg
  Intubation for airway protection (if bulbar paralysis present) and to minimize aspiration risk

Incentive spirometry
Chest physiotherapy
Aggressive suctioning to maintain airway
Routine chest x-ray and sputum monitoring (as indicated)

Foley catheter

Limb repositioning to minimize decubitus ulcers
Air mattress

Deep venous thrombosis and pulmonary embolism prophylaxis
  Subcutaneous heparin sulfate
  Venodyne boots

Gastrointestinal bleeding prophylaxis
Bowel regimen to avoid ileus
Nutritional support: nasogastric tube feedings or total parenteral nutrition
Monitoring of albumin, prealbumin, blood urea nitrogen, calcium levels

Adequate pain and sleep management

SPECIFIC IMMUNE MODULATING THERAPY
Intravenous immune globulin (IVIG)
400 mg/kg/day for 5 days
Plasma exchange
250 ml/kg over 4–5 sessions

diaphragmatic weakness in GBS patients. Vital capacity, tidal volume, and negative inspiratory force (NIF) are better measures of strength of the diaphragm, and progressive decline in these values indicate the need for ventilatory support. In general, intubation and mechanical ventilation are advised if the vital capacity drops below 15 ml/kg, but additional factors such as age, pre-existing lung disease, and risk of aspiration need to be considered.[1,73] Respiratory mechanics should be monitored every 4 to 6 hours initially, and if the values remain stable (vital capacity consistently above approximately 1.5 L, and negative inspiratory force > –40 cm H_2O) for several consecutive measurements, the frequency of measurement may be reduced.

Incentive spirometry is useful in the early stages of the illness to prevent atelectasis. Frequent suctioning and chest physiotherapy clear secretions and reduce the risk of aspiration. Patients with bulbar weakness who cannot protect their airway also require intubation. Persons with severe GBS who require prolonged ventilator support benefit from tracheostomy to avoid tracheal stenosis and maximize comfort.[91]

Many of the features of dysautonomia are transient and require no intervention. Hypertension usually does not require therapy unless there is sustained blood pressure elevation; angiotensin-converting enzyme inhibitors or beta-blocking agents are generally effective. Severe, labile high blood pressure can be treated with short-acting intravenous agents, such as nitroprusside or esmolol. Minor position changes may trigger postural hypotension that responds to intravenous fluids or repositioning. Vasopressors should be avoided because of the risk of rebound hypertension. Tachycardia is common in patients with GBS and does not require treatment except in those with unstable angina. Sudden bradycardia or asystole has been observed after invasive procedures or administration of cholinergic medications and has been attributed to excessive discharges from the vagus nerve (termed vagal spells).[1,92] These episodes are usually transient, but treatment with atropine or cardiac pacing may be necessary. Some patients develop urinary retention and require chronic intermittent catheterization or an indwelling catheter.

Pulmonary and urinary tract infections are common medical problems encountered in GBS patients in the intensive care unit. Routine monitoring of the chest x-ray and sputum and urine cultures may be helpful, but bacterial colonization in intubated patients is common, and patients should be treated with antibiotics only when there is clinical evidence of an infection. Sinusitis and tracheitis are other considerations in intubated patients who have a persistent fever and no apparent source of infection.

Immobilization increases the risk of deep venous thrombosis and pulmonary embolism. Subcutaneous heparin and intermittent pneumatic compression boots are routine prophylactic measures, and chronic anticoagulation with warfarin may be considered for those who remain paralyzed for long periods. Low-molecular-weight heparin has become an alternative, but its value over traditional preventive measures has not been studied in patients with GBS. Any unexplained episode of sudden hypoxia requires evaluation for pulmonary embolism.

Nasogastric tube feedings should be initiated in ventilated patients and those with dysphagia for short-term nutritional support. A gastrostomy tube can be endoscopically placed in patients with dysphagia persisting beyond a few weeks. Those with prolonged immobilization or dysautonomia often develop an ileus, and parenteral nutrition may be necessary.

Pain is a common symptom in patients with GBS and is often unrecognized by caregivers.[1,42] Narcotics are almost always required for effective pain management. Epidural analgesia is a useful alternative for patients with severe pain in the back or legs that is refractory to narcotics. Most patients benefit from early physical and occupational therapy, including range of motion exercises and frequent turning to reduce the potential for skin breakdown. Depression and anxiety are other common features in GBS patients and should be treated.

Immune Therapy

The benefits of plasma exchange have been substantiated in three randomized controlled trials.[82,93,94] In the North American study, 245 patients were randomized to receive plasma exchange (200 to 250 ml/kg over 5 sessions), or best medical care.[82] Treated patients in the exchange group regained the ability to walk after an average of 53 days compared with 85 days in controls, a statistically significant difference. Those on ventilators also could be weaned earlier (mean, 24 days) than untreated patients (mean, 48 days). Comparable benefits were confirmed by other large plasma exchange trials.[93,94] The efficacy of exchange was less impressive in patients who were treated 3 or more weeks after onset of symptoms. A recent randomized study demonstrated that two exchanges were better than no treatment in patients with mild disease, and six exchanges were no better than four in those with moderate or severe weakness.[95] Treatment-associated complications are rare and include hypotension due to rapid fluid shifts, pneumothorax and infection from central venous lines, and cardiac arrhythmias.[1,82,93–95] Plasma exchange is relatively contraindicated in patients with unstable cardiac disease or severe dysautonomia.

Intravenous immune globulin (IVIG) has been used successfully in other immune-mediated conditions and was introduced as an alternative therapy for GBS almost a decade ago.[83,96] The treatment is easy to administer and generally well tolerated. A Dutch trial of 150 GBS patients showed that IVIG is an effective therapy with benefits similar to plasma exchange.[83] The patients randomized to the plasma exchange arm of the trial, however, did not fare as well as those in prior studies (only 34% of the plasma exchange group improved one dis-

ability grade, compared to 54% of patients in the North American trial), raising concerns about the validity of the study. However, a small pilot trial from one center also indicated that the efficacy of IVIG was similar to that of plasma exchange.[97] This issue has been resolved following completion of an international randomized, controlled trial that compared IVIG (400 mg/kg/d for 5 days), plasma exchange (50 ml/kg exchanges over 8 to 13 days), and plasma exchange followed by IVIG in patients with GBS.[84] This study has confirmed that IVIG and plasma exchange provide similar benefits and that combined treatment offers no additional efficacy. Specifically, functional disability scores were similar among the treatment groups at 4 weeks and 1 year after therapy. Furthermore, the number of days to walk and duration of mechanical ventilation were also similar among the groups. Serious complications developed in approximately 5% of patients and also were evenly distributed among the various therapies.[84]

Headache is probably the most common side effect of IVIG and is usually related to the rate of the infusion. Other complications include transient fever, malaise, aseptic meningitis, renal insufficiency, and a hyperviscosity state with risk of myocardial infarction or stroke, especially in patients with risk factors for vascular disease.[96] IVIG should not be administered to patients with IgA deficiency because of a high risk of developing an anaphylactic reaction. Transmission of HIV has not been reported. Infection with hepatitis C virus has been documented, but this risk has been virtually eliminated with better purification techniques. Similar to plasma exchange, IVIG can be administered safely to pregnant patients.[98] IVIG is less cumbersome than plasma exchange and is currently the preferred therapy for GBS.[84]

Approximately 10% of treated GBS patients experience a relapse, usually worsening of limb weakness in muscles that were initially weak and had improved after therapy. The large prospective trials have shown that the frequency of relapse is similar for IVIG and plasma exchange.[83,84] The reason for relapse is not known but may be initiated by a medical complication (e.g., sepsis, pulmonary embolus) or by an increase in antibody production related to ongoing immune activation.[99] Most patients improve with a repeated course of the initial therapy.[99]

Early reports suggested that corticosteroids might be effective in GBS, but careful meta-analysis has demonstrated that corticosteroids offer no benefit to patients with GBS.[100] The efficacy of combined therapy with corticosteroids and IVIG is being tested with a randomized controlled trial.[100,101]

PROGNOSIS

Most patients with GBS have a progressive phase that reaches a nadir within 4 weeks, followed by a plateau phase of variable duration. Approximately 15% of patients have a mild condition manifested by slight limb weakness and paresthesias but do not lose the ability to walk; all recover uneventfully, with or without treatment, within weeks.[102] Conversely, the disorder is devastating in 10% to 20% of cases, in which patients develop flaccid paralysis and require ventilator assistance within days from the onset of symptoms.[103] In this group most have severe residual deficits. At the time of the maximum deficit, approximately one-third of patients require assisted ventilation and 50% are nonambulatory.

One recent study showed that at 1 year follow-up, 62% had recovered completely, 17% could not run, 9% could not walk without assistance, 4% remained ventilated, and 8% had died.[104] Poor recovery has been associated with a fulminant course, need for ventilator assistance, EMG features of low motor potential amplitudes or inexcitable nerves, and age greater than 60 years.[105,106] Most studies have demonstrated a mortality rate of 5% to 10%.[104–107]

REFERENCES

1. Ropper AH, Wijdicks EFM, Truax BT: Guillain-Barré Syndrome. Philadelphia, FA Davis, 1991.
2. Winer JB, Hughes RAC, Anderson MJ, et al: A prospective study of acute idiopathic neuropathy. II Antecedent events. J Neurol Neurosurg Psychiatry 1988;51:613–618.
3. Hadden RD, Karch H, Hartung HP, et al: Preceding infections, immune factors, and outcome in Guillain-Barré syndrome. Neurology 2001;56:758–765.
4. Jacobs B, Rothbarth P, van der Meché F: The spectrum of antecedent infections in Guillain-Barré syndrome. Neurology 1998;51:1110–1115.
5. Rees J, Soudain S, Gregson N, et al: *Campylobacter jejuni* infection and Guillain-Barré syndrome. N Engl J Med 1995;333:1374–1379.
6. Mishu B, Ilyas AA, Koski CL, et al: Serologic evidence of previous *Campylobacter jejuni* infection in patients with Guillain-Barré syndrome. Ann Intern Med 1993;118:947–953.
7. Jacobs BC, van Doorn PA, Schmitz PI, et al: *Campylobacter jejuni* infections and anti-GM1 antibodies in Guillain-Barré syndrome. Ann Neurol 1996;40:181–187.
8. Feasby TE, Hughes RAC: *Campylobacter jejuni*, anti-ganglioside antibodies, and Guillain-Barré syndrome. Neurology 1998;51:340–342.
9. McCarthy N, Giesecke J: Incidence of Guillain-Barré syndrome following infection with *Campylobacter jejuni*. Am J Epidemiol 2001;153:610–614.
10. Kuroki S, Saida T, Nukina M, et al: *Campylobacter jejuni* strains from patients with Guillain-Barré syndrome belong mostly to Penner serogroup 19 and contain beta-N-acetylglucosamine residues. Ann Neurol 1993;33:243–247.
11. Sheikh KA, Ho TW, Nachamkin I, et al: Molecular mimicry in Guillain-Barré syndrome. Ann NY Acad Sci 1998;845:307–321.
12. Ang C, Jacobs B, Bradenburg A, et al: Cross reactive antibodies against GM2 and CMV infected fibroblasts in Guillain-Barré syndrome. Neurology 2000;54:1453–1458.
13. Kaida K, Kusunoki S, Kamakura K, et al: Guillain-Barré syndrome with antibody to a ganglioside, *N*-acetylgalactosaminyl GD1a. Brain 2000;123:116–124.
14. Ang CW, Yuki N, Jacobs BC, et al: Rapidly progressive predominantly motor Guillain-Barré syndrome with anti-GalNac-GD1a antibodies. Neurology 1999;53:2122–2127.
15. Mori M, Kuwabara S, Miyake M, et al: *Haemophilus influenzae* infection and Guillain-Barré syndrome. Brain 2000;123:2171–2178.
16. Meseguer M, Aparicio M, Calvo A, et al: *Mycoplasma pneumoniae* antigen detection in Guillain-Barré syndrome. Eur J Pediatr 1998;157:1034.
17. Khouri SA: Guillain-Barré syndrome: Epidemiology of an outbreak. Am J Epidemiol 1978;107:433–438.
18. Berger JR, Ayyar DR, Kaszovitz B: Guillain-Barré syndrome complicating typhoid fever. Ann Neurol 1986;20:649–650.
19. Al Deeb SM, Yaqub BA, Sharif HS, et al: Neurobrucellosis: Clinical characteristics, diagnosis, and outcome. Neurology 1989;39:498–501.
20. Faraq SS, Gelles BD: *Yersinia* arthritis and Guillain-Barré syndrome [letter]. N Engl J Med 1982;307:755.
21. Logigian EL, Steere AC: Clinical and electrophysiologic findings in chronic neuropathy of Lyme disease. Neurology 1992;42:303–311.
22. Wulff CH, Hansen K, Strange P, et al: Multiple mononeuritis and radiculitis with erythema, pain, elevated CSF protein and pleocytosis (Bannwarth's syndrome). J Neurol Neurosurg Psychiatry 1983;46:485–490.
23. Sterman AB, Nelson S, Barclay P: Demyelinating neuropathy accompanying Lyme disease. Neurology 1982;32:1302–1305.
24. Visser LH, van der Meché FGA, Meulstee J, et al: Cytomegalovirus infection and Guillain-Barré syndrome: The clinical, electrophysiologic, and prognostic features. Dutch Guillain-Barré study group. Neurology 1996;47:668–673.
25. Kaida K, Kusunoki S, Kamakura K, et al: Guillain-Barré syndrome with IgM antibody to the ganglioside Ga1NAc-GD1a. J Neuroimmunol 2001;113:260–267.
26. Parry GJ: Peripheral neuropathies associated with human immunodeficiency virus infection. Ann Neurol 1988;23 (Suppl):549–553.
27. Cornblath DR, McArthur JC, Kennedy PGE, et al: Inflammatory demyelinating peripheral neuropathies associated with human T-cell lymphotrophic virus type III infection. Ann Neurol 1987;21:32–40.
28. Dalakas MC, Cupler EJ: Neuropathies in HIV infection. Baillieres Clin Neurol 1996;5:199–218.
29. Thornton C, Latif A, Emmanuel J: Guillain-Barré syndrome associated with human immunodeficiency virus infection in Zimbabwe. Neurology 1991;41:812–815.
30. Bosch V, Dowling P, Cook S: Hepatitis A virus immunoglobulin M antibody in acute neurological disease. Ann Neurol 1983;14:685–687.
31. Roccatagliata L, Ucceli A, Murialdo A: Guillain-Barré syndrome after reactivation of varicella zoster virus. N Engl J Med 2001;344:65–66.
32. Ahmed S, Libman R, Wesson K, et al: Guillain-Barré syndrome: An unusual presentation of West Nile virus infection. Neurology 2000;55:144–146.
33. Schonberger L, Bregman D, Sullivan-Bolyai J, et al: Guillain-Barré syndrome following vaccination in the national influenza immunization program, United States, 1976–1977. Am J Epidemiol 1979;110:105–123.
34. Wijdicks E, Fletcher D, Lawn N: Influenza vaccine and the risk of relapse of Guillain-Barré syndrome. Neurology 2000;55:452–453.
35. Lasky T, Terracciano GJ, Magder L, et al: The Guillain-Barré syndrome and the 1992–1993 and 1993–1994 influenza vaccines. N Engl J Med 1998;339:1797–1802.
36. Patja A, Paunio M, Kinnunen E, et al: Risk of Guillain-Barré syndrome after measles-mumps-rubella vaccination. J Pediatri 2001;138:250–254.
37. Stratton K, Howe C, Johnston R: Adverse effects associated with childhood vaccines other than pertussis and rubella.

Summary of report from the Institute of Medicine. JAMA 1994;271:1602–1605.

38. Gorson KC, Allam G, Ropper AH: Chronic inflammatory demyelinating polyneuropathy: Clinical features and response to treatment in 67 patients with and without a monoclonal gammopathy. Neurology 1997;48:321–328.

39. Bolton C, Laverty D, Brown J, et al: Critically ill polyneuropathy: Electrophysiological studies and differentiation from Guillain-Barré syndrome. J Neurol Neurosurg Psychiatry 1986;49:563–573.

40. Cheng Q, Jiang G, Fredrikson S, et al: Increased incidence of Guillain-Barré syndrome post-partum. Epidemiology 1998; 9:601–604.

41. Ropper AH: Unusual clinical variants and signs in Guillain-Barré syndrome. Arch Neurol 1986;43:1150–1152.

42. Moulin DE, Hagen N, Feasby TE, et al: Pain in Guillain-Barré syndrome. Neurology 1997;48:328–331.

43. Gracey DR, McMichan JC, Divertie MB, et al: Respiratory failure in Guillain-Barré syndrome. A 6-year experience. Mayo Clin Proc 1982;57:742–746.

44. Ropper AH, Kehne S: Guillain-Barré syndrome: Management of respiratory failure. Neurology 1985;35:1662–1665.

45. The Italian Guillain-Barré Study Group: The prognosis and main prognostic indicators of Guillain-Barré syndrome. A multicentre prospective study of 297 patients. Brain 1996;119:2053–2061.

46. Truax BT: Autonomic disturbances in the Guillain-Barré syndrome. Semin Neurol 1984;4:462–468.

47. Tuck RR, McLeod JG: Autonomic dysfunction in Guillain-Barré syndrome. J Neurol Neurosurg Psychiatry 1981;44:983–990.

48. Feasby TE, Gilbert JJ, Brown WF, et al: An acute axonal form of Guillain-Barré polyneuropathy. Brain 1986;109:1115–1126.

49. Feasby T, Hahn A, Brown WF, et al: Severe axonal degeneration in acute Guillain-Barré syndrome: Evidence of two different mechanisms. J Neurol Sci 1993;116:185–192.

50. Griffin J, Li C, Ho T, et al: Pathology of the motor-sensory axonal Guillain-Barré syndrome. Ann Neurol 1996;39:17–28.

51. McKann G, Cornblath D, Ho T, et al: Clinical and electrophysiological aspects of acute paralytic disease of children and young adults in northern China. Lancet 1991;338:593–597.

52. McKann GM, Cornblath DR, Griffin JW, et al: Acute motor axonal neuropathy: A frequent cause of acute flaccid paralysis in China. Ann Neurol 1993;33:333–342.

53. Hafer-Macko C, Hsieh S, Li C, et al: Acute motor axonal neuropathy: An antibody-mediated attack on axolemma. Ann Neurol 1996;40:635–644.

54. Ho TW, Li CY, Cornblath DR, et al: Patterns of recovery in the Guillain-Barré syndromes. Neurology 1997;48:695–700.

55. Fisher CM: An unusual variant of acute idiopathic polyneuritis (syndrome of ophthalmoplegia, ataxia and areflexia). N Engl J Med 1956;255:57–65.

56. ter Bruggen JP, van der Meché FGA, de Jager AEJ, et al: Ophthalmoplegic and lower cranial nerve variants merge into each other and into classical Guillain-Barré syndrome. Muscle Nerve 1998;21:239–242.

57. Ropper AH: Miller Fisher syndrome and other acute variants of Guillain-Barré syndrome. Baillieres Clin Neurol 1994;1:95–106.

58. Chiba A, Kusunoki S, Obata H, et al: Serum anti-GQ1b IgG antibody is associated with ophthalmoplegia in Miller Fisher syndrome and Guillain-Barré syndrome: Clinical and immunohistochemical studies. Neurology 1993;43:1911–1917.

59. Chiba A, Kusunoki S, Obata H, et al: Ganglioside composition of the human cranial nerves, with special reference to pathophysiology of Miller Fisher syndrome. Brain Res 1997;745:32–36.

60. Visser LH, van der Meché FGA, van Doorn PA, et al: Guillain-Barré syndrome without sensory loss (acute motor neuropathy). A subgroup with specific clinical, electrodiagnostic and laboratory features. Brain 1995;118:841–847.

61. Oh SJ, LaGanke C, Claussen GC: Sensory Guillain-Barré syndrome. Neurology 2001;56:82–86.

62. Dawson D, Samuels M, Morris J: Sensory form of acute polyneuritis. Neurology 1988;38:1728–1731.

63. Kanter M, Nori S: Sensory Guillain-Barré syndrome. Arch Phys Med Rehabil 1995;76:882–883.

64. Ropper A: Further regional variants of acute immune polyneuropathy. Bifacial weakness or sixth nerve palsies with paresthesias, lumbar polyradiculopathy, and ataxia with pharyngeal-cervical-brachial weakness. Arch Neurol 1994;51:671–675.

65. Ropper AH, Wijdicks EFM, Shahani BT: Electrodiagnostic changes in early Guillain-Barré. A prospective study in 113 patients. Arch Neurol 1990;47:881–887.

66. Albers JW, Donofrio PD, McGonagle TK: Sequential electrodiagnostic abnormalities in acute inflammatory demyelinating polyradiculoneuropathy. Muscle Nerve 1985;8:528–539.

67. Hadden RD, Cornblath DR, Hughes RAC, et al: Electrophysiological classification of Guillain-Barré syndrome: Clinical associations and outcome. Ann Neurol 1998; 44:780–788.

68. Weiss GB, Bajwa ZH, Mehler MF: Co-occurrence of pseudotumor cerebri and Guillain-Barré syndrome in an adult. Neurology 1991;41:603–604.

69. Rees JH, Gregson NA, Hughes RAC: Anti-ganglioside GM1 antibodies in Guillain-Barré syndrome and their relationship to Campylobacter jejuni infection. Ann Neurol 1995;38:809–816.

70. Wohrle JC, Spengos K, Steinke W, et al: Alcohol-related acute axonal polyneuropathy: A differential diagnosis of Guillain-Barré syndrome. Arch Neurol 1998;55:1329–1334.

71. Gorson K, Ropper A: Nonpoliovirus poliomyelitis simulating Guillain-Barré syndrome. Arch Neurol 2001;58:1460–1464.

72. Hartung HP, Pollard JD, Harvey GK, et al: Immunopathogenesis and treatment of the Guillain-Barré syndrome—Part I. Muscle Nerve 1995;18:137–153.

73. Hughes RAC: Guillain-Barré Syndrome. London, Springer-Verlag, 1990.

74. Hughes RA, Hadden RD, Gregson NA, et al: Pathogenesis of Guillain-Barré syndrome. J Neuroimmunol 1999;100:74–97.

75. Sharief MK, Ingram DA, Swash M: Circulating tumor necrosis factor-alpha correlates with electrodiagnostic abnormalities in Guillain-Barré syndrome. Ann Neurol 1997;42:68–73.

76. Zhu J, Mix E, Link H: Cytokine production and the pathogenesis of experimental autoimmune neuritis and Guillain-Barré syndrome. J Neuroimmunol 1998;84:40–52.

77. Waksman B, Adams R: Allergic neuritis: Experimental disease of rabbits induced by the injection of peripheral nervous tissue and adjuvants. J Exp Med 1955;102:213–225.

78. Hafer-Macko C, Sheikh K, Li C, et al: Immune attack on the Schwann cell surface in acute inflammatory demyelinating polyneuropathy. Ann Neurol 1996;39:625–635.

79. Brown M, Rosen J, Lisak R: Demyelination in vivo by Guillain-Barré syndrome and other human serum. Muscle Nerve 1987;10:263–271.

80. Koski CL: Characterization of complement-fixing antibodies to peripheral nerve myelin in Guillain-Barré syndrome. Ann Neurol 1990;27(Suppl):S44–S47.

81. Koski CL: Humoral mechanisms in immune neuropathies. Neurol Clin 1992;10:629–649.

82. Guillain-Barré Syndrome Study Group: Plasmapheresis and acute Guillain-Barré syndrome. Neurology 1985; 35:1096–1104.

83. van der Meché FGA, Schmitz PIM, and the Dutch Guillain-Barré Study Group: A randomized trial comparing intravenous immune globulin and plasma exchange in Guillain-Barré syndrome. N Engl J Med 1992;326:1123–1129.

84. Plasma Exchange/Sandoglobulin Guillain-Barré Syndrome Study Group: Comparison of plasma exchange, intravenous gammaglobulin, and plasma exchange followed by intravenous gammaglobulin in the treatment of Guillain-Barré syndrome. Lancet 1997;349:225–230.

85. Prineas J: Pathology of the Guillain-Barré syndrome. Ann Neurol 1981;9(Suppl):6–19.

86. Honovar M, Tharakan J, Hughes R, et al: A clinicopathological study of the Guillain-Barré syndrome. Nine cases and literature review. Brain 1991;114:1245–1269.

87. Griffin JW, Li CY, Macko C, et al: Early nodal changes in the acute motor axonal neuropathy pattern of the Guillain-Barré syndrome. J Neurocytol 1996;25:33–51.

88. Griffin JW, Li CY, Ho TW, et al: Guillain-Barré syndrome in northern China. The spectrum of neuropathological changes in clinically defined cases. Brain 1995;118:577–595.

89. Gregson N, Jones D, Thomas P, et al: Acute motor neuropathy with antibodies to GM1 ganglioside. J Neurol 1991;238:447–451.

90. Kuwabara S, Asahina M, Koga M, et al: Two patterns of clinical recovery in Guillain-Barré syndrome with IgG anti-GM1 antibody. Neurology 1998;51:1656–1660.

91. Lawn ND, Wijdicks EFM: Tracheostomy in Guillain-Barré syndrome. Muscle Nerve 1999;22:1058–1062.

92. Minahan RE, Bhardwaj A, Traill TA, et al: Stimulus-evoked sinus arrest in severe Guillain-Barré syndrome: A case report. Neurology 1996;47:1239–1242.

93. French Cooperative Group on plasma exchange in Guillain-Barré syndrome: Role of replacement fluids. Ann Neurol 1987;22:753–761.

94. Osterman PO, Lundemo G, Pirskanen R, et al: Beneficial effects of plasma exchange in acute inflammatory polyradiculoneuropathy. Lancet 1984;2:1296–1312.

95. The French Cooperative Group on Plasma Exchange in Guillain-Barré Syndrome: Appropriate number of plasma exchanges in Guillain-Barré syndrome. Ann Neurol 1997;41:298–306.

96. Dalakas MC: Intravenous immune globulin therapy for neurologic diseases. Ann Intern Med 1997;126:721–730.

97. Bril V, Allenby K, Midroni G, et al: IVIG in neurology—evidence and recommendations. Can J Neurol Sci 1999; 26:139–152.

98. Clark A: Clinical uses of intravenous immunoglobulin in pregnancy. Clin Obstet Gynecol 1999;42:368–380.

99. Kleyweg RP, van der Meché FGA: Treatment related fluctuations in Guillain-Barré syndrome after high dose immunoglobulin or plasma exchange. J Neurol Neurosurg Psychiatry 1991;54:957–960.

100. Hughes RA, van der Meché FG: Corticosteroids for treating Guillain-Barré syndrome. Cochrane Database Sys Rev 2000;2:CD001446.

101. The Dutch Guillain-Barré Study Group: Treatment of Guillain-Barré syndrome with high-dose immune globulins combined with methylprednisolone: A pilot study. Ann Neurol 1994;35:749–752.

102. Green DM, Ropper AH: Mild Guillain-Barré syndrome. Arch Neurol 2001;58:109–110.

103. Ropper AH: Severe acute Guillain-Barré syndrome. Neurology 1986;36:429–432.

104. Rees JH, Thompson RD, Smeeton NC, et al: Epidemiological study of Guillain-Barré syndrome in south east England. J Neurol Neurosurg Psychiatry 1998;64:74–77.

105. Vedeler CA, Wik E, Nyland H: The long-term prognosis of Guillain-Barré syndrome. Evaluation of prognostic factors including plasma exchange. Acta Neurol Scand 1997; 95:298–302.

106. Visser LH, Schmitz PIM, Meulstee J, et al: Prognostic factors of Guillain-Barré syndrome after intravenous immunoglobulin or plasma exchange. Neurology 1999;53:598–604.

107. Lawn ND, Widjicks EFM: Fatal Guillain-Barré syndrome. Neurology 1999;52:635–638.

Tetanus and Botulism

BARNETT NATHAN, MD

Tetanus and botulism are a result of the effects of protein neurotoxins produced by two related species of *Clostridium*. The toxins are similar in structure and function but differ dramatically in their clinical effects because they target different cells in the nervous system. Tetanus toxin affects the inhibitory cells of the central nervous system and primarily manifests as rigidity and spasm. Botulinum neurotoxins primarily affect the peripheral neuromuscular junction (NMJ) and autonomic synapses and primarily manifest as weakness. Both conditions have potentially high fatality rates, and both are preventable through education and public health measures. Tetanus remains a significant health concern in the developing world; there are between 800,000 and 1 million deaths from tetanus each year, of which 400,000 are due to neonatal tetanus.[1] By and large, most of the deaths occurred in Africa and Southeast Asia, and tetanus continues to be endemic in close to 100 countries worldwide.[2] Botulism too remains a considerable public health problem, although the absolute number of cases in the United States remains small. Since 1973 the median number of reported cases per type is infant, 71; food-borne, 24; and wound, 3.[3] The cost of care per botulism patient in Canada and the United States was estimated to be $340,000 in 1989.[4]

MICROBIOLOGY

Clostridium tetani

C. tetani is a slender, obligately anaerobic bacillus, and although it is classified as a gram-positive organism, it may stain variably, especially in tissue or older cultures.[5] Most strains are slightly motile, and they have abundant flagellae during growth. The mature organism loses its flagellae and forms a spherical terminal spore,[6] producing a profile like that of a tennis or squash racket. The spores resist extremes of temperature and moisture, are stable at atmospheric oxygen tension, can survive indefinitely, and are viable after exposure to ethanol, phenol, or formalin. Death of the spores can be accomplished by exposure to 100°C for 4 hours, autoclaving at 121°C and 103 kPa (15 psi) for 15 minutes, or by exposure to iodine, glutaraldehyde, or hydrogen peroxide. Spores can be isolated from animal feces and therefore are ubiquitous in the environment. In culture, the bacterium grows best at 37°C and will grow on a variety of media as long as oxygen is excluded. Standard anaerobic isolation techniques, such as placing the sample in an anaerobic transport system, is important in the culture of the organism. Diagnostic and therapeutic decisions should not be based on the culture, however, as cultures are frequently negative in patients with clinical tetanus, and routine bacteriologic studies do not indicate whether a strain of *C. tetani* carries the plasmid required for toxin production.

Clostridium botulinum

C. botulinum is a large, usually gram-positive, strictly anaerobic bacillus that forms a subterminal spore. The species is divided into four physiologic groups:

- Group I organisms are proteolytic in culture and can produce toxin types A, B, or F.
- Group II organisms are nonproteolytic and can produce toxin types B, E, or F.
- Group III organisms produce toxin types C or D.
- Group IV produces type G toxin.

A single strain almost always produces only one toxin type. Group II organisms grow optimally between 25°C and 30°C, whereas the other groups grow best between 30°C and 37°C. Although each strain of the organism typically contains several plasmids, only type G toxin is encoded on one.[7] *C. botulinum* spores are found worldwide and inhabit soil samples and marine sediments. These spores are able to tolerate 100°C at 1 atm for several hours, and since boiling renders solutions more anaerobic, it may actually favor the growth of *C. botulinum*.[8] Proper preparation of food in a pressure cooker (>1 atm) will kill spores.

PATHOPHYSIOLOGY

Tetanus

The spores of *C. tetani* will germinate and the bacteria proliferate when the oxygen tension of the tissue is low. Once growing, two exotoxins are produced: tetanospasmin and tetanolysin. The clinical significance of tetanolysin is not fully understood. It may aid in the damage of viable tissue near the wound site, lowering the redox potential and allowing for continued growth of anaerobes, perhaps by disrupting membrane channels.[9,10] Tetanolysin has been found to cause electrocardiographic abnormalities and disseminated intravascular coagulation when given systemically in experimental animals.[11]

Tetanospasmin, or "tetanus toxin," is felt to cause all the typical clinical manifestations of tetanus. It is synthesized as a single 151-kDa (1315 amino acid) chain.[12] This molecule is then cleaved by a bacterial protease[13] into a heavy chain and a light chain, connected by a disulfide bridge. The disulfide bridge is necessary for the activity of the toxin.[14] The DNA for this polypeptide resides on a single plasmid[15]; strains of *C. tetani* that do not have this plasmid have no toxogenic properties. Tetanospasmin inhibits neurotransmitter release at the presynaptic nerve terminal,[16] and this is what accounts for the clinical presentation of tetanus. The toxin first binds to the presynaptic membrane (as reviewed by Middlebrook[17]) and then must pass through the cell membrane and into the cytoplasm. Once in the cytoplasm of the presynaptic terminal, tetanospasmin inactivates synaptobrevin,[18] a neuronal protein that "docks" the neurotransmitter filled vesicle to the membrane. Because synaptobrevin is inactivated, the vesicle is unable to fuse with the membrane, and neurotransmitter cannot be released.

Tetanospasmin travels via retrograde transport back to the cell body and can then cross several orders of synaptically connected neurons. This process allows the toxin to move from the NMJ of alpha motor neurons, to the spinal cord, and ultimately to the brain. This may explain its effects on the NMJ, autonomic function, and the central nervous system. Tetanospasmin also is hematogenously spread but ultimately must still enter the nervous system via neurons and retrograde transport. Any toxin that has not entered a neuron (i.e., in the blood or the intracellular space) is potentially accessible to antitoxin antibody; however, toxin that is intraneuronal or intra-axonal is not. This may be the explanation for the delay in improvement for several days after initiation of treatment.

Once transported to the spinal cord, tetanospasmin primarily affects the inhibitory neurons. These inhibitory neurons use either glycine or gamma-aminobutyric acid (GABA) as neurotransmitters. Without these neurons the motor neuron increases its firing rate, ultimately causing rigidity of the muscle innervated by this neuron. More clinically relevant is the fact that without this inhibition the normal inhibition of antagonist muscles is impaired, and in response to movement or stimulation the characteristic tetanic spasm occurs.

Tetanospasmin decreases the inhibition of sympathetic reflexes at the spinal cord level, implying hyperadrenergic findings do not depend on the hypothalamus or brainstem. The development of the syndrome of inappropriate antidiuretic hormone secretion, however, may support hypothalamic involvement.[19] Patients with tetanus occasionally develop bradycardia, hypotension,[20] and disruptions in gastric motility, raising the likelihood that parasympathetic function is also disrupted.

Recent studies on the effect of tetanospasmin on the NMJ show a presynaptic defect in the release of acetylcholine (similar to botulism) as demonstrated by single fiber electromyography.[21] The NMJ may be permanently poisoned by tetanospasmin, and return of muscle fiber function is dependent on sprouting of new synapses at the NMJ. Muscular weakness may be seen at times in tetanus, and the effect of tetanospasmin on the NMJ is likely the reason.

Botulism

Botulinum toxin is synthesized as a single polypeptide chain of low potency. It is then nicked by a bacterial protease to produce two chains, with the light chain constituting approximately one-third of the total mass. As with tetanospasmin, the chains remain connected by a disulfide bond and are zinc-dependent metalloproteinases.[22] The nicked toxin type A is on a molecular weight basis, the most potent toxin found in nature. In contrast to the spores, the toxin is destroyed by high temperatures. The different toxin types may undergo different postsynthetic processing.[23]

Once present at the synapse, the toxin ultimately prevents the release of acetylcholine. The toxin enters the cell by receptor-mediated endocytosis.[24] Once inside the neuron, the toxin types differ in the mechanisms by which they inhibit acetylcholine vesicle release.[25] Tetanospasmin, along with botulinum neurotoxins B, D, F, and G, cleaves synaptobrevin.[18] Tetanospasmin and botulinum neurotoxin B also appear to share the same cleavage site on synaptobrevin.[26] The result is that stimulation of the presynaptic cell (e.g., the alpha motor neuron) fails to produce transmitter release, thus producing paralysis in the motor system, or autonomic dysfunction when parasympathetic nerve terminals or autonomic ganglia are involved. The toxins only affect the free proteins; once vesicular and synaptic proteins have formed a complex to cause transmitter release, they are not subject to attack.

Once damaged, the synapse is apparently permanently affected. The recovery of function requires sprouting of the presynaptic axon and the subsequent formation of a new synapse. Botulinum toxin is also transported within nerves in a manner analogous to that of tetanospasmin and thereby can gain access to the central nervous system. However, although symptomatic central nervous system involvement is reported, it is rare.[27]

In food-borne botulism, toxin is ingested with the food in which it was produced. It is absorbed primarily in the duodenum and jejunum and passes into the bloodstream, by which it reaches peripheral cholinergic synapses (including the NMJ). In cases of wound botulism, spores are introduced into a wound, where they germinate and produce toxin. Infant botulism and probably adult botulism of unknown cause follow ingestion of spores. Gastric acid–lowering agents and antibiotic use may predispose to gastrointestinal colonization with *C. botulinum*. The clinical manifestations of botulism depend on the type of toxin produced, not on the site of its production.

CLINICAL MANIFESTATIONS

Tetanus

Tetanus is classified into four clinical types: generalized, localized, cephalic, and neonatal. These four clinical subtypes represent the site of toxin action; either predominantly at the NMJ or the inhibitory neurons in the central nervous system. Incubation time (the time from spore inoculation to first symptoms) for all clinical types depends on severity and distance of injury or inoculum

site to the central nervous system, with more severe disease developing more quickly (8.3 ± 4.7 days) and mild disease taking longer (11 ± 6.7 days).[28]

Generalized Tetanus

Generalized tetanus is the most commonly recognized form of the disease with trismus, or lockjaw, the most common presenting sign. Trismus is caused by rigidity of the masseter muscles, which prevents the opening of the mouth. The more severe it is, the smaller the opening between the upper and lower jaw. Trismus results in a facial expression called risus sardonicus, which consists of lateral extension of the corners of the mouth, raised eyelids, and wrinkling of the forehead. These facial features may at times be subtle. Involvement of other muscle groups can then follow the onset of trismus; first the neck, then the thorax and abdomen, and finally the extremities. Tetanospasms, or generalized spasms that superficially resemble opisthotonus, decerebrate posturing, or seizures, are elicited by external or internal stimuli or both. Since full consciousness is retained, the spasms are extremely painful. This maintenance of consciousness helps to differentiate them from seizures or decerebrate posturing. Respiratory compromise, due to spasm of the glottis, diaphragm, or abdominal muscles, is the most serious early problem in generalized tetanus. Later in the illness, defects in autonomic dysfunction, usually as manifested by increased sympathetic tone, are frequently noted in patients with severe tetanus. Autonomic dysfunction is now the chief cause of death in tetanus patients.[29] It is characterized by labile hypertension (and sometimes hypotension) and tachycardia, arrhythmias, peripheral vascular constriction, diaphoresis, pyrexia, increased carbon dioxide output, and increased urinary catecholamine excretion.

The progression of the disease may last for 10 to 14 days This reflects the time it takes for the toxin to be transported to the central nervous system. Recovery may take 4 weeks or more. Without antitoxin the disease persists for as long as the toxin is produced, and because toxin is produced in insufficient quantities to stimulate an immune response, recurrent tetanus is documented.[30,31]

Neonatal Tetanus

Neonatal tetanus is a generalized form of the disease and is far more common in underdeveloped countries than in the developed world. It is the leading cause of neonatal mortality in many parts of the world, and of the diseases that can be vaccinated against, it is second only to measles as a cause of childhood death.[32] It usually follows an infection of the umbilical stump, often because of improper wound care. A lack of maternal immunity to tetanus is also necessary for the development of this disease. The incubation period is anywhere from 1 to 10 days postpartum. The infants usually present with weakness, irritability, and inability to suck. Tetanic spasms occur later, and the opisthotonic posturing can be confused with neonatal seizures or other metabolic or congenital abnormalities that cause posturing in this age group. The hypersympathetic state described above is also common and is frequently the cause of death. The mortality is up to 90%, and developmental retardation is common in those that survive.[33]

Localized and Cephalic Tetanus

Localized and cephalic tetanus is characterized by fixed rigidity of the muscles at or near the site of injury. This may be mild or painful and may persist for months, sometimes resolving spontaneously. Partial immunity to the toxin may be the mechanism responsible for preventing further spread and generalized tetanus[34]; however, unless treated, localized tetanus can evolve into the generalized form. The cephalic form is an unusual type of localized tetanus and occurs with injuries to the head or at times is associated with *C. tetani* infections of the middle ear.[35] Patients on presentation have weakness of the facial musculature, dysphagia,[36] and extraocular muscle[37] involvement. Both cephalic and localized forms of tetanus can spread to become the generalized form.

Botulism

The classic presentation of botulism is that of a patient who develops acute, bilateral cranial neuropathies associated with symmetrical descending weakness.

Food-Borne Botulism

Food-borne botulism usually develops between 12 and 36 hours after toxin ingestion. The patient initially complains of nausea and a dry mouth and at times diarrhea. Cranial nerve dysfunction most commonly starts with the eyes, including blurred vision due to pupillary dilation (reflecting parasympathetic dysfunction) or diplopia (reflecting dysfunction of nerves III, IV, or VI.[38] Pupils are either dilated or unreactive in less than 50% of patients. The absence of these signs in no way diminishes the likelihood of botulism. Lower cranial nerve dysfunction manifests as dysphagia, dysarthria, and hypoglossal weakness. Weakness then spreads to the upper extremities, the trunk, and the lower extremities. Respiratory dysfunction and failure may result from either upper airway obstruction from a weakened glottis or diaphragmatic weakness. Autonomic problems may include gastrointestinal dysfunction, alterations in resting heart rate, loss of responsiveness to hypotension or postural change, hypothermia, or urinary retention,[39] although these are not usually as common or severe as that seen in tetanus. Recovery may not begin for up to 100 days.[40]

Infantile Botulism

Infantile botulism presents with constipation, which may be followed by feeding difficulties, hypotonia, increased drooling, and a weak cry.[41] Upper airway obstruction may be the initial sign[42] and is the major indication for intubation.[43] In severe cases the condition progresses to include cranial neuropathies and respiratory weakness, with ventilatory failure occurring in about 50% of diagnosed patients. The condition progresses for 1 to 2 weeks and then stabilizes for another 2 to 3 weeks before recovery starts.

Wound Botulism

Wound botulism lacks the prodromal gastrointestinal disorder of the food-borne form but is otherwise similar in presentation. Fever, if present, reflects wound infection rather than botulism. Rarely the wound itself appears to be healing well while neurologic manifestations are occurring. The incubation period varies from 4 to 14 days.

DIAGNOSIS

Tetanus

The diagnosis of tetanus is primarily clinical. A clinical picture of trismus, muscle rigidity, stimulus-induced tetany, and a history of a wound or injury within the last 3 weeks is highly suggestive of generalized tetanus. Likewise a newborn with a poor suck and increased muscle rigidity and spasms, in the setting of poor umbilical hygiene and a mother with no immunization history, likely has neonatal tetanus. An electromyogram may demonstrate findings consistent with increased excitability of the motor neurons and NMJ blockade, although this is not specific for tetanus. *C. tetani* rarely is cultured from the wound, and in any case a positive culture does not prove the presence of the disease, nor does a negative culture disprove it. Blood and serum studies are usually normal or nonspecific, and cerebrospinal fluid is usually normal. For the most part, laboratory studies help evaluate for other entities in the differential diagnosis.

Botulism

As with tetanus a history appropriate to the type of botulism suspected is the most important diagnostic test. If other people are already affected who have ingested the contaminated food source, the condition is easily recognized. However, since the toxin may not be evenly distributed in food, the absence of other patients does not eliminate the diagnosis.

Laboratory evaluation includes anaerobic cultures and toxin assays of serum, stool, and the implicated food if available. Confirmation and toxin typing is obtained in almost 75% of cases.[44] Early cases are more likely to be diagnosed by the toxin assay, whereas those studied later in the disease are more likely to have a positive culture than a positive toxin assay.[45] Specimens should be obtained and sent for consultation with the appropriate officials (in the United States, the Centers for Disease Control and Prevention [CDC]). Toxin excretion may continue up to 1 month after the onset of illness, and stool cultures may remain positive for a similar period.

Electrophysiologic studies reveal normal nerve conduction velocities; the amplitude of compound muscle action potentials is reduced in 85% of cases, although not all motor units may demonstrate this abnormality.[46] Repetitive nerve stimulation at high rates (20 Hz or greater, compared with the 4 Hz rate used in the diagnosis of myasthenia gravis) may reveal a small increment in the motor response. This test is uncomfortable and should not be requested unless botulism or the Lambert-Eaton myasthenic syndrome are serious considerations. In infant botulism the increments may be dramatic; however, there is currently some debate regarding the sensitivity of electrodiagnostic techniques in cases of infant botulism.[47]

TREATMENT

Tetanus

A patient with generalized tetanus or neonatal tetanus will require the facilities and the expertise of an intensive care unit (ICU) to survive. A review of 335 consecutive tetanus patients revealed that survival drastically improved after the development of ICUs (44% mortality vs. 15%) and that the major improvement came from the prevention of death from respiratory failure.[48] The mainstays of treatment include the following:

1. Neutralization of existing toxin before it enters the nervous system
2. Inhibition of further production of tetanus toxin
3. Muscle relaxation and sedation
4. Management of autonomic instability
5. Ventilatory, nutritional, and general ICU support

Treatment of generalized tetanus should begin with administration of human tetanus immunoglobulin (HTIG). Blake et al[49] have demonstrated that a single dose of 500 IU is as effective as the standard 3000- to 5000-IU dose. This smaller amount can be given as a single dose; this is important as each intramuscular injection is a potential stimulus for a tetanic spasm. Equine antitetanus serum may be more readily available, particularly in underdeveloped regions; however, it is associated with a much higher incidence of adverse reactions such as anaphylaxis and serum sickness. It is dosed at 10,000 to 100,000 units intramuscularly. Once the tetanus toxin has entered the motor neuron, it can no longer be neutralized with the antibody. Therefore intrathecal administration of HTIG has been attempted. Intrathecal administration of HTIG is not approved by the United States Food and Drug Administration. Some report that it may be advantageous[50,51]; however, a meta-analysis failed to demonstrate a benefit.[52] Corticosteroids may be of some benefit in the treatment of tetanus, although studies demonstrating their efficacy have been small or not adequately controlled.[53–55] Because of the uncertain role of an anti-inflammatory agent in tetanus, corticosteroids are not currently recommended. Débriding the portal of entry does not change the course of the disease, although it may help prevent secondary infection.

Antibiotic treatment should be initiated at the outset, although it likely plays a minor role in the treatment of the disease. In the only study comparing metronidazole and penicillin, metronidazole was superior, with significantly less progression of the disease, shorter hospitalization, and improved survival.[56] Penicillin, although more readily available than metronidazole, has a potential for more adverse effects, as it is a competitive antagonist of GABA and in high enough doses can cause central nervous system hyperexcitability. Metronidazole 500 mg IV is given every 6 hours for 7 to 10 days. Muscle relaxation is best accomplished with benzodiazapines or baclofen. Diazepam, lorazepam, and midazolam are all effective. With all three agents, large doses are required to control spasms; doses in excess of 500 mg/24 h of diazepam, 200 mg/24 h of lorazepam, and 0.1–0.3 mg/kg/h of midazolam may be required. Other drugs such as phenothiazines (e.g., chlorpromazine), phenobarbital, and morphine have also been used for their sedative effects. Intrathecal administration of baclofen has also proven to be effective[57,58] but may have a more limited role because intrathecal administration is more difficult than intravenous administration and has the potential for epidural complications. Magnesium sulfate has been used both in ventilated patients to reduce autonomic disturbance and in nonventilated patients to control spasms.[59–62]

Magnesium has a variety of physiologic effects: it is a presynaptic neuromuscular blocker; it blocks catecholamine release from nerves and the adrenal medulla; it reduces receptor responsiveness to released catecholamines and is an anticonvulsant and vasodilator. It is difficult to maintain constant serum concentrations of magnesium, making its dosing complicated; however, infusion rates of magnesium sulfate sufficient to maintain serum concentrations of 3 to 4 mmol/L may be adequate if it is used as an adjunct therapy.[63] Ventilatory support must be available when administering such high doses of magnesium sulfate. If GABA receptor agonists, such as benzodiazapines or baclofen, are unsuccessful in controlling the muscle spasms, neuromuscular blockade is necessary. Vecuronium (6 to 8 mg/h) or pancuronium bromide (bolus of 0.1 mg/kg, then infusion of 0.3 to 0.6 μg/kg/min) can be used. Vecuronium is preferred, as it is less likely to cause autonomic instability. A recent case report demonstrated the ineffectiveness of rocuronium in controlling tetany and spasms.[64] Of course, once paralytic agents are used, the patient must be intubated and mechanically ventilated. It is likely, however, that the patient will have been intubated before the administration of paralytic agents; this is done both to protect the airway and to provide ventilatory support.

Control of autonomic instability can be achieved with a variety of agents. Intravenous labetalol, a combined alpha- and beta-blocker is the treatment of choice. Esmolol, clonidine,[65] and morphine sulfate have also been shown to be effective. A recent retrospective report demonstrated the efficacy of epidural infusion of bupivacaine and sufentanil for control of blood pressure swings[66]; however, complications, such as an epidural abscess, were noted. For bradycardia a temporary pacemaker may be necessary, and for hypotension, fluid boluses and sympathomimetics (e.g., dopamine) may be necessary. The nutritional requirements of tetanus patients may be extraordinary until they have been sedated appropriately. Then their nutritional requirements are similar to those of other critically ill patients. Gastric emptying may be impaired; therefore central venous nutrition may be necessary.

There is no agreed upon specific regimen for the treatment of neonatal tetanus; however, it is treated much like the generalized variety is. Tetanus antitoxin should be administered to neutralize the tetanospasmin that has not yet entered neurons. A single intramuscular injection of 500 U of HTIG is sufficient to neutralize systemic tetanus toxin, but doses as high as 3000 to 6000 U are also recommended. Infiltration of HTIG into the wound is now considered unnecessary. If HTIG is unavailable, human intravenous immune globulin (IVIG), which contains 4 to 90 U/ml of TIG, or equine- or bovine-derived tetanus antitoxin may be necessary. The optimal dosage of IVIG, however, is not known, and it is not approved for this usage.[67] Equine antitoxin is more widely used because of its availability; however, serum sickness or allergic reactions are, of course, a significant concern. A single dose of 5000 U of equine antiserum is appropriate. A recent study in neonatal tetanus failed to show any advantage for intrathecal administration of antitoxin.[68] Although débridement of the wound or the removal of the infected umbilical stump may be surgically indicated, there is no evidence that this helps prevent the progression of the disease. Eradication of the organism can be accomplished with penicillin (100,000 U/kg daily), although penicillin, being a GABA antagonist, can theoretically act synergistically with tetanospasmin and worsen spasms. Metronidazole may be a better choice. In patients with generalized tetanus (no distinction between neonatal or generalized tetanus cases), those treated with metronidazole (500 mg PO every 6 hours or 1 g PR every 8 hours) fared better than those treated with penicillin.[56] Sedation and muscle relaxation of the neonate can be accomplished with a variety of agents including the following:

- Acute control of spasms: paraldehyde 0.3 ml/kg IM or diazepam 1 to 2 mg/kg IM or IV
- Chronic sedation: phenobarbital 5 mg/kg every 6 hours, chlorpromazine 2 mg/kg every 6 hours, or diazepam 1 to 2 mg/kg every 6 hours

Long-term ICU support must also be maintained as described above for generalized tetanus. Pyridoxine (vitamin B_6) is a coenzyme in the synthesis of GABA. In a controlled trial of 31 children, pyridoxine 100 mg IM or IV on day 1 was followed by 25 mg PO on the next days. The pyridoxine group had significantly better outcomes than the control group had.[69] Others have not demonstrated the usefulness of pyridoxine.[70]

Botulism

In contrast to tetanus, the autonomic dysfunction of botulism is rarely life-threatening, and patients who receive appropriate airway and ventilator management should recover unless there are other complications. Survival rates in patients with botulism have improved as critical care medicine has improved, particularly in the arena of ventilatory support. The decision to intubate is similar to that for most cases of neuromuscular respiratory failure (e.g., Guillain-Barré, myasthenia gravis) and should be based on (1) assessment of upper airway competence, (2) a vital capacity, in general, below 12 ml/kg, or (3) a rapidly declining vital capacity. Do not wait for the P_{CO_2} to rise or the oxygen saturation to fall before intubating the patient.

If contaminated food may still reside in the gastrointestinal tract, purgatives may be useful unless ileus has occurred, in which case gastric lavage may prove valuable.

Antitoxin therapy is usually carried out with a trivalent (types A, B, and E) equine serum; in the United States it is obtained from state health departments or the CDC. Its use is supported by inferential studies; controlled clinical trials are lacking. Reported hypersensitivity rates are about 9%.[71] Skin testing is performed before the antitoxin is administered; a regimen for desensitization is included in the package insert. The standard antitoxin dose is one vial intravenously and one vial intramuscularly; although the package insert recommends repeating the dose in 4 hours in severe or progressive cases, this is not necessary.[71] Human botulinum immune globulin may be available in California for clinical trials in infant botulism.[71] In contrast to tetanus, patients with wound botulism should also undergo débridement, and anaerobic cultures should be obtained at the time of surgery. The value of local instillation of antitoxin is unknown. The role of antibiotic treatment is untested, but penicillin G, 10 to 20 MU daily, is frequently recommended. Metronidazole may be an effective alternative. The use of local antibiotics, such as penicillin G or metronidazole, may be helpful in eradicating *C. botulinum* in wound botulism. Antibiotic use, however, is not recommended for infant botulism because cell death and lysis may result in the release of more toxin. Aminoglycoside antibiotics and tetracyclines in particular may increase the degree of neuromuscular blockade by impairing neuronal calcium entry. This effect has not been reported in adult cases but should be considered when gastrointestinal infection is considered. Drugs that may improve acetylcholine release at the NMJ, such as guanidine,[72,73] have been tried in botulism without tremendous success. Other drugs, such as 3,4-diaminopyridine, have been of limited usefulness.[74]

Although the greatest improvement in muscle strength occurs in the first 3 months of recovery from botulism, patients still show improvements in strength and endurance for up to 1 year after disease onset.[75] Recovery from botulism may also be followed by persistent psychological dysfunction, which may require mental health intervention.[76]

PREVENTION

Tetanus

Active immunization with tetanus toxoid is one of the most effective preventive measures in medicine. Preventing one case of tetanus saves enough health care expense to immunize several thousand people.[77] Active immunization with three intramuscular injections of alum-adsorbed tetanus toxoid (10 lyophilized units, 0.5 ml) provides almost complete immunity for 5 years. Routine immunization in the infant begins at 6 weeks to 2 months of age, with two other immunizations at 1- or 2-month intervals. A fourth vaccination should be given 1 year after the third, and a fifth at 4 to 6 years of age. Children under 7 years of age should receive the combined diphtheria-tetanus-pertussis (DTP) vaccine, and in those over 7 the tetanus-diphtheria vaccine is recommended. The pertussis component of the vaccine can be given in acellular rather than cellular form with fewer side effects and better efficacy in preventing pertussis. The complete series must be given to ensure adequate antibody titers. Routine boosters should be administered every 10 years.

In the developing world neonatal tetanus remains a significant problem because large numbers of women of child-bearing age are not immunized. To improve compliance and lower costs a single dose of tetanus toxoid was administered to unimmunized pregnant women in their third trimester; the study demonstrated that both the mothers and their babies developed protective antibody titers.[78]

In human immunodeficiency virus (HIV)-infected adults and infants, protective tetanus antibody titers can develop.[79,80]

Immunization after an injury that is tetanus prone (contaminated wounds, punctures, burns, frostbite, avulsions, and crush injuries) should be performed if no tetanus booster has been given within the last 5 years, and any injured patient should be boosted with the adsorbed tetanus-diphtheria (Td) vaccine if none has been administered within the last 10 years. If prior immunization history is unavailable or unclear, a series of three monthly Td injections should be administered. HTIG should also be administered (250 to 500 U) in a patient with no clear previous vaccination history, particularly if the wound is at high risk to develop tetanus. Both HTIG and tetanus toxoid can be given simultaneously as long as different injection sites are used.

On the horizon are other methods of immunization, most notabley the ability to dose the immunization by other routes. Sustained release, orally dosed tetanus toxoid,[81] oral immunization with a genetically engineered live mutant *Salmonella typhi* strain to carry a fragment of the tetanospasmin gene (fragment C),[82] and nasal administration of liposome-incorporated tetanus toxoid may also be possible.[83]

Botulism

The most important aspect of botulism prevention is proper food handling and preparation. It is impractical or undesirable to treat all foods in a manner to eliminate *C. botulinum* spores. Methods for the control of botulism focus on the inhibition of bacterial growth and toxin production.[71] Since the toxin is heat labile, boiling or similarly intense heating of food will inactivate it. Food containers that appear to bulge may contain gas produced by *C. botulinum* and should not be opened.

In contrast to tetanus, immunization for botulism is not practical. Humans can be vaccinated with the use of the toxoids corresponding to each of the serologic types of the neurotoxin, but the disease is so rare that vaccination is typically not done. Technicians and researchers working with the toxin can be vaccinated with a pentavalent toxoid available through the CDC Drug Service Office.[71] Immunity to botulinum toxin does not develop even with severe disease, and its repeated occurrence has been reported.[84]

CONCLUSIONS

Tetanus and botulism are manifestations of toxins expressed by two different species in the genus *Clostridium*. The toxins have significant similarities; however, their ultimate site of action and the clinical consequences of each are quite different. Tetanus toxin primarily affects the inhibitory neurons in the central nervous system, causing a potentially fatal increase in muscle tone and muscle spasms. Botulinum toxin's target is the NMJ, which when inhibited manifests as profound muscle weakness. Both can ultimately lead to respiratory failure, and critical care management is essential in their treatment. Tetanus responds well to treatment with immunoglobulin antitoxin, but the usefulness of antibotulinum in botulism is not well documented. Both are preventable diseases, with immunization for tetanus the keystone in the control of the disease, and improved food handling is the key to preventing botulism. Much work remains in the attempt to reduce fatalities and to eradicate tetanus worldwide. Botulinum toxin on the other hand has become a mainstay therapeutic agent in the treatment of dystonia and other muscle spasms.[85]

REFERENCES

1. Dietz V, Milstien JB, van Loon F, et al: Performance and potency of tetanus toxoid: Implications for eliminating neonatal tetanus. Bull World Health Organ 1996;74:619–628.
2. Whitman C, Belgharbi L, Gasse F, et al: Progress towards the global elimination of neonatal tetanus. World Health Stat Q 1992;45(2–3):248–256.
3. Shapiro RL, Hatheway C, Swerdlow DL: Botulism in the United States: A clinical and epidemiologic review. Ann Intern Med 1998;129:221–228.
4. Todd EC: Costs of acute bacterial foodborne disease in Canada and the United States. Int J Food Microbiol 1989;9(4):313–326.
5. Hatheway CL: Bacterial sources of clostridial neurotoxins. In Simpson LL (ed): Botulinum Neurotoxin and Tetanus Toxin. San Diego, Academic Press, 1989, pp 4–24.
6. Hoeniger JF, Tauschel HD: Sequence of structural changes in cultures of *Clostridium tetani* grown on a solid medium. J Med Microbiol 1974;7:425–432.
7. Eklund MW, Poysky FT, Habig WH: Bacteriophages and plasmids in *Clostridium botulinum* and *Clostridium tetani* and their relationship to the production of toxin. In Simpson LL (ed): Botulinum Neurotoxin and Tetanus Toxin. San Diego, Academic Press, 1989, pp 25–51.
8. Tacket CO, Rogawski MA: Botulism. In Simpson LL (ed): Botulinum Neurotoxin and Tetanus Toxin. San Diego, Academic Press, 1989, pp 351–378.
9. Rottem S, Groover K, Habig WH, et al: Transmembrane diffusion channels in *Mycoplasma gallisepticum* induced by tetanolysin. Infect Immun 1990;58:598–602.
10. Blumenthal R, Habig WH: Mechanism of tetanolysin-induced membrane damage: Studies with black lipid membranes. J Bacteriol 1984;157(1):321–323.
11. Hardegree MC, Palmer AE, Duffin N: Tetanolysin: In-vivo effects in animals. J Infect Dis 1971;123:51–60.
12. Matsuda M: The structure of tetanus toxin. In Simpson LL (ed): Botulinum Neurotoxin and Tetanus Toxin. San Diego, Academic Press, 1989, pp 69–92.
13. Bergey GK, Habig WH, Bennett JI, Lin CS: Proteolytic cleavage of tetanus toxin increases activity. J Neurochem, 1989;53:155–161.
14. Krieglstein K, Henschen A, Weller U, Habermann E: Arrangement of disulfide bridges and positions of sulfhydryl groups in tetanus toxin. Eur J Biochem 1990;188:39–45.
15. Eisel U, Jarausch W, Goretzki K, et al: Tetanus toxin: Primary structure, expression in E. coli, and homology with botulinum toxins. EMBO J 1986;5:2495–2502.
16. Bleck TP: Pharmacology of tetanus. Clin Neuropharmacol 1986;9(2):103–120.
17. Middlebrook JL: Cell surface receptors for protein toxins. In Simpson LL (ed): Botulinum neurotoxin and tetanus toxin. San Diego, Academic Press, 1989, pp 95–119.
18. Schiavo G, Benfenati F, Poulain B, et al: Tetanus and botulinum-B neurotoxins block neurotransmitter release by proteolytic cleavage of synaptobrevin. Nature 1992;359:832–835.
19. Potgieter PD: Inappropriate ADH secretion in tetanus. Crit Care Med 1983;11:417–418.
20. Ambache N, Lippold OCH: Bradycardia of central origin produced by injections of tetanus toxin into the vagus nerve. J Physiol (Lond) 1949;108:186–196.
21. Fernandez JM, Ferrandiz M, Lorrea L, et al: Cephalic tetanus studied with single fibre EMG. J Neurol Neurosurg Psychiatry 1983;46:862–866.

22. Fu FN, Lomneth RB, Cai S, Singh BR: Role of zinc in the structure and toxic activity of botulinum neurotoxin. Biochemistry 1998;37:5267–5278.
23. Critchley EM, Mitchell JD: Human botulism. Br J Hosp Med 1990;43(4):290–292.
24. Black JD, Dolly JO: Interaction of ^{125}I-labeled botulinum neurotoxins with nerve terminals. II. Autoradiographic evidence for its uptake into motor nerves by acceptor-mediated endocytosis. J Cell Biol 1986;103:535–544.
25. Simpson LL: Peripheral actions of the botulinum toxins. In Simpson LL (ed): Botulinum Neurotoxin and Tetanus Toxin. San Diego, Academic Press, 1989, pp 153–178.
26. Foran P, Shone CC, Dolly JO: Differences in the protease activities of tetanus and botulinum B toxins revealed by the cleavage of vesicle-associated membrane protein and various sized fragments. Biochemistry 1994;33:15365–15374.
27. Jones S, Huma Z, Haugh C, et al: Central nervous system involvement in infantile botulism. Lancet 1990;335:228.
28. Vieira SRR, Brauner JS: Tetanus: Following up 176 patients in the ICU. In VI World Congress on Intensive and Critical Care Medicine, 1993, Madrid.
29. Luisto M, Iivanainen M: Tetanus of immunized children. Dev Med Child Neurol, 1993;35:351–355.
30. Spenney JG, Lamb RN, Cobbs CG: Recurrent tetanus. South Med J 1971;64:859 passim.
31. Kimura F, Sasaki N, Uehara H: Long-term recurrent infection of tetanus in an elderly patient. Am J Emerg Med 2001;19:168.
32. Progress towards the global elimination of neonatal tetanus, 1989–1993. MMWR Morb Mortal Wkly Rep 1994;43:885–887.
33. Anlar B, Yalaz K, Dizmen R: Long-term prognosis after neonatal tetanus. Dev Med Child Neurol, 1989;31:76–80.
34. Risk WS, et al: Chronic tetanus: Clinical report and histochemistry of muscle. Muscle Nerve, 1981;4:363–366.
35. Patel JC, Kale PA, Mehta BC: Otogenic tetanus: Study of 922 cases. In Patel JC (ed): Proceedings of an International Conference on Tetanus. Bombay, 1965, pp 640–644.
36. Lathrop DL, Griebel M, Horner J: Dysphagia in tetanus: Evaluation and outcome. Dysphagia 1989;4:173–175.
37. Saltissi S, Hakin RN, Pearce J: Ophthalmoplegic tetanus. BMJ, 1976;1:437.
38. Terranova W, Palumbo JN, Breman JG: Ocular findings in botulism type B. JAMA 1979;241:475–477.
39. Vita G, Girlanda P, Puglisi RM, et al: Cardiovascular-reflex testing and single-fiber electromyography in botulism. A longitudinal study. Arch Neurol 1987;44:202–206.
40. Colebatch JG, Wolff AH, Gilbert RJ, et al: Slow recovery from severe foodborne botulism. Lancet, 1989;2:1216–1217.
41. Cornblath DR, Sladky JT, Sumner AJ: Clinical electrophysiology of infantile botulism. Muscle Nerve 1983;6:448–452.
42. Oken A, Barnes S, Rock P, Maxwell L: Upper airway obstruction and infant botulism. Anesth Analg 1992;75:136–138.
43. Schreiner MS, Field E, Ruddy R: Infant botulism: A review of 12 years' experience at the Children's Hospital of Philadelphia. Pediatrics 1991;87:159–165.
44. Dowell VR Jr, McCroskey LM, Hatheway CL, et al: Coproexamination for botulinal toxin and *Clostridium* botulinum. A new procedure for laboratory diagnosis of botulism. JAMA 1977;238:1829–1832.
45. Woodruff BA, Griffin PM, McCroskey LM, et al: Clinical and laboratory comparison of botulism from toxin types A, B, and E in the United States, 1975–1988. J Infect Dis 1992; 166:1281–1286.
46. Cherington M: Electrophysiologic methods as an aid in diagnosis of botulism: A review. Muscle Nerve 1982; 5(9S):S28–S29.
47. Graf WD, Hays RM, Astley SJ, Mendelman PM: Electrodiagnosis reliability in the diagnosis of infant botulism. J Pediatr 1992;120:747–749.

48. Trujillo MH, Castillo A, Espana J, et al: Impact of intensive care management on the prognosis of tetanus. Analysis of 641 cases. Chest 1987;92:63–65.

49. Blake PA, Feldman RA, Buchanan TM, et al: Serologic therapy of tetanus in the United States, 1965–1971. JAMA 1976;235:42–44.

50. Sun KO, Chan YW, Cheung RT, et al: Management of tetanus: A review of 18 cases [see comments]. J R Soc Med 1994;87:135–137.

51. Agarwal M, Thomas K, Peter JV, et al: A randomized double-blind sham-controlled study of intrathecal human anti-tetanus immunoglobulin in the management of tetanus. Natl Med J India 1998;11:209–212.

52. Abrutyn E, Berlin JA: Intrathecal therapy in tetanus. A meta-analysis. JAMA 1991;266:2262–2267.

53. Sanders RK, Strong TN, Peacock ML: The treatment of tetanus with special reference to betamethasone. Trans R Soc Trop Med Hyg 1969;63:746–754.

54. Chandy ST, Peter JV, John L, et al: Betamethasone in tetanus patients: An evaluation of its effect on the mortality and morbidity. J Assoc Physicians India 1992;40:373–376.

55. Paydas S, Akoglu TF, Akkiz H, et al: Mortality-lowering effect of systemic corticosteroid therapy in severe tetanus. Clin Ther 1988;10:276–280.

56. Ahmadsyah I, Salim A: Treatment of tetanus: An open study to compare the efficacy of procaine penicillin and metronidazole. BMJ (Clin Res Ed) 1985;291:648–650.

57. Boots RJ, Lipman J, O'Callaghan J, et al: The treatment of tetanus with intrathecal baclofen. Anaesth Intensive Care, 2000;28:438–442.

58. Dressnandt J, Konstanger A, Weinzierl FX, et al: Intrathecal baclofen in tetanus: Four cases and a review of reported cases. Intensive Care Med 1997;23:896–902.

59. James MF: Magnesium sulphate for the control of spasms in severe tetanus. Anaesthesia 1998;53:605–606.

60. Attygalle D, Rodrigo N: Magnesium sulphate for control of spasms in severe tetanus. Can we avoid sedation and artificial ventilation? Anaesthesia 1997;52:956–962.

61. Attygalle D: Magnesium sulphate in the management of severe tetanus averts artificial ventilation and sedation. Ceylon Med J 1996;41(3):120.

62. Lipman J, James MF, Erskine J, et al: Autonomic dysfunction in severe tetanus: Magnesium sulfate as an adjunct to deep sedation. Crit Care Med 1987;15:987–988.

63. Ho HS, Lim SH, Loo S: The use of magnesium sulphate in the intensive care management of an Asian patient with tetanus. Ann Acad Med Singapore 1999;28:586–589.

64. Anandaciva S, Koay CW: Tetanus and rocuronium in the intensive care unit [letter]. Anaesthesia 1996;51:505–506.

65. Sutton DN, Tremlett MR, Woodcock TE, Nielsen MS: Management of autonomic dysfunction in severe tetanus: the use of magnesium sulphate and clonidine. Intensive Care Med 1990;16(2):75–80.

66. Bhagwanjee S, Bosenberg AT, Muckart DJ: Management of sympathetic overactivity in tetanus with epidural bupivacaine and sufentanil: Experience with 11 patients [see comments]. Crit Care Med 1999;27:1721–1725.

67. Arnon S: Tetanus. In Behrman R, Kliegman R, Jenson H (eds): Nelson Textbook of Pediatrics, 16th ed. Philadelphia, WB Saunders, 2000, pp 879–880.

68. Begue RE, Lindo-Soriano I: Failure of intrathecal tetanus antitoxin in the treatment of tetanus neonatorum. J Infect Dis 1991;164:619–620.

69. Dianto Mustadjab I: The influence of pyridoxin in the treatment of tetanus neonatorum. Paediatr Indones 1991;31:165–169.

70. Caglar MK: Pyridoxine in the treatment of tetanus neonatorum. Paediatr Indones 1989;29:233–236.

71. Centers for Disease Control and Prevention: Botulism in the United States, 1899–1996. Handbook for Epidemiologists, Clinicians, and Laboratory Workers. Atlanta, Centers for Disease Control and Prevention, 1998.

72. Neal KR, Dunbar EM: Improvement in bulbar weakness with guanoxan in type B botulism. Lancet 1990;335:1286–1287.

73. Roblot P, Roblot F, Fouchere JL, et al: Retrospective study of 108 cases of botulism in Poitiers, France. J Med Microbiol 1994;40:379–384.

74. Siegel LS, Price JI: Ineffectiveness of 3,4-diaminopyridine as a therapy for type C botulism. Toxicon 1987;25:1015–1018.

75. Wilcox PG, Morrison NJ, Pardy RL: Recovery of the ventilatory and upper airway muscles and exercise performance after type A botulism. Chest 1990;98:620–626.

76. Cohen FL, Hardin SB, Nehring W, et al: Physical and psychosocial health status 3 years after catastrophic illness—botulism. Issues Ment Health Nurs 1988;9:387–398.

77. Bleck TP: Tetanus: Pathophysiology, management, and prophylaxis. Dis Mon 1991;37:545–603.

78. Dastur FD, Awatramani VP, Chitre SK, D'Sa JA: A single dose vaccine to prevent neonatal tetanus. J Assoc Physicians India 1993;41:97–99.

79. Barbi M, Biffi MR, Binda S, et al: Immunization in children with HIV seropositivity at birth: Antibody response to polio vaccine and tetanus toxoid. AIDS 1992;6:1465–1469.

80. Kurtzhals JA, Kjeldsen K, Heron I, Skinkoj P: Immunity against diphtheria and tetanus in human immunodeficiency virus–infected Danish men born 1950–59. APMIS, 1992; 100:803–808.

81. Higaki M, Azechi Y, Takase T, et al: Collagen minipellet as a controlled release delivery system for tetanus and diphtheria toxoid. Vaccine 2001;19:3091–3096.

82. Fairweather NF, Chatfield SN, Makoff AJ, et al: Oral vaccination of mice against tetanus by use of a live attenuated Salmonella carrier. Infect Immun 1990;58:1323–1326.

83. Eyles JE, Williamson ED, Alpar HO: Immunological responses to nasal delivery of free and encapsulated tetanus toxoid: Studies on the effect of vehicle volume. Int J Pharm 1999;189:75–79.

84. Beller M, Middaugh JP: Repeated type E botulism in an Alaskan Eskimo. N Engl J Med 1990;322:855.

85. Bell MS, Vermeulen LC, Sperling KB: Pharmacotherapy with botulinum toxin: Harnessing nature's most potent neurotoxin. Pharmacotherapy 2000;20:1079–1091.

section

7

Skin and Supporting Structure Infections

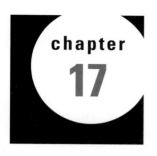

chapter
17

Skin and Soft Tissue Infections

SHERWOOD L. GORBACH, MD

SUPERFICIAL SKIN AND SOFT TISSUE INFECTIONS

Superficial skin and soft tissue infections are among the most common infections seen in clinical practice.[1] These infections occur in three sites within the skin structures:

- Just below the stratum corneum (impetigo)
- In the hair follicles (furuncles) or apocrine glands (hidradenitis suppurativa)
- Below the epidermis, penetrating the dermis to subcutaneous tissues (cellulitis)

They do not involve the fascia (as in necrotizing fasciitis) or muscle. It is necessary to make the diagnosis of these superficial skin lesions by direct inspection

- To initiate appropriate antimicrobial drugs immediately, if indicated
- Because many lesions will not yield a positive culture (cellulitis), or it is unnecessary to order a culture since the result is predictable (furunculosis)
- To avoid surgery (erysipelas) or recommend surgery (carbuncle)

Pyodermas: *Staphylococcus aureus* Infections

S. aureus is present in the anterior nares in 10% to 40% of people, depending on their underlying health, association with hospitals, and age; it also, although less commonly, colonizes the skin. *S. aureus* skin infections are more common in persons with diabetes and immunocompromised hosts.

Clinical Manifestations

Folliculitis involves the ostium of a hair follicle, usually on the face or extensor surface of an extremity; it has an uncomplicated evolution from a vesicle that points to the outside, to drainage, encrustment, and finally spontaneous healing. (*Pseudomonas aeruginosa* can cause extensive folliculitis 2 days after exposure to a contaminated swimming pool or whirlpool. Pruritic papulourticarial lesions that progress to vesicle formation are seen in various stages at multiple sites, sparing the palms and soles.)

A furuncle (boil) develops from folliculitis, spreading to the subcutaneous layers of the skin. There is a firm, discrete nodule with purulent drainage. Systemic manifestations are not seen.

Carbuncle, a more extensive, multiloculated lesion involving subcutaneous fat, occurs in skin that is thick and inelastic, as on the back of the neck, the back, or thighs. Abundant pus drains along hair follicles from deep, septated pockets. It is painful, indurated, and often associated with systemic signs of fever, headache, and malaise.

Recurrent furunculosis occurs most often in otherwise healthy persons. The strain of *S. aureus* is usually identical on each recurrence and does not display antibiotic resistance or special virulence factors. The organism usually is carried in the anterior nares or on the skin.

Differential Diagnosis

It is important to distinguish these staphylococcal infections from acne vulgaris, which involves the sebaceous follicles and is infected with *Propionibacterium acnes* and *Staphylococcus epidermidis*, but rarely *S. aureus*, and from hidradenitis suppurativa, which is an inflammation of the apocrine glands of the axilla or perineal and inguinal areas.

Management

Folliculitis and milder furuncles are treated with warm, moist packs to encourage localization and drainage. No medical or surgical therapy is necessary. More severe furuncles and localized carbuncles require judicious incision and drainage.

Extensive, multiloculated carbuncles should be drained with a small wick inserted to encourage drainage and to prevent closure of the incision. Drainage, although often necessary, also carries some risk of spreading infection to distant sites, since the incision destroys the demarcation by pyogenic membranes, which can lead to dissemination and septicemia.

Antibiotics are indicated for furuncles when they are drained and for carbuncles. Oral drugs are usually sufficient. The preferred treatment is an antistaphylococcal penicillin (cloxacillin, by mouth, or oxacillin or nafcillin, by the parenteral route) or a cephalosporin. For methicillin-resistant *S. aureus*, vancomycin or linezolid is preferred.

Recurrent furunculosis is difficult to manage. An attempt should be made to eliminate nasal carriage by intranasal application of 2% mupirocin for 5 days. Prolonged antistaphylococcal treatment (for 2 months) is sometimes helpful. A mostly successful, although admittedly difficult, treatment is use of low dose (150 mg/d) oral clindamycin for 3 months.

Pyodermas: *Streptococcus pyogenes* Infections

Group A *S. pyogenes* is the most common strain, although some cases are caused by organisms in group C or G, and in newborns, in group B.[2] Rarely, *S. aureus* can produce erysipelas. The incriminated *Streptococcus* is carried in the nasopharynx or on the skin. It is acquired from the host or by person-to-person transmission from a carrier.

Erysipelas

Clinical Manifestations

More common in children, especially infants, and in the elderly, erysipelas presents as a hyperacute cellulitis with involvement of underlying lymphatics.[3] It is a painful condition that starts as a raised, bright red, indurated lesion that spreads circumferentially over a period of minutes to hours, with an advancing red border that sometimes shows small streaks from the edge. Because of underlying lymphatic obstruction, the lesion is edematous, with a peau d'orange appearance. The extremities are the most common sites of involvement, followed by the face, especially over the bridge of the nose ("butterfly") or the cheeks. Some cases occur spontaneously, but most cases are associated with traumatic wounds, skin ulcers, psoriatic lesions, or the umbilical stump of newborns. Facial erysipelas is often preceded by a respiratory infection. Patients at risk are those with diabetes, venous stasis, underlying skin ulcers, alcohol abuse, and nephrotic syndrome. Systemic findings are prominent, with high fever and shaking chills and altered mental status. Erysipelas before the antibiotic era was associated with a high mortality.

Diagnosis

The diagnosis is based on clinical findings, since it is uncommon for a positive culture to be obtained. An open skin lesion is usually absent; needle aspiration from the advancing edge is a fruitless exercise, being positive in <10% of cases. Blood cultures are rarely positive. Serology for streptococcal infection is usually positive, but this is retrospective.

Differential diagnosis includes cellulitis and necrotizing fasciitis, which have a more leisurely course and are not associated with such systemic toxicity at the onset, and streptococcal gangrene (see below), which is a more localized condition. Contact dermatitis and giant urticaria deserve consideration, but they are pruritic and do not have the systemic manifestations. Erythema chronicum migrans of Lyme disease is another consideration, but it generally has the central zone of clearing, moves more slowly, and is associated with only low-grade fever.

Treatment

Penicillin is the preferred treatment, orally (as penicillin V-K) or by intramuscular injection (as procaine penicillin). Most cases are severe enough to require hospitalization, where intravenous penicillin can be given in high doses (2 to 4 μ every 4 to 6 hours). Erythromycin can be used but is often unsatisfactory in terms of therapeutic response. Treatment should be continued for 2 to 3 weeks, usually with oral penicillin to complete the course. There is risk of relapse, so the patient should be warned of this possibility and followed at least by phone. Surgery is not a consideration in erysipelas.

Recurrent Erysipelas

Recurrent erysipelas is associated with chronic edema due to lymphatic or venous obstruction in a limb: axillary dissection secondary to breast cancer surgery or any lymph node resection for cancer or trauma, Milroy's disease, or chronic venous stasis. In persons with an initial attack the recurrence rate is about 10% per year, but in some persons it can recur several times a year. Each event is rather stereotypic for that person; it usually begins with some pain or discomfort in the limb at a specific site, where within hours, a red, tender lesion appears, which rapidly advances up the limb, often with lymphatic streaking. The patient experiences pain and fever with shaking chills. Blood cultures are, as a rule, negative. Aspiration of the lesion does not yield a microbiologic diagnosis. In the rare cases in which positive cultures have been obtained, they are invariably *Streptococcus* but not necessarily group A. Added weight to the association with *Streptococcus* is the rapid and universal response to penicillin.

Penicillin G, administered in high doses intravenously, is the treatment of choice. The treatment should be extended to 2 to 4 weeks depending on the rapidity of the initial response. Oral penicillin can be given in the final phase. Cephalosporins are also effective, and erythromycin or clindamycin can be used in allergic persons.

Preventive measures are sometimes effective. Pressure devices are available to "milk" the affected limb during the night to reduce edema. Physiotherapy to improve muscle tone can also be effective in selected cases. Suppression by antibiotics can be tried in cases involving multiple relapses. Low-dose, oral penicillin (penicillin V-K, 250 mg/d) is given for 3 to 6 months and then stopped. If recurrences continue after medication is stopped, continuous oral penicillin should be given.

Streptococcal Gangrene

Caused in the main by group A *Streptococcus*, although rarely by group C or G, streptococcal gangrene starts at the site of previous skin damage, trauma, which may be minor, puncture wound, or surgical incision. The initial lesion is painful and erythematous and may have surrounding edema and an advancing edge. Within 1 to 2 days the center of the lesion becomes dark red, then blue-black, with frank necrosis. Bullae that contain dark red fluid are sometimes present. Deeper fascia and muscle may also be involved, and if the condition is untreated, septicemia and shock can ensue.

Surgical management involves débridement of the gangrenous skin and incision and drainage of the surrounding tissues and fascial planes. As it is important to release the pressure on the skin and subcutaneous tissues, the incisions should be extended beyond the areas of gangrene and far enough into the superficial fascia to establish good drainage. The limb should be elevated to promote drainage and dressed with moist packs for superficial débridement. High-dose, intravenous penicillin G is administered in doses of 2 to 4 μ every 4 to 6 hours.

Impetigo

Either together or separately, group A *Streptococcus* and *S. aureus* cause this most superficial of the skin infections. Although the streptococcal and mixed forms predominated in the past, recent studies suggest that the pure staphylococcal form is becoming the most common.

Clinical Manifestations
- Bullous impetigo: superficial flaccid bullae containing neutrophils and gram-positive cocci; upon rupture of the bullae the fluid dries on the skin surface to form a brown lacquered patina.
- Nonbullous impetigo: thin-walled vesicles and pustules form on an erythematous base.

The lesions appear on the face or on extremities (at the site of minor trauma or insect bites or eczema). Impetigo is most common during the hot, humid summer season and is related to skin colonization by the microorganisms. They can also be spread from nasopharyngeal colonization during any season. The condition is highly contagious and is spread by direct person-to-person contact, often in school or day care facilities. Poor hygiene and crowded living conditions can facilitate spread. Because the lesions are pruritic, scratching can spread the infection to uninvolved sites or to other persons.

Treatment
Antimicrobial therapy is the preferred approach to impetigo. Oral drugs active against *S. aureus* should be used. Dicloxacillin, amoxicillin-clavulanate, or a cephalosporin is preferred, although erythromycin can also be used in allergic children. Penicillin or ampicillin treatment was used in the past but may be associated with failures because of the presence of resistant staphylococcal strains. Treatment should be given for 1 week.

A topical antimicrobial is an alternative in some patients. Mupirocin is the preferred agent, given 3 times daily for 7 days. Disadvantages of the topical regimen are the inconvenience of application when lesions are widespread on the skin, less effectiveness in bullous impetigo, and the inability to eradicate the site of colonization in the respiratory tract.

Mechanical débridement with soaps or antibacterial soaks may produce a satisfactory cosmetic effect, but there is little evidence that it hastens healing.

Cellulitis

Cellulitis is a spreading inflammatory process involving the deep dermis and subcutaneous fat.[4] It can occur acutely and then proceed to a chronic phase. The infection is caused mainly by *S. pyogenes* or *S. aureus* in normal hosts. Several other bacteria can cause cellulitis, often with distinguishing physical findings and in special clinical settings.

Clinical Manifestations

The infection often develops in association with an initial portal of entry.

- Local: a traumatic injury, puncture wound, insect bite, or surgical incision
- Distant: a foot lesion, such as interdigital tinea pedis or skin fissures, or a hand wound, which spreads to cause cellulitis of the limb

Intense erythema, pain, and advancing edema develop within a few days after the inciting event. Cellulitis moves more slowly, over days, than erysipelas does. The progression of erysipelas is measured in hours. The appearance of cellulitis is also different from that of erysipelas, which has a discrete, expanding red margin. The advancing edge of cellulitis is elevated but is not well demarcated. Systemic complaints—chills, fever, and malaise—are common. Bacteremia is seen in a minority of patients, usually those with more aggressive infection. A more indolent form of cellulitis can develop in the lower leg in association with chronic edema and venous insufficiency.

Streptococcal Cellulitis

Group A *S. pyogenes* (GAS) is a major cause of cellulitis. It occurs acutely but often is associated with a previous injury. The appearance is a diffuse, intense erythema with pain, tenderness, and swelling of the entire area of skin. Patients with dependent edema due to venous insufficiency or lymphatic obstruction are at high risk of streptococcal cellulitis.

Postoperative wound infection with GAS is a life-threatening occurrence. The incubation period is shorter than with most such wounds, ranging from 6 to 48 hours, often in the first postoperative day. In most cases there is no drainage, at best only a minimal amount of serous discharge that contains polymorphonuclear leukocytes (PMNs) and abundant gram-positive cocci in chains. Systemic manifestations, such as high fever, tachycardia, and hypotension, are profound. Bacteremia, which may be accompanied by hemolysis, is common in this setting, and the associated hypotension may be the heralding event. The route of spread is direct inoculation into the wound from a carrier of the organism, usually someone in direct contact with the patient during or just after the operation.

Streptococcal cellulitis can be the presenting condition in a more ominous infection, necrotizing fasciitis with septic shock (see below).

Non-group A streptococci, such as those belonging to groups B, C, and G, can cause cellulitis, particularly in the presence of a chronic condition such as lymphatic obstruction or fissures between the toes. Such organisms have been associated with postoperative cellulitis at the saphenous vein donor site in patients who have undergone cardiac bypass surgery.

Staphylococcal Cellulitis

S. aureus is the main pathogen. Other staphylococci, such as *S. epidermidis*, can cause cellulitis in immunocompromised hosts. Most strains of community-acquired *S. aureus* are sensitive to methicillin (MSSA), although an increasing number of methicillin-resistant strains (MRSA) are causing infections that arise in the community in otherwise-healthy persons. Staphylococci tend to spread through the subcutaneous tissues of the skin in a circumferential, slowly progressive fashion over a period of days. The usual appearance is different from that of streptococcal cellulitis, although there is enough overlap that the cause cannot be distinguished with certainty even when a "classic" lesion is present. This organism is still the major cause of postoperative wound infection, which usually is transferred by person-to-person contact either on the hands of medical personnel or from a carrier who harbors the organism in the nares. Clinically a staphylococcal wound infection becomes obvious 3 to 4 days after the procedure. The suture line becomes reddened, tender, and somewhat tense. A slow ooze of odorless, yellow pus can be discerned at the edges and on the dressing. MRSA infections are rather common in many United States hospitals, with rates of 40% to 80% of all staphylococcal infections.

Other Gram-Positive Organisms Causing Cellulitis

Erysipelothrix rhusiopathiae, a gram-positive bacillus, causes a distinctive form of cellulitis known as erysipeloid. It occurs mostly on the fingers and hands, presenting as purplish red, indurated, painful or burning lesions with a sharp margin that spread peripherally with some central clearing. The surrounding area of skin is rather swollen. The organism is ubiquitous in nature, found in fish, mammals, birds, insects, organic matter, and contaminated water, and the patient invariably has a history of contact with a known source.

Streptococcus pneumoniae is a rare cause of cellulitis and is a result of bacteremia from a primary site, usually in the lung.

Gram-Negative Organisms Causing Cellulitis

P. aeruginosa can cause several types of cellulitis in healthy as well as immunocompromised hosts. Its usual habitat is water, so the infection is often associated with exposure to water sources or moist sites. Besides its intrinsic virulence, invading small arterioles leading to avascular necrosis of skin and soft tissues, *Pseudomonas* is difficult to treat because of its resistance to many antibiotics.

Swimmer's ear, paronychia, and aggressive interdigital infections are caused by *Pseudomonas* in persons who have prolonged contact with a contaminated water source. Exposure to hot tubs, spas, or whirlpools can cause a diffuse, pruritic, maculopapular, or vesiculopustular eruption caused by *Pseudomonas*. The bathing suit area is often spared. Outbreaks of such infections are common because of contamination of the water and poor environmental control. The condition is self-limited, without need for medical intervention.

A severe form of cellulitis known as malignant external otitis involves the ear pinna in diabetic persons and usually is preceded by a chronic otitis externa or trauma from a hearing aid or irrigation of the ear canal to remove cerumen. The condition advances rapidly, destroying cartilage and bone locally and invading the central nervous system. Puncture wounds in persons wearing sneakers or old shoes, which harbor *Pseudomonas* in their moist, warm crevices, can lead to cellulitis of the sole of the foot with underlying osteomyelitis. In immuno-compromised hosts *Pseudomonas* bacteremia can produce cellulitis, as well as discrete, necrotic ulcers (ecthyma gangrenosum).

Aeromonas is found in fresh or brackish waters. It causes cellulitis in persons with previous lacerations or traumatic injuries who are exposed to such conditions.

Vibrio spp, which are found in sea water, can cause cellulitis and ear infections. The following species have been incriminated:

- *V. cholerae* non-0:1*
- *V. parahaemolyticus**
- *V. vulnificus**
- *V. mimicus*

V. vulnificus is particularly virulent. It can cause severe cellulitis in persons who develop skin injuries while swimming in sea water or who have prior lacerations. A life-threatening form of cellulitis develops from bacteremia associated with eating raw oysters in persons with underlying liver disease.

Haemophilus influenzae type b can cause cellulitis of the face, neck, or arms in young children with bacteremia from a primary site in the middle ear or upper respiratory tract. This infection can also occur in adults with epiglottis or lower respiratory tract infections. The classic form has a purple or blue hue, but most cases in fact have an erythematous appearance that is indistinguishable from other forms of cellulitis.

Diagnosis

When cellulitis is associated with an open wound, there is usually an exudate that can be used for Gram stain and culture. In the setting of cellulitis with unbroken skin a needle aspiration from the advancing edge can sometimes (10%) yield a positive diagnosis. A positive blood culture is diagnostic. Bacteremia is uncommon in staphylococcal cellulitis but is common in cellulitis caused by *Streptococcus* or gram-negative bacteria. Clues can be gleaned from the patient's underlying disease (diabetes, cirrhosis, malignancy), recent exposures

(swimming in fresh or salt water), or occupation (commercial fishing).

Management

As a rule cellulitis is not treated by surgical intervention. Antimicrobial therapy is required, often administered on an empiric basis awaiting laboratory confirmation:

- Streptococcal infection: large doses of intravenous penicillin or ampicillin
- Staphylococcal infection: oxacillin or nafcillin or a first-generation cephalosporin, for example, cefazolin.
- When the diagnosis of streptococcal vs. staphylococcal infection is unclear: a combination of ampicillin and oxacillin or a first-generation cephalosporin should be used.
- *Pseudomonas* infection: a quinolone with an aminoglycoside (for more serious infections such as malignant external otitis).
- Swimmer's ear and hot tub folliculitis do not require antibiotics.
- *Aeromonas* and *Vibrio* infections: a quinolone or a tetracycline. The life-threatening forms should be given an intravenous quinolone with an aminoglycoside.

Streptococcal Necrotizing Fasciitis with Toxic Shock

In the past decade there has been a dramatic increase in the number of severe, life-threatening cases of GAS infections associated with necrotizing fasciitis and toxic shock syndrome.[5] In 1995 it was estimated that 10,000 to 15,000 cases of severe GAS infections occur annually in the United States, of which 5% to 10% are cases of necrotizing fasciitis with toxic shock.

Definitions

CONFIRMED. Necrosis of subcutaneous tissue together with severe systemic illness (including one or more of the following: sudden death, shock with a systolic blood pressure <90 mm Hg, disseminated intravascular coagulation, and system failure such as respiratory, hepatic, or renal failure) and with GAS isolated from the affected site or a normally sterile site.

PROBABLE. Clinical criteria above and with serologic or histologic evidence of streptococcal infection but without a culture of GAS from the affected site or a normally sterile site.

Clinical Manifestations

The age range is 20 to 50 years. There is usually no underlying disease. The portal of entry is found in 50% of cases, often the local skin site. A mucous membrane (throat, vagina) site of GAS infection is uncommon. The initial symptom is abrupt, severe pain (in 85%).

---

*Also causes septicemia.

Signs and symptoms	Percent
Fever >38°C	70
Confusion	55
Heart rate >100/min	80
Hypotension	100
Skin changes	80
Swelling	10
Swelling and erythema	65
Bullae	5
Desquamation (late)	20

Laboratory findings	Mean values on admission/ at 48 hours
Leukocytes	11,765/...
Immature granulocytes	43%/...
Platelets	216,000/129,000
Creatinine	2.5/3.4
Calcium	8.1/6.6
Albumin	3.3/2.3
Creatine phosphokinase	3000/100,000

Microbiology

Bacteremia is present in 60% of cases. When available, culture from the skin site is positive for GAS. GAS M types are 1, 3, 28, 12. Mucoid colonies are rare. The strains contain streptococcal pyrogenic exotoxins A (SPEA) or B (SPEB) or both.

Complications

Condition	Percent
Shock	95
ARDS	55
Renal impairment	80
Irreversible	10
Reversible	70
Death	30

Management

Penicillin G is the treatment of choice; however, failures are noted in humans and experimental animals. In experimental animals with GAS infections results are as follows: clindamycin better than erythromycin better than penicillin. Results may be related to inhibition of M protein and toxin production. Ceftriaxone has a greater affinity for streptococcal penicillin-binding proteins. On the basis of experimental results, clindamycin should be used with either penicillin or ceftriaxone. Treatment with intravenous immunoglobulin G (IVIGG) is recommended for severe cases. Surgery—drainage, débridement, fasciotomy, amputation—is determined by the clinical situation.

NECROTIZING SKIN AND SOFT TISSUE INFECTIONS

Severe skin and soft tissue infections differ from the milder, superficial infections by clinical presentation, coexisting systemic manifestations, and treatment strategies.[6,7] They are often deep and devastating: deep because they involve the fascial or muscle compartments or both and devastating because they cause major destruction of tissue and can cause death. These conditions are usually "secondary" infections in that they develop from an initial break in the skin related to trauma or surgery. They can be *monomicrobial*, usually streptococci or staphylococci, or *polymicrobial*, involving a mixed aerobe-anaerobe bacterial flora.

Five clinical features suggest the presence of a deep and severe infection of the skin and its deeper structures:

1. Severe pain, which is constantly present.
2. Bullous lesions, related to occlusion of deep blood vessels that traverse the fascia or muscle compartments. Bullae are not diagnostic of deep infections, since they can also be found in association with superficial infections (erysipelas, cellulitis, toxic shock syndrome, disseminated intravascular coagulation, purpura fulminans), some toxins (e.g., brown recluse spider bites), and primary dermatologic conditions (e.g., pyoderma gangrenosum).
3. Gas in the soft tissues, which is detected by palpation, roentgenograms, or scanning. Gas is produced by metabolic activity of the aerobic or anaerobic bacteria. When anaerobes are present, there is also a distinctive odor of putrefaction.
4. Systemic toxicity, manifested by fever, leukocytosis, delirium, and renal failure.
5. Rapid spread centrally along fascial planes.

Another distinction from the milder skin infections is that necrotizing deep infections usually require surgical intervention along with antimicrobial drugs for cure. While attempting to preserve as much viable tissue as possible, it is necessary to perform bold resection of all necrotic material and to incise the fascial planes until the full extent of purulence is realized.

The choice of antimicrobial drugs is based on the specific organisms present (Table 17–1).

Necrotizing Fasciitis

Necrotizing fasciitis is a relatively rare infection involving subcutaneous tissues with extensive undermining and tracking along fascial planes.[8,9]

Clinical Features

Extension from a skin lesion is seen in 80% of cases. The initial lesion often is trivial, such as a minor abrasion, insect bite, injection site (in the case of heroin addicts), or boil. Rare cases have arisen in Bartholin's gland abscess or perianal abscess, from which the infection spreads to fascial planes of the perineum, thigh, groin, and abdomen. The remaining 20% of patients have no visible skin lesion. The initial presentation is that of cellulitis, which advances rather

TABLE 17–1 ■ Treatment of Necrotizing Infection of the Skin, Fascia, and Muscle

First-line	Second-line or penicillin allergic persons
MIXED INFECTIONS	
Imipenem-cilastatin	Cefoxitin, clindamycin, or
Ticarcillin-clavulanate	metronidazole and an
Ampicillin-sulbactam	aminoglycoside
Piperacillin-tazobactam	
STREPTOCOCCUS	
Penicillin (and clindamycin for toxic shock or necrotizing fasciitis)	Cefazolin Vancomycin
STAPHYLOCOCCUS AUREUS	
Nafcillin	
Cloxacillin	Cefazolin
Vancomycin (for resistant strains)	Vancomycin

slowly. Over the next 2 to 4 days, however, there is systemic toxicity with high temperatures. The patient is disoriented and lethargic. The local site shows the following features: cellulitis (90%), edema (80%), skin discoloration or gangrene (70%), and anesthesia of involved skin (common, but true incidence is unknown).

The most distinguishing clinical feature is the wooden-hard feel of the subcutaneous tissues. In cellulitis or erysipelas the subcutaneous tissues can be palpated and are yielding. But in fasciitis the underlying tissues are firm, and the fascial planes and muscle groups cannot be discerned by palpation. It is often possible to observe a broad erythematous tract in the skin along the route of the fascial plane as the infection advances cephalad in an extremity. If there is an open wound, probing the edges with a blunt instrument permits ready dissection of the superficial fascial planes well beyond the wound margins. There is remarkably little pain associated with this procedure.

Bacteriology

MONOMICROBIAL FORM. Pathogens in this group are group A ß-hemolytic *S. pyogenes*, *S. aureus*, and anaerobic streptococci (*Peptostreptococcus*). Staphylococci and hemolytic streptococci occur in about equal frequency, and approximately one-third of patients will have both pathogens simultaneously. Most patients acquire their infection outside the hospital. Most of these infections present in the extremities, approximately two-thirds in the lower extremity. There is often an underlying cause, such as diabetes, arteriosclerotic vascular disease, or venous insufficiency with edema. In some instances a chronic vascular ulcer changes into a more acute process. The mortality in this group is high, approaching 50% in patients with severe vascular disease.

POLYMICROBIAL FORM. An array of anaerobic and aerobic organisms can be cultured from the involved fascial plane: from 1 to 15 bacteria, with an average of five pathogens in each wound. Most of the organisms originate from the bowel flora, for example, coliforms and anaerobic bacteria. The polymicrobial infection is associated with four clinical settings:

1. Surgical procedures, especially bowel resections and penetrating trauma, can be complicated by cellulitis, leading to a superficial fascial dissection.
2. An infection proceeding from a decubitus ulcer, minor trauma, or a perianal abscess can involve the buttocks and perineum. Because of the proximity of the anus, contamination by fecal bacteria is universally present.
3. In intravenous drug users the upper extremities are frequently involved at the site of injection. Because the needles and "works" are contaminated, unusual organisms such as *Pseudomonas* and *Citrobacter* can be isolated, sometimes in association with anaerobes.
4. The lesion can spread from a Bartholin's gland abscess or a minor vulvovaginal infection. Some cases have been associated with pudendal block anesthesia during delivery. Although mixed infections are usually noted in this setting, some cases are caused by a single pathogen, particularly anaerobic *Streptococcus*.

Diagnosis

It may not be possible to diagnose fasciitis upon first seeing the patient. Overlying cellulitis is a frequent accompaniment. That the process involves the deeper fascial planes is suggested by the following features: Failure to respond to initial antibiotic therapy. Cellulitis usually improves, with lowering of fever and reduction in local signs, within 24 to 48 hours. Fasciitis is a more stubborn infection and shows little improvement in the initial few days. The hard, wooden feel of the subcutaneous tissue, extending beyond the area of apparent skin involvement. Systemic toxicity, often with altered mental status.

A computed tomography (CT) scan or magnetic resonance imaging may show exudate extending along the fascial plane. The most important diagnostic feature of necrotizing fasciitis is the appearance of the fascial planes at surgery. Upon direct inspection the fascia is swollen and dull gray, with stringy areas of necrosis. A thin, brownish exudate emerges from the wound. Even upon deep dissection there is no true pus. Extensive undermining of surrounding tissues is present, and the fascial planes can be dissected with a gloved finger or a blunt instrument. A Gram stain of the exudate demonstrates the pathogens and provides an early clue to therapy. Gram-positive cocci in chains suggest *Streptococcus* (either group A or anaerobic). Large gram-positive cocci in clumps suggest *S. aureus*. A mixed flora suggests polymicrobial infection. Cultures are best obtained from the deep tissues. If the infection has emanated from a contaminated skin wound, such as a vascular ulcer, the bacteriology of the superficial wound is not necessarily indicative of the deep tissue infection. An array of coliforms, staphylococci, and various streptococci can be isolated from the ulcer, but the fascia may have a pure culture or single organism, such as anaerobic streptococci or *S. aureus*. Direct needle aspiration of the advancing edge has been advocated as a means of obtaining material for culture, but this technique is nearly always unproductive. A definitive bacteriologic diagnosis can be established only by culture of the fascia at surgery or by a positive blood culture.

Treatment

Surgical intervention is the major therapeutic modality in cases of necrotizing fasciitis. It should be emphasized, however, that some patients can be treated with large doses of appropriate antibiotics and thereby avoid potentially mutilating surgery. The decision to undertake aggressive surgery should be based on the following:

1. Failure to respond to antibiotics after a reasonable trial is the most common index. A response to antibiotics should be judged by reduction in fever and toxicity and lack of advancement.
2. Profound toxicity, fever, hypotension, or advancement of the skin and soft tissue infection during antibiotic therapy is an indication for surgical intervention.
3. When the local wound shows extensive necrosis with easy dissection along the fascia by a blunt instrument, more complete incision and drainage are required.

With the patient under general anesthesia the skin is incised or the wound is widened down to the fascial plane for complete inspection. Finger dissection along the fascial plane determines the extent of the linear incision. Usually multiple incisions or "filets" are required to delineate adequately the extent of involvement. Loose gauze dressings are packed into the wound and changed every 6 hours or as required. Wet-to-dry dressings are used to facilitate mechanical débridement. As the dressings are removed, the depth of the wound should be inspected by a gloved finger to determine any extension that requires further incision. The first procedure is almost never sufficient to determine the extent of involvement. As further tracts are discovered, the patient is returned to the operating room for additional incision and débridement. Although no discrete pus is encountered, these wounds can discharge copious amounts of tissue fluid; aggressive fluid and colloid therapy is a necessary adjunct.

Antimicrobial therapy can minimize the extent of, and even avert, surgical intervention, especially in those cases in which the distinction between cellulitis and fasciitis is difficult. The medications must be directed at the pathogens and used in high doses for a prolonged period, usually 2 to 3 weeks (Table 17–1).

Outcome

The overall mortality in necrotizing fasciitis is 20% to 30%. Adverse risk factors include diabetes, advanced arteriosclerotic vascular disease, and lesions that involve an extremity and progress into the buttocks or back muscles or onto the chest wall.

Anaerobic Streptococcal Myositis

Anaerobic streptococci cause a more indolent process than other streptococcal infections. Involvement of the muscle and fascial planes by anaerobic streptococci usually is associated with trauma or a surgical procedure.

Clinical Features

There may be severe local pain. The overlying skin appears as a gangrenous wound that emits a foul, watery, brown discharge. Bleb formation is common. Crepitus may be apparent in the surrounding tissue. The gas formation can be extensive, with tracking into the adjacent healthy tissues. Inspection of the muscle reveals redness and edema with some local destruction. There is no myonecrosis, however, and the muscle contracts under the scalpel. Although there is generalized toxicity and fever and even organ failure, the patient is not so ill as someone with gas gangrene.

Diagnosis

The initial approach to a crepitant skin infection is to obtain a sample of exudate for Gram stain and to open the wound for inspection of muscle and soft tissue. The major distinctions between the disease caused by anaerobic streptococci and clostridia are as follows:

1. Systemic effects are less prominent with the streptococcal form. This infection does not cause hypotension and renal failure, as does the clostridial disease.
2. The involved muscle remains viable in the streptococcal disease, although there may be inflammatory reaction and edema. True myonecrosis is not found.
3. Considerable gas is produced, occurring early in the course, whereas clostridial infections tend to have less gas and usually as a late development.
4. The discharge from the wound is thin, brown ooze that shows gram-positive cocci and multiple PMNs in the Gram stain slide. By contrast, the discharge in gas gangrene shows gram-positive rods but few PMNs.

Treatment

Incision and drainage are critical. Necrotic tissue and debris are resected, but the inflamed muscle should not be removed, since it can heal and become functionally useful. The incision should be packed with moist dressings. Antibiotic treatment is highly effective. These organisms are all sensitive to penicillin or ampicillin, which should be administered in high doses.

Streptococcal Gangrene (Meleney's Streptococcal Gangrene, ß-Hemolytic Streptococcal Gangrene)

A superficial streptococcal infection can progress to cause severe destruction of the superficial layers of skin. This condition occurs most frequently in the extremities, associated with minor trauma, puncture wound, or surgical incision, but can occur in postoperative abdominal incisions. The initial event is erysipelas, with the typical findings of pain, erythema, edema, and advancing border. Within 1 to 2 days the center of the lesion becomes dark red, then blue-black, with formation of bullae and gangrene of the skin and subcutaneous tissues. The surrounding tissue is fiery red, abraded, and edematous. Deeper fascia and muscle may also be involved.

Surgical management involves débridement of the gangrenous skin and incision and drainage of the surrounding tissues and fascial planes. It is important to release the pressure on the skin and subcutaneous tissues; so incisions should be extended beyond the areas of gangrene and far enough into the superficial fascia to establish good drainage. The limb should be elevated to promote drainage and dressed with moist packs for superficial débridement. Although no discrete pockets of pus are found, there is significant oozing of tissue fluid, which must be made up by appropriate intravenous administration of fluid and colloids. High-dose penicillin or ampicillin is also given.

Progressive Bacterial Synergistic Gangrene (Meleney's Gangrene)

Meleney's synergistic gangrene is an indolent process characterized by poor wound healing, with elevation and erythema of the surrounding skin. This is a postoperative infection that typically occurs in the vicinity of retention suture or in a drain site following an abdominal operation or an incision of the chest wall. In recent years this infection is rare because postoperative antibiotics are administered at the earliest sign of infection in the wound. In the classic presentation the diagnosis is recognized 1 to 2 weeks after surgery, when the lesion has extended circumferentially with three zones of involvement: a central area of necrosis, a middle zone of violaceous, tender, edematous tissue, and an outer zone of bright erythema. Local pain and tenderness are nearly always present; however, fever and systemic toxicity usually are absent.

The condition is caused by synergistic (cooperative) association between *S. aureus* and a microaerophilic or anaerobic *Streptococcus*. These organisms can be isolated from the outer zone of infection; sampling the central zone of necrosis, however, yields a mixed flora of coliforms that does not reflect the essential pathologic process. In experimental studies, synergy has been demonstrated in mixed infections of *S. aureus* and *S. pyogenes* and of various aerobes and anaerobes.

In the preantibiotic era, Meleney advocated extensive resection of all nonviable tissue, as well as extension of the incision beyond the area of induration and necrosis to include some healthy tissue. The availability of antibiotics has eliminated the requirement for such radical excision. It is now recommended that all necrotic tissue be removed, with inspection of subcutaneous structures for burrowing tracks. Wet-to-dry dressings should then be applied. Daily inspection should reveal any extension of the process that requires additional débridement. A xenograft or allograft may be necessary to cover the wound. Antimicrobial therapy should be directed at the two major pathogens, *S. aureus* and the anaerobic streptococcus. A semisynthetic penicillin (nafcillin or oxacillin) or a cephalosporin can be used.

Pyomyositis

Pyomyositis is a discrete abscess within an individual muscle group caused in the main by *S. aureus*.[10] Occasionally *S. pneumoniae* or a gram-negative enteric rod is the responsible pathogen. Blood cultures are positive in 5% to 30% of cases. Because of its geographic distribution, pyomyositis is often referred to as "tropical pyomyositis," but cases are increasingly recognized in temperate climates, especially in patients with HIV infection or diabetes. Presenting findings are localized pain in a single muscle group, muscle spasm, and fever. The disease occurs most often in an extremity, but any muscle group can be involved, including the psoas or muscles of the trunk. Initially it may not be possible to palpate a discrete abscess because the infection is localized deep within the muscle, but the area has a firm, "woody" feel on palpation, along with pain and tenderness. In the early stages an ultrasound or CT scan is needed to make the diagnosis, which can be confused with deep vein thrombosis, but in more advanced cases a bulging abscess is apparent. Surgical incision and drainage are required, along with appropriate antibiotics.

Synergistic Necrotizing Cellulitis

Synergistic necrotizing cellulitis is a highly lethal polymicrobial infection that produces extensive necrosis of skin and soft tissues with progressive undermining along fascial planes.[11-13] The process may be rather indolent at first, presenting after 7 to 10 days of mild symptoms. Patients are often afebrile or have only low-grade fever, lacking systemic toxicity in the early stages. The initial lesion in the skin is a small area of necrotic or reddish brown bleb with extreme local tenderness; however, the superficial appearance belies the widespread destruction of the deeper tissues. By direct inspection through skin incisions there is extensive gangrene of the superficial tissues and fat, with gelatinous necrosis of fascia and muscle. Gas can be palpated in the tissues in 25% of patients. The most common site of involvement is the perineum, seen in one-half of patients. The major predisposing causes are perirectal abscess and ischiorectal abscess; these conditions track to the deeper structures of the pelvis, leading to a severe form of the disease. A more superficial form involves the buttocks without extension to deeper muscles. In approximately 40% of patients the thigh and leg are involved. Some infections arise in the adductor compartment of the thigh, often extending from an infected amputation stump or diabetic gangrene. Lesions in the lower leg usually are associated with vascular disease or diabetic foot ulcers. The remaining 10% of cases occur in the upper extremities or in the neck, most frequently in patients with vascular disease or diabetes. Seventy-five percent of patients have diabetes mellitus, which may be relatively mild and only discovered at the time of admission. Some patients present with ketoacidosis. Cardiovascular and renal disease are seen in 50% of patients. Obesity is common, found in over 50% of patients.

Bacteriology

The discharge is brown, rather thin and watery, with a foul odor; such exudate has been labeled "dishwater pus." This is a mixed aerobic-anaerobic infection, consisting of organisms that have their origin in the intestinal tract. Gram stain reveals a mixed flora with abundant PMNs. Among the aerobes, coliforms are most common, such as *Escherichia coli, Klebsiella*, and *Proteus*. Anaerobes are usually abundant, including *Bacteroides, Peptostreptococcus, Clostridium*, and *Fusobacterium*. Approximately one-third of patients have positive blood cultures, usually a coliform, *Bacteroides* or *Peptostreptococcus*.

Treatment

Surgical management of synergistic necrotizing cellulitis involves radical débridement of involved tissues, followed by wet-to-dry dressing and mechanical débridement. When the lower extremity is involved, as in diabetes, an amputation usually is required. In the perineum, infection that is confined to the buttocks can be managed with complete surgical excision; however, deeper infection in the pelvis, extending from perirectal disease, is difficult to approach by complete resection and may require repeated sessions of débridement in the operating room to achieve adequate drainage. Antibiotic therapy involves a spectrum broad enough to cover both aerobes and anaerobes.

Outcome

There is 50% mortality in this disease. The patient usually succumbs to septic shock and circulatory collapse. Adverse risk factors include diabetes, especially ketoacidosis, severe renal disease, and involvement of deep tissues of the pelvis and perineum.

Nonclostridial Crepitant Cellulitis

Nonclostridial crepitant cellulitis is caused by gas-forming bacteria that involve the skin, either primarily or as an extension from deeper structures. The origin of infection is an abdominal wound, perianal disease, or operative incisions that have become secondarily infected. Tracking of gas-forming organisms from deeper sites of infection may also present as crepitant cellulitis without a break in the skin. Infection of the perineal area is associated with ischiorectal abscess, whereas infections in the flank generally communicate with a perinephric abscess. Persons with diabetes are more likely to acquire such infections, especially in the lower extremities. These emphysematous infections generally are not so serious as those associated with clostridia, since the nonclostridial pathogens do not liberate systemic toxins. Among the bacteria isolated are anaerobic organisms, such as *Bacteroides* or anaerobic streptococci (*Peptostreptococcus*), and coliform bacteria, especially *E. coli* and *Klebsiella*.

Treatment

The surgical approach should be aggressive but tailored specifically to the underlying cause of infection. Extensive resection usually is not required, since the gas is not an index of underlying necrosis but rather reflects tracking of the infection along the fascial or lymphatic planes. Antibiotic therapy is directed at a mixed aerobic-anaerobic flora until culture reports are available.

Differential Diagnosis

Noninfectious processes can be associated with gas in subcutaneous tissues. On the chest wall at the site of thoracentesis, chest tube insertion, or a thoracic procedure, there may be subcutaneous emphysema that tracks extensively along subcutaneous tissues. A tracheotomy provides a portal for air to track along the tissues of the neck, even to the anterior chest wall. Transtracheal aspiration by a needle produces local emphysema in approximately 10% of cases. On rare occasions a thin column of gas is palpated or seen by x-ray examination along the course of an intravenous catheter in the arm. This is most likely caused by a central venous pressure line or a Swan-Ganz catheter and is a benign condition, not associated with infection in the lines or the surrounding veins

Fournier's Gangrene

Fournier's gangrene is a variant of synergistic gangrene that involves the scrotum and penis and has an explosive onset.[14,15] The average age of onset is 50 to 60 years. Most have significant underlying disease, particularly diabetes. Twenty percent of patients have no preceding cause. The remaining persons have one of the following conditions: ischiorectal abscess, perianal fistula, erysipelas of the perineum, bowel disease (rectal carcinoma, diverticulitis), scrotal trauma, prior urogenital surgery, especially involving the periurethral glands, rarely in alcoholics who develop pressure sores of the scrotum and perineum by sitting in the same position in a drunken stupor, or dissection of pancreatic juice through the retroperitoneum and into the scrotum.

The infection can begin insidiously with a discrete area of necrosis on the scrotum, which can then move rapidly with skin necrosis advancing over 1 to 2 days. The route of infection is via Buck's fascia, spreading along the planes of the dartos fascia of the scrotum and penis. The infection may then extend to Colles' fascia of the perineum and even to Scarpa's fascia of the abdominal wall. At the outset it tends to be superficial gangrene, limited to skin and subcutaneous tissue, extending to the base of the scrotum. The testes, glans penis, and spermatic cord usually are spared, since they have a separate blood supply. There may be extension to the perineum and the anterior abdominal wall through the fascial planes.

Bacteriology

Most cases are caused by a mixed flora of aerobic and anaerobic bacteria, similar to those noted in synergistic necrotizing cellulitis. Staphylococci are frequently present, usually in mixed culture but occasionally as a single pathogen. *Pseudomonas* is another common organism in the mixed culture.

Treatment

Prompt and aggressive surgical débridement should be instituted with removal of all necrotic tissue, sparing the deeper structures when possible. It is often necessary to return to the operating room on several occasions for the necessary resection of necrotic tissue. Diversion of the fecal or urinary stream is necessary in some but not all cases. Antibiotic therapy should cover the range of organisms in the mixed culture. Special attention is paid to *Staphylococcus* and *Pseudomonas*.

Outcome

Even with optimal surgical and medical therapy, mortality ranges from 10% to 40%.

REFERENCES

1. File TM Jr, Tan JS: Treatment of skin and soft-tissue infections. Am J Surg 1995;169:27S–33S.
2. Bisno AL, Stevens DL: Streptococcal infections of skin and soft tissues. N Engl J Med 1996;334:240–245.
3. Chartier C, Grosshans E: Erysipelas: An update. Int J Dermatol 1996;35:779–781.
4. Brook I, Frazier EH: Clinical features and aerobic and anaerobic microbiological characteristics of cellulitis. Arch Surg 1995;130:786–792.
5. Stevens DL: Streptococcal toxic shock syndrome associated with necrotizing fasciitis. Ann Rev Med 2000;51:271–288.
6. Ahrenholz DH: Necrotizing soft-tissue infections. Surg Clin North Am 1988;68:199–214.
7. Lewis RT: Necrotizing soft-tissue infections. Infect Dis Clin North Am 1992;6:693–703.
8. Rea WJ, Wyrick WJ Jr: Necrotizing fasciitis. Ann Surg 1970;172:957–964.
9. Giuliano A, Lewis F Jr, Hadley K, Blaisdell FW: Bacteriology of necrotizing fasciitis. Am J Surg 1977;134:52–57.
10. Sissolak D, Weir WR: Tropical pyomyositis. J Infect 1994;29:121–127.
11. Stone HH, Martin JD Jr: Synergistic necrotizing cellulitis. Ann Surg 1972;175:702–711.
12. Kingston D, Seal DV: Current hypotheses on synergistic microbial gangrene. Br J Surg 1990;77:260–264.
13. Salvino C, Harford FJ, Dobrin PB: Necrotizing infections of the perineum. South Med J 1993;86:908–911.
14. Eke N: Fournier's gangrene: A review of 1726 cases. Br J Surg 2000;87:718–728.
15. Laucks SS II: Fournier's gangrene. Surg Clin North Am 1994;74:1339–1352.

Animal and Human Bites

FREDRICK M. ABRAHAMIAN, DO
ELLIE J. C. GOLDSTEIN, MD

Animal and human bites are common injuries in patients seeking medical attention. Of all the animal species, dog and cat bites account for most animal bite injuries in the United States. Annually in the United States more than 4.7 million people are bitten by dogs. Approximately 20 deaths per year are attributed to dog bites.[1,2] A survey conducted in emergency departments (ED) across the United States from 1992 to 1994 estimated that for each dog-bite fatality there were about 670 hospitalizations and 16,000 ED visits, making dog bite–related injuries responsible for 0.4% of all ED visits.[3] Since physicians are more likely to encounter bites from land-based animals (mainly dogs and cats) and other humans, this chapter focuses mainly on principles of bite wound therapy and injuries sustained from these species.

ANIMAL BITES

Initial evaluation of an injured patient begins by obtaining a history. The history should include information about the victim, animal, time of the injury, and the circumstances leading to the injury. Important elements in a patient's history include identification of comorbidities (e.g., splenectomy, diabetes, liver disease, cancer, human immunodeficiency virus (HIV) infection, chronic steroid use), previous history of tetanus and rabies immunizations, and drug allergies. For hand injuries the patient's occupation and hand dominance are important information for determining further disability. Essential information about the animal includes its behavior patterns, circumstances of the attack (e.g., provoked), and if known, its status of rabies immunization.

The spectrum of injuries resulting from animal bites ranges from minor wounds where minimal external signs of a bite are evident to injuries in which the victim is left with avulsions, large lacerations, fractures, and crush injuries. Dogs can exert bite forces as high as 2000 pounds per square inch and often produce several types of tissue injuries including punctures, lacerations, and avulsions.[4] Because of their sharp, thin teeth, cats often produce small puncture wounds rather than avulsions.[5] Some species of bats have small, thin, sharp teeth and may leave minimal if any external signs of a bite, making these wounds difficult to detect.[6]

The physical examination should include evaluation for signs of infection and injuries to deeper structures. It is best to draw a picture on the medical chart specifying the location, type of injury (e.g., avulsion, puncture, laceration, crush), depth of the wound, presence and extent of edema, fluctuance, or erythema. Other important elements of physical examination include a description of an infected wound (e.g., abscess, purulent, nonpurulent), presence of lymphadenopathy or lymphangitis, and assessment of the integrity of neurovascular and musculoskeletal structures. It is best to demarcate the areas of fluctuance or erythema with a pen. The demarcation can visually aid in identifying improvement or progression of infection.

The appearance of the wound alone should not deter one from excluding injuries to tendons, joint capsule, bones, and neurovascular structures. Cats' long sharp teeth often penetrate the bone cortices. Because of their small stature, children are especially susceptible to injuries around the face and head regions. Skull and facial fractures may accompany cranial injuries.[7] Joints should be taken through their full range of motion both actively and passively. Careful exploration of the wound, especially those on the hands, by a trained specialist may be necessary for exclusion of involvement of deeper anatomic structures.

Pain out of proportion to physical findings should raise suspicion for joint and bone injuries, compartment syndrome, and necrotizing infection. Other clues suggestive of compartment syndrome include increased pain on passive stretching or active contraction of involved muscle groups and paresthesia or hypoesthesia in the distribution of the nerves crossing the involved compartment. Necrotizing infection should be suspected with a rapid development and progression of infection or the presence of crepitus, blistering, or subcutaneous emphysema.[8]

Unless there are clinical indications, routine blood cultures and other laboratory tests such as white blood cell counts, hemoglobin and hematocrit levels, platelet count, and prothrombin time often are not performed on bite victims. Routine culturing of noninfected wounds is also unnecessary. Cultures of such wounds do not yield much information with respect to predicting the bacteriology of subsequent infection.[9] Because of the polymicrobial nature of bite wounds, however, infected wounds should be cultured for both aerobic and anaerobic organisms.[10]

Viral cultures are indicated for bites by primates potentially infected with B virus (also known as Cercopithecine herpesvirus 1). B-virus infections have been commonly reported among rhesus (*Macaca mulatta*) and cynomolgus monkeys (*Macaca fascicularis*). It is recommended that B-virus culture specimens be obtained after thorough cleansing of the wound. Patients potentially infected with B virus also require two serologic studies 3 weeks apart for acute B virus–specific antibody.[11]

The Gram stain also has limited clinical usefulness because of the polymicrobial nature of bite wounds.[9] In suspected cases of septicemia due to *Capnocytophaga canimorsus* following dog bites, however, a provisional diagnosis can be made by Gram stain of the buffy coat. In such circumstances a Gram stain of the buffy coat becomes a useful diagnostic test, since *C. canimorsus* demonstrates slow growth in blood cultures (range, 1 to 14 days).[12,13]

Plain radiographs are also an important diagnostic tool in the evaluation of bite wounds. They can reveal cortical injuries, fractures, foreign bodies (e.g., tooth), and subcutaneus air. Initial films can also serve as a baseline for the further evaluation of osteomyelitis. Computed tomography scanning utilizing bone windows is the preferred modality for the evaluation of bone injuries to the cranium.[14]

Treatment of bite wounds should begin by thorough cleansing of the wound with soap and water. This initial decontamination is an important step in the management of wounds from any source but is more important in those potentially infected with rabies or B viruses.[11,15] Local wound care should be followed with high-pressure (5 to 8 psi) irrigation of the wound.[16] When done properly, irrigation is an effective means of reducing the concentration of microorganisms in a wound, hence reducing the possibility of subsequent infection.[17] High-pressure irrigation is commonly done with sterile saline using a 30- to 60-cc syringe attached to a 19-gauge catheter.[18] Other solutions such as povidone-iodine surgical scrub, ethyl alcohol, and hydrogen peroxide are not recommended as irrigating solutions, since they can cause further tissue irritation and damage.[19] High-pressure irrigation should be avoided around the eye.[18] The amount of irrigating fluid used is dependent on the extent of the injury.

Abscesses should undergo incision and drainage. Débridement of necrotic and devitalized tissues, when appropriate, is also an important factor in minimizing the risk of infection. Débridement should always be kept to a minimum, as unnecessary removal of tissue may create a larger defect requiring more complicated surgical repairs.

There are no reliable prospective data to support standardized guidelines for primary repair (e.g., suturing) of bite wounds. Each wound should be considered separately. Factors such as the relative risk of infection, time from injury to presentation, location of the wound, cosmetic appearance, and functional status play a role in the decision to close a wound.[18] The risk of infection is determined by host factors, wound type, location of the wound, and local wound care (Table 18–1).[14] With respect to cat and dog bites, cat bites generally have a higher incidence of infections.

As a general rule, bite wounds should be left open and reevaluated within 48 to 72 hours. They can be treated by secondary intention or delayed primary closure after 3 to 5 days. Primary closure should be avoided in clinically infected wounds, puncture wounds, crush injuries, and wounds over the hands and wrists.[17,20,21] Despite the absence of prospective studies, wound closure is not recommended in injuries more than 24 hours old, extremity wounds more than 12 hours old, and facial wounds more than 24 hours old.[10,17] If closure is indicated for either cosmetic or functional reasons, wound edges can be loosely approximated using adhesive strips. Facial lacerations less than 24 hours old can be closed primarily if there is no evidence of infection. The use of

TABLE 18–1 ■ Factors Predisposing Patients to Wound Infection

HOST FACTORS
Age <2 and >50 years
Comorbid conditions (e.g., liver disease, splenectomy, diabetes mellitus, malignancy, and other immunocompromising conditions)
Pre-existing edema in the area of the bite
Chronic alcohol consumption
Use of immunosuppressive drugs (including chronic steroid use)

WOUND TYPE
Moderate-to-severe wounds
Cat and human bites
Puncture wound, crush injury
Presence of foreign material

WOUND LOCATION
Hand, wrist, foot
Scalp or face in infants and young children
Penetration of bone, joint, tendon sheath, or neurovascular structure
Proximity to a prosthetic joint

WOUND CARE
Delay in treatment >24 hours
Improper wound cleansing or débridement
Noncompliance with prescribed antibiotics

Adapted from Abrahamian FM: Dog bites: Bacteriology, management, and prevention. Curr Infect Dis Rep 2000;2:446–453.

TABLE 18–2 ■ Common Organisms Recovered from Infected Dog and Cat Bites

Organism	Dog bites (%)	Cat bites (%)
Pasteurella spp	50	75
Pasteurella canis	26	2
Pasteurella multocida subspecies *multocida*	12	54
Pasteurella multocida subspecies *septica*	10	28
Pasteurella stomatis	12	4
Streptococcus spp	46	46
Streptococcus mitis	22	23
Streptococcus mutans	12	11
Staphylococcus spp	46	35
Staphylococcus aureus	20	4
Staphylococcus epidermidis	18	18
Staphylococcus warneri	6	11
Corynebacterium spp	12	28
Neisseria spp	16	19
Moraxella spp	10	35
Fusobacterium spp	32	33
Fusobacterium nucleatum	16	25
Bacteroides spp	30	28
Bacteroides tectum	14	28
Porphyromonas spp	28	30
Prevotella spp	28	19

subcutaneous sutures should be kept to a minimum, since the presence of foreign material can increase the risk of infection.

Antibiotics should be initiated in patients with infected wounds or with conditions predisposing them to wound infection (Table 18–1), patients undergoing primary wound closure, and those with cat bites.[10,14,17,22] Initiation of antibiotics for dog bites with no evidence of infection not meeting the preceding criterion is somewhat controversial.[23–25] Initial empiric antibiotic therapy should demonstrate activity against the normal oral flora of the biting animal and the skin flora of the victim. The bacteriology of bite wounds is typically a complex microbiologic mix of aerobic and anaerobic organisms.[9,22,26–28] Table 18–2 presents common organisms recovered from 107 infected dog and cat bites. Less common organisms isolated from infected cat and dog bites include *Pseudomonas vesicularis*, *Bacillus firmus*, *Actinomyces viscosus*, *Propionibacterium acnes*, and *Peptostreptococcus anaerobius*. Unusual pathogens isolated from infected cat bites include *Erysipelothrix rhusiopathiae*, *Reimerella anatipestifer*, *Rothia dentocariosa*, *Pantoea agglomerans*, and *Weeksella virosa*.[28]

Single antimicrobial therapy may include a combination of β-lactam antibiotic and a β-lactamase inhibitor (e.g., amoxicillin-clavulanate or ampicillin-sulbactam) or a second-generation cephalosporin with anaerobic activity (e.g., cefoxitin or cefotetan). Combination antimicrobial therapy may include clindamycin with either penicillin or a fluoroquinolone, or trimethoprim/sulfamethoxazole (TMP-SMX). Table 18–3 outlines some examples of single and combination antimicrobial therapies for bite wounds. Because of inconsistent antimicrobial activity against *Pasteurella* species, first-generation cephalosporins (e.g., cephalexin), macrolides, clindamycin, and dicloxacillin should not be used as single agents. In vitro activities of the newer fluoroquinolones (e.g., levofloxacin) or the ketolide antibiotics have also been shown to be excellent against common bite wound isolates.[22] Specific antimicrobial coverage can later be tailored to wound culture results.

The duration of therapy typically ranges from 10 to 14 days, although other factors such as extent of injury, complications (e.g., septic arthritis or osteomyelitis), comorbid conditions, and rate of improvement need to be considered also. For patients undergoing prophylaxis the course is usually 3 to 5 days. Basic guidelines for hospital admission are outlined in Table 18–4. It is important to realize that these are only guidelines, and decisions should be individualized.

Significant hand wounds may require evaluation by a physician familiar with hand injuries. Elevation of the injured extremity during the first 48 to 72 hours is also an important component in the overall management of extremity wounds. Noncompliance with elevation of an injured extremity is a common cause of therapeutic failure. Outpatient management of patients with bite wounds requires close follow-up. Patients should return for clinical re-evaluation within 48 hours after the initial visit.

TABLE 18–3 ■ **Some Examples of Single and Combination Antimicrobial Therapies for Animal and Human Bite Wounds**

Drug(s)	Dosage/route/frequency*
Amoxicillin/clavulanate[†]	**Adult dosage:** 875/125 mg PO q12h or 500/125 mg PO q8h **Pediatric dosage** (base dose on amoxicillin component): <12 wk of age: 30 mg/kg/d PO in 2 divided doses q12h (use 125 mg/5 ml suspension) ≥12 wk (<40 kg): 25–45 mg/kg/d PO in 2 divided doses q12h ≥40 kg: same as adults
Ampicillin-sulbactam[†]	**Adult dosage:** 1.5–3 g IV q6h **Pediatric dosage:** (based on ampicillin component) <1 y: not recommended ≥1 y (<40 kg): 100–300 mg/kg/d IV in 4 equally divided doses q6h (max. 8 g/d ampicillin) ≥40 kg: same as adults
Cefotetan[†]	**Adult dosage:** 1–3 g IV q12h (maximum daily dosage should not exceed 6 g) **Pediatric dosage:** Not recommended
Cefoxitin[†]	**Adult dosage:** 1–2 g IV q6–8h **Pediatric dosage:** <3 mo: not recommended ≥3 mo: 80–160 mg/kg/d IV in equally divided doses q4–6h (The total daily dose should not exceed 12 g)
Clindamycin with TMP-SMX	**Clindamycin** **Adult dosage:** 150–450 mg PO q6h or 0.6–2.7 g/d IV divided equally in 2, 3, or 4 doses **Pediatric dosage:** 8–20 mg/kg/d PO divided into 3 or 4 equal doses <1 mo: 15–20 mg/kg/d IV in 3 or 4 equal doses ≥1 mo: 20–40 mg/kg/d IV in 3 or 4 equal doses **TMP-SMX**[†] **Adult dosage:** 160 mg trimethoprim–800 mg sulfamethoxazole (1 DS tablet) PO q12h; 8 mg/kg/d (based on the trimethoprim component) IV in 2 divided doses q12h **Pediatric dosage:** <2 mo: not recommended ≥2 mo: 8 mg/kg/d (based on the trimethoprim component) PO or IV in 2 divided doses q12h

TMP-SMX, trimethoprim/sulfamethoxazole.

*Readers are encouraged to refer to a drug reference manual for further details on dosage, dose adjustments, drug interactions, adverse reactions, precautions, and contraindications.

[†]Dosage needs to be adjusted based on creatinine clearance.

Complications

Complications of bites penetrating bones, joints, or tendons can include osteomyelitis, septic arthritis, and tenosynovitis. Compartment syndrome and necrotizing infection are other potential complications of bite wounds.[29] Vascular injuries can be complicated by subsequent dissection, thrombosis, and embolism.[30] Bites to the head and face can result in skull fractures, cerebral contusions, intracranial hemorrhage, and brain

TABLE 18–4 ■ **Basic Guidelines for Hospital Admission**

Multiple and severe injuries (especially hand wounds)
Moderate-to-severe local infection
Signs of systemic infection (e.g., fever, hypotension)
Wounds complicated by injuries to bone, joints, or tendons
Wounds with cranial perforation
Severe underlying illnesses or immunocompromising conditions
Failure of outpatient therapy
Social reasons

Adapted from Abrahamian FM: Dog bites: Bacteriology, management, and prevention. Curr Infect Dis Rep 2000;2:446–453.

abscess.[7,31] Cat-scratch disease may also develop following a bite or a scratch from a cat or a dog.

Rarely, fulminant septicemia, endocarditis, or meningitis may develop after a bite injury. *C. canimorsus* is often implicated as the cause of overwhelming septicemia following dog bite injuries, which has a latency period ranging from 1 to 8 days.[12,13,32,33] Initial manifestations of the *C. canimorsus* septicemia are nonspecific and include symptoms such as fever, chills, myalgias, vomiting, diarrhea, and abdominal pain.[32] *C. canimorsus* should be strongly suspected if the patient presents with symmetrical, peripheral gangrenous lesions. Other clinical manifestations of *C. canimorsus* sepsis can include local wound necrosis, purpura fulminans, endocarditis, meningitis, brain abscess, renal insufficiency, disseminated intravascular coagulation, and adult respiratory distress syndrome.[12] Conditions predisposing to *C. canimorsus* sepsis include asplenia, liver disease, compromised immune system, and use of immunosuppressive drugs (e.g., long-term steroid use).[10,12,13,32] The case fatality rate associated with *C. canimorsus* septicemia is 28%.[12]

C. canimorsus is typically susceptible to penicillins, clindamycin, and fluoroquinolones, and has a variable resistance to TMP-SMX and aminoglycosides.[12,32,34]

HUMAN BITES

The principal elements (e.g., history, physical examination, laboratory evaluation) of human bite wound therapy are similar to those of animal bites. The history should focus on features that would help identify patients at higher risk for complications (Table 18–1). A history of HIV or hepatitis B or C infection should be elicited for bites inflicted by other humans. The physical examination should include evaluation for signs and symptoms of infection and injuries to deeper structures.

Examination of human bites sustained while striking another person with a clenched fist deserves special consideration. In these injuries the wound is often found over the third, fourth, or fifth metacarpal head. The tooth may penetrate the extensor tendon, joint capsule, and the metacarpal head. Injuries to these structures may be overlooked if the hand is examined in an open position. In an open-hand position the skin and the tendon retract proximally with respect to the metacarpal head. Upon inspection of the wound with the hand in this position the tendon will appear intact, leading to the conclusion that the joint capsule and metacarpal head are not violated. However, since the site of the skin perforation is relative to the position of the hand at the time of the impact, the wound should be examined with the hand in a clenched-fist position. Careful exploration and direct visualization by a physician familiar with hand injuries may be necessary to evaluate the depth of the wound and to exclude underlying tendon, joint capsule, or bone injuries.[35,36]

As with animal bites, routine Gram stain and bacterial cultures are not necessary for noninfected human bites. However, both aerobic and anaerobic cultures are indicated for infected wounds. Radiographs can serve as a baseline for evaluation of osteomyelitis from bites that cause bone injuries.

Treatment of human bite wounds begins by washing the wound with soap and water and high-pressure (5 to 8 psi) irrigation with a copious volume of normal saline. Necrotic and devitalized tissues should undergo débridement, and abscesses should be incised and drained. Primary closure of human bite wounds is frequently avoided.[17] Closure is most often accomplished by secondary intention or delayed primary closure after 3 to 5 days. Primary closure should also be avoided in clinically infected wounds, puncture wounds, crush injuries, and wounds over the hands and wrists.

Antimicrobial therapy should be initiated for infected wounds and in persons at high risk of wound infection (Table 18–1). Patients undergoing primary wound closure and patients with noninfected hand bite wounds may also benefit from antimicrobial therapy.[37] The initial empiric therapy should be directed against *Staphylococcus aureus*, *Haemophilus influenzae*, and β-lactamase-producing oral anaerobic bacteria.[10] Table 18–5 presents common organisms recovered from infected human bites. *Eikenella corrodens* and α-hemolytic streptococci often coexist and demonstrate a synergistic relationship.[38] *E. corrodens* is more commonly cultured from dental scrapings than from saliva and as a result is more often present in clenched-fist injuries.[39]

Proper choices of antibiotics include amoxicillin-clavulanic acid, ampicillin-sulbactam, cefoxitin, cefotetan, imipenem, meropenem, or piperacillin-tazobactam. Combination therapy can include cefuroxime with clindamycin or metronidazole. Other alternatives can include clindamycin with either ciprofloxacin or TMP-SMX (Table 18–3). *E. corrodens* typically is resistant to penicillinase-resistant penicillins (e.g., oxacillin, methicillin, dicloxacillin, and nafcillin), most aminoglycosides, clindamycin, erythromycin, metronidazole, and first-generation cephalosporins. Generally it is susceptible to second- or third-generation cephalosporins, penicillin, amoxicillin-clavulanic acid, tetracycline, TMP-SMX, and ciprofloxacin.[35,38]

Indications for hospital admission are similar to those for animal bites (Table 18–4). Significant hand wounds, especially clenched-fist injuries, may require evaluation by a physician familiar with hand injuries. Hand wounds benefit from 3 to 5 days of immobilization in a splint in the position of function and with elevation. Outpatient management requires close follow-up, and patients should return for re-evaluation within 48 hours after the initial visit.

Human bites are associated with a higher rate of infection than animal bites are. Other complications can include arthritis, osteomyelitis, toxic shock syndrome, and septicemia.[40]

TETANUS AND RABIES IMMUNOPROPHYLAXIS

Tetanus immunization is important to consider in bites of all types. Table 18–6 provides a summary guide to tetanus prophylaxis in routine wound management.[41,42]

Rabies prophylaxis should also be considered with animal bites. Although human rabies is rare in the United

TABLE 18–5 ■ Common Organisms Recovered from Infected Human Bite Wounds

α-Hemolytic streptococci
Staphylococcus aureus
Staphylococcus epidermidis
Corynebacterium spp
Eikenella corrodens
Haemophilus influenzae
Prevotella melaninogenica
Fusobacterium nucleatum
Peptostreptococcus spp

TABLE 18–6 ■ Current Summary Guide to Tetanus Prophylaxis in Routine Wound Management

History of adsorbed tetanus toxoid (doses)	Clean, minor wounds* (nontetanus-prone wounds)		All other wounds† (tetanus-prone wounds)	
	Td‡ (0.5 ml IM)	TIG (250 U IM)	Td‡ (0.5 ml IM)	TIG (250 U IM)
Unknown or <3	Yes§	No	Yes§	Yes
Three or more	No‖	No	No¶	No

Td, diphtheria-tetanus vaccine adsorbed; DTaP, diphtheria-tetanus-acellular pertussis vaccine adsorbed; TIG, tetanus immune globulin.

*Typically superficial, clean, linear with sharp edges, recent (<6 h old), neurovascularly intact, and not infected.

†Tetanus-prone wounds include, but are not limited to, contaminated wounds (e.g., with dirt, feces, soil, or saliva); puncture wounds; avulsions; and wounds resulting from missiles, crushing, burn, or frost bite. Other wound characteristics can include deep (>1 cm); >6 h old; infection; neurovascularly compromised (e.g., necrotic tissue).

‡Use DTaP for children <7 y old.

§The primary immunization series should be completed at recommended monthly intervals. Primary immunization is recommended to start during infancy with IM injections of DTaP at 2, 4, 6, and 15 mo of age, with a booster at 4 to 6 y of age. Additional boosters are given with Td once every 10 y after the last dose. For adults and children >7 y old, the first two doses of Td are given 4 to 8 wk apart, and the third dose of Td is given 6 to 12 mo after the second dose.

‖Yes if >10 y have elapsed since the last dose.

¶Yes if >5 y have elapsed since the last dose.

States, approximately 16,000 to 39,000 patients receive rabies postexposure prophylaxis (RPEP) every year.[43] A recent multicenter, prospective study of patients presenting to the ED with an animal exposure demonstrated that RPEP is often used inappropriately.[44] The decision to initiate RPEP is dependent on several key factors: type of exposure, animal type, availability of the animal for brain testing or observation, the location of the incident (i.e., the probability of rabies for that animal in that particular region), animal's history of immunization, and circumstances of the attack (i.e., provoked).

The animal's behavior and circumstances of an attack are sometimes factors to assess when considering RPEP. Rabid animals tend to be agitated and attack indiscriminately. Normal behavior in an animal makes the possibility of rabies less likely, although assessment of "normal" behavior in wild terrestrial carnivores is difficult. Typically most animals avoid humans, and often bites are provoked. Feeding or handling a healthy animal is considered provocation. A history of current rabies vaccination in any animal makes it less likely that the animal has acquired an infection.[45]

A summary algorithm of current RPEP recommended by the Advisory Committee on Immunization Practices (ACIP) is depicted in Figure 18–1.[45,46] It is imperative to realize that regions can have slightly different approaches to RPEP because of geographic variations in the prevalence of rabies. Physicians should be familiar with their own local rabies epidemiology and site-specific practice and reporting guidelines. The local health department should be consulted for current information.

RPEP should always include the administration of both active and passive immunization, except in persons who have been previously immunized. Active immunization commonly is achieved by human diploid cell vaccine (HDCV). Other preparations available in the United States include rabies vaccine adsorbed (RVA) and puri-

fied chick embryo cell vaccine (PCEC). All three types of vaccine are equally safe and efficacious when used properly.[45] The development of antibodies by active immunization takes 7 to 10 days and usually persists for 2 years or longer. For the purpose of RPEP a regimen of five 1 ml doses of any of the vaccines should be given intramuscularly. The first dose should be given as soon as possible after exposure (day 0), with the remaining four doses administered on days 3, 7, 14, and 28 after the first vaccination. Patients with a prior history of vaccination should only receive intramuscular injections of the vaccine on days 0 and 3. The preferred site for intramuscular injections for adults is the deltoid area and for children is the anterolateral aspect of the thigh. There is also an intradermal preparation of HDCV; however, the intradermal route is reserved only for pre-exposure (primary or booster) vaccination. The gluteal region should be avoided for rabies vaccine injections because of diminished antibody response in that area.[47]

To provide protection while awaiting the immune response from vaccination, passive immunization is achieved by the administration of human rabies immune globulin (RIG). RIG provides rapid protection with a serum half-life of 21 days. The recommended dose of RIG is 20 IU/kg of body weight. Adherence to this dosage is important, since higher doses have the potential for suppressing active antibody production. If possible, a full dose should be infiltrated into the areas around and into the wound.[48] If it is not possible to inject the full dose around the wound (e.g., finger wound) the remaining dose should be administered intramuscularly at a location distant from the site of the vaccine injection. Repeated injections of RIG are not necessary. RIG should not be administered to persons with a prior history of rabies immunization. If the rabies vaccine and RIG were not administered on the same day, RIG may be given through the seventh day after the first dose of vaccine. Beyond

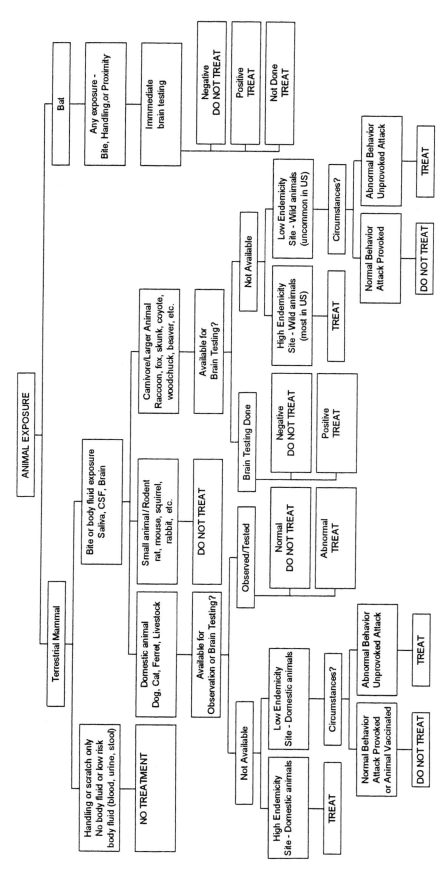

FIGURE 18–1. Summary algorithm for determining need for rabies postexposure prophylaxis in the United States. Local health department should be consulted for advice regarding rabies endemicity. Rabies postexposure prophylaxis should be initiated if there is reasonable probability of a bat bite, scratch, or mucous membrane exposure. Postexposure prophylaxis is also warranted if a bat is found in the room of a person who is unable to or incapable of attesting to a direct contact (e.g., a sleeping person awakens to find a bat in the room or a bat is found in a room occupied by an unattended child or a mentally disabled or intoxicated person).

this period, since active immunization has taken effect, RIG is no longer indicated. To prevent antigen-antibody antagonism, RIG and rabies vaccine should not be administered at the same site or by the same syringe.

SUMMARY

Bite wounds are common injuries, and physicians need to be familiar with the various elements of therapy. Principles of bite wound therapy include thorough cleansing of the wound, copious irrigation, cautious débridement, and drainage of abscesses when indicated. In addition, proper antibiotics, elevation of extremity wounds, attention to tetanus and rabies prophylaxis, and close follow-up are also integral components of bite wound therapy.

REFERENCES

1. Sacks JJ, Kresnow M, Houston B: Dog bites: How big a problem? Injury Prev 1996;2:52–54.
2. Sacks JJ, Lockwood R, Hornreich J, et al: Fatal dog attacks, 1989–1994. Pediatrics 1996;97:891–895.
3. Weiss HB, Friedman DI, Coben JH: Incidence of dog bite injuries treated in emergency departments. JAMA 1998; 279:51–53.
4. Huston HR, Anglin D, Pineda GV, et al: Law enforcement K-9 dog bites: Injuries, complications, and trends. Ann Emerg Med 1997;29:637–642.
5. Snyder CC: Animal bite infections of the hand. Hand Clin 1998;14:691–711.
6. Feder HM, Nelson R, Reiher HW: Bat bite? Lancet 1997; 350:1300.
7. Brogan TV, Bratton SL, Dowd D, et al: Severe dog bites in children. Pediatrics 1995;96:947–950.
8. Elliott DC, Kufera JA, Myers RAM: Necrotizing soft tissue infections. Risk factors for mortality and strategies for management. Ann Surg 1996;224:672–683.
9. Ordog GJ: The bacteriology of dog bite wounds on initial presentation. Ann Emerg Med 1986;15:1324–1329.
10. Goldstein EJC: Bite wounds and infection. Clin Infect Dis 1992;14:633–640.
11. Holmes GP, Chapman LE, Stewart J, et al: B Virus Working Group. Guidelines for the prevention and treatment of B virus infections in exposed persons. Clin Infect Dis 1995; 20:421–439.
12. Kullberg BJ, Westendorp RJ, van't Wout JW, et al: Purpura fulminans and symmetrical peripheral gangrene caused by *Capnocytophaga canimorsus* (Formerly DF-2) septicemia—A complication of dog bite. Medicine 1991;70:287–292.
13. Mellor DJ, Bhandari S, Kerr K, et al: Man's best friend: Life threatening sepsis after minor dog bite. BMJ 1997; 314:129–130.
14. Abrahamian FM: Dog bites: Bacteriology, management, and prevention. Curr Infect Dis Rep 2000;2:446–453.
15. Dean DJ, Baer GM, Thompson WR: Studies on the local treatment of rabies-infected wounds. Bull World Health Organ 1963;28:477–486.
16. Edlich RF, Rodeheaver GT, Morgan RF, et al: Principles of emergency wound management. Ann Emerg Med 1988; 17:1284–1302.
17. Fleisher GR: The management of bite wounds. N Engl J Med 1999;340:138–140.
18. Hollander JE, Singer AJ: Laceration management. Ann Emerg Med 1999;34:356–367.
19. Oberg MS, Lindsey D: Do not put hydrogen peroxide or povidone iodine into wounds. J Trauma 1980;20:323–324.
20. Garcia VF: Animal bites and Pasteurella infections. Pediatr Rev 1997;18:127–130.
21. Wiggins ME, Akelman E, Weiss APC: The management of dog bites and dog bite infections to the hand. Orthopedics 1994;17:617–623.
22. Goldstein EJC: Current concepts on animal bites: Bacteriology and therapy. Curr Clin Top Infect Dis 1999;19:99–111.
23. Dire DJ, Hogan DE, Walker JS: Prophylactic oral antibiotic for low-risk dog bite wounds. Pediatr Emerg Care 1992; 8:194–199.
24. Cummings P: Antibiotics to prevent infection in patients with dog bite wounds: A meta-analysis of randomized trials. Ann Emerg Med 1994;23:535–540.
25. Callaham M: Prophylactic antibiotics in dog bite wounds: Nipping at the heels of progress. Ann Emerg Med 1994; 23:577–579.
26. Goldstein EJC, Citron DM, Wield B, et al: Bacteriology of human and animal bite wounds. J Clin Microbiol 1978; 8:667–672.
27. Brook I: Microbiology of human and animal bite wounds in children. Pediatr Infect Dis J 1987;6:29–32.
28. Talan DA, Citron DM, Abrahamian FM, et al: Bacteriologic analysis of infected dog and cat bites. N Engl J Med 1999;340:85–92.
29. Anderson PJ, Zafar I, Nizam M, et al: Compartment syndrome in victims of dog bites. Injury 1997;28:717.
30. Meuli M, Glarner H: Delayed cerebral infarction after dog bites: Case report. J Trauma 1994;37:848–849.
31. Jones N, Khoosal M: Infected dog and cat bites. N Engl J Med 1999;340:1841.
32. Pers C, Gahrn-Hansen B, Frederiksen W: *Capnocytophaga canimorsus* septicemia in Denmark, 1982–1995: Review of 39 cases. Clin Infect Dis 1996;23:71–75.
33. Hovenga S, Tulleken JE, Möller LVM, et al: Dog-bite induced sepsis: A report of four cases. Intensive Care Med 1997; 23:1179–1180.
34. Verghese A, Hamati F, Berk S, et al: Susceptibility of dysgonic fermenter 2 to antimicrobial agents in vitro. Antimicrob Agents Chemother 1988;32:78–80.
35. Faciszewski T, Coleman DA: Human bite infections of the hand. Hand Clinics 1998;14:683–690.
36. Fremling MA, Francel T, Weeks PM: Evaluation of hand injuries. In Martin DS, Collins ED (eds): Manual of Acute Hand Injuries, St Louis, Mosby–Year Book, 1998, pp 34–94.
37. Zubowicz VN, Gravier M: Management of early human bites of the hand: A prospective randomized study. Plast Reconstr Surg 1991;88:111–114.
38. Griego RD, Rosen T, Orengo IF, et al: Dog, cat, and human bites: A review. J Am Acad Dermatol 1995;33:1019–1029.
39. Rayan GM, Putnam JL, Cahill SL: *Eikenella corrodens* in human mouth flora. Am J Hand Surg 1988;13:953–956.
40. Long WT, Filler BC, Cox E II, et al: Toxic shock syndrome after a human bite to the hand. Am J Hand Surg 1988; 13:957–959.
41. CDC surveillance summaries: Tetanus surveillance-US, 1995–1997. MMWR Morb Mortal Wkly Rep 1998;7(SS- 2): 1–13.
42. Abrahamian FM: Tetanus: An update on an ancient disease. Infect Dis Clin Pract 2000;9:228–235.
43. Krebs JW, Long-Martin SC, Childs JE: Causes, costs and estimates of rabies postexposure prophylaxis treatments in the United States. J Public Health Manag Pract 1998;4(5):56–62.

44. Moran GJ, Talan DA, Mower W, et al: Appropriateness of rabies postexposure prophylaxis treatment for animal exposures. JAMA 2000;284:1001–1007.

45. Human rabies prevention—United States, 1999. MMWR Morb Mortal Wkly Rep 1999;48(RR-1):1–21.

46. Human rabies—California, Georgia, Minnesota, New York, and Wisconsin, 2000. MMWR Morb Mortal Wkly Rep 2000;49:1111–1115.

47. Fishbein DB, Sawyer LA, Reid Sanden FL, et al: Administration of human diploid-cell rabies vaccine in the gluteal area. N Engl J Med 1988;318:124–125.

48. Wilde H, Sirikawin S, Sabcharoen A, et al: Failure of postexposure treatment of rabies in children. Clin Infect Dis 1996;22:228–232.

ELIE BERBARI, MD
DOUGLAS R. OSMON, MD, MPH
JAMES M. STECKELBERG, MD

Osteomyelitis and Infectious Arthritis

chapter 19

OSTEOMYELITIS

Osteomyelitis, an ancient disease found in dinosaur bones, remains a challenging clinical problem.[1-3] Osteomyelitis is due to a variety of different microorganisms (Table 19–1). Certain organisms such as *Staphylococcus aureus*, a colonizer of the skin and the anterior nares in 30% to 50% of the population, preferentially cause osteomyelitis because they bind to bone through the expression of receptors for fibronectin, laminin, collagen, or sialoglycoprotein present on the bone surface. Osteomyelitis can be produced by several mechanisms: hematogenous seeding, contiguous spread from adjacent soft tissues and joints, and direct inoculation of microorganisms into the bone through trauma or surgery. Once infection becomes established, the bacteria produce a local inflammatory reaction that promotes bone necrosis and the formation of sequestra.

Several authorities have tried to classify osteomyelitis. Waldvogel's classification of osteomyelitis is based on the duration of illness (acute vs. chronic), the mechanism of infection (hematogenous vs. contiguous), and the presence of vascular insufficiency. Cierny and Mader's classification of osteomyelitis is based on the part of the bone affected and the physiologic status of the host.

Hematogenous osteomyelitis occurs most often in children and the elderly. In children it frequently occurs in the metaphysis of the femur, tibia, and humerus. Hematogenous osteomyelitis in adults often seeds the intervertebral disc space and two adjacent vertebrae. Bacteria will lodge more commonly in the hypervascularized anterior end plates. The infection eventually will inhibit the supply of nutrients to the nucleus pulposus, leading to necrosis and disc space narrowing.

Contiguous focus osteomyelitis is much more common in adults than in children and is typically seen in persons more than 50 years of age who have diabetes or severe peripheral vascular disease. Contiguous focus osteomyelitis is due to spread of infection from adjacent soft tissue or joints or to direct inoculation of microorganisms through trauma or surgery.

Management of Osteomyelitis

The optimal management of osteomyelitis requires a multidisciplinary team of physicians that might include (depending on the infected bone) an orthopedic surgeon, neurosurgeon, oral surgeon, plastic surgeon, vascular surgeon, invasive radiologist, and an infectious disease specialist. The usual goals of therapy are the eradication of the infection and the restoration of function. Treatment of established chronic osteomyelitis requires aggressive surgical débridement and prolonged antimicrobial therapy.[1-3] Long-bone osteomyelitis in children and vertebral osteomyelitis in adults are successfully

TABLE 19–1 ■ Microbiology of Osteomyelitis

COMMON
Staphylococcus aureus
Coagulase-negative staphylococcus
β-hemolytic streptococci
Enterobacteriaceae
Pseudomonas aeruginosa
Anaerobic

RARE
Atypical mycobacteria
  Mycobacterium kansasii
  Mycobacterium fortuitum
  Mycobacterium avium-intracellulare complex
Gemella haemolysans
Mycoplasma spp
Aspergillus spp
Candida spp
Actinomycosis
Eikenella corrodens

treated medically without surgery in most cases. If treatment is delayed, osteomyelitis can progress from superficial to diffuse disease or from Cierny Mader stage 1 or 2 to stage 3 or 4 and thus become much more difficult to eradicate. Untreated acute hematogenous osteomyelitis in children can spread to adjacent joints and cause infectious arthritis. If untreated, vertebral osteomyelitis can have neurologic sequelae including paralysis either through extension to the epidural space or through spinal column instability. Long-term complications of untreated osteomyelitis include systemic amyloidosis and squamous cell carcinoma of the skin at the exit site of a sinus tract.

Medical Therapy

Selection of the optimal antimicrobial agent for the treatment of osteomyelitis depends on definitive identification of the microorganism(s) causing the infection and knowledge of its antimicrobial susceptibilities. Other factors that might influence the choice of a specific antimicrobial include drug interactions, toxicities, and cost. Suggested antimicrobials for specific pathogens causing osteomyelitis are shown in Table 19–2. Quinolones have

TABLE 19–2 ■ Antibiotic Therapy of Chronic Osteomyelitis in Adults for Selected Microorganisms

Microorganisms	First choice	Alternative choice

Staphylococci
  Oxacillin sensitive
	Nafcillin sodium or oxacillin sodium 1.5–2 g
	  IV q4 h × 4–6 wk
	or
	Cefazolin 1 g IV q8h × 4–6 wk
		Vancomycin* 15 mg/kg IV q12h × 4–6 wk

Oxacillin resistant	Vancomycin* 15 mg/kg IV q12h × 4–6 wk	Linezolid 600 mg PO or IV q12h × 6 wk or Levofloxacin 400 mg/d PO and rifampin 600 mg/d PO × 6 wk

Penicillin-sensitive
streptococci
	Aqueous crystalline penicillin G 20 MU/24 h
	  IV continuously or in 6 equally divided
	  doses for 4–6 wk
	or
	Ceftriaxone 2 g IV or IM q24h × 4–6 wk
	or
	Cefazolin 1 g IV q8h × 4–6 wk
		Vancomycin 15 mg/kg IV q12h × 4–6 wk

Enterococci or
streptococci with an
MIC ≥ 0.5 µg/ml or
nutritionally variant
streptococci
	Aqueous crystalline penicillin G 20 MU/24h
	  IV continuously or in 6 equally divided
	  doses × 4–6 wk
	or
	Ampicillin sodium 12 g/24 h IV continuously
	  or in 6 equally divided doses
	- - - - - - - -
	The addition of gentamicin sulfate 1 mg/kg IV
	  or IM q8h × 1–2 wk is optional
		Vancomycin* 15 mg/kg IV q12h × 4–6 wk
		- - - - - - - -
		The addition of gentamicin sulfate 1 mg/kg IV or
		  IM q8h × 1–2 wk is optional

Enterobacteriaceae	Ceftriaxone 2 g IV q24h × 4–6 wk	Ciprofloxacin 500–750 mg PO q12h × 4–6 wk
Pseudomonas aeruginosa or Enterobacter spp	Cefepime 1 g IV q12h × 4–6 wk or Meropenem 1 g IV q8h × 4–6 wk	Ciprofloxacin 750 mg PO q12h × 4–6 wk or Ceftazidime 2 g IV q8h

*Dosages recommended are for patients with normal renal function.

been shown to impair fracture healing in vitro and in vivo in animal models.[4] Therefore, if possible, they should be avoided in patients with an infected nonunion.

In patients with chronic osteomyelitis and no acute soft tissue infection or sepsis syndrome, antimicrobial therapy should be withheld until deep bone cultures have been obtained. In the group of patients already receiving antimicrobial therapy, antimicrobials should be withheld for a period of at least 1 week before surgical débridement and culture ascertainment. Tissue and purulent material should be sent at the time of bone biopsy or surgical débridement for aerobic and anaerobic cultures. The microorganism(s) obtained from sinus tract swab cultures are not accurate in predicting the microbiology of deep infection. The isolation of S. aureus from a swab culture of the sinus tract, however, correlates highly with an associated deep infection. It is important to obtain a culture for anaerobic bacteria, especially in contiguous osteomyelitis in diabetic patients and osteomyelitis due to animal bites. Tissue specimens should be sent to both the pathology laboratory and the microbiology laboratory. Review of tissue for pathogenic organisms is important to document the presence of osteomyelitis, to exclude the presence of squamous cell carcinoma (in patient with long-standing sinus tract), and to diagnose unusual infections such as fungi and mycobacteria. The microbiologist should perform a Gram stain and cultures on all specimens. In selected cases, special culturing techniques for organisms such as fungi, mycobacteria, *Mycoplasma*, or *Brucella* may be required. Certain microorganisms are more prevalent in some patient groups (Table 19–3). Unused surgical specimen(s) may be saved in the microbiology laboratory at 4°C to 6°C for a short time. Specialized cultures can be added if the aerobic and the anaerobic cultures do not yield pathogenic organisms.

Once the microorganism responsible for the infection has been identified, antimicrobial susceptibility tests should be performed and appropriate antimicrobial therapy commenced (Table 19–2). Data from experimental animal models of osteomyelitis and some human studies suggest that the addition of rifampin to β-lactams, vancomycin, or quinolone for S. aureus osteomyelitis may be superior to monotherapy, particularly in the presence of foreign bodies.[1] Because no large clinical trials have confirmed this superiority and because of some contradictory data in animal models,[5] we have not routinely implemented this therapy in our orthopedic infectious diseases practice at the Mayo Clinic.

The availability of newer antimicrobial agents (quinolones, oxazolidinone) with high oral bioavailability offering concentrations in serum and tissue comparable to concentrations following parenteral administration has led some experts to study the efficacy of orally administered antimicrobials in osteomyelitis. Oral quinolones have been studied most.[6] In selected populations with infection due to susceptible organisms, outcomes of patients treated with oral quinolones were not significantly different statistically from outcomes of conventionally treated patients. Unfortunately these trials have lacked sufficient statistical power to establish equivalency, especially when particular

TABLE 19–3 ■ Osteomyelitis in Special Groups

Mechanism	Special groups	Microbiology
Hematogenous	Most common cause in children and adults	*Staphylococcus aureus*
	Neonates	Enterobacteriaceae, group B streptococci
	Sickle cell disease	*Salmonella* spp, *S. aureus*
	Injection drug users	*Pseudomonas aeruginosa*, *S. aureus*, Candida sp
	Infants and children*	*Haemophilus influenzae*
Vertebral osteomyelitis	Most common in adults	*S. aureus*
	Urinary tract infection	Aerobic gram-negative bacilli, *Enterococcus* spp
	Injection drug users	*P. aeruginosa*, *S. aureus*, Candida sp
	Spine surgery with or without spinal hardware implantation	Coagulase-negative staphylococci, *S. aureus*, and aerobic gram-negative bacilli
	Candidemia due to infections of intravascular devices	*Candida* spp
Contiguous focus osteomyelitis	Diabetes mellitus or vascular insufficiency or osteomyelitis of the long bones following a contaminated open fracture	Polymicrobial: *S. aureus*, β-hemolytic streptococci, enterococci, aerobic gram-negative bacilli
	Soil contamination	*Clostridium* spp, *Bacillus* spp, *Stenotrophomonas maltophilia*, *Nocardia* spp, atypical mycobacteria, *Aspergillus* spp
	Orthopedic fixation devices	*S. aureus* or coagulase-negative staphylococci
	Cat bites	*Pasteurella multocida*
	Osteomyelitis of the foot following puncture injuries by nails or other sharp objects	*P. aeruginosa*
	Mandibular or skull osteomyelitis following periodontal infection	*Actinomyces* spp

*The incidence of invasive disease due to *H. influenzae* is decreasing because of the *H. influenzae* b conjugated vaccine that is now administered routinely to children.

organisms such as *S. aureus* are evaluated. In addition the frequent development of resistance to specific antimicrobials by some organisms during therapy precludes their use as monotherapy (e.g., the use of rifampin or ciprofloxacin for *S. aureus* osteomyelitis).[7,8]

The optimal duration of therapy in osteomyelitis has been the subject of great debate, largely because there are no prospective randomized human trials assessing the length of antimicrobial therapy in patients with osteomyelitis. Because it takes 4 to 6 weeks for the débrided bone to be covered by vascularized soft tissue, because of the high relapse rate of 20%, and because of anecdotal experiences suggesting a higher relapse rate with a shorter duration of therapy, many experts advocate a total duration of 4 to 6 weeks of parenteral antimicrobial therapy. Other authors have suggested longer treatment of 6 to 8 weeks followed by 3 months of oral antimicrobial therapy.[9] We believe that 4 to 6 weeks of directed antimicrobial therapy is sufficient for osteomyelitis due to most common organisms, given an adequate surgical débridement. If multiple débridements are required, then 4 to 6 weeks of antimicrobial therapy should be given after the last débridement. Administration of antimicrobial therapy for longer periods might promote antimicrobial resistance and drug toxicity. This therapy can be administered on an outpatient basis in most cases.

Acute hematogenous osteomyelitis of the long bones in children and vertebral osteomyelitis in adults may be cured with antimicrobial therapy alone. The duration of therapy for acute hematogenous osteomyelitis of the long bones in children is 3 to 4 weeks. After 7 to 10 days of intravenous antimicrobial therapy the intravenous antimicrobial agents are switched to an oral agent for the remaining 2 to 3 weeks.[10] In this case, surgical intervention would be indicated when the femoral head is involved, when efforts to make a specific microbiologic diagnosis with noninvasive techniques have failed, when there are neurologic complications and sequestra, or when appropriate antimicrobial therapy has failed to improve the condition. The duration of antimicrobial therapy for vertebral osteomyelitis in adults is usually 4 to 6 weeks of parenteral antimicrobial therapy. In cases with extensive epidural abscess that is not surgically débrided, longer use of antimicrobials may be warranted. Surgical intervention would be warranted in cases in which diagnosis is required or when there is neurologic compromise or failure to improve on medical therapy alone.[11]

Surgical Therapy

Surgical débridement and resection of dead and infected bone, removal of foreign bodies, rigid fixation of fractures, local antimicrobial therapy with antibiotic-impregnated polymethylmethacrylate beads or spacers, and prolonged systemic directed antimicrobial therapy are often warranted.[1–3] In difficult cases, partial or complete amputation of a limb may be required to control the spread of the infectious process. In such a case discontinuation of antimicrobial therapy shortly after the amputation is warranted. In occasional cases, delayed reconstructive orthopedic surgery such as bone grafting and distraction osteogenesis (Ilizarov technique) are also necessary. To reduce the risk of recurrence after medical and surgical therapy, physiologic factors (Table 19–1) that may promote treatment failure should be modified (e.g., cessation of smoking, enhancement of the local blood supply in the area of the infection, and improved control of diabetes mellitus).

Adjunctive Therapy

Hyperbaric oxygen has been used as an adjunctive measure for patients with chronic refractory osteomyelitis.[12] Hyperbaric oxygen increases the oxygen tension in infected tissue, including bone. An adequate oxygen tension is necessary for oxygen-dependent killing of organisms by the polymorphonuclear leukocytes and for fibroblast activity leading to angiogenesis and wound healing. In addition, hyperbaric oxygen has a direct bactericidal or bacteriostatic effect on anaerobic organisms. Randomized studies in animals showed that adjunctive hyperbaric oxygen therapy reduced the number of bacterial colonies more than antimicrobial therapy alone did.[13,14] Anecdotal experience in humans includes patients with recurrent and refractory osteomyelitis. To our knowledge there are no randomized trials assessing the efficacy of adjunctive hyperbaric oxygen therapy in humans. Hyperbaric oxygen has been administered once daily for 90 to 120 minutes at 2 to 3 atmospheres at 100% oxygen tension for 15 to 20 separate sessions.

Outcome and Complications

Despite advancement in antimicrobial therapy and surgical techniques, infection recurs in 22% of cases. Recurrence can occur years after treatment.

In some difficult to treat cases the consequences of aggressive surgical and medical treatment for osteomyelitis may be more detrimental than the disease itself. In these cases, palliative therapy with local wound care and oral antimicrobial suppressive therapy is warranted. Close monitoring for squamous cell carcinoma, systemic amyloidosis, pathologic fracture, and drug toxicities is needed.

INFECTIOUS ARTHRITIS

Native Joint Infectious Arthritis

Infectious arthritis is an inflammatory disease of a joint. Hematogenous seeding of the joint is the most common mechanism of infection, followed by direct traumatic or surgical seeding of the joint. The tropism of bacteria to the synovial tissue is due to its rich vascular supply and the absence of basement membrane. *S. aureus* is the most common cause of infection, in part because of its ability to bind to sialoprotein, a glycoprotein found in joints. Direct inoculation of microorganisms through trauma, arthrotomy, arthroscopy, or arthrocentesis also occurs.

Infection due to contiguous soft tissue infection or periarticular osteomyelitis is rare. Biochemical changes in the cartilage occur within hours following microbial invasion of the synovium. Locally produced cytokines and proteolytic enzymes cause hydrolysis of the cartilage proteoglycans and collagens, eventually narrowing the joint space. Polymorphonuclear cells infiltrate the synovium within 3 days. Mononuclear cells are seen afterward. The degree of cartilage destruction is in part microorganism dependent. Microorganisms such as *S. aureus* have a tendency to cause greater cartilage damage, whereas others such as *Neisseria gonorrheae* have little effect on the cartilage. Coagulase-negative staphylococci, rarely implicated in monoarticular hematogenous infectious arthritis, are commonly encountered after arthroscopic procedures. *Propionibacterium acnes* is often encountered in infectious arthritis of the shoulder following arthroscopic procedures and rotator cuff repair.[15]

Variables that have been associated with an increased risk of native infectious arthritis include rheumatoid arthritis, diabetes mellitus, malignancy, prior surgery on the joint, and old age.[16] Prior joint damage that compromised local host defenses can also predispose the joint to hematogenous infection. In addition, factors that increase the risk of bacteremia such as intravenous drug use and chronic skin infection or that allow direct inoculation of microorganisms such as therapeutic arthrocentesis predispose to infection.

A causative microorganism is documented in 70% to 90% of cases in monoarticular infectious arthritis. Culture-negative cases (aerobic cultures) are usually the result of prior use of antimicrobials, fastidious organisms, and crystal-induced arthritis (Fig. 19–1). In polyarticular disease the differential includes viral, reactive, and noninfectious arthritides (Fig. 19–1). Lidocaine used to anesthetize the skin before a diagnostic aspiration has been found to have an antimicrobial effect[17]. This observation could potentially explain some culture-negative cases. Culture of synovial fluid for aerobes and anaerobes and other organisms should depend on the clinical circumstances. The Bactec system might be superior to standard culturing techniques. Molecular testing using polymerase chain reaction is now the test of choice for detecting *Borrelia burgdorferi* and *Tropheryma whippleii*. In addition synovial tissue culture is superior to synovial fluid culture in detecting mycobacteria and fungi. Synovial fluid from adults should be examined under a polarized microscope for the presence of monosodium urate and calcium pyrophosphate crystals. It is often difficult to distinguish infection from inflammatory arthritis using radiographic methods in the setting of rheumatoid arthritis when the development of a rapid, destructive arthritis in one or two joints suggests infection. Computed tomography (CT) scans, magnetic resonance imaging (MRI), and indium bone scans are useful for making the diagnosis of infectious arthritis in deep-seated joints such as hips and sacroiliacs joints. Sacroiliac or sternoclavicular joint disease can be evaluated with all three radiographic modalities.

The differential diagnosis of patients with an acute onset of fever, chills, and an inflammatory arthritis of one or more joints revolves around three groups of diseases: infectious arthritis, crystal-induced arthritis, and a rheumatologic disorder (Fig. 19–1).

Management of Patient with Infectious Arthritis

Infectious arthritis is a medical emergency. Any delay of the diagnosis and subsequent therapy will jeopardize the function of the joint. Prompt therapy has been found to be the major determinant of good functional outcome.[18] The goals of therapy are to prevent irreversible cartilage destruction and to eradicate infection. To achieve that goal, antimicrobial therapy, drainage, and early articular rest should go hand in hand.

Medical Therapy

Antimicrobial therapy should be started as soon as the diagnosis is suspected and after obtaining blood and synovial fluid cultures. The initial empiric choice of antimicrobial therapy is based on the Gram stain results and the clinical scenario (Table 19–4). Once the microorganism is isolated and the in vitro antimicrobial susceptibility determined, antimicrobial therapy should be adjusted. The choice of a specific antimicrobial agent depends on the pathogen isolated and its susceptibility profile, pharmacokinetics, tissue penetration, and potential toxicities. Integration of this knowledge with information about drug allergies, current medications, concurrent remote infection, and hepatic and renal insufficiency allows for selection of an optimal antimicrobial agent and dosage. Suggested antimicrobials for specific pathogens causing infective arthritis are shown in Table 19–2. Intrasynovial joint injection of antimicrobials, frequently done in the past, is not recommended, since most of the antimicrobials used achieve bactericidal

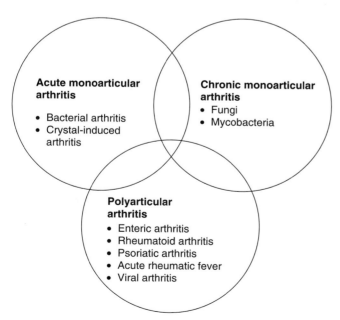

FIGURE 19–1. Arthritis Syndromes. (© Mayo Clinic)

TABLE 19–4 ■ Management of Patient Suspected of Having Infectious Arthritis on the Basis of Clinical, Laboratory, and Radiologic Findings[*]

Gram stain	First choice	Alternative choice
GRAM STAIN POSITIVE		
Gram-positive cocci	First-generation cephalosporin: cefazolin 1 g IV q8h	Vancomycin 15 mg/kg IV q12h
Gram-negative bacilli	Ceftazidime 1 g IV q8h or Fourth-generation cephalosporin: cefepime 1 g IV q12h	Ciprofloxacin 500 mg PO q12h
GRAM STAIN NEGATIVE		
Young, sexually active, characteristic rash	Cefepime 1 g IV q12h	Levofloxacin 500 mg IV or PO q24h
Rheumatoid arthritis, multiple joints	Cefepime 1 g IV q12h	Vancomycin 15 mg/kg IV q12h
Monoarticular arthritis; elderly, diabetes mellitus, end-stage renal disease	Cefepime 1 g IV q12h	Vancomycin 15 mg/kg IV q12h or Ciprofloxacin 500 mg PO q12h

[*]All dosing schedules are in adults with normal renal function.

levels in the inflamed synovial fluid. In addition, some data suggest that locally instilled antimicrobials can cause chemical synovitis.[19] Most experts recommend 2 to 4 weeks of parenteral antimicrobial therapy for nongonococcal infectious arthritis instead of the usual 4 to 6 weeks recommended for osteomyelitis. This therapy can be administered on an outpatient basis after an initial period of hospitalization in most cases. Oral antimicrobial therapy with an effective agent with excellent bioavailability such as ciprofloxacin or cotrimoxazole is also acceptable for appropriate microorganisms, particularly if the patient has rapidly improved on intravenous therapy and if compliance with oral therapy can be assured.

Up-to-date treatment guidelines for gonococcal infectious arthritis can be obtained from the Centers for Disease Control and Prevention (CDC) (www.cdc.gov/publications.htm). In patients without β-lactam allergy, ceftriaxone at a daily dose of 1 g intravenously or cefotaxime at a dose of 1 g intravenously every 8 hours is recommended. Intravenous regimens should be continued for 24 to 48 hours after improvement begins, at which time therapy may be switched to oral cefixime at a dose of 400 mg twice daily or ciprofloxacin at a dose of 500 mg twice daily to complete a full week of antimicrobial therapy. Compliance with therapy must be assured. Patients who are allergic to β-lactam are usually treated with a quinolone. Hospitalization is recommended for initial therapy. Patients treated for gonococcal infectious arthritis should be treated concurrently for *Chlamydia trachomatis* infection unless it is excluded by appropriate testing.

Surgical Therapy

Despite the paucity of human and animal data supporting the use of systematic drainage in patients with infectious joints, there is a general agreement among experts regarding its necessity and its importance.[19,20] This position is supported by many theoretical reasons such as the relief of pressure on the cartilage, early symptomatic relief promoting early mobilization, and reduction of the microorganism's burden and of the autolytic enzymes present with the reduction of the parallel inflammatory reaction and adhesions.

The optimal method of drainage of an infectious joint is a matter of great controversy. To date there are no well-controlled randomized trials to guide the best choice of drainage. Children (except with infectious arthritis of the hip) and patients with gonococcal infection do not require repeated therapeutic joint aspirations or arthrotomy. Until recently, most adults with infectious arthritis have been managed with repeated joint aspirations. Broy et al in a summary analysis of all published series involving 371 infected joints revealed a significantly better outcome among medically treated patients (aspirations) than among surgically treated patients (66% vs. 57%). In the medically treated group however, more deaths were observed (7.3% vs. 3.4%).[21] These data were derived solely from retrospective case series, and there is a potential for selection bias. In addition newer arthroscopic techniques were not evaluated. Arthrotomy should be reserved to the following situations: (1) cases that failed to improve within 7 days of conservative therapy, (2) an inability to adequately drain the infected joint by aspiration either because of location, such as the hip or the shoulder, or the loculations of purulence within the joint, (3) patients with a history of symptoms longer than 3 days.[22] The use of arthroscopic drainage has expanded in recent years because of the minimal associated morbidity and because purulent material can be drained from the joint better than with joint aspiration.[23–38] A review of all studies that evaluated the efficacy of arthroscopic débridement published to date is tabulated in Table 19–5. The overall high success rate of 90.2% likely represents an optimistic estimate, which is probably the result of a reporting bias in these series.

Several other potential methods to effectively drain infected joints have been described. These include a

TABLE 19–5 ■ Reports of Arthroscopic Débridement of Infectious Arthritis

Year	Reference	No. of patients	Hip/knee	Success (%)
1981	Jarrett et al[23]	1	0/1	1/1 (100%)
1982	Mitchell et al[24]	1	0/1	1/1 (100%)
1983	Lurie & Musil[25]	1	0/1	1/1 (100%)
1984	Gainor[26]	3	0/4	2/3 (77%)
1984	Mason[27]	23	0/23	20/23 (91.3%)
1985	Jackson[28]	14	14	14/14 (100%)
1985	Nottage[29]	4	4	3/4 (75%)
1985	Ivey and Clark[30]	10	0/11	11/11 (100%)
1986	Smith[31]	30	0/30	28/30 (93.3%)
1987	Skyhar and Mubarak[32]	15	0/15	15/15 (100%)
1989	Thiery[33]	46	0/46	36/46 (78.3%)
1992	Parisien and Shaffer[34]	16	13/0	16/16 (100%)
1993	Chung et al[35]	9	9/0	9/9 (100 %)
1993	Blitzer[36]	4	4/0	4/4 (100%)
1995	Jerosch et al[37]	12	0/9	10/12 (83%)
1997	Sanchez and Hennrikus[38]	5	0/5	5/5 (100%)
	Total			176/195 (90%)

distention-irrigation method or placement of a continuous irrigation or suction tube in a septic joint using minimal arthroscopic guidance or under fluoroscopic guidance.[39] These techniques have not achieved acceptance because there is no randomized trial affirming them and because of the wide availability of improved arthroscopic techniques.

Comparison of these methods is difficult because of the lack of standardization of case definitions, the differences in follow-up, and the variables that were not studied in each group.

Adjunctive Therapy

The practice of joint immobilization and elevation has been derived solely from a study performed before the availability of effective antimicrobial therapy and effective drainage. In Phemister's observation, cartilage destruction was noted at points of contact between joint surfaces.[40] A clinical corollary then became common practice, which is to immobilize the joint to avoid surface contact. Recently this practice has been challenged. Animal studies in rabbits actually showed evidence of regeneration of the cartilage with the use of intermittent pressure as well as better functional outcomes.[41,42] In addition some studies had showed a high rate of decreased range of motion among immobilized patients with infectious arthritis.[43] Therefore immobilization can be used for symptomatic relief early in the course of the infection. Active range of motion exercises should be started as soon as the pain subsides for a beneficial functional outcome.

Outcome and Complications

Patients with infectious arthritis have an estimated case-fatality rate of 9%, but in patients with polyarticular infectious arthritis and rheumatoid arthritis it is as high as 56%. In as many as 42% of patients who survive, loss of joint function is permanent. Total joint arthroplasty could be considered after successful therapy. Patients should be thoroughly assessed to exclude any residual infection prior to total joint arthroplasty. The risk of prosthetic joint infection after total joint arthroplasty in patients with treated native infectious arthritis is two times higher[44] than in their counterparts without native infectious arthritis. Predictors of morbidity and mortality include older age, rheumatoid arthritis, infection in the hip or shoulder, time between appearance of symptoms and initiation of treatment longer than 1 week, involvement of more than four joints, persistently positive cultures after 7 days of appropriate therapy, and bacteremia.[45]

Prosthetic Joint Infection

The cumulative incidence of prosthetic joint infection (PJI) among the approximately 500,000 total hip and knee arthroplasties performed in the United States of America each year varies between 0.5% to 15% over the lifetime of the prosthetic joint. The rate is highest in the first 6 months after surgery and declines thereafter.[46] Most PJI are acquired in the operating room through direct inoculation during prosthesis implantation or as a result of airborne or contiguous contamination of the wound.[46] Hematogenous seeding during a bacteremia or through direct contiguous spread from an adjacent focus of infection is much less common. Most PJI occur in immunocompetent hosts. Risk factors for PJI include prior joint surgery, malignancy, a high national nosocomial infection score (NNIS), and postoperative wound complications such as hematoma formation and superficial wound infection.[44] Other less well documented risk factors include rheumatoid arthritis, diabetes mellitus, the use of steroids, obesity, extreme age, joint dislocation, poor nutrition, distant infection, psoriasis, hemophilia, sickle cell hemoglobinopathy, joint implantation for malignancy, prior infectious arthritis, total elbow arthroplasty, and hinged knee prostheses.

Coagulase-negative staphylococci and *S. aureus* account for almost 60% of PJIs. Aerobic gram-negative bacteria, streptococci, and anaerobes cause PJI in 11%, 10% and 6% of cases, respectively. Almost 14% of PJIs are polymicrobial.[46] A common characteristic among the microorganisms that cause PJI is their ability to adhere to foreign materials. Certain settings would increase the risk of specific microorganisms. For instance, patients with rheumatoid arthritis are at increased risk for *S. aureus* PJI. *P. acnes* PJI is more commonly encountered in patients with an infected total shoulder arthroplasty.[47] In addition, patients with diabetes mellitus and malignancy are at increased risk for *Streptococcus agalactiae*.

A PJI classification could be based on the mechanism of infection (intraoperative vs. hematogenous) or on the joint age (early vs. late). A more useful classification by Tsukayama et al divided PJI into 4 categories: intraoperative positive-culture infection, early postoperative infection, late postoperative infection, and hematogenous infection.[48,49]

When an infection is acute or if a sinus tract is draining, the diagnosis of PJI is clear. If chronic pain is the only symptom, infection must be distinguished from aseptic loosening or mechanical prosthesis failure.

Management of Patients with Prosthetic Joint Infection

The successful treatment of patients with PJI relies on close cooperation between the orthopedic surgeon and the infectious disease specialist. The therapeutic strategies used in patients with PJI are different from those used in patients with septic native arthritis. The goal of treatment is a pain-free functional joint. Eradication of infection is the most direct method for achieving this goal but may not be possible in certain instances.

Surgical Therapy

Surgical approaches include débridement of the affected prosthesis, one-stage exchange, two-stage exchange, removal of the prosthetic joint without reimplantation, amputation of the affected limb, or antimicrobial suppression only.

Depending on the microorganism, débridement and retention of the prosthetic joint is ultimately successful in less than 30% of selected patients without long-term antimicrobial suppression.[50,51] This modality should be reserved for patients with a well-seated prosthesis débrided within a short time after the onset of symptoms and with an infection due to low-virulence bacteria such as coagulase-negative staphylococci. Other circumstances in which this modality may be useful include elderly patients at high risk for cardiopulmonary events after anesthesia and when the removal of the prosthesis is not surgically feasible without joint amputation.

In addition, selected patients with early postoperative wound infection can benefit from this therapeutic strategy. Tsukayama et al reported a success rate of 50% to 71% when patients with early postoperative wound infection or

postoperative hematoma infection of the wound underwent extensive surgical débridement followed by a course of parenteral antimicrobial therapy.[48,49] This surgical modality should be used with great caution in patients with bacteremia or sepsis or in patients with prosthetic implants elsewhere. Long-term suppression with an oral antimicrobial was not used in this study. After the initial débridement the patient is placed on a course of antimicrobial therapy as outlined in Table 19–6 (induction phase). The need for subsequent long-term oral antimicrobial suppression therapy has not been established. The optimal duration of suppression is unknown.[51,52] If it is used, we favor continuing long-term suppression for as long as the patient is doing well and there is no side effect from the use of antimicrobial agents.

The two-stage exchange procedure offers a success rate of more than 90% in experienced hands.[48,53] It is the most widely used procedure in the United States to treat patients with PJIs. It requires at least two major operations separated by 4 to 6 weeks of intravenous antimicrobial therapy (Table 19–6). The débridement should be extensive to ensure that all the periprosthetic cement has been removed, as retained cement or incomplete débridement has been in our experience the most common reason for persistent infection. One of the major disadvantages in two-stage exchange arthroplasty is that the interval between stages is often associated with impaired mobility, limited stability, and pain. The length of time before reimplantation depends on the site of the prosthesis. There are no controlled trials to guide clinicians in terms of the optimal reimplantation time. At the Mayo clinic the reimplantation of total knee arthroplasty usually occurs 6 weeks after resection arthroplasty. For the hip joint, reimplantation is commonly performed after 3 months.[53] If a cemented prosthesis is used, antimicrobial-impregnated cement may be used.[54] Reimplantation is often difficult because of arthrofibrosis. To preserve the length of the limb and to minimize soft-tissue contractures the use of nonarticulating antibiotic-loaded cement spacers between stages has been advocated.[55]

One-stage exchange refers to removal of the infected prosthesis, surgical débridement, and reimplantation of a new prosthesis in a single surgical procedure.[46,48] Preferentially this procedure should be performed in a healthy patient with good soft tissues, minimal femoral bone loss, and a responsible organism identified preoperatively as antibiotic sensitive and gram positive.[56] In one study, only 11% of patients seen with PJI were deemed potential candidates for this procedure.[57] This procedure is widely used in selected centers in Europe. The reported success rate of this strategy is 70% to 80%. A course of antimicrobials is usually recommended. Most cases of infection due to coagulase-negative staphylococci do not require long-term suppression. This surgical strategy is unintentionally used in the United States in cases in which the infection was not suspected but was diagnosed later on culture results. These are most commonly due to organisms such as coagulase-negative staphylococci.

TABLE 19–6 ■ Medical Treatment of Patients with Prosthetic Joint Infection

Microbiology	First choice	Alternative choice	Comments
Staphylococcus, coagulase negative MIC for oxacillin sensitive	Cefazolin 1 g IV q8h × 4 wk	Vancomycin 15 mg/kg IV q12h × 4 wk or Levofloxacin 500 mg PO or IV and rifampin 600 mg/d × 4 wk	
Staphylococcus, coagulase negative MIC for oxacillin resistant	Vancomycin 15 mg/kg IV q12h × 4 wk	Linezolid 600 mg PO or IV q12h or Levofloxacin 500 mg PO or IV and rifampin 600 mg/d × 4 wk	
Staphylococcus aureus MIC for oxacillin sensitive	Cefazolin 1 g IV q8h × 6 wk	Vancomycin 15 mg/kg IV q12h × 6 wk or Levofloxacin 500 mg PO or IV and rifampin 600 mg/d × 6 wk	
S. aureus MIC for oxacillin resistant	Vancomycin 15 mg/kg IV q12h × 6 wk	Linezolid 600 mg PO or IV q12h or Levofloxacin 500 mg PO or IV and rifampin 600 mg/d × 6 wk	
Enterococcus spp Penicillin sensitive	Ampicillin sodium 12 g/24h IV continuously or in 6 equally divided doses × 4 wk	Vancomycin 15 mg/kg IV q12h × 4 wk	Addition of an aminoglycoside is optional
Enterococcus spp Penicillin resistant	Vancomycin 15 mg/kg IV q12h × 4 wk	Linezolid 600 mg PO or IV q12h × 4 wk	Addition of an aminoglycoside is optional
Pseudomonas aeruginosa	Cefepime 1 g IV q12h × 6 wk or Meropenem 1 g IV q8h × 6 wk	Levofloxacin 500 mg PO or IV × 6 wk or Ceftazidime 1 g IV q8h × 6 wk	
Enterobacter spp	Cefepime 1 g IV q24h × 4–6 wk	Ciprofloxacin 500 mg PO or IV × 6 wk	
β-hemolytic streptococci	Aqueous crystalline penicillin G20 MU/24 h IV continuously or in 6 equally divided doses × 4–6 wk or Ceftriaxone 1 g/d IV × 4 wk	Vancomycin 15 mg/kg IV q12h × 4 wk	
Propionibacterium acnes	Aqueous crystalline penicillin G 20 MU/24 h IV continuously or in 6 equally divided doses × 4 wk or Ceftriaxone 1 g/d IV × 4 wk	Vancomycin 15 mg /kg IV q12h for 4 weeks	

Resection arthroplasty without subsequent reimplantation of a new prosthesis was originally used by Girdlestone to treat patients with infected hip joints. Currently this strategy is often used in patients with severe bone loss where reimplantation of a new prosthesis is not technically better or in patients with recurrent infection. For a better functional outcome, arthrodesis of the knee is performed. Although internal arthrodesis may provide better stability and fixation, it might be associated with a higher infection rate than external arthrodesis is.

Amputation of a limb is reserved for extremely difficult to treat infections or patients with life-threatening infection.

Medical Therapy

Antimicrobial therapy for the treatment of PJI is tabulated in Table 19–6. Rifampin, a cornerstone antimycobacterial, has received a fair amount of attention in studies of orthopedic hardware infections.[58–60] Its ability to kill microorganisms that are in the stationary phase has made it an attractive agent to treat patients with orthopedic hardware infection without removal of the hardware. In addition rifampin has a minimum inhibitory concentrations range from 0.004 to 0.03 mg/L against most isolates of both methicillin-sensitive and methicillin-resistant *Staphylococcus aureus* (MSSA, MRSA, respectively), and methicillin-sensitive and methicillin-resistant *Staphylococcus epidermidis*. Because of its pharmacologic properties, rifampin achieves excellent concentrations in soft tissues, bone, and abscess cavities. The use of rifampin monotherapy against these infections, however, is usually associated with the rapid emergence of resistance. Therefore rifampin combined with a second antimicrobial is warranted to avoid the emergence of resistance. Quinolones share similar pharmacologic properties with rifampin. Cohort studies on combination therapy given to patients with orthopedic implant–related infection in whom the device could not be removed showed a success rate of 74% to 82%.[58,59] Recently Zimmerli et al examined the potential role for rifampin in the successful treatment of implant-related staphylococcal infections with salvage of stable prosthetic devices in a randomized, prospective, controlled clinical trial.[60] Patients who received quinolones and rifampin had a significantly higher success rate than those who received quinolones alone (100% vs. 58%). Given the increasing emergence of quinolone resistance among staphylococci and the lack of data derived from large studies, this practice has not yet achieved wide acceptance. Future studies looking at the efficacy of newer quinolones in association with rifampin are warranted

Local antimicrobial delivery devices such as antimicrobial beads or spacers, which are used rarely in patients with native joint infectious arthritis, are common practice in patients with PJI. In addition to the theoretical advantage of attaining an extremely high concentration of the antimicrobial locally in dead space management, some of these techniques are believed to maintain a functional joint space and improve the ease of reimplantation.[55] Vancomycin, aminoglycosides, or both have been used most commonly with polymethylmethacrylate beads or spacers. In occasional cases such as vancomycin-resistant enterococci and *Candida* and multidrug-resistant Enterobacteriaceae, beads might serve as foreign bodies and should be avoided.

Prevention

Because of the high morbidity and mortality associated with PJI, prevention is highly desirable. Antimicrobial prophylaxis given within 120 minutes before incision has been shown to reduce the risk of PJI.[61] Prophylactic antimicrobial agents should be directed against staphylo-

cocci and streptococci. First-generation cephalosporins are often used. Recent studies also suggest that antibiotic-impregnated cement may be effective in the prophylaxis of deep wound infection following total joint replacement.[46,54] Further studies with longer follow-up periods are needed before this practice can be endorsed. The use of laminar airflow devices in preventing prosthetic joint infection remains controversial.[62]

Hematogenous Infection

The microorganisms that cause hematogenous PJI are similar to the microorganisms that are acquired intraoperatively and postoperatively. Paradoxically, viridans group streptococci, a common cause of infective endocarditis, is rarely encountered in PJI. Urinary tract and respiratory tract infections have also been implicated as sources of infection. Therefore it seems prudent to aggressively diagnose and treat significant bacterial infections in patients with a total joint arthroplasty. Prevention of hematogenous PJI should begin with identification of potential sources of remote infection prior to prosthesis insertion to avoid hematogenous infection in the high-risk period immediately after prosthesis insertion (e.g., dental review preoperatively if poor dentition, urologic review if recurrent UTI). In addition, optimization of the host risk factors (e.g., immunosuppressive drugs, diabetes mellitus, tobacco abuse, skin diseases, vaccination status) and local factors (e.g., lymphedema, tinea pedis, venous insufficiency, vascular supply) should be undertaken before total joint arthroplasty. In the postoperative period the treating physician should aggressively treat remote infection when it occurs.

A consensus panel formed by the American Academy of Orthopaedic Surgeons and the American Dental Association has recommended that routine antimicrobial prophylaxis before invasive dental procedures for all patients with a total joint arthroplasty is not necessary.[64] The panel recommended, however, that prophylaxis be considered in high-risk patients undergoing high-risk dental procedures (Table 19–7). A single antibiotic dose within 60 minutes of the procedure was recommended. This statement provides guidelines to supplement practitioners in their clinical judgment regarding antibiotic

TABLE 19–7 ■ Suggested Antimicrobial Prophylaxis Regimens for High-Risk Patient with Total Joint Arthroplasty Undergoing High-Risk Dental Procedure

- Patients not allergic to penicillin:
  Amoxicillin, cephalexin, or cephadrine: 2 g PO 1 h before the procedure
- Patients not allergic to penicillin and unable to take oral medication:
  Ampicillin 2 g or cefazolin 1 g IM or IV 1 h before the procedure
- Patients allergic to penicillin:
  Clindamycin 600 mg PO 1 h before the procedure
- Patients allergic to penicillin and unable to take oral medication:
  Clindamycin 600 mg IV 1 h before the procedure

Adapted from Advisory statement: Antibiotic prophylaxis for dental patients with total joint replacements. American Dental Association; American Academy of Orthopaedic Surgeons. J Am Dent Assoc 1997;128:1004–1008.

prophylaxis for dental patients. It is not intended as the standard of care or as a substitute for clinical judgment.

There are no data to provide a rational basis for any recommendation regarding antimicrobial prophylaxis prior to invasive gastrointestinal and genitourinary procedures.[64,66] The American Society of Colon and Rectal Surgeons and the American Society for Gastrointestinal Endoscopy do not recommend antibiotic prophylaxis for endoscopy.[66]

REFERENCES

1. Lew DP, Waldvogel FA: Osteomyelitis. N Engl J Med 1997;336:999–1007.
2. Mader JT, Ortiz M, Calhoun JH: Update on the diagnosis and management of osteomyelitis. Clin Podiatr Med Surg 1996;13:701–724.
3. Haas DW, McAndrew MP: Bacterial osteomyelitis in adults: Evolving considerations in diagnosis and treatment. Am J Med 1996;101:550.
4. Huddleston PM, Steckelberg JM, Hanssen AD, et al: Ciprofloxacin inhibition of experimental fracture healing. J Bone Joint Surg Am 2000;82:161–173.
5. Brandt CM, Rouse MS, Tallan BM, et al: Failure of time-kill synergy studies using subinhibitory antimicrobial concentrations to predict in vivo antagonism of cephalosporin-rifampin combinations against Staphylococcus aureus. Antimicrob Agents Chemother 1994;38:2191–2193.
6. Lew DP, Waldvogel FA: Use of quinolones in osteomyelitis and infected orthopaedic prosthesis. Drugs 1999;58 (Suppl 2):85–91.
7. Mader JT, Cantrell JS, Calhoun JH: Oral ciprofloxacin compared with standard parenteral antibiotic therapy for chronic osteomyelitis in adults. J Bone Joint Surg Am 1990;72:104–110.
8. Gentry LO, Rodriguez GG: Oral ciprofloxacin compared with parenteral antibiotics in the treatment of osteomyelitis. Antimicrob Agents Chemother 1990;34:40–43.
9. Waldvogel FA, Medoff G, Swartz MN: Treatment of osteomyelitis. N Engl J Med 1970;283:822.
10. Wall EJ: Childhood osteomyelitis and septic arthritis. Curr Opin Pediatr 1998;10:73–76.
11. Lehovsky J: Pyogenic vertebral osteomyelitis/disc infection. Baillieres Best Pract Res Clin Rheumatol 1999;13:59–75.
12. Morrey BF, Dunn JM, Heimbach RD, Davis J: Hyperbaric oxygen and chronic osteomyelitis. Clin Orthop 1979;144:121–127.
13. Mendel V, Reichert B, Simanowski HJ, Scholz HC: Therapy with hyperbaric oxygen and cefazolin for experimental osteomyelitis due to Staphylococcus aureus in rats. Undersea Hyperb Med 1999;26:169–174.
14. Mader JT, Adams KR, Wallace WR, Calhoun JH: Hyperbaric oxygen as adjunctive therapy for osteomyelitis. Infect Dis Clin North Am 1990;4:433–440.
15. Settecerri JJ, Pitner MA, Rock MG, et al: Infection after rotator cuff repair. J Shoulder Elbow Surg 1999;8:1–5.
16. Kaandorp CJ, Van Schaardenburg D, Krijnen P, et al: Risk factors for septic arthritis in patients with joint disease. A prospective study. Arthritis Rheum 1995;38:1819–1825.
17. Dory MA, Wautelet MJ: Arthroscopy in septic arthritis. Lidocaine- and iodine-containing contrast media are bacteriostatic. Arthritis Rheum 1985;28:198–203.
18. Smith JW: Infectious arthritis. Infect Dis Clin North Am. 1990;4:523–538.
19. Goldenberg DL, Cohen AS: Acute infectious arthritis. A review of patients with nongonococcal joint infections (with emphasis on therapy and prognosis). Am J Med 1976;60:369–377.
20. Jackson RW: The minimally invasive treatment of septic arthritis. J Rheumatol 1993;20:12.
21. Broy SB, Schmid FR: A comparison of medical drainage (needle aspiration) and surgical drainage (arthrotomy or arthroscopy) in the initial treatment of infected joints. Clin Rheum Dis 1986;12:501–522.
22. Esterhai JL Jr, Gelb I: Adult septic arthritis. Orthop Clin North Am 1991;22:503–514.
23. Jarrett MP, Grossman L, Sadler AH, Grayzel AI: The role of arthroscopy in the treatment of septic arthritis. Arthritis Rheum 1981;24:737–739.
24. Mitchell H, Travers R, Barraclough D: Septic arthritis caused by Pasteurella multocida. Med J Aust 1982;1:137.
25. Lurie DP, Musil G: Staphylococcal septic arthritis presenting as acute flare of pseudogout: Clinical, pathological and arthroscopic findings with a review of the literature. J Rheumatol 1983;10:503–506.
26. Gainor BJ: Instillation of continuous tube irrigation in the septic knee at arthroscopy. A technique. Clin Orthop 1984;183:96–98.
27. Mason L: Arthroscopic management of the infected knee. In Grana W (ed.): Update in arthroscopic techniques. Baltimore, University Park Press, 1984, pp 67–77.
28. Jackson RW: The septic knee—arthroscopic treatment. Arthroscopy 1985;1:194–197.
29. Nottage WM: Arthroscopic management of the septic knee. In Shahriaree H (ed): O'Connor's Textbook of Arthroscopic Surgery. Philadelphia, JB Lippincott, 1985, pp 299–302.
30. Ivey M, Clark R: Arthroscopic débridement of the knee for septic arthritis. Clin Orthop 1985;199:201–206.
31. Smith MJ: Arthroscopic treatment of the septic knee. Arthroscopy 1986;2:30–34.
32. Skyhar MJ, Mubarak SJ: Arthroscopic treatment of septic knees in children. J Pediatr Orthop 1987;7:647–651.
33. Thiery JA: Arthroscopic drainage in septic arthritides of the knee: A multicenter study. Arthroscopy 1989;5:65–69.
34. Parisien JS, Shaffer B: Arthroscopic management of pyarthrosis. Clin Orthop 1992;275:243–247.
35. Chung WK, Slater GL, Bates EH: Treatment of septic arthritis of the hip by arthroscopic lavage. J Pediatr Orthop 1993;13:444–446.
36. Blitzer CM: Arthroscopic management of septic arthritis of the hip. Arthroscopy 1993;9:414–416.
37. Jerosch J, Hoffstetter I, Schroder M, Castro WH: Septic arthritis: Arthroscopic management with local antibiotic treatment. Acta Orthop Belgica 1995;61:126–134.
38. Sanchez AA, Hennrikus WL: Arthroscopically assisted treatment of acute septic knees in infants using the Micro-Joint Arthroscope. Arthroscopy 1997;13:350–354.
39. Ike RW: Tidal irrigation in septic arthritis of the knee: A potential alternative to surgical drainage. J Rheumatol 1993;20:2104–2111.
40. Phemister DB: The effect of pressure on articular surfaces in pyogenic and tuberculous arthritis and its bearing on treatment. Ann Surg 1924;80:481.
41. Salter RB: The biologic concept of continuous passive motion of synovial joints. The first 18 years of basic research and its clinical application. Clin Orthop 1989;242:12–25.
42. Trias A: Effect of persistent pressure on the articular cartilage: An experimental study. J Bone Joint Surg 1961;43B:376.
43. Insall JN: Intra-articular surgery for degenerative arthritis of the knee. A report of the work of the late K. H. Pridie. J Bone Joint Surg Br 1967;49:211–228.
44. Berbari EF, Hanssen AD, Duffy MC, et al: Risk factors for prosthetic joint infection: Case-control study. Clin Infect Dis 1998;27:1247–1254.
45. Smith JW, Piercy EA: Infectious arthritis. Clin Infect Dis 1995;20:225.
46. Steckelberg JM, Osmon DR: Prosthetic joint infection. In Bisno AL, Waldvogel FA (eds): Infections Associated with

Indwelling Medical Devices, 3rd ed. Washington DC, American Society of Microbiology, 2000.

47. Sperling JW, Kozak TKW, Hanssen AD, Cofield RH: Infection after shoulder arthroplasty. Clin Orthop 2001;382:206–216.

48. Tsukayama DT, Estrada R, Gustilo RB: Infection after total hip arthroplasty: A study of the treatment of one hundred and six infections. J Bone Joint Surg Am 1996;78:512–523.

49. Segawa H, Tsukayama DT, Kyle RF, et al: Infection after total knee arthroplasty. A retrospective study of the treatment of eighty-one infections. J Bone Joint Surg Am 1999; 81:1434–1445.

50. Tattevin P, Cremieux AC, Pottier P, et al: Prosthetic joint infection: When can prosthesis salvage be considered? Clin Infect Dis 1999;29:292–295.

51. Brandt CM, Sistrunk WW, Duffy MC, et al: *Staphylococcus aureus* prosthetic joint infection treated with débridement and prosthesis retention. Clin Infect Dis 1997;24:914–919.

52. Segreti J, Nelson JA, Trenholme GM: Prolonged suppressive antibiotic therapy for infected orthopedic prostheses. Clin Infect Dis 1998;27:711–713.

53. Brandt CM, Duffy MC, Berbari EF, et al: *Staphylococcus aureus* prosthetic joint infection treated with prosthesis removal and delayed reimplantation arthroplasty. Mayo Clin Proc 1999;74:553–558.

54. Hanssen AD, Rand JA, Osmon DR: Treatment of the infected total knee arthroplasty with insertion of another prosthesis. The effect of antibiotic-impregnated bone cement. Clin Orthop 1994;309:44–55.

55. Haddad FS, Masri BA, Campbell D, et al: The PROSTALAC functional spacer in two-stage revision for infected knee replacements. Prosthesis of antibiotic-loaded acrylic cement. J Bone Joint Surg Br 2000;82:807–812.

56. Schmalzried TP: Careful patient selection is the key for direct exchange in the infected THA. Orthopedics 1999;22:919.

57. Hanssen AD, Osmon DR: Assessment of patient selection criteria for treatment of the infected hip arthroplasty. Clin Orthop 2000;381:91–100.

58. Widmer AF, Gaechter A, Ochsner PE, Zimmerli W: Antimicrobial treatment of orthopedic implant-related infections with rifampin combinations. Clin Infect Dis 1992;14:1251–1253.

59. Drancourt M, Stein A, Argenson JN, et al: Oral rifampin plus ofloxacin for treatment of staphylococcus-infected orthopedic implants. Antimicrob Agents Chemother 1993;37:1214–1218.

60. Zimmerli W, Widmer AF, Blatter M, et al: Role of rifampin for treatment of orthopedic implant-related staphylococcal infections: A randomized controlled trial. Foreign-Body Infection (FBI) Study Group. JAMA 1998;279:1537–1541.

61. Classen DC, Evans RS, Pestotnik SL, et al: The timing of prophylactic administration of antibiotics and the risk of surgical-wound infection. N Engl J Med 1992;326:281–286.

62. Hanssen AD, Osmon DR: Prevention of deep periprosthetic joint infection. J Bone Joint Surg Am 1996;78:458–471.

63. Advisory statement: Antibiotic prophylaxis for dental patients with total joint replacements. American Dental Association;American Academy of Orthopaedic Surgeons. J Am Dent Assoc 1997;128:1004–1008.

64. Antibiotic prophylaxis for gastrointestinal endoscopy. Gastrointest Endosc 1995;42:630–635.

65. LaPorte DM, Waldman BJ, Mont MA, Hungerford DS: Infections associated with dental procedures in total hip arthroplasty. J Bone Joint Surg Br 1999;81:56–59.

66. Oliver G, Lowry A, Vernava A, et al: Practice parameters for antibiotic prophylaxis—supporting documentation. The Standards Task Force. The American Society of Colon and Rectal Surgeons. Dis Colon Rectum 2000;43:1194–1200.

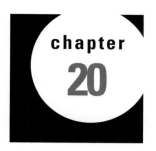

Foot Infections in the Diabetic Patient and Infections Associated with Pressure Sores

FRANCISCO L. SAPICO, MD, FACP

FOOT INFECTIONS IN THE DIABETIC PATIENT

The economic, social, and personal costs of foot infections in diabetic patients are considerable. In the United States alone at least 20% of hospital admissions among diabetic patients are for foot problems. Of all nontraumatic amputations, 50% to 70% are performed on patients with diabetes.[1–3] This increased susceptibility to foot infection has been attributed to several factors: immune dysfunction, neuropathy, and vascular insufficiency. The same factors also play important roles in the poor healing often observed in this population of patients.

Pathogenesis and Microbiology

Minor foot trauma and improperly fitting footwear contribute to the initiation and perpetuation of early lesions (Table 20–1). Early lesions are characterized by local cellulitis, non-foul-smelling drainage, and poorly healing tissue defects without tissue necrosis and gangrene. These infections are usually monomicrobial (e.g., *Staphylococcus aureus*, coagulase-negative staphylococci, enterococci, and aerobic streptococci).[4,5] Moderate-to-severe infections (especially when tissue necrosis or gangrene is present) are usually characterized by a polymicrobial picture, generally a mixture of aerobic and anaerobic organisms.[6,7] The organisms most commonly isolated from blood cultures in diabetic patients with foot infections have been *Bacteroides fragilis* and *S. aureus*.[8]

Collection of specimens for culture necessitates removal of superficial necrotic tissue overlying the base of the ulcer (usually by sharp débridement). Bits of tissue can be obtained from the underlying surface with a dermal curette or a scalpel 9 and should be sent for aerobic and anaerobic cultures in appropriate transport media. Pus obtained by needle aspiration is excellent for culture, but results obtained after injection of nonbacteriostatic normal saline and subsequent reaspiration have been disappointing.[7]

Certain variants of necrotizing soft tissue infections have been shown to be more prevalent in diabetic patients. Necrotizing fasciitis (usually polymicrobial), nonclostridial anaerobic myonecrosis, spontaneous (hematogenous) clostridial myonecrosis (usually caused by *Clostridium septicum*), and crepitant anaerobic cellulitis have been observed with greater frequency in the diabetic than in the general population.[10]

Diagnostic Evaluation

The status of the neurologic and vascular systems should be evaluated thoroughly in diabetic patients with foot infections. Noninvasive tests, such as Doppler

TABLE 20–1 ■ **Basic Foot Care Principles for the Diabetic Patient**

1. Feet should be washed daily with soap and water and dried thoroughly afterward (especially between toes).
2. Mild lubricants may be applied daily.
3. Feet should be kept dry and warm (use woolen socks; never hot water bags).
4. Feet should be inspected daily for lesions (may use mirrors; relatives and friends should be asked to help if patient has visual impairment).
5. Shoes should be well fitting (made of soft leather or "running" shoes); special footwear is needed if there is foot deformity and if sensation is impaired. Shoes should be broken in gradually. If possible, at least 3 pairs should be worn alternately.
6. Lipid disorders or an overweight condition should be corrected by diet or medically.
7. Feet should be examined regularly during outpatient clinic visits.
8. New lesions should be immediately reported to the health care professional.
9. Corns or calluses should be taken care of by a health care professional or podiatrist.
10. Open-toed footwear should not be worn.
11. Heating pads, hot packs, or hot water bags should not be used.
12. Smoking is contraindicated.

ultrasonography with waveform analysis and transcutaneous oximetry, can help assess the vascular status. Plain radiographs, computed tomographic scans, technetium bone scans, gallium scans, and white blood cell scans have problems with lack of sensitivity or specificity for the diagnosis of osteomyelitis. Enthusiasm for magnetic resonance imaging has been generated by some studies.[11,12] Another promising diagnostic modality is the monoclonal antibody scan.[13]

Management

Antimicrobial therapy should be directed at the most likely organisms involved. Milder cases of localized cellulitis or infected ulcers (without gangrene, tissue necrosis, or foul smell) generally necessitate therapy directed primarily at gram-positive aerobic cocci (i.e., *S. aureus*). A first-generation cephalosporin such as cefazolin may be used if there are no contraindications. Moderate to more severe infections may require broader spectrum coverage such as parenteral ampicillin-sulbactam,[14] ticarcillin-clavulanate, piperacillin-tazobactam,[15] or imipenem.[13] Vancomycin may be added if there is a good possibility of oxacillin-resistant staphylococcus. The presence of vancomycin-resistant enterococci may necessitate use of quinupristin-dalfopristin or of linezolid. The antimicrobial regimen may be changed on the basis of the culture results. The reliability of anaerobic cultures depends on the techniques of culture collection and may vary from one laboratory to another. Gangrene, tissue necrosis, or foul-smelling discharge strongly suggests the presence of anaerobes regardless of culture results. The length of therapy depends on the severity of the infection, lasting from 7 to 10 days for mild cellulitis to several weeks for more severe infections. Osteomyelitis dictates longer therapy if ablation of infected bone is not complete. A minimum of 4 weeks of parenteral therapy or a combination of parenteral and oral therapy totaling 10 weeks has been suggested for osteomyelitis.[16]

Surgical removal of necrotic, devitalized tissue and drainage of pus are essential. Limited ablative surgery removing all infected bone and soft tissue (e.g., toe amputation, metatarsal ray resection) may shorten the course of antibiotic therapy and hospital stay.[17] The level of surgical amputation is dictated by the extent of soft tissue and bone involvement and the vascular status of the extremity. Vascular reconstruction may be necessary to ameliorate vascular insufficiency; healing of some persistent ulcers may be accelerated by this surgical procedure.

No form of local therapy appears to have clear-cut superiority over the others. Normal saline wet-to-dry dressings following surgical débridement, removal of external pressures, and avoidance of the dependent position will accelerate wound healing.

Other treatments have included hyperbaric oxygen, bioengineered tissue grafts, and recombinant platelet-derived growth factors.[18] More controlled studies, especially in infected wounds, are needed for these treatments.

INFECTED PRESSURE SORES

It has been estimated that more than 1 million patients in hospitals and nursing homes in the United States suffer from pressure sores and that at least 3% of patients in acute care hospitals are similarly afflicted.[19,20]

The pathophysiology of pressure sore formation involves an interplay of pressure, shearing forces, friction, excess moisture, local spasticity, and a local blood supply deficiency.[19–21] Because more than 90% of pressure sores are located on the lower part of the body (usually sacral, trochanteric, and ischial) and especially since patients are often fecally incontinent, these sores are colonized by a variety of microorganisms. Continued worsening of tissue necrosis may lead to soft tissue infection, osteomyelitis, and septic complications.

Microbiology

Moderately to severely infected pressure sores show polymicrobial flora similar to that seen in infected feet in diabetic patients.[22–24] The dominant microorganisms are microorganisms that constitute fecal flora. *Escherichia coli* and *Proteus mirabilis* are the gram-negative, aerobic, enteric bacilli most commonly seen. Among the gram-positive aerobic cocci, *S. aureus, Enterococcus* spp., and coagulase-negative staphylococci are the most common. Anaerobes, such as *Bacteroides* and *Peptostreptococcus* spp. are clearly dominant organisms in this disease entity, especially when the sores are close to the perianal area.[24]

Bacteremic sepsis associated with infected pressure sores is most often associated with *B. fragilis, P. mirabilis, Peptostreptococcus* spp., and *S. aureus*.[22,25] As the pressure sore heals and necrotic and gangrenous tissue are eliminated, anaerobic microorganisms gradually disappear, but gram-negative bacilli and gram-positive cocci may persist. When the sore is almost healed and a smaller lesion with healthy granulation tissue remains, fewer microorganisms may be seen, primarily *Pseudomonas aeruginosa* and *Enterococcus* spp.[23]

Proper anaerobic culture collection using proper transport media includes submission of material such as aspirated pus or deep tissue or bone obtained after overlying superficial necrotic tissue is removed.

Diagnostic Evaluation

Pressure sores may be classified into four stages.

- Stage I represents nonblanchable erythema of intact skin.
- Stage II involves partial-thickness skin loss involving epidermis or dermis or both.

- Stage III involves full-thickness skin loss with damage or necrosis of subcutaneous tissue down to but not through underlying fascia.
- Stage IV represents extensive destruction with damage to muscle, bone, or supporting structures (Table 20–2).[26]

As with the evaluation for osteomyelitis in foot infections, plain radiographs may be limited in sensitivity and specificity. Lack of specificity has also hampered radionuclide scans, and more is needed with magnetic resonance imaging for this disease entity. Bone biopsy for histologic examination is still considered to be the "gold standard" for the diagnosis of osteomyelitis.[27–29] Quantitative microbiology of bone was disappointing in one study.[29]

Management

Surgical removal of dead, necrotic tissue is paramount in the management of infected pressure sores. These surgical procedures may have to be performed repeatedly to keep up with continuing advance of tissue necrosis. Liquid purulent material should be drained as completely as possible. Infected bone should be surgically removed until healthy bone is encountered.

Empiric antimicrobial coverage before culture results are received should address the potential for polymicrobial flora. The choice of antimicrobial agents for

---

TABLE 20–2 ■ Pressure Sore Stages

I. Nonblanchable erythema of intact skin (may or may not be associated with discoloration, warmth, edema, induration, or hardness)
II. Partial-thickness skin loss involving epidermis, dermis, or both (may be in the form of an abrasion, blister, or shallow crater)
III. Full-thickness skin loss involving subcutaneous tissue that may extend down, but not through, fascia (with or without undermining of adjacent tissue)
IV. Full-thickness skin loss with destruction, tissue necrosis, or damage to muscle, bone, or supporting structures such as tendon or joint capsule.

Adapted from the agency for Health Care Policy and Research Guidelines.

TABLE 20–3 ■ Management of Pressure Sores

I. Débridement
  A. Mechanical
  B. Autolytic (using the body's own enzymes and white blood cells)
  C. Chemical
II. Wound cleansing
III. Dressings
  A. Vapor-permeable, transparent adhesive
  B. Hydrocolloid
  C. Nonadhesive, semipermeable polyurethane foam dressings
  D. Alginates
  E. Hydrogel
  F. Gauze
IV. Other modalities: hyperbaric oxygen, electrical stimulation, growth factors
V. Surgery and plastic reconstruction
VI. Antimicrobial agents

moderate-to-severe infections would be similar to the choice in the case of moderate-to-severe foot infections in diabetic patients. The antimicrobial regimen can be changed later in accordance with the culture results. Tissue gangrene, necrosis, and foul smell strongly suggest the presence of anaerobes. There is no consensus on the length of antimicrobial therapy. One study found no necessity to treat longer than 3 weeks as long as surgical removal of infected bone is thorough.[28] Another recommended 6 weeks of antimicrobial therapy.[29]

There is also no clear consensus on the most efficacious type of local therapy.[30] As with diabetic foot ulcers, normal saline wet-to-dry dressings are often used. Recently, the use of silver sulfadiazine has achieved some popularity.[31] Frequent turning, proper positioning, pressure dispersion, and specialized beds and mattresses are requisites in the prevention and therapy of pressure sores. Control of muscle spasticity and surgical release of flexion contractures are likewise important measures in preventing and alleviating pressure sores.

Besides removal of necrotic tissue, infected bone, and bony prominences, surgical management includes the use of a variety of myocutaneous flaps once the wound is clean and shows healthy granulation tissue.[32,33]

Innovative or unconventional modalities of management have included those discussed in diabetic foot ulcer management, a vacuum-sealing technique, and maggot therapy.[34,35] More studies are needed for the vacuum-seal technique. Patient and physician acceptance are limiting factors for widespread adoption of maggot therapy.

REFERENCES

1. Sapico FL: Foot infections in patients with diabetes mellitus. J Am Podiatr Med Assoc 1989;79:482–485.
2. Levin ME, O'Neal LW (eds): Preface. In The Diabetic Foot, ed 4. St. Louis, Mosby, 1988, pp ix and x.
3. Gibbons GW, Eliopoulos GM: Infections of the diabetic foot. In Kozak GP, Hoar CS, Rawbottom JL, et al (eds): Management of Diabetic Foot Problems. Philadelphia, WB Saunders, 1984, p 97.
4. Leslie CA, Sapico FL, Ginunas VJ, et al: Randomized, controlled trial of topical hyperbaric oxygen for the treatment of diabetic foot ulcers. Diabetes Care 1988;11:111–115.
5. Lipsky BA, Pecoraro RE, Larson SA, et al: Outpatient management of uncomplicated lower-extremity infections in diabetic patients. Arch Intern Med 1990;150:790–797.
6. Sapico FL, Canawati HN, Witte JL, et al: Quantitative aerobic and anaerobic bacteriology of infected diabetic feet. J Clin Microbiol 1980;12:413–420.
7. Sapico FL, Witte JL, Canawati HN, et al: The infected foot of the diabetic patient: Quantitative microbiology and analysis of clinical features. Rev Infect Dis 1984;6(Suppl 1):171–176.
8. Sapico FL, Bessman AN, Canawati HN: Bacteremia in diabetic patients with infected lower extremities. Diabetes Care 1982;5:101–104.
9. Louie TJ, Bartlett JG, Tally FP, et al: Aerobic and anaerobic bacteria in diabetic foot ulcers. Ann Intern Med 1976;85:461–463.
10. Leslie CA, Sapico FL, Bessman AN: Infections in the diabetic host. Compr Ther 1989;15(7):23–32.
11. Yuh WTC, Corson JD, Baraniewski HM, et al: Osteomyelitis of the foot in diabetic patients: Evaluation with plain film, 99mTc-MDP bone scintigraphy, and MR imaging. AJR Am J Roentgenol 1989;152:795–800.
12. Wang A, Weinstein D, Greenfield L, et al: MRI and diabetic foot infections. Magn Reson Imaging 1990;8:805–809.
13. Hakki S, Harwood SJ, Morisey MA, et al: Comparative study of monoclonal antibody scan in diagnosing orthopaedic infection. Clin Orthop 1997;335:275–285.
14. Grayson ML, Gibbons GW, Habershaw GM, et al: Use of ampicillin/sulbactam versus imipenem/cilastatin in the treatment of limb-threatening foot infections in diabetic patients. Clin Infect Dis 1994;18:683–693.
15. Tan JS, Wishnow RM, Talan DA, et al: Treatment of hospitalized patients with complicated skin and skin structure infections: Double-blind randomized multicenter study of piperacillin-tazobactam versus ticarcillin-clavulanate. Antimicrob Agents Chemother 1993;37:1580–1586.
16. Bamberger DM, Dans GP, Gerding DN: Osteomyelitis in the feet of diabetic patients: Long-term results, prognostic factors, and the role of antimicrobial and surgical therapy. Am J Med 1987;83:653–660.
17. Tan JS, Miller C, File TM, et al: Can aggressive therapeutic intervention of diabetic foot infection reduce the length of hospitalization? Clin Infect Dis 1994;23:286–291.
18. Millington JT, Norris TW: Effective treatment strategies for diabetic foot wounds. J Fam Pract 2000;49:S40–S48.
19. Reuler JB, Coonoy TG: The pressure sore: Pathophysiology and principles of management. Ann Intern Med 1981;94:661–666.
20. Allman RM, Laprade CA, Noel LB, et al: Pressure sores among hospitalized patients. Ann Intern Med 1986;105:337–342.
21. Cooney TG, Reuler JB: Pressure sores. West J Med 1984;940:622–624.
22. Galpin JE, Chow AW, Bayer AS, et al: Sepsis associated with decubitus ulcers. Am J Med 1975;61:345–350.
23. Sapico FL, Ginunas VJ, Thornhill-Joynes M, et al: Quantitative microbiology of pressure sores in different stages of healing. Diagn Microbiol Infect Dis 1986;5:31–38.
24. Brook I: Microbiological studies of decubitus ulcers in children. J Pediatr Surg 1991;26:207–209.
25. Bryan CS, Dew CE, Reynolds KL: Bacteremia associated with decubitus ulcers. Arch Intern Med 1983;143:2093–2095.
26. Pressure ulcer prevalence, cost and risk assessment: Consensus development conference statement—The National Pressure Ulcer Advisory Panel. Decubitus 1989;2:24–28.
27. Sugarman B, Hawes S, Musher DM, et al: Osteomyelitis beneath pressure sores. Arch Intern Med 1983;143:683–688.
28. Thornhill-Joynes M, Gonzales F, Stewart CA, et al: Osteomyelitis associated with pressure sores. Arch Phys Med Rehab 1986;67:314–318.
29. Darouiche RO, Landon GF, Klima M, et al: Osteomyelitis associated with pressure sores. Arch Intern Med 1994;154:753–758.
30. DeLisa JA, Mikulic MH: Pressure ulcers: What to do if preventive management fails. Postgrad Med 1985;77:209–220.
31. Kucan JO, Robson MC, Heggers JP, Ko F: Comparison of silver sulfadiazine, povidone-iodine and physiologic saline in the treatment of chronic pressure ulcers. J Am Geriatr Soc 1981;29:232–235.
32. Mathes SJ, Nahai F: Clinical Applications for Muscle and Musculocutaneous Flaps. St. Louis, Mosby, 1982.
33. Rubayi S, Cousins S, Valentine WA: Myocutaneous flaps. Surgical treatment of severe pressure ulcers. AORN J 1990;52:40–55.
34. Müllner T, Mrkonjic L, Kwasny O, Vecsei V: The use of negative pressure to promote the healing of tissue defects: A clinical trial using the vacuum sealing technique. Br J Plast Surg 1997;50:194–199.
35. Sherman RA: A new dressing design for use with maggot therapy. Plast Reconstr Surg 1997;100:451–456.

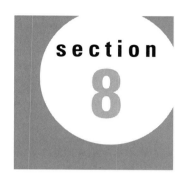

section

8

Toxin-Mediated Infections

chapter 21

Scarlet Fever and Toxic Shock Syndromes

DENNIS L. STEVENS, PhD, MD

SCARLET FEVER

Clinical Course

The mortality and morbidity of scarlet fever have declined dramatically since the end of the 19th century and well before the availability of penicillin. The best descriptions of scarlet fever, therefore, are those of the 19th century physician Osler. He described three types of malignant scarlet fever: atactic, hemorrhagic, and anginose.[1] The anginose form was basically membranous exudation of the throat, with necrosis of the soft tissues of the pharynx and soft palate. Exudation could continue into the trachea, bronchi, eustachian tubes, and middle ear. He noted that in some cases necrosis and sloughing of tissue about the tonsils was so severe that necrosis of the carotid artery occurred with fatal hemorrhage. Osler did not specify the time course of this form, although Holt[2] subsequently stated that the duration of the symptoms in fatal cases was from six to fourteen days. In the second variety, hemorrhages into the skin, hematuria, and epistaxis occurred. "Enfeebled children" were the most common group associated with this form, and death when it occurred was usually within the first 2 to 3 days of illness.[1,2] The third form was atactic scarlet fever, in which children presented with the characteristics of an acute intoxication.[1] The disease began with great severity, high fever, extreme restlessness, headache, and delirium.[1] Temperatures were frequently 107°F to 108°F (41.6°C to 42.2°C), and Osler[1] stated, "rare cases have been observed in which the thermometer has registered even higher." Convulsions, coma, severe dyspnea, and rapid feeble pulse was the most common presentation.[1] Patients died within 24 to 48 hours.[1]

Weaver[3] combined all these definitions into the following groups: mild, moderate, toxic, and septic. Thus, benign scarlet fever could be either mild or moderate, and the fatal or malignant form of scarlet fever could be either septic or toxic. The toxic cases invariably began with a severe sore throat, marked fever (107°F to 108°F), delirium, skin rash, and painful cervical lymph nodes.[1] In severe cases (similar to the malignant scarlet fever described by Osler[1] and Rotch[4]), fulminating fevers to 107°F to 108°F, pulse rates of 130 to 160, severe headache, delirium, convulsions, little if any skin rash, and death within 24 hours were the usual findings. These cases occurred before the advent of antibiotics, antipyretics, and anticonvulsants. The septic cases were similar to those described by Wood[5] as scarlatina anginosa, and by Osler[1] as the anginose form of scarlet fever. Here, local invasion of the soft tissues of the neck were the prominent features with subsequent upper airway obstruction, otitis media with perforation, profuse mucopurulent drainage from the nose, bronchopneumonia, and death. Note that necrotizing fasciitis and myositis were not described in association with scarlet fever. The only exception being locally invasive infection of the soft tissues of the neck as a complication of pharyngitis. In modern times, scarlet fever has been of the benign form and could be described as streptococcal pharyngitis with skin rash.

Demographics

Scarlet fever is most prevalent in children 4 to 8 years of age and is uncommon in adults. The primary infection most commonly associated with scarlet fever is pharyngitis, although soft tissue infection at a surgical site has been described (surgical scarlet fever). Scarlet fever is characterized by high fever, circumoral pallor, and a diffuse erythematous rash over the neck, trunk, face, and limbs. There is a sandpaper consistency to the rash, which blanches with pressure. A white coating over the tongue resolves quickly, leaving a strawberry appearance to the tongue owing to the swollen papillae. In modern times the illness resolves in 5 to 7 days, and by 10 to 14 days there may be impressive desquamation of the skin, particularly over the hands and feet.

Epidemiology

Large epidemics of scarlet fever have been reported in the literature since the 12th and 13th centuries in association with childbed fever, nonpasteurized milk, surgical wards, schools, day care centers, and certainly among family members. The transmission in nonhospitalized patients is usually via the oral route from droplets from primary cases or from ingestion of milk contaminated with toxin-producing strains of group A streptococci.

The Organism and Its Toxins

Group A streptococcus of M-types 1, 3, 4, 6, 12, and 18 have been the most common strains isolated from patients with scarlet fever, and currently M-4 is most common. In the 1920s, workers demonstrated that an extracellular protein produced by group A streptococci was responsible for scarlet fever, and they named this material scarlatina toxin. Over the years the name has been changed to erythrogenic toxin and finally to pyrogenic exotoxin. Filtrate from toxin-producing cultures could cause erythroderma (Dick test) and in high concentrations caused scarlet fever. Antibody raised against this crude material could blanch the rash of scarlet fever

(Schultz-Charlton reaction) and could attenuate the course of scarlet fever. It has also been observed that some children had more than one course of scarlet fever, and consequently we now know that 6 or 7 different pyrogenic exotoxins exist.

Treatment

Antimicrobial Therapy

Appropriate treatment of the primary streptococcal infection is the main objective, and penicillin, cephalosporins, erythromycin, or clindamycin is a good antibiotic choice (Table 21–1). In all fairness, there has never been a clinical trial comparing the efficacy of antibiotics in the treatment of scarlet fever. Thus antibiotic treatment recommendations are based upon treatment of streptococcal pharyngitis. Because all strains of group A streptococcus remain susceptible to penicillin, it is still the drug of choice, although cephalosporins, erythromycin, and clindamycin are at least as effective as penicillin.

Antipyretics

The fever associated with scarlet fever may be dramatic, and certainly temperatures above 104°F (40°C) or rapid changes in temperature warrant treatment with antipyretic agents. Acetaminophen (Tylenol) may be preferable to nonsteroidal agents, since the latter may also alter the host response to infection.[6] Aspirin should be avoided because of its association with Reye's syndrome.

Surgical Drainage

Some patients may require surgical intervention if they have postoperative, postpartum, or incisional scarlet fever or if a primary pharyngeal infection extends into the soft tissues of the neck or peritonsillar areas. In these cases surgical exploration and appropriate débridement may be necessary.

Prevention

Because group A streptococcus is highly contagious, appropriate measures should be taken in the home, day care center, school, or hospital to prevent secondary cases. Patients with surgical or nosocomial scarlet fever, although rare in modern times, should be placed in isolation and universal precautions implemented. Most cases of scarlet fever occur in school-age children. Thus the

TABLE 21–1 ■ Treatment of Streptococcal Pharyngitis and Tonsillitis

	Children	Adults
First choice	<60 lb (27 kg): Benzathine penicillin 600,000 U IM	>60 lb: Benzathine penicillin 1.2 MU IM
Second choice	Ampicillin plus clavulanic acid 20–40 mg/kg/d PO (may require IV treatment)	Ampicillin plus clavulanic acid 20–40 mg/kg/d PO (may require IV treatment)
Options for penicillin-allergic patients	Clindamycin 10 mg/kg/d PO	Clindamycin 10 mg/kg/d PO

school nurse or local health authority should be notified, since epidemics may develop rapidly. It should be noted that because of the recent benign nature of scarlet fever, reporting of cases to state health authorities has not been mandatory, although reporting of invasive cases of group A streptococcal infections is required.

STREPTOCOCCAL TOXIC SHOCK SYNDROME

Emergence and Persistence

In the 15 years since the first description of the streptococcal toxic shock syndrome (strepTSS), reports have documented the presence of these invasive infections in all corners of the world, in all races, sexes, and age groups. The strains responsible for these infections have been similar, suggesting a global spread of infection. As might be expected, identical strains have also accounted for less serious infections, such as cellulitis, pharyngitis, and even asymptomatic carriage. Thus host factors and comorbid conditions must account for the different diseases caused by identical strains.

The most prevalent M type associated with strepTSS has been, and continues to be, M-1. Interestingly M-3 strains have always been in second place, and together M-1 and M-3 account for approximately 50% of cases. Recent studies in the Netherlands found M-1 and M-3 strains each accounted for 25% of cases of invasive group A streptococcal infection.[7] In some geographic areas, M-1 strains have accounted for 70% of invasive infections.[8,9] In contrast, in the epidemic that occurred in Winnamango, Minnesota, 100% of the strains were M-3.[10] Other strains less commonly associated with strepTSS include M-types 4, 6, 11, 18, and 28 and nontypeable strains (reviewed in Stevens[11]). In most geographic settings a mixture of strains is responsible for sporadic cases.

As remarkable as the emergence of invasive group A streptococcal infections was in the mid-1980s, the continued persistence of such infections worldwide is equally unusual. The strains most commonly associated with these infections over the past 15 years have been M-1 and M-3 strains. From the theoretical perspective the high prevalence and persistence of such strains could be due to an absence of protective immunity in a significant portion of the human population (i.e., no herd immunity) or to changes in protective epitopes in the organism analogous to antigenic drift among influenza viruses. Although restriction fragment length polymorphism (RFLP) patterns of M-1 strains suggest that these strains have remained identical over a 10-year period, biophysical studies imply that this may not be the case. For example, de Malmanche and Martin, using functional studies of opsonophagocytosis, demonstrated that immunity may only be strain and not M-type specific.[12] In some of these strains, marked differences in the amino acid sequence of M-1 strains were apparent despite the fact that these strains were serologically typed as M-1. In addition, Villasenor et al have demonstrated that among 75 strains of M-1 group A streptococci, susceptibility to opsonophagocytosis in the presence of polyclonal anti-M-1 sera followed a normal distribution curve.[13] In fact some M-1 strains were no better opsonized than heterologous, non-M-1 strains.[14] In representative strains selected on the basis of their susceptibility to phagocytosis, differences were found in the sequence of M-protein in both the hypervariable region and the A-repeat regions of the molecule. Clearly these changes did not affect the structure enough to alter the serologic determination of M-type but were enough to affect opsonization with convalescent sera. Thus subtle differences in the surface structure of M-1 protein renders some strains resistant to immune sera, suggesting that antigenic drift could account for the high prevalence and persistence of M-1 strains over the last 15 years.

The apparent increase in the incidence of invasive group A streptococcal infections also suggests a change in the virulence of the organism. M-protein, streptolysin O (SLO), and streptococcal pyrogenic exotoxins A and B (SPEA, SPEB) have been implicated as important virulence factors. None of these, however, have been associated with all invasive cases. For example, although M-1 and M-3 have been most common, M-12, M-28, and nontypeable strains have also been associated with invasive streptococcal infection.[15] Similarly in the United States, M-1 strains containing the gene for SPEA have been commonly associated with strepTSS; however, only about 50% of these strains produce SPEA.[16] Recently streptococcal superantigen (SSA), a novel pyrogenic exotoxin, has been isolated from an M-3 strain, albeit in small concentrations.[17] In addition, mitogenic factor (MF) has been demonstrated in many different M-types of group A streptococcus.[18,19] Therefore no single surface component or extracellular toxin has thus far been identified that correlates with the recent increase in virulence in group A streptococcus. In 1997 we reported a strong association between isolates from invasive disease, regardless of M-type, and the production of nicotinamide adenine dinucleotide glycohydrolase (NADase).[20] In contrast, isolates that were most commonly associated with rheumatic fever (i.e., M-5 and M-18) did not produce NADase.[20] Throat isolates associated with uncomplicated symptomatic pharyngitis were most commonly M-1, M-12, and M-4,[15] and 100% of these isolates from the early 1980s to the present time were NADase producers.[20] This is not surprising, since the source of bacteria in invasive streptococcal infections is frequently the throat.

It is of special interest that M-1 strains isolated from recent (circa 1980) invasive cases were NADase producers,[20] since historically M-1 group A streptococci have been characteristically non-NADase producers.[21,22] This observed shift in NADase production has also been reported by Karasawa et al[23] among M-1 isolates in Japan and most recently by Ajdic et al[24] at the University of

Oklahoma, where the group A streptococcal genome has been elucidated. Our genetic analysis demonstrated that all strains of group A streptococci, regardless of their ability to produce NADase, possess the NADase gene, *nga*, and that all isolates examined were more than 96% identical in *nga* and upstream regulatory sequences.[25] Further, because NADase-negative strains did not produce any immunoreactive protein or peptide fragment, we concluded that additional regulatory element(s) control NADase production.[25] Taken together, these findings suggest that in the early 1980s, serotype M-1 underwent a stable genetic change resulting in the ability to produce NADase. Further, acquisition of this trait occurred in temporal association with the emergence of M-1 group A streptococcus as the predominant serotype associated with severe invasive infections.[15,26,27] NADase's role in pathogenesis is currently under study.

Epidemiology

Several population-based studies of strepTSS have documented the annual incidence of 1 to 5 cases per 100,000 population,[28] with most cases being sporadic occurrences; however, larger epidemics of invasive group A streptococcal infections have also been described in some settings. In 1994 an epidemic of related invasive infections occurred in Wannamingo, Minnesota,[10] with an annualized prevalence of 24 cases per 100,000 population. In Missoula, Montana, in 1999 the incidence of invasive infections reached 30 cases per 100,000 population. In addition to community-based infections, invasive group A streptococcal infections have been described in hospitals and convalescent centers and among hospital employees and family contacts of patients with invasive infections.[16,29,30] Some of these studies have documented the same M-type and identical RFLP patterns in strains from primary and index cases.[16,29–31] In addition, carriage of group A streptococcus by health care personnel has been associated with the spread of life-threatening group A streptococcal infections in the obstetrics-gynecology and ear-nose-throat wards of American hospitals.[32] Such infections have also originated in outpatient surgical settings and within the home environment.

It has been estimated that the risk of secondary cases may be approximately 200 times greater than the risk among the general population.[33] There is ample data from studies conducted over several decades that group A streptococcus is quickly and efficiently transmitted from index cases to susceptible individuals and that transmission may result in colonization, pharyngitis, scarlet fever, rheumatic fever, or invasive group A streptococcal infections. The risk for secondary cases is likely related to close or intimate contact, crowding, and such host factors as the following:

1. Active viral infections such as varicella or influenza
2. Recent surgical wounds or childbirth (my unpublished observations)

3. Absence of type-specific opsonic antibody against the group A streptococcus causing the index case
4. Absence of neutralizing antibody against SPEA or SPEB.[7]

Acquisition of Group A Streptococcus

The portals of entry for streptococci are the vagina, pharynx, mucosa, and skin in 50% of cases.[26] Interestingly a portal of entry cannot be defined in the remaining 50%.[26] Rarely, patients with symptomatic pharyngitis develop strepTSS. Surgical procedures such as suction lipectomy, hysterectomy, vaginal delivery, bunionectomy, and bone pinning provide a portal of entry in some cases. Numerous cases have developed within 24 to 72 hours of minor nonpenetrating trauma resulting in hematoma or a deep bruise to the calf and even following muscle strain.[26] Virus infections such as varicella and influenza have provided portals in other cases.[26] In some cases the use of nonsteroidal anti-inflammatory agents may have masked the presenting symptoms or predisposed the person to more severe streptococcal infection and shock.[26] Most cases of strepTSS occur sporadically, although outbreaks of severe group A streptococcal infections have been described in closed environments such as nursing homes[34,35] and hospital environments.[29,30]

Symptoms and Signs

Twenty percent of strepTSS patients have an influenza-like syndrome characterized by fever, chills, myalgia, nausea, vomiting, and diarrhea (Table 21–2).[26] Fever is the most common presenting sign, although hypothermia may be present in patients in shock.[26] Confusion is present in 55% of patients, and in some, coma or combativeness are manifest.[26] Pain—the most common initial symptom of strepTSS—starts abruptly, is severe,[26] and usually precedes tenderness or physical findings. The pain usually involves an extremity but may also mimic peritonitis, pelvic inflammatory disease, pneumonia, acute myocardial infarction, or pericarditis.[26] Eighty percent of patients have clinical signs of soft tissue infection such as localized swelling and erythema, which progresses to necrotizing fasciitis or myositis in 70% of those cases, requiring surgical débridement, fasciotomy, or amputation.[26] Of the 20% of cases without soft tissue findings, various clinical presentations were observed, including endophthalmitis, myositis, perihepatitis, peritonitis, myocarditis, and overwhelming sepsis.[26] A diffuse, scarlatina-like erythema is uncommon, occurring in only 10% of cases.

Laboratory Evaluation of Patients with StrepTSS

The serum creatinine phosphokinase level is useful in detecting the presence of deeper soft-tissue infections, and when the level is elevated or rising, there is a good

TABLE 21-2 ■ Defining the Streptococcal Toxic Shock Syndrome

An acute, febrile illness that begins with a mild viral-like prodrome and involves minor soft tissue infection that may progress to shock, multiorgan failure, and death.

SYMPTOMS
Early symptoms are vague:
  Viral-like prodrome
  Severe pain and erythema of an extremity
  Mental confusion

SIGNS
  Hypotension, systolic
  Fever >38°C
  Soft tissue swelling
  Tenderness
  Respiratory failure, rales, cyanosis, tachypnea

LABORATORY FEATURES
Hematologic:
  Marked left shift
  Decline in hematocrit
  Thrombocytopenia
Renal azotemia (2.5 × normal on admission) and hematuria
Hypocalcemia
Hypoalbuminemia
Creatinine phosphokinase elevation
Pulmonary abnormalities:
  Pulmonary infiltrate on chest radiograph
  Hypoxia

---

correlation with necrotizing fasciitis or myositis.[26] Although the initial laboratory studies may demonstrate only mild leukocytosis, the mean percentage of immature neutrophils (including band forms, metamyelocytes, and myelocytes) is striking, reaching 40% to 50%.[26] Hemoglobinuria and elevated serum creatinine values are evidence of renal involvement. It is important to note that renal impairment precedes hypotension in 40% to 50% of cases.[26] Hypoalbuminemia and hypocalcemia occur early and become profound within 24 to 48 hours of admission.

Clinical Course

The rapidity with which shock and multiorgan failure can progress is impressive, and many patients may die within 24 to 48 hours of hospitalization.[26] Shock was apparent at the time of admission or within 4 to 8 hours in virtually all patients. In only 10% of patients did systolic blood pressure become normal 4 to 8 hours after administration of antibiotics, albumin, and electrolyte solutions containing salts or dopamine; in all other patients shock persisted. Interestingly, renal dysfunction preceded shock in many cases and was apparent on admission in most patients. Renal failure progressed or persisted in all patients for 48 to 72 hours, and several patients required dialysis for 10 to 20 days.[26] In patients who survived, serum creatinine values returned to normal within 4 to 6 weeks. Acute respiratory distress syndrome (ARDS) occurred in 55% of patients and generally developed after the onset of hypotension.[26] The severity of ARDS was

such that supplemental oxygen, intubation, and mechanical ventilation was necessary in 90% of those who developed this syndrome.[26] Mortality has varied from 30% to 70%[26,36,37]; however, morbidity is also high: 13 of 20 patients in one series underwent major surgical procedures, which included fasciotomy, surgical débridement, exploratory laparotomy, intraocular aspiration, amputation, or hysterectomy.[26]

Pathogenic Mechanisms

The role of adherence and penetration of pharyngeal epithelial cells has been the subject of intense research recently to determine what surface components of the group A streptococcus are involved and to determine if penetration of such cells correlates with the ability of a strain to cause invasive infection. Lapenta et al[38] demonstrated that M-1 strains efficiently adhered to and penetrated respiratory epithelial cells. Dombeck et al[39] then demonstrated that a clonal variant of M-1 group A streptococcus linked to invasive infections (designated M1inv+) was internalized with high frequency by cultured HeLa cells and that this internalization depended on M-protein. In contrast, others have demonstrated that M-1 strains adhered to and invaded epithelial cells less efficiently than other M-types did.[40,41] In addition Molinari and Chhatwal[40] have demonstrated that regardless of M-type, strains isolated from invasive cases (blood isolates) exhibited poorer attachment and internalization of epithelial cells than strains isolated from throat or skin.

Kawabata et al[42] demonstrated that the hyaluronic acid capsule of group A streptococci hampered their invasion efficiency. Tsai et al[43] investigated the role of SPEB in the invasion of respiratory epithelial cells (A-549) and found that SPEB knockout strains' ability to invade cells was reduced and that exogenous addition of SPEB spurred invasion by the SPEB knockout mutants. In other studies, SPEB knockout mutants' ability to invade epithelial cells was not affected.[44] This discrepancy could in part be explained by the recent work of Woischnik, Buttaro, and Podbielski,[45] who demonstrated that inactivation of the SPEB structural gene (speB) decreased hyaluronic acid capsule production but did not affect other virulence factors. These findings demonstrate that interpretation of data from experiments using isogenic mutants may not always be straightforward.

Talay et al[46] and Hanski and Caparon[47] demonstrated that streptococcal fibronectin binding protein I (SfbI) mediated binding of group A streptococcus to epithelial cells in the presence of fibronectin. Subsequently Okada et al[48] using strains lacking prtF1 gene have conclusively demonstrated that (SfbI) mediates attachment of group A streptococcus to HeLa cells. Molinari and Chhatwal[40] demonstrated that the distribution of SfbI was lowest among blood isolates (27%) and highest among skin and throat isolates (95%). These authors concluded that reduced SfbI expression is responsible for the reduced attachment to and invasion of tissue culture cells by blood isolates of group A streptococcus.

As described under the discussion on keratinocyte adherence and penetration, M-protein may serve as a ligand in specific strains of group A streptococcus. Recent studies by Jadoun et al[49] suggest that both M-protein (M-6) and SfbI may participate in adherence and invasion of epithelial cells. This is supported by the observation that type-specific sIgA and IgG antibody prevented adherence and invasion, respectively, of human pharyngeal cells challenged with M-6 strains.[50]

In summary, adherence and penetration of epithelial cells by group A streptococcus is a complex process that is dependent upon the cell type, state of differentiation (e.g., keratinocyte), strain of group A streptococcus, the immune status of the host, and the inflammatory milieu of the host environment. The importance of these latter points is substantiated by the observation that tumor necrosis factor (TNF) and interleukin (IL)-1 reduce the adherence of group A streptococcus to keratinocytes[51] and by the demonstration that SfbI-vaccinated animals showed protection against 80% of homologous and 90% of heterologous viable group A streptococcus when challenged intranasally.[52] Finally, SfbI was found in 64% and SfbII in 36% of strains in the northern territory of Australia, and high levels of IgG antibody were found in the sera of 80 subjects with defined streptococcal infections such as pharyngitis or pyoderma.[53]

Mechanisms of Shock

Pyrogenic exotoxins induce fever in humans and animals and also participate in shock by lowering the threshold to exogenous endotoxin.[27] SPEA and SPEB induce human mononuclear cells to synthesize not only TNF-α[54] but also IL-1β[55] and IL-6,[55–57] suggesting that TNF could mediate the fever, shock, and organ failure observed in patients with strepTSS.[26] Pyrogenic exotoxin C (SPEC) has been associated with mild cases of scarlet fever in the United States (my observations) and in England.[58] The roles of newly described pyrogenic exotoxins, such as SSA[17] and MF,[19] in the pathogenesis of strepTSS have not been elucidated.

There is strong evidence suggesting that SPEA, SPEB, SPEC, and a number of toxic shock staphylococcal toxins (TSST-1 and staphylococcal enterotoxins A, B, and C) act as superantigens and stimulate T cell responses through their ability to bind to both the class II major histocompatibility complex (MHC) of APCs and the Vβ region of the T cell receptor.[59] The net effect is induction of T cell proliferation (via an IL-2 mechanism) with concomitant production of cytokines (e.g., IL-1, TNF-α, TNF-β, IL-6, interferon-gamma [IFN-γ] that mediate shock and tissue injury. Recently, Hackett and Stevens demonstrated that SPEA induced both TNF-α and TNF-β from mixed cultures of monocytes and lymphocytes,[60] supporting the role of lymphokines (TNF-β)

in shock associated with strains producing SPEA. Kotb et al have[61] shown that a digest of M-protein type 6 can also stimulate T cell responses by this mechanism. Interestingly, quantitation of such Vβ T cell subsets in patients with acute strepTSS demonstrated deletion rather than expansion, suggesting that perhaps the life span of the expanded subset was shortened by a process of apoptosis.[62] In addition, the subsets deleted were not specific for SPEA, SPEB, SPEC, or MF, suggesting that perhaps an as yet undefined superantigen may play a role in strepTSS.[62]

Cytokine production by less exotic mechanisms may also contribute to the genesis of shock and organ failure. Peptidoglycan, lipoteichoic acid,[63] and killed organisms[64,65] are capable of inducing TNF-α production by mononuclear cells in vitro.[27,65,66] Exotoxins such as SLO are also potent inducers of TNF-α and IL-1β. SPEB, a proteinase precursor, has the ability to cleave pre-IL-1β to release preformed IL-1β.[67] Finally, SLO and SPEA together have additive effects in the induction of IL-1β by human mononuclear cells.[60] Whatever the mechanisms, induction of cytokines in vivo is likely the cause of shock, and, for example, SLO, SPEA, SPEB, SPEC, and cell wall components are potent inducers of TNF and IL-1.[16] Finally, a cysteine protease formed from cleavage of SPEB may play an important role in pathogenesis by the release of bradykinin from endogenous kininogen and by activating metalloproteases involved in coagulation.[68]

The mere presence of virulence factors, such as M-protein or pyrogenic exotoxins, may be less important in strepTSS than the dynamics of their production invivo. For example, Chaussee et al[16] have demonstrated that among strains from patients with necrotizing fasciitis and strepTSS, SPEA was produced by approximately 40% and SPEB by approximately 75%. In addition, the quantity of SPEA but not SPEB was higher for strains from strepTSS patients than from patients with noninvasive cases.[16] Recently, Clearly et al have proposed a regulon in group A streptococcus that controls the expression of a group of virulence genes coding for virulence factors such as M-protein and C5-peptidase.[69] DNA fingerprinting showed differences between M-1 strains isolated from patients with invasive disease and M-1 strains from patients with noninvasive group A streptococcal infections.[70] Such strains of group A streptococci could acquire genetic information coding for SPEA via specific bacteriophage. Multilocus enzyme electrophoresis demonstrates two patterns that correspond to M-1 and M-3 organisms that produce SPEA, a finding that fits epidemiologic studies implicating these strains in invasive group A streptococcal infections[71] in the United States.

Numerous studies have demonstrated that SPEA potentiates the action of lipopolysaccharide (LPS) in inducing shock.[72] Interestingly this effect is largely the result of T cell activation, and the "potentiating activity," which can be passively transferred to rabbits by infusing supernatants from SPEA-stimulated lymphocytes,[73] is likely mediated by INF-γ and TNF-β. In contrast the timing of pretreatment with SPEA is crucial, since we have shown that pretreatment of mice with SPEA 96 hours before LPS challenge gives protection from LPS-induced shock,[74] probably through the production of immunosuppressive cytokines such as IL-10. Finally, Sriskandan et al have demonstrated that animals immunized with recombinant SPEA have a higher mortality when challenged with an SPEA-producing strain of group A streptococcus than animals that are sham immunized.[75] Further, Sriskandan et al have demonstrated that animals challenged with an SPEA knockout strain of group A streptococcus had greater mortality and more tissue destruction than animals challenged with the wild-type parent strain.[76]

Thus the roles of the pyrogenic exotoxins in the pathogenesis of severe group A streptococcal infections are complex and remain to be fully elucidated. However, the importance of cytokine induction in group A streptococcal infections cannot be denied. Hackett et al have shown that cell wall components from killed invasive and noninvasive strains of group A streptococci elicit significant TNF-α production by mononuclear cells,[64] exceeding that elicited by SPEA, SPEB, or SLO.[64] Further, viable SLO-deficient, but not viable wild-type, group A streptococci stimulated high levels of TNF-α, suggesting that SLO suppresses induction of this cytokine, perhaps in part because of its cytotoxic effect on host cells. Cytokine induction by cell wall components of the group A streptococcus has also been demonstrated by Muller-Alouf et al.[65]

An important role for TNF-α in shock associated with severe group A streptococcal infections is also suggested by the remarkable efficacy of a neutralizing monoclonal antibody against TNF-α in an experimental streptococcal bacteremia model in nonhuman primates.[77] Survival of animals was increased by 50%, and markers of organ failure such as serum creatinine and lactate were also significantly improved.[77]

Other Mechanisms of Shock and Organ Failure

Recently, Chatellier and Kotb demonstrated the CpG-CG–rich motifs of *emm1* functioned as superantigens and induced T cell proliferation.[78] Sriskandan et al have also demonstrated that inducible nitric oxide (iNOS) may play a role in shock associated with a group A streptococcal necrotizing soft tissue infection.[79] In that model, *N*-monomethyl-L-arginine (L-NMMA) administration reduced nitrate levels in serum but did not reduce mortality.[79]

The role of streptokinase in invasive group A streptococcal infections has not been extensively studied; however, recent studies demonstrate that certain alleles of streptokinase (*ska2*) have three energetic folding units that change the tertiary structure of *ska* into a more lipophilic molecule with high affinity for glomeruli. Only *ska2* isogenic mutants are capable of causing kidney lesions with polymorphonuclear leukocyte influx into the glomeruli as well as deposition of C3.[80]

Streptolysin S (SLS) has been known for a long time to be a potent cytotoxin for many different cell types, although its role as a significant virulence factor has only recently been implicated. Betschel et al[81] have demonstrated that insertional activation of the gene controlling SLS reduced the virulence in a mouse model. Recently Nizet et al have demonstrated that SLS production is controlled by a contiguous nine-gene locus (*sagA* to *sagI*) and that the gene product SLS likely has a structure similar to that of the bacteriocin family of microbial toxins.[82]

Treatment and Experimental Therapeutics

Antibiotic Therapy—Importance of the Mechanism of Action

Streptococcus pyogenes remains exquisitely susceptible to β-lactam antibiotics, and penicillin has excellent efficacy in the treatment of erysipelas, impetigo, and cellulitis and in the prevention of acute rheumatic fever. Nonetheless, clinical failures of penicillin treatment of streptococcal infection do occur, and penicillin fails to eradicate bacteria from the pharynx of patients with documented streptococcal pharyngitis in 5% to 20% of patients.[83–85] Finally, more aggressive group A streptococcal infections (such as necrotizing fasciitis, empyema, burn wound sepsis, subcutaneous gangrene, and myositis) do not respond well to penicillin and continue to be associated with high mortality and extensive morbidity.[8,26,27,86–89] For example, a recent report of 25 cases of streptococcal myositis reported an overall mortality of 85% despite penicillin therapy.[86]

Studies in experimental infection have demonstrated that penicillin fails when large numbers of organisms are present.[90,91] For example, in a mouse model of myositis due to *S. pyogenes*, penicillin was ineffective when treatment was delayed for 2 hours or longer after initiation of infection.[91] Mice receiving clindamycin, however, had survival rates of 100%, 100%, 80%, and 70% when treatment was delayed 0, 2, 6, and 16.5 hours, respectively.[91,92] Eagle suggested that penicillin failed in this type of infection because of the "physiologic state of the organism."[90] This phenomenon has recently been attributed to inoculum effects, both in vitro and in vivo.[93,94] It has also been observed that penicillin and other β-lactam antibiotics are most efficacious against rapidly growing bacteria. Early in the stages of infection or in mild infections, organisms grow rapidly in vivo but are present in rather small numbers. With delays in treatment, higher concentrations of group A streptococci accumulate, and growth begins to slow to a stationary phase. That high concentrations of *S. pyogenes* accumulate in deep seated infection is supported by data from Eagle.[90]

Why should penicillin lose its efficacy when large numbers of group A streptococci are present or when they are making the transition from logarithmic to stationary growth? Since penicillin mediates its antibacterial action against group A streptococci by intimately interacting with the expressed penicillin-binding proteins (PBPs), we compared the PBP patterns from membrane proteins of group A streptococci isolated from different stages of growth, that is, mid-log phase and stationary phase. Binding of radiolabeled penicillin by all PBPs was lower in stationary cells. In fact, PBPs 1 and 4 were undetectable at 36 hours.[93] Thus the loss of certain PBPs during stationary-phase growth in vitro may be responsible for the inoculum effect observed in vivo and may account for the failure of penicillin in both experimental and human cases of severe streptococcal infection.

The greater efficacy of clindamycin in severe group A streptococcal infections is due to many factors. First, its efficacy is not affected by inoculum size or stage of growth.[93,95] Second, clindamycin suppresses bacterial toxin synthesis.[96,97] Third, clindamycin facilitates phagocytosis of *S. pyogenes* by inhibiting M-protein synthesis.[97] Fourth, clindamycin suppresses synthesis of PBPs, which, in addition to being targets for penicillin, are also enzymes involved in cell wall synthesis and degradation.[95] Fifth, clindamycin has a longer postantibiotic effect than β-lactams such as penicillin. Lastly, we have recently shown that clindamycin suppresses LPS-induced monocyte synthesis of TNF-α.[98] Thus clindamycin's efficacy may also be related to its ability to modulate the immune response to group A streptococcal infection. Interestingly in a recent retrospective analysis of strepTSS cases, Zimbelman et al demonstrated significantly better survival in patients receiving clindamycin than in those treated with β-lactam antibiotics.[99]

Other Treatment Measures

Prompt and aggressive exploration and débridement of suspected deep-seated *S. pyogenes* infection is crucial to limiting complications and to preventing extension to vital areas that may be impossible to débride (i.e., the head and neck, thorax, or abdomen). Since definite cutaneous evidence of necrotizing fasciitis and myositis may not appear until late in the course of the disease, the index of suspicion should be high in patients with fever, excruciating pain, and systemic toxicity. Radiographs, computed tomography (CT) and magnetic resonance imaging (MRI) scans in patients with strepTSS show soft tissue swelling and an absence of gas, thus providing clues to the site of the deep infection. Prompt surgical exploration with visualization of muscle and fascia and timely Gram stain of surgically obtained material provide the earliest and most definitive etiologic diagnosis.[100] Clearly, evidence of muscle necrosis and necrotizing fasciitis requires extensive, and often multiple, surgical débridements.

Because of intractable hypotension and diffuse capillary leak, massive amounts of intravenous fluids (10 to 20 L/d) are often necessary, and about 10% of patients have significant clinical improvement after hydration.

Pressors such as dopamine are used frequently, although no controlled trials have been performed in strepTSS. In patients with intractable hypotension, vasoconstrictors such as epinephrine have been used, but often symmetrical gangrene of digits results (my unpublished observations). Loss of all digits on both hands and feet or loss of both arms and legs has occurred in this setting. In these cases it is difficult to determine if symmetrical gangrene is due to pressors or infection or both.

Neutralization of circulating toxins would be a desirable therapeutic modality, yet hyperimmune sera are not commercially available in the United States or Europe. Case reports[101,102] and one nonrandomized clinical trial[103] report that commercial intravenous immune globulin (IVIG) may be useful for treating strepTSS. A double-blind study using IVIG is currently under way in northern Europe. Because cytokines are important mediators of shock in strepTSS, strategies to inhibit or neutralize their effects may also provide useful treatments. Recently a monoclonal antibody against TNF-α showed promising efficacy in a baboon model of strepTSS.[77] Finally, anecdotal reports suggest that hyperbaric oxygen may be helpful; however, no controlled studies are under way, and it is not clear if this treatment is useful.

Prevention

Vaccine

Currently, there are several group A streptococcal virulence factors being investigated as potential vaccine candidates. These include group A polysaccharide, C5a peptidase, SPEB, SPEA, the conserved segment of the M-protein molecule, and a cassette of peptides representing the hypervariable regions of M-protein from strains commonly encountered. At the present time, none have been studied in humans.

Prophylaxis and the Risk of Secondary Cases of StrepTSS

The incidence of primary cases of strepTSS is low (3.5 cases per 100,000 population per year; Centers for Disease Control and Prevention [CDC] unpublished results) despite the high prevalence of "virulent strains of group A streptococci" in the population at large.[10] Yet clusters of group A streptococcal invasive infections have been described in nursing homes,[34,35,104] in health care workers,[30,105] and among family members.[30,104] Patients may acquire group A streptococci from hospital personnel, and this was best demonstrated by Semmelwise in Vienna and Holme in the United States, although even in modern times such transmission is well documented.[30,105,106] Epidemiologic investigation of clusters of cases is important, and treatment of contacts may be necessary despite the low risk of secondary invasive infection.[107] Primary care physicians must consider the extent of exposure, the type of exposure, and the risk factors of the contact. For example, a contact of a case of strepTSS with risk factors such as chickenpox, leukemia, burns, recent surgery, or any open skin lesion should receive prophylaxis with penicillin, erythromycin, or clindamycin.[107]

The principles that should guide use of secondary prophylaxis are the observations that group A streptococcus is highly transmissible in closed environments such as hospital wards and family homes. Thus secondary cases of streptococcal colonization are common, but development of invasive disease remains rare. However, the risk of development of invasive disease following contact with a primary case is higher than in the general population. The goal should be to reduce the incidence of secondary cases and to investigate the cause of hospital-acquired cases. Hospital workers who are pharyngeal, rectal, or vaginal carriers of group A streptococcus have been implicated in disease transmission on surgical and obstetrics and gynecology wards.

STAPHYLOCOCCAL TOXIC SHOCK SYNDROME

Epidemiology

Toxic shock syndrome associated with *Staphylococcus aureus* infections originally was referred to as TSS,[108] although in this paper this syndrome is designated staphTSS to clearly distinguish it from strepTSS. Between 77% and 93% of cases of staphTSS have occurred in females, and most (greater than 90%) of them were 15- to 19-year-old white girls.[109–114] The incidence of staphTSS was highest in 1980 and ranged from 2.4 to 16/100,000 population.[112,113,115–118] Because most of these studies were performed using similar techniques and case definitions, the differences in the incidence of disease likely represented bona fide epidemiologic variations, with northern California having the lowest[118] and Colorado[117] having the highest infection rates. The peak of reported cases of staphTSS occurred during 1980, followed by a marked and persistent decline. Numerous epidemiologic studies established that the illness was associated with females during their menstrual cycles and that *S. aureus* colonization or infection within the vagina played a significant role.[109–117] A novel toxin, called toxic shock syndrome toxin-1 (TSST-1), was isolated from *S. aureus*[119,120] and was found to be produced by over 90% of *S. aureus* strains isolated from menstrual cases of staphTSS.[121]

The marked decline in the incidence of staphTSS that occurred in 1981 has many possible explanations. First, there may have been enhanced reporting of cases in 1980 because of extensive media coverage. Second, there may have been a true decline in the incidence because of education of the patients at risk, loss of virulence of the microbe, or acquisition of immunity to the putative toxins. Alternatively, subsequent under-reporting of cases after the 1980 peak in staphTSS may have contributed to a falsely apparent decline in prevalence. Last, some suggest that the reduced prevalence was due to removal of Rely tampons from the marketplace. Clearly the removal of one brand of tampon from stores does not explain this epidemiologic phenomenon fully since menstrual cases of staphTSS continue to occur. Excellent articles about the epidemiologic studies implicating tampons and Rely brand in particular have been published.[109–112,122,123]

Also in the early 1980s it was established that nonmenstrual cases of staphTSS occurred among both sexes, regardless of age, and were associated with surgical procedures such as rhinoplasty with Teflon stents or nasal packing.[124] Nonmenstrual cases have also been described in association with a variety of primary *S. aureus* infections including cutaneous infection, postsurgical or postpartum infection, focal tissue infection, and pneumonia with or without antecedent influenza infection.[125] In contrast to menstrual cases of staphTSS, TSST-1 has been detected in only half of strains isolated from patients with nonmenstrual staphTSS.[121,124] Finally, staphylococcal enterotoxin B (SEB) and to a lesser extent enterotoxins A (SEA) and C (SEC) have been found in the remaining strains.[126–129] In addition, case reports suggest that strains that produce TSST-1 together with SEC may be more likely to cause fatalities,[127,128] although both toxins are rarely found together in the same strain.[129]

Clinical Presentation of StaphTSS

A prodromal period of 2 to 3 days precedes the physical manifestations of staphTSS and consists of malaise, myalgia, and chills.[130] Fever begins soon thereafter and immediately before lightheadedness, modest confusion, and lethargy appear. Most patients develop diarrhea early in the course of staphTSS. Symptoms of hypovolemia, due in part to capillary leak and diarrhea, then predominate and include hyperventilation, palpitations, and dizziness on standing. Confusion, a prominent feature of staphTSS, may affect some patients' ability to recognize the seriousness of their illness, resulting in delayed treatment.

When patients are first examined, fever, tachycardia, tachypnea, and hypotension are usually present. A transient, erythematous rash has been observed in over 50% of patients and may be either diffuse or patchy in distribution.[130] Many patients have marked peripheral vasodilation associated with high cardiac output, and thus erythematous skin may represent maximal capillary dilatation due to toxins or endogenous mediators. The capillary leak mentioned above may not be apparent until fluid resuscitation has been undertaken. Desquamation of skin, particularly at sites of a previous erythematous rash, occurs between 7 and 14 days after the fever began.[130]

Pathogenesis of StaphTSS

There is little doubt that TSST-1 and staphylococcal enterotoxins are the major virulence factors associated with cases of staphTSS. There is substantial evidence that the genetic determinants for TSST-1 and SEB are neither plasmid- nor bacteriophage-mediated and that the gene is a variably expressed mobile element, likely a transposon.[131] Because the gene is variably expressed, there has been intense research to elucidate the environmental and genetic control mechanisms responsible for enhanced toxin production. Clearly, neutral pH, iron, trace elements such as magnesium and calcium, and oxygen enhance TSST-1 production (reviewed in Bergdoll and Chesney[123]). Toxin is produced mainly during the late-log phase and early stationary phase of growth.

Extrapolation of these findings to the apparent increased risk of menstrual staphTSS with tampon use in 1980 has been more difficult if not controversial. Some suggest that tampons could (1) increase vaginal partial oxygen pressure, at least during placement, thereby stimulating toxin synthesis by colonizing strains of *S. aureus*, (2) supply surfactants that could increase toxin production, and (3) bind magnesium and shift the growth kinetics of staphylococci toward enhanced toxin production.[125] Thus modest quantities of these toxins, locally produced, interact with the immune system first at the site of infection and then systemically.

Monocytes and a mononuclear cell line have the ability to bind TSST-1 and staphylococcal enterotoxins. In addition these toxins bind to specific sites on the Vβ region of the T lymphocyte receptor (TCR). Simultaneous binding to both monocyte and T lymphocyte results in T cell proliferation (blastogenesis) and activation of both cell types via the superantigen mechanism.[132] Recent studies have shown that activation of the T cell via this mechanism requires the appropriate toxin, viable T lymphocytes bearing a specific Vβ repertoire, and either a viable APC, a nonviable APC, or a fragment of the MHC class II receptor.[133]

Other accessory molecules may also participate in the docking between MHC class II and TCR. One of the T lymphocyte binding sites for enterotoxin appears to be CD4.[134] This could serve to stabilize the complex between the TCR and MHC class II. Further, blocking of other surface molecules such as ICAM-1, CD11a, CD28, or CD2 with monoclonal antibodies effectively prevented T cell proliferation in the presence of SEB.[135]

The consequences of superantigen stimulation of the immune system is T lymphocyte proliferation and generation of vast quantities of lymphokines (IL-2, INF-γ, and TNF-β)[56,66,132] and monokines (TNF-α, IL-1, and IL-6),[54,66] yet the dynamics of production are quite different for each. Specifically, during the first 24 hours, production of TNF-α by peripheral blood mononuclear cells (PBMC) predominates. By 48 hours, TNF-β is detectable, and at 72 hours, equal quantities of TNF-α and TNF-β can be measured.[66]

The control mechanisms of cytokine production via the superantigen mechanism is poorly understood; however, both counter-regulator cytokines and accelerated programmed cell death are likely involved. For example,

the conventional wisdom regarding T cell proliferation describes the initial proliferation of T cells in response to superantigens followed by the rapid depletion of T cell subsets bearing the specific Vβ repertoire through accelerated programmed cell death or apoptosis.[132] Recently T lymphocyte dynamics were studied in a mouse model of SEB-induced shock.[136,137] There was clear evidence of Vβ-selective clonal expansion 24 to 48 hours after administration of SEB.[136,137] On day 3, clonally expanding cells became depleted through accelerated programmed cell death (apoptosis), resulting in anergy.[136,137] McCormack et al[138] demonstrated that this expansion-deletion sequence occurred predictably in vivo when high concentrations of a superantigen are used. However, deletions also occur with low dosages. In fact, concentrations insufficient to cause T cell blastogenesis in vivo were still capable of depleting specific Vβ subsets of T lymphocytes.[138] Using sublethal concentrations of a superantigen, Miethke et al recently demonstrated that 4 to 6 hours after in vivo challenge with SEB, BALB/c mice became resistant to an otherwise lethal dose of SEB plus D-galactosamine.[139] These authors demonstrated that PBMC harvested from such animals during this time lost the ability to release lymphokines such as TNF and IL-2.[139] They hypothesized that endogenous corticosteroids released in response to the first wave of lymphokines induced by SEB may have suppressed T cell responsiveness. Although this might be an adequate explanation, counter-regulatory cytokines likely play a more important role. For example, 10 ng/ml of IL-10, a regulatory cytokine produced by the Th2 subset of CD4+ helper T lymphocytes, inhibited synthesis of TNF-α and INF-γ production by TSST-1-stimulated PBMC by 68% and 86% respectively.[140] The relevance of this endogenous control mechanism in vivo is uncertain, since only 72 pg/ml of IL-10 was produced in vitro by PBMC stimulated with TSST-1,[140] a concentration well below that used in the in vitro studies. Regardless of whether IL-10 contributes as an autocrine or paracrine endogenous inhibitor of PBMC synthesis of TNF-α or TNF-β, Krakauer points out that exogenous administration of recombinant IL-10 might be a rational treatment for superantigen-induced disease.[140] Recent studies showing that IL-10 protected animals from lethal challenge supports this hypothesis[141] (see also discussion under Treatment). Interestingly, IL-10 did not inhibit T lymphocyte blastogenesis,[140] suggesting that IL-10 works largely by inhibiting transcriptional events.

Although the previously described animal models of superantigen injection demonstrate lethality, what is the evidence that *S. aureus* toxins such as TSST-1 or the enterotoxins cause an illness resembling staphTSS? The animal model that has been best studied in this regard is the rabbit wiffle ball model. Briefly, sterile plastic chambers are implanted beneath the skin of rabbits and allowed to mature over the course of 3 to 4 weeks. Strains of *S. aureus* are then inoculated into these chambers, and physiologic measurements of blood chemistries, blood pressure, pulse, and temperature and mortality are recorded. Scott and coworkers[142] and Rasheed et al[143] using this model and De Azevedo et al[144] using an implanted uterine diffusion chamber model, demonstrated that strains producing TSST-1 were more likely to induce a toxic shock–like syndrome than were strains that did not produce TSST-1. Recently strains of *S. aureus* that produced altered TSST-1 toxins lacking the ability to induce mitogenicity were nontoxic in the rabbit wiffle ball chamber model,[145] although the reason for the loss of mitogenicity was unexplained. Subsequently, using both genetically altered SEC mutants and peptide fragments of SEC to stimulate lymphocyte proliferation in vitro, it was determined that toxin binding to the alpha helix of the MHC class II portion of the APC was critical in the induction of lymphocyte blastogenesis.[146]

The role of TSST-1 in inducing a TSS-like illness is also supported by the demonstration that a neutralizing monoclonal antibody prevented illness in rabbits challenged with a TSST-1-producing strain of *S. aureus*.[147] Parsonnet et al[148] developed a slow infusion model that allows the investigation of purified, recombinant, and genetically altered toxins.

Staphylococcal Infections

Patients diagnosed as having staphTSS will be profoundly hypotensive, tachycardic, and febrile and may have evidence of coagulopathy (see Table 21–3). The general supportive measures described in the previous discussion apply to staphTSS as well. Clearly in menstrual cases early removal of the tampon and irrigation of the vaginal vault are important. Similarly in nonmenstrual cases, surgical débridement, drainage, and removal of stents and packing are vital.[149]

Antibiotic treatment based on in vitro susceptibility would suggest that nafcillin, first- or second-generation cephalosporins, vancomycin, clindamycin, erythromycin, and fluoroquinolones would be reasonable choices. Various of these antibiotics have been used in the last 15

years, and the mortality of staphTSS remains at about 3% for menstrual cases and is twofold to threefold higher for nonmenstrual cases.[123]

As is the case with strepTSS, shock and organ failure in patients with staphTSS are clearly the consequence of extracellular proteinaceous toxins' deleterious effects upon the immune system. Thus antibiotics that suppress protein (toxin) synthesis might be more efficacious than cell wall–active antibiotics. Clindamycin in concentrations that were either above the minimal inhibitory concentration[150] or below it[151] suppressed TSST-1 synthesis by strains of *S. aureus*. Parsonnet et al[152] demonstrated that clindamycin, erythromycin, rifampin, and fluoroquinolones all suppressed TSST-1 synthesis by greater than 90%. In addition, they demonstrated that 5 different β-lactam antibiotics including nafcillin and cephalosporins increased measurable TSST-1 in culture supernatants, probably by lysing or at least increasing the permeability of the cell membrane.[152] Unfortunately there has been no controlled clinical trial to compare different antibiotics; however, these results suggest that antibiotic susceptibility alone may not be all the information needed. Because of the high incidence of *S. aureus* strains that are resistant to methicillin, appropriate cultures and sensitivities become more important in the new millennium. Thus treatment should be based on definitive sensitivities, and if methicillin-resistant *S. aureus* is encountered, quinupristin-dalfopristin (Synercid), linezolid (Zyvox), or vancomycin may be necessary.[153]

The potential use of immunoglobulin to treat staphTSS has a sound basis (see also Treatment of strepTSS). First, many investigators have demonstrated that patients who develop staphTSS have low-to-absent antibody titers against TSST-1 and enterotoxins (reviewed by Bergdoll and Chesney[123]). Second, the general population in both the United States and Europe has significant antibody titers against these toxins, and titers increase with age.[123] That titers increase with age is supported by the observation that pooled immunoglobulin preparations have high antibody titers against TSST-1.[123] Finally, recent data in experimental animals indicates that

---

TABLE 21–3 ■ Comparison of Staphylococcal and Streptococcal Toxic Shock Syndromes

Feature	Staphylococcal	Streptococcal
Age	Primarily 15–35 y	Primarily 20–50 y
Sex	Greatest in women	Either
Severe pain	Rare	Common
Hypotension	100%	100%
Erythroderma rash	Very common	Less common
Renal failure	Common	Common
Bacteremia	Low	60%
Tissue necrosis	Rare	Common
Predisposing factors	Tampons, packing, NSAID use?	Cuts, burns, bruises, varicella, NSAID use?
Thrombocytopenia	Common	Common
Mortality	<3%	30%–70%

NSAID, nonsteroidal anti-inflammatory drug.

antibody that neutralizes TSST-1 is therapeutic.[154,155] There have been no prospective studies done in humans.

The usefulness of corticosteroids in shock has been studied for many years and is not currently considered to be an effective treatment in the United States, although some centers in Europe currently use this treatment. Todd advocates corticosteroids for patients with "severe staphTSS unresponsive to initial antibiotic therapy."[149]

Prevention of StaphTSS

Prevention of first episodes of menstrual staphTSS requires minimal use of high-absorbency tampons, careful placement of tampons according to the manufacturer's directions, and reduction in the time that a particular tampon is left in place. Prevention of recurrence is best accomplished by aggressively treating the initial infection with parenteral antibiotics, education of the patient about the preceding factors, and avoidance of tampons in general.

Clinical Clues and Differential Diagnosis of Toxic Shock Syndromes

The abrupt onset of shock in a previously healthy person has a limited number of causes. In addition to strepTSS, staphTSS must be considered, particularly in females during menstruation or in either sex in association with recent surgery or any localized staphylococcal abscess (Table 21–3). Gram-negative sepsis can mimic strepTSS, yet it is uncommon in nonhospitalized, non-neutropenic patients. The exception is typhoid fever, which certainly attacks healthy people. Although sporadic cases of bacteremia due to *Salmonella* occur in association with foodborne illnesses, typhoid fever is usually related to natural disasters such as hurricanes, floods, and earthquakes. Renal impairment frequently precedes hypotension in strepTSS, whereas in gram-negative shock, renal failure (acute tubular necrosis) develops only after hypotension. Similarly the white blood cell count is generally normal or elevated with a marked left shift in strepTSS and to a lesser extent in staphTSS, whereas in gram-negative shock, and typhoid fever in particular, the white blood cell count is usually low. Rocky Mountain spotted fever (RMSF) must be distinguished from staphTSS and strepTSS because all three cause shock in otherwise healthy persons. In RMSF the rash is most commonly petechial, whereas in staphTSS and strepTSS it is diffusely erythematous. Most patients with RMSF have severe headache and rash, whereas in strepTSS, headache is rare, and rash is present in only 10% of patients. If rash is not present, distinguishing these two causes would be difficult. Meningococcemia could be confused with either staphTSS or strepTSS, although the rash resembles RMSF to a much greater extent. Meningitis, although common in meningococcemia, is uncommon in either staphTSS or

strepTSS. Some persons with strepTSS have respiratory symptoms and on presentation to the hospital have lobar consolidation and empyema. When such patients present with shock, it may be difficult to distinguish them from those with overwhelming *Streptococcus pneumoniae* sepsis. Finally, heat stroke has been confused with some cases of strepTSS, largely because of the patients' elevated temperature, dehydration with evidence of renal impairment, confusion, hypotension, and sunburn rash.

The differential diagnosis of deep soft tissue infection with or without shock includes the following clinical entities. Acute hemorrhage in the form of a retroperitoneal, intra-abdominal, or deep soft tissue bleed can result in increasing pain at the site of previous injury or surgery and, if blood loss is massive, hypotension. The absence of fever and a normal white blood cell count and differential would weigh against a diagnosis of staphTSS or strepTSS. In cases in which necrotizing fasciitis develops following a penetrating injury, progression of the cutaneous infection to necrotizing fasciitis is more obvious. In situations in which necrotizing fasciitis develops in the deep tissue following nonpenetrating trauma, there may be no cutaneous signs of infection until late in the course of the disease when violaceous bullae may appear. Thus in these cases, increasing pain at the site of injury, fever, marked left shift, and elevated creatine phosphokinase may be clues to the diagnosis of strepTSS. At this stage the symptoms frequently are attributed to a putative thrombophlebitis secondary to prior trauma. Venograms are invariably normal, and soft tissue radiograph and CT scan results usually demonstrate diffuse soft tissue swelling, moderate fluid accumulation in the muscle compartments, no abscess formation, and no gas. Frequently the interpretation is "results compatible with prior muscle injury, hematoma, or deep vein thrombophlebitis." In the setting of chills, fever, and marked left shift, such an interpretation is inappropriate and frequently delays surgical exploration. In contrast, necrotizing fasciitis and myonecrosis caused by mixed aerobic and anaerobic bacteria or *Clostridium* spp. are associated with gas in the tissues, and thus soft tissue radiographs are of more value. MRI and CT scans are useful to localize the site of infection, but they do not provide specificity that is clinically useful.

Once the site of infection has been localized, either by clinical clues or radiographic techniques, surgical intervention not only is useful for diagnostic purposes but also is of major therapeutic importance. A decision to surgically explore a patient is easy when there is cutaneous evidence of an infectious process and the patient is either not responding to medical management or is clinically deteriorating. It is more difficult to suspect necrotizing fasciitis in a patient with only increasing pain and fever and no cutaneous evidence of infection. Since about 50% of patients with strepTSS have deep-seated soft tissue infections and only about 50% have obvious portals of entry, the aforementioned presentation is quite common.

The physician's job gets even more difficult when patients are taking nonsteroidal anti-inflammatory agents (e.g., aspirin) or acetaminophen, since these agents reduce pain and suppress fever. Some of these agents may predispose patients to a more severe type of infection by their abilities to suppress phagocytic killing of bacteria and to alter the host's response.[6] Still, necrotizing fasciitis due to *S. pyogenes* progresses rapidly, and a delay in diagnosis for any reason is associated with a worse prognosis. In addition, the greater the delay, the greater the need for more extensive surgery. In some cases the rapid onset of shock and organ failure may preclude surgical intervention.

REFERENCES

1. Osler W: Practice of Medicine, 2nd ed. New York, D Appleton and Co, 1895.
2. Holt LE: Scarlet fever. In Holt LE (ed): The Diseases of Infancy and Childhood. New York, D Appleton and Co, 1897, pp 888–910.
3. Weaver GH: Scarlet fever. In Abt IA (ed): Pediatrics. Philadelphia, WB Saunders, 1925, pp 298–362.
4. Rotch TM: Pediatrics: The Hygienic and Medical Treatment of Children. Philadelphia, JB Lippincott, 1896.
5. Wood GB: A Treatise on the Practice of Medicine, 5th ed. Philadelphia, JB Lippincott, 1858.
6. Stevens DL: Could nonsteroidal anti-inflammatory drugs (NSAIDs) enhance the progression of bacterial infections to toxic shock syndrome? Clin Infect Dis 1995;21:977–980.
7. Mascini EM, Jansze M, Schellenkens JFP, et al: Invasive group A streptococcal disease in the Netherlands: Evidence for a protective role of anti-exotoxin A antibodies. J Infect Dis 2000;181:631–638.
8. Martin PR, Hoiby EA: Streptococcal serogroup A epidemic in Norway 1987–1988. Scand J Infect Dis 1990;22:421–429.
9. Eriksson BK, Andersson J, Holm ED, Norgren M: Invasive group A streptococcal infections: T1M1 isolates expressing pyrogenic exotoxins A and B in combination with selective lack of toxin-neutralizing antibodies are associated with increased risk of streptococcal toxic shock syndrome. J Infect Dis 1999;180:410–418.
10. Cockerill FR, MacDonald KL, Thompson RL, et al: An outbreak of invasive group A streptococcal disease associated with high carriage rates of the invasive clone among school-aged children. JAMA 1997;277:38–43.
11. Stevens DL: Streptococcal toxic shock syndrome: Spectrum of disease, pathogenesis and new concepts in treatment. Emerg Infect Dis 1995;1:69–78.
12. de Malmanche SA, Martin DR: Protective immunity to the group A streptococcus may be only strain specific. Med Microbiol Immunol 1994;183:299–306.
13. Villasenor-Sierra A, McShan WM, Salmi D, et al: Variable susceptibility to opsonophagocytosis of group A streptococcus M-1 strains by human immune sera. J Infect Dis 1999;180:1921–1928.
14. Villasenor A: Hetereogeneous opsonic activity of convalescence serum against M-1 strains of group A streptococci (GAS). In Proceedings and Abstracts of the 37th Interscience Conference on Antimicrobial Agents and Chemotherapy, Toronto. Washington, DC, American Society for Microbiology, 1997.
15. Johnson DR, Stevens DL, Kaplan EL: Epidemiologic analysis of group A streptococcal serotypes associated with severe systemic infections, rheumatic fever, or uncomplicated pharyngitis. J Infect Dis 1992;166:374–382.
16. Chaussee MS, Liu J, Stevens DL, Ferretti JJ: Genetic and phenotypic diversity among isolates of Streptococcus pyogenes from invasive infections. J Infect Dis 1996;173:901–908.
17. Mollick JA, Miller GG, Musser JM, et al: A novel superantigen isolated from pathogenic strains of Streptococcus pyogenes with amino terminal homology to staphylococcal enterotoxins B and C. J Clin Invest 1993;92:710–719.
18. Iwasaki M, Igarashi H, Hinuma Y, Yutsudo T: Cloning, characterization and overexpression of a Streptococcus pyogenes gene encoding a new type of mitogenic factor. FEBS Lett 1993;331:187–192.
19. Norrby-Teglund A, Newton D, Kotb M, et al: Superantigenic properties of the group A streptococcal exotoxin SpeF (MF). Infect Immun 1994;62:5227–5233.
20. Stevens DL, McIndoo E, Bryant AE, Zuckerman D: Production of NADase in clinical isolates of Streptococcus pyogenes. In Program and Abstracts of the 37th Interscience Conference on Antimicrobial Agents and Chemotherapy, Toronto. Washington, DC, American Society for Microbiology, 1997.
21. Bernheimer AW, Lazarides PD, Wilson AT: Diphosphopyridine nucleotidase as an extracellular product of streptococcal growth and its possible relationship to leukotoxicity. J Exp Med 1957;106:27–37.
22. Lutticken R, Lutticken D, Johnson DR, Wannamaker LW: Application of a new method for detecting streptococcal nicotinamide adenine dinucleotide glycohydrolase to various M types of Streptococcus pyogenes. J Clin Microbiol 1976;3:533–536.
23. Karasawa T, Yamakawa K, Tanaka D, et al: NAD$^+$-glycohydrolase productivity of haemolytic streptococci assayed by a simple fluorescent method and its relation to T serotype. FEMS Microbiol Lett 1995;128:289–292.
24. Ajdic D, McShan WM, Savic DJ, et al: The NAD-glycohydrolase (nga) gene of Streptococcus pyogenes. FEMS Microbiol Lett 2000;191:235–241.
25. Stevens DL, Salmi DB, McIndoo ER, Bryant AE: Molecular epidemiology of nga and NAD glycohydrolase/ADP-ribosyltransferase activity among Streptococcus pyogenes causing streptococcal toxic shock syndrome. J Infect Dis 2000;182:1117–1128.
26. Stevens DL, Tanner MH, Winship J, et al: Reappearance of scarlet fever toxin A among streptococci in the Rocky Mountain West: Severe group A streptococcal infections associated with a toxic shock–like syndrome. N Engl J Med 1989;321:1–7.
27. Stevens DL: Invasive group A streptococcus infections. Clin Infect Dis 1992;14:2–13.
28. Schwartz B, Facklam RR, Brieman RF: Changing epidemiology of group A streptococcal infection in the USA. Lancet 1990;336:1167–1171.
29. Gamba MA, Martinelli M, Schaad HJ, et al: Familial transmission of a serious disease-producing group A streptococcus clone: Case reports and review. Clin Infect Dis 1997;24:1118–1121.
30. Dipersio JR, File TM, Stevens DL, et al: Spread of serious disease-producing M3 clones of group A streptococcus among family members and health care workers. Clin Infect Dis 1996;22:490–495.
31. Ichiyama S, Nakashima K, Shimokata K, et al: Transmission of Streptococcus pyogenes causing toxic shock–like syndrome among family members and confirmation by DNA macrorestriction analysis. J Infect Dis 1997;175:723–726.
32. Nosocomial group A streptococcal infections associated with asymptomatic health-care workers—Maryland and California. MMWR Morb Mortal Wkly Rep 1997;48:163–165.
33. Davies HD, McGeer A, Schwartz B, et al: Invasive group A streptococcal infections in Ontario, Canada. N Engl J Med 1996;335:547–554.

34. Auerbach SB, Schwartz B, Williams D, et al: Outbreak of invasive group A streptococcal infections in a nursing home. Lessons on prevention and control. Arch Intern Med 1992;152:1017–1022.

35. Hohenboken JJ, Anderson F, Kaplan EL: Invasive group A streptococcal (GAS) serotype M-1 outbreak in a long-term care facility (LTCF) with mortality. In Program and Abstracts of the Interscience Conference on Antimicrobial Agents and Chemotherapy, Orlando, Fla, Abstract J189, 1994.

36. Demers B, Simor AE, Vellend H, et al: Severe invasive group A streptococcal infections in Ontario, Canada: 1987–1991. Clin Infect Dis 1993;16:792–800.

37. Stegmayr B, Bjorck S, Holm S, et al: Septic shock induced by group A streptococcal infections: Clinical and therapeutic aspects. Scand J Infect Dis 1992;24:589–597.

38. Lapenta D, Rubens C, Chi E, Cleary PP: Group A streptococci efficiently invade human respiratory epithelial cells. Proc Natl Acad Sci USA 1994;91:12115–12119.

39. Dombek PE, Cue D, Sedgewick J, et al: High-frequency intracellular invasion of epithelial cells by serotype M1 group A streptococci: M1 protein-mediated invasion and cytoskeletal rearrangements. Mol Microbiol 1999;31:859–870.

40. Molinari G, Chhatwal GS: Invasion and survival of Streptococcus pyogenes in eukaryotic cells correlates with the source of clinical isolates. J Infect Dis 1998;177:1600–1607.

41. Hagman MM, Stevens DL: Comparison of adherence to and penetration of a human laryngeal epithelial cell line by group A streptococci of various M protein types. FEMS Immunol Med Microbiol 1999;23:195–204.

42. Kawabata S, Kuwata H, Nakagawa I, et al: Capsular hyaluronic acid of group A streptococci hampers their invasion into human pharyngeal epithelial cells. Microb Pathog 1999;27:71–80.

43. Tsai PJ, Kuo CF, Lin KY, et al: Effect of group A streptococcal cysteine protease on invasion of epithelial cells. Infect Immun 1998;66:1460–1466.

44. Darmstadt GI, Mentele L, Podbielski A, Rubens CE: Role of group A streptococcal virulence factors in adherence to keratinocytes. Infect Immun 2000;68:1215–1221.

45. Woischnik M, Buttaro BA, Podbielski A: Inactivation of the cysteine protease SpeB affects hyaluronic acid capsule expression in group A streptococci. Microb Pathog 2000;28:221–226.

46. Talay SR, Valentin-Weigand P, Jerlström PG, et al: Fibronectin-binding protein of Streptococcus pyogenes: Sequence of the binding domain involved in adherence of streptococci to epithelial cells. Infect Immun 1992;60:3837–3844.

47. Hanski E, Caparon M: Protein F, a fibronectin-binding protein, is an adhesin of the group A streptococcus Streptococcus pyogenes. Proc Natl Acad Sci USA 1992;89:6172–6176.

48. Okada N, Tatsuno I, Hanski E, et al: Streptococcus pyogenes protein F promotes invasion of HeLa cells. Microbiol 1998;144:3079–3086.

49. Jadoun J, Ozeri V, Burstein E, et al: Protein F1 is required for efficient entry of Streptococcus pyogenes into epithelial cells. J Infect Dis 1998;178:147–158.

50. Fluckiger U, Jones KF, Fischetti VA: Immunoglobulins to group A streptococcal surface molecules decrease adherence to and invasion of human pharyngeal cells. Infect Immun 1998;66:974–979.

51. Darmstadt GL, Fleckman P, Rubens CE: Tumor necrosis factor-alpha and interleukin-1-alpha decrease the adherence of Streptococcus pyogenes to cultured keratinocytes. J Infect Dis 1999;180:1718–1721.

52. Guzman CA, Talay SR, Molinari G, et al: Protective immune response against Streptococcus pyogenes in mice after intranasal vaccination with the fibronectin-binding protein SfbI. J Infect Dis 1999;179:901–906.

53. Goodfellow AM, Hibble M, Talay SR, et al: Distribution and antigenicity of fibronectin binding proteins (SfbI and SfbII) of Streptococcus pyogenes clinical isolates from the northern territory, Australia. J Clin Microbiol 2000;38:389–392.

54. Fast DJ, Schlievert PM, Nelson RD: Toxic shock syndrome–associated staphylococcal and streptococcal pyrogenic toxins are potent inducers of tumor necrosis factor production. Infect Immun 1989;57:291–294.

55. Hackett SP, Schlievert PM, Stevens DL: Cytokine production by human mononuclear cells in response to streptococcal exotoxins. Clin Res. 1991; 39.

56. Norrby-Teglund A, Norgren M, Holm SE, et al: Similar cytokine induction profiles of a novel streptococcal exotoxin, MF, and pyrogenic exotoxins A and B. Infect Immun 1994;62:3731–3738.

57. Muller-Alouf H, Alouf JE, Gerlach D, et al: Cytokine production by murine cells activated by erythrogenic toxin type A superantigen of Streptococcus pyogenes. Immunobiology 1992;186:435–448.

58. Hallas G: The production of pyrogenic exotoxins by group A streptococci. J Hyg (Camb) 1985;95:47–57.

59. Mollick JA, Rich RR: Characterization of a superantigen from a pathogenic strain of Streptococcus pyogenes. Clin Res 1991;39:213A.

60. Hackett SP, Stevens DL: Streptococcal toxic shock syndrome: Synthesis of tumor necrosis factor and interleukin-1 by monocytes stimulated with pyrogenic exotoxin A and streptolysin O. J Infect Dis 1992;165:879–885.

61. Kotb M, Tomai M, Majumdar G, et al: Cellular and biochemical responses of human T lymphocytes stimulated with streptococcal M protein. In 11th Lancefield International Symposium on Streptococcal Diseases, Sienna, Italy. Abstract L77, 1990.

62. Watanabe-Ohnishi R, Low DE, McGeer A, et al: Selective depletion of Vβ-bearing T cells in patients with severe invasive group A streptococcal infections and streptococcal toxic shock syndrome. J Infect Dis 1995;171:74–84.

63. Stevens DL, Bryant AE, Hackett SP: Gram-positive shock. Curr Opin Infect Dis 1992;5:355–363.

64. Hackett S, Ferretti J, Stevens D: Cytokine induction by viable group A streptococci: Suppression by streptolysin O. In Program and Abstracts of the American Society for Microbiology, Las Vegas, Nev. Abstract B-249, 1994.

65. Muller-Alouf H, Alouf JE, Gerlach D, et al: Comparative study of cytokine release by human peripheral blood mononuclear cells stimulated with Streptococcus pyogenes superantigenic erythrogenic toxins, heat-killed streptococci and lipopolysaccharide. Infect Immun 1994;62:4915–4921.

66. Hackett SP, Stevens DL: Superantigens associated with staphylococcal and streptococcal toxic shock syndromes are potent inducers of tumor necrosis factor beta synthesis. J Infect Dis 1993;168:232–235.

67. Kappur V, Majesky MW, Li LL, et al: Cleavage of interleukin 1β (IL-1β) precursor to produce active IL-1β by a conserved extracellular cysteine protease from Streptococcus pyogenes. Proc Natl Acad Sci USA 1993;90:7676–7680.

68. Burns EH, Marciel AM, Musser JM: Activation of a 66-kilodalton human endothelial cell matrix metalloprotease by Streptococcus pyogenes extracellular cysteine protease. Infect Immun 1996;64:4744–4750.

69. Cleary P, Chen C, Lapenta D, et al: A virulence regulon in Streptococcus pyogenes. In Program and Abstracts of the Third International ASM Conference on Streptococcal Genetics, Minneapolis, Minn, Abstract 19, 1990.

70. Cleary PP, Kaplan EL, Handley JP, et al: Clonal basis for resurgence of serious Streptococcus pyogenes disease in the 1980s. Lancet 1992;339:518–521.

71. Musser JM, Hauser AR, Kim MH, et al: Streptococcus pyogenes causing toxic-shock-like syndrome and other invasive

diseases: Clonal diversity and pyrogenic exotoxin expression. Proc Natl Acad Sci USA 1991;88:2668–2672.

72. Schlievert PM, Watson DW: Group A streptococcal pyrogenic exotoxin: Pyrogenicity, alteration of blood-brain barrier, and separation of sites for pyrogenicity, and enhancement of lethal endotoxin shock. Infect Immun 1978;21:753–763.

73. Murai T, Ogawa Y, Kawasaki H: Macrophage hyperreactivity to endotoxin induced by streptococcal pyrogenic exotoxin in rabbits. FEMS Microbiol Lett 1990;68:61–64.

74. Stevens DL, Bryant AE, Hackett SP: Pretreatment with either endotoxin (LPS), tumor necrosis factor α (TNFα) or streptococcal pyrogenic exotoxin A (SPEA) protects mice from lethal streptococcal infection. In Program and Abstracts of the American Society for Microbiology, Atlanta, Ga. Abstract B369, 1993.

75. Sriskandan S, Moyes D, Buttery LK, et al: Streptococcal pyrogenic exotoxin A release, distribution, and role in a murine model of fasciitis and multiorgan failure due to Streptococcus pyogenes. J Infect Dis 1996;173:1399–1407.

76. Sriskandan S, Unnikrishnan M, Cohen J: Streptococcal pyrogenic exotoxin A (SPEA) can augment neutrophil recruitment to sites of inflammation. In Proceedings and Abstracts of Interscience Conference on Antimicrobial Agents and Chemotherapy (ICAAC), San Francisco. Washington, DC, American Society for Microbiology, 1999.

77. Stevens DL, Bryant AE, Hackett SP, et al: Group A streptococcal bacteremia: The role of tumor necrosis factor in shock and organ failure. J Infect Dis 1996;173:619–626.

78. Chatellier S, Kotb M: Identification of DNA CpG sequence motifs in group A streptococcal virulent genes that preferentially stimulate human lymphocytes: Evidence for differential host reponsiveness. In Proceedings and Abstracts of Interscience Conference on Antimicrobial Agents and Chemotherapy (ICAAC), San Francisco. Washington, DC, American Society for Microbiology, 1999.

79. Sriskandan S, Moyes D, Buttery LK, et al: The role of nitric oxide in experimental murine sepsis due to pyrogenic exotoxin A–producing Streptococcus pyogenes. Infect Immun 1997;65:1767–1772.

80. Nordstrand A, McShan WM, Ferretti JJ, et al: Allele substitution of the streptokinase gene reduces the nephritogenic capacity of group A streptococcal strain NZ131. Infect Immun 2000;68:1019–1025.

81. Betschel SD, Borgia SM, Barg NL, et al: Reduced virulence of group A streptococcal Tn916 mutants that do not produce streptolysin S. Infect Immun 1998;66:1671–1679.

82. Nizet V, Beall B, Bast DJ, et al: Genetic locus for streptolysin S production by group A streptococcus. Infect Immun 2000;68:4245–4254.

83. Kim KS, Kaplan EL: Association of penicillin tolerance with failure to eradicate group A streptococci from patients with pharyngitis. J Pediatr 1985;107:681–684.

84. Gatanaduy AS, Kaplan EL, Huwe BB, et al: Failure of penicillin to eradicate group A streptococci during an outbreak of pharyngitis. Lancet 1980;2:498–502.

85. Brook I: Role of beta-lactamase-producing bacteria in the failure of penicillin to eradicate group A streptococci. Pediatr Infect Dis 1985;4:491–495.

86. Adams EM, Gudmundsson S, Yocum DE, et al: Streptococcal myositis. Arch Intern Med 1985;145:1020–1023.

87. Kohler W: Streptococcal toxic shock syndrome. Zentralbl Bakteriol 1990;272:257–264.

88. Hribalova V: Streptococcus pyogenes and the toxic shock syndrome. Ann Intern Med 1988;108:772.

89. Gaworzewska ET, Coleman G: Correspondence: Group A streptococcal infections and a toxic shock–like syndrome. N Engl J Med 1989;321:1546.

90. Eagle H: Experimental approach to the problem of treatment failure with penicillin. I. Group A streptococcal infection in mice. Am J Med 1952;13:389–399.

91. Stevens DL, Bryant-Gibbons AE, Bergstrom R, Winn V: The Eagle effect revisited: Efficacy of clindamycin, erythromycin, and penicillin in the treatment of streptococcal myositis. J Infect Dis 1988;158:23–28.

92. Stevens DL, Bryant AE, Yan S: Invasive group A streptococcal infection: New concepts in antibiotic treatment. Int J Antimicrob Agents 1994;4:297–301.

93. Stevens DL, Yan S, Bryant AE: Penicillin binding protein expression at different growth stages determines penicillin efficacy in vitro and in vivo: An explanation for the inoculum effect. J Infect Dis 1993;167:1401–1405.

94. Yan S, Mendelman PM, Stevens DL: The in vitro antibacterial activity of ceftriaxone against Streptococcus pyogenes is unrelated to penicillin-binding protein 4. FEMS Microbiol Lett 1993;110:313–318.

95. Yan S, Bohach GA, Stevens DL: Persistent acylation of high-molecular-weight penicillin binding proteins by penicillin induces the post antibiotic effect in Streptococcus pyogenes. J Infect Dis 1994;170:609–614.

96. Stevens DL, Maier KA, Mitten JE: Effect of antibiotics on toxin production and viability of Clostridium perfringens. Antimicrob Agents Chemother 1987;31:213–218.

97. Gemmell CG, Peterson PK, Schmeling D, et al: Potentiation of opsonization and phagocytosis of Streptococcus pyogenes following growth in the presence of clindamycin. J Clin Invest 1981;67:1249–1256.

98. Stevens DL, Bryant AE, Hackett SP: Antibiotic effects on bacterial viability, toxin production, and host response. Clin Infect Dis 1995;20:S154–S157.

99. Zimbelman J, Palmer A, Todd J: Improved outcome of clindamycin compared with beta-lactam antibiotic treatment for invasive Streptococcus pyogenes infection. Pediatr Infect Dis J 1999;18:1096–1100.

100. Bisno AL, Stevens DL: Streptococcal infections in skin and soft tissues. N Engl J Med 1996;334:240–245.

101. Barry W, Hudgins L, Donta S, Pesanti E: Intravenous immunoglobulin therapy for toxic shock syndrome. JAMA 1992;267:3315–3316.

102. Yong JM. Letter. Lancet 1994;343:1427.

103. Kaul R, McGeer A, Norrby-Teglund A, et al: Intravenous immunoglobulin therapy for streptococcal toxic shock syndrome—A comparative observational study. Clin Infect Dis 1999;28:800–807.

104. Schwartz B, Elliot JA, Butler JC, et al: Clusters of invasive group A streptococcal infections in family, hospital, and nursing home settings. Clin Infect Dis 1992;15:277–284.

105. Valenzuela TD, Hooton TM, Kaplan EL, Schlievert PM: Transmission of 'toxic strep' syndrome from an infected child to a firefighter during CPR. Ann Emerg Med 1991;20:90–92.

106. Stamm WE, Feeley JC, Facklam RR: Wound infections due to group A streptococcus traced to a vaginal carrier. J Infect Dis 1978;138:287–292.

107. The Working Group on Prevention of Invasive Group A Streptococcal Infections: The working group on prevention of invasive group A streptococcal infections. Prevention of invasive group A streptococcal diseases among household contacts of case-patients: Is prophylaxis warranted? JAMA 1998;279:1206–1210.

108. Todd J, Fishaut M: Toxic-shock syndrome associated with phage-group-1 staphylococci. Lancet 1978;2:1116–1118.

109. Broome CV: Epidemiology of toxic shock syndrome in the United States: Overview. Rev Infect Dis 1989;11(Suppl 1):S14–S21.

110. Davis JP, Chesney PJ, Wand PJ, LaVenture M, the Investigation and Laboratory Team: Toxic shock syndrome: Epidemiologic features, recurrence, risk factors, and prevention. N Engl J Med 1980;303:1429–1435.

111. Shands KN, Schmidt GP, Dan BB, et al: Toxic shock syndrome in menstruating women. N Engl J Med 1980;303:1436–1442.

112. Schlech WF, Shands KN, Reingold AL, et al: Risk factors for the development of toxic shock syndrome: Association with a tampon brand. JAMA 1982;248:835–839.

113. Osterholm MT, Davis JP, Gibson RW, et al: Tri-state toxic-shock syndrome study. I. Epidemiologic findings. J Infect Dis 1982;145:431–440.

114. Latham RH, Kehrberg MW, Jacobson JA, Smith CB: Toxic shock syndrome in Utah: A case-control and surveillance study. Ann Intern Med 1982;96:906–908.

115. Helgerson SD, Foster LR: Toxic shock syndrome in Oregon. Ann Intern Med 1982;96:909–911.

116. Osterholm MT, Forfang JC: Toxic shock syndrome in Minnesota: Results of an active-passive surveillance system. J Infect Dis 1982;145:458–464.

117. Todd JK, Wiesenthal AM, Ressman M, et al: Toxic shock syndrome. II. Estimated occurrence in Colorado as influenced by case ascertainment methods. Am J Epidemiol 1985;122:857–867.

118. Petitti DB, Reingold AL, Chin J: The incidence of toxic shock syndrome in northern California: 1972–1983. JAMA 1986;255:368–372.

119. Schlievert PM, Shands KN, Dan BB, et al: Identification and characterization of an exotoxin from Staphylococcus aureus associated with toxic-shock syndrome. J Infect Dis 1981;143:509–516.

120. Bergdoll MS, Crass BA, Reiser RF, et al: A new staphylococcal enterotoxin, enterotoxin F, associated with toxic-shock-syndrome Staphylococcus aureus isolates. Lancet 1981;1:1017–1021.

121. Bonventre PF, Weckbach L, Harth G, Haidaris C: Distribution and expression of toxic shock syndrome toxin 1 gene among Staphylococcus aureus isolates of toxic shock syndrome and non-toxic shock syndrome origin. Rev Infect Dis 1989;11:S90–S95.

122. Mittag H-C: Toxic Shock Syndrome and the Other Staphylococcal Toxicoses. Stuttgart, Schattauer, 1988.

123. Bergdoll MS, Chesney PJ: Toxic Shock Syndrome. Boca Raton, Fla, CRC Press, 1991.

124. Jacobson JA, Kasworm E, Daly JA: Risk of developing toxic shock syndrome associated with toxic shock syndrome toxin 1 following nongenital staphylococcal infection. Rev Infect Dis 1989;11:S8–S13.

125. Murray DL, Ohlendorf DH, Schlievert PM: Staphylococcal and streptococcal superantigens: Their role in human diseases. ASM News 1995;61:229–235.

126. Crass BA, Bergdoll MS: Involvement of staphylococcal enterotoxins in nonmenstrual toxic shock syndrome. J Clin Microbiol 1986;23:1138–1139.

127. Schlievert PM: Staphylococcal entertoxin B and toxic shock syndrome toxin 1 are significantly associated with non-menstrual TSS. Lancet 1986;1:1149–1150.

128. Crass BA, Bergdoll MS: Toxin involvement in toxic shock syndrome. J Infect Dis 1986;153:918–926.

129. Bohach GA, Kreiswirth BN, Novick RP, Schlievert PM: Analysis of toxic shock syndrome isolates producing staphylococcal enterotoxins B and C1 with use of southern hybridization and immunologic assays. Rev Infect Dis 1989;11:S75–S81.

130. Chesney PJ: Clinical aspects and spectrum of illness of toxic shock syndrome: Overview. Rev Infect Dis 1989;11:S1–S13.

131. Kreiswirth BN, Projan SJ, Schlievert PM, Novick RP: Toxic shock syndrome toxin 1 is encoded by a variable genetic element. Rev Infect Dis 1989;11:S83–S88.

132. Marrack P, Kappler JW: The staphylococcal enterotoxins and their relatives. Science 1990;248:705–711.

133. See RH, Kum WWS, Chang AH, et al: Induction of tumor necrosis factor and interleukin-1 by purified staphylococcal toxic shock syndrome toxin 1 requires the presence of both monocytes and T lymphocytes. Infect Immun 1992;60:2612–2618.

134. Bavari S, Ulrich RG: Staphylococcal entertoxin A and toxic shock syndrome toxin compete with CD4 for human major histocompatibility complex class II binding. Infect Immun 1995;63:423–429.

135. Krakauer T: Costimulatory receptors for the superantigen staphylococcal entertoxin B on human vascular endothelial cells and T cells. J Leuk Biol 1994;56:458–463.

136. MacDonald HR, Baschieri S, Lees RK: Clonal expansion precedes anergy and death of Vbeta8+ peripheral T cells responding to staphylococcal entertoxin B in vivo. Eur J Immunol 1991;21:1963–1966.

137. Kawabe Y, Ochi A: Programmed cell death and extrathymic reduction of Vbeta8+ CD4 T cells in mice tolerant to Staphylococcus aureus entertoxin B. Nature 1991;349:245.

138. McCormack JE, Callahan JE, Kappler J, Marrack PC: Profound deletion of mature T cells in vivo by chronic exposure to exogenous superantigen. J Immunol 1993;150:3785–3792.

139. Miethke T, Wahl C, Heeg K, Wagner H: Acquired resistance to superantigen-induced T cell shock. Vβ selective T cell unresponsiveness unfolds directly from a transient state of hyperreactivity. J Immunol 1993;150:3776–3784.

140. Krakauer T: Inhibition of toxic shock syndrome toxin-1-induced cytokine production and T cell activation by interleukin-10, interleukin-4, and dexamethasone. J Infect Dis 1995;172:988–992.

141. Bean AGD, Freiberg RA, Andrade S, et al: Interleukin 10 protects mice against staphylococcal enterotoxin B–induced lethal shock. Infect Immun 1993;61:4937–4939.

142. Scott DF, Kling JM, Kirkland JJ, Best GK: Characterization of Staphylococcus aureus isolates from patients with toxic shock syndrome, using polyethylene infection chambers in rabbits. Infect Immun 1983;39:383–387.

143. Rasheed JK, Arko RJ, Feeley JC, et al: Acquired ability of Staphylococcus aureus to produce toxic shock–associated protein and resulting illness in a rabbit model. Infect Immun 1985;47:598–604.

144. De Azavedo JCS, Foster TJ, Hartigan PJ, et al: Expression of the cloned toxic shock syndrome toxin 1 gene (tst) in vivo with a rabbit uterine model. Infect Immun 1985;50:304–309.

145. Bonventre PF, Heeg H, Cullen C, Lian C-J: Toxicity of recombinant toxic shock syndrome toxin 1 and mutant toxins produced by Staphylococcus aureus in a rabbit infection model of toxic shock syndrome. Infect Immun 1993;61:793–799.

146. Hoffmann ML, Jablonski LM, Crum KK, et al: Predictions of T-cell receptor– and major histocompatibility complex–binding sites on staphylococcal enterotoxin C1. Infect Immun 1994;62:3396–3407.

147. Best GK, Scott DF, Kling JM, et al: Protection of rabbits in an infection model of toxic shock syndrome (TSS) by a TSS toxin-1-specific monoclonal antibody. Infect Immun 1988;56:998–999.

148. Parsonnet J, Gillis ZA, Richter AG, Pier GB: A rabbit model of toxic shock syndrome that uses a constant, subcutaneous infusion of toxic shock syndrome toxin 1. Infect Immun 1987;55:1070–1076.

149. Todd JK: Therapy of toxic shock syndrome. Drugs 1990;39:856–861.

150. Wexler DE, Nelson RD, Cleary PP: Human neutrophil chemotactic response to group A streptococci: Bacteria-mediated interference with complement-derived factors. Infect Immun 1983;39:239–246.

151. Dickgiesser N, Wallach U: Toxic shock syndrome toxin-1 (TSST-1): Influence of its production by subinhibitory antibiotic concentrations. Infect Immunol 1996;15:351.

152. Parsonnet J, Modern PA, Giacobbe K: Effect of subinhibitory concentrations of antibiotics on production of toxic shock syndrome toxin-1 (TSST-1). In 32nd Meeting of the Infectious Disease Society of America. Abstract 29, 1994.

153. Stevens DL, Smith LG, Bruss JB, et al: Randomized comparison of linezolid (PNU-100766) versus oxacillin-dicloxacillin for treatment of complicated skin and soft tissue infections. Antimicrob Agents Chemother 2000;44:3408–3413.

154. Bonventre PF, Thompson MR, Adinolfi LE, et al: Neutralization of toxic shock syndrome toxin 1 by monoclonal antibodies in vitro and in vivo. Infect Immun 1988;56:135–141.

155. Melish ME, Frogner KS, Hirata SA, Murata MS: Human gamma globulin therapy in experimental toxic shock syndrome (TSS). In Program and Abstracts of the American Society for Microbiology. Abstract B194, 1987.

section

9

Miscellaneous Infections

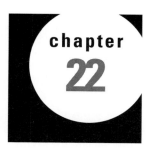

chapter
22

Kawasaki Syndrome

H. CODY MEISSNER, MD
DONALD Y.M. LEUNG, MD, PhD

Kawasaki syndrome is an acute vasculitis that primarily affects infants and young children under 5 years of age. The illness was first described by Tomisaku Kawasaki in 1967 in Japanese in the *Journal of Allergology*.[1] Although Kawasaki syndrome originally was described as a benign illness of early childhood, it is now recognized that this disease is a leading cause of acquired heart disease in children in the United States and western Europe.[2,3] Children with Kawasaki syndrome who do not receive treatment with intravenous immune globulin (IVIG) and aspirin within the first 10 days of onset of fever have a 20% to 25% risk of developing coronary artery abnormalities. Early recognition and prompt treatment reduce the incidence of coronary artery abnormalities to less than 5% of those who have Kawasaki syndrome, which emphasizes the need for early diagnosis and treatment.[4–7] A diagnosis of Kawasaki syndrome is based on fever plus at least four of five criteria, just as a diagnosis of rheumatic fever is based on the Jones criteria. Although the cause of Kawasaki syndrome is not fully defined, features of this syndrome are similar to those found in certain illnesses known to be caused by toxin-producing bacteria, such as toxic shock syndrome and scarlet fever.

EPIDEMIOLOGY

Kawasaki syndrome has been reported from countries throughout the world, although the highest rates of disease are found in Japan and children of Japanese ancestry living outside of Japan. In the United States the incidence of Kawasaki syndrome is highest in Asians, intermediate in blacks, and lowest in whites. The hospitalization rate for Kawasaki syndrome among American Indians and Alaskan natives appears to be lower than among whites.[8] Disease occurs in boys about 1.5 times more often than in girls.[2] The peak age at which disease occurs is 12 to 24 months. More than 80% of cases occur in children under 5 years of age, and most cases occur before the child is 2 years old. The onset of disease after 8 years of age is rare, representing less than 10% of cases reported to the Center for Disease Control and Prevention (CDC). Kawasaki syndrome recurs in fewer than 2% of patients. Some reports suggest that cardiac sequelae may be more common in children who are 8 years of age or older.[9,10] It is not clear whether older patients are predisposed to more severe disease or whether in older patients there is more likely to be a delay in diagnosis and initiation of treatment until later in the course of their illness with correspondingly greater morbidity. Infants less than 12 months of age and particularly those less than 6 months of age also appear to be at greater risk of developing coronary artery abnormalities.[11]

Person-to-person transmission of Kawasaki syndrome is uncommon, although one Japanese study suggested a second case in a family may be more likely than in the general population. Three national epidemics have occurred in Japan in 1979, 1987, and in 1985–86.[2] One well-documented epidemiologic study demonstrated spread of disease outward from Tokyo during an epidemic in a manner clearly suggesting transmission of an infectious agent. Endemic Kawasaki syndrome occurs in Japan with an annual incidence of 67 cases per 100,000 children less than 5 years of age. In industrialized countries there is a seasonality of disease with a peak in activity in late winter and spring.

CLINICAL DISEASE

The possibility of Kawasaki syndrome should be considered in any patient with a fever lasting 5 or more days without an alternative explanation and the presence of at least four of the five clinical criteria listed in Table 22–1.[12] Kawasaki syndrome typically has an acute onset with daily fevers to 40°C or greater in a toxic-appearing child. Fever may last 2 weeks or longer without treatment. It is important to consider Kawasaki syndrome in the differential diagnosis of a child who presents with fever of unknown origin.

The mucocutaneous manifestations of Kawasaki syndrome are varied, and not all patients will exhibit each feature. In the first days of acute febrile illness, approximately 90% of children with Kawasaki syndrome develop a polymorphous exanthem, which may demonstrate a variety of forms. The eruption tends to be most prominent on the trunk and extremities. The rash is rarely vesicular, pustular, or bullous. One early sign may be accentuation of a perineal rash.[13] This may occur before the rash appears on the trunk or extremities.

In most patients a nonexudative, bilateral conjunctival injection begins shortly after the onset of fever and generally involves the bulbar conjunctiva to a greater extent than the palpebral conjunctiva. Conjunctival vessels become engorged and dilated. Purulent discharge is generally not present. Conjunctival injection is associated with anterior uveitis in about 80% of patients.[14]

Oral mucosal findings occur in almost all typical cases. The lips become red, dry, and often cracked, producing small hemorrhagic fissures. There are no punctate ulcerations such as those seen in herpes gingivostomatitis and no erosions suggestive of Stevens-Johnson syndrome. The tongue is often "strawberry" in appearance

with hypertrophied papillae and hyperemia, similar to that seen with streptococcal infections. A generalized erythema of the oropharynx is common, although ulceration of the mucosal surface is not characteristic.

Changes in the extremities may be the most distinctive finding among the five criteria. Erythema and edema of the hands and feet with fusiform swelling of the fingers and toes are often observed. Swelling usually begins within a few days of the onset of illness. The hyperemic areas desquamate during the second or third week. The desquamation characteristically begins at the tips of the fingers and toes (the periungual region) and may extend to involve the palms and soles in a manner similar to that seen in scarlet fever. Lymphadenopathy is the least common finding and is seen in only 50% to 75% of patients. It is most often unilateral, and the nodes are firm and nontender.

Other associated clinical features of Kawasaki syndrome are listed in Table 22–2. Polyarticular arthralgia and arthritis may occur soon after the onset of fever and involve the small joints.[15] Pauciarticular arthritis involving the large weight-bearing joints (hips, knees, and ankles) may occur in the second or third week of illness. Urethritis associated with sterile pyuria is common. A mononuclear cell pleocytosis of the cerebrospinal fluid with normal glucose and protein levels occurs in approximately one-third of patients who undergo lumbar puncture.[16] It should be remembered that a small number of patients will develop aseptic meningitis (fever, headache, vomiting, nuchal rigidity) within 48 h following IVIG infusion.[17] Hydrops of the gallbladder may be present with or without obstructive jaundice. Diarrhea, vomiting, abdominal pain, cranial nerve palsies, tympanitis, and infarction of organs whose vascular supply is compromised by thrombosis may also be presenting symptoms.

CARDIAC INVOLVEMENT

Cardiac abnormalities are the major complication of Kawasaki syndrome and constitute the most serious complication of this disease.[18] Myocarditis may develop during the first few days following the onset of fever and is manifest by tachycardia out of proportion to fever elevation, conduction irregularities, a gallop rhythm, or electrocardiogram changes.[19] Pericardial effusion may develop as a manifestation of carditis. Congestive heart

TABLE 22–1 ■ Diagnostic Criteria for Kawasaki Syndrome

Fever for ≥5 d without other explanation and at least 4 of the following 5 criteria:
1. Nonexudative bulbar conjunctival injection
2. Oropharyngeal changes, including injected or fissured lips, injected pharynx, or strawberry tongue
3. Extremity changes, including erythema of the palms or soles, edema of the hands or feet, or periungual desquamation
4. Polymorphous rash
5. Acute nonsuppurative cervical lymphadenopathy

A diagnosis of atypical Kawasaki syndrome can be made when <4 criteria are met but coronary artery aneurysms are present

TABLE 22–2 ■ Associated Features of Kawasaki Syndrome

Cardiovascular abnormalities including myocarditis, arterial aneurysms, pericarditis, aortic or mitral regurgitation, ventricular arrhythmias
Arthralgia and arthritis
Hepatic dysfunction
Urethritis with sterile pyuria
Aseptic meningitis
Hydrops of the gallbladder
Diarrhea, vomiting, or abdominal pain
Peripheral gangrene
Uveitis
Sensorineural hearing loss

failure may develop as a complication of myocardial dysfunction secondary to ischemia or infarct.

Coronary artery abnormalities occur in 20% to 25% of untreated patients. Dilatation of the coronary arteries can be detected by echocardiography soon after the onset of fever. Aneurysms of the coronary arteries may be demonstrable by echocardiography as soon as a few days after the onset of illness but more typically occur between 1 and 4 weeks after onset of illness. Rarely patients experience aortic regurgitation or mitral regurgitation due to valvulitis, transient papillary muscle dysfunction, or myocardial infarction. Occasionally aneurysm of the brachial, renal, or iliac arteries develops.[20] This usually occurs in association with coronary artery abnormalities.

Factors associated with an increased risk for coronary artery involvement include male sex, age younger than 12 months, and prolonged signs of inflammation such as fever lasting longer than 10 days. The major complication of aneurysms is thrombosis and stenosis leading to myocardial infarction. Aneurysms greater than 8 mm in diameter (giant aneurysms) pose the greatest risk for myocardial infarction and sudden death. Infarction most commonly occurs within 1 year after the onset of disease. Approximately 50% of aneurysms regress within 1 year because of intimal proliferation as assessed by angiography. In those children with aneurysms that do not regress, long-term studies suggest that most will continue to show normal blood flow and normal myocardial function during stress testing.

During the acute stage, two-dimensional echocardiography should be performed as soon as possible in an appropriately sedated child to assess ventricular function, coronary artery structure, and valvular function and for the presence of pericardial effusion. Follow-up echocardiography is generally performed 6 to 8 weeks later if the initial study shows no aneurysm formation and inflammation promptly subsides with treatment. The next echocardiogram should be performed 12 months later if the earlier studies remain normal. If the initial echocardiogram is abnormal, management involves therapy to reduce the risk for thrombosis, restrictions on physical activity, and consideration of cardiac catheterization.

Such management should be conducted by a physician experienced in pediatric cardiology.

DIFFERENTIAL DIAGNOSIS

The clinical manifestations of Kawasaki syndrome are not specific for this disease and occur in a number of other infectious and rheumatologic diseases. Other diseases that may resemble Kawasaki syndrome are shown in Table 22–3. A firm diagnosis of Kawasaki syndrome is often difficult because the symptoms are not unique to this disease and because not all symptoms are seen in all patients. Because therapy within the first 10 days of onset of fever is clearly desirable in terms of reducing the risk for cardiac complications, rapid diagnosis and treatment are important. In many patients, differentiation of Kawasaki syndrome from other illnesses that resemble this syndrome may be difficult. When measles is common in the community, this diagnosis may be among the most difficult to exclude. Considerations that may eliminate measles from the differential diagnosis include local epidemiology, vaccination history, and culture results. Other viral illnesses that may enter the differential diagnosis include Epstein-Barr virus, adenovirus, and influenza virus infections. Nasal secretions should be cultured in a patient whose symptoms include evidence of an upper respiratory tract infection, especially to rule out adenovirus infection. Group A β-hemolytic streptococcus and *Staphylococcus aureus* infections may also mimic Kawasaki syndrome. Noninfectious diseases that frequently appear in the differential diagnosis include drug reactions and juvenile rheumatoid arthritis. Findings on physical examination that are not typical of Kawasaki syndrome include discrete intraoral ulcerations, exudative conjunctivitis, and generalized lymphadenopathy.

LABORATORY FINDINGS

Patients develop a leukocytosis with a predominance of neutrophils and an increase in band counts in the first

TABLE 22–3 ■ Differential Diagnosis of Kawasaki Syndrome

Measles
Scarlet fever
Drug reactions
Toxic shock syndrome
Staphylococcal scalded skin syndrome
Stevens-Johnson syndrome
Rocky Mountain spotted fever
Viral exanthems
Leptospirosis
Juvenile rheumatoid arthritis
Adenovirus infection
Epstein-Barr virus infection

week of illness. A normocytic, normochromic anemia may also be present. Thrombocytosis is generally present by the end of the first week of illness. A mild elevation of liver transaminase levels is common, usually with elevated bilirubin and alkaline phosphatase. Sterile pyuria due to urethritis occurs in about 75% of patients during the first week of illness. Early in the disease, acute-phase reactants are elevated and remain high for 1 to 2 months.

Electrocardiographic changes include prolonged PR or QT intervals, ST segment depression, T wave changes, evidence of left ventricular hypertrophy, and ventricular arrhythmias. A baseline two-dimensional echocardiogram should be obtained at the time of diagnosis. If the results are abnormal, a pediatric cardiology consultation and serial echocardiograms are indicated.

ATYPICAL KAWASAKI SYNDROME

Kawasaki syndrome is based on diagnostic criteria that use clinical signs and symptoms that overlap with other illnesses. This can result in diagnostic dilemmas, particularly in atypical cases that do not completely fulfill the diagnostic criteria but are associated with the development of coronary artery abnormalities. Reports of atypical Kawasaki syndrome have increased in recent years.[21] In certain cases the decision to treat with IVIG and aspirin can be a difficult diagnostic dilemma. The risk of coronary artery abnormalities increases in direct proportion to the interval of time between the onset of fever and the administration of IVIG. Instances of atypical Kawasaki syndrome are most common in infants, the age group that is at greatest risk of coronary artery abnormalities. The decision to initiate therapy in children who do not satisfy the American Heart Association criteria can be supported by laboratory results showing acute-phase reactants (elevated white bloodcell count, elevated sedimentation rate), an ultrasound showing a pericardial effusion, or a slit lamp examination showing anterior uveitis.

TREATMENT

Management of patients with Kawasaki syndrome is directed at reducing inflammation in the myocardium and coronary artery wall during the acute phase.[12] Once the acute stage has passed, therapy is directed at prevention of coronary artery thrombosis. Aspirin in combination with high-dose IVIG forms the basis of current therapy (Table 22–4). Aspirin is used for both anti-inflammatory and antithrombotic actions, although convincing data that aspirin reduces coronary artery abnormalities are not available. Aspirin is administered at a dose of 80 to 100 mg/kg/d in four divided doses to achieve a serum salicylate level of 20 to 25 mg/dl during the acute phase of the illness.[4–7] This is the only dose of aspirin that has been carefully studied in the United States. Lower doses of aspirin

TABLE 22–4 ■ Treatment of Kawasaki Syndrome

Acute phase
   Intravenous immune gloubin 2 g/kg over 10–12 h
   Aspirin, 80–100 mg/kg/d in 4 divided doses until patient is afebrile
Convalescent phase in patients with uncomplicated Kawasaki syndrome
   Aspirin 3–5 mg/kg/d once daily for 6–8 w
For patients with coronary artery disease
   Aspirin 3–5 mg/kg/d once daily
   Dipyridamole 1 mg/kg/d in selected patients
   Anticoagulant therapy as needed in patients with arterial thrombosis

may have equal efficacy, but a minimum of 30 to 50 mg/kg/d in combination with IVIG should be used.[22,23] Efficacy from IVIG therapy has only been demonstrated when it is administered within the first 10 days of the illness. Patients who present beyond the 10th day of fever should still be treated with IVIG and aspirin, although supporting data are not available. It is not clear whether different preparations of IVIG have similar efficacy in the prevention of coronary artery abnormalities. In afebrile children the aspirin dose is reduced to 3 to 5 mg/kg/d to continue antithrombosis activity. Aspirin is discontinued if no coronary abnormalities have been detected by 6 to 8 weeks after the onset of the illness. Aspirin therapy is continued indefinitely if coronary artery aneurysms develop.

Several studies have demonstrated that high-dose IVIG in combination with aspirin therapy is safe and effective in reducing the incidence of coronary artery abnormalities in Kawasaki syndrome.[5,6] Rowley et al demonstrated that IVIG and aspirin not only reduce the overall incidence of coronary artery abnormalities but also prevent the formation of giant aneurysms, the most serious coronary abnormality caused by Kawasaki syndrome.[7] Newburger et al have found also that abnormalities of left ventricular systolic function and contractility abate more rapidly in children treated in the acute phase with high-dose IVIG together with aspirin than in those treated with aspirin alone.[24]

At present the treatment of choice for acute Kawasaki syndrome is a single dose of IVIG at 2 g/kg administered over 10 to 12 hours in combination with aspirin. With this regimen the incidence of coronary artery abnormalities falls to less than 5% of patients with Kawasaki syndrome. Compared with multiple-dose regimens of approximately equivalent total dose, this single high dose of IVIG has been associated with a lower incidence of coronary abnormalities, more rapid resolution of fever and laboratory indexes of acute inflammation, less hospitalization time, and higher peak serum IgG levels. Peak adjusted serum globulin levels are lower among patients who subsequently develop coronary artery abnormalities and are inversely related to fever duration and laboratory indexes of acute inflammation.

Other symptoms are treated symptomatically. Digitalis and diuretics are used as needed in the patient with congestive heart failure. In patients at risk of cardiovascular complications, some physicians add dipyridamole 1 mg/kg/d to further inhibit platelet aggregation. Treatment of the mucocutaneous manifestations of the disease includes emollients for desquamation and antihistamines for pruritus.

All children diagnosed with Kawasaki syndrome should have two-dimensional echocardiography at the time of diagnosis. Repeat studies are recommended at 4 to 6 weeks and again at 6 to 12 months.[12]

RE-TREATMENT

Approximately 5% to 10% of patients who receive IVIG have persistent fever 48 hours after completion of the infusion. Other patients may demonstrate initial defervescence but then experience recurrence of fever after being afebrile for 24 hours or more. Because of concern that persistent fever correlates with elevated levels of proinflammatory cytokines, which are associated with increased risk for the development of coronary artery abnormalities, re-treatment with 2 g/kg of IVIG is often provided for both groups of patients.

CORTICOSTEROID THERAPY

At present the use of systemic steroids in the treatment of Kawasaki syndrome is controversial.[25] Several studies from Japan have reported that patients treated with steroids alone or in combination with aspirin have a higher frequency of coronary artery aneurysms and of subsequent myocardial infarction and death. Therefore, despite the use of corticosteroids in other forms of vasculitis, there has been a reluctance to use steroids in children with Kawasaki syndrome. A more recent uncontrolled study of four patients with Kawasaki syndrome resistant to repeat doses of IVIG suggested a response to high-dose pulse methylprednisolone (30 mg/kg/d for 1 to 3 days) therapy.[26] In 1999, Shinohara et al reviewed the experience with prednisolone in children with Kawasaki syndrome.[27] They concluded that prednisolone curtailed the duration of fever and lowered the incidence of coronary artery aneurysms. This study, however, was a retrospective review of patients who received different doses and different schedules of IVIG than are currently used in the United States. Case reports of either oral or intravenous corticosteroid use in patients with unresponsive disease despite at least two adequate doses of IVIG suggest a possible role in the reduction of the acute inflammatory phase and control of the vasculitis.[28] Before steroid use can be recommended for treatment of Kawasaki syndrome, both the efficacy and safety of steroid therapy should be evaluated in randomized, controlled trials.

MECHANISM OF ACTION OF IVIG

The mechanism by which high-dose IVIG works to reduce the vasculitis associated with Kawasaki syndrome is unknown. The observation that IVIG works rapidly in reducing the laboratory parameters of the acute-phase response associated with Kawasaki syndrome suggests a generalized anti-inflammatory effect. In this regard it has been reported that before initiation of IVIG therapy, peripheral blood mononuclear cells from patients with acute Kawasaki syndrome secrete high levels of IL-1, an endogenous pyrogen, and tissue vascular endothelial cells express IL-1-inducible endothelial activation antigens. IL-1 secretion remained elevated in IVIG-treated patients in whom coronary artery abnormalities developed. However, IL-1 secretion levels fell to normal in patients who responded to IVIG therapy. These data support the notion that IVIG may work in Kawasaki syndrome by reducing cytokine-inducible endothelial activation.

Takei et al have demonstrated that IVIG contains high concentrations of neutralizing antibodies that inhibit the T cell response to staphylococcal superantigens.[29] With the use of affinity absorption techniques it was shown that this T cell–inhibiting effect was mediated by antitoxin-specific antibodies in IVIG. Thus the beneficial effect of IVIG may be partially due to antibodies that inhibit bacterial toxin–induced stimulation of the immune response.

The following hypothesis has been proposed to explain the pathogenesis of this illness[30]: a genetically susceptible host becomes colonized on the mucous membranes of the gastrointestinal tract by an organism that produces a toxin that behaves as a superantigen. Toxin is absorbed through the inflamed mucosal surface and stimulates local or circulating mononuclear cells to produce proinflammatory cytokines, which in turn produce fever and the clinical picture of Kawasaki syndrome. In response to cytokine-induced stimulation, antigens are expressed on the surface of vascular endothelial cells, rendering them susceptible to attack by cytotoxic antibodies and activated T cells. Neoantigens on endothelial cells render the vessels more thrombogenic.

LONG-TERM MANAGEMENT

Patients who develop cardiovascular disease must be monitored closely.[31] Stress echocardiography and coronary angiography may be indicated for patients with evidence of myocardial ischemia. For patients with obstructive changes in their coronary arteries, anticoagulation therapy may be required. For more severe cardiovascular symptoms the options include intravenous streptokinase when a thrombus is present, balloon angioplasty, or coronary artery bypass grafting. Long-term patency of saphenous vein grafts has been a problem, but it has been reported that internal mammary artery grafts give better results.

The major long-term morbidity in Kawasaki syndrome is related to cardiovascular complications. Approximately 50% of children with arterial aneurysms will show angiographic regression within 6 months to 2 years after onset of their disease. The likelihood of resolution of the aneurysm is determined by the initial size of the aneurysm, with smaller aneurysms having a greater likelihood of regression. Patients with giant aneurysms (diameter >8 mm) have the worst prognosis. Approximately 70% of patients with giant aneurysms progress to stenosis or obstruction over an 11-month follow-up period.[4] Thirty percent of giant aneurysms develop obstruction at a mean follow-up of 32 months. Nearly all late deaths from Kawasaki syndrome occur in patients with this complication. Cardiac transplantation for patients with severe ischemic heart disease has been completed in a small number of patients.

Understanding the cause of Kawasaki syndrome remains a major unresolved issue of pediatrics. It is important that the cause of this illness be resolved so that a definitive test can be developed to identify children with typical Kawasaki syndrome as well as those who present with atypical disease and who do not satisfy the diagnostic criteria but are still at risk for coronary artery disease. In addition it is unlikely that a more specific form of therapy than IVIG will be found until the cause is known.

REFERENCES

1. Kawasaki T: Acute febrile mucocutaneous syndrome with lymphoid involvement with specific desquamation of the fingers and toes in children: Clinical observations of 50 cases. Jpn J Allergol 1967;16:178–222.
2. Yanagawa H, Nakamura Y, Yashiro M, et al: A nationwide incidence survey of Kawasaki disease in 1985–1986 in Japan. J Infect Dis 1988;158:1296–1301.
3. Taubert K, Rowely A, Shulman S: A nationwide survey of Kawasaki disease and acute rheumatic fever. J Pediatr 1991;119:279–282.
4. Furusho K, Kamiya T, Nakano H, et al: High-dose intravenous gammaglobulin for Kawasaki disease. Lancet 1984;2:1055–1058.
5. Newburger JW, Takahashi M, Burns JC, et al: The treatment of Kawasaki syndrome with intravenous gammaglobulin. N Engl J Med 1986;315:341–347.
6. Newburger JW, Takahashi M, Beiser AS, et al: A single intravenous infusion of gamma globulin as compared with four infusions in the treatment of acute Kawasaki syndrome. N Engl J Med 1991;324:1633–1639.
7. Rowley AH, Duffy CE, Shulman ST: Prevention of giant coronary artery aneurysms in Kawasaki disease by intravenous gamma globulin therapy. J Pediatr 1989;114:1065–1066.
8. Holman RC, Belay ED, Clarke MJ, et al: Kawasaki syndrome among American Indian and Alaska native children, 1980 through 1995. Pediatr Infect Dis J 1999;18:451–455.
9. Stockbeim JA, Innocentini N, Shulman ST: Kawasaki disease in older children and adolescents. J Pediatr 2000;137:250–252.
10. Momenah T, Sanatani S, Potts J, et al: Kawasaki disease in the older child. Pediatrics 1998;102:e7.
11. Rosenfield EA, Corydon KE, Shulman ST: Kawasaki disease in infants less than one year of age. J Pediatr 1995;126:524–529.
12. Dajani AS, Taubert KA, Gerber MA, et al: Diagnosis and therapy of Kawasaki disease in children. Circulation 1993;87:1776–1780.
13. Friter BS, Lucky AW: The perineal eruption of Kawasaki syndrome. Arch Dermatol 1988;124:1805–1810.
14. Burns JC, Joffe L, Sargent RA, Glode MP: Anterior uveitis associated with Kawasaki syndrome. Pediatr Infect Dis 1985;4:258–261.
15. Hicks RV, Melish ME: Kawasaki Disease. Pediatr Clin North Am 1986;33:1151–1175.
16. Dengler LD, Capparelli EV, Bastian JF, et al: CSF profile in Kawasaki disease. Pediatr Infect Dis J 1998;17:478–481.
17. Boyce TG, Spearman P: Acute aseptic meningitis in a patient with Kawasaki syndrome. Pediatr Infect Dis J 1998;17:1054–1056.
18. Kato H, Ichinose E, Kawasaki Y: Myocardial infarction in Kawasaki disease: Clincal analyses in 195 cases. J Pediatr 1986;108:923–927.
19. Yutani C, Okano K, Kamiya T, et al: Histopathological study on right endomyocardial biopsy of Kawasaki disease. Br Heart J 1980;43:589–592.
20. Fukushige J, Nihill MR, McNamara DG: Spectrum of cardiovascular lesions in mucocutaneous lymph node syndrome: Analysis of eight cases. Am J Cardiol 1980;45:98–107.
21. Witt MT, Minich LL, Bohnsack JF, Young PC: Kawasaki disease: More patients are being diagnosed who do not meet American Heart Association Criteria. Pediatrics 1999;104:e10.
22. Terai M, Shulman ST: Prevalence of coronary artery abnormalities in Kawasaki disease is highly dependent on gamma globulin dose but independent of salicylate dose. J Pediatr 1997;131:888–893.
23. Durongpisitkul K, Gururaj VJ, Park JM, Martin CF: Prevention of coronary artery aneurysms in Kawasaki disease: A meta-analysis on the efficacy of aspirin and immunoglobulin treatment. Pediatrics 1995;96:1057–1061.
24. Newburger JW, Sanders SP, Burns JC, et al: Left ventricular end function in Kawasaki syndrome: Effect of intravenous gammaglobulin. Circulation 1989;79:1237–1246.
25. Newburger JW: Treatment of Kawasaki disease: Corticosteroids revisited. J Pediatr 1999;135:411–413.
26. Wright DA, Newburger JW, Baker A, Sundel RP: Treatment of immune globulin–resistant Kawasaki disease with pulsed doses of corticosteroids. J Pediatr 1996;128:146–149.
27. Shinohara M, Sone K, Tomomasa T, Morikawa A: Corticosteroids in the treatment of the acute phase of Kawasaki disease. J Pediatr 1999;135:465–469.
28. Dale R, Saleem MA, Daw S, Dillon MJ: Treatment of severe complicated Kawasaki disease with oral prednisolone and aspirin. J Pediatr 2000;137:723–726.
29. Takei S, Arora YK, Walker SM: Intravenous immunoglobulin contains specific antibodies inhibitory to activation of T cells by staphylococcal toxin superantigens. J Clin Invest 1993;91:602–607.
30. Meissner HC, Leung DYM: Superantigen, conventional antigens and the etiology of Kawasaki syndrome. Pediatr Infect Dis J 2000;19:91–94.
31. Dajani AS, Taubert KA, Takahashi M, et al: Guidelines for long-term management of patients with Kawasaki disease. Circulation 1994;89:916–922.

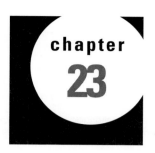

Fever of Unknown Origin

JEFFREY A. GELFAND, MD

MICHAEL V. CALLAHAN, MD, MSPH, DTM&H

DEFINITION OF FEVER OF UNKNOWN ORIGIN

The appelation fever of unknown origin (FUO) was proposed by Petersdorf and Beeson[1] in 1961 to describe a febrile illness that met specific criteria: (1) temperature greater than 38.3°C (101°F) on several occasions, (2) duration of fever longer than 3 weeks, and (3) failure to reach a diagnosis despite 1 week of inpatient investigation. Over the last 40 years the development of new diseases, new medical conditions, and new methods of managing patients challenges the relevance of this definition. Understandably this original definition could not have anticipated the causes of persistent fever in patients with human immunodeficiency virus (HIV), neutropenia, or immunosuppression or in patients receiving chemotherapy or treatment with new therapeutic modalities such as implantable materials.

In 1991 Durack and Street proposed that FUO be categorized to reflect specific medical conditions.[2] Their description of FUO included four categories:

1. Classic FUO, similar to the original definition proposed in 1961
2. Nosocomial FUO, reflecting the risks associated with surgery and hospitalization
3. Neutropenia-associated FUO
4. HIV-associated FUO (Table 23–1).

This chapter will use this categorization as the framework to describe an approach to the evaluation and treatment of FUO.

TYPES OF FEVER OF UNKNOWN ORIGIN

Classic Fever of Unknown Origin

Classic FUO accounts for most FUO cases seen in general hospitals and nonspecialty clinics. The newer definition for classic FUO differs from the original definition in that the period of inpatient evaluation is shortened from 1 week to 3 days, and close investigation in the ambulatory setting may be substituted for inpatient evaluation. The new definition is also broader, stipulating that a diagnosis of FUO may be applied if the clinician is unable to establish the cause of fever after three outpatient visits, 3 days in the hospital, or 1 week of aggressive and thorough investigation in the ambulatory setting.

Causes of Classic Fever of Unknown Origin

Table 23–2 summarizes underlying causes of classic FUO in several studies performed since the advent of the antibiotic era. Traditionally the leading causes of

TABLE 23–1 ■ Categories of Fever of Unknown Origin*

Nosocomial	Neutropenic	HIV-associated	Classic
Hospitalized, acute care, no infection when admitted	Neutrophil count either <500 μl or expected to reach that level in 1–2 d	Confirmed HIV-positive	All others with fevers for ≥ 3 wk
3 d[†]	3 d[†]	3 d[†] (or 4 wk as outpatient)	3 d[†] or 3 outpatient visits
Septic thrombophlebitis, sinusitis, *Clostridium difficile* colitis, drug fever	Perianal infection, aspergillosis, candidemia	MAI[‡] infection, tuberculosis, non-Hodgkin's lymphoma, drug fever	Infections, malignancy, inflammatory diseases, drug fever

*All require temperatures of ≥38.3°C (101°F) on several occasions.
[†]Includes at least 2 days' incubation of microbiology cultures.
[‡]*Mycobacterium avium-intracellulare.*
Modified from Durack DT, Street AC, Remington JS, Swartz MN (eds): Current Clinical Topics in Infectious Diseases. Cambridge, Mass, Blackwell, 1991.

TABLE 23–2 ■ Major Causes of Classic Fever of Unknown Origin in Adults

Authors (year of publication)	Years of study	No. of cases	Infections (%)	Neoplasms (%)	Noninfectious inflammatory diseases (%)	Miscellaneous causes (%)	Undiagnosed causes (%)
Petersdorf and Beeson (1961)[1]	1952–1957	100	36	19	19*	19*	7
Larson et al (1982)[15]	1970–1980	105	32	20	16*	11*	7
Knockaert et al (1992)[70]	1980–1989	199	22.5	7	23*	21.5*	25.5
de Kleijn et al (1997, part I)[44]	1992–1994	167	26	12.5	24	8	30

*Authors' raw data retabulated to conform to altered diagnostic categories.
Modified from de Kleijn EM, Vandenbroucke JP, van der Meer JWM: Fever of unknown origin (FUO) I. A prospective multicenter study of 167 patients with FUO using fixed epidemiologic entry criteria. The Netherlands FUO Study Group. Medicine (Baltimore) 1997;76:392–400.

FUO in young and middle-aged patients have been infectious diseases.[3] In several recent studies, however, the leading causes have been malignancies.[4] These studies demonstrate both the changing patterns of disease and the role that modern diagnostic techniques play in eliminating patients with specific illness from the category of classic FUO.[5] In recent years the ubiquitous use of microbiologic cultures, serologic and molecular diagnostic techniques, and dramatic advances in imaging such as computed tomography (CT), magnetic resonance imaging (MRI), and ultrasonography have enhanced the ability to diagnose indolent infections, autoimmune diseases, and occult malignancies in patients with FUO.[6–8]

Infectious Causes of Classic Fever of Unknown Origin

The primary cause of classic FUO in patients under 65 years of age is still infection.[9] It is also axiomatic that the longer the fever persists, the less likely infection is the cause. Miliary and extrapulmonary tuberculosis, in particular renal tuberculosis, is a leading infectious cause of diagnosable FUO.[10] Other causes are chronic infection with Epstein-Barr virus (EBV), cytomegalovirus (CMV), and HIV,[11] all of which may result in either a delayed or a low-titer antibody response. This observation underscores the need to repeat previously negative serology

studies or to change the immunoassay to increase the likelihood of timely diagnosis.

FUO may also result from poorly localized infections. Typical causes include osteomyelitis, especially in association with prosthetic devices; retroperitoneal, intra-abdominal, and paraspinal abscesses; and prostatic and urinary tract infections.[12,13] Less commonly, atypical cholangitis, sinusitis, periapical dental abscesses of the anterior maxilla, and brain abscesses may be the cause of FUO.

Infections associated with FUO may also occur in patients with underlying defects in humoral or cellular-mediated immunity. Renal malacoplakia, for example, is a coliform infection of the urinary tract that results in the formation of submucosal plaques in the proximal urinary collection system.[14] The condition is often fatal if untreated and should be considered in the workup of any patient with FUO who has a known defect in intracellular killing. Renal malacoplakia is treated with antibiotics active against coliforms; examples include the newer fluoroquinolones and TMP-SMZ.

Native and prosthetic valve endocarditis should be considered in any patients presenting with FUO who have prior risk factors, such as valvular abnormalities.[15] Since true culture-negative endocarditis is rare, the clinician may be misled by delayed bacterial growth in blood cultures that contain trace antibiotics. Similarly, culture-negative endocarditis may be suggested when incubation of blood cultures is terminated before slow-growing organisms are identified. Therefore an absolute minimum of 14 days of culture is required to exclude fever due to endocarditis caused by members of the HACEK group (*Haemophilus aphrophilus*, *Actinobacillus actinomycetemcomitans*, *Cardiobacterium hominis*, *Eikenella corrodens*, and *Kingella kingae*: see Chapter 7, Baddour, and 8, Tilles). FUO associated with true culture-negative endocarditis is rare; when it occurs, it is often caused by *Coxiella burnetii*[16,17] and *Brucella* spp.[18] Infections caused by intracellular or zoonotic microorganisms such as *Bartonella* (previously *Rochalimaea*), *Coxiella*, *Chlamydia*, and *Legionella* also present as classic FUO.[19–21] These infections are likely to be associated with travel to an endemic region or a history suggesting a specific environmental or animal exposure.

Advances in viral culture techniques and improvements in serologic diagnosis in recent years have increased recognition of FUO caused by chronic CMV and EBV infection. Infections caused by dimorphic fungi, such as histoplasmosis infection of the reticuloendothelial system,[22,23] and occasionally mold infections may also be the cause of FUO in debilitated patients. Identification of these pathogens requires careful tissue biopsy with specialized staining or culture by a specialty laboratory. FUO in the presence of headache should prompt immediate examination of the spinal fluid for meningitis caused by atypical pathogens or by *Cryptococcus neoformans*.

Infectious causes of FUO vary markedly with population, travel history, and environmental exposure. In one Mediterranean study of FUO, visceral leishmaniasis accounted for 8% of all cases of unexplained fever.[24] Migration and travel between undeveloped and developed countries has increased the number of tropical infections diagnosed in the West. Improved ease of air travel to and from tropical regions has increased the number of patients who return home before the onset of symptoms of travel-acquired infections.[25,26] Protozoan infections remain a leading cause of fever in travelers, returning expatriate employees, immigrants, and foreign-born visitors. *Plasmodium falciparum*, however, is rarely a cause of FUO because the infection proceeds so quickly in nonimmune patients, and the association with a history of recent travel is well established. Conversely, indolent infections from *Plasmodium malariae* and recrudescence *of Plasmodium vivax* and *Plasmodium ovale* hypnozoites occasionally are implicated in FUO and should be considered in any febrile patient who presents with a history of malaria exposure, however remote. In Western laboratories the diagnosis of malaria may be delayed by improper preparation or examination of blood films. In recent years several sensitive finger-stick blood tests against antigens unique to *P. falciparum*, *P. vivax,* and *P. ovale* have become available, providing an additional method of establishing diagnosis.[27]

Babesia microti, a protozoan endemic to the New England coast, the U.S. Great Lakes region, Missouri, and the Pacific Northwest may present as FUO.[28] *Ixodid* ticks, the vector for babesiosis, may also cotransmit *Borrelia burgdorferi*, another organism associated with FUO.[29]

A comprehensive list of infections associated with FUO is provided in Table 23–3. Although this list applies to the United States, the frequency of global travel underscores the need for a detailed travel history, and the continuing emergence of new infectious diseases makes this potentially incomplete.

Noninfectious Causes of Classic Fever of Unknown Origin

The differential diagnosis of FUO includes a large number of noninfectious disorders. As with infections, noninfectious causes of FUO may be associated with specific epidemiologic features such as age, and its overall incidence has changed in response to improved diagnostic techniques. In recent years the percentage of FUO attributed to malignancy has decreased as a result of improved invasive and noninvasive diagnostic techniques.[30] However, this observation does not diminish the importance of considering neoplasms in the initial diagnosis of any patient with fever.

Leukemia-related FUO may also be associated with mild symptoms such as fatigue, vague pain of the pelvic girdle, scapula, or sternum.[31] In the case of monocytic leukemias, automated complete blood counts or even manual blood smears may not demonstrate blast cells until the disease is advanced. Early diagnosis is most readily obtained using bone marrow biopsy.

Retroperitoneal and small-bowel lymphomas are other malignancies presenting as FUO.[32] In contrast with the leukemias, lymphomas may produce fevers that present as chaotic and near-circadian (Pel-Ebstein). Associated complaints include malaise and weight loss. As a result of their location, these lymphomas may not cause appreciable lymphadenopathy or hepatosplenomegaly. Laboratory findings associated with lymphoma include unexplained elevation of alkaline phosphatase, elevated basophils or eosinophils, and an elevated erythrocyte sedimentation rate (ESR). Definitive diagnosis is achieved using high-resolution CT or MRI followed by careful biopsy of suspicious lymph nodes. One recent study demonstrated that for isolated inguinal or cervical lymphadenopathy, biopsy was of little diagnostic value as compared to biopsy of these nodes in patients who have generalized lymphadenopathy.[33] Small-bowel lymphomas occasionally are identified by biopsy using esophagogastroduodenoscopy.

FUO may be a symptom of either luminal or metastatic adenocarcinoma of the colon.[30] Adenocarcinomas of the right colon may be particularly challenging to diagnose if the physical examination is normal and the stool character unchanged. The incidence of FUO related to gastrointestinal cancers has decreased in recent years because of improvements in cancer screening and imaging techniques.

TABLE 23–3 ■ **Infectious Causes of Fever of Unknown Origin in Adults in the United States**

LOCALIZED PYOGENIC INFECTIONS
Appendicitis
Cat-scratch disease
Cholangitis
Cholecystitis
Dental abscess
Diverticulitis/abscess
Lesser sac abscess
Liver abscess
Mesenteric lymphadenitis
Pancreatic abscess
Pelvic inflammatory disease
Perinephric/intrarenal abscess
Prostatic abscess
Renal malacoplakia
Sinusitis
Subphrenic abscess
Suppurative thrombophlebitis
Tubo-ovarian abscess

INTRAVASCULAR INFECTIONS
Bacterial aortitis
Bacterial endocarditis
Vascular catheter infection

SYSTEMIC BACTERIAL INFECTIONS
Bartonellosis
Brucellosis
Campylobacter infection
Cat-scratch disease (bacillary angiomatosis) (*Bartonella henselae*)
Gonococcemia
Legionnaires' disease
Leptospirosis
Listeriosis
Lyme disease
Melioidosis
Meningococcemia
Rat-bite fever
Relapsing fever
Syphilis
Tularemia
Typhoid fever
Vibriosis
Yersinia infection

MYCOBACTERIAL INFECTIONS
Mycobacterium avium-intracellulare infections
Other atypical mycobacterial infections
Tuberculosis

FUNGAL INFECTIONS
Aspergillosis
Blastomycosis

Candidiasis
Coccidioidomycosis
Cryptococcosis
Histoplasmosis
Mucormycosis/zygomycosis
Paracoccidioidomycosis
Sporotrichosis

OTHER BACTERIAL INFECTIONS
Actinomycosis
Nocardiosis
Whipple's disease

RICKETTSIAL INFECTIONS
Ehrlichiosis
Murine typhus
Q fever
Rickettsialpox
Rocky Mountain spotted fever
Mycoplasmal infections
Chlamydial infections
Lymphogranuloma venereum
Psittacosis
TWAR (*Chlamydia pneumoniae*) infection

VIRAL INFECTIONS
Colorado tick fever
Coxsackievirus group B infection
Cytomegalovirus infection
Dengue fever
Epstein-Barr virus infection
Hepatitis A, B, C, D, and E
Human herpesvirus 6 infection
Human immunodeficiency virus infection
Lymphocytic choriomeningitis
Parvovirus B19 infection

PARASITIC INFECTIONS
Amebiasis
Babesiosis
Chagas' disease
Leishmaniasis
Malaria
Pneumocystis carinii infection
Strongyloidiasis
Toxocariasis
Toxoplasmosis
Trichinosis

PRESUMED INFECTIONS, AGENT UNDETERMINED
Kawasaki syndrome (mucocutaneous lymph node syndrome)
Kikuchi's disease (necrotizing lymphadenitis)

Primary liver cancers may be associated with hepatitis B or C infection and are suggested by right upper quadrant tenderness and elevation or discomfort of the right hemidiaphragm. This diagnosis is supported by elevated α-fetoprotein and alkaline phosphatase levels, as well as an elevated ESR.

Pancreatic carcinoma may also cause FUO, and the diagnosis is suggested by dull pain localized to the middle of the back, fatigue, weight loss, and anorexia. Small tumors of the pancreatic head may result in extrahepatic jaundice, which is present in 50% of patients at the time of diagnosis.[34] The combination of FUO and jaundice suggests either pancreatic or biliary disease and should trigger a high-contrast CT or MRI. Biliary malignancies may be associated with FUO when they are complicated by secondary bacterial infection.

Renal cell carcinoma (hypernephroma) is a cytokine-inducing tumor and a rare cause of FUO. Clinical clues include gross hematuria, an abdominal mass, and, occasionally, a dry cough. Supportive laboratory studies include an elevated ESR, microscopic hematuria, and anemia of chronic disease. Erythrocytosis, due to unregulated erythropoietin production, is a rare finding.

In recent years the term "noninfectious inflammatory diseases" has been favored to describe the broad range of systemic rheumatologic or vasculitic diseases such as polymyalgia rheumatica, lupus, adult Still's disease, acute rheumatic fever, and granulomatous diseases such as sarcoidosis, Crohn's disease, and granulomatous hepatitis.

The leading causes of FUO among the noninfectious, inflammatory disorders are rheumatic. As with malignancies, rheumatic disorders vary with age. Differentiating rheumatologic disorders from chronic infections may be challenging, as the syndromes often induce inflammation in a similar manner. In particular, Takayasu's arteritis and the granulomatous arteritis syndromes may both present with features typical of infectious processes.[35,36] Of these, giant cell arteritis is the most common cause of inflammatory FUO in the elderly, and a critical diagnosis to establish because of the threat to vision and neurologic function that it poses. Symptoms may include headache, blurred vision (possibly bilateral), and tenderness over the affected artery. If the diagnosis is suspected, an ESR should be obtained, a temporal artery biopsy performed, and corticosteroid treatment promptly initiated. An elevated ESR should prompt continuation of steroid therapy until a definitive diagnosis is established by biopsy of the affected vessel. In the absence of a positive biopsy for temporal arteritis, a brisk defervescence with prednisone (20 mg PO) and a rapid fall in ESR may signal polymyalgia rheumatica as the cause of chronic low-grade fever.

Polyarteritis nodosa is a necrotizing vasculitis that affects small and midsized vessels. In association with FUO this inflammatory vasculitis occasionally presents with widely divergent symptoms.[37] The syndrome has a predisposition for arteries of the renal and mesenteric plexus. In contrast with giant cell arteritis, granulomas and peripheral eosinophilia are rarely present. Polyarteritis nodosa should be ruled out in any FUO case that has a history of arthritis, congestive heart failure, or renal failure.

Adult Still's disease, the adult variant of juvenile rheumatoid arthritis, is a cause of FUO and should be considered when patients present with joint discomfort, history of a truncal rash, and a negative rheumatoid factor. The diagnosis of adult Still's disease is suggested by an appropriate clinical picture that may include various combinations of sore throat, faint erythematous rash (usually over the trunk), splenomegaly, lymphadenopathy, and polyserositis, with the systematic exclusion of other causes.

Miscellaneous Causes of Classic Fever of Unknown Origin

Many causes of classic FUO are not easily categorized. This miscellaneous category includes drug fever and the neuroleptic malignant syndrome, factitious fever,

pulmonary embolism, dissecting abdominal aortic aneurysm, and Fabry's disease.

A drug-related cause must be considered in any case of prolonged fever. The febrile pattern associated with drugs typically is constant and not associated with the pharmacologic half-life of the offending drug. Eosinophilia or rash or both are found in only one-fifth of patients with drug fever, and relative bradycardia and hypotension are uncommon presentations.[38] Fever associated with drugs usually begins 1 to 3 weeks after the start of therapy and begins to remit 2 to 3 days after therapy is stopped. Virtually all classes of drugs cause fever, but antimicrobials (especially β-lactam antibiotics), cardiovascular drugs (e.g., quinidine and other class I agents), antineoplastic drugs, and drugs acting on the central nervous system (e.g., phenytoin) are frequently implicated in FUO. Among the elderly in nursing homes and among intensive care unit patients, the widespread use of sedating antipsychotics and anticonvulsants is associated with neuroleptic malignant syndrome.[39]

Patients with periodic fever must be carefully evaluated to differentiate the rare patient with hereditary febrile disorders such as familial Hibernian fever, familial Mediterranean fever, and hyperimmunoglobulinemia D syndrome (HIDS).

When FUO is of long duration, the major causes may be quite different than would normally be expected. In a series of 347 patients with fevers lasting longer than 6 months referred to the National Institutes of Health over a 16-year period[40] (Table 23–4), only 6% of the cases were due to an infection and only 7% due to neoplasms. A significant number of these patients (9%) were diagnosed with factitious fever, that is, fever due either to false elevations of temperature or to self-induced disease. Many of these factitious cases involved young women working in the health professions.[41] It is worth noting that 8% of the patients, some of whom had completely normal liver function studies, had granulomatous hepatitis, and 6% had adult Still's disease. After prolonged investigation, 19% of the cases still had no specific diagnosis. A total of 27% of patients had either an exaggerated circadian temperature without chills, elevated pulse, or other abnormalities and had no actual fever during the weeks of inpatient observation.

A list of other miscellaneous conditions that should be considered in a differential diagnosis of classic FUO in adults is listed in Table 23–3.

Epidemiology of Classic Fever of Unknown Origin

The major underlying causes of classic FUO vary with age. In patients older than 65 years of age, temporal arteritis and inflammatory connective tissue diseases displace infection as the leading cause of FUO, accounting for up to 31% of cases.[42] Tuberculosis is the most common infection causing FUO in this age group, and colon cancer is the primary cause of FUO associated with malignancy. Older patients presenting with FUO have a

TABLE 23–4 ■ Examples of Rare Miscellaneous Causes of Fever

Alcoholic hepatitis
Allergic alveolitis
Aortitis
Aortic dissection
Atrial myxoma
Behçet's syndrome
Castleman's disease
Chronic meningitis
Cirrhotic fever
Carcinomatous meningitis
Cyclic neutropenia
Drug fever and other hypersensitivities
Erythema multiforme
Fabry's disease
Factitious fever
Familial Hibernian fever
Familial Mediterranean fever
Granulomatous hepatitis
Granulomatous peritonitis
Hemoglobinopathies
Hemolytic anemias
Histiocytosis X
Hypereosinophilic syndrome
Immunoblastic lymphadenopathy
Inflammatory bowel disease
Kikuchi-Fujimoto disease
Lymphomatoid granulomatosis
Metal fume fever
Myeloproliferative syndromes
Pancreatitis
Paroxysmal hemoglobinurias
Pericarditis
Periodic fever
Pheochromocytoma
Pulmonary emboli
Postpericardiotomy syndrome
Retroperitoneal fibrosis
Sarcoidosis
Schnitzler's syndrome
Serum sickness
Sjögren's syndrome
Subacute necrotizing lymphadenitis
Thrombotic thrombocytopenic purpura
Thyroiditis and thyrotoxicosis
Veno-occlusive disease
Wegener's granulomatosis
Whipple's disease

decidedly poorer prognosis because of the higher percentage of malignancies in this age group. Conversely, in younger patients, persistent fever is more likely to resolve spontaneously. In one study of pediatric patients with FUO, 43% of the cases diagnosed were due to infections; 7.5% were due to autoimmune disorders; and 2.7% were due to malignancies.[43] In smaller children, FUO may also be caused by allergy to dairy products or heavy metal poisoning.

It is generally true that the cause of the FUO is more likely to be identified in older patients. In one study of patients over 65 years of age the underlying cause of FUO remained undiagnosed in only 8% of the patients.[42]

In a corresponding study in patients less than 65 years of age the underlying cause of FUO could not be established in 30% of patients,[44] and in one series of pediatric patients with FUO, the cause was not identified in 42% of patients.[45]

Nosocomial Fever of Unknown Origin

The characteristics of nosocomial FUO are temperatures greater than or equal to 38.3°C (101°F) on several occasions in a hospitalized patient who is receiving acute medical care and in whom infection was not manifest at the time of admission. The diagnosis of nosocomial FUO is given only after 3 days of inpatient investigation, including incubation of blood cultures for more than 48 hours.

The primary considerations in the evaluation of nosocomial FUO are the underlying susceptibility of the patient and the potential complications resulting from hospitalization or surgery. Over 50% of patients diagnosed with nosocomial FUO are ultimately found to be infected, with the most common sources of infection being intravascular lines, prostheses, and septic phlebitis.[46] *Clostridium difficile* colitis may be associated with fever and leukocytosis before diarrhea appears. In this setting the recommended diagnostic approach focuses on sites where occult infections might be sequestered, such as the ethmoid or frontal sinuses of intubated patients or prostatic abscesses in males with urinary catheters. For the post-surgery patient the original procedural field is the place to begin directed physical and laboratory examinations for abscesses, hematomas, or infected foreign bodies.

In an additional 25% of patients, noninfectious causes of nosocomial FUO are determined,[47] including acalculus cholecystitis, deep vein thrombophlebitis, and pulmonary embolism, all complications of the "hypercoagulable state" following surgery, trauma, and immobilization. Drug fever, transfusion reactions, alcohol or drug withdrawal, adrenal insufficiency, thyroiditis, pancreatitis, gout, and pseudogout are among the many other causes to be considered. As with classic FUO, repeated meticulous physical examination and focused diagnostic techniques are imperative. Multiple blood, wound, and fluid cultures are mandatory. The pace of decision making must be accelerated, and the threshold for invoking procedures— CT scans, ultrasonography, indium 111 white blood cell scans, noninvasive venous studies—is low, as is the threshold for instituting empiric therapies. Even so, up to 20% of the cases may go undiagnosed.

As with diagnosis, therapeutic maneuvers must be swift and decisive, as patients are often critically ill. Intravenous lines must be changed (and tips cultured), noncritical medication stopped for 72 hours, and empiric therapy started if bacteremia is a threat. In many hospital settings, empiric antibiotic coverage for nosocomial FUO must now include vancomycin for methicillin-resistant *Staphylococcus aureus* (MRSA) and broad-spectrum, gram-negative coverage with piperacillin-tazobactam, ticarcillin-clavulanate, imipenem, or meropenem. Practice guidelines covering many of these issues were recently published jointly by the Infectious Diseases Society of America (IDSA) and the Society for Critical Care Medicine and can be accessed on the web at http://www.journals.uchicago.edu/idsa/guidelines.

HIV-Associated Fever of Unknown Origin

Patients infected with HIV may present with persistent fevers directly caused by HIV or by a wide array of opportunistic pathogens.[48] During the acute phase of HIV infection, patients develop fever, which routinely precedes lymphadenopathy, a truncal rash, and seroconversion. The fever typically lasts 3 to 9 days but may last for weeks. In the months following infection the return of fever most likely indicates infection by an opportunistic organism or onset of an HIV-related disease such as non-Hodgkin's lymphoma.

As the patient's immune system becomes increasingly compromised by HIV infection, the potential causes of fever become more diverse. In many cases the symptoms of the infection are altered by derangement in the immune system or by concomitant use of antiviral therapies or antibiotic chemoprophylaxis agents.[49] HIV-positive patients also have heightened sensitivity to sulfa-containing agents such as TMP-SMZ used in the prophylaxis against *Pneumocystis carinii* pneumonia.[50]

In areas where HIV is increasing, the number of opportunistic infections implicated in FUO is also on the rise.[51,52] It should be emphasized that patients with HIV are highly susceptible to *Leishmania* and often exhibit low-titer or aberrant antibodies in response to infection.[53,54] Diagnosis of *Leishmania* infection, particularly visceral leishmaniasis caused by *Leishmania infantum*, may be difficult to confirm using conventional serologic assays. Since current antileishmanial therapies are toxic, more aggressive methods of establishing the diagnosis may need to be performed. For this reason the physician caring for the febrile HIV patient with a tropical or Mediterranean travel history should consider imaging studies of the liver and spleen and early bone marrow biopsy to maximize the chance of timely diagnosis. Recently a polymerase chain reaction (PCR) assay has been developed that shows promise in the diagnosis of *L. infantum* in patients infected with HIV.[55]

Neutropenic Fever of Unknown Origin

The increased use of chemotherapy, bone marrow, and stem-cell transplantation to manage patients with malignancies has also increased the number of patients presenting with FUO. Of these immunosuppressed patients the largest group—and the one at greatest risk of sudden deterioration—are patients with neutropenia who also present with FUO. Neutropenia, defined as an absolute neutrophil count less then 500/mm^3, may result from chemotherapy, side effects to medication, or infiltrative or myelodysplastic syndromes.

All neutropenic patients with fever require prompt and careful evaluation, even if that fever has persisted long enough to meet the definition of FUO. The workup should be aggressive because patients may deteriorate with little warning. It should also be stressed that neutropenia not only raises the risk of infection but also may blunt or delay symptoms associated with life-threatening infection.

The leading cause of infection in neutropenic patients who do not have indwelling catheters is gram-negative bacteria. If the neutropenic patient has recently been hospitalized or has received antibiotics, the bacteria may be resistant to many first-line antibiotics. For this reason, empiric treatment should make use of antibiotics that are both bactericidal and broad spectrum. Neutropenic patients who are already on antibiotics directed against gram-negative and gram-positive organisms will need to be closely evaluated for fungal infections such as *Candida*, and the use of anti-fungal therapy should be considered.

As new therapies become available for treating malignancies, inflammatory diseases, and solid organ rejection, distinct forms of immunosuppression arise. Cyclosporin and antithymocyte immunoglobin, used in transplantation immunology, may cause quantitative or functional lymphopenia. Patients treated with these therapies may present with FUO resulting from infections normally controlled by T lymphocytes and natural killer cells. In a 1998 study of FUO in solid organ transplant patients treated with cyclosporine and steroids, 5(42%) of the 12 cases were due to human herpesvirus 6 or varicella-zoster infection.[56]

Many patients undergoing chemotherapy or bone marrow transplantation are also at risk of infection from invasive fungal pathogens. Fungal infections may progress quickly in the immunocompromised patient with FUO, which has prompted widespread use of empiric antifungal therapy using liposomal and traditional amphotericin B.[57] A recent multicenter trial suggests that voriconazole, a new generation triazole, is a cost-effective alternative to liposomal amphotericin B in treating patients with neutropenia and persistent fever.[58] As use of new immune modulators becomes more widespread, such as anti-tumor necrosis factor (TNF) immunotherapy with etanercept in rheumatoid arthritis or Crohn's disease, it is likely that an increasing number of FUO syndromes associated with intracellular pathogens will be observed in patients treated with these therapies.

EVALUATION OF FEVER OF UNKNOWN ORIGIN

The evaluation of any patient with FUO includes a comprehensive history and physical examination and critical evaluation of all prior data and test results. The most efficient and cost-effective approach is to follow the history and physical with directed diagnostic studies.[59]

An in-depth travel history should be repeated with an emphasis on overlooked airline connections in endemic areas, interruption of malaria chemoprophylaxis, and participation in dining adventures involving uncooked meat, seafood, or invertebrates. Assessment of environmental exposures should include detailed questions regarding animal contact, unusual hobbies, contact with new flora, and consumption of food prepared by others. Occupational risk factors should be evaluated with extreme care. Workers should be carefully questioned about rodent exposure and contact with air-conditioning filters or standing water. Recent bioterrorist attacks using *Bacillus anthracis* endospores delivered through the U.S. mail are a sobering example of a dangerous new occupational hazard that will now have to be considered in febrile patients. Several microorganisms considered suitable for weaponization, such as *Brucella suis* and *C. burnetii*,[60,61] are also known to cause FUO. Mail handlers, currency counters, celebrities, political figures, and military personnel should be questioned about receipt of suspicious packages or events and about illness in colleagues. Risk factors for HIV should be discussed and carefully readdressed at several points in the history. A thorough family history should be obtained to uncover potential hereditary causes of fever.

Physical findings may become more obvious as the underlying cause of FUO persists. For this reason, physical examination should be repeated with particular attention directed toward identifying changes in the liver, spleen, joints, skin, and eyes. Abnormalities detected on physical examination should inspire specific tests.

The patient may benefit from knowing in advance that the cause of FUO is often established only after repetitive studies and a prolonged period of evaluation.[62] Certain specific diagnostic maneuvers become critical in the early evaluation of FUO. If completely normal laboratory values are noted, factitious fever should be suspected, but factitious fever may be part of factitiously induced inflammation or infection. The diagnosis may be difficult to exclude without thorough inpatient observation coupled with temperature measurements obtained by tympanic infrared thermometry. In suspected factitious fevers, temperature assessments should be supervised and compared to simultaneous urine and stool temperatures if possible. In general the pattern of fever is of limited diagnostic utility, although possible exceptions include Pel-Ebstein fever of lymphoma, synchronous schizogeny of malaria, and low pulse-to-temperature ratio observed in infections from intracellular microorganisms such as *Salmonella typhi*.

Tissue biopsies obtained from prior relevant surgery should be requested, and if necessary, paraffin-fixed tissue samples should be re-examined and the value of repeating special stains considered. Relevant imaging studies should be re-examined by a radiologist with the appropriate skills; reliance on prior radiologic reports may be insufficient. Serum should be obtained and frozen as soon as possible for future comparison with convalescent antibody titers.

When a travel history is obtained, the blood smear should be examined for *Plasmodium*, *Babesia*, *Trypanosoma*, *Leishmania*, *Borrelia*, microfilaria, and inclusion artifacts suggesting *Bartonella* infection. Rising antibody titers to *Brucella* are merely supportive rather than confirmatory, since false-positive results have been observed in yersinial infections, typhoid fever, and tularemia.[63] Infection with *Brucella canis* may be missed when the standard antibody panel is used to diagnose Brucellosis. Acute *Salmonella* infection typically elevates antibody titers to both H and O antigens. High titers of antibody to H antigen persist for years, however, and may reflect either prior immunization or infection.[64]

Serologic tests for *Yersinia enterocolitica* are more specific than those for *Salmonella* and thus tend to be more useful. The measurement of specific antirickettsial titers should be requested for the diagnosis of Rocky Mountain spotted fever, tropical rickettsia, or Q fever.

Infection with fastidious and anaerobic organisms requires that multiple blood cultures be obtained using primary venipuncture. At least three, and rarely more than six, blood cultures should be incubated for at least 2 weeks to ensure that any HACEK-group microorganisms have had sufficient time to grow. If the patient received antibiotics, lysis-centrifugation blood cultures should be obtained, a technique usually reserved for the identification of fungal or atypical mycobacterial infections.

Fever caused by infection with nutritionally variant streptococci is difficult to confirm without the use of blood culture media supplemented with both L-cysteine and pyridoxal. Immaculate polymicrobial bacteremia without an apparent source may reflect self-injection of contaminated substances. Urine cultures, including cultures for mycobacteria, fungi, and CMV, may be indicated. PCR is now widely available for detecting the viral nucleic acid from hepatitis C, CMV, HIV, and various herpesvirus infections.[65]

If the patient is stable, tissue biopsy studies should be delayed until all blood cultures and imaging and serology studies are known to be negative. Liver biopsy, even when liver function studies are normal, should be considered and pursued if the diagnosis remains elusive. Liver tissue should be processed to allow both culture of mycobacteria and fungi and special staining to be performed. Likewise, bone marrow biopsy (not simple aspiration) should be used to obtain specimens for histology and culture.

An early step in the workup of FUO is determination of the ESR. Striking elevation of the ESR and anemia of chronic disease are frequently seen in association with giant cell arteritis or polymyalgia rheumatica, common causes of FUO in patients over 50 years of age.[66] Still's disease is suggested by elevations of the ESR, leukocytosis, and anemia and often is accompanied by arthralgias, polyserositis (pleuritis, pericarditis), lymphadenopathy, splenomegaly, and rash.[67] Antinuclear antibody, antineutrophil cytoplasmic antibody, rheumatoid factor, and serum for cryoglobulins should be measured to rule out other collagen vascular diseases and vasculitis. Another cause of an extremely high ESR may be a false-positive value attributable to a cold agglutinin with a broad thermal amplitude. The ESR test is nonspecific, yielding values that depend on certain serum proteins (most notably fibrinogen) known to interfere with the zeta potential that keeps erythrocytes from clumping. When fibrinogen levels go up, the zeta potential is inhibited, erythrocytes clump, and the ESR is high. A cold agglutinin, by binding to erythrocytes, can produce a false-positive agglutinin that mimics an acute-phase response; cold agglutinins may be seen in *Mycoplasma* and EBV infections and in lymphomas.[68]

The intermediate-strength purified protein derivative (PPD) skin test should be used to screen for tuberculosis in virtually all patients with classic FUO. Concurrent control tests for anergy, such as the CMI test (Pasteur Merieux Connaught, Swiftwater, PA), which is especially effective, should also be used. It should be kept in mind that a negative PPD skin test with anergy may be seen with miliary tuberculosis, sarcoidosis, Hodgkin's disease, malnutrition, or AIDS.

Noninvasive procedures should include an upper gastrointestinal contrast study with small-bowel follow-through and barium enema to include the terminal ileum and cecum. Chest radiographs should be repeated if new symptoms arise. In some cases, pulmonary function studies may be necessary. A diminished carbon monoxide diffusing capacity (DLCO) may indicate a restrictive lung disease such as sarcoidosis, even with a normal chest radiograph. In such cases, transbronchial biopsy may prove diagnostic. Flexible colonoscopy may be advisable, since colon carcinoma is a cause of FUO and easily escapes detection by ultrasound and CT.

CT of the chest and abdomen should be obtained. If a spinal or paraspinal lesion is suspected, however, MRI is preferred. MRI may be superior to CT in demonstrating intra-abdominal abscesses and aortic dissection, but the relative utility of MRI and CT in the diagnosis of FUO is unknown. At present it would appear that abdominal CT, with oral and intravenous contrast, should be used unless MRI is specifically indicated. Ultrasonography of the abdomen is useful for the investigation of the hepatobiliary tract, kidneys, spleen, and pelvis. Echocardiography may be helpful in an evaluation for bacterial endocarditis, pericarditis, nonbacterial thrombotic endocarditis, and atrial myxomas. Transesophageal echocardiography is especially sensitive for these lesions.

Radionuclide scanning procedures using technetium Tc 99m sulfur colloid, gallium citrate, or indium In 111–labeled leukocytes or immunoglobulin may be useful in identifying or localizing inflammatory processes. In a recent study, gallium scintigraphy yielded useful diagnostic information in almost one-third of cases, and it was suggested that this procedure might actually be used before other imaging techniques if no specific organ is suspected of being abnormal.[69] Technetium bone scan should be undertaken to look for osteomyelitis or bony metastases; gallium scan may be used to identify sarcoidosis, *P. carinii* in the lungs, or Crohn's disease in the abdomen. ^{111}In-labeled white blood cell scan may be used to locate abscesses; ^{111}In-labeled immunoglobulin scan also shows promise in this regard. With both gallium and indium white blood cell and immunoglobulin scans, false-positive and false-negative findings are common. There is general agreement that gallium scans should be used earlier in the workup of FUO.[70] More recently, positron emission tomography (PET) scanning has been proposed as useful but is not yet widespread.

Biopsy of the liver and bone marrow should be considered routine in the workup of FUO if the studies mentioned above are unrevealing or if fever is prolonged. It goes without saying that areas of suspected abnormality should be sampled for pathologic examination whenever practical. When it is possible, a section of the tissue block should be retained for further sections or stains. PCR makes it possible to identify and speciate mycobacterial DNA in paraffin-embedded, fixed tissues. Thus in some cases it is possible to make a retrospective diagnosis based on studies of long-fixed pathologic tissues. In a patient over age 50 or occasionally in a younger patient with a suspicious history and supportive laboratory findings, blind biopsy of one or both temporal arteries may yield a diagnosis of arteritis. If noted, tenderness or decreased pulsation should guide the selection of a site for biopsy. Lymph node biopsy may be helpful if nodes are enlarged, but inguinal nodes are often palpable and are seldom diagnostically useful.

Exploratory laparotomy has been performed when all other diagnostic procedures fail but has largely been replaced by modern imaging and guided-biopsy techniques. Laparoscopic biopsy may provide more adequate, guided sampling of lymph nodes or liver.

TREATMENT OF FEVER OF UNKNOWN ORIGIN

It is beyond the scope of this chapter to outline the therapies for all causes of infectious and noninfectious FUO. Instead this discussion will be directed at the generalized approach to treating FUO.

In most cases, management of FUO is directed at the underlying cause rather than at the fever itself. Exceptions to this approach include rare situations in which the fever directly endangers the patient. Management of fever without a diagnosis should be reserved for patients with cardiac or pulmonary disease, convulsions or mental status changes, or prolonged hypercatabolic states and for any fever exceeding 41°C (105.8°F).

Treating fever without diagnosing the underlying cause is a last resort. Injudicious use of glucocorticoids or nonsteroidal anti-inflammatory drugs may mask fever during the spread of infection. These therapies should be avoided unless infection has been ruled out and inflammatory disease is likely. External cooling has no effect on the hypothalamus and thus should be used only as an interim method of controlling life-threatening fever. This technique should be reserved for hyperthermic emergencies and should not be viewed as routine.

The guiding principles for treating patients with classic FUO are careful investigation, continued observation, and re-examination. Empiric treatment should be avoided whenever possible unless the patient is deteriorating or there are specific reasons to invoke a diagnosis. Every patient with FUO should undergo comprehensive evaluation for tuberculosis. If the PPD skin test is positive or if granulomatous hepatitis or other granulomatous disease is present with anergy, a 6-week therapeutic trial with isoniazid, rifampin, and pyrazinamide should be initiated. The clinician should remember that rifampin has activity against a large number of bacteria, so defervescence in this setting does not necessarily confirm TB as the diagnosis. Conversely, failure of FUO to respond to this therapy suggests another cause.

The response of adult Still's disease and rheumatic fever to nonsteroidal anti-inflammatory agents and aspirin may be dramatic. Glucocorticoids have a rapid and powerful effect on temporal arteritis, polymyalgia rheumatica, and granulomatous hepatitis. Colchicine, which impairs leukocyte chemotaxis and phagocytosis, is highly effective in preventing attacks in familial Mediterranean fever but is of little benefit once an attack is under way. Physicians who initiate therapy using these medications will also need to monitor the patient for evidence of infection.

When no underlying source of FUO is identified after more than 6 months of observation, the prognosis is generally favorable. Under these conditions, debilitated patients and patients with profound subjective complaints may be treated with NSAIDs, with glucocorticoids a last resort. Initiation of empiric therapy does not mark the end of the diagnostic workup; rather it commits the physician to continued and thoughtful re-examination and evaluation.

REFERENCES

1. Petersdorf RG, Beeson PB: Fever of unexplained origin: Report on 100 cases. Medicine 1961;40:1–30.
2. Durack DT, Street AC: Fever of unknown origin reexamined and redefined. Curr Clin Top Infect Dis 1991;11:35–51.
3. Tumulty PA: Topics in clinical medicine. The patient with fever of undetermined origin: A diagnostic challenge. Johns Hopkins Med J 1967;120:95–106.
4. Shoji S, Imamura A, Imai Y, et al: Fever of unknown origin: A review of 80 patients from the Shin'etsu area of Japan from 1986–1992. Intern Med 1994;33:74–76.
5. Iikuni Y, Okada J, Kondo H, Kashirvazaki S: Current fever of unknown origin, 1982–1992. Intern Med 1994;33:67–73.
6. Gartner JC Jr: Fever of unknown origin. Adv Pediatr Infect Dis 1992;7:166–169.
7. Volk EE, Miller ML, Kirkley BA, Washington JA: The diagnostic usefulness of bone marrow cultures in patients with fever of unknown origin. Am J Clin Pathol 1998;110:150–153.
8. Knockaert DC, Mortelmans LA, De Roo MC, Bobbaers HJ: Clinical value of gallium-67 scintigraphy in evaluation of fever of unknown origin. Clin Infect Dis 1994;18:601–605.
9. Kazanjian PH: Fever of unknown origin: Review of 86 patients treated in community hospitals. Clin Infect Dis 1992;15:968–973.
10. Harris HW, Menitove S: Miliary tuberculosis. In Schlossberg D (ed): Tuberculosis, 3rd ed. New York, Springer-Verlag, 1994, pp 233–245.
11. Hirschmann JV: Fever of unknown origin in adults. Clin Infect Dis 1997;24:291–300.
12. Larson EB, Featherstone HJ, Petersdorf RG: Fever of undetermined origin: Diagnosis and follow-up of 105 cases, 1970–80. Medicine 1982;61:269–292.
13. Kazanjian PH: Fever of unknown origin: Review of 86 patients treated in community hospitals. Clin Infect Dis 1992;15:968–973.
14. Mitchell MA, Markovitz DM, Killen PD, Braun DK: Bilateral renal parenchymal malacoplakia presenting as fever of unknown origin: Case report and review. Clin Infect Dis 1994;18:704–718.
15. Hoen B, Beguinot I, Rabaud C, et al: The Duke criteria for diagnosing infective endocarditis are specific: Analysis of 100 patients with acute fever or fever of unknown origin. Clin Infect Dis 1996;23:298–302.
16. Petersdorf RG: FUO: How it has changed in 20 years. Hosp Pract 1985;20:84I–84M.
17. Knockaert DC: Fever of unknown origin: A literature survey. Acta Clin Belg 1992;47:100–116.
18. Keles C, Bozbuga N, Sismanoglu M: Surgical treatment of Brucella endocarditis. Ann Thorac Surg 2001;71:1160–1163.
19. Numazaki K, Ueno H, Yokoo K, et al: Detection of serum antibodies to Bartonella henselae and Coxiella burnetii from Japanese children and pregnant women. Microbes Infect 2000;2:1431–1434.
20. Boldur I, Kahana H, Kazak R, et al: Western blot analysis of immune response to Legionella bozemanii antigens. J Clin Pathol 1991;44:932–935.
21. Orr PH, Peeling RW, Fast M, et al: Serological study of responses to selected pathogens causing respiratory tract infection in the institutionalized elderly. Clin Infect Dis 1996;23:1240–1245.
22. Zoutman DE, Ralph ED, Frei JV: Granulomatous hepatitis and fever of unknown origin. An 11-year experience of 23 cases with three years' follow-up. J Clin Gastroenterol 1991;13:69–75.
23. Burke DS, Churchill FE Jr, Gaydos JC, et al: Epidemic histoplasmosis in patients with undifferentiated fever. Mil Med 1982;147:466–467.
24. Benito N, Nunez A, de Gorgolas M, et al: Bone marrow biopsy in the diagnosis of fever of unknown origin in patients with acquired immunodeficiency syndrome. Arch Intern Med 1997;157:1577–1580.
25. Zenilman JM: Typhoid fever. JAMA 1997;278:847–850.
26. Liu LX, Weller PF: Approach to the febrile traveler returning from Southeast Asia and Oceania. Curr Clin Top Infect Dis 1992;12:138–164.
27. Moody A: Rapid diagnostic tests for malaria parasites. Clin Microbiol Rev 2002;15:66–78.
28. Falagas ME, Klempner MS: Babesiosis in patients with AIDS: A chronic infection presenting as fever of unknown origin. Clin Infect Dis 1996;22:809–812.
29. Kazanjian PH: Fever of unknown origin: Review of 86 patients treated in community hospitals. Clin Infect Dis 1992;15:968–973.

30. Knockaert DC, Vaneste LJ, Bobbaers HJ: Recurrent or episodic fever of unknown origin. Review of 45 cases and survey of the literature. Medicine (Baltimore) 1993;72:184–196.

31. Majeed HA: Differential diagnosis of fever of unknown origin in children. Curr Opin Rheumatol 2000;12: 439–444.

32. Chim CS, Au WY, Shek TW, et al: Primary CD56 positive lymphomas of the gastrointestinal tract. Cancer 2001; 91:525–533.

33. de Kleijn EM, van Lier HJ, van der Meer JW: Fever of unknown origin (FUO) II. Diagnostic procedures in a prospective multicenter study of 167 patients. The Netherlands FUO Study Group. Medicine 1997;76:401–414.

34. Bakkevold KE, Arnesjo B, Kambestad B: Carcinoma of the pancreas and papilla of Vater: Presenting symptoms, signs, and diagnosis related to stage and tumour site. Scand J Gastroenerol 1992;27:317–325.

35. Uthman IW, Bizri AR, Hajj Ali RA, et al: Takayasu's arteritis presenting as fever of unknown origin: Report of two cases and literature review. Semin Arthritis Rheum 1999;28:280–285.

36. Wu YJ, Martin BR, Ong K, et al: Takayasu's arteritis as a cause of fever of unknown origin. Am J Med 1989; 87:476–477.

37. Tsunoda K, Akaogi J, Ohya N, et al: Sensorineural hearing loss as the initial manifestation of polyarteritis nodosa. J Laryngol Otol 2001;115:311–312.

38. Mackowiak PA, LeMaistre CF: Drug fever: A critical appraisal of conventional concepts. An analysis of 51 episodes diagnosed in two Dallas hospitals and 97 episodes reported in the English literature. Ann Intern Med 1987;106: 728–733.

39. Rosenberg MR, Green M: Neuroleptic malignant syndrome. Arch Intern Med 1927;149:1989.

40. Aduan RP, Fauci AS, Dale DC, Wolff SM: Prolonged fever of unknown origin. Clin Res 1978;26:558A.

41. Aduan RP, Fauci AS, Dale DC, et al: Factitious fever and self-induced infection: A report of 32 cases and review of the literature. Ann Intern Med 1979;90:230–242.

42. Knockaert DC, Vaneste LJ, Bobbaers HJ: Fever of unknown origin in elderly patients. J Am Geriatr Soc 1993;41:1187–1192.

43. Jacobs RF, Schutze GE: *Bartonella henselae* as a cause of prolonged fever and fever of unknown origin in children. Clin Infect Dis 1998;26:80–84.

44. de Kleijn EM, Vandenbroucke JP, van der Meer JWM: Fever of unknown origin (FUO): I. A prospective multicenter study of 167 patients with FUO using fixed epidemiologic entry criteria. The Netherlands FUO Study Group. Medicine (Baltimore) 1997;76:392–400.

45. Jacobs RF, Schutze GE: *Bartonella henselae* as a cause of prolonged fever and fever of unknown origin in children. Clin Infect Dis 1998;26:80–84.

46. O'Grady NP, Barie PS, Bartlett JG, et al: Practice guidelines for evaluating new fever in critically ill adult patients. Task Force of the Society of Critical Care Medicine and the Infectious Diseases Society of America. Clin Infect Dis 1998;26:1042–1059.

47. Murray HW, Ellis GC, Blumenthal DS, Sos TA: Fever and pulmonary thromboembolism. Am J Med 1979;67:232–235.

48. Bissuel F, Leport C, Perrone C, et al: Fever of unknown origin in HIV-infected patients: A critical analysis of a retrospective series of 57 cases. J Intern Med 1994;236: 529–535.

49. Sepkowitz KA: Effect of prophylaxis on the clinical manifestation of AIDS related opportunistic infections. Clin Infect Dis 1998;26:806–810.

50. Sattler FR, Cowan R, Nielsen DM, Ruskin J: Trimethoprim-sulfamethoxazole compared with pentamidine for treatment of *Pneumocystis carinii* pneumonia in the acquired immunodeficiency syndrome. A prospective, non-crossover study. Ann Intern Med 1988;109:280–287.

51. Mayo J, Collazos J, Martinez E: Fever of unknown origin in the HIV-infected patient: New scenario for an old problem. Scand J Infect Dis 1997;29:327–336.

52. Handa R, Bhatia S, Wali JP: Meliodosis: A rare but not forgotten cause of fever of unknown origin. Br J Clin Pathol 1996;50:116–117.

53. Consensus report (no authors): Conclusions and recommendations of the IVth Joint Meeting on Leishmania/HIV Co-Infections. Parasite 2001;8:376–379.

54. Ritmeijer K, Veeken H, Melaku Y: Ethiopian visceral leishmaniasis: Generic and proprietary sodium stibogluconate are equivalent; HIV co-infected patients have a poor outcome. Trans R Soc Trop Med Hyg 2001;95: 668–672.

55. Martin-Sanchez J, Lopez-Lopez MC, Acedo-Sanchez C, et al: Diagnosis of infections with *Leishmania infantum* using PCR-ELISA. Parasitology 2001;122(Pt 6):607–615.

56. Chang FY, Singh N, Gayowski T, et al: Fever in liver transplant recipients: Changing spectrum of etiologic agents. Clin Infect Dis 1998;26:59–65.

57. Hughes WT, Armstrong D, Bodey GP, et al: 1997 Guidelines for the use of antimicrobial agents in neutropenic patients with unexplained fever. Clin Infect Dis 1997;25(3): 551–572.

58. Walsh TH, Pappas, P, Winston, DJ: Voriconazole compared with liposomal amphotericin B for empirical antifungal therapy in patients with neutropenia and persistent fever. N Engl J Med 2002;346:225–234.

59. Murray HW: FUO. In Murray HW (ed): FUO: Fever of Undetermined Origin. Mount Kisco, NY, Futura Publishing, 1983, pp. 87–88.

60. Christopher GW, Cieslak TJ, Pavlin JA, et al: Biological warfare: A historical perspective. JAMA 1997;278: 412–417.

61. Henderson DA: Bioterrorism as a public health threat. Emerg Infect Dis 1998;4:488–492.

62. Arnow PM, Flaherty JP: Fever of unknown origin. Lancet 1997;350:575–580.

63. Walker DH, Barbour AG, Oliver JH, et al: Emerging bacterial zoonotic and vector-borne diseases. Ecological and epidemiological factors. JAMA 1996;14:275:463–469.

64. Levine MM, Ferreccio C, Abrego P, et al: Duration of efficacy of Ty21a, attenuated *Salmonella typhi* live oral vaccine. Vaccine 1999;17(Suppl 2):S22–S27.

65. Kelley VA, Caliendo AM: Successful testing protocols in virology. Clin Chem 2001;47(8):1559–1562.

66. Hazleman B: Laboratory investigations useful in the evaluation of polymyalgia rheumatica (PMR) and giant cell arteritis (GCA). Clin Exp Rheumatol 2000;18(Suppl 20):S29–S31.

67. Evans, RH: Pyrexia of unknown origin, grand rounds—University Hospital of Wales. BMJ 1997;314(7080): 583–586.

68. McNicholl FP: Clinical syndromes associated with cold agglutinins. Transfus Sci 2000;22:125–133.

69. Sfakianakis GN, Al-Sheikh W, Heal A, et al: Comparison of scintigraphy with ^{111}In leukocytes and ^{67}Ga in the diagnosis of occult sepsis. J Nucl Med 1982;23:618–626.

70. Knockaert DC, Vaneste LJ, Vaneste SB, Bobbaers HJ: Fever of unknown origin in the 1980s. An update of the diagnostic spectrum. Arch Intern Med 1992;152:51–55.

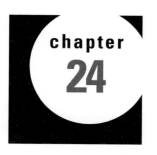

Fever in the Neutropenic Host

JERRY L. SHENEP, MD

MONITORING THE NEUTROPENIC HOST AND INITIAL EVALUATION OF FEVER

The neutropenic host (absolute neutrophil count [ANC] <500/μl or <1000/μl and decreasing) is at significant risk for developing bacteremia, especially if neutropenia is accompanied by mucositis.[1] In the absence of an immune system, some bacterial pathogens can double every 20 minutes in human plasma at 37°C. Given this potential for fulminant infection and the neutropenic host's risk for developing bacteremia, vigilant monitoring of these patients is paramount. Although there are exceptions, elevated temperature is typically the earliest and most reliable warning of an infection in the neutropenic patient. The neutropenic patient's temperature should be monitored at least every 4 hours if the patient is not perfectly well. In contrast to management of the immunocompetent host a new fever (≥38.3°C orally or oral equivalent, e.g., axillary temperature plus 0.6°C; or ≥38°C orally over 1 hour) in a neutropenic host warrants evaluation regardless of how healthy the patient appears. In many cases initiation of empiric antibiotic therapy is indicated. An ill-appearing neutropenic patient also warrants evaluation, and empiric therapy may be indicated regardless of the presence of fever.

For the higher risk patient and for neutropenic patients following the development of fever a daily interval history with particular attention to oral, abdominal, or perirectal pain, diarrhea, cough, chills, rash, and any notable change is warranted. Daily physical examination should likewise focus on the oral cavity, chest, skin and nails, pericatheter skin, abdomen, perirectal area, bone marrow aspiration sites, and any lesion or focal complaint. The clinician must be especially vigilant because inflammation is attenuated in the neutropenic host, and the clinical manifestations of infection may be markedly diminished. For example, meningismus can be absent in the neutropenic patient with meningitis, headache being perhaps the only clue of central nervous system infection.

If fever or illness occurs, blood specimens should be obtained for culture. For patients with catheters a specimen from each catheter lumen should be collected because the source of an infection can be limited to a single lumen of a multiple-lumen catheter. By collecting simultaneous specimens via a peripheral venipuncture and catheter lumens and culturing blood specimens quantitatively, the role of the catheter as a focus of infection can be determined.[2,3] Comparative quantitative blood cultures may influence the decision to remove a catheter if bacteremia persists and may also influence the duration and route of treatment (see Catheter-Related Infections). For patients with suspected abdominal infections or other infections in which anaerobic bacteria are suspected, a specific request to culture blood for anaerobes may be

This work was supported by National Cancer Institute Cancer Center CORE Support Grant P30 CA 21765, and by the American Lebanese Syrian Associated Charities.

appropriate depending on the local institutional blood culture methodologies. Likewise, some institutions may require specific requests to culture blood for fungi. Baseline renal and hepatic function blood tests should be obtained, and these parameters should then be monitored every 3 to 5 days during empiric therapy. A baseline chest radiograph has low yield in the absence of any respiratory signs or symptoms after careful examination[4-6]; however, a chest radiograph is indicated in the presence of respiratory signs or symptoms. If diarrhea is present, stool should be tested for *Clostridium difficile* toxin, rotavirus, and *Cryptosporidium* species and cultured for bacteria (species of *Salmonella*, *Shigella*, *Campylobacter*, and *Yersinia*). If diarrhea is persistent and no cause is determined on initial workup, stool should be examined for ova and parasites and cultured for cytomegalovirus (CMV), *Aeromonas*, enteropathogenic *Escherichia coli*, or other uncommon pathogens.

The value of routine surveillance cultures is controversial. Because most infections in neutropenic patients are derived from the patient's own microbial flora, the composition of that flora is relevant. Known colonization by antibiotic-resistant *Pseudomonas aeruginosa* or *Staphylococcus aureus* or fluconazole-resistant *Candida krusei* may lead to alteration of empiric therapy regimens. In addition, colonization with a pathogenic species of *Aspergillus* (especially *A. flavus*, *A. fumigatus*, *A. niger*, *A. versicolor*, or *A. terreus*) may encourage earlier empiric use of amphotericin B. Febrile neutropenic patients treated with empiric antibiotics and colonized with *Candida tropicalis* are at about a 10-fold higher risk to develop disseminated candidiasis than patients colonized with *Candida albicans*, roughly a risk of 10% versus 1%.[7] Thus detection of *C. tropicalis* colonization may also be an indication for earlier empiric antifungal therapy. Despite these potentials for guiding therapy,[8-10] the use of surveillance cultures to predict infecting organisms is not universally practiced, in large part because of the substantial costs of processing surveillance cultures.

Fungal infections and infections with multiresistant bacteria of low pathogenic potential typically are preceded by several days of antibiotic therapy. Consequently the microorganisms most frequently encountered in the neutropenic patient vary during the course of neutropenia. The organisms most likely to be isolated according to whether the patient is experiencing a new fever or a fever that is occurring during or soon after a course of empiric antibiotic therapy are summarized in Table 24–1. This pattern should be considered in selecting an initial empiric antimicrobial regimen and in modifying the regimen when response is suboptimal.

ASSESSING RISK FOR INFECTION

Among febrile neutropenic patients not presenting with sepsis or other signs and symptoms of infection, about

TABLE 24–1 ■ Most Likely Pathogens in the Neutropenic Patient

Initial fever	During or soon after empiric antibiotics
GRAM-POSITIVE BACTERIA	**FUNGI**
Coagulase-negative staphylococci	*Candida* spp
Viridans streptococci	*Aspergillus* spp
Staphylococcus aureus	*Fusarium* spp
Enterococcus spp	*Mucor* spp
Streptococcus pneumoniae	*Rhizopus* spp
Bacillus cereus	*Pseudallescheria boydii*
Clostridium septicum	
	VIRUSES
GRAM-NEGATIVE BACTERIA	Cytomegalovirus
Escherichia coli	Herpes simplex
Pseudomonas aeruginosa	Adenovirus
Klebsiella spp	
Enterobacter spp	**GRAM-NEGATIVE BACTERIA**
	Escherichia coli
VIRUSES	*Pseudomonas aeruginosa*
Enterovirus	*Klebsiella* spp
Coxsackievirus	*Enterobacter* spp
Influenza virus	*Acinetobacter* spp
Parainfluenza virus	
Respiratory syncytial virus	**GRAM-POSITIVE BACTERIA**
Adenovirus	Coagulase-negative staphylococci
	Viridans streptococci
FUNGI	*Enterococcus* spp
Pneumocystis carinii	
Candida spp	
Cryptococcus neoformans	
Histoplasma capsulatum	

10% to 15% will have bacteria isolated from their blood. Consequently the febrile neutropenic patient traditionally has been hospitalized and treated empirically with broad-spectrum antibiotics. This strategy significantly reduces morbidity and mortality but also is expensive empiric therapy for many patients who would fare well with no treatment. The advent of managed care and renewed appreciation of the limitations and risks of hospitalization prompted by the Institute of Medicine's report "To Err is Human: Building a Safer Health Care System"[11] have led clinicians to attempt to target both hospitalization and empiric therapy to the patients who are most likely to derive benefit. The approach employed usually has been one of classifying patients according to projected risk for infection and limiting treatment for the lower risk patient.

The more stringent the definition of lower risk, the smaller the group of patients to benefit from limited treatment, necessitating efforts to balance between the competing priorities of identifying all patients at risk and keeping the intensively treated population small. Neutropenia and mucositis are cardinal risk factors; the greater the severity of these conditions, the higher the risk of infection.[1,12] Gradually developing neutropenia has less risk than rapidly developing neutropenia. Chemotherapy-induced neutropenia is higher risk than cyclic neutropenia.[12,13] The longer the period of neutropenia, the greater the incremental risk, indicating that the risk is highest near the time of resolution of neutropenia.[14–16] In addition the probability of prompt response to treatment is less with prolonged versus early neutropenia.[17] Patients receiving induction therapy or in whom their cancer has recurred are at significantly greater risk of infection than patients in remission of their cancer.[12] Malnutrition is an independent risk factor for infection but is associated with an even greater risk in the patient with cancer. Moreover, efforts to manage malnutrition in the cancer patient with parenteral nutrition increase the risk of catheter-related infections.[18] Risk factors for infection in the cancer patient that have been cited in various clinical studies are summarized in Table 24–2.[19–34]

Patients without identified risk factors other than neutropenia and fever are candidates for less stringent management than the traditional approach of intravenous broad-spectrum antibiotic therapy in an inpatient setting until neutropenia resolves. Among the less stringent approaches that have been advocated are outpatient intravenous therapy, short-course intravenous therapy with switch to oral therapy or discontinuance of antibiotics, inpatient oral therapy, outpatient oral therapy, and outpatient observation with no empiric therapy. There are currently no widely accepted endorsements of any of these approaches for well-defined patient groups. This reluctance is in part because assessing the risk to the patient is based on probabilities, in essence predicting an occasional failure. Also limiting this approach, some institutions do not have an adequate infrastructure to support outpatient care of the patient. Reliable outpatient monitoring of the patient, usually by the patient's family or friends, must also be assured. Although not yet routine practice, when all of these requirements can be met and the patient has no risk factors, there is increasing but cautious acceptance of outpatient management and oral antibiotic therapy.[23,32–34]

TABLE 24–2 ■ Risk Factors for Infection in the Patient with Cancer

Neutropenia
    Severe, especially absolute neutrophil count <100/µl
    Prolonged duration
    Rapid onset
No evidence of marrow recovery
    Monocytopenia
    Thrombocytopenia
Mucositis in the presence of neutropenia
    Chemotherapy-induced, especially by ara C
    Herpetic
    Diarrhea
Indwelling catheter
Relapsed or induction status of cancer
Malnutrition
    Parenteral nutrition
Abdominal pain
High fever or rigors
Unexplained signs or symptoms

Omission of antibiotics and early discontinuance of therapy are less widely practiced, despite substantial literature favoring these approaches.[20,21,24,25,28]

BALANCING INDIVIDUALIZED AND STANDARD MANAGEMENT

Treatment of the neutropenic host with unexplained fever should reflect the spectrum of infections characteristic of the patient's specific underlying disease and cancer therapy protocol as well as the patient's individual risk factors. The need for individualized therapy notwithstanding, there is clinical value in using a standard management plan. Practicing according to a standard management plan allows the clinician to analyze unfavorable outcomes in a framework that facilitates identification of deficiencies in treatment strategies. The greater the variability in management, the more difficult it is to attribute unfavorable outcomes to a particular practice. The optimal strategy is to individualize treatment only to the degree necessary to meet specific therapeutic objectives. Aggregate patient outcomes should be constantly assessed in relation to the management plan to identify therapeutic shortcomings and excesses, modifying the plan as warranted. Issues occasionally may be raised that can be addressed most appropriately by clinical trial.

INITIAL THERAPY FOR THE HIGHER RISK PATIENT

Management of the higher risk neutropenic patient with unexplained fever is in one sense easier than managing the lower risk patient. There is little controversy regarding the approach to management and no need to painstakingly weigh the benefits and costs of inpatient empiric intravenous therapy. Admission to the hospital and prompt administration of broad-spectrum antibiotics is mandatory. To emphasize the need for prompt administration of therapy, it is worth repeating that many bacterial pathogens will grow in fresh human blood at 37°C with a doubling time of less than 30 minutes. Most likely there is a level of bacteremia that once attained will inevitably be fatal. This threshold level presumably can be exceeded during a given 30-minute interval. Consequently blood cultures should be obtained, but no substantial delay of therapy to obtain cultures or to elicit and record a detailed history can be tolerated.

For patients with suspected sepsis, broad coverage, as with a combination of a third-generation cephalosporin, an aminoglycoside, and vancomycin, is advisable pending culture results. The specific choice of antimicrobial agents should reflect the bacterial antibiotic susceptibility patterns and epidemiology of the local institution. If an abdominal infection or other potential source of anaerobic bacteria is suspected, substitution of meropenem or imipenem for the third-generation cephalosporin is suggested. Most bacterial pathogens encountered in the blood of the neutropenic host will be demonstrated in the first 48 hours of incubation in the microbiology laboratory. Antibiotic therapy may be reevaluated and modified at that time, depending on the culture results and the patient's hospital course. Fungi are unusual causes of initial fever. If the patient has been receiving antibiotic therapy, however, regardless of whether oral or intravenous or administered as inpatient or outpatient, the risk is significantly increased. Empiric antifungal therapy with amphotericin B, fluconazole, or itraconazole is not routine for the initial empiric therapy but should be considered especially in seriously ill patients who recently had received antibiotic therapy. Although most of the bacterial infections in the neutropenic host are derived from the patient's resident flora,[35] one should be alert for unusual epidemiologic considerations that may alter the selection of an empiric therapy regimen (e.g., recent tick exposure in an area endemic for Rocky Mountain spotted fever). An approach to the patient with suspected sepsis is summarized in Figure 24–1.

For higher risk patients who do not have clinically apparent sepsis or suspected anaerobic or fungal infection, two pivotal questions should be addressed in deciding upon an empiric antibiotic regimen. First, Is there a need to provide coverage for gram-negative bacteria beyond the institution's standard regimen? And second, Is there a need to add vancomycin empirically for expanded gram-positive coverage beyond that provided by the institution's standard regimen?

Currently many institutions use monotherapy for routine empiric therapy of neutropenic patients with unexplained fever. Because of its safety and extensive gram-negative bacterial coverage, including *P. aeruginosa*, ceftazidime was among the first drugs advocated for use as monotherapy. Three other antibiotics have challenged ceftazidime as the preferred monotherapy drug. Imipenem and meropenem offer safety and broader spectrum coverage including gram-positive bacteria, although at greater expense and with potentially more disturbance of normal anaerobic flora, favoring colonization with *Candida* and antibiotic-resistant bacteria. Imipenem may induce seizures, especially in patients with renal dysfunction, and also causes significant nausea in many patients. Meropenem is generally well tolerated. Cefepime, a fourth-generation cephalosporin, has gained increasing favor because it provides broad-spectrum coverage including gram-positive bacteria and is well tolerated, but this so-called fourth-generation cephalosporin does not target anaerobic bacterial flora that could provide colonization resistance against more pathogenic microorganisms. Cefepime also provides increased activity against most strains of *Enterobacter* spp compared to ceftazidime,[36] although its bacteriocidal activity against *P. aeruginosa* is frequently about a twofold dilution lower than that of ceftazidime. In general, results have been satisfactory with any of the four aforementioned monotherapy drugs; however, although definitive trials are lacking, imipenem, meropenem, and cefepime have tended to fare better than ceftazidime or combination therapies overall.[37–48] For institutions routinely managing febrile neutropenic patients with monotherapy the addition of an aminoglycoside should be considered if the patient is known to be colonized with *P. aeruginosa* or resistant gram-negative organisms. The combination of an aminoglycoside and a β-lactam antibiotic or two β-lactam antibiotics has fallen out of favor other than for treating *P. aeruginosa* infection because of no demonstrated advantages over monotherapy and the greater expense of administration.

Reduction in empiric vancomycin usage has been advocated because of the concern regarding development of resistance and the studies showing that vancomycin can be added on the basis of the results of initial cultures with little risk to the patient.[49,50] In select patients, however, inclusion of vancomycin in the initial regimen may be justified. Factors that favor the addition of vancomycin to the initial empiric regimen are moderate-to-severe oral mucositis, especially due to cytarabine, suspected catheter-related infection, suspected *Bacillus cereus* infection (e.g., vesicular skin lesions during warm months),[51] known colonization with methicillin-resistant *S. aureus* or cephalosporin-resistant *Streptococcus pneumoniae*, or demonstration of gram-positive bacteria in a local site of infection or in blood culture media by Gram's stain, pending identification and susceptibility testing.

Sepsis in the Neutropenic Host

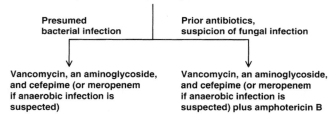

Consider using G-CSF or GM-CSF to shorten the duration of neutropenia if the infection is not readily controlled.

Alter the antimicrobial regimen as appropriate for patient-specific factors (tick exposure, for example).

FIGURE 24–1. Management depends on the risk of fungal infection, which is determined by preceding antibiotic therapy (oral or intravenous, including outpatient therapy) and other epidemiologic exposures. The use of colony-stimulating factors (CSF) should be considered unless the infection can be readily managed. Reassess the therapy on the basis of culture results and the patient's course. (G, granulocyte; GM, granulocyte-macrophage.)

The initial empiric therapy approach to the higher risk febrile patient is summarized in Figure 24–2.

INITIAL THERAPY FOR THE LOWER RISK PATIENT

The lower risk patient can be managed as an inpatient with empiric monotherapy similar to that for the higher risk patient, and this pathway is preferable if there is any concern regarding the ability to provide close monitoring or prompt evaluation of a neutropenic outpatient. For patients who are lower risk and for whom close monitoring and prompt evaluation can be assured, however, there are alternative approaches that increase the patient's quality of life during the febrile neutropenic episode and potentially prevent nosocomial infection. The best candidates for outpatient management are patients with an ANC >100 μl, evidence of marrow recovery, and none of the risk factors listed in Table 24–2. Outpatient intravenous therapy is the safest outpatient approach, but this tactic requires a sophisticated outpatient therapy team, the ability to self-administer intravenous antibiotics or the availability of programmable drug delivery systems, or a visiting home health care staff. Oral antibiotics with broad-spectrum activity provide an alternative to intravenous antibiotics. Two approaches have been studied: initial oral therapy and switch from initial intravenous therapy to oral therapy after pretreatment blood cultures have demonstrated no growth for at least 48 hours of incubation in the microbiology laboratory. Quinolones are not recommended for general use in febrile neutropenia because their outcomes in some studies were inferior to those of third-generation cephalosporins or carbapenems,[52,53] but quinolones may be considered for outpatient use in the lower risk patient. In general, the clinical outcomes of lower risk neutropenic adults managed with initial oral quinolones have not been significantly different from those of comparable patients managed with intravenous antibiotics.[29,52,54–57] Nonetheless clinicians should be cognizant that quinolones are generally less effective against gram-positive bacteria than cefepime, meropenem, or imipenem is and may even predispose the patient to the development of viridans streptococcal sepsis.[58] For this reason some clinicians have used a quinolone in combination with amoxicillin-clavulanate. Quinolones are not approved for use in children because of concern about the demonstrated adverse effects of this drug class on cartilage following experimental administration to several species of growing animals. Limited experience indicates that cartilage problems are infrequent or mild if such events occur at all following quinolone use in children.[59] Lower risk neutropenic children have been successfully switched to oral cefixime after 48 hours of intravenous therapy,[32,33] but initial oral therapy has not been extensively studied in neutropenic children.

Some clinical investigators have argued that empiric therapy can be discontinued early or not started in lower risk patients,[20,21,24,25,28] but acceptance of these approaches has been appropriately cautious because of the known risks accompanying febrile neutropenia and the exceptionally high rate of favorable outcomes currently attained using empiric therapy.

The initial empiric therapy approach to the lower risk febrile patient is summarized in Figure 24–3.

CATHETER-RELATED INFECTIONS

Central venous catheter–related infections may be classified into four basic categories: exit site infections of the

Fever in the Higher Risk Neutropenic Host

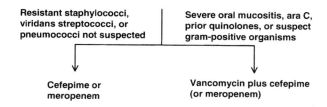

FIGURE 24–2. Management with cefepime or meropenem monotherapy is appropriate unless gram-positive bacterial infection is suspected (add vancomycin) or *Pseudomas aeruginosa* or other resistant gram-negative bacteria are suspected (add an aminoglycoside). The regimen should be reassessed after 48 hours.

Fever in the Lower Risk Neutropenic Host

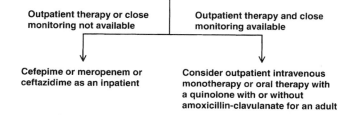

For lower risk children, switching to cefixime after a 48-hour inpatient stay with negative blood cultures has been successful.

If fever recurs or the patient becomes higher risk, admission for intravenous antibiotics and amphotericin B when appropriate is recommended.

FIGURE 24–3. Patients should be considered for outpatient therapy only if appropriate monitoring is assured and support for outpatient management is available continuously. Outpatient intravenous therapy can provide antimicrobial coverage equivalent to inpatient therapy. Oral antibiotic therapy has also been successfully used, although coverage may not be as extensive as with intravenous therapy. Patients with new fevers should be evaluated promptly and admitted for intravenous therapy. Antifungal therapy is indicated if the patient has been on antibiotics for 5 days or longer.

skin, tunnel tract or pocket infections, intraluminal infections, and pericatheter infections.

Exit site infections are localized skin infections, often due to *S. aureus* or *Candida* spp. These infections generally can be managed with appropriate intravenous, oral, or even topical therapy.

Tunnel tract infections are infections of the soft tissues adjacent to the tunnel tract, at least 2 cm from the exit site, and often extending beyond the catheter cuff. In the case of totally implanted catheters, so-called pocket infections are the equivalent of tunnel tract infections. Generally these infections require catheter removal combined with parenteral therapy for 7 to 10 days. However, successful in situ therapy is occasionally possible. Atypical mycobacteria may cause tunnel tract infections, particularly in warm climates, and are characterized by a discharge of green pus and poor response to therapy.[60] Recognition of these infections is particularly important because in this case the catheter should be removed along with wide excision of the involved tissue. Antimicrobial therapy may include agents such as clarithromycin, rifampin, and aminoglycosides as guided by susceptibility testing.

In cancer patients with indwelling catheters a substantial proportion of documented bacteremias are catheter-related intraluminal infections. The use of quantitative cultures is helpful in establishing the catheter lumen as a source of infection. A fivefold or greater concentration of organisms in blood obtained from the catheter compared to the concentration in blood simultaneously obtained from a peripheral vein is considered evidence of a catheter-related infection. Distinction of catheter-related bacteremia from bacteremia unrelated to the catheter is important because therapy can be directed at eradicating the catheter-related infection. New fever in cancer patients who are not neutropenic is the most common presentation. Often the patient reports an abrupt fever, sometimes associated with rigors, about 30 to 60 minutes after the catheter is flushed. This interval is apparently due to the delay required for cytokine response following exposure to microbial toxins. The patient may experience hypotension if the bacterial load is high.[61] Shock related to suspected catheter-related intraluminal infection is an indication to discontinue infusion through the catheter and to remove it as soon as feasible. In general, uncomplicated intraluminal infections not causing vascular instability can be cured by infusing antibiotics through the catheter for at least 10 days.[2] In the case of multiple lumen catheters, antibiotic administration should be alternated through the lumens to avoid a sequestered site of infection. Flushing the catheter between infusions with a heparin solution containing antibiotics at a concentration equivalent to that prepared for intravenous infusion allows high concentrations of antibiotics to be delivered to the site of infection constantly (referred to as dwell or antibiotic-lock therapy). Antibiotic-lock therapy has been found to achieve a significantly better rate of cure of intraluminal catheter-related infections than parenteral therapy alone achieves.[62-64] Care must be taken to avoid incompatible mixtures of antibiotics and heparin. Certain bacteria such as *Bacillus* spp are difficult to eradicate and are an indication for catheter removal. *Candida* intraluminal infections are also an indication for catheter removal, although eradication without catheter removal is possible. Management of intraluminal catheter-related infections is summarized in Figure 24–4.

Pericatheter infections reside in fibrin clot around the external surface of the distal catheter. Such infections are not readily recognized, explaining in part the rarity of their diagnosis. This condition should be suspected when patients have persistent bacteremia and a pericatheter clot can be demonstrated by radiographic study such as a fluoroscopic examination in conjunction with injecting dye through the catheter. Catheter removal may be necessary to cure the infection; however, the clinician should be alert to the possibility that the clot may be dislodged in the process, creating emboli.

PERSISTENT AND RECURRENT FEVER

Most neutropenic patients with unexplained fever will defervesce within the first 5 days of empiric antibiotic therapy. For patients who fail to defervesce, daily reassessment is warranted. Most neutropenic patients with prolonged fever will have an infection, and fever may persist until there is marrow recovery. Drug fever is less common in the immunosuppressed patient than in the nonimmunosuppressed patient. On day 3 of treatment the antimicrobial regimen should be reassessed. If vancomycin or aminoglycosides were included in the initial empiric regimen, their use should be reevaluated in light of admission culture results and the patient's clinical course. If there is no specific indication, these drugs should be discontinued to

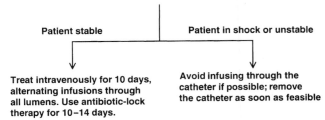

Catheter-related Intraluminal Infection

Patient stable → Treat intravenously for 10 days, alternating infusions through all lumens. Use antibiotic-lock therapy for 10–14 days.

Patient in shock or unstable → Avoid infusing through the catheter if possible; remove the catheter as soon as feasible

Candida and *Bacillus* species are less likely to respond. Removal of the catheter is advisable if catheter-infection is due to these organisms.

FIGURE 24–4. If the patient is in shock or is unstable, avoid infusing solutions through the catheter if feasible, as organisms and microbial toxins may be infused into the circulation. If the patient is stable, most infections can be cured using a combination of intravenous and antibiotic-lock therapy.

reduce toxicity and avoid unnecessarily inducing antibiotic resistance. Conversely, if vancomycin was not started initially and the patient has mucositis or another indication for vancomycin, addition of this drug may be warranted. Likewise, abdominal findings or isolation of *P. aeruginosa* may be an indication for the addition of an aminoglycoside, a carbapenem, or both. If the patient is clinically well other than persistent fever, monotherapy may be continued with close monitoring of the patient.

Persistent fever despite 5 days of broad-spectrum antibiotic therapy is an indication for empiric antifungal therapy. Despite significant nephrotoxicity, most clinicians prefer to start amphotericin B as empiric therapy because of its activity against a broad range of fungi, including *Aspergillus* spp. Fluconazole, which has good activity against *Candida* spp, is ineffective against *Aspergillus* spp and other molds. Empiric therapy with fluconazole can be considered only in a setting where the risk of mold infection is low. Itraconazole, which is active against *Aspergillus* spp, is less active against *Candida* spp than fluconazole is. However, use of itraconazole is also limited because of an impression that it has less clinical efficacy against molds like *Aspergillus* spp than amphotericin B has. A liposomal preparation of amphotericin B (AmBisome) is as effective as conventional amphotericin B or amphotericin B lipid complex (Nelcet) but is significantly less toxic than either agent.[65,66] The liposomal preparation, however, costs 20- to 60-fold more than conventional amphotericin B, creating a medical management dilemma.

At the time antifungal therapy is initiated, consideration should be given to obtaining a computed tomography (CT) scan of the chest. The primary justification is to identify occult pulmonary mold infections so that immediate resection of lesions can be considered. Early surgical resection, in conjunction with maximal antifungal therapy and possibly granulocyte transfusions, is perhaps the best hope for survival of the neutropenic cancer patient with a pulmonary mold infection, a group with a high mortality when managed with conventional treatment.[67] Candidal lesions can also be demonstrated by CT of the chest and abdomen, but early identification of these lesions is generally not essential because no additional treatment other than antifungal therapy is usually warranted, and the diagnostic yield of the test will be improved when neutropenia is resolved. Thus CT of the abdomen can be delayed until marrow function is recovering and assessment is needed to determine if continued antifungal therapy is indicated. CT of the chest should also be obtained after marrow recovery to assess the need for continuation of antifungal therapy.

A patient whose fever recurs on continued antibiotic therapy should be managed similarly to a patient who never defervesced. Fungal infections are again the primary concern. If the patient was treated for a recent episode of febrile neutropenia, perhaps with only a few intervening days off antibiotic therapy, management as a recurrent fever rather than an initial fever is advisable.

Prolonged or recurrent fever has the same implications regardless of whether the patient is being managed as an inpatient or outpatient. To optimize monitoring and timely interventions, outpatients should be considered for admission in the presence of prolonged or recurrent fever.

Management of the neutropenic patient with persistent fever is summarized in Figure 24–5.

DURATION OF THERAPY

Many cancer patients experience brief episodes of neutropenia, rendering moot the decision of when to discontinue empiric antibiotic therapy. If there is no evidence of infection, therapy may generally be discontinued as soon as the fever and neutropenia resolve. Occasionally patients have continued fever despite resolution of neutropenia. A CT of the chest and abdomen after the ANC is >500/μl may reveal evidence of disseminated candidiasis. Another common cause of fever after resolution of neutropenia is CMV infection, although even with blood isolation of the virus, distinguishing between latent and active infection may be difficult. Histoplasmosis and occult catheter-related infection should also be considered.

Higher risk patients with persistent fever accompanying prolonged neutropenia generally should be continued on therapy until neutropenia resolves. Amphotericin B should be initiated empirically after 5 days of fever. Because fever is the most consistent early indicator of bacterial infection in the neutropenic patient, stopping therapy in such patients creates a dilemma. If fever is disregarded as an indicator of empiric therapy initiation, bacterial infection may be far advanced before detected. Persistent fever in the lower risk neutropenic patient with a projected prolonged course of neutropenia presents a quandary. Some clinicians advocate stopping empiric therapy after 14 days with close observation.

The patients who have prolonged neutropenia and defervesce after initiation of empiric therapy are the

Persistent Fever in the Neutropenic Host

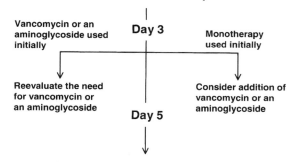

FIGURE 24–5. Reassess the patient after 3 days of empiric therapy and consider altering the regimen. After 5 days of persistent fever or with recurrent fever after more than 5 days of antibiotics, add amphotericin B empirically. Computed tomography of the chest to check for mold disease is suggested for patients considered at risk.

patients who generally require a clinical judgment regarding the relative benefits and risks of continued therapy. Unless there is evidence that defervescence was not a response to antibiotic therapy, a minimum course of 7 days is warranted. Following a 7-day course of antibiotics, factors that favor continuing therapy are severe neutropenia (ANC <100/µl) without evidence of marrow recovery, a suspected or documented focus of infection including mucositis, a history of a previous serious infection, a regimen that is well tolerated, and an inability to assure careful follow-up. In the absence of specific indications, empiric antibiotic therapy may be discontinued after the patient has been afebrile for at least 5 days and a minimum course of 7 days of therapy has been completed. Discontinuing antibiotics in these patients may reduce the risk of fungal infection or infection with antibiotic-resistant bacteria. With fever recurrence, prompt resumption of antibiotic therapy is essential, and consideration should be given to initiation of antifungal therapy at this time.

Recommended duration of treatment of the neutropenic host is summarized in Figure 24–6.

CHRONIC NEUTROPENIA UNRELATED TO CHEMOTHERAPY

Patients with chronic neutropenia unrelated to chemotherapy, such as patients with congenital neutropenia or aplastic anemia, generally have less risk of infection per time interval of neutropenia. The same principles used to manage the neutropenic cancer patient are applicable, but there is generally no anticipation of marrow function recovery. Empiric therapy courses of 2 weeks are often used, with this endpoint in part reflecting the perceived

Duration of Therapy in the Neutropenic Host

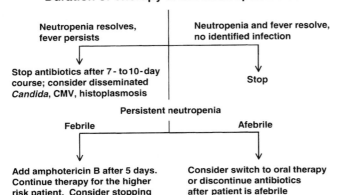

FIGURE 24–6. If neutropenia resolves, antibiotics can be stopped immediately if the patient is afebrile with no evidence of infection or after a 7- to 10-day course if fever persists. If neutropenia persists, continue antibiotics and amphotericin B in the higher risk patient. Consider stopping therapy after 2 weeks in the lower risk patient with no evidence of infection including negative computed tomography scans of the chest and abdomen.

futility of continuing empiric therapy beyond this time without a specific indication. Despite marked advances in managing the neutropenic patient, irreversible absolute neutropenia ultimately has a poor outcome.

NEUTROPENIA IN THE BONE MARROW TRANSPLANT PATIENT

It is important to recognize that patients in the early postallogeneic bone marrow transplantation period have all the risks that attend the neutropenic patient plus profound risks of infection unique to transplantation. In particular, the bone marrow transplant patient is at greatly increased risk of fungal infection (especially molds like *Aspergillus* spp) and viral infections (especially CMV; respiratory viruses including influenza, parainfluenza, and respiratory syncytial virus; and adenovirus).

Comprehensive guidelines on the management of opportunistic infections in hematopoietic stem cell transplant patients were recently published jointly by the Centers for Disease Control and Prevention (CDC), the Infectious Diseases Society of America, and the American Society of Blood and Marrow Transplantation.[68] Prophylaxis in bone marrow transplant patients against *Pneumocystis carinii* pneumonia is warranted.[68] Trimethoprim sulfamethoxazole (TMP-SMX) is usually preferred, although dapsone and atovaquone may be considered, the latter only in patients who don't have diarrhea, which leads to inadequate absorption of atovaquone. Either prophylaxis or pre-emptive therapy with ganciclovir is indicated for the prevention of CMV infection in bone marrow transplantation patients who are at risk.[68] If pre-emptive therapy is used, careful monitoring, optimally using both CMV pp65 antigen and CMV-DNA plasma polymerase chain reaction (PCR), should be performed at least weekly. Fluconazole prophylaxis against candidal infections is practiced at most bone marrow transplant centers and has been endorsed by the CDC.[68] Clinicians should be alert for the potential emergence of fluconazole-resistant *C. krusei* or *Candida (Torulopsis) glabrata* in patients receiving fluconazole. Gut decontamination to prevent infection is not recommended,[68] although some investigators believe, on the basis of limited data, that gut decontamination can reduce the risk of graft-versus-host disease.

The risk of infection remains high in the post–bone marrow transplant period despite resolution of neutropenia. Thus unexplained fever in the non-neutropenic transplant patient is often managed with empiric antibiotic therapy, and if fever persists, antifungal therapy may be added empirically. The possibility of viral infection must also be pursued.

In the cancer patient, respiratory virus infections have variable severity, but in the bone marrow transplant patient, these infections must always be considered life threatening, although initially the infection may not appear to be serious. Among the viruses most likely to be encountered are adenovirus, influenza virus, parainfluenza virus, and respiratory syncytial virus. Consultation with an infectious diseases specialist to help identify the most promising marketed or experimental agents is suggested.

PROPHYLAXIS

The use of nonabsorbable prophylactic antibiotics in the neutropenic cancer patient has declined in recent years because of concerns regarding the induction of antibiotic resistance and the appreciation that widespread use of antimicrobials frequently will shift the pattern of infecting microorganisms or induce resistance in the targeted microbes. Two absorbable antibiotics, TMP-SMX and oral quinolones, have had limited use as prophylactic agents for patients with febrile neutropenia. Three days per week administration of TMP-SMX is highly effective in preventing *P. carinii* pneumonia, and its use is warranted for this purpose in all cancer patients at risk. There is evidence that both TMP-SMX (including 3 days per week administration) and quinolones can decrease the risk of bacterial infections, but concerns about the development of resistance have discouraged their use for this purpose. Penicillin is sometimes administered along with a quinolone because quinolone administration may predispose the patient to the development of viridans streptococcal infections.[58] Many viridans streptococcal isolates are now penicillin resistant, however, underscoring the limitations of antibiotic prophylaxis. Vancomycin should rarely, if ever, be used for prophylaxis because if resistance to this antibiotic becomes extensive among gram-positive bacteria, the medical consequences would be substantial.

Some studies support the use of fluconazole in selected higher risk neutropenic patients to prevent candidal infections. However, outbreaks of *C. krusei*, which is intrinsically resistant to fluconazole, have been reported in the setting of widespread use of fluconazole.[69] Itraconazole has activity against *Candida* and *Aspergillus* spp, but the oral capsule does not produce predictable blood levels.[68] The intravenous formulation may circumvent this problem, but this drug has a number of concerning drug interactions including with vinca alkaloids, cyclosporin, and methylprednisolone.[68] The potential benefits in the local institution must be weighed against the possible adverse effects and drug interactions, the development of resistance, and the cost of prophylaxis.

Viral chemoprophylaxis is routinely indicated only to prevent CMV infection in bone marrow transplantation patients. Influenza vaccine is recommended for prevention of influenza disease in immunocompromised hosts.

COLONY-STIMULATING FACTORS

Granulocyte and granulocyte-monocyte colony-stimulating factors (G-CSF and GM-CSF) can significantly shorten the duration of a chemotherapy-induced neutropenic episode, which would seemingly reduce the risk of infection. The results of clinical trials, however, have not consistently shown morbidity benefit from the use of colony-stimulating factors,[70-75] and no trial has demonstrated a survival benefit. Current guidelines from the American Society of Clinical Oncology therefore do not recommend routine use of these agents.[76] Nonetheless, use of G-CSF or GM-CSF in selected patients should be considered when the benefit of reduced duration of neutropenia might be substantial.[77] Examples include patients with bacterial infections not readily managed with antibiotics; patients with fungal infections, especially molds; and patients at extraordinary risk of infection, such as patients known to be colonized with highly resistant microorganisms.

COST CONTAINMENT

Cost containment is not the primary concern of the clinician caring for the febrile neutropenic patient, but the reality is that in the absence of unlimited resources, cost containment must be addressed. Cost containment can be accomplished without compromising patient care in a few key areas. First, the use of a standardized monotherapy such as cefepime or meropenem for empiric therapy of the febrile neutropenic patient is cost effective in that administration is efficient, toxicity is low, and there is no need to monitor drug levels. Outpatient management of lower risk patients with intravenous or oral empiric therapy is highly cost effective but requires some investment to build a supporting infrastructure.[78] In the general absence of evidence of overall improvement in outcomes, prophylaxis and experimental therapies such as granulocyte transfusions should be used only in carefully selected patient populations, such as allogeneic bone marrow transplant patients with mold infections.

One of the greatest dilemmas faced today in the management of the neutropenic patient is the selection of empiric antifungal therapy. Liposomal amphotericin B (AmBisome) has been shown to have efficacy comparable to that of conventional amphotericin B but is less toxic.[65] Nonetheless the cost differential between liposomal and conventional amphotericin B, 20- to 60-fold, has restrained the use of this drug. Hopefully, competition from new antifungal agents will lower prices and reduce the impact of cost as a factor in medical management recommendations.

Use of standardized treatment plans should be encouraged because this approach facilitates both medical and financial management of the neutropenic patient, fostering optimal use of limited resources.

REFERENCES

1. Shenep JL: Combination and single agent empirical antibacterial therapy for febrile cancer patients with neutropenia and mucositis. NCI Monogr 1990;(9):117–122.

2. Flynn PM, Shenep JL, Stokes DC, et al: In situ management of confirmed central venous catheter–related bacteremia. Pediatr Infect Dis J 1987;(6):729–734.

3. Benezra D, Kiehn TE, Gold JW, et al: Retrospective study of infections in indwelling central venous catheters using quantitative blood cultures. Am J Med 1988;(85):495–498.

4. Korones DN, Hussong MR, Gullace MA: Routine chest radiography of children with cancer hospitalized for fever and neutropenia. Cancer 1997;(80):1160–1164.

5. Donowitz GR, Harman C, Pope T, et al: The role of the chest roentgenogram in febrile neutropenic patients. Arch Intern Med 1991:(151);701–704.

6. Katz JA, Bash R, Rollins N, et al: The yield of routine chest radiography in children with cancer hospitalized for fever and neutropenia. Cancer 1991;(68):940–943.

7. Marina NM, Flynn PM, Rivera GK, et al: *Candida tropicalis* and *Candida albicans* fungemia in children with leukemia. Cancer 1991;(68):594–599.

8. Editorial: Surveillance cultures in neutropenia. Lancet 1989;(1):1238.

9. Aisner J, Murillo J, Schimpff SC, et al: Invasive aspergillosis in acute leukemia: Correlation with nose cultures and antibiotic use. Ann Intern Med 1979;(90):4–9.

10. Yu VL, Muder RR, Poorsattar A: Significance of isolation of *Aspergillus* from the respiratory tract in diagnosis of invasive pulmonary aspergillosis. Results from a three-year prospective study. Am J Med 1986;(81):249–254.

11. Committee on Quality of Health Care in America, Institute of Medicine: In Kohn LT, Corrigan JM, Molla SD (eds): To Err is Human: Building a Safer Health Care System. Washington DC, National Academy Press, 2000, p 312.

12. Bodey GP, Buckley M, Sathe YS, et al: Quantitative relationships between circulating leukocytes and infection in patients with acute leukemia. Ann Intern Med 1966;(64):328–340.

13. Dale DC, Guerry D IV, Wewerka JR, et al: Chronic neutropenia. Medicine (Baltimore) 1979;(58):128–144.

14. Bodey GP, Fainstein V, Elting LS, et al: Beta-lactam regimens for the febrile neutropenic patient. Cancer 1990;(65):9–16.

15. Jones PG, Rolston KV, Fainstein V, et al: Aztreonam therapy in neutropenic patients with cancer. Am J Med 1986;(81):243–248.

16. Rolston KV, Berkley P, Bodey GP, et al: A comparison of imipenem to ceftazidime with or without amikacin as empiric therapy in febrile neutropenic patients. Arch Intern Med 1992;(152):283–291.

17. Rubin M, Hathorn JW, Pizzo PA: Controversies in the management of febrile neutropenic cancer patients. Cancer Invest 1988;(6):167–184.

18. Danzig LE, Short LJ, Collins K, et al: Bloodstream infections associated with a needleless intravenous infusion system in patients receiving home infusion therapy. JAMA 1995;(273):1862–1864.

19. Talcott JA, Finberg R, Mayer RJ, et al: The medical course of cancer patients with fever and neutropenia. Clinical identification of a low-risk subgroup at presentation. Arch Intern Med 1988;(148):2561–2568.

20. Mullen CA, Buchanan GR: Early hospital discharge of children with cancer treated for fever and neutropenia: Identification and management of the low-risk patient. J Clin Oncol 1990;(8):1998–2004.

21. Griffin TC, Buchanan GR: Hematologic predictors of bone marrow recovery in neutropenic patients hospitalized for fever: Implications for discontinuation of antibiotics and early discharge from the hospital. J Pediatr 1992;(121):28–33.

22. Talcott JA, Siegel RD, Finberg R, et al: Risk assessment in cancer patients with fever and neutropenia: A prospective, two-center validation of a prediction rule. J Clin Oncol 1992;(10):316–322.

23. Talcott JA, Whalen A, Clark J, et al: Home antibiotic therapy for low-risk cancer patients with fever and neutropenia: A pilot study of 30 patients based on a validated prediction rule. J Clin Oncol 1994;(12):107–114.

24. Jones GR, Konsler GK, Dunaway RP, et al: Risk factors for recurrent fever after the discontinuation of empiric antibiotic therapy for fever and neutropenia in pediatric patients with a malignancy or hematologic condition. J Pediatr 1994;(124):703–708.

25. Bash RO, Katz JA, Cash JV, et al: Safety and cost effectiveness of early hospital discharge of lower risk children with cancer admitted for fever and neutropenia. Cancer 1994;(74):189–196.

26. Lucas KG, Brown AE, Armstrong D, et al: The identification of febrile, neutropenic children with neoplastic disease at low risk for bacteremia and complications of sepsis. Cancer 1996;(77):791–798.

27. Rackoff WR, Gonin R, Robinson C, et al: Predicting the risk of bacteremia in children with fever and neutropenia. J Clin Oncol 1996;(14):919–924.

28. Aquino VM, Tkaczewski I, Buchanan GR: Early discharge of low-risk febrile neutropenic children and adolescents with cancer. Clin Infect Dis 1997;(25):74–78.

29. Rolston KVI: New trends in patient management: Risk-based therapy for febrile patients with neutropenia. Clin Infect Dis 1999;(29):515–521.

30. Klaassen RJ, Goodman TR, Pham B, Doyle JJ: "Low-risk" prediction rule for pediatric oncology patients presenting with fever and neutropenia. J Clin Oncol 2000;(18):1012–1019.

31. Klastersky J, Paaesmans M, Rubenstein EB, et al and the Study Section on Infections of Multinational Association for Supportive Care in Cancer: The multinational association for supportive care in cancer risk index: A multinational scoring system for identifying low-risk febrile neutropenic cancer patients. J Clin Oncol 2000;(18):3038–3051.

32. Shenep JL, Flynn PM, Baker DK, et al: Oral cefixime is comparable to continued intravenous antibiotics in the empirical treatment of febrile, neutropenic children with cancer. Clin Infect Dis 2001;(32):36–43.

33. Paganini HR, Sarkis CM, Demartino MG, et al: Oral administration of cefixime to lower risk febrile children with cancer. Cancer 2000;(88):2848–2852.

34. Hughes WT, Armstrong D, Body GP, et al: 1997 Guidelines for the use of antimicrobial agents in neutropenic patients with unexplained fever. Clin Infect Dis 1997;(25):551–573.

35. Schimpff SC, Young VM, Greene WH, et al: Origins of infection in acute nonlymphocytic leukemia: Significance of hospital acquisition of potential pathogens. Ann Intern Med 1972;(77):707–714.

36. Johnson MP, Ramphal R: Beta-lactam-resistant *Enterobacter* bacteremia in febrile neutropenic patients receiving monotherapy. J Infect Dis 1990;(162):981–983.

37. Ramphal R, Gucalp R, Rotstein C, et al: Clinical experience with single agent and combination regimens in the management of infection in the febrile neutropenic patient. Am J Med 1996;100(suppl 6A):83S–89S.

38. Cometta A, Calandra T, Gaya H, et al: Monotherapy with meropenem versus combination therapy with ceftazidime plus amikacin as empiric therapy for fever in granulocytopenic patients with cancer. Antimicrob Agents Chemother 1996;(40):1108–1115.

39. Yamamura D, Gacalp R, Carlisle P, et al: Open randomized study of cefepime versus piperacillin-gentamicin for treatment of febrile neutropenic cancer patients. Antimicrob Agents Chemother 1997;(41):1704–1708.

40. Pfaller MA, Marshall SA, Jones RN: In vitro activity of cefepime and ceftazidime against 197 nosocomial blood stream isolates of streptococci: A multicenter sample. Diagn Microbiol Infect Dis 1997;(29):273–276.

41. Raad II, Abi-Said D, Rolston KV, et al: How should imipenem-cilastatin be used in the treatment of fever and infection in neutropenic cancer patients? Cancer 1998;(82):2449–2458.

42. Lindblad R, Rödjer S, Adriansson M, et al: Empiric monotherapy for febrile neutropenia — a randomized study comparing meropenem with ceftazidime. Scand J Infect Dis 1998; (30):237–243.

43. Biron P, Fuhrmann C, Cure H, et al: Cefepime versus imipenem-cilastin as empirical monotherapy in 400 febrile patients with short duration neutropenia. J Antimicrob Chemother 1998;(42):511–518.

44. Ramphal R: Is monotherapy for febrile neutropenia still a viable alternative? Clin Infect Dis 1999;(29):508–514.

45. Akova M, Akan H, Korten V, et al: Comparison of meropenem with amikacin plus ceftazidime in the empirical treatment of febrile neutropenia: A prospective randomized multicentre trial in patients without previous prophylactic antibiotics. Meropenem Study Group of Turkey. Int J Antimicrob Agents 1999;(13):15–19.

46. Wang FD, Liu CY, Hsu HC, et al: A comparative study of cefepime versus ceftazidime as empiric therapy of febrile episodes in neutropenic patients. Chemotherapy 1999;(45):370–379.

47. Feld R, DePauw B, Berman S, et al: Meropenem versus ceftazidime in the treatment of cancer patients with febrile neutropenia: A randomized, double-blind trial. J Clin Oncol 2000;(18):3690–3698.

48. Vandercam B, Gerain J, Humblet Y, et al: Meropenem versus ceftazidime as empirical monotherapy for febrile neutropenic cancer patients. Ann Hematol 2000;(79):152–157.

49. Rubin M, Hathorn JW, Marshall D, et al: Gram-positive infections and the use of vancomycin in 550 episodes of fever and neutropenia. Ann Intern Med 1988;(108):30–35.

50. European Organization for Research and Treatment of Cancer (EORTC) International Antimicrobial Therapy Cooperative Group, and The National Cancer Institute of Canada—Clinical Trials Group: Vancomycin added to empirical combination antibiotic therapy for fever in granulocytopenic cancer patients. J Infect Dis 1991;(163):951–958.

51. Henrickson KJ, Shenep JL, Flynn PM, et al: Primary cutaneous *Bacillus cereus* infection in neutropenic children. Lancet 1989;(1):601–603.

52. Malik IA, Abbas Z, Karim M: Randomized comparison of oral ofloxacin alone with combination of parenteral antibiotics in neutropenic febrile patients. Lancet 1992;(339):1092–1096.

53. Meunier F, Zinner SH, Gaya H, et al: Prospective randomized evaluation of ciprofloxacin versus piperacillin plus amikacin for empiric antibiotic therapy of febrile granulocytopenic cancer patients with lymphomas and solid tumors. The European Organization for Research on Treatment of Cancer International Antimicrobial Therapy Cooperative Group. Antimicrob Agents Chemother 1991;(35):873–878.

54. Malik IA, Khan WA, Karim M, et al: Feasibility of outpatient management of fever in cancer patients with low-risk neutropenia: Results of a prospective randomized trial. Am J Med 1995;(98):224–231.

55. Garcia-Carbonero R, Cortes-Funes H: Outpatient therapy with oral ofloxacin for patients with low risk neutropenia and fever: A prospective, randomized clinical trial. Cancer 1999;(85):213–219.

56. Freifeld A, Marchigiani D, Walsh T, et al: A double-blind comparison of empirical oral and intravenous antibiotic therapy for low-risk febrile patients with neutropenia during cancer chemotherapy. N Engl J Med 1999;(341):305–311.

57. Kern WV, Cometta A, DeBock R, et al: Oral versus intravenous empirical antimicrobial therapy for fever in patients with granulocytopenia who are receiving cancer chemotherapy. N Engl J Med 1999;(341):312–318.

58. Elting LS, Bodey GP, Keefe BH: Septicemia and shock syndrome due to viridans streptococci: A case-control study of predisposing factors. Clin Infect Dis 1992;(14):1201–1207.

59. Freifeld A, Pizzo P: Use of fluoroquinolones for empirical management of febrile neutropenia in pediatric cancer patients. Pediatr Infect Dis J 1997;(16):140–146.

60. Flynn PM, Van Hooser B, Gigliotti F: Atypical mycobacterial infections of Hickman catheter exit sites. Pediatr Infect Dis J 1998;(7):510–513.

61. Henrickson KJ, Shenep JL: Fulminating *Staphylococcus epidermidis* bacteremia. South Med J 1990;(83):231–234.

62. Capdevila JA: Catheter-related infection: An update on diagnosis, treatment, and prevention. Int J Infect Dis 1998;(2):230–236.

63. Krzywda EA, Andris DA, Edmiston CE Jr, Quebbeman EJ: Treatment of Hickman catheter sepsis using antibiotic lock technique. Infect Control Hosp Epidemiol 1995;(16):596–598.

64. Mermel LA, Farr BM, Sherertz RJ, et al: Guidelines for the management of intravascular catheter-related infections. Clin Infect Dis 2001;(32):1249–1272.

65. Walsh TJ, Finberg RW, Arndt C, et al: Liposomal amphotericin B for empirical therapy in patients with persistent fever and neutropenia. N Engl J Med 1999;764–771.

66. Wingard JR, White MH, Anaissie E, et al: A randomized, double-blind comparative trial evaluating the safety of liposomal amphotericin B versus amphotericin lipid complex in the empirical treatment of febrile neutropenia. Clin Infect Dis 2000;(31):1155–1163.

67. Abbasi S, Shenep JL, Hughes WT, et al: Aspergillosis in children with cancer: A 34-year experience. Clin Infect Dis 1999;(29):1210–1219.

68. Centers for Disease Control and Prevention: Guidelines for Preventing Opportunistic Infections Among Hematopoietic Stem Cell Transplant Recipients. Recommendations of CDC, the Infectious Disease Society of America, and the American Society of Blood and Marrow Transplantation. MMWR Morb Mortal Wkly Rep 2000;49(RR-10):1–95.

69. Wingard JR, Merz WG, Rinaldi MG, et al: Increase in *Candida krusei* infection among patients with bone marrow transplantation and neutropenia treated prophylactically with fluconazole. N Engl J Med 1991;(325):1274–1277.

70. Riikonen P, Saarinen UM, Makipernaa A: Recombinant human granulocyte-macrophage colony-stimulating factor in the treatment of febrile neutropenia: A double blind placebo-controlled study in children. Pediatr Infect Dis J 1994;(13):197–202.

71. Maher DW, Lieschke GJ, Green M, et al: Filgrastim in patients with chemotherapy-induced febrile neutropenia—a double-blind, placebo-controlled trial. Ann Intern Med 1994;(121):492–501.

72. Anaissie EJ, Vartivarian S, Bodey GP, et al: Randomized comparison between antibiotics alone and antibiotics plus granulocyte-macrophage colony-stimulating factor (*Escherichia coli*–derived) in cancer patients with fever and neutropenia. Am J Med 1996;(100):17–23.

73. Vellenga E, Uyl-de Groot CA, de Wit R, et al: Randomized placebo-controlled trial of granulocyte-macrophage colony-stimulating factor in patients with chemotherapy related febrile neutropenia. J Clin Oncol 1996;(14):619–627.

74. Michon JM, Hartmann O, Boufett E, et al: An open-label, multicentre, randomised phase 2 study of recombinant human granulocyte colony-stimulating factor (filgrastim) as an adjunct to combination chemotherapy in paediatric patients with metastatic neuroblastoma. Eur J Cancer 1998;(34):1063–1069.

75. Mitchell PL, Morland B, Stevens MC, et al: Granulocyte colony-stimulating factor in established febrile neutropenia: A

randomized study of pediatric patients. J Clin Oncol 1997;(15):1163–1170.

76. Ozer H, Armitage JO, Bennett CL, et al: For the American Society of Clinical Oncology Growth Factors Expert Panel. 2000 Update of recommendations for the use of hematopoietic colony-stimulating factors: Evidence-based clinical practice guidelines. J Clin Oncol 2000;(18):3558–3585.

77. Liang DC, Chen SH, Lean SF: Role of granulocyte colony-stimulating factor as adjunct therapy for septicemia in children with acute leukemia. Am J Hematol 1995;(48):76–81.

78. Talcott JA, Whalen A, Clark J, et al: Home antibiotic therapy for low-risk cancer patients with fever and neutropenia: A pilot study of 30 patients based on a validated prediction rule. J Clin Oncol 1994;(12):107–114.

Bacterial and Viral Diarrhea

DAVIDSON H. HAMER, MD, FACP

Diarrheal disease remains a significant cause of morbidity and mortality in industrialized countries, where its greatest impact is seen in infants and children. A child less than 5 years old experiences an average of two episodes of diarrhea per year in the United States. In developing countries the burden of disease due to diarrhea is generally much greater, with young children experiencing diarrhea rates that are two to three times higher than in industrialized nations. In fact, diarrheal disease is one of the top three causes of death for infants and young children in most developing countries.

In the United States an average of 300 deaths per year is recorded for children under 5 years of age, mostly related to dehydration.[1] Adults generally have fewer episodes of diarrheal disease, with the important exception of human immunodeficiency virus (HIV)–infected persons. The elderly, however, are susceptible to more complications, especially when dehydration occurs.[2] The treatment of diarrhea in patients with HIV infection has been reviewed elsewhere[3] and therefore will not be addressed in this chapter.

Physicians in the United States are consulted annually for 8.2 million diarrheal episodes.[4] Medical costs and loss of productivity due to infectious diarrhea amount to 23 billion a year. Given the extensive morbidity and cost of diarrheal disease, prompt appropriate therapy is vital for the prevention of complications and death due to this common problem. As most episodes of infectious diarrhea are self-limited, the main goals of treatment should be rehydration and the relief of symptoms.

FLUID THERAPY

The most devastating consequences of acute infectious diarrhea result from fluid and electrolyte losses.[5] Toxigenic bacteria, such as *Vibrio cholerae* and certain strains of *Escherichia coli*, are associated with extreme forms of dehydration caused by the production of large amounts of isotonic fluid in the small bowel that overwhelm the ability of the lower intestine to reabsorb (Table 25–1). Children with toxigenic diarrhea lose slightly less sodium and bicarbonate in their feces than do adults, but they excrete significantly more potassium. "Nonspecific" diarrhea, usually caused by viruses, is associated with less fluid loss and lower fecal electrolyte concentrations.

The major aim of treatment is the replacement of fluid and electrolytes. Although the traditional route of administration has been intravenous, in recent years oral rehydration solutions (ORS) have proven equally effective physiologically[5] and more practical logistically in developing countries.[6–8] Even in industrialized countries, ORS is the treatment of choice for mild-to-moderate diarrhea in both children and adults, and it can be used in severe diarrhea after initial parenteral fluid replacement.[8,9] ORS is based on the physiologic principle that glucose enhances sodium absorption in the

TABLE 25–1 ■ Fluid Compositions in Infectious Diarrhea and Hydration Solutions

STOOL OR HYDRATION FLUID	Electrolyte concentrations (mmol/L)			
	SODIUM	POTASSIUM	CHLORIDE	BICARBONATE
Cholera, adult	124	16	90	48
Cholera, child	101	27	92	32
Nonspecific diarrhea, child	56	25	55	14
Ringer's lactated solution	130	4	109	28*
Oral rehydration therapy (WHO formula)†	90	20	80	30

*Equivalent from lactate conversion.
†Includes glucose, 110 mmol/L (20 g/L).
WHO, World Health Organization.

TABLE 25–2 ■ Oral Rehydration Solutions

Components	WHO Formula*	Ricelyte†	Pedialyte‡	Rehydralyte§	Ceralyte‖
Sodium (q/L)	90	50	45	75	70
Potassium (q/L)	20	25	20	20	20
Chloride (q/L)	80	45	35	65	60
Citrate (q/L)	30	34	30	30	30
Glucose (g/L)	20		25	25	
Sucrose (g/L)					
Rice syrup solid (g/L)		30			40

*Not available at most pharmacies but can be ordered in bulk from the Jianas Brothers Packaging Company, Kansas City, MO; telephone (816) 421–2880.
†Mead Johnson Nutritionals, Evansville, IN.
‡Ross Laboratories, Columbus, OH.
§Not available at most pharmacies. May be ordered from Ross Laboratories in cases of 8-oz (240 ml) bottles.
‖Available as packets of powder that must be reconstituted in 1 L of drinking water. Manufactured by Cera Products, Columbia, MO; telephone 1-888-CERALYTE.
WHO, World Health Organization.

small intestine, even in the presence of secretory losses caused by bacterial toxins. Formulations of ORS available in the United States are listed in Table 25–2.

Although there is agreement on the value of ORS in treating dehydrating diarrhea, the formulation of electrolytes remains in dispute, particularly in treating well-nourished children in industrialized countries with mild-to-moderate diarrhea. Some authorities have expressed concern about what is considered a high concentration of sodium (90 mmol/L) in the standard ORS formulation because it might cause hypernatremia and lead to seizures.[7,8,10] This issue was examined in a Scottish study in which children with acute diarrhea with mild dehydration were treated in a randomized fashion with solutions containing sodium concentrations of 35, 50, or 90 mmol/L and glucose concentrations of 200, 111, and 110 mmol/L, respectively; all three formulations proved to be equally safe and effective.[11] On the basis of these and other studies, several authorities have recommended lower concentrations of sodium and a reduced osmolarity in ORS for children with diarrhea living in a developed country.[8,10] A multicenter study of male children with acute, noncholera diarrhea found that rehydration with a reduced osmolarity, reduced sodium ORS (Table 25–2) was associated with a lower total stool output, less total ORS intake, and a shortened duration of diarrhea than in

the standard ORS group.[12] After treatment, patients who had received the reduced osmolarity ORS had a lower mean serum sodium; however, this was not associated with any adverse clinical events. Similar findings were encountered in a trial of adults with severe cholera, which compared reduced osmolarity ORS with standard ORS.[13] This study found no difference in clinical outcomes between the two forms of ORS. As in the pediatric study, reduced osmolarity ORS was associated with an increased incidence of asymptomatic hyponatremia.

Additional criticisms of the traditional glucose-based ORS center around its failure to decrease the quantity and duration of diarrhea and the fact that ORS provides little nutrition along with the rehydration.[8] An inexpensive alternative to glucose-based ORS is the substitution of starch derived from rice or cereals for glucose. Rice-based salt solutions produce lower stool losses, shorter duration of diarrhea, and greater fluid and electrolyte absorption and retention than do glucose-based ORS in treating childhood and adult diarrhea.[14,15] Improved growth and weight gain are also observed with rice-based ORS. Using a novel approach, it was recently demonstrated that the addition of an amylase-resistant starch to ORS is even more effective in reducing the duration of diarrhea and fecal weight than a rice flour–based ORS in patients with cholera.[16]

DIET

In the past the traditional approach to any diarrheal illness included dietary abstinence, with the restricted intake of necessary calories, fluids, and electrolytes. Certainly during an acute attack the patient often finds it more comfortable to avoid high-fiber foods, fats, and spices, all of which can increase stool volume and intestinal motility. In fact any oral consumption can provide a stimulus to defecation. Although giving the bowel a rest provides symptomatic relief, the patient must maintain intake with oral fluids containing some calories and appropriate concentrations of electrolytes. It is better to eat judiciously during an attack of diarrhea than to severely restrict oral intake. In children it is particularly important to restart feeding immediately after the child is able to accept oral intake to avoid the potential complication of malnutrition.

It is wise to avoid milk and dairy products during the acute episode because ingestion of such items in this setting could potentiate fluid secretion and increase stool volume. Beverages that contain caffeine or methylxanthine products such as coffee, strong tea, cocoa, and certain soft drinks all should be avoided as these agents increase intestinal motility. Alcohol similarly affects the gut, and therefore abstinence is recommended. In addition to the oral rehydration therapy described, acceptable beverages for mildly dehydrated adults include fruit juices and bottled soft drinks. It is advisable to "de-fizz" a carbonated drink by letting it stand in a glass before it is consumed.

ANTIMICROBIAL THERAPY

Treatment with antimicrobial agents provides minimal to no benefit in most patients with acute diarrhea. Among the types of diarrhea that should be treated with such drugs are shigellosis, cholera, typhoid fever, moderate-to-severe traveler's diarrhea, *E. coli* diarrhea in infants, and *Clostridium difficile* colitis (Table 25–3). There are conflicting reports regarding the efficacy of antibiotics in certain important infections, notably those due to *Campylobacter jejuni*, and there is insufficient data for infections caused by *Yersinia*, *Aeromonas*, noncholera vibrios, and several forms of *E. coli*. An algorithm for the diagnosis and treatment of acute diarrhea is provided in Figure 25–1.

The issue of when antimicrobial therapy is appropriate for the management of acute diarrhea remains a vexing problem. This issue was addressed in a placebo-controlled study with empiric ciprofloxacin treatment of severe, acute community-acquired gastroenteritis.[17] This study included patients who had had more than three stools per day for more than 3 days with at least one associated symptom. Treatment with ciprofloxacin, 500 mg twice daily for 5 days, was associated with a reduction in the duration of diarrhea and other symptoms by more than 2 days, fewer failures, and significant clearing of pathogens when compared to placebo. Six weeks later there was no difference in stool carriage of the original pathogen (12%) nor any evidence of demonstrable antibiotic resistance emerging during therapy. A study in Chicago, of adults with acute diarrhea, which compared outpatient treatment with ciprofloxacin vs. TMP-SMX vs. placebo, found that ciprofloxacin, but not TMP-SMX, shortened the duration of diarrhea.[18] Similar results have been noted in other studies of the empiric therapy of diarrhea.[19]

On the basis of the findings of these studies, patients with severe community-acquired diarrhea, defined as diarrhea (four or more unformed stools per day) lasting at least 3 days in an otherwise healthy person with at least one of the following symptoms: abdominal pain, fever, vomiting, myalgia, or headache should receive an antimicrobial drug, preferably a fluoroquinolone (Fig. 25–1). In this subset of patients with severe acute diarrhea there is a high likelihood of isolating a bacterial pathogen, and treatment with an antibiotic will most likely provide prompt relief of symptoms with a low risk of adverse effects.

In patients with bloody diarrhea it is not possible to distinguish between *Shigella, C. jejuni,* and enterohemorrhagic *E. coli* (EHEC) on clinical grounds. If dysentery symptoms predominate, then therapy with a fluoroquinolone is indicated (Fig. 25–1). In the absence of dysentery and if there is a reasonable possibility, based on epidemiologic evidence, that EHEC is the responsible pathogen, antimicrobial therapy should be withheld until a microbiologic diagnosis can be established (see treatment of EHEC).[20]

The choice of antimicrobial drugs, when indicated, should be based on in vitro sensitivity patterns; these are affected by the local prevalence of resistant organisms. The fluoroquinolones, including norfloxacin, ciprofloxacin, and ofloxacin, have broad-spectrum activity against virtually all important diarrheal pathogens (except *C. difficile*) and thus represent one of the best choices for treatment.

The optimal duration of antimicrobial therapy for acute diarrhea has not been well defined. Some authors recommend 3 days of treatment for diarrhea, others 5 days, and others 10 days. Despite these varying recommendations, several studies of relatively severe forms of diarrhea suggest a single dose of an antimicrobial agent is as effective as more prolonged therapy. For example, single-dose tetracycline produced the same results in treating cholera as the standard 2-day regimen.[21] Similarly a single dose of trimethoprim had the same efficacy in shigellosis as a standard 5-day course.[22] Single-dose fluoroquinolone therapy has been demonstrated to be highly effective for infections due to *V. cholerae, Vibrio parahaemolyticus,* and most *Shigella* spp.[23,24] On the other hand, short-course treatment of gastroenteritis due to *Salmonella* with fleroxacin was not found to be clinically beneficial.[23]

TABLE 25–3 ■ Therapy of Bacterial Infectious Diarrhea

	Antibiotic of choice	Dose, route, and duration	Alternative drugs
RECOMMENDED IN SYMPTOMATIC CASES			
Shigella	Ampicillin	500 mg PO qid or 1 g IV q6h × 3 d 50–100 mg/kg/d for children	Fluoroquinolones, nalidixic acid
	Ampicillin-resistant strains: TMP-SMX	One double-strength tablet PO bid, for children, 10 mg/kg/d TMP and 50 mg/kg/d SMX × 3 d (max 320 mg/ 1600 mg/d)	
Travelers' diarrhea	Ciprofloxacin	500 mg PO bid × 3 d	TMP-SMX, other fluoroquinolones, azithromycin
Enteropathogenic *Escherichia coli* (EPEC) Enteroaggregative *E. coli* (EAggEC) Diffusely adherent *E. coli* (DAEC) in infants; Enteroinvasive *E. coli* (EIEC)	TMP-SMX	As for shigellosis	Fluoroquinolones
Typhoid fever	Chloramphenicol	500 mg PO or IV qid × 14 d	Amoxicillin 1 g PO qid × 14 d; ciprofloxacin 500 mg PO bid × 7 d; TMP-SMX; azithromycin; third-generation cephalosporins
Cholera	Tetracycline*	500 mg PO qid; for children, 40 mg/kg/d in 4 doses (max 4 g/d) × 3 d	Ciprofloxacin, TMP-SMX, furazolidinone
	Doxycycline	100 mg PO bid × 3 d	
Salmonella (unusual cases)	Ampicillin	50–100 mg/kg/d in 4 doses × 10–14 d	Ciprofloxacin 500 mg PO bid × 14 d
	Ampicillin-resistant strains: TMP-SMX	One double-strength tablet PO bid, for children, 8 mg/kg/d TMP and 40 mg/kg/d TMP and 40 mg/kg/d SMX (max 320 mg/1600 mg/d) × 14 d	
NOT GENERALLY RECOMMENDED BECAUSE OF LACK OF CONCLUSIVE FINDINGS OR NO STUDIES			
Campylobacter jejuni	Erythromycin	500 mg PO bid × 5 d	Ciprofloxacin 500 mg PO bid × 5 d Azithromycin 500 mg PO on day 1, 250 mg/d PO days 2–5
Yersinia enterocolitica	Fluoroquinolones, TMP-SMX, chloramphenicol,		Aminoglycosides, tetracycline
Aeromonas spp	TMP-SMX, third-generation cephalosporins, fluoroquinolones		Tetracycline, chloramphenicol
Vibrio, noncholera species	Tetracycline		
EPEC, EAggEC, or DAEC in adults, enterohemorrhagic *E. coli*	TMP-SMX		
NOT RECOMMENDED (EXCEPT IN UNUSUAL CASES)			
Nontyphoidal *Salmonella* Enterotoxigenic *E. coli*			

*Should not be administered to children younger than 8 years old.

NONSPECIFIC THERAPY

Certain antimotility drugs such as loperamide and diphenoxylate are particularly useful in controlling moderate-to-severe diarrhea (Table 25–4). These agents decrease jejunal motor activity, thereby disrupting forward propulsive motility.[25,26] Opiates may decrease fluid secretion, enhance mucosal absorption, and increase rectal sphincter tone. The overall effect is to normalize fluid transport, slow transit time, reduce fluid losses, and diminish abdominal cramping.

Loperamide is one of the best antimotility drugs because it neither crosses the blood-brain barrier, and thus does not lead to habituation, nor carries the risk of

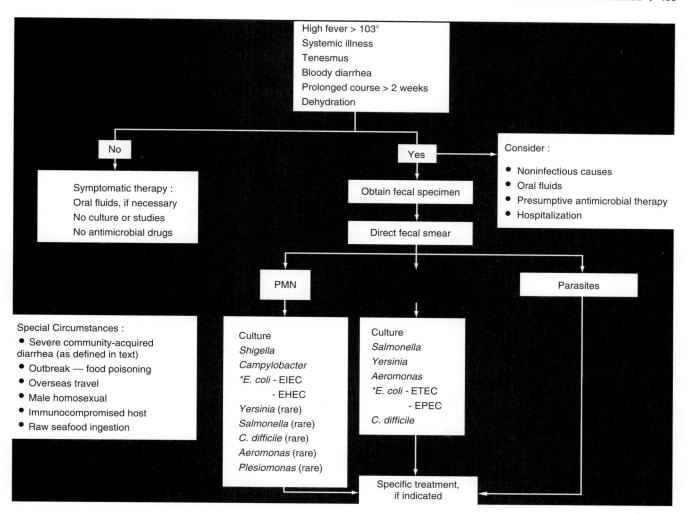

FIGURE 25–1. Algorithm for the diagnosis and treatment of acute diarrhea. EHEC, enterohemorrhagic *Eschericia coli*; EIEC, enteroinvasive *E. coli*; EPEC, enteropathogenic *E. coli*; ETEC, enterotoxigenic *E. coli*; PMN, polymorphonuclear neutrophil; *special tests required for diagnosis. (Modified from Hamer DH, Gorbach SL: Infectious diarrhea. In Feldman, Friedman, and Sleisenger: Sleisenger and Fordtran's Gastrointestinal and Liver Disease, 7th ed. Philadelphia, Elseiver, In press.)

depressing the respiratory center. Treatment with loperamide produces rapid improvement, often within the first 24 hours of therapy.[27] Racecadotril, an enkephalinase inhibitor that has both antisecretory and antidiarrheal properties, has been shown to be effective and safe for the treatment of acute watery diarrhea.[28] Early studies raised the concern that use of an antimotility agent in a patient with dysentery might worsen the infection,[29] but this concern has largely been dispelled by clinical experience. Patients suffering from shigellosis, including *Shigella dysenteriae* type I, have been treated inadvertently with loperamide as the only drug and have had a normal resolution of symptoms without prolonging the illness or delaying excretion of the pathogen.[30,31] Nevertheless these drugs generally should not be used in a patient with acute, severe colitis, either infectious or noninfectious in origin, which is suggested on clinical grounds by the presence of bloody, mucoid diarrhea or by endoscopy.

Bismuth subsalicylate (BSS), an insoluble complex of trivalent bismuth and salicylate, is effective therapy for mild-to-moderate forms of diarrhea.[32] The bismuth component of BSS possesses antimicrobial properties, and there are antisecretory properties related to the salicylate moiety. In studies of traveler's diarrhea among visitors to Mexico or West Africa, BSS reduced the frequency of diarrhea significantly more than placebo did; results were usually better when a high dose (4.2 g/d) was used.[33]

The combination of an antimicrobial drug and an antimotility drug provides the most rapid relief of diarrhea. In a study of travelers to Mexico, the combined use of loperamide and TMP-SMX resolved the diarrhea in 1 hour, compared to 30 hours with either drug alone or 59 hours with placebo.[27] Even in the most severe forms of diarrhea (i.e., those with fecal leukocytes or blood-tinged stool) the median duration of illness was 4.5 hours. In a similar study of United States military personnel in

TABLE 25–4 ■ Nonspecific Therapy of Infectious Diarrhea

EFFECTIVE
Fluids
    Intravenous
    Oral rehydration therapy
Food
    Continue nutrition intake
    Avoid lactose, caffeine, and methylxanthines
Antimotility drugs
    Codeine, paregoric, tincture of opium
    Loperamide
    Diphenoxylate
    Bismuth subsalicyclate
Antisecretory drug
    Zaldaride maleate
Other approach
    Lactobacillus GG

NOT EFFECTIVE
Lactobacilli
Kaolin, pectin, charcoal
Anticholinergics
Cholestyramine
Hydroxyquinolones* (enterovioform, diiodohydroxyquin)

*Warning: hydroxyquinolones may be harmful.

Egypt, loperamide added little to the efficacy of ciprofloxacin except in the initial 24 hours, when the combination was slightly better than the antibiotic alone.[34] The addition of loperamide to ciprofloxacin for the treatment of invasive diarrhea, however, significantly shortened the duration of diarrhea and decreased the median number of diarrheal stools.[35]

Hundreds of different kinds of antidiarrheal remedies can be found in pharmacies, apothecary shops, herbal medicine stores, and assorted medical establishments around the world. Each country has its own brand names and labeling requirements. Many products contain a combination of drugs, most of them therapeutically ineffective, others potentially dangerous. Various starches, talcs, and chalks have been prescribed for diarrheal illnesses for as long as recorded history. Kaolin and pectin, alone or in combination, are popular treatments, but there is no evidence that these preparations reduce intestinal fluid losses.[25,26]

Since most cases of infectious diarrhea, even those with an identified pathogen, have a mild, self-limited course, neither a stool culture nor specific treatment is required. For more severe cases as defined above, empiric antimicrobial therapy with a fluoroquinolone should be instituted, pending results of stool and blood cultures (Fig. 25–1).

TREATMENT OF SPECIFIC PATHOGENS

Cholera

Both the restoration of fluid and electrolyte balance and the maintenance of intravascular volume are cen-

tral to the successful treatment of cholera. This can be accomplished with intravenous solutions or oral rehydration therapy. Particular attention should be paid to the administration of bicarbonate and potassium, as these electrolytes are lost excessively in the stool of patients with cholera. ORS was developed for treating mild-to-moderate cases and is especially useful in developing countries.[6]

Although oral or parenteral hydration is crucial, antimicrobial agents are useful as ancillary therapeutic measures, since their use reduces stool output, duration of diarrhea, fluid requirements, and *Vibrio* excretion.[36] In the absence of resistance, tetracycline represents an effective, inexpensive choice. Intravenous therapy is indicated for patients unable to take medication by mouth. There is no proven value in lengthening the duration of treatment to 4 days or longer. In fact, single-dose therapy with ciprofloxacin produces a successful clinical response in more than 90% of patients infected with *V. cholerae*.[37] As a result of rising rates of resistance, tetracycline and doxycyline are often less effective than the fluoroquinolones.[37,38] TMP-SMX and furazolidone represent potential alternatives (Table 25–3).

The quinolones are highly effective for the treatment of cholera.[38,39] A double-blind, randomized, placebo-controlled trial of adults with cholera in India found that a 5-day course of norfloxacin was superior to TMP-SMX and placebo in reducing stool output, duration of diarrhea, fluid requirements, and *Vibrio* excretion.[40] A study that compared 3-day courses of ciprofloxacin, erythromycin, nalidixic acid, pivmecillinam, and tetracycline found that ciprofloxacin with concomitant fluid therapy was the most effective treatment for adults infected with tetracycline-resistant strains of *V. cholerae*.[41] Diarrhea resolved within 72 hours in 93% of patients treated with ciprofloxacin but in only 42% of those receiving tetracycline. As little as 250 mg of ciprofloxacin given daily for 3 days has been found to be as effective as a standard 3-day course of tetracycline for the treatment of moderate-to-severe cholera.[42]

Simplifying antimicrobial therapy even further, recent studies have demonstrated that single-dose fluoroquinolone therapy is highly effective for the treatment of cholera. A study carried out in Bangladesh found that a single 1-g dose of ciprofloxacin had a successful clinical response in 94% of patients infected with *V. cholerae* O1 as opposed to only 73% of those who received single-dose therapy with doxycycline.[37] In this study, ciprofloxacin also had excellent clinical and bacteriologic responses in patients infected with *V. cholerae* O139. Tetracycline-resistant strains of *V. cholerae* O1 were associated with treatment failure in 52% of patients treated with doxycyline. Fortunately to date, resistance to the quinolones has not been observed in any studies that have used these agents for the treatment of cholera.

Vibrio parahaemolyticus and Other Noncholera Vibrios

Although explosive in onset, disease due to *V. parahaemolyticus* is generally rather short lived. Oral rehydration is the mainstay of therapy for this infection. The organism is sensitive to several antibiotics, including tetracycline and the fluoroquinolones. Although antimicrobial therapy is generally unnecessary, treatment with a fluoroquinolone will lead to a more rapid resolution of diarrhea than placebo will.[23] Gastroenteritis caused by other *Vibrio* strains is also treated supportively without antibiotics except when complicated by bacteremia or wound infections.

Aeromonas and Plesiomonas

As is the case with noncholera vibrios, rehydration is often all that is needed for the treatment of infections due to *Aeromonas* or *Plesiomonas shigelloides*. Strains of *Aeromonas* are consistently resistant to β-lactam antibiotics such as penicillin, ampicillin, and first- or second-generation cephalosporins.[43] *Aeromonas* spp are usually susceptible to TMP-SMX, third-generation cephalosporins, fluoroquinolones, tetracycline, and chloramphenicol. There is no convincing evidence that mild cases are improved by antibiotic treatment, but it may be possible to shorten a chronic infection by appropriate use of these drugs.

P. shigelloides is also a member of the family Vibrionaceae, but it is isolated less frequently than *Aeromonas*. Its antibiotic sensitivity pattern is similar to that of *Aeromonas*, but little information is available on the efficacy of treatment.

Shigellosis

As is the case for other diarrhea-causing pathogens, rehydration plays a central role in the management of shigellosis. General supportive measures require attention; children with shigellosis may have electrolyte imbalances, altered mental status, meningismus, and seizures.[44] In general, narcotic-related drugs should be avoided, including tincture of opium, paregoric, diphenoxylate (Lomotil), and loperamide (Imodium).[39] Antibiotic treatment is indicated for most patients with shigellosis.

Most patients with shigellosis can be managed with oral rehydration. Indications for parenteral fluid replacement include marked diarrhea associated with moderate-to-severe dehydration and severe vomiting that prevents oral replacement. High-volume diarrhea occasionally is seen with shigellosis, even to the point of severe dehydration and hypovolemia. Intravenous fluid replacement is indicated in this situation. Fluid losses usually can be replenished within a few hours by intravenous solutions, and then, as soon as possible, oral rehydration therapy should be started (see Table 25–2). Careful attention

should be paid to the monitoring and management of electrolyte abnormalities, including hypoglycemia, hyponatremia, and hypokalemia. High fever in children should be managed with lukewarm water sponges or baths. Short-term use of phenobarbital is recommended for children with seizures or meningismus.

Moderate-to-severe cases of dysentery should receive antimicrobial therapy. Mild cases often pass as self-limited events, without coming to a physician's attention. If such cases are seen in the clinic or in the doctor's office, antibiotic therapy may not be necessary, given the relatively benign course. By the time a culture report returns positive for *Shigella*, the diarrhea often has already ceased. Patients with persistent symptoms, however, should receive antibiotics.

Ampicillin is preferred for drug-sensitive strains when a decision is made to begin therapy (Table 25–3). When isolates in a community are known to be resistant to ampicillin, TMP-SMX is a good alternative in the United States. The latter agent also should be used for patients with penicillin allergy. Plasmid-mediated resistance of *Shigella* strains to ampicillin, particularly *S. dysenteriae* type 1, *Shigella sonnei*, and *Shigella flexneri*, is widespread in some areas. Although the rates of resistance to ampicillin or TMP-SMX of *Shigella* strains identified in the United States used to be relatively low, recent data from Oregon reveal increasing rates of resistance to both of these antibiotics.[45] The situation outside the United States is often worse. For example, in Pakistan more than 90% of *Shigella* isolates are resistant to both TMP-SMX and ampicillin.[46] Because *Shigella* strains acquired during travel outside the United States have a higher incidence of antibiotic resistance, therapy with a fluoroquinolone should be considered for recent travelers with diarrhea. Fortunately quinolone resistance has been found in less than 1% of imported strains.[47]

The fluoroquinolones, such as ciprofloxacin, ofloxacin, and norfloxacin, are highly active in vitro against *Shigella*. A clinical trial of ciprofloxacin vs. ampicillin in Bangladeshi men with shigellosis found that ampicillin failed in two-thirds of the participants who had ampicillin-resistant isolates.[48] Although 60% of the isolates were resistant to ampicillin, all strains were susceptible to ciprofloxacin. In addition to the lack of resistance, ciprofloxacin also produced better clinical results than ampicillin did, even in patients with ampicillin-sensitive strains. A subsequent study found that single-dose therapy with 1 g of ciprofloxacin was as effective as two doses or a 5-day standard regimen in patients with *Shigella*, although single-dose therapy was less effective for patients with *S. dysenteriae* type 1.[49]

As there is now increasing evidence of the skeletal safety of quinolones in children,[50] these drugs are being increasingly evaluated in pediatric populations. During an outbreak in Burundi of multidrug-resistant *S. dysenteriae* type 1, single-dose therapy of infected children with pefloxacin resulted in 91% of treated children becoming completely symptom free by day 5, and the remainder were substantially improved.[51] None of the children experienced and joint problems during the 4-week period of follow-up. Similarly a double-blind trial of pivmecillinam vs. ciprofloxacin suspension for childhood shigellosis found that ciprofloxacin had clinical responses in 80% of children and no evidence of treatment-related arthropathy.[52]

Although the use of antimotility agents in the treatment of invasive diarrhea may lead to prolonged fever and pathogen carriage,[29] a recent study challenges this dictum. In a study of dysenteric patients, treatment with a combination of loperamide and ciprofloxacin resulted in a shorter duration of diarrhea and a lower number of stools than ciprofloxacin alone did.[53] In this study, loperamide was not associated with prolonged fever or excretion of *Shigella* or other pathogenic bacilli. However, because the number of patients studied was relatively small and there have been reports of children with diarrhea who developed shock and necrotizing enterocolitis after treatment with loperamide, this antimotility drug should be used with caution,[54,55] especially in children with invasive diarrhea.

Antibiotics for shigellosis must be absorbed to reach the population of organisms within the intestinal wall and lamina propria; thus the most effective delivery system is the bloodstream.[56] Nonabsorbable drugs, such as neomycin, paromomycin, and colistin, are clinically ineffective, despite in vitro activity against *Shigella*. Surprisingly amoxicillin, which is well absorbed and achieves higher serum levels than ampicillin does, is not effective therapy for shigellosis.[57]

Chronic *Shigella* carriage is unusual. After an acute episode of shigellosis, carriage of the organism generally lasts less than 3 to 4 weeks and rarely exceeds 3 to 4 months. In circumstances in which eradication of the carrier state is deemed necessary, TMP-SMX is effective, as a prolonged course (i.e., 4 weeks) of this agent eliminates the carrier state in about 90% of patients.

Nontyphoidal Salmonellosis

Nontyphoidal salmonellosis is caused by serotypes of the genus *Salmonella*, with the exception of *Salmonella enterica* subspecies Typhi and *Salmonella enterica* subspecies paratyphi, the causes of enteric fever. There are roughly 2000 serotypes and variants, which are all potentially pathogenic for animals and humans. *Salmonella* can cause large outbreaks, often associated with common-source routes of spread. Nonhuman reservoirs, especially animal or animal products such as poultry, eggs, dairy products, and meat, play an important role in the transmission of the disease.

Clinical syndromes seen with *Salmonella* include gastroenteritis; bacteremia, with or without gastrointestinal involvement; typhoidal or "enteric fever," seen with all *S.* Typhi and *S.* Paratyphi strains; localized infections

(e.g., septic arthritis, osteomyelitis, meningitis); and a carrier state in asymptomatic people (in which the organism is usually harbored in the gallbladder). The most common syndrome is gastroenteritis.

Patients become chronic carriers (defined as persistence for more than 1 year) of nontyphoidal *Salmonella* as a consequence of either symptomatic or asymptomatic infections. The overall carrier rate ranges from 2 to 6 per 1000 infected people. Children, especially neonates, and patients over 60 years old more commonly become carriers. In addition, structural abnormalities of the biliary or urinary tract predispose to the carrier state and perpetuate it.[58]

Numerous studies have evaluated antibiotics for the treatment of nontyphoidal *Salmonella* gastroenteritis, but all have failed to alter the rate of clinical recovery. In fact, antimicrobial therapy increases the incidence and duration of intestinal carriage of these organisms. In a study of 185 patients with *Salmonella* Typhimurium gastroenteritis who were treated with either chloramphenicol or ampicillin, stools from 65.4% were still positive for the organism 12 days after antibiotic exposure, and 27% were positive at 31 days. In contrast, among 87 patients who were not treated, only 42.5% and 11.5% of stool cultures were positive at 12 and 31 days, respectively.[59] A systematic review of 12 randomized trials found no differences in the duration of illness, diarrhea, or fever between the antibiotic regimen and placebo.[60] Relapses were more common in those treated with antimicrobial agents, as were adverse drug reactions. It thus appears that antimicrobial therapy should not be used in most cases of *Salmonella* gastroenteritis.

Despite this general rule, however, antibiotics should be used for the treatment of *Salmonella* gastroenteritis in certain high-risk patients including those with lymphoproliferative disorders; malignancy; immunosuppression (HIV infection and congenital or acquired immunodeficiency syndrome [AIDS]); solid organ or bone marrow transplantation; known or suspected abnormalities of the cardiovascular system such as prosthetic heart valves, vascular grafts, aneurysms, and rheumatic or congenital valvular heart disease; foreign bodies implanted in the skeletal system; hemolytic anemias; and patients at the extreme ages of life.[61] In addition, treatment should be initiated in patients with *Salmonella* gastroenteritis if findings of severe sepsis are present, for example, high fever, rigors, hypotension, decreased renal function, and systemic toxicity.

If therapy is deemed necessary, the choice of drug may be problematic because of high levels of resistance to ampicillin or TMP-SMX. For patients with sensitive strains, ampicillin or TMP-SMX can be used (Table 25–3). The fluoroquinolones, particularly ciprofloxacin, which has been studied most intensely, are highly active in vitro and have provided good results in patients with enteric fever[62] and in chronic *Salmonella* carriers.[63] However, patients with uncomplicated *Salmonella* gastroenteritis who were treated with ciprofloxacin have had an unacceptably high relapse rate and more prolonged fecal excretion of salmonellae than placebo-treated controls have had.[64] As might be expected, resistance to ciprofloxacin has developed during therapy.[65]

During the last decade in Europe the isolation of quinolone-resistant *Salmonella* isolates, especially from cattle, has increased.[66] The rise in resistance has been blamed on the use of quinolones in farm animals. The definitive phage type 104 (DT104) strain of *S.* Typhimurium is often multidrug resistant, but until recently this strain remained susceptible to the quinolones. However, a community outbreak of salmonellosis in Denmark in 1998, which appeared to arise from a Danish swineherd, was caused by a strain of DT104 that was nalidixic acid resistant and that exhibited decreased susceptibility to fluoroquinolones in vitro.[67] The epidemiologic investigation of this outbreak found a decrease in the clinical effectiveness of the fluoroquinolones in the treatment of these *Salmonella* infections. In the United States a *Salmonella* strain resistant to third-generation cephalosporins was recently isolated from a child with acute gastroenteritis; an isolate with identical characteristics was found in local livestock.[68] Because of rising levels of drug resistance, both domestically and internationally, antimicrobial therapy of *Salmonella* infections must be limited to high-risk patients and should be based on susceptibility testing.

Typhoid Fever

Typhoid fever is a febrile illness of prolonged duration characterized by high fever, delirium, persistent bacteremia, splenomegaly, abdominal pain, and numerous systemic manifestations. Typhoidal disease is not truly an intestinal disease, having more systemic symptoms than just those related to the bowel; it clearly differs from the usual form of gastroenteritis produced by nontyphoidal strains of *Salmonella*. While *S.* Typhi is the main cause of typhoid fever, other *Salmonella* serotypes, particularly *S.* Paratyphi, occasionally produce a similar clinical picture, which is known variously as enteric fever, typhoidal disease, or paratyphoid fever.

Plasmid-mediated drug resistance is common among strains of S. Typhi. In the seventies and eighties most strains were susceptible to chloramphenicol and ampicillin, but epidemics with strains resistant to either or both of these drugs were reported in more recent years. Consequently an effort should be made in each case to isolate the organism and to perform susceptibility testing. Chloramphenicol has good in vitro activity against most clinical isolates of typhoid bacilli. In the absence of resistance the response to therapy is remarkably constant: defervescence regularly occurs 3 to 5 days after treatment is initiated.[69] The patient's clinical condition usually improves within 1 to 2 days, with decreased toxemia and slowly declining fever. Chloramphenicol is well absorbed

from the intestinal tract but is rather poorly absorbed from intramuscular sites. Thus the intramuscular route should be avoided. In adults, chloramphenicol can generally be administered by mouth (Table 25–3), although very sick patients occasionally may need to receive the drug by the intravenous route. Oral therapy can then be given after improvement in the clinical status. The usual duration of treatment is 2 weeks; more prolonged therapy does not reduce the incidence of complications or chronic carriage. Intestinal perforation and hemorrhage can occur during what is apparently successful treatment. Relapse may follow an otherwise uneventful course. This can be treated with the same drug.

Although ampicillin has been recommended as alternative therapy, it has been somewhat diappointing in comparison with chloramphenicol.[70] On the other hand, amoxicillin, which is better absorbed, has been demonstrated to have good activity for the treatment of typhoid fever in several studies. Similarly, TMP-SMX also has been used in the therapy of typhoid fever with good results.

Chloramphenicol and TMP-SMX were the treatments of choice for many years, but the advent of plasmid-mediated multidrug resistance and newer, potentially more effective antimicrobial agents, including the fluoroquinolones and third-generation cephalosporins, has led to a re-evaluation of the role of these two antibiotics in the treatment of typhoid fever. The fluoroquinolones ciprofloxacin and ofloxacin have been found to be highly effective therapy for infections due to multidrug-resistant *S.* Typhi and *S.* Paratyphi. In addition, long-term fecal carriage of *S.* Typhi rarely occurs in patients treated with fluoroquinolones. A 10- to 14-day course of a fluoroquinolone is highly effective for the treatment of enteric fever, with cure rates consistently near 100%.[38] The one exception is norfloxacin; it has had slightly lower cure rates of 83% to 90%.[38] Fever generally resolves within 3 to 5 days from the start of therapy. When treatment of enteric fever with a fluoroquinolone was compared to treatment with chloramphenicol or TMP-SMX, no significant difference in clinical or microbiologic efficacy was found.

The optimal duration of fluoroquinolone therapy for typhoid fever has not been fully clarified but appears to be on the order of 7 to 14 days. Numerous studies have shown that courses of therapy ranging from 7 to 14 days provide a high degree of success. Therapeutic courses shorter than 5 to 6 days, however, have been associated with unacceptable levels of failure.[38] Factors that must be taken into consideration when one is determining the duration of fluoroquinolone therapy in a patient with enteric fever include the duration of fever prior to treatment initiation, severity of infection at the time of initial presentation, and amount of time until defervescence.

During the last decade, *S.* Typhi resistance to ciprofloxacin has been gradually increasing, especially in the Indian subcontinent, central Asia, and Vietnam.[71–73]

In a study conducted in India in the early nineties, no strains of *S.* Typhi or *S.* Paratyphi were isolated that had a minimum inhibitory concentration (MIC) for ciprofloxacin of 0.25 μg/ml or greater.[72] In the period 1998 to 1999, however, 60% of isolates tested had a MIC of 2 μg/ml or greater. In association with a rise in nalidixic acid resistance and decreased in vitro susceptibility to ciprofloxacin, clinicians in India and Vietnam have observed a longer time to defervescence and more patients requiring alternative treatments in recent years.[72,73]

Azithromycin, an azalide, has moderate in vitro activity against *S.* Typhi, and it achieves high intracellular concentrations.[74] After initially promising results from pilot studies, azithromycin has been compared in a number of randomized controlled trials to antimicrobial agents that have been previously demonstrated to be effective for the treatment of typhoid fever. Results with azithromycin were equivalent to those of chloramphenicol in a randomized, multicenter trial of patients with enteric fever.[75] Azithromycin was also shown to have equivalent efficacy to ciprofloxacin, even for multidrug-resistant isolates of *S.* Typhi.[76] More recently a 5-day course of high-dose azithromycin (1 g once daily) had a similar overall cure rate to a 5-day course of ofloxacin.[77] Also, azithromycin performed better than ofloxacin in terms of fever clearance time and positive fecal cultures at the end of therapy in those patients who had nalidixic acid–resistant strains of *S.* Typhi. All three of these studies involved adults. A study that compared azithromycin to ceftriaxone for the therapy of typhoid fever in children found that a 7-day course of either agent had equivalent clinical results, although a small proportion of the children treated with ceftriaxone had a relapse as opposed to none of those who received azithromycin.[78] Based on these studies, azithromycin appears to be an excellent alternative to the fluoroquinolones for the treatment of typhoid fever.

Parenteral third-generation cephalosporins such as cefotaxime, ceftriaxone, and cefoperazone have also been used successfully to treat typhoid fever, with courses as brief as 3 days showing efficacy similar to the usual 10- to 14-day regimens.[79,80] However, a recent trial that compared a 5-day course of ofloxacin to a 7-day course of cefixime found that the median fever clearance time was significantly longer and the proportion of treatment failures or relapses was higher in children treated with cefixime.[81] On the basis of these studies, short courses of parenteral third-generation cephalosporins can be endorsed for the treatment of typhoid fever, whereas we need more information, particularly studies involving longer duration of therapy with oral cephalosporins, before the oral agents can be used routinely in this disease. Resistance to the cephalosporins has not yet been a meaningful problem, but it should be noted that a strain of *S.* Typhi highly resistant to ceftriaxone has been isolated in Bangladesh.[82]

Good nursing care plays a major role in the recovery from typhoid fever. The fevers can be managed with tepid baths and sponging. Salicylates and antipyretics should be avoided, as they can cause severe sweating and lower the blood pressure.

Corticosteroids administered to patients with severe toxemia and fever may produce a dramatic response.[83] The treatment should be given in high dosages, 60 mg of prednisone divided into four doses on day 1, and rapidly tapered over the following 3 days. The broad experience with steroid treatment has failed to show any adverse effects, although the potential for masking intestinal perforation is always of concern. Steroids are thus best reserved for patients with severe toxicity.

Intestinal perforation should be managed by standard operative approaches. Indications for surgery include progressive peritoneal signs or abscess formation. Simple closure of the perforation is the treatment of choice. The ileum may be riddled with multiple perforations, however; under these circumstances, resection or exteriorization of the intestinal loop may be required. Recent studies have emphasized the importance of aggressive surgical intervention in typhoid fever.[84,85] Double-layer closure of the perforation coupled with broad-spectrum antibiotics has reduced mortality from this dreaded complication.[85]

Chronic carriers, that is, those who have been excreting *S.* Typhi for longer than 1 year, can be treated with antimicrobials in an attempt to eliminate the infection. The fluoroquinolones, particularly ciprofloxacin and norfloxacin, have become the treatment of choice in eradicating the carrier state.[86] Reappearance of the carrier state following such treatment is generally associated with gallbladder disease. Cholecystectomy eliminates the carrier state in about 85% of persons with gallstones or chronic cholecystitis. However, this procedure is recommended only for those whose profession is not compatible with the typhoid carrier state, such as food handlers and health care providers.

Campylobacter

The *Campylobacter* spp that cause human infections are chiefly *C. jejuni*, a major cause of diarrhea; *C. fetus*, generally found in immunocompromised patients; *C. coli*, a rare cause of gastroenteritis; and two new species, *C. cinaedi* and *C. fennelliae*, which have been found in male homosexuals. Other species that cause diarrhea on rare occasions are *C. hyointestinalis*, *C. upsaliensis*, and *C. laridis*. During the last 2 decades the importance of human *Campylobacter* gastroenteritis has been increasingly recognized. Approximately 4% to 11% of all diarrhea cases in the United States are caused by *C. jejuni*; in fact, the isolation of *Campylobacter* often exceeds that of *Salmonella* and *Shigella*.[87]

The most common route of transmission appears to be from infected animals and food products to humans.

Although the reservoir for *Campylobacter* is enormous, most human infections are related to consumption of improperly cooked or contaminated foodstuffs, with chickens serving as a major source of infections.

Although *C. jejuni* is susceptible to erythromycin in vitro, three controlled therapeutic trials demonstrated that erythromycin had no more effect on the clinical course than placebo had.[88] One study did show some clinical benefit when the antibiotic was started within 3 days of symptom onset. Therapy started more than 4 days after symptom onset produces no clinical improvement. However, fecal excretion of the organism is reduced by erythromycin (Table 25–3). The fluoroquinolone antibiotics, such as ciprofloxacin, are also active in vitro against *C. jejuni*, and clinical trials have shown encouraging results.[89] Fluoroquinolone resistance has been observed during the course of treatment for *Campylobacter* diarrhea.[90,91] The penicillins, cephalosporins, and sulfonamides are not effective for the treatment of *Campylobacter*.

Resistance to the quinolones has become a major problem in some parts of the world. In Thailand a study of United States military personnel found that 50% of isolates were resistant to ciprofloxacin, whereas none were resistant to azithromycin.[92] In Thailand, coresistance to both azithromycin and ciprofloxacin has been encountered in *Campylobacter* isolates, thus leaving no effective antimicrobial regimen available.[93] In the United States, fluoroquinolone resistance is also on the rise. A large study of human *Campylobacter* isolates in Minnesota found an increase in quinolone resistance from 1.3% to 10.2% between 1992 and 1998.[94] Factors associated with *Campylobacter* spp resistance to quinolone include foreign travel and local patterns of fluoroquinolone use, especially if these agents are used in animal husbandry.[94–96] In areas where fluoroquinolone resistance is common, azithromycin has been shown to be superior to ciprofloxacin in decreasing the excretion of *Campylobacter* spp and to be equivalent in terms of symptom duration.[92]

Milder cases of *Campylobacter* do not benefit from antibiotic therapy, and therefore only supportive treatment with oral rehydration is necessary. Treatment should be administered, early if possible, however, to patients with dysentery and to those suspected of having bacteremia. Because of the difficulty in making an etiologic diagnosis on clinical grounds, a fluoroquinolone such as ciprofloxacin should be used because it would be active against *Shigella* and *Campylobacter*, as well as other enteric pathogens.

Yersinia

Yersinia enterocolitica is a ubiquitous intestinal pathogen that causes a spectrum of clinical illnesses ranging from acute gastroenteritis to invasive ileitis and colitis.[97] *Yersinia* can be found in stream and lake water, and it has been isolated from many species of animals, which either as pets or food sources have been implicated in the transmission of this disease.

Strains of *Y. enterocolitica* are susceptible to several antimicrobial agents, including chloramphenicol, tetracycline, TMP-SMX, gentamicin, and quinolones, but they are resistant to penicillins and cephalosporins. There is no substantial evidence that antibiotics alter the course of the gastrointestinal infection[98]; indeed the diagnosis often is established rather late in the course when the patient is improving spontaneously. Antibiotics should be used in more severe intestinal infections, however, particularly those that mimic appendicitis. Antibiotic therapy is not useful for the chronic, relapsing form of diarrhea. Septicemia in the immunocompromised patient is associated with a high mortality; no apparent benefit is gained from antibiotics, although treatment is mandatory in this setting.

Escherichia coli

At least six types of *E. coli* intestinal pathogens have been recognized. The type of illness that they cause and the epidemiology vary from strain to strain as a result of different virulence factors, for example, toxin production, adherence to epithelial cells, and invasiveness, which are each encoded by specific genetic elements that determine pathogenicity.

Enteroinvasive E. coli (EIEC)
EIEC is a rare cause of a dysenteric syndrome. Options for treatment include TMP-SMX or the fluoroquinolones (Table 25–3).[35,99]

Enteropathogenic E. coli (EPEC)
EPEC strains are relatively uncommon causes of diarrhea in developed countries, but they appear to be common pathogens in many developing countries, particularly in children in the first 2 years of life.[100] Resistance to antimicrobial drugs is common in classic EPEC strains, which are EPEC adherence factor probe positive.[101] Since many of these infections are self-limited, there is no indication for antibiotic treatment, although nonabsorbable antibiotics such as neomycin have been used in the past for neonates with severe EPEC diarrhea.

Enterotoxigenic E. coli (ETEC)
ETEC diarrhea generally only causes mild dehydration, although in children and older people, even loss of small amounts of intestinal fluid can have serious consequences. Fecal electrolyte losses in ETEC diarrhea are similar to those in cholera, so fluid replacement should follow the same principles. Although these organisms are usually sensitive to many antimicrobial drugs including tetracycline, ampicillin, and TMP-SMX, resistant isolates increasingly are being encountered.[102] Studies of patients with acute traveler's diarrhea, which is often due to ETEC, have demonstrated shortening of the duration of

diarrhea when effective antimicrobial therapy is initiated early in the course of illness.[103] Since most episodes of ETEC diarrhea are self-limited, however, treatment with antibiotics is generally not necessary.

Enteroaggregative (EaggEC) and Diffusely Adherent *E. coli* (DAEC)

Conflicting results have been encountered in epidemiologic studies of EaggEC and DAEC, with some studies implicating these strains as a cause of acute or persistent diarrhea but others finding no evidence of its pathogenicity. To date there have been no controlled trials of therapy of either of these types of *E. coli* infections in children. In a study of HIV-seropositive patients with diarrhea due to EaggEC, treatment with ciprofloxacin resulted in a 50% reduction in stool output, fewer intestinal symptoms, and microbiologic eradication of the organism.[104] Similarly ciprofloxacin reduced the duration of diarrhea in patients with traveler's diarrhea caused by EAggEC.[105] More epidemiologic and clinical data are needed before concrete recommendations can be made regarding the treatment of these two strains of *E. coli*.

Enterohemorrhagic *E. coli* (EHEC)

The urge to treat EHEC infections is understandable given the presence of bloody diarrhea and the concern that hemolytic uremic syndrome (HUS) will develop. However, antimicrobial therapy has not been shown to benefit the acute diarrheal portion of the illness and may even increase the risk of HUS.

In a mouse model of infection, treatment with certain antibiotics, notably ciprofloxacin, enhanced the production of Shigalike toxin by *E. coli* O157:H7, which was associated with increased death rates in the treated mice.[106] This was shown in vitro to occur via the induction of a bacteriophage-encoded gene.

Several studies have suggested that antimicrobial therapy of EHEC colitis in humans does not appear to provide much benefit and may even be harmful. Treatment with antibiotics had a detrimental effect on development of HUS in one study,[107] whereas others have found that treatment during the prodromal illness led to a milder course with fewer complications.[108] In contrast to these uncontrolled studies a randomized, controlled trial of TMP-SMX in children with O157:H7 enteritis found treatment had no effect on the duration of symptoms, pathogen excretion, or incidence of HUS.[109]

A recent prospective cohort study identified 71 children with acute gastroenteritis caused by *E. coli* O157:H7, of whom only 9 had been treated with antibiotics.[20] Five of the ten children who developed HUS had been treated with either TMP-SMX or a cephalosporin. In this study antimicrobial therapy was associated with a 14-fold increased risk for the development of HUS.

Since antibiotics have not been shown to decrease morbidity due to EHEC and appear to increase the risk of HUS, antibiotic treatment should not be initiated in patients with gastroenteritis that is suspected to be due to *E. coli* O157:H7. In addition, antimotility agents should be avoided in patients with known or suspected EHEC infections.[39] All patients with confirmed *E. coli* O157:H7 infections should be followed closely for the development of HUS, so that appropriate supportive therapy can be initiated early.

Viral Diarrhea

Viruses are major causes of acute gastroenteritis in the United States and in the rest of the world as well, accounting for 30% to 40% of episodes.[110] Viral diarrheal pathogens can be grouped into five categories: rotavirus, enteric adenovirus, calicivirus including Norwalk virus, astrovirus, and torovirus.[111] No specific antimicrobial therapy is yet available for the treatment of viral diarrhea, so oral rehydration therapy remains the mainstay of treatment.

Because rotavirus infections can cause moderate-to-severe dehydration, replacement of fluid and electrolyte losses is integral to its treatment. Field studies have shown that ORS (Table 25–2) is effective in restoring fluid balance.[112] Bovine colostral antirotavirus immunoglobulin has been found to be effective in reducing the duration of rotavirus diarrhea and the amount of oral rehydration therapy required.[113]

Acute gastroenteritis caused by caliciviruses including the Norwalk family of viruses tend to cause illnesses that are usually mild, although they can produce dehydration in elderly patients that occasionally requires hospitalization. BSS was unimpressive in a controlled trial of treatment of disease induced in volunteers; there was a decrease in abdominal cramping, but vomiting, the rate of purging, and other symptoms were unaffected.[114]

Treatment of diarrhea due to enteric adenovirus or astrovirus is supportive with an emphasis on oral rehydration. The same is true of infections caused by toroviruses, although fluid replacement is often required for as long as a week.[115]

SPECIAL SITUATIONS

Traveler's Diarrhea

Severe dehydration is rarely encountered in cases of traveler's diarrhea, and consequently fluid losses can generally be replaced with fruit juices, soft drinks, and clear liquids. Drug treatment is directed at either eliminating the pathogen, as with antibiotics, or at reducing fluid and electrolyte losses with antisecretory agents.

Several antibiotics have been used successfully for the treatment of traveler's diarrhea. In one study TMP-SMZ or TMP alone reduced the duration of diarrhea from 93 hours to approximately 30 hours.[116] Ciprofloxacin was as effective as TMP-SMX[117]; in fact, results with single-dose therapy of acute diarrhea with fluoroquinolones have been encouraging.[118] In patients with *Campylobacter* enteritis, however, the development of ciprofloxacin resistance has been associated with clinical relapse after treatment.[119] In areas where fluoroquinolone-resistant *C. jejuni* has become more commonplace, such as Thailand, azithromycin should be used for treatment of traveler's diarrhea rather than ciprofloxacin.[92]

Antimotility drugs are often used by tourists to provide relief from the intestinal indignities of travel, and their approbation is supported by good scientific studies.[30,31] Loperamide rapidly improves the situation, even on the first day of therapy, providing significantly better early results than either placebo or BSS.[30] BSS is an alternative treatment that is effective in treating mild-to-moderate traveler's diarrhea.[32] The combination of an antimicrobial drug and an antimotility drug appears to provide the most effective relief from symptoms. In a study of travelers to Mexico the combination of loperamide and TMP-SMX curtailed diarrhea in 1 hour, as opposed to 30 hours with either drug alone or 59 hours with placebo.[27] A study carried out in Egypt, however, failed to show much benefit for the combination over the antibiotic alone.[34]

Current recommendations for treatment are based on clinical evidence that has accrued over the last 20 years. For mild-to-moderate diarrhea, generally less than four bowel movements per day without blood or fever, either loperamide or BSS is an effective therapeutic option. For more severe forms of diarrhea the optimal therapy seems to be a combination of an antimotility drug and an effective antimicrobial drug.[120] Because in many patients with bacterial diarrhea the symptoms will completely resolve after only one dose of antimicrobial therapy,[37,42,49,118] the following approach can be taken. If a patient has moderate-to-severe diarrhea, especially if accompanied by fever or bloody stools, a single-day course of antibiotic treatment (with or without an antimotility agent) should be taken. If there are no further symptoms the following day, no further therapy is necessary. If there are still gastrointestinal symptoms, however, another day's course of treatment should be taken. If after 3 days of treatment there is no improvement, diagnostic testing for parasites or resistant bacteria should be undertaken.

Food Poisoning

The major recognized causes of bacterial food poisoning are limited to 12 bacteria: *Clostridium perfringens, Staphylococcus aureus, Vibrio* (including *V. cholerae* and *V. parahaemolyticus*), *Bacillus cereus, Salmonella, Clostridium botulinum, Shigella,* toxigenic *E. coli,* and certain species of *Campylobacter, Yersinia, Listeria,* and *Aeromonas.* Viral causes of food poisoning include hepatitis A and caliciviruses, including the Norwalk agent.

Most episodes of toxin-mediated food poisoning are self-limited, with symptoms rarely lasting longer than 24 to 36 hours. No specific treatment is required for illness due to *C. perfringens* or *B. cereus.* People with staphylococcal food poisoning usually suffer in silence, without reporting their symptoms to a physician. Fatalities are unusual, and recovery is complete within 24 to 48 hours. More severe cases may require supportive care in the form of rehydration and correction of alkalosis. No specific therapy is available.

Invasive *Listeria monocytogenes* infections should be treated with parenteral ampicillin, with gentamicin added for more serious infections.[121] TMP-SMX may be used for penicillin-allergic patients.

Botulism

Food-borne botulism represents a unique situation: it is the most deadly of all the bacterial toxin-mediated food-borne diseases and is also the only one for which specific effective therapy is available. In the United States, trivalent equine botulinum antitoxin is available only through the Centers for Disease Control and Prevention (CDC), which maintains supplies of the antitoxin at sites around the United States for immediate release in an emergency. To obtain the antitoxin, physicians need to contact their state health department's emergency hotline or the CDC directly.

Once botulism is suspected or confirmed, speed is of the essence, since the antitoxin cannot displace the toxin once it has bound to the presynaptic nerve terminal; instead it acts by binding up free toxin in circulation. Once symptoms have developed, the antitoxin's utility is greatly reduced. In a large retrospective analysis of 134 cases of botulinum toxin A–mediated disease, patients who received early antitoxin therapy had a 10% mortality, as opposed to 15% in those who received the antitoxin more than 24 hours after symptom onset, and 46% for those who did not receive antitoxin at all.[122] The duration of hospitalization also differed markedly: treated patients spent an average of 10 days in the hospital, compared with 56 days for the untreated group.

Since antitoxin has the greatest benefit for asymptomatic patients or those with symptoms at an early stage, a systematic approach to the treatment of botulism should be followed. First, the diagnosis of botulism must be considered early in any case of unexplained paralysis and antitoxin administered if the diagnosis is credible. Second, a list of the potential offending food vehicles must be made. Third, on the basis of this list the cohort of potentially exposed but still asymptomatic patients should be identified. Finally, prophylactic antitoxin should be promptly administered to these people.

The current recommendation is for a single 10-ml dose of intravenous antitoxin for each exposed person. This recommendation is based on the calculation that each vial has enough neutralizing antibody to bind up toxin titer 100 times greater than the highest titer documented to date by the CDC.[123] Multidose protocols are no longer recommended, as they have been associated with a 9% risk of a hypersensitivity reaction; it is hoped (though as yet unproven) that the single-dose protocol will decrease the rate of this complication.

REFERENCES

1. Glass RI, Lew JF, Gangarosa RE, et al: Estimates of morbidity and mortality rates for diarrheal diseases in American children. J Pediatr 1991;118:S27.
2. Warren JL, Bacon E, Harris T, et al: The burden and outcomes associated with dehydration among US elderly, 1991. Am J Public Health 1994;84:1265.
3. Bellosillo NA, Gorbach SL: Diarrhea and HIV infection. Infect Dis Clin Pract 1998;7:213.
4. Gorbach SL: Infectious diarrhea. Infect Dis Clin North Am 1988;2:557.
5. Hamer DH, Cash RA: Cholera and enterotoxigenic *Escherichia coli*. In Armstrong D, Cohen J (eds): Infectious Diseases. London, Harcourt Brace, 1999.
6. World Health Organization: Guidelines for cholera control. Geneva, Switzerland, World Health Organization, Programme for control of diarrhoeal disease. WHO/CCD/SER/80.4 Rev. 2, 1991.
7. Avery ME, Snyder JD: Oral therapy for acute diarrhea: The underused simple solution. N Engl J Med 1990;13:891.
8. Duggan C, Santosham M, Glass RI: The management of acute diarrhea in children: Oral rehydration, maintenance, and nutritional therapy. MMWR Morb Mortal Wkly Rep 1992;41(RR-16):1.
9. Santosham M, Daum AS, Dillman L, et al: Oral rehydration therapy of infantile diarrhea. A controlled study of well-nourished children hospitalized in the United States and Panama. N Engl J Med 1982;306:1071.
10. Santosham M, Burns B, Nadkarni V, et al: Oral rehydration therapy for acute diarrhea in ambulatory children in the United States: A double-blind comparison of four different solutions. Pediatrics 1985;76:159.
11. Cutting WA, Belton NR, Gray JA, et al: Safety and efficacy of three oral rehydration solutions for children with diarrhoea (Edinburgh 1984–1985). Acta Paediatr Scand 1989;78:253.
12. International Study Group on Reduced-Osmolarity ORS solutions: Multicentre evaluation of reduced-osmolarity oral rehydration salts solution. Lancet 1995;345:282.
13. Alam NH, Majumder RN, Fuchs GJ, et al: Efficacy and safety of oral rehydration solution with reduced osmolarity in adults with cholera: A randomised double-blind clinical trial. Lancet 1999;354:296.
14. Khin-Maung W, Greenough WB III: Cereal-based oral rehydration therapy. I. Clinical studies. J Pediatr 1991;118:S72.
15. Gore SM, Fontaine O, Pierce NF: Impact of rice based oral rehydration solution on stool output and duration of diarrhoea: Meta-analysis of 13 clinical trials. BMJ 1992;304:287.
16. Ramakrishna BS, Venkataraman S, Srinivasan P, et al: Amylase-resistant starch plus oral rehydration solutions for cholera. N Engl J Med 2000;342:308.
17. Dryden MS, Gabb RJ, Wright SK: Empirical treatment of severe acute community-acquired gastroenteritis with ciprofloxacin. Clin Infect Dis 1996;22:1019.
18. Goodman LJ, Trenholme GM, Kaplan RL, et al: Empiric antimicrobial therapy of domestically acquired acute diarrhea in urban adults. Arch Intern Med 1990;150:541.
19. Wistrom J, Norrby SR: Fluoroquinolones and bacterial enteritis, when and for whom? J Antimicrob Chemother 1995;36:23.
20. Wong CS, Srdjan J, Habeeb RL, et al: The risk of hemolytic-uremic syndrome after antibiotic treatment of *Escherichia coli* O157:H7 infections. N Engl J Med 2000;342:1930.
21. Islam MR: Single dose tetracycline in cholera. Gut 1987;28:1029.
22. Oldfield EC III, Bourgeois AL, Omar AK, et al: Empirical treatment of *Shigella* dysentery with trimethoprim: Five-day course vs. single dose. Am J Trop Med Hyg 1986;37:616.
23. Butler T, Lolekha S, Rasidi C, et al: Treatment of acute bacterial diarrhea: A multicenter international trial comparing placebo with fleroxacin given as a single dose or once daily for 3 days. Am J Med 1993;94(Suppl. 3A):187S.
24. Bennish ML, Salam MA, Khan WA, et al: Treatment of shigellosis. III. Comparison of one- or two-dose ciprofloxacin with standard 5-day therapy. A randomized, blinded trial. Ann Intern Med 1992;117:727.
25. Ericsson CD, DuPont HL, Johnson PC: Nonantibiotic therapy for travelers' diarrhea. Rev Infect Dis 1986;8:S202.
26. DuPont HL: Nonfluid therapy and selected chemoprophylaxis of acute diarrhea. Am J Med 1985;78(Suppl. 6B):8.
27. Ericsson CD, DuPont HL, Mathewson JJ, et al: Treatment of travelers' diarrhea with sulfamethoxazole and trimethoprim and loperamide. JAMA 1990;263:257.
28. Salazar-Lindo E, Santisteban-Ponce J, Chea-Woo E, et al: Racecadotril in the treatment of acute watery diarrhea in children. N Engl J Med 2000;343:463.
29. DuPont HL, Hornick RB: Adverse effect of lomotil therapy in shigellosis. JAMA 1973;226:1525.
30. Johnson PC, Ericsson CD, DuPont HL, et al: Comparison of loperamide with bismuth subsalicylate for the treatment of acute travelers' diarrhea. JAMA 1986;255:757.
31. Van Loon FPL, Bennish ML, Speelman P, et al: Double-blind trial of loperamide for treating acute watery diarrhoea in expatriates in Bangladesh. Gut 1989;30:492.
32. Gorbach SL: Bismuth therapy in gastrointestinal diseases. Gastroenterology 1990;99:863.
33. DuPont HL, Sullivan P, Pickering LK, et al: Symptomatic treatment of diarrhea with bismuth subsalicy late among students attending a Mexican university. Gastroenterology 1977;73:715.
34. Taylor DN, Sanchez JL, Candler W, et al: Treatment of travelers' diarrhea: Ciprofloxacin plus loperamide compared with ciprofloxacin alone. Ann Intern Med 1991;114:731.
35. Murphy GS, Bodhidatta L, Echeverria P, et al: Ciprofloxacin and loperamide in the treatment of bacillary dysentery. Ann Intern Med 1993;118:582.
36. Centers for Disease Control. Update: Cholera—Western Hemisphere, and recommendations for treatment of cholera. MMWR Morb Mortal Wkly Rep 1991;40:562.
37. Khan WA, Bennish ML, Seas C, et al: Randomised controlled comparison of single-dose ciprofloxacin and doxycycline for cholera caused by *Vibrio cholerae* O1 or O139. Lancet 1996;48:296.
38. Hamer DH, Gorbach SL: Use of the quinolones for the treatment and prophylaxis of bacterial infections. In Andriole VT (ed): The Quinolones, 3rd ed. San Diego, Academic Press, 2000.
39. Guerrant RL, Van Gilder T, Steiner TS, et al: Practice guidelines for the management of infectious diarrhea. Clin Infect Dis 2001;32:331–350.
40. Bhattacharya SK, Bhattacharya MK, Dutta P, et al: Double-blind, randomized, controlled trial of norfloxacin for cholera. Antimicrob Agents Chemother 1990;34:939.
41. Khan WA, Begum M, Salam MA, et al: Comparative trial of five antimicrobial compounds in the treatment of cholera in adults. Trans R Soc Trop Med Hyg 1995;89:103.
42. Gotuzzo E, Seas C, Echevarria J, et al: Ciprofloxacin for the treatment of cholera: A randomized, double-blind, controlled clinical trial of a single daily dose in Peruvian adults. Clin Infect Dis 1995;20:1485.
43. Jones BL, Wilcox MH: *Aeromonas* infections and their treatment. J Antimicrob Chemother 1995;35:453.
44. Khan WA, Dhar U, Salam MA, et al: Central nervous system manifestations of childhood shigellosis: Prevalence, risk factors, and outcome. Pediatrics 1999;103:E18. [www.pediatrics.org/cgi/content/full/103/e18].

45. Replogle ML, Fleming DW, Cieslak PR: Emergence of antimicrobial-resistant shigellosis in Oregon. Clin Infect Dis 2000;30:515.

46. Khalil K, Khan SR, Mazhar K, et al: Occurrence and susceptibility to antibiotics of *Shigella* species in stools of hospitalized children with bloody diarrhea in Pakistan. Am J Trop Med Hyg 1998;58:800.

47. Tauxe RV, Puhr ND, Wells JG, et al: Antimicrobial resistance of *Shigella* isolates in the USA: The importance of international travelers. J Infect Dis 1990;162:1107.

48. Bennish ML, Salam MA, Haider R, Barza M: Therapy for shigellosis. II. Randomized, double-blind comparison of ciprofloxacin and ampicillin. J Infect Dis 1990;162:711.

49. Bennish ML, Salam MA, Khan WA, Khan AM: Treatment of shigellosis. III. Comparison of one- or two-dose ciprofloxacin with standard 5-day therapy. A randomized, blinded trial. Ann Intern Med 1992;117:727.

50. Burkhardt JE, Walterspiel JN, Schaad UB: Quinolone arthropathy in animals versus children. Clin Infect Dis 1997;25:1196.

51. Gendrel D, Moreno JL, Nduwimana M, et al: One-dose treatment of pefloxacin for infection due to multidrug-resistant *Shigella dysenteriae* type 1 in Burundi. Clin Infect Dis 1997;24:83.

52. Salam MA, Dhar U, Khan AK, Bennish ML: Randomised comparison of ciprofloxacin suspension and pivmecillinam for childhood shigellosis. Lancet 1998;352:522.

53. Murphy GS, Bodhidatta L, Echeverria P, et al: Ciprofloxacin and loperamide in the treatment of bacillary dysentery. Ann Intern Med 1993;118:582.

54. Chow CB, Li SH, Leung NK: Loperamide-associated necrotising enterocolitis. Acta Paediatr Scand 1986;75:1034.

55. Minton NA, Smith PG: Loperamide toxicity in a child after a single dose. BMJ 1987;294:1383.

56. Haltalin KC, Nelson JD, Hinton LV, et al: Comparison of orally absorbable and nonabsorbable antibiotics in shigellosis. J Pediatr 1968;2:708.

57. Nelson JD, Haltalin KC: Amoxicillin less effective than ampicillin against *Shigella* in vitro and in vivo: Relationship of efficacy to activity in serum. J Infect Dis 1974;129:S222.

58. Musher DN, Rubenstein AD: Permanent carriers of nontyphosa salmonellae. Arch Intern Med 1973;132:869.

59. Askerkoff B, Bennett JV: Effect of antibiotic therapy in acute salmonellosis on the fecal excretion of salmonellae. N Engl J Med 1969;281:636.

60. Sirinavin S, Garner P: Antibiotics for treating *Salmonella* gut infections. The Cochrane Library, 2000.

61. Hohmann EL: Nontyphoidal salmonellosis. Clin Infect Dis 2001;32:263.

62. Stanley PJ, Flegg PJ, Mandal BK, Geddes AM: Open study of ciprofloxacin in enteric fever. J Antimicrob Chemother 1989;23:789.

63. Cherubin CE, Kowalski J: Nontyphoidal *Salmonella* carrier state treated with norfloxacin. Ann Intern Med 1990;85:100.

64. Neill MA, Opal SM, Heelan J, et al: Failure of ciprofloxacin in convalescent fecal excretion after acute salmonellosis: Experience during an outbreak in health care workers. Ann Intern Med 1991;114:195.

65. Piddock LJV, Whale K, Wise R: Quinolone resistance in *Salmonella*: Clinical experience. Lancet 1990;1:1459.

66. Malorny B, Schroeter A, Helmuth R: Incidence of quinolone resistance over the period 1986 to 1998 in veterinary *Salmonella* isolates from Germany. Antimicrob Agents Chemother 1999;43:2278.

67. Molbak K, Baggesen DL, Aarestrup FM, et al: An outbreak of multidrug-resistant, quinolone-resistant *Salmonella enterica* serotype typhimurium DT104. N Engl J Med 1999;341:1420.

68. Fey PD, Safranek TJ, Rupp ME, et al: Ceftriaxone-resistant *Salmonella* infection acquired by a child from cattle. N Engl J Med 2000;342:1242.

69. Woodward TE, Smadel JE: Management of typhoid fever and its complications. Ann Intern Med 1964;60:144.

70. Robertson RP, Wahab MFA, Raasch FO: Evaluation of chloramphenicol and ampicillin in *Salmonella* enteric fever. N Engl J Med 1968;278:171.

71. Tarr PE, Kuppens L, Jones TC, et al: Considerations regarding mass vaccination against typhoid fever as an adjunct to sanitation and public health measures: Potential use in an epidemic in Tajikistan. Am J Trop Med Hyg 1999;61:163.

72. Chitnis V, Chitnis D, Verma S, Hemvani N: Multidrug-resistant *Salmonella typhi* in India. Lancet 1999;354:514.

73. Wain J, Hoa NTT, Chinh NT, et al: Quinolone-resistant *Salmonella typhi* in Vietnam: Molecular basis of resistance and clinical response to treatment. Clin Infect Dis 1997;25:1404.

74. Metchock B: In vitro activity of azithromycin compared with other macrolides and oral antibiotics against *Salmonella typhi*. J Antimicrob Chemother 1990;25(Suppl A):29.

75. Butler T, Sridhar CB, Daga MK, et al: Treatment of typhoid fever with azithromycin versus chloramphenicol in a randomized multicentre trial in India. J Antimicrob Chemother 1999;44:243.

76. Girgis NI, Butler T, Frenck RW, et al: Azithromycin versus ciprofloxacin for treatment of uncomplicated typhoid fever in a randomized trial in Egypt that included patients with multidrug resistance. Antimicrob Agents Chemother 1999;43:1441.

77. Chinh NT, Parry CM, Li NT, et al: A randomized controlled comparison of azithromycin and ofloxacin for treatment of multidrug-resistant or nalidixic acid–resistant enteric fever. Antimicrob Agents Chemother 2000;44:1855.

78. Frenck RW, Nakhla I, Sultan Y, et al: Azithromycin versus ceftriaxone for the treatment of uncomplicated typhoid fever in children. Clin Infect Dis 2000;31:1134.

79. Soe GB, Overturf GD: Treatment of typhoid fever and other systemic salmonelloses with cefotaxime, ceftriaxone, cefoperazone, and other new cephalosporins. Rev Infect Dis 1987;9:719.

80. Acharya G, Butler T, Ho M, et al: Treatment of typhoid fever: Randomized trial of a three-day course of ceftriaxone versus a fourteen-day course of chloramphenicol. Am J Trop Med Hyg 1995;52:162.

81. Phuong CXT, Kneen R, Anh NT, et al: A comparative study of ofloxacin and cefixime for treatment of typhoid fever in children. Pediatr Infect Dis J 1999;18:245.

82. Samir SK, Talukder SY, Islam M, Saha S: A highly ceftriaxone-resistant *Salmonella typhi* in Bangladesh. Pediatr Infect Dis J 1999;18:387.

83. Hoffman SL, Punjabi NH, Kumala S, et al: Reduction of mortality in chloramphenicol-treated severe typhoid fever by high-dose dexamethasone. N Engl J Med 1984;310:83.

84. Bitar R, Tarpley J: Intestinal perforation in typhoid fever: An historical and state-of-the-art review. Rev Infect Dis 1985;7:257.

85. Mock CN, Amaral J, Visser LE: Improvement in survival from typhoid ileal perforation. Results of 221 operative cases. Ann Surg 1992;215:244.

86. Rodriguez-Noriega E, Andrade-Villanueva J, Amaya-Tapia G: Quinolones in the treatment of *Salmonella* carriers. Rev Infect Dis 1989;11:S1179.

87. Altekruse SF, Stern NJ, Fields PI, Swerdlow DL: *Campylobacter jejuni*—an emerging foodborne pathogen. Emerg Infect Dis 1999;5:28.

88. Levine MM: Antimicrobial therapy for infectious diarrhea. Rev Infect Dis 1986;8:S207.

89. Pichler HET, Diridl G, Stickler K, et al: Clinical efficacy of ciprofloxacin compared with placebo in bacterial diarrhea. Am J Med 1987;82(S4A):329.

90. Segreti J, Gootz TD, Goodman LJ, et al: High-level quinolone resistance in clinical isolates of Campylobacter jejuni. J Infect Dis 1992;165:667.

91. Wretlind B, Stromberg A, Ostlund L, et al: Rapid emergence of quinolone resistance in *Campylobacter jejuni* in patients treated with norfloxacin. Scand J Infect Dis 1992;24:685.

92. Kuschner RA, Trofa AF, Thomas RJ, et al: Use of azithromycin for the treatment of *Campylobacter* enteritis in travelers to Thailand, an area where ciprofloxacin resistance is prevalent. Clin Infect Dis 1995;21:536.

93. Hoge CW, Gambel JM, Srijan A, et al: Trends in antibiotic resistance among diarrheal pathogens isolated in Thailand over 15 years. Clin Infect Dis 1998;26:341.

94. Smith KE, Besser JM, Hedberg CW, et al: Quinolone-resistant *Campylobacter jejuni* infections in Minnesota, 1992–1998. N Engl J Med 1999;340:1525.

95. Talsma E, Goettsch WG, Nieste HLJ, et al: Resistance in *Campylobacter* species: Increased resistance to fluoroquinolones and seasonal variation. Clin Infect Dis 1999;29:845.

96. Endtz HP, Ruijs GJ, van Klingeren B, et al: Quinolone resistance in *Campylobacter* isolated from man and poultry following the introduction of fluoroquinolones in veterinary medicine. J Antimicrob Chemother 1991;27:199.

97. Naktin J, Beavis KG: *Yersinia enterocolitica* and *Yersinia pseudotuberculosis*. Clin Lab Med 1999;19:523.

98. Paim CH, Gillis F, Tuomanen E, et al: Placebo-controlled double-blind evaluation of trimethoprim-sulfamethoxazole treatment of *Yersinia enterocolitica* gastroenteritis. J Pediatr 1984;104:308.

99. Prado D, Lopez E, Liu H, et al: Ceftibuten and trimethoprim-sulfamethoxazole for treatment of shigella and enteroinvasive *Escherichia coli* disease. Pediatr Infect Dis J 1992;11:644.

100. Levine MM, Ferreccio C, Prado V, et al: Epidemiologic studies of *Escherichia coli* diarrheal infections in a low socioeconomic level peri-urban community in Santiago, Chile. Am J Epidemiol 1993;138:849.

101. Tardelli TA, Rassi V, MacDonald KL, et al: Enteropathogens associated with acute diarrheal disease in urban infants in Sao Paulo, Brazil. J Infect Dis 1991;164:331.

102. Daniels NA, Neimann J, Karpati A, et al: Traveler's diarrhea at sea: Three outbreaks of waterborne enterotoxigenic *Escherichia coli* on cruise ships. J Infect Dis 2000;181:1491.

103. Mattila L, Peltola H, Siitonen A, et al: Short-term treatment of traveler's diarrhea with norfloxacin: A double-blind, placebo-controlled study during two seasons. Clin Infect Dis 1993;17:779.

104. Wanke CA, Gerrior J, Blais V, et al: Successful treatment of diarrheal disease with enteroaggregative *Escherichia coli* in adults infected with human immunodeficiency virus. J Infect Dis 1998;178:1369.

105. Glandt M, Adachi JA, Mathewson JJ, et al: Enteroaggregative *Escherichia coli* as a cause of traveler's diarrhea: Clinical response to ciprofloxacin. Clin Infect Dis 1999;29:335.

106. Zhang X, McDaniel AD, Wolf LE, et al: Quinolone antibiotics induce Shiga toxin–encoding bacteriophages, toxin production, and death in mice. J Infect Dis 2000;181:664.

107. Carter AO, Borczyk AA, Carlson JAK, et al: A severe outbreak of *Escherichia coli* O157:H7-associated hemorrhagic colitis in a nursing home. N Engl J Med 1987;317:1496.

108. Martin DL, MacDonald KL, White KE, et al: The epidemiology and clinical aspects of the hemolytic uremic syndrome in Minnesota. N Engl J Med 1990;323:1161.

109. Proulx F, Turgeon JP, Delage G, et al: Randomized, controlled trial of antibiotic therapy for *Escherichia coli* O157:H7 enteritis. J Pediatr 1992;121:299.

110. Kotloff KL, Wasserman SS, Steciak JY, et al: Acute diarrhea in Baltimore children attending an outpatient clinic. Pediatr Infect Dis J 1988;7:753.

111. Blacklow NR, Greenberg HB: Viral gastroenteritis. N Engl J Med 1991;325:252.

112. Santosham M, Burns B, Nadkarni V, et al: Oral rehydration therapy for acute diarrhea in ambulatory children in the United States: A double-blind comparison of four different solutions. Pediatrics 1985;76:159.

113. Sarker SA, Casswall TH, Mahalanabis D, et al: Successful treatment of rotavirus diarrhea in children with immunoglobulin from immunized bovine colostrum. Pediatr Infect Dis J 1998;17:1149.

114. Steinhoff MC, Douglas RG, Greenberg HB, Callahan DR: Bismuth subsalicylate therapy of viral gastroenteritis. Gastroenterology 1980;78:1495.

115. Jamieson FB, Wang EEL, Bain C, et al: Human torovirus: A new nosocomial gastrointestinal pathogen. J Infect Dis 1998;178:1263.

116. DuPont HL, Evans DG, Rios N, et al: Prevention of travelers' diarrhea with trimethoprim-sulfamethoxazole. Rev Infect Dis 1982;4:533.

117. Ericsson CD, Johnson PC, DuPont HL, et al: Ciprofloxacin or trimethoprim-sulfamethoxazole as initial therapy for travelers' diarrhea. A placebo-controlled, randomized trial. Ann Intern Med 1987;106:216.

118. Salam I, Katelaris P, Leigh-Smith S, Farthing MJG: Randomised trial of single-dose ciprofloxacin for travellers' diarrhoea. Lancet 1994;344:1537.

119. Petruccelli BP, Murphy GS, Sanchez JL, et al: Treatment of traveler's diarrhea with ciprofloxacin and loperamide. J Infect Dis 1992;165:557.

120. Adachi JA, Ostrosky-Zeichner L, DuPont HL, Ericsson CD: Empirical antimicrobial therapy for traveler's diarrhea. Clin Infect Dis 2000;31:1079.

121. Schlech WF III: Foodborne listeriosis. Clin Infect Dis 2000;31:770.

122. Tacket CO, Shandera W, Mann J, et al: Equine antitoxin use and other factors that predict outcome in type A foodborne botulism. Am J Med 1984;76:794.

123. Hatheway CL, Snyder JD, Seals JE, et al: Antitoxin levels in botulism patients treated with trivalent equine botulism antitoxin to toxin types A, B, and E. J Infect Dis 1984;150:407.

Protozoal Diarrhea

LISA A. GREISMAN, MD

DAVID GLEMBOCKI, MD

WILLIAM A. PETRI, JR, MD, PhD

The diverse group of protozoa that infect the gastrointestinal tract are generally more common in tropical and underdeveloped countries than in the United States. Expanding globalization, however, is increasing the incidence of these infections in the United States. American physicians therefore need to be familiar with the presentation, diagnosis, and treatment of these protozoa and the illnesses they cause.

Giardiasis

Giardia lamblia is a prevalent enteric parasite and the most common cause of waterborne diarrheal illness in the United States.[1] Although first identified by van Leeuwenhoek in 1681, *Giardia* was believed to be a commensal of the human intestine until relatively recently.[2] Its importance as a disease-causing pathogen is underscored by the fact that between 1978 and 1991, 34 water-borne outbreaks of *Giardia lamblia* were reported in the United States. Most occurred in the Northeast, Northwest, and Rocky Mountain regions of the United States.[3,4]

Life Cycle

Giardia lamblia infection begins with ingestion of the cyst form of the protozoan. Excystation occurs in the duodenum after exposure to the gastric acid and pancreatic enzymes. Two trophozoites are released and replicate asexually via binary fission in the duodenum and upper jejunum.[2] The trophozoites attach to enterocytes via a ventral adhesive disk but do not invade the epithelial cells (Fig. 26–1).[5] *Giardia* requires host bile acids for growth, which likely explains its tropism for the upper small intestine.[6] This may also explain the syndrome of fat malabsorption often observed in symptomatic patients.[7] Some trophozoites encyst in the ileum and pass with feces to the external environment.[2]

Epidemiology

Giardia cysts can survive several months in the environment under favorable conditions. They are resistant to chlorination levels found in municipal water supplies and can endure freezing for several days.[2] Boiling can inactivate cysts.[2] In addition, municipal water filtration methods are believed to be effective in removing *Giardia* cysts. The Environmental Protection Agency (EPA), however, reported that 17% of filtered municipal water samples were contaminated by *Giardia* cysts in 1991.[8]

Giardiasis is caused by fecal-oral spread of cysts via contaminated food or water as well as by direct person-to-person transmission.[1,2,4,5] In the United States those

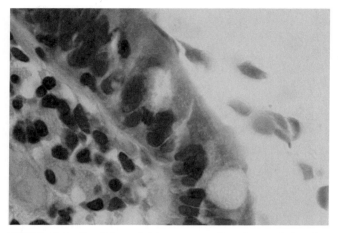

FIGURE 26–1. Small-bowel biopsy revealing intracellular but extracytoplasmic inclusions of *Cryptosporidium parvum*. (See Color Plate 1.)

most at risk include day care providers, homosexual men, institutionalized persons, and travelers to developing countries (Table 26–1). *Giardia* is found worldwide but is most prominent in the developing world. Evaluation by microscopy of stool samples from natives in developing countries show 20% to 30% are infected with *Giardia* vs. 2% to 5% of stool samples in industrialized nations.[2] Hikers and campers who drink from contaminated streams or ponds are also at risk for giardiasis.[4] Water may also be contaminated by domestic and wild animals (such as beavers and muskrats).[4] Ingestion of as few as 10 to 25 cysts may cause symptomatic disease.[1,2,4,5]

Clinical Features

Approximately 60% of those infected with *Giardia* remain asymptomatic.[2] Symptoms develop in the remainder of those infected after an incubation period of 1 to 2 weeks.[1,2] Common symptoms include diarrhea, fatigue, malaise, abdominal cramps, bloating, malodorous stool, and flatulence (Table 26–2). Over 50% will have weight loss, but fever is uncommon. Most patients have diarrhea for 1 to 2 weeks before seeking care. Without treatment, diarrhea may resolve spontaneously after weeks to months. Alternatively, giardiasis may become chronic, which manifests as profound malaise and an often intermittent course of diarrhea alternating with periods of normal bowel habits and even constipation.[1,2,4,5] Neither acute nor chronic giardiasis is associated with fecal blood or leukocytes. AIDS patients do not differ from immunocompetent patients in terms of disease severity.[1]

Diagnosis

Giardiasis should always be considered in patients with prolonged diarrhea and known risk factors. Stool antigen detection via enzyme-linked immunosorbent assay (ELISA) and immunofluorescence are now considered first-line diagnostic techniques (Table 26–3). These tests

TABLE 26–1 ■ Risk Factors

Organism	Risk factors
Giardia lamblia	Travel to underdeveloped countries
	Day care workers and children
	Homosexual men
	Campers and hikers
	Institutionalized persons
Entamoeba histolytica	Travel to or immigration from Mexico, India, East and South Africa, Central and South America
	Homosexual men
	HIV infection
	Chronic infections
	Malnutrition
	Pregnancy
	Heavy alcohol use
	Cancer
Cryptosporidium parvum	HIV infection
	Day care workers and children
	Elderly
	Children
Isospora belli	HIV infection
	Travel to or immigration from Africa, Asia, South America
	Day care workers and children
	Institutionalized persons
	Cancer
Cyclospora cayetanensis	Same as for *Isospora belli*
Microspora	Advanced HIV infection
	Organ transplantation
	Homosexual men
	Nonpiped household water
Sarcocystis	Eating undercooked pork or beef
Balantidium coli	Achlorhydria
	Poor nutrition
	Travel to Latin America, Southeast Asia, or New Guinea
Blastocystis hominis	Unknown

HIV, human immunodeficiency virus.

are 85% to 100% sensitive and 90% to 100% specific vs. microscopy, which is approximately 83% sensitive and 100% specific.[9,10] Microscopy is performed by preserving feces in polyvinyl alcohol, then staining it with trichrome or iron hematoxylin, which is taken up by cysts. Because cysts are passed sporadically, evaluating several stool specimens optimizes diagnostic yield. In addition, wet mounts of fresh stool specimens may be observed for motile trophozoites, although this is a less sensitive technique. The string test or endoscopy with small-bowel biopsy can be performed if the diagnosis remains in doubt.[1,2,4,5]

Treatment

Treatment of choice for adults with giardiasis is metronidazole, which is 80% to 95% effective (Table 26–4).[1,2,5,11] If this is unsuccessful, some experts advocate repeating the course of treatment with a higher dose of metronidazole.[5] Side effects of metronidazole include nausea, dizziness, metallic taste, a disulfiram reaction with ingestion of alcohol, and rarely, reversible neutropenia.[1]

TABLE 26–2 ■ Clinical Features

Organism	Signs and symptoms
Giardia lamblia	Diarrhea Malodorous stools Nausea or vomiting or both Fatigue and malaise Abdominal cramps Bloating Flatulence Weight loss Anorexia Low-grade fever
Entamoeba histolytica (amebic dysentery)	Gradual onset Diarrhea Heme-positive stools Weight loss Abdominal pain Fever
Entamoeba histolytica (amebic liver abscess)	Abdominal pain Abdominal tenderness Fever Nausea or vomiting or both Anorexia Pleurisy, shortness of breath or cough or both Decreased breath sounds Hepatomegaly Diarrhea
Cryptosporidium parvum	Watery, nonbloody diarrhea Abdominal cramping Nausea or vomiting or both Anorexia Headache Myalgias Low-grade fevers Extraintestinal*
Isospora belli	Watery Abdominal cramping Nausea or vomiting or both

*Primarily in immunosuppressed patients.

TABLE 26–3 ■ Diagnosis

Organism	Diagnostic methods
Giardia lamblia	Stool antigen detection by ELISA or immunofluorescence* Microscopy using trichrome or hematoxylin stains Endoscopy with small-bowel biopsy String test
Entamoeba histolytica Colitis	TechLab *E. histolytica* II stool antigen test* Microscopy Serology Colonoscopy with biopsy
Hepatic abscess	TechLab *E. histolytica* II serum antigen test* Radiologic imaging Aspiration
Cryptosporidium parvum	Stool antigen detection by ELISA or immunofluorescence* Microscopy using modified acid-fast staining Endoscopy with small-bowel biopsy
Isospora belli	Microscopy using modified acid-fast staining Duodenal aspirate String test Endoscopy with small-bowel biopsy
Cyclospora cayetanensis	Same as for *Isospora belli*
Microspora	Microscopy using modified trichrome stain Biopsy of infected organ
Sarcocystis	Microscopy
Balantidium coli	Microscopy
Blastocystis hominis	Microscopy

ELISA, enzyme-linked immunosorbent assay.

*Diagnostic method of choice.

Use in the pediatric population is debated because of concerns about mutagenicity, but this has never been documented in humans.[12] Tinidazole is widely used in other countries as a single-dose preparation, but it is not yet approved in the United States Quinacrine HCl is also effective but is no longer available in the United States. Furazolidone is less effective against *Giardia* but commonly is used in children because it is available in liquid form.[1,2] Its side effects include gastrointestinal distress, brown discoloration of urine, and mild hemolysis in glucose-6-phosphate dehydrogenase (G6PD)-deficient patients. Albenedazole, which has been found to be effective against giardiasis in children, has an efficacy similar to that of metronidazole and fewer side effects.[13]

The pregnant woman with giardiasis is of special concern because of theoretical adverse effects of the aforementioned drugs on the fetus. Therefore if she has mild symptoms, treatment should be delayed until after delivery or at least until after the first trimester. If she must be treated, paromomycin is recommended, as it is a nonabsorbed aminoglycoside and is 60% to 70% effective.[1] Metronidazole is generally avoided in pregnancy because of concern over possible teratogenic effects, but its teratogenicity has not been proven.[14,15]

Prevention

To prevent *Giardia* infection, fecal-oral spread needs to be interrupted. This is best accomplished by proper handwashing, boiling possibly contaminated water, and avoiding uncooked foods that may have been in contact with contaminated water.[1] Treatment of infected patients is also important to prevent further spread of the disease.

Amebiasis

Amebiasis, caused by the protozoan *Entamoeba histolytica*, is the third most common parasitic cause of death worldwide.[16] It is responsible for both amebic dysentery and extraintestinal disease, which primarily manifests as amebic liver abscess.

TABLE 26–4 ▪ Treatment

Organism	Agent	Adult dose
Giardia lamblia	Metronidazole*	250 mg tid × 5 d
	Tinidazole	50 mg/kg × 1 dose
	Quinacrine	100 mg tid × 5–7 d
	Albendazole	400 mg qd × 5 d
	Furazolidone[†]	100 mg qid × 7–10 d
	Paromomycin[‡]	25–35 mg/kg/d in 3 divided doses × 7 d
Entamoeba histolytica		
Asymptomatic	Paromomycin	25–35 mg/kg/d in 3 divided doses × 7 d
	Iodoquinol	650 mg tid × 20 d
	Diloxanide furoate	500 mg tid × 10 d
Mild-to-moderate intestinal disease	Metronidazole*	500–750 mg tid × 10 d
	Tinidazole[†]	2 g qd × 3 d
	Doxycycline[‡]	250 mg bid × 14 d
Severe intestinal disease	Metronidazole*	750 mg tid × 10 d
or liver abscess or both	Tinidazole[†]	600 mg bid or 800 mg tid × 5 d
Cryptosporidium parvum	HAART	
	Paromomycin	25–35 mg/kg/d in 3 divided doses × 14–28 d
	Nitazoxanide	Not approved in the United States
Isospora belli	TMP-SMX[§]	160 mg TMP, 800 mg SMX qid × 10 d, then bid × 3 wk
	Ciprofloxacin	500 mg bid × 7–10 d
	Pyrimethamine and folinic acid	75 mg qd pyrimethamine, 10–25 mg qd of folinic acid × 2–4 wk
Cyclospora cayetanensis	TMP-SMX[§]	160 mg TMP, 800 mg SMX qid × 7 d
Microspora	HAART	
	Albendazole	400 mg bid × 2–4 wk
	Nitazoxanide	Not approved in the United States
Sarcocystis	No known treatment	
Balantidium coli	Tetracycline*	500 mg qid × 10 d
	Iodoquinol	650 mg tid × 20 d
	Metronidazole	750 mg tid × 5 d
Blastocystis hominis	Iodoquinol	650 mg tid × 20 d
	Metronidazole	750 mg tid × 10 d

HAART, highly active antiretroviral therapy.

*Drug of choice.

[†]Second-line drug.

[‡]Recommended in pregnant patients.

[§]AIDS patients need lifelong suppression with TMP-SMX three times a week.

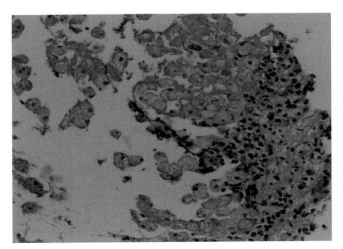

FIGURE 26–2. Small-bowel biopsy of extracellular *Giardia lamblia* adherent to the intestinal epithelium. (See Color Plate 1.)

Life Cycle and Pathogenesis

E. histolytica exists in both cyst and trophozoite forms. Humans are the primary reservoirs of *E. histolytica*. The organism is spread via fecal-oral contamination. Cysts pass with feces and, much like *Giardia lamblia*, can survive low levels of chlorination.[17] Cysts are ingested orally and resist gastric acid degradation in the stomach. In the small intestine a cyst releases eight trophozoites. The trophozoites pass to the large intestine, where they adhere to the mucosal epithelium via a galactose and *N*-acetyl-D-galactosamine (Gal/GalNAc) lectin receptor (Fig. 26–2). Besides its role in attachment, this receptor is also important to the virulence of the ameba, for it appears to induce apoptosis in the host cell.[18] This same lectin receptor also protects the parasite by inhibiting the host's terminal complement cascade (the membrane attack complex). In the large intestine the trophozoites cause either an asymptomatic carrier state, amebic dysentery, or extraintestinal disease (primarily amebic liver abscess).[16–18]

Epidemiology

E. histolytica is endemic in Mexico, India, East and South Africa, and certain areas of Central and South America.[16–18] Amebic dysentery and liver abscess are increasing in the United States for several reasons (Table 26–1). There is a rise in immigration from and travel to endemic areas. In addition the reported homosexual population is increasing in the United States, and amebiasis is increasing in both human immunodeficiency virus (HIV)-positive and HIV-negative gay men.[19] The other primary risk factor is immunosuppression from such causes as HIV, other chronic infections, cancer, pregnancy, immunosuppressant medications, and heavy alcohol use.[16,18,20] Men and women are equally affected by amebic dysentery; however, amebic liver abscess is 7 to 12 times more common in men.[18]

Clinical Features

Colonization with *E. histolytica* can be asymptomatic and is found primarily in high-risk populations and endemic areas.[18] The related protozoan *Entamoeba dispar* is a more common cause of asymptomatic infection. *E. dispar* infections should not be treated, however, as they do not cause symptomatic illness (even in AIDS patients).

The onset of amebic dysentery is gradual, with abdominal pain, diarrhea, and heme-positive stools (Table 26–2). Patients also often complain of weight loss, but fever is uncommon.[16,18] In 0.5% of cases, patients develop fulminant colitis with fever, abdominal pain with distension, and rebound tenderness. These patients have a mortality of greater than 40% and often require surgical intervention.[16,18] Several other complications of amebic dysentery are notable. Toxic megacolon is a rare but often fatal complication seen primarily in patients given steroids for presumed inflammatory bowel disease.[19] An ameboma is a localized mass of granulation tissue in the large intestine which causes a tender, palpable mass that can mimic colon cancer on physical examination.[17,19] Amebic strictures can occur in the anus, rectum, or sigmoid colon.[19] Rarely, cutaneous amebiasis develops in the perineum and genitalia.[17,19]

Unlike amebic dysentery, 90% of amebic liver abscess patients in the United States are men.[18] They frequently report travel to or emigration from Central or South America, and a history of alcohol abuse is common.[18,20] Patients present with fever, chills, nausea, and abdominal pain. They may also have weight loss and cough.[16,17,19,20] Surprisingly, diarrhea is present in only about one-third of patients.[16] Physical examination findings include right upper quadrant tenderness, occasional hepatomegaly, and rarely jaundice.[19] Typically patients have an elevated white blood cell count and an elevated alkaline phosphatase (sometimes occurring with elevated transaminases) and may have an elevated right hemidiaphragm on chest radiographs.[19] *E. histolytica* most commonly causes a single right lobe abscess.

Complications of amebic liver abscess include rupture and extension of infection to the pericardium, peritoneum, or pleural cavity. Mechanical compression of the biliary tree can cause jaundice. Pleural effusion, empyema, and acute respiratory distress syndrome can also occur. The abscess can become superinfected with bacteria, which is more likely if it is aspirated. Brain abscess occurs rarely.[16,18–21]

One challenging aspect of amebic liver abscess is differentiating it from pyogenic abscess. Pyogenic abscess is more likely in patients over 50 years of age and with comorbidities, such as diabetes. They commonly have signs and symptoms of biliary tract disease including jaundice, pruritus, and elevated liver function tests (bilirubin, alkaline phosphatase, and aspartate transaminase [AST]). In addition these patients are more likely to have multiple abscesses in the right hepatic lobe.[19] Hepatoma and echinococcal cyst should also be considered in the differential diagnosis.[18]

Diagnosis

The most accurate method of diagnosing amebic dysentery is by the TechLab *E. histolytica* II stool antigen test (Table 26–3).[21,22] It has a sensitivity and specificity of over 90% and has the added advantage of detecting only *E. histolytica*.[22] Microscopy misses one-half to two-thirds of amebae found by culture and cannot distinguish between *E. histolytica* and *E. dispar* (which should not be treated).[18] The same antigen test should be used to test serum in patients suspected of having amebic liver abscess, as it has a nearly 100% sensitivity.[21] Most patients develop antiamebic antibodies, but serology can be negative early in the course of the disease. In addition, antibody tests fail to distinguish past from present infection.[18] Colonoscopy with biopsy is sometimes needed to confirm a diagnosis of amebic dysentery. Inflammation can be localized or involve the entire large intestine and often has the appearance of inflammatory bowel disease.[16,18,21] Amebic liver abscess requires radiologic imaging. Ultrasound, computed tomography (CT), and magnetic resonance imaging (MRI) are equally sensitive in detection but cannot distinguish amebic from pyogenic abscess.[19] Aspiration of amebic abscess may be required in an unusually large abscess or to rule out pyogenic abscess.[19]

Treatment

Symptomatic colonization with *E. histolytica* should be treated with a luminal agent (Table 26–4). Paromomycin is often used, as iodoquinol is difficult to obtain. Diloxanide furoate is available only through the Centers for Disease Control and Prevention (CDC).[11] The stool antigen test can be used to test for cure 1 to 2 weeks after treatment.[21]

Amebic colitis and liver abscess require metronidazole therapy for 10 days. Approximately one-third of patients develop nausea, vomiting, and anorexia with the

750 mg dose.[21] If 750 mg is intolerable, 500 mg tid may be effective for dysentery and has fewer side effects.[21] Tinidazole and doxycycline are other alternatives.[11,21] Diarrhea, fever, and right upper quadrant pain usually resolve within 2 to 5 days.[16–18,21] Treatment should be followed by a luminal agent as described for asymptomatic infection to eradicate intestinal carriage.[11,16–18,21] Patients with amebic liver abscess should not have radiologic imaging in follow-up, as resolution of the abscess varies from 6 to 12 months and is not associated with clinical response.[19]

Fulminant amebic colitis requires broad-spectrum antibiotics. Surgery is required for complications of toxic megacolon and acute necrotizing colitis.[21]

Pregnant patients with invasive disease may be treated with paromomycin for mild colitis in the first trimester. For moderate-to-severe disease and after the first trimester, however, patients should probably be treated with metronidazole, as pregnant women are at increased risk for fulminant colitis.[16,21] There are conflicting reports on the teratogenicity of metronidazole.[14]

Prevention

Interrupting the fecal-oral spread of *E. histoytica* is the only current method of preventing amebiasis. In endemic areas this includes boiling water and washing fresh vegetables with soap followed by vinegar. A vaccine is currently in development, which, once available, could eradicate *E. histolytica*.

SPORE-FORMING PROTOZOA

The four spore-forming protozoa that cause human intestinal disease are named for the infectious form of the parasite—the spore. In general they cause self-limited disease in immunocompetent hosts but can cause chronic or relapsing diarrhea in immunosuppressed individuals.

Cryptosporidiosis

Cryptosporidium parvum is the most common of the spore-forming protozoa in the United States.[23] It was first recognized as causing human disease in 1976 and was identified as a major cause of diarrhea in AIDS patients in the 1980s.[24]

Life Cycle

Cryptosporidial infection is acquired by ingestion of oocysts. The oocysts release four sporozoites, which attach to the small intestine epithelium. They then form a vacuole derived from both epithelial and parasite membranes and mature asexually inside the protected vacuole (Fig. 26–3). Mature asexual organisms either reinvade epithelial cells, continuing the cycle, or sexually mature and form oocysts. The oocysts are excreted with feces and can remain viable in the environment for months.[25]

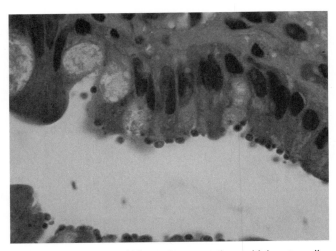

FIGURE 26–3. Large-bowel biopsy demonstrating multiple extracellular trophozoites of *Entamoeba histolytica* and extensive destruction of the intestinal epithelium and lamina propria. (See Color Plate 1.)

Epidemiology

Cryptosporidium is most prevalent in Asia and Africa, where 5% to 10% of the population is infected. It is less common in Europe and North American, where the prevalence is 1% to 3%.[26]

Cryptosporidial oocysts can be transmitted via person-to-person or animal-to-person contact or by food and water contamination (Table 26–1). Water becomes contaminated by runoff from grazing lands used by infected cattle, which serve as a reservoir for *Cryptosporidium*.[27] The oocysts are resistant to chlorination and can survive modern water treatment methods.[24] In the largest water-borne outbreak, which occurred in Milwaukee in 1993, approximately 400,000 people experienced diarrhea.[28] Cryptosporidiosis is caused by food-borne transmission as well. One outbreak occurred via unpasteurized apple juice made from fallen apples contaminated with infected manure.[27] Day care centers and hospitals have also been centers of *Cryptosporidium* outbreaks.[27]

Clinical Features

AIDS patients are at highest risk of acquiring cryptosporidiosis, which accounts for 9% to 32.5% of chronic diarrhea cases in AIDS patients.[24] Symptoms begin about 7 days after ingestion of oocysts. Persons with normal immunity develop watery, nonbloody diarrhea for up to several weeks, but then the infection clears spontaneously (Table 26–2). The diarrhea may be accompanied by abdominal cramping, nausea, vomiting, anorexia, headache, myalgias, weakness, and low-grade fevers.[29] HIV patients have similar symptoms, but the diarrhea tends to be persistent, especially with CD4 counts less than 200/μl.[23,30] Extraintestinal disease occurs primarily in the immunosuppressed and includes cholecystitis, hepatitis, pancreatitis, reactive arthritis, and respiratory symptoms of shortness of breath, cough, or wheezing.[25]

Approximately 10% of AIDS patients with cryptosporidiosis develop gallbladder involvement, manifesting as either acalculous cholecystitis or sclerosing cholangitis.[25]

Diagnosis

Both ELISA and direct immunofluorescence tests are now available to detect *Cryptosporidium* in stool samples (Table 26–3). They have a sensitivity and specificity of over 90%.[24] Small-bowel biopsy is rarely needed to make a diagnosis now that ELISA methods are available.

Treatment

Unfortunately there is presently no cure for cryptosporidiosis. In immunocompetent persons, treatment is probably unnecessary, as their illness resolves spontaneously.[28] Several studies in HIV patients have shown that reconstitution of the immune system using highly active antiretroviral therapy (HAART) may completely resolve symptoms.[31,32] Therefore HAART is the optimum treatment for HIV-infected patients (Table 26–4). Paromomycin can lessen symptoms temporarily but does not eradicate infection.[24] Paromomycin used in combination with azithromycin has been found to produce a greater reduction in symptoms.[33] In addition, nitazoxanide, especially when used with azithromycin and rifabutin, significantly decreases cryptosporidial growth in vitro.[34] In a clinical study involving AIDS patients in Mexico, diarrhea completely resolved in 19 of 22 subjects after 28 days of nitazoxanide.[35] Nitazoxanide currently is not approved by the United States Food and Drug administration (FDA).

Isosporiasis

Life Cycle

Isospora belli is thought to only infect humans.[36] Infection is acquired by ingestion of oocysts. Oocysts release four sporozoites that penetrate the proximal small intestine and become trophozoites. Trophozoites multiply asexually, which is followed by a sexual maturation stage in which they become unsporulated oocysts. Oocysts pass with feces and sporulate 2 to 3 days later.[36]

Epidemiology

Isospora is spread by contaminated food and water.[36] It is endemic in parts of Africa, Asia, and South America.[26] In the United States it is primarily seen in HIV-infected patients, immigrants from or travelers to endemic areas, and in day care centers and mental institutions (Table 26–1).[36] It is a common cause of diarrhea in AIDS patients living in endemic countries. It is the cause of chronic diarrhea in 15% of Haitian AIDS patients and 16% of Zambian AIDS patients, whereas only 2% of American or European AIDS patients with chronic diarrhea are infected with *Isospora*.[26] Its low prevalence in United States AIDS patients is likely due to the widespread use of TMP-SMX prophylaxis, as TMP-SMX is also effective against *Isospora*.[24] Patients with cancer are also at increased risk of acquiring isosporiasis.[24]

Clinical Features

In immunocompetent patients, *Isospora* causes watery, nonbloody diarrhea that typically persists for 2 to 3 weeks before spontaneously resolving (Table 26–2).[24] It may be associated with abdominal cramps, malaise, anorexia, nausea, vomiting, headache, myalgias, weakness, and low-grade fever.[29,36] In AIDS and cancer patients it causes protracted diarrhea that can lead to wasting.[24] In severe cases it can result in hemorrhagic colitis.[36] Acalculous cholecystitis and reactive arthritis are rare.[36]

Diagnosis

There is currently no antigen-based assay to detect *Isospora* in stool samples. Therefore diagnosis is based on microscopy using a modified acid-fast stain to view the oocysts (Table 26–3). Multiple stool samples and fluorescence microscopy increases sensitivity.[24,26,36] Duodenal aspirate, the string test, or small-bowel biopsy is occasionally needed for definitive diagnosis.[36]

Treatment

Immunosuppressed patients respond well to TMP-SMX double strength four times a day for 10 days followed by twice a day for 3 weeks (Table 26–4). This needs to be followed by lifelong suppression 3 times a week.[11,24,27] Diarrhea usually resolves within several days of starting therapy.[24] AIDS patients have a 50% chance of recurrence within 6 to 8 weeks if they discontinue TMP-SMX.[36] In sulfa-allergic patients, either ciprofloxacin or pyrimethamine can be used.[11,37,38]

Cyclosporiasis

Life Cycle

Cyclospora cayetanensis appears closely related to *Isospora*.[39] Infection is acquired by ingestion of oocysts that release four sporozoites. The sporozoites invade small intestine epithelial cells and undergo maturation and asexual replication. Similar to *Isospora*, a sexual maturation stage follows, producing unsporulated oocysts that are passed with feces. Like *Isospora*, they require several days outside of the host to sporulate and become infectious.[40]

Epidemiology

Cyclospora is transmitted via contaminated food and water (Table 26–1).[36] The largest outbreak in North America occurred in the spring and summer of 1996 and 1997 when over 3000 persons developed cyclosporiasis traced to contaminated raspberries imported from Guatemala.[41,42] *Cyclospora*, similar to *Isospora*, appears to be endemic in tropical underdeveloped countries.[39] Like *Isospora*, it accounts for a much larger proportion of chronic diarrhea in AIDS patients living in endemic countries than living in the United States.[24] This is likely due to the widespread use of TMP-SMX prophylaxis, which is effective against both *Isospora* and *Cyclospora*.[24] Travelers to and immigrants from endemic areas are also at risk for infection.[37]

Clinical Features

Cyclospora has an incubation period of 2 to 11 days.[39] It then causes a watery, nonbloody diarrheal illness often accompanied by low-grade fever, nausea, vomiting, anorexia, abdominal cramping, and fatigue (Table 26–2).[40] Immunocompetent persons have a self-limiting illness lasting up to several weeks, whereas HIV-infected persons usually have a chronic, persistent diarrhea.[40] AIDS patients may develop biliary tract disease as well.[36]

Diagnosis

As is the case with *Isospora*, diagnosis rests on identification of the organism by microscopy using modified acid-fast stains (Table 26–3).[40] Evaluating multiple stool samples and using fluorescence microscopy increases sensitivity.[40] A small intestine aspirate or biopsy may be needed if microscopy fails to make the diagnosis.[36]

Treatment

Immunosuppressed patients can be treated with TMP-SMX double strength once a day for 7 days (Table 26–4).[11,36,40] As with *Isospora*, this should be followed with lifelong suppression using TMP-SMX three times a week.[24,27] Ciprofloxacin may be used for sulfa-allergic patients.[38] Azithromycin is ineffective against *Cyclospora*. Some drugs, including metronidazole, quinacrine, and tinidazole, actually prolong symptoms when compared to placebo.[40]

Microsporidiosis

The phylum Microspora includes over 1000 protozoan species, 12 of which infect humans.[43] Only two species, however, are responsible for most human disease, *Enterocytozoon bieneusi* and *Encephalitozoon intestinalis*, and of these, *E. bieneusi* is responsible for approximately 90% of cases of microsporidioses.[24]

Life Cycle

Infection by microsporidia is acquired by ingestion or inhalation of spores that excyst and multiply in epithelial cells of either the small intestine or the respiratory tract.[43,44] Depending on the species, microsporidia divide by binary fission or multiple fission to form meronts. The meront cell membranes thicken and form sporonts. The sporonts develop into mature spores. Spores accumulate and expand the epithelial cell until it bursts, releasing the spores. Spores then either reinfect epithelial cells or are passed to the environment via stool, urine, or respiratory secretions.[44] *E. intestinalis* differs from other spore-forming protozoa in that it also infects macrophages that can disseminate and cause illness in virtually every organ of the body.[43]

Epidemiology

Human microsporidia spread via the fecal oral or urinary oral route (Table 26–1).[43] Water outbreaks have occurred, but no food outbreak has yet been reported.[43] It is unclear if transmission occurs sexually, but microsporidia have been found in prostatic and urethral fluid.[44] Infection is associated with homosexuality, nonpiped household water, and diarrhea among household members.[24] Microsporidia appear to cause disease only in the immunocompromised, including transplant and AIDS patients.[24] In the United States, microsporidia are the cause of chronic diarrhea in 5% to 50% of AIDS patients, primarily affecting those with a CD4 counts less than 100/μl.[24,26,27,43,44]

Clinical Features

Both *E. bieneusi* and *E. intestinalis* cause watery, nonbloody, chronic diarrhea that may be associated with fever, anorexia, weight loss, and eventually wasting (Table 26–2).[43] *E. bieneusi* may also infect the biliary system, leading to cholangitis or cholecystitis.[43] *E. intestinalis*, however, can cause widely disseminated disease, including sinusitis, keratoconjunctivitis, pneumonia, hepatitis, peritonitis, nephritis, and encephalitis.[29,43,44]

Diagnosis

The diagnosis of microsporidiosis relies on microscopy, which has a sensitivity of 67% (Table 26–3).[34] A modified trichrome stain is used to view the spores from fluid samples.[24,43] Biopsy of infected tissue may be required to definitively make the diagnosis.[44] Polymerase chain reaction (PCR) and immune methods of diagnosis should be available in the future that will likely obviate the need for biopsy.[24]

Treatment

As is the case with the other spore-forming protozoa, reconstituting the immune system with HAART resolves symptoms (Table 26–4).[43] For those who are resistant to HAART or cannot take these medications, albendazole effectively treats symptoms due to *E. intestinalis*.[24,43,44] Unfortunately, *E. bienuesi* is only partially responsive to albendazole.[24,43,44] Nitazoxanide may be an effective alternative for AIDS patients infected with *E. bieneusi*.[45]

Sarcocystis, *Balantidium coli*, and *Blastocystis hominis*

Sarcocystis, *B. coli*, and *B. hominis* are protozoa that less commonly cause gastrointestinal illness in humans.

Sarcocystis species

Sarcocystis is a protozoa transmitted to humans via undercooked pork and beef. It is found worldwide, but most cases of the disease have been reported from Southeast Asia. Symptoms include myalgias and fever, often with eosinophilia. In addition, self-limited mild diarrhea may occur. Diagnosis is based on microscopy. There is no known treatment for *Sarcocystis*.[30]

Balantidium coli

B. coli is probably the least common protozoan to cause human illness. It is found most commonly in Latin America, Southeast Asia, and Papua, New Guinea. Pigs are the main reservoir for human infection. Risk factors for infection include achlorhydria and poor nutrition. Most infections are asymptomatic, but a chronic illness consisting of intermittent diarrhea, abdominal pain, and weight loss may also occur. Fulminant colitis is rare. *B. coli* is diagnosed by microscopy. Tetracycline 500 mg four times a day for 10 days is the treatment of choice, but iodoquinol and metronidazole may also be used.[36]

Blastocystis hominis

B. hominis is more prevalent in developing countries than in industrialized nations. Infection may cause diarrhea, bloating, flatulence, abdominal cramps, and fatigue. Infections can also be asymptomatic. Microscopy is used to diagnose *B. hominis* from stool samples. As evidence for the pathogenic role of *B. hominis* is conflicting it is recommended that other causes of gastrointestinal illness be ruled out before treating *B. hominis*. There is no definitive therapy, but metronidazole and iodoquinol have been used with varying results.[36]

REFERENCES

1. Hill DR: *Giardia lamblia*. In Mandell GJ, Bennett JE, Dolin R (eds): Mandell, Douglas, and Bennett's Principles and Practice of Infectious Diseases, 5th ed. Philadelphia, Churchill Livingstone, 2000, pp 2888–2894.
2. Ortega YR, Adam RD: *Giardia*: Overview and update. Clin Infect Dis 1997;25:545–549.
3. Marshall MM, Naumovitz D, Ortega Y, Sterling CR: Waterborne protozoa pathogens. Clin Microbiol Rev 1997;10:67–85.
4. Petri WJ: Protozoan parasites that infect the gastrointestinal tract. Curr Opin Gastroenterol 2000;16:18–23.
5. Vesy CJ, Peterson WL: Review article: The management of giardiasis. Aliment Pharmacol Ther 1999;13:843–850.
6. Farthing MJ, Keusch GT, Carey MC: Effects of bile and bile salts on growth and membrane lipid uptake by *Giardia lamblia*: Possible implications for pathogenesis of intestinal disease. J Clin Invest 1985;76:1727–1732.
7. Tewari SG, Tandon BN: Functional and histological changes of small bowel in patients with *Giardia lamblia* infestation. Indian J Med Res 1974;62:689–695.
8. LeChevallier MW, Norton WD, Lee RG: *Giardia* and *Cryptosporidium* spp. in filtered drinking water supplies. Appl Environ Microbiol 1991;57:2617–2622.
9. Addiss DG, Mathews HM, Stewart JM, et al: Evaluation of a commercially available enzyme-linked immunosorbent assay for *Giardia lamblia* antigen in stool. J Clin Microbiol 1991;29:1137–1142.
10. Garcia LS, Shimizu RY: Evaluation of nine immunoassay kits (enzyme immunoassay and direct fluorescence) for detection of *Giardia lamblia* and *Cryptosporidium parvum* in human fecal specimens. J Clin Microbiol 1997;35:1526–1529.
11. Abramowicz M: Drugs for parasitic infections. Med Lett Drugs Ther 1998;40:1–12.
12. Beard CM, Noller KL, O'Fallon WM: Cancer after exposure to metronidazole. Mayo Clin Proc 1998;63:147–153.
13. Dutta AK, Phadke MA, Bagade AC, et al: A randomised multicentre study to compare the safety and efficacy of albendazole and metronidazole in the treatment of giardiasis in children. Indian J Pediatr 1994;61:689–693.
14. Burton P, Taddio A, Ariburno O, et al: Safety of metronidazole in pregnancy: A meta-analysis. Am J Gynecol 1995;172:525–529.
15. Rosenblatt JE: Antiparasitic agents. Mayo Clin Proc 1999;74:1161–1175.
16. Li E, Stanley SL: Amebiasis. Gastroenterol Clin 1996;25:471–492.
17. Ravdin J: *Entamoeba histolytica* (amebiasis). In Mandell GL, Bennett JE, Dolin R (eds): Mandell, Douglas, and Bennett's Principles and Practice of Infectious Diseases, 5th ed. Philadelphia, Churchill Livingstone, 2000, pp 2798–2810.
18. Petri WA, Singh U: Diagnosis and management of Amebiasis. CID 1999;29.
19. Hughes MA, Petri WA: Amebic liver abscess. Infect Dis Clin North Am 2000;38:3235–3239.
20. Seeto RK: Amebic liver abscess: epidemiology, clinical features, and outcome. West J Med 1999;70:104–109.
21. Huston CD, Petri WA, Haque R: Amebiasis. In Rakel RE, Bope ET (eds): Conn's Current Therapy. Philadelphia, WB Saunders, 2001, pp 50–54.
22. Haque R, Mollah NU, Ali IK et al: Diagnosis of amebic liver abscess and intestinal infection with the Techlab *Entamoeba histolytica* II antigen detection and antibody tests. J Clin Microbiol 2000;38:3235–3239.
23. Petri WA: Protozoan parasites that infect the gastrointestinal tract. Curr Opin Gastroenterol 2000;16:18–23.
24. Huston CD, Petri WA: Emerging and reemerging intestinal protozoa. Curr Opin Gastroenterol 2001;17:17–23.
25. Ungar BL: *Cryptosporidium*. In Mandell GL, Bennett JE, Dolin R (eds): Mandell, Douglas, and Bennett's Principles and Practice of Infectious Diseases, 5th ed. Philadelphia, Churchill Livingstone, 2000, pp 2903–2915.
26. Goodgame RW: Understanding intestinal spore-forming protozoa: *Cryptosporidia*, microsporidia, *Isospora*, and *Cyclospora*. Ann Intern Med 1996;124:429–441.
27. Petri WA: Spore-forming protozoan diarrheal diseases. Cortlandt Forum 1998, pp 182–186.
28. MacKenzie WR, Hoxie NJ, Proctor ME, et al: A massive outbreak in Milwaukee of *Cryptosporidum* infection transmitted through the public water supply. N Engl J Med 1994;331;161–167.
29. Flynn PM: Emerging diarrheal pathogens: *Cryptosporidium parvum*, *Isospora belli*, *Cyclospora* species, and Microsporidia. Pediatr Ann 1996;25:480–487.
30. Clark DP: New insights into human cryptosporidiosis. Clin Microbiol Rev 1999;12:554–563.
31. Foudraine NA, Weverling GJ, VanGool T, et al: Improvement of chronic diarrhea in patients with advanced HIV-1 infection during potent antiretroviral therapy. AIDS 1998;12:35–41.
32. Maggi P, Larocca AM, Quarto M, et al: Effect of antiretroviral therapy on cryptosporidiosis and microsporidiosis in patients infected with human immunodeficiency virus type 1. Eur J Clin Microbiol Infect Dis 2000;19:213–217.
33. Smith NH, Cron S, Valdez LM, et al. Combination drug therapy for cryptosporidiosis in AIDS. J Infect Dis 1998;178:900–903.
34. Giacometti A, Cirioni O, Barchiesi F, et al. Activity of nitazoxanide alone and in combination with azithromycin and

rifabutin against *Cryptosporidium parvum* in cell culture. J Antimicrob Chemother 2000;45:453–456.

35. Rossignol JF, Hidalgo H, Feregrino M, et al: A double-blind placebo controlled study of nitazoxanide in the treatment of cryptosporidial diarrhea in AIDS patients in Mexico. Trans R Soc Trop Med Hyg 1998;92:663–666.

36. Keystone HS, Kozarsky P: Isospora belli, Sarcocystis species, Blastocystis hominis and Cyclospora. In Mandell GL, Bennett JE, Dolin R (eds): Mandell, Douglas, and Bennett's Principles and Practice of Infectious Diseases, 5th ed. Philadelphia, Churchill Livingstone, 2000, pp 2915–2920.

37. Weiss LM, Perlman DC, Sherman J, et al: *Isospora belli* infection: treatment with pyrimethamine. Ann Intern Med 1988;109:474–475.

38. Verdier RI, Fitzgerald DW, Johnson WD, et al: Trimethoprim-sulfamethoxazole compared with ciprofloxacin for treatment and prophylaxis of *Isospora belli* and *Cyclospora cayetanensis* infection in HIV-infected patients: a randomized, controlled trial. Ann Intern Med 2000;132:885–888.

39. Soave R. Cyclospora: an overview. CID 1996;23:429–437.

40. Brown GH, Rotshafer JC. Cyclospora: review of an emerging parasite. Pharmacotherapy 1999;19:70–75.

41. Herwaldt BL, Ackers ML and the Cyclospora Working Group. An outbreak in 1996 of cyclosporiasis associated with imported raspberries. N Engl J Med 1997;336:1548–1556.

42. Centers for Disease Control and Prevention. Outbreak of cyclosporiasis: United States and Canada. MMWR Morb Mortal Wkly Rep 1997;46:689–691.

43. Didier ES. Microsporidiosis. CID 1998;27:1–8.

44. Weber R, Schwartz DA, Bryan RT: Microsporidia. In Mandell GL, Bennett JE, Dolin R (eds): Mandell, Douglas, and Bennett's Principles and Practices of Infectious Diseases, 5th ed. Philadelphia, Churchill Livingstone, 2000, pp 2920–2933.

45. Bicart-See A, Massip P, Linas MD, et al: Successful treatment with nitazoxanide of *Enterocyozoan bieneusi* microsporidiosis in a patient with AIDS. Antimicrob Agents Chemother 2000;44:167–168.

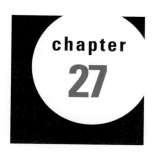

Obstetric-Gynecologic Infections

WILLIAM J. LEDGER, MD

Writing a chapter on obstetric-gynecologic infections in this new century is a challenge because of the revolutionary changes in daily practice patterns. Over the last three decades this specialty has changed from one whose main emphasis was inpatient hospital care to an outpatient practice setting. Today our emphases and concerns are different. In the past the main focus was on the seriously ill patient with a pelvic abscess who required myriad intravenous antibiotics and, if these failed, the dramatic trip to the operating room, with the scalpel as the final arbiter for cure. Not so today, for our preventive techniques are so effective that these patients who were often so seriously ill in the past are now limited to the elderly oncology patient after radical surgery or immunosuppressive therapy or the immunocompromised patient, a result of human immunodeficiency virus (HIV) infection. Predominantly outpatient prevention and treatment comprise most of the daily practice decisions about infection for the 21st century obstetrician-gynecologist.

OUTPATIENT PREVENTIVE MEDICINE

A major source of the focus upon outpatient preventive care has been the reaffirmation of obstetrics and gynecology as a primary care specialty. This has burdened the obstetrician-gynecologist with a series of practice concerns that were foreign to me as a resident in training in the early 1960s.

To provide a framework for discussion of preventive care, I want to use the mnemonic STORCH[6] (Table 27–1). This is my modification of the old TORCH mnemonic, which stood for *t*oxoplasmosis, *o*ther, *r*ubella, *c*ytomegalovirus, and *her*pes. These organisms caused some problems for the mother-to-be but could be devastating for the fetus in utero. The designation "other" was just too large because it covered too many organisms for the physician to keep in mind. To simplify the doctor's recollections, we have added "*s*" for *s*yphilis. This should be easy to remember, for *storch* is German for stork, the universal symbol of pregnancy. *H* has been enlarged to H[6], because of the number of potentially harmful organisms that have "H" as a part of their name. In addition to herpes, the original *H*, we have added H[2], hepatitis B; H[3], HIV; H[4], human papillomavirus; H[5], human parvovirus (a fitting designation, since human parvovirus causes fifth disease in children), and H[6], hepatitis C virus. With this as a framework, what are the preventive strategies against infectious disease employed by obstetrician-gynecologists in their encounters with a patient?

Syphilis

The risk of syphilis varies with the social strata of patients and their living sites. In the United States this is primarily a problem of urban poor women in New York, Florida,

TABLE 27–1 ■ STORCH[6]

S Syphilis
T Toxoplasmosis
O Other
R Rubella
C Cytomegalovirus
H[1] Herpes
H[2] Hepatitis B
H[3] Human immunodeficiency virus
H[4] Human papillomavirus
H[5] Human parvovirus
H[6] Hepatitis C

Texas, and California.[1] Particularly at risk populations are those women who attempt to support a crack cocaine habit through prostitution.

The problem in diagnosis for the practitioner is that the clinical symptoms are so mild that the patient does not seek medical attention. A chancre is usually painless and heals, lulling the patient into believing that she is cured, and the rash of secondary syphilis is mild and transient. In nearly every case the diagnosis is made by serologic screening. In the United States, serologic screening is done with a reagin test, a nonspecific test that is positive in patients with syphilis but that can be biologically false positive in other conditions. More specific tests, for example, a fluorescent treponemal antibody-absorption test (FTA-ABS), should be done to confirm the diagnosis in patients who are reagin antibody positive. For the patient with syphilis the treatment strategy is to prevent infection of the fetus in utero as well as to prevent any long-term problems such as cardiovascular or central nervous system syphilis for the mother. The spirochete *Treponema pallidum* is sensitive to penicillin and replicates slowly, approximately once a day. A long-acting penicillin, benzathine, is used to achieve a cure. A single intramuscular injection of 2.4 MU if the patient has evidence of having acquired the disease in the past year (i.e., physical signs: chancre, the rash of secondary syphilis, or evidence of recent serologic conversion from nonreactive to reactive) is usually sufficient for cure. If the disease was acquired more than a year ago or the date of acquisition is unknown, the initial dose of 2.4 MU is followed by two more 2.4 MU doses at weekly intervals.[2]

Although this strategy effectively treats syphilis, there are two important subgroups of patients who may require different approaches. The first is the patient allergic to penicillin. Because penicillin effectively crosses the placenta and treats and cures the fetus in utero, women with a history of penicillin allergy should be evaluated to see if they have a true allergy, and if they do, they should be desensitized to penicillin and then treated.[2] The final group are those women who are HIV positive. In this population the low levels of penicillin achieved in the central nervous system with benzathine penicillin may not be enough to achieve a cure. One study of adults with or without HIV infection, however,

found no benefit with a 10-day course of amoxicillin and probenecid.[3] More studies are needed in the new era of combination antiviral therapy for HIV-infected patients.

Toxoplasmosis

There is controversy about routine screening for toxoplasmosis in the United States. The suggested practice patterns in a publication of the American College of Obstetricians and Gynecologists do not recommend it because it is such an uncommon disease.[4] It *is* uncommon. One survey of New York City obstetric patients found that only 6 of 4,048 patients surveyed acquired the disease during pregnancy.[5] Another study of neonatal screening for toxoplasmosis confirmed congenital infection in 52 of 635,000 patients who were screened.[6] Of particular interest, only two would have been detected by clinical examination. Although it is uncommon, this infection cannot be ignored. It can have serious long-term central nervous system implications for the newborn. The disease in utero can be detected and treated, but even more important, there are effective methods of prevention for the susceptible female. Since only 10% of pregnant women who acquire this infection are symptomatic,[7] a program of universal serologic screening is needed. There can be problems of interpretation, and the U.S. Food and Drug Administration (FDA) issued a warning about the reliability of the *Toxoplasma* IgM test kits used by commercial laboratories in 1997.[8] If there are concerns about the screening examination, another sample should be sent to Jack Remington's laboratory in Palo Alto, California. In the patient who has evidence of serologic conversion, an amniocentesis between 16 and 20 weeks' gestation with polymerase chain reaction (PCR) testing of the amniotic fluid for *Toxoplasma gondii* identifies the patient who needs treatment.[9] Spiramycin and sulfonamides in combination yield good results, although many women will opt for a pregnancy termination.[10] More important is a program of prevention because it involves so many more patients. For the susceptible patient a program of prevention markedly reduces the risk of infection (Table 27–2).[11] A nationwide program in Belgium has significantly reduced the incidence of toxoplasmosis infection in pregnant women.[12]

Other

This category encompasses a wide variety of infections that can be prevented through education, vaccines, or therapeutic intervention.

Tetanus and Diphtheria

Tetanus and diphtheria are linked because there is a toxoid vaccine available that contains these two components.

Tetanus is an uncommon disease in the United States with fewer than 100 cases reported annually.[13] It has significance for the obstetrician-gynecologist because it is

TABLE 27-2 ■ Prevention of Toxoplasmosis Infection During Pregnancy

1. Patients are advised not to eat raw or undercooked meat, particularly pork, lamb, or venison. Specifically, meat should be cooked to an internal temperature of 150°F; meat cooked until no longer pink inside generally has an internal temperature of 165°F.
2. Patients should wash their hands after contact with raw meat and after gardening or other contact with soil; in addition, they should wash fruit and vegetables well before eating them raw.
3. If the patient owns a cat, someone else should change the litter box daily; alternatively the patient should wash her hands after changing the litter box. Patients should be encouraged to keep their cats inside and not to adopt or handle stray cats.

preventable with immunization and occurs most commonly in elderly women.[13] Patients should be reimmunized with tetanus toxoid if this has not been done within the past 10 years.

For most obstetrician-gynecologists, diphtheria seems to be a disease worthy of historic note only. Not so. In the 1990s there were outbreaks of diphtheria involving thousands of patients in Eastern Europe, particularly in portions of the former Soviet Union.[14] A few cases have been reported among United States tourists to the former Soviet Union.[15] Travelers to this area of the world should receive diphtheria toxoid before leaving the United States. If more cases are reported in the United States, more widespread immunization should be instituted.

Varicella

I have screened my prenatal patients for the presence of varicella antibody for two decades. Originally I did it to avoid the hysteria of a large subgroup of patients when a varicella outbreak occurred in New York and they were not sure whether they had had "chickenpox" as children. Prior testing and the presence of antibody denoted immunity. This avoided a crush of many patients coming to the office to get blood antibody studies and their anxiety-laden wait for results.

The availability of a live varicella vaccination has added another dimension to this screening. Varicella can be a serious, life-threatening infection for pregnant women,[16] and acquisition of the infection during pregnancy poses a risk of infection to the fetus in utero.[17] Problems in the newborn from this infection are uncommon, but when they occur, they can result in lifelong impairment for the newborn.[17] For the pregnant patient who acquires varicella and who has any respiratory symptoms, the antiviral medication acyclovir may help reduce the risk of varicella pneumonia.[18] Whether this benefits the fetus in utero is not known. Identifying the susceptible women by antepartum antibody testing targets a population for postpartum immunization,[19] and one study suggested this approach was cost effective.[20]

Influenza

There is historic evidence that pregnant women with influenza have a poorer prognosis than nonpregnant women.[21,22] This increased risk is most marked in the third trimester. Because of this, pregnant women who will be in the second or third trimester in the winter

months should receive the influenza vaccine in late fall after they have passed the first trimester.[23]

Pneumococcal Pneumonia

Pulmonary infections due to *Streptococcus pneumoniae* have brought a resurgence of concern to obstetrician-gynecologists. In the preantibiotic era, pregnant women with a pneumococcal infection, particularly those in the third trimester, had a much higher mortality rate than nonpregnant women had.[24] With the advent of antibiotics effective against these aerobic gram-positive cocci, this problem seemed under control. In the last decade there has been an emergence of *S. pneumoniae* resistance to penicillin in the United States.[25] One strategy of prevention would be the use of the multivalent pneumococcal vaccine in pregnant women. This vaccine has been recommended for high-risk populations, such as patients over the age of 65.[26] I think all pregnant women would qualify as a high-risk population, but to date recommendations have been made targeting high-risk subgroups such as those who are HIV positive or who have sickle cell disease or functional asplenia.[26]

Group B Streptococcus

Prevention of group B streptococcus infections in the newborn is an important obstetric goal. It was estimated in 1990 that 8000 cases of early onset neonatal sepsis occurred each year in the United States with over 300 deaths.[27] In any preventive program a variety of problems must be dealt with. Maternal carriage of the group B streptococcus is the source for most subsequent neonatal infection. Over 10% of pregnant women in labor carry this organism, so there is a much higher maternal carriage rate than newborn infection rate.[27] An additional problem is that maternal carriage of the group B streptococcus is highly variable. A positive first trimester or 26- to 28-week culture is a poor predictor of the presence or absence of vaginal group B streptococcus when the patient goes into labor at term.[28] The incidence of vaginal culture–positive patients varies with both the technique used and the site of culture. The lower third of the vagina and the rectum yield a higher number of positive cultures than the more traditional endocervical sample does;[29] the use of a selective broth for initial culture can increase the yield of positive cultures by as much as 50%.[30] Successful intervention to prevent infection prescribes antibiotics for the mother prior to delivery. This timing is more effective than dosages given only to the newborn.[31]

With input from the obstetric and pediatric communities, the Centers for Disease Control and Prevention (CDC) published its recommendations for prevention in 1996.[29] Two prevention strategies were suggested. The first was a risk strategy that administered antibiotics prior to labor to mothers who had any one of five identified high risk factors: (1) the delivery of a previous infant with neonatal group B streptococcus sepsis, (2) a maternal history of group B streptococcus bacteriuria, (3) delivery at less than 37 weeks' gestation, (4) an oral temperature of 38°C (100.4°F) or greater during labor, and (5) membranes ruptured for 18 hours or more at time of delivery. The second strategy adds lower vaginal and rectal culture for group B streptococcus at 35 to 37 weeks' gestation. Those who are culture positive are treated with antibiotics in labor. The suggested antibiotic regimens are (1) penicillin G 5 MU IV followed by 2.5 MU IV every 4 hours until delivery, (2) ampicillin 2 g loading dose followed by 1 g IV every 4 hours until delivery. For those patients allergic to penicillin, two alternate regimens are recommended: (1) clindamycin 900 mg IV followed by 900 mg IV every 8 hours until delivery, (2) erythromycin 500 mg IV followed by 500 mg every 6 hours until delivery.[29]

A recent report suggested some modifications to the protocol.[30] Several observations were made that might modify approaches. The microbiologic screening strategy seemed more effective than the risk-based method in lowering attack rates in the newborn. Both strategies used intrapartum antibiotics to prevent early-onset group B streptococcal sepsis but had no impact on the incidence of late-onset group B sepsis.[30] The authors noted clinical observations of a large number of patients from Dallas. The women undergoing a repeat cesarean section, not in labor, with membranes intact did not need antibiotics, even if the patient was vaginal culture positive for the group B streptococcus. The Dallas group had no early onset group B streptococcal newborn sepsis in this population when they reviewed their database.

A number of questions remain about these CDC guidelines. This sole reliance upon antibiotics as a preventive strategy means that over 1 million women will receive antibiotics in labor to reduce the 1990 baseline rates of 8000 cases of newborn sepsis and over 300 cases of newborn mortality due to early onset sepsis caused by this organism.[27,32] This huge number of intrapartum patients exposed to antibiotics places a selection pressure on obstetrical services that in the future could result in organisms other than the group B streptococcus causing newborn sepsis. There has already been one report that linked the extensive use of ampicillin on an obstetric service with the emergence of *Escherichia coli* newborn infection.[33] In addition, another study found increasing levels of group B streptococcus resistance to the alternative antibiotics, clindamycin and erythromycin.[34] All these trends will have to be closely monitored and could lead to changes in the antibiotic profile.

With these concerns, are there any future alternatives? I think so. At least one study in Europe found a lower rate of newborn group B streptococcal infection when a dilute hexachlorophene douche was given to all women admitted to the obstetrical unit in labor.[35] This technique needs further evaluation. Finally, the development of an effective group B streptococcal vaccine would be a major advance in patient care.[30]

Listeria monocytogenes

Listeriosis, caused by *L. monocytogenes*, can be a serious disease in pregnant women. Pregnant women are particularly susceptible to *Listeria* bacteremia. They present clinically with an acute febrile illness with myalgias, arthralgias, headache, and backache. Loss of the pregnancy is common, with spontaneous abortion and either intrauterine or neonatal death. In an epidemic of *Listeria* infections in Los Angeles in 1985, 93 cases occurred in pregnant women, who had 20 stillbirths and 10 neonatal deaths.[36] If listeriosis is recognized, treatment with ampicillin and gentamicin should be given.[37] A strategy of prevention should be employed. Pregnant women should be informed that many foods can be contaminated with *L. monocytogenes*, including soft cheeses and fresh and processed chicken and beef available, for example, at a New York City delicatessen. Obstetric patients should be advised to avoid soft cheeses and to heat or microwave take-out sandwiches and other take-out foods.

Rubella

Rubella represents one of the success stories of modern medicine. In 1941, Gregg, an Australian ophthalmologist, reported this to be a teratogen for humans.[38] In 1965–1968 the last major rubella epidemic occurred in the United States, and it was estimated that more than 20,000 children were born with congenital rubella syndrome (CRS).[39] In contrast, from 1969 to 1979 there was an average of 39 CRS cases per year, and from 1985 to 1996, only 106 confirmed CRS cases and 16 probable cases were reported.[39] This dramatic reduction happened because of three related events: In 1962 the rubella virus was isolated; in 1966 the rubella virus was attenuated; and in 1969 a live attenuated virus vaccine was licensed in the United States.[39] A strategy of herd immunity in the United States was followed with a focus upon young children. Currently it is recommended that all children between 12 and 15 months of age should receive the measles-mumps-rubella vaccine. Current obstetric practice in the United States includes routine screening for the presence of rubella antibodies at the time of the first prenatal visit. Patients likely to be susceptible include members of religious sects who do not favor immunization[40] and recent immigrants to the United States from the Caribbean and Central American and South American countries, where universal rubella immunization policies are not in place.[39] Although the attenuated virus has not been associated with CRS, immunization with a live virus vaccine during pregnancy is not recommended. The vaccine can be given to susceptible women after delivery, but they should be warned that the incidence of transient arthritis is more common in adult women than in men.[41] The fact that the arthritis is transient is reassuring, but I am impressed that this is one symptom to be avoided for a new mother attempting to handle the sleep deprivation of the early postpartum period. Because of this, I do my rubella immunization of susceptible women 6 to 12 months after delivery.

Cytomegalovirus

American obstetricians have had a schizophrenic attitude toward cytomegalovirus (CMV) infections in pregnancy. On the one hand, they acknowledge the seriousness of the problem. This virus infects more newborns than does any other infectious agent in the United States. It is estimated that each year 30,000 to 40,000 infants are infected with CMV and that 9000 of these infants suffer permanent sequelae.[42] On the other hand, there is no American College of Obstetricians and Gynecologists' plan of intervention because no treatments are available.[4]

This attitude is misguided, because preventive strategies based upon our knowledge of the natural progression of CMV infections in pregnancy can be devised. It is clear that primary CMV infection in pregnancy is associated with much more frequent clinically apparent disease in the newborn.[43] In addition, most CMV infections in adults are asymptomatic. The virus can be contracted by intimate contact with infected body fluids such as saliva, urine, ejaculate, and vaginal secretions. Any plan of prevention requires blood antibody screening of the pregnant patient at the first prenatal visit. For those women who are discovered to be susceptible by the absence of antibodies, the methods of prevention outlined in Table 27–3 should be employed by the pregnant patient.[11]

H[1]: Herpes Simplex Virus

Our understanding of the pathophysiology of genital herpes simplex virus (HSV) infections has undergone a major transformation in the last two decades. Before this, it was assumed that the first genital herpes outbreak was a symptomatic event for a woman and that a patient could recognize prodromal symptoms of recurrent outbreaks to inform her obstetrician that an outbreak was impending so that a cesarean section could be performed to reduce

the risk of a neonatal infection. This strategy, based upon clinical recognition of HSV infection, was severely flawed. It is now apparent from a number of studies that most women with evidence of prior genital tract herpes as documented by positive HSV 2 antibody status are either asymptomatic or so mildly symptomatic that they have no awareness they have the disease.[44] These patients can shed virus without symptoms at the time of delivery[45] and are the source of the large number of asymptomatic women who deliver infants who subsequently develop a newborn herpetic infection. These new insights into the pathophysiology of this problem necessitate new preventive strategies for physicians caring for pregnant women. Two problems remain with all of our recommendations: Neonatal herpes infections are uncommon, with rates estimated between 1:2500 to 1:15,000 deliveries. In addition, prospective studies with the large numbers of patients necessary to demonstrate efficacy have not yet been done. With this in mind there are two categories of patients in whom some preventive strategies can be used to lower the incidence of newborn herpes infections.

For the patient with a history of symptomatic genital HSV infections, some guidelines are in place. If these women become symptomatic during pregnancy, they should be treated with an oral antiviral agent such as acyclovir. During labor, if they are asymptomatic, fetal invasive diagnostic techniques, such as an intrauterine scalp electrode or intrauterine fetal scalp blood sampling, should not be used. During labor if they have developed prodromal symptoms or are discovered to have genital lesions, a cesarean section should be performed as soon as possible.[4] If the lesions are remote from the genitalia, for example, on the buttocks, a cesarean section is not necessary.[46] Although studies support the use of suppressive acyclovir therapy during the last few weeks of pregnancy,[47] a large controlled study to determine benefit has not yet been done.

For the patient with no history of genital herpes, there are no established guidelines. Antibody testing for HSV antibodies establishes those patients with prior exposure to the virus. Knowing who is HSV 1 or HSV 2 antibody positive could be used to determine whether a scalp electrode or fetal blood scalp sampling should be done. The problem is that large numbers of women have HSV antibodies,[44] but the incidence of HSV newborn infection is low. Another possible preventive measure involves susceptible women who are living with HSV antibody–positive men. Patients who are seronegative early in pregnancy have a 13% chance of acquiring genital herpes

---

TABLE 27–3 ■ Prevention of Cytomegalovirus (CMV) Infections During Pregnancy

1. Those pregnant patients who are not in a monogamous sexual relationship should have their sexual partners wear a condom.
2. Providers of child care or parents of children in child care centers should be informed that they are at increased risk of acquiring a CMV infection. The risk of CMV infection can be diminished by avoiding mouth-to-mouth kissing and by hand washing, particularly after changing diapers.
3. If a blood transfusion is needed, these patients should receive only CMV antibody–negative blood or leukocyte-reduced cellular blood products in nonemergency situations.

by the time of labor if their partner is HSV 2 antibody positive.[48] Whether condoms, acyclovir, or abstinence will be effective preventive techniques in these couples has not been studied to date.

H²: Hepatitis B

Currently there is a program designed to prevent hepatitis B infection in the newborn that is recommended for use in the United States.[49] Pregnant women are screened for the presence of hepatitis B surface antigen. The newborns of women who are hepatitis B antigen positive receive hepatitis B immune globulin (HBIG) and hepatitis B vaccine (Table 27–4).[49] Although this does not eliminate all newborn hepatitis B infections, it does markedly reduce the incidence of newborn infection.[50]

This policy of prevention of hepatitis B infection should be expanded. A number of reasons justify this. Hepatitis B can be transmitted by blood and through sexual contact without barrier methods with a hepatitis B antigen–positive partner. It is still a common infection in the United States, and most new infections occur in the 15- to 39-year-old age group, with the highest incidence in the 20- to 29-year age group.[51] All new hepatitis B infections in adults carry with them a risk of chronic infection that places the future mother at risk for future serious liver disease, creating the possibility of a chronic hepatitis B infection for her newborn through a vertical transmission of the virus. Since the number of new hepatitis B infections in the United States is so much greater than new rubella infections, it seems logical to expand preventive immunization of adults to include hepatitis B as well as rubella.

The starting point in this new preventive policy is to screen pregnant women for the presence of hepatitis B antibody and antigen. Those patients whose tests are negative are susceptible, and they are candidates for immunization. Since this is not a live virus vaccine, there are two possible immunization strategies, either antepartum or postpartum. The antepartum strategy takes advantage of the pregnant woman's repeated antepartum visits, which provide the opportunity to

TABLE 27–4 ▪ **Prevention of Hepatitis B in Newborns**

MOTHERS WHO ARE HEPATITIS B ANTIGEN POSITIVE

Hepatitis B immune globulin		
(0.5 ml) IM		Within 12 h of birth
Hepatitis B vaccine	Dose 1	Within 12 h of birth
	Dose 2	1–2 mo after birth
	Dose 3	6 mo after birth

MOTHERS NOT SCREENED FOR HEPATITIS B ANTIGEN

Hepatitis B immune globulin		
(0.5 ml) IM		Within 12 h of birth
Hepatitis B vaccine	Dose 1	Within 12 h of birth
	Dose 2	1–2 mo after birth
	Dose 3	6–18 mo

administer the recommended three-dose immunization scheme over a 6-month interval. The problems noted in one report are daunting and include both compliance and efficacy.[52] Only 9 of 80 (11%) of the study population received the recommended three doses of the vaccine, and the seroconversion rate for the 80 study patients was lower (49%) than has been reported in nonpregnant adults.[52] In contrast a study of postpartum immunization at Cornell had a much better record of compliance: 104 of 113 (92%) patients received at least two immunization injections, and the seroconversion rate after three injections of 66 of 69 (95.7%) was comparable to that of nonpregnant adults undergoing immunization.[53] The problem with this postpartum strategy involves getting three postpartum visits from harried, exhausted, postpartum women to complete their immunization series. The benefits are obvious, for their immunization, when successful, protects these women and their subsequent newborns from hepatitis B infection.

H³: Human Immunodeficiency Virus

The management of HIV infection in pregnant women has undergone a dramatic transformation in the past decade. New effective antiviral agents have changed most of the previously held stances toward screening and potential treatment regimens. Today identification of the HIV-infected pregnant woman permits the use of new treatment initiatives that lower the incidence of newborn HIV infection.

The prevention of newborn infection with HIV can be achieved by a number of physician interventions. The obvious starting point is maternal blood antibody testing to determine if the patient has an HIV infection. For those women who are HIV antibody positive, strategies are in place to reduce newborn infection rates. Zidovidine (ZDV) given to pregnant women before and during labor and to the newborn infant significantly lowers the transmission rate.[54] The CDC has recommended this regimen to reduce HIV transmission (Table 27–5)[55] During labor, obstetric interventions that might breach the integrity of the fetus's skin, such as fetal scalp electrode application, amniotomy, fetal scalp blood sampling, and forceps, should be avoided.[56] There is also evidence that elective cesarean section prior to the onset of labor lowers the risk of fetal HIV infection.[57] Postpartum breast-feeding can transfer maternal infection to the infant.[56] All these strategies will probably be supplanted in the next few years. No infectious disease physician in America treating a newly discovered HIV-infected adult would consider ZDV monotherapy as an option,[58] and yet this is the current recommendation for obstetricians.[55] The effectiveness of combination antiviral chemotherapy,[59] our ability to measure viral load, and the evidence that viral load is an important risk factor in maternal-fetal HIV transfer[60] should spawn studies to see if in the future combination antiviral treatment can be used in pregnant women to

TABLE 27–5 ■ Centers for Disease Control and Prevention Recommendations on the Use of Zidovudine (ZDV) to Prevent Transmission of Human Immunodeficiency Virus

Antepartum	At 14 wk gestation and afterward: ZDV 100 mg PO five times daily (alternatively, 200 mg tid or 300 mg bid)
Intrapartum	A loading dose of ZDV 2 mg/kg IV the first hour and then 1 mg IV each hour until delivery
Postpartum	For the neonate: oral ZDV syrup 2 mg/kg qid × 6 wk

reduce the HIV viral load. With a reduced viral load the intrapartum delivery and postpartum standards of care could be less stringently modified for the HIV anti-body–positive pregnant patient.

H⁴: Human Papillomavirus

Our knowledge of the role of human papilloma virus (HPV) infection has expanded exponentially in the past decade. Prior to this, clinician focus was upon visible warts, caused by HPV 6 and HPV 11. The major obstetric concern was that these large visible warts might complicate the vaginal delivery process for the mother and increase the risk of laryngeal papillomatosis in the newborn. In these uncommon and untreated cases, cesarean section was a good option.[61] Prevention techniques in the antepartum period focused upon ablating these large, visible genital growths. Recently it has become evident that there are now strains of HPV called high-risk because they are associated with intraepithelial lesions of the cervix and invasive cancer of the cervix.[62] Newer techniques of detecting HPV infections, including hybrid capture of DNA[63] and PCR,[64] make it possible to detect the presence of HPV in an asymptomatic woman who has no visible lesions.

There will be a role for the prevention of HPV infection. Animal studies demonstrate the ability of a single HPV-type surface antigen to produce blood and local tissue antibodies.[65] An effective HPV vaccine would be a boon to womankind. Until such a vaccine has been tested and approved, preventive measures using HPV testing can be employed. One of the most difficult therapeutic decisions is the management of the pregnant patient with an abnormal Papanicolaou smear. It is a difficult clinical situation because many Pap smear reports suggest more advanced tissue changes than are demonstrated by the subsequent tissue biopsy. This is an important therapeutic consideration because biopsy and conization during pregnancy are associated with high bleeding and infection risks as well as with the possible loss of the pregnancy. One future strategy may include the use of sensitive HPV testing in patients with a Pap smear reading of atypical squamous cells of uncertain significance (ASCUS).[66] I think patients in this category with a negative result from a test sensitive for HPV such as a Digene HPV test could be followed throughout the pregnancy with repeated cytology and PCR testing, avoiding biopsy or conization intervention. Patients with the possibility of a high grade lesion on Pap smear should have biopsy, no matter what the HPV test results are. My own experience with such patients is limited, but this protocol has been successful. Future studies will be needed to determine if this option to prevent cervical biopsy or conization will be safe for those patients with an ASCUS cytology report who are negative for HPV.

H⁵: Human Parvovirus (Fifth Disease)

Human parvovirus is an infrequent cause of fetal death and fetal hydrops, despite the fact that this is a common infection of children.[67]

The only preventive strategy that might be used in the future would be to identify susceptible women. This could be done by obtaining antibody studies at the first prenatal visit. This information would be particularly useful in the pregnant woman working with young children, such as an elementary school teacher or day care center worker. The susceptible woman should be retested when any subsequent outbreaks of fifth disease are noted in the classroom or day care center.

H⁶: Hepatitis C

Hepatitis C was identified in 1990 as the viral cause of hepatitis that in the past usually had been identified as non-A non-B hepatitis.[68] It can be a serious problem for adults who are chronic carriers of the virus, for it has been the cause of most liver transplantations in some series.[69] Infection with this virus in adults is marked by a high percentage of chronic virus carriers.[70] In contrast, young children who acquired the virus through blood transfusions for open heart surgery had a lower level of chronic viral carriage.[71]

The main concern for the obstetrician is transfer of the virus from the mother to the newborn. The risk seems greater, the higher the maternal hepatitis C viral load. Hepatitis C is seen most often in women who are HIV positive.[72] It seems prudent to avoid invasive fetal techniques during labor, such as fetal scalp electrodes and fetal scalp blood sampling. The role of elective cesarean section in preventing transmission has not been studied, and the risk with breast-feeding seems low.[73] As hepatitis C antibody sampling of pregnant women becomes more widespread, more data about the risk of hepatitis C transmission will be obtained.

OTHER PREVENTIVE STRATEGIES IN OBSTETRICS

Pyelonephritis

Prevention of urinary tract infections in pregnant women is an important part of prenatal care. This population is at increased risk for urinary tract infections because of the delayed transit time of urine from the kidneys to the bladder and the increasing capacity of the urinary tract for residual urine during pregnancy. An important component of obstetric care is screening for asymptomatic bacteriuria at the first prenatal visit and treating those patients who have it. There is evidence that this lowers the incidence of pyelonephritis later in pregnancy.[74] Preventive treatment is a simple task for the practitioner. Various antibiotic regimens are available (Table 27–6).[75] The difficulty is that no studies have been done to determine length of therapy. The short 3-day course of antibiotics usually will be completed in the asymptomatic pregnant patient, and follow-up culture should be done to see if the bacteria have been eliminated. Although patients with asymptomatic bacteriuria in the first trimester have a higher than expected rate of preterm labor and delivery, there is no evidence that antibiotic eradication of the bacteriuria lowers the rate of preterm delivery.[76]

Preterm Labor and Delivery

Over the last three decades there has been a search to determine infectious causes of preterm labor. Associations were noted between the recovery of either a specific organism or a high level of organisms from a culture site and preterm labor and delivery. The recovery of these potential bacterial instigators of preterm labor generated enthusiasm for antibiotic intervention to eliminate the detected organism. Some of the associated conditions are asymptomatic bacteriuria,[77] *Ureaplasma urealyticum* infection of the placenta,[78] group B streptococcal colonization in the first trimester,[79] asymptomatic bacterial vaginosis,[80] and *Trichomonas vaginalis* vaginal colonization.[81] To date, antibacterial intervention studies for these entities have not lowered the preterm delivery rate. Despite these repeated failed therapeutic trials, interest in the detection and treatment of vaginal microbiologic abnormalities has not waned.

Screening for the presence of *Neisseria gonorrhoeae* and treatment are an accepted part of preventive prenatal care. Although the observations are few in number, one study suggested that detection and treatment of this bacterial pathogen might lower the prematurity rate.[82] The CDC-recommended treatments include a single dose of intramuscular ceftriaxone 125 mg or oral cefixime 400 mg plus oral erythromycin base 500 mg four times a day for 7 days.[2] For the penicillin-allergic patient, spectinomycin 2 g IM plus the previously noted erythromycin base regimen for 7 days.[2]

The treatment of pregnant patients with bacterial vaginosis to prevent prematurity remains a work in progress. There have been a number of conflicting studies regarding the benefits, or lack of benefit, of antibiotic treatment in different patient populations. In one study by Hauth et al, combination treatment with oral metronidazole 250 mg three times a day for 7 days plus oral erythromycin base 333 mg three times a day for 14 days in women with a history of prior preterm deliveries lowered the prematurity rate.[83] In contrast a multicenter study of oral metronidazole treatment in asymptomatic pregnant women with bacterial vaginosis showed no improvement in the rate of prematurity in the antibiotic-treated arm of the study.[84] Unfortunately this study of a large pregnant patient population was seriously flawed. There were many pluses. The multicenter study garnered a large number of patients, and the individual physician chief investigators at the separate centers were competent obstetricians, and I have no doubt the protocol was adhered to at each site. Two questions remain. The dose of metronidazole, 2 g initially and then repeated 4 days later, may not be the best for this intervention scheme. It certainly differs from the successful Hauth et al regimen.[83] There is another major concern. The scientific emphasis in this study was on a central laboratory confirmation of the diagnosis by the evaluation of the Gram stain of vaginal secretions. This delayed treatment in all cases by several days. In addition, restrictions on antibiotic interventions by the dating of the pregnancy also meant further delays in the initiation of treatment by days or weeks. Certainly the experience with prophylactic antibiotics in gynecologic operations[85] and in laboratory investigations of the ability of systemic antibiotics to lessen the severity of local infection caused by bacterial contamination[86] suggest to me that any delay in the treatment of bacterial vaginosis is the mark of a flawed investigation. Would more immediate antibiotic intervention give better results? This will require more study, but one German investigation using biweekly patient determination of the vaginal pH followed by immediate physician evaluation and treatment of those with bacterial vaginosis has lowered the prematurity rate. The treatment for women at less than 12 weeks' gestation was clindamycin vaginal cream for 7 days, and for those beyond 12 weeks', oral metronidazole 1 g a day for 7 days.[87] Obviously, further study is needed.

TABLE 27–6 ■ Oral Treatments for Asymptomatic Bacteriuria

Ampicillin 500 mg qid × 3 d
Amoxicillin 500 mg tid × 3 d
Cephalexin 500 mg qid × 3 d
Nitrofurantoin (Macrodantin) 50 mg qid × 3 d
Nitrofurantoin (Macrobid) 100 mg bid × 3 d

Postdelivery Infection in Newborns

Eye infections of the newborn (Ophthalmia neonatorum) usually are caused by *Neisseria gonorrhoeae* or *Chlamydia trachomatis*. Although antepartum screening for these organisms is a standard of antepartum care and detection always results in maternal treatment, some asymptomatic women will remain positive at delivery because their treatment was inadequate, they have been reinfected, or the diagnostic screening test, for example, the DNA probe, is less sensitive than PCR,[88] and the infection has not been detected. For this reason, treatment of the eyes is routine at birth. For years the delivery room routine in the United States was the immediate application to the eyes of silver nitrate drops. Two treatment problems have led to the abandonment of this method in most United States centers. There were questions about its effectiveness against *C. trachomatis* conjunctivitis. A more important concern was the frequent chemical conjunctivitis caused by this topical antiseptic. Today most services use a single-use tube of ophthalmic ointment containing 0.5% erythromycin or 1% tetracycline. This is much better tolerated, but the effectiveness of this treatment has not been well documented.[89] In this study, most newborn ocular gonococcal infections occurred when the mother had not received any prenatal care. For most women, antepartum screening followed by maternal treatment should be of benefit. If *C. trachomatis* is identified before delivery, antibiotic treatment can be given to the mother.[90]

Postpartum Infection in Mothers

Any strategy for the prevention of postpartum infection requires a delineation of risk factors, that is, those patients most likely to develop a postdelivery infection. In any evaluation of postpartum infectious morbidity, some high-risk groups are clearly identified. Cesarean section of a patient in labor, particularly a patient from a lower socio-economic class, increases the risk of infection.[91]

To date the most effective method for reducing the rate of postpartum infection of the uterus (endomyometritis) and abdominal wound infection is the intraoperative use of systemic prophylactic antibiotics in the mother. Experimental studies in animals of the role of parenteral antibiotics in reducing infection caused by local bacterial contamination had the best results when the intravenous antibiotics were administered prior to the local bacterial contamination.[86] Those findings introduce a therapeutic dilemma for the obstetrician. If intravenous prophylactic antibiotics for the patient undergoing a cesarean section are given just prior to the initial abdominal incision, the dynamics of the distribution of antibiotics from the maternal intravascular space means that high levels of antibiotics will be achieved in the fetal circulation.[92] This is a problem. Since the clinical diagnosis of newborn sepsis is difficult, much neonatology diagnostic emphasis is placed upon positive blood cultures, and this preoperative maternal antibiotic administration could lower the sensitivity of this important screening test. Because of this, prophylactic antibiotics for cesarean section are administered after the cord is clamped. Fortunately there is good evidence that this approach is still protective.[93,94] A number of regimens have been used with success. These agents include first- and second-generation cephalosporins, penicillins with and without a β-lactam inhibitor, and clindamycin and gentamicin. All have reduced the rate of postoperative site infections, and one study with 10 treatment arms had the best results with cefazolin 2 g, cefotetan 1 g, ampicillin 2 g, and piperacillin 4 g as the treatment selection.[95] Concerns about hospital costs led to a comparison of single- vs. multiple-dose antibiotic prophylaxis. To the delight of cost-conscious administrators, the single dose yielded results comparable to the multiple-dose regimen.[96] Since first-generation cephalosporins are inexpensive and seem to yield results comparable to those of more expensive antibiotics,[95] there has been much momentum to focus on these agents for prophylaxis. I still have concerns about first-generation cephalosporins because of their poor gram-negative anaerobic activity. In one study at Cornell we had better results, although not statistically significant, with an ampicillin-sulbactam combination as compared to cefazolin.[97] In addition to this intravenous antibiotic prophylaxis strategy, an alternative method has been to apply an antibiotic solution lavage to the uterine incision after the delivery of the baby. There is appeal to this approach because of the two-pronged attack to prevent infection. There is the local impact of antibiotics upon the contaminating uterine bacterial flora, and the antibiotics are absorbed through the peritoneum, which achieves systemic levels and fulfills the role of intravenously administered antibiotics.[98] This method of prevention is effective[99] but is not now widely used in the United States. It is messy, prolongs the operation, and has not been universally effective, possibly because of too rapid suction removal of the antibiotic solution.[100] The standard of care now is a single-dose intravenous administration of one of the antibiotics noted in Table 27–7 after delivery of the baby and clamping of the cord.

Infection in Gynecology

The starting point for the prevention of infection in nonpregnant women requires a basic change in the attitudes

TABLE 27–7 ■ Intravenous Drugs for Cesarean Section Prophylaxis

Cefazolin 2 g
Cefotetan 1–2 g
Cefoxitin 2 g
Ampicillin 2 g
Piperacillin 4 g
For the penicillin-allergic patient: Clindamycin 900 mg

of both physician and patient. Preventive gynecologic care has focused upon the avoidance of unwanted pregnancies. For sexually active women in childbearing years, oral contraceptives have been a boon, eliminating the occasional failures of barrier methods of contraception. This is good, but physicians and patients have to add to the equation the prevention of infection. The new standard of care should pair oral contraceptives to prevent pregnancy and the condom to reduce the risk of such sexually transmitted organisms as *N. gonorrhoeae, C. trachomatis*, HIV, herpes, hepatitis B and C, CMV, and human papillomavirus.

Screening techniques should be used to detect infection in women with few or no symptoms in the early stages of disease when antibiotic treatment provides the best opportunity for care without any residual damage to the pelvic organs. Patients in the early stages of *N. gonorrhoeae* infection may present with symptoms of cystitis, abnormal uterine bleeding, or a new vaginal discharge.[101] Sexually active women with these symptoms should be screened for *N. gonorrhoeae* with a DNA probe or PCR test. Silent infection with *C. trachomatis* should be considered at the first examination of a sexually active woman who is not using a condom or who has a new sexual partner. Since PCR is so much more sensitive and specific than a DNA probe test, it should be used.[88] I believe these same test methods should be used to screen for the high-risk human papillomavirus.[64] It identifies a population at risk for developing abnormal cervical cellular changes, and it is a population that should be rescreened at intervals of less than a year to determine if the virus has been eliminated and the Pap smear has remained normal.

Postoperative Infections in Gynecology: Prehospital Admission Care

A number of important care priorities have to be assessed by the gynecologist prior to the care of the patient in the operating room. These were summarized in an excellent review article by Nichols in 1991 on surgical wound infection[102]:

1. Preoperative hospital stay. There is a direct correlation between prolonged preoperative stay in the hospital and abdominal wound infections. Same-day operative admissions eliminate this concern, but occasionally, on consultation, a medical inpatient will be discovered who should have elective operative care. If at all possible, these operations should not be done during this hospital course but should be scheduled for later.
2. No preoperative shaving should be done the night before the scheduled operation. Years ago, Cruse and Foord found this associated with a significantly higher wound infection rate.[103] Instead, remove the hair adjacent to the operative site with a clipper or a razor in the operating room, just before the skin preparation.[104]
3. The longer the operation, the greater the risk of postoperative infection. This is one of the following

three components of a risk index for postoperative infections:

a. A patient with an American Society of Anesthesiologists preoperative assessment score of 3, 4, or 5
b. An operation classified as contaminated or dirty infected
c. An operation lasting over T hours, which for abdominal and vaginal hysterectomy is 2 hours[105]

The postoperative wound infection rate for score zero is 1.5%, score 1 is 2.9%, score 2 is 6.8%, and score 3 is 13%. Obviously, haste makes waste, but efficient use of skilled operative care is important.

4. Abdominal drains should be avoided if possible. If abdominal drainage is indicated, a closed suction drainage system should be used through a drainage site separate from the incisional wound.[106]
5. Preoperative showering with antiseptic-containing soaps lowers the postoperative wound infection rate. This can be done the evening before operation for an inpatient or in the morning for same-day admission patients.
6. The presence of an active infection in a remote site such as the urinary tract, skin, or respiratory tract increases the rate of postoperative infections. These should be effectively treated more than 24 hours before the planned operation.

Another area of preventive care for the gynecologist is the use of antibiotics to lower the incidence of infection after operations, that is, prophylactic antibiotics. In the past there were many theoretical concerns about this strategy. One dominant theme supported by one general surgical study[107] was that antibiotics used this way would not work. Another concern again documented by a neurosurgical study was that widespread use of prophylactic antibiotics would cause the emergence of difficult to treat, antibiotic-resistant organisms on a service.[108] These concerns are real, but a number of studies have shown their benefit to patients if guidelines of care are established that are based upon an experimental design of antibiotic prophylaxis.[86]

These guidelines are modifications of a set published over 25 years ago,[85] but they remain standards for care in the 21st century:

1. The operation should have a significant risk of postoperative site infection. The key word is "significant." Significant infections can be the frequent postoperative vaginal cuff infection following vaginal or abdominal hysterectomy[109] or the less frequent, but more serious postoperative adnexal abscess usually following vaginal hysterectomy but on occasion an abdominal hysterectomy as well.[110] In addition, one recent study found the same rate of febrile morbidity following abdominal myomectomy as was seen after abdominal hysterectomy.[111] Significant can also mean

the infrequent infection that follows pregnancy termination but that is a threat to the future patency of tubes[112] and the infrequent but serious infections that can follow hysterosalpingography.[113] All these procedures are candidates for antibiotic prophylaxis.

2. The operation should be associated with significant endogenous bacterial contamination. For the gynecologist the vagina and cervix are the sites of this bacterial contamination. One type of vaginitis, bacterial vaginosis, is characterized by a marked increase in the numbers of bacteria in the vagina and has been associated with a higher incidence of vaginal cuff infections following abdominal hysterectomy.[114]

3. The antibiotic used for prophylaxis should have exhibited clinical effectiveness. This guideline marks the major divergence in therapeutic strategy between prophylaxis and treatment. Treatment of soft tissue pelvic infections has been characterized by broad-spectrum antimicrobial coverage, usually achieved by a combination of antibiotics. In contrast, successful prophylactic antibiotic regimens in gynecology are single agent and do not cover all the potential infectious agents present in the vaginal flora.

4. The antibiotic should be present in the tissue of the potential wound at the time of incision. This is crucial, because it has great significance for the timing of the administration of the antibiotics. This was first demonstrated by Burke in his experimental study of prophylaxis; antibiotics administered 1 hour before or at the time of bacterial contamination had the highest rates of success.[86] All successful prophylactic antibiotic regimens in gynecology have been associated with preoperative administration. There is another portion of this antibiotic administration timing. If antibiotics with a short half-life are used for preoperative prophylaxis, a second dose should be administered in the operating room if the procedure lasts 4 hours or more. Those long operations without this antibiotic administration policy had higher rates of infection.[115]

5. A short-term prophylactic antibiotic regimen should be used. This is another deviation from most therapeutic antibiotic strategies in which those agents are prescribed for several days. There are many justifications for this short-term approach. The experimental study of Burke showed no benefit from antibiotics given 4 hours or more after the bacterial contamination had occurred.[86] Clinically studies have shown that single-dose antibiotic prophylaxis is effective. In abdominal hysterectomy, cefamandole and cefotaxime, given as a single dose, were effective in lowering the rates of postoperative pelvic infections.[116] Similarly, in pregnancy termination a single dose of oral doxycycline given preoperatively significantly lowered the postprocedure infection rate.[117] In patients undergoing abdominal and vaginal hysterectomy a study comparing a single preoperative dose of cefote-

tan to a regimen with a preoperative dose of cefoxitin plus two subsequent postoperative doses had equivalent results.[118] This is good evidence that this short-term strategy is effective. Why does this need to be emphasized? Operatively oriented physicians have a tendency to prolong prophylactic antibiotic treatment with the misguided logic that if a short course of antibiotics is good, a longer course will be even better. In one study of surgical antibiotic prophylaxis published in 1979, 80% of prophylactic antimicrobial drugs were given for at least 48 hours after an operation.[119] Fortunately the diagnosis-related group (DRG) reimbursement formulas have curtailed this practice. What are the concerns of prolonged antibiotic prophylaxis? The first is theoretical and is related to the assumption that prolonged exposure of the patient to antibiotics increases the likelihood that an allergy will develop or that the antibiotic will have a toxic effect on a susceptible organ system, such as the kidney, liver, or gastrointestinal tract. Of equal concern is that prolonged use of antibiotics could result in patient colonization and subsequent infection with more resistant organisms. This was seen on a neurosurgical service where prolonged prophylaxis increased resistant gram-negative aerobic infections,[108] and prolonged use of prophylactic antibiotics in unconscious patients on a medical service increased *Staphylococcus aureus* and gram-negative aerobic infections.[120] In at least one study of short-term use of antibiotic prophylaxis in gynecologic patients, no significant changes in bacterial flora were seen.[121]

6. Antibiotics with extensive broad-spectrum antibacterial action or specific activity against dangerous more resistant pathogens need not be used for prophylaxis. There are two reasons for this. Antibiotics with a lesser antibacterial spectrum were just as effective as prophylactic agents in abdominal hysterectomy as were those with a broader spectrum.[122] Additionally a cephalosporin with a longer half-life had no better results than the cephalosporin with a shorter half-life.[116] If they are demonstrated to be effective, antibiotics can be employed for prophylaxis that would not be the physician's first choice for treatment of a severe pelvic infection. This defines a strategy of limiting the use of new effective agents for those patients with a serious infection.

7. The benefits of prophylactic antibiotics must outweigh the dangers of the use of antibiotics. Adverse events do occur. In 1974 two deaths were reported following an anaphylactoid reaction to intravenous cephalothin.[123] One of these patients had a history of a penicillin allergy, which should highlight the avoidance of cephalosporins for prophylaxis in patients with a history of a penicillin allergy. The second case in this report, however, had no such history, and three cases of cefotetan-induced anaphylaxis occurred in women with no history of a penicillin allergy.[124] In addition to

these adverse events, two fatal cases of pseudomembranous colitis occurred in patients receiving multiple doses of prophylactic antibiotics.[125] It should be acknowledged that postoperative colitis occurred in the preantibiotic era.[126] Despite these serious complications the benefits of prophylactic antibiotics outweigh the risks for their use with abdominal hysterectomy, vaginal hysterectomy, pregnancy termination, and hysterosalpingography. No comparative study on antibiotic prophylaxis has been reported in women undergoing laparoscopic assisted vaginal hysterectomy and in those undergoing abdominal myomectomy.

8. There should be a rational strategy for antibiotic prophylaxis in patients undergoing gynecologic operative procedures.

   a. Abdominal hysterectomy. The predominant finding in women undergoing abdominal hysterectomy is the weak impact of prophylactic antibiotics in some studies[122] and the paucity of serious postoperative pelvic or wound infections in patients who have received prophylactic antibiotics. With this background there are a variety of effective prophylactic antibiotic regimens available. The following antibiotics can be given intravenously in the operating room just prior to the incision.

      (1) For the patient not allergic to penicillin:
         (a) Ampicillin 1–2 g
         (b) Cefazolin 1–2 g
         (c) Cefoxitin 1–2 g
         (d) Cefotetan 1–2 g
      (2) For the patient allergic to penicillin:
         (a) Clindamycin 900 mg
         (b) Metronidazole 1 g

   b. Vaginal hysterectomy: Most prophylactic regimens are effective, yet infrequent but serious postoperative adnexal abscesses have been reported with a first-generation cephalosporin, cefazolin,[127] cefamandole,[128] doxycycline,[127,128] and ampicillin.[129] Because of this, I believe antibiotics for prophylaxis should have good activity against gram-negative anaerobes. The following antibiotics can be given intravenously in the operating room just prior to the incision:

      (1) For the patient not allergic to penicillin:
         (a) Piperacillin 4 g
         (b) Cefoxitin 1–2 g
         (c) Cefotetan 1–2 g
      (2) For the patient allergic to penicillin:
         (a) Clindamycin 900 mg
         (b) Metronidazole 1 g

   c. Pregnancy termination: There are two important considerations for antibiotic prophylaxis for pregnancy termination. Most are done early in pregnancy as an outpatient office procedure without intravenous fluids. This requires reliance upon oral antibiotic prophylaxis. There is evidence that women colonized with either N. gonorrhoeae[130] or C. trachomatis[131] can have an increased rate of infectious complications. It is important that a culture screen of the lower genital tract be done before the procedure to identify patients who will need more than a single preoperative antibiotic dose. The following regimens can be given just prior to the procedure:

      (1) For the patient culture negative for N. gonorrhoeae and C. trachomatis:
         (a) Doxycycline 100 mg
         (b) Metronidazole 500 mg
      (2) For the patient culture positive for N. gonorrhoeae: ceftriaxone 250 mg IM
      (3) For the patient positive for C. trachomatis: doxycycline 100 mg PO prior to the procedure followed by 100 mg twice daily for 10 to 14 days

   d. Hysterosalpingography: The same regimen as used for pregnancy termination.

TREATMENT OF INFECTION: OBSTETRICS

Vaginitis

Many pregnant women have an irritating excessive vaginal discharge. This medical problem is poorly handled by many practitioners because it is not accurately diagnosed. There are many reasons for this: Physicians have been taught that vaginal yeast infections are more common in pregnancy; many physicians do not have a microscope in their office; and because of the pressure of the volume of antepartum patients to be seen in each practice session, many practitioners avoid a vaginal examination that delays the turnover of patients. Instead physicians or patient care helpers advise the patient to empirically use an over-the-counter (OTC) antiyeast preparation. This is inappropriate, for there are other causes of vaginitis, and one, bacterial vaginosis, has been associated with a higher rate of preterm labor.[80] To properly diagnose the cause of an excessive vaginal discharge in a pregnant woman requires a pH determination of vaginal fluids, a "whiff" test after vaginal secretions are placed in dilute potassium hydroxide (KOH) solution, and microscopic examination of vaginal secretions in saline and KOH. If the diagnosis remains in doubt after this immediate office evaluation, cultures or PCR tests can be done for Candida and Trichomonas. When a specific diagnosis is made, the following therapeutic interventions should be employed:

1. Candida vaginitis: This can be a troubling symptom complex for a pregnant woman. Local antifungal preparations containing azoles are usually effective and are safe for use during pregnancy. The oral agent, fluconazole (Diflucan), should not be used, however, because of reported fetal developmental abnormalities in pregnant women taking this drug.[132]

2. Bacterial vaginosis: All aspects of treatment have not yet been confirmed. There is good evidence that bacterial vaginosis is associated with preterm delivery,[80] but in the largest study reported to date, metronidazole treatment did not reduce the incidence of prematurity.[84] Bacterial vaginosis also is associated with a higher rate of postpartum endomyometritis.[133] For the patient less than 12 weeks' gestation the treatment of choice is clindamycin vaginal cream 2% 5 g intravaginally for 7 days; for the woman beyond 12 weeks' gestation, oral metronidazole 250 mg three times a day for 7 days.

3. *Trichomonas* vaginalis: This is another controversial area. Vaginal colonization with *Trichomonas* is associated with a higher incidence of preterm delivery.[81] Treatment with oral metronidazole, however, was associated with an even higher rate of prematurity. Until more definitive studies are done, oral metronidazole treatment should be avoided, if possible, in the *Trichomonas*-positive patient.[134]

Urinary Tract Infections

Bacteriuria

Despite screening for asymptomatic bacteriuria and treating those patients who have positive tests, urinary tract infections are the most common bacterial infection seen by the obstetrician. There is good evidence that this asymptomatic bacteriuria screening and antibiotic eradication do not alter the incidence of cystitis in antepartum patients.[74] The diagnosis should be confirmed with a clean voided urine culture with the proviso that colony counts of less than 10^5 E. coli are significant in symptomatic women.[135] Fortunately there is a wide choice of effective antibiotics that can be used:

1. Ampicillin 500 mg PO four times a day, before meals and at bedtime, for 3 days.
2. Cephalexin 500 mg PO four times a day, before meals and at bedtime, for 3 days.

As an alternative,

1. Trimethoprim/sulfamethoxazole (TMP-SMX) 160/800 mg PO twice a day for 3 days. This is a category C drug for pregnant patients, and it should be discontinued if the patient goes into labor.
2. Nitrofurantoin: Macrodantin 50 mg four times a day for 3 days or Macrobid 100 mg twice a day for 3 days.

The quinolones are contraindicated during pregnancy because they have been associated with cartilage erosions in the weight-bearing joints of young animals.[136]

Pyelonephritis

Patients with pyelonephritis present a more complex set of therapeutic problems for the physician. They are usually sicker, and they need to be closely monitored for any indications of preterm labor. In fact, one study showed increased uterine activity in the first hour or two after the administration of antibiotics in these patients.[137] Fortunately with treatment and hydration these contractions usually cease. Occasionally patients become seriously ill and present with septic shock and acute respiratory distress syndrome.[138] These patients are appropriately cared for in intensive care units. These problems seem to be associated with the use of tocolytic agents and overhydration, so tocolytic agents should be reserved for the patient with documented cervical changes.[138] There is a wide spectrum of clinical presentations in patients with pyelonephritis of pregnancy and few controlled studies of treatment, so that treatments of necessity are empiric. One study defined low-risk patients as those without any evidence of labor during a 2-hour observation period and no other underlying disease.[139] These women were given 2 g of intravenous ceftriaxone, followed by a daily intramuscular 2-g dose of ceftriaxone until they were afebrile and flank tenderness was gone, and then on the basis of sensitivity studies, oral antibiotics were given for 10 days.[139] Of 34 patients treated this way, four required hospital admission, and one had a recurrent upper urinary tract infection. On most services, patients with pyelonephritis will be admitted, given sufficient hydration to ensure a urine output of greater than 30 ml per hour, and treated with intravenous antibiotics. This is an important therapeutic consideration. At least one study documented diminished renal function in women with acute pyelonephritis that was probably related to excessive insensible fluid loss prior to hospital admission.[140] I personally have never favored combination antibiotics for the usual single bacterial species pyelonephritis infection. Ampicillin plus gentamicin has been suggested because of concerns about E. coli resistance to ampicillin,[141] but this disregards the higher levels of antibiotics achieved in the kidneys and urine than are accounted for by standard laboratory susceptibility testing. At least one study demonstrated higher rates of cure in urinary infections with a lower rate of serum bacteriostatic activity than was necessary in other sites of infection.[142] My choices of treatment would be

1. Ampicillin 2 g IV every 6 hours or
2. Cefazolin 1 g IV every 8 hours

For the seriously ill patient it would be appropriate to add gentamicin 1.5 mg/kg IV every 8 hours, with the option that one of the antibiotics can be discontinued when sensitivity tests are available. The choices for the penicillin-allergic patient are limited, but if necessary, TMP-SMX should be given in pregnancy, although not to the patient in labor, and the quinolones are contraindicated in pregnancy.[136] The best alternatives are the aminoglycosides alone or in combination with erythromycin on the slim chance that you can keep this seriously ill patient's urine alkaline and thus increase the effectiveness of erythromycin.[143]

Respiratory Tract Infections

Respiratory tract infections occur with some frequency in pregnant women, particularly in the winter months. Pneumonia is uncommon; one recent study noted 1.5 cases per 1000 deliveries.[144] It is hard to document specific treatment strategies because controlled studies have not been done, and therapeutic considerations are changing because of the increasing resistance of *Streptococcus pneumoniae* to antibiotics.[25] There are a number of indicated diagnostic and therapeutic approaches for the pregnant patient with pneumonia. Until specific guidelines are established by prospective study, these patients should be treated as inpatients. Attempts should be made to determine the microbiologic cause of the disease. Recommended diagnostic studies include blood cultures and Gram stain and culture of expectorated sputum.[145] These cultures should be obtained before any antibiotic treatment is started if possible, because prior antibiotic treatment eliminates the chance of isolation of the pneumococcus.[146] In addition there is a scoring system that assigns risk and can be used to determine what patients should be admitted.[145] Women patients get lower scores than men, but pregnancy was not considered in this scheme. In contrast to this approach, one recent obstetric study had excellent results with a regimen of intravenous erythromycin 500 mg every 6 hours.[144] Another contemporary study, however, found erythromycin resistance to the pneumococcus in 15% of the isolates.[25] This is the reason that adequate expectorated sputum should be obtained for culture with alternate antibiotics used if a resistant strain is recovered in a patient not responding to therapy.

Chorioamnionitis

Chorioamnionitis does occur in pregnant women, usually after prolonged rupture of the membranes. The availability of antibiotics effective against the organisms that most commonly cause newborn infections, that is, the group B streptococcus, *E. coli*, *Haemophilus influenzae*, and *L. monocytogenes*, has resulted in reports in which there were good survival figures in newborns and mothers with this disease.[147] New concerns have been raised, however, by the reports of an increased incidence of cerebral palsy among the term infants delivered by mothers with chorioamnionitis.[148] How this will influence future therapy is a work in progress. Options to be analyzed include immediate cesarean section or the addition of steroids that cross the placenta to be used with antibiotics in these patients. When the diagnosis of chorioamnionitis is made, intravenous antibiotics should be administered with the strategy of covering the previously cited organisms most commonly involved with newborn infection. My therapy of choice is a combination of intravenous antibiotics:

1. Ampicillin 2 g initially followed by 1 g every 4 hours until delivery plus gentamicin 1.5 mg/kg every 8 hours until delivery
2. For the penicillin-allergic patient: cefoxitin 2 g initially followed by 1 g every 8 hours until delivery
3. For the penicillin-allergic patient in whom *L. monocytogenes* is suspected: erythromycin 500 mg every 6 hours until delivery

Postpartum Infections

Recent trends in obstetric care have altered the presentations of postpartum infection and have modified strategies of care. Many of these infections will first be manifested after the patient has been discharged from the hospital. After an uncomplicated vaginal delivery, patients go home 1 to 2 days later, and after an uncomplicated cesarean section, women are home 2 to 4 days after delivery. In addition large numbers of patients, over 1 million a year, receive antibiotics before delivery to prevent early onset newborn sepsis caused by the group B streptococcus,[32] and nearly all of the more than 20% of pregnant women who undergo cesarean section receive prophylactic antibiotics after the cord is clamped. A prolonged course of antibiotics is given to most women with premature rupture of the membranes, and this decreases the incidence of postpartum endomyometritis, even when corticosteroids are given as well.[149] Some patients will still become infected, and most of these postpartum infections will be manifested by a temperature elevation at night[150] so that empiric oral antibiotic therapy is the rule, not the exception.

Mastitis

With these current practice realities in mind, there are observations about postpartum infections that should help to guide treatment strategies. For the obstetrician with a high percentage of women breast-feeding, mastitis is a common problem. Diagnosis over the phone is seldom difficult, for these women usually are febrile with an inflamed, tender breast. Although a wide spectrum of many different organisms can be recovered by culture, my concern is the coagulase-positive staphylococcus. Patients should be encouraged to continue breast-feeding and should receive these oral treatment options:

1. Cephalexin 500 mg four times a day for 10 days
2. For the penicillin-allergic patients: clindamycin 150 mg four times a day for 10 days

I recommend these regimens because they offer good coverage against the coagulase-positive staphylococcus and offer the best protection against the development of a breast abscess. There is one study, however, comparing cephradine with good activity against staphylococci to amoxicillin with poor antistaphylococci activity, and the results were equivalent.[151]

Endomyometritis

Another common postpartum infection is an endomyometritis. Risk factors for this infection are well known. These uterine infections following vaginal delivery are less frequent[91] and less severe[152] than those following a cesarean section performed on a patient in labor. This will have an influence on our choice of antibiotics in these patients.

All of these new practice trends have to be acknowledged and accounted for in any strategy of antibiotic treatment of a patient with postpartum endomyometritis. A starting point would be to avoid retreatment of the patient with the same antibiotic or family of antibiotics given to the patient in labor or at the time of delivery. This is a theoretical concern because no large-scale clinical studies have been done. It is based upon the awareness that in this patient the endomyometritis occurred despite prior exposure to these antibiotics, raising the possibility of an infection due to an organism resistant to that antibiotic. With this safeguard in mind, there are four groups of women who can develop an endomyometritis:

1. Low-risk patients who manifest the first signs of infection as an inpatient. These include women who have had an uncomplicated vaginal delivery or an elective cesarean section, not in labor, with a presenting temperature spike of 39.4°C (103°F) orally or less. They should have a complete physical examination, including a pelvic examination, and cultures of the lochia for aerobic bacteria. Single-agent intravenous antibiotics can be given for 3 to 5 days until the patient has been afebrile for more than 24 hours. These women should not be sent home on oral antibiotics, for there is no evidence this improves the outcome.[153] The following antibiotic regimens can be used:

   a. Cefoxitin 2 g every 6 hours*
   b. Cefotetan 2 g every 12 hours*
   c. Ampicillin-sulbactam 3 g every 6 hours†
   d. Ticarillin-clavulanic acid, 3.1 g every 6 hours†

   For the penicillin-allergic patient:

   a. Clindamycin 900 mg plus gentamicin 1.5 mg/kg every 8 hours
   b. Metronidazole 500 mg every 12 hours plus gentamicin 1.5 mg/kg every 8 hours

2. High-risk patients who manifest the first signs of infection as an inpatient. These include women who have had an operative vaginal delivery, a cesarean section in labor or with ruptured membranes, excessive bleeding postpartum, a vaginal hematoma, or a presenting fever above 39.4°C (103°F). These women should be examined and have lochia culture and a blood culture for aerobic organisms. A recent article questioned the value of blood culture in patients with chorioamnionitis,[154] but for me any blood isolate helps to provide a focus for the antibiotic therapy. A number of intravenous antibiotic regimens are acceptable. These can be given for 3 to 5 days, and no oral antibiotics are necessary.[155]

   a. Clindamycin 900 mg every 8 hours and gentamicin 1.5 mg/kg every 8 hours. One recent study indicated that once daily dosing of gentamicin is effective in obstetric patients.[156]

   Single antibiotic regimens are effective if the agents have good gram-negative anaerobic coverage.[157] Acceptable regimens include the following:

   b. Cefoxitin 2 g every 6 hours*
   c. Cefotetan 2 g every 12 hours*
   d. Ampicillin-sulbactam 3 g every 6 hours†
   e. Ticarcillin-clavulanic acid 3.1 g every 6 hours†

   For the patient presenting with a high fever, greater than 40°C (104°F) the physician should consider the possibility of a group A streptococcal infection.[158] The drug of choice in this situation is clindamycin, not penicillin, for it avoids the Eagle effect, the inhibition of penicillin activity caused by the high numbers of organisms at the infection site.[159]

3. Low-risk patients who manifest the first signs of infection after discharge from the hospital. These are the same patients as noted in no.1. Oral antibiotics can be started with the proviso that the patient will soon be examined. Again, an antibiotic different from any given during labor or at the time of delivery should be prescribed.

   a. Metronidazole 500 mg twice daily
   b. Clindamycin 300 mg four times a day

   For regimen "a," ceftriaxone 250 mg IM can be given as well when the patient is first seen in the office. The office examination is particularly important in women who have had a cesarean section. A frequent cause of a late developing postpartum infection is an abdominal wound infection.[160] Identification of the infection, followed by incision and drainage, usually achieves a cure.

4. High-risk patients who manifest the first signs of infection after discharge from the hospital require more focused care. These include all the high-risk patients noted in group 2. They should be examined to determine the site and the extent of infection with intravenous antibiotics even after appropriate cultures have been obtained. I favor hospital admission with the same antibiotic choices as noted in 2, but if home intravenous therapy is available, this can be used to avoid separation of the mother and the newborn.[161]

---

*Should not be prescribed for women who received cephalosporin prophylaxis.

†Should not be prescribed for women who received penicillin prophylaxis in labor.

TREATMENT OF INFECTION: GYNECOLOGIC

Vaginitis

The infection most frequently seen by the gynecologist in office practice is vaginitis. Some have estimated that patients with a complaint of an abnormal vaginal discharge comprise up to one-third of the patients seen in an outpatient setting.

Patients with a vaginitis too often have an incomplete workup and inappropriate care. There are many reasons for this: Many physicians do not have a microscope in their office, and an equivalent number do not have testing paper to determine vaginal pH. Too many depend on the gross appearance of the vaginal discharge or a phone description to initiate treatment. A major problem is that vaginitis does not have a high diagnostic or therapeutic priority among most practicing physicians. This is unfortunate, for an accurate diagnosis gives the best opportunity for a clinical cure.

Candida Vaginitis

Physicians have many misconceptions about *Candida* vaginitis. They believe it is easy to diagnose, and they have communicated to patients the belief that self-diagnosis by the patient is accurate as well. In fact two studies of health care workers showed a low specificity for the accuracy of an office microscopic diagnosis of vaginal candidiasis, 42%[162] and 50.8%.[163] More cultures for *Candida* should be done by physicians, particularly in the patient with recurrent infections. The culture confirms the accuracy of the office diagnosis, and it can be a great help for the detection of the patient with non-*albicans* vaginitis. Fortunately there are a number of effective treatment regimens for the patient with *Candida albicans* vaginitis. These include vaginal creams, suppositories, and tablets containing azoles and the oral agent fluconazole (Diflucan), which is effective with a single oral dose of 150 mg.[2] The patient with *Candida glabrata* vaginitis is a more difficult therapeutic problem. The most effective regimen is 600 mg of boric acid in a gelatin capsule inserted vaginally at bedtime for 14 days.[164] For all patients with a yeast vaginitis, treatment of the male is usually not necessary, but in a woman with documented recurrent yeast infections, the male should be examined, cultured, and treated with local azole cream, particularly if the male has symptomatic balanitis or penile dermatitis.[2]

Bacterial Vaginosis

Bacterial vaginosis is an easy diagnosis to confirm if the patient has any three findings of a homogeneous discharge: alkaline vaginal pH, a positive whiff test when vaginal secretions are added to potassium hydroxide, and on microscopic examination of the saline preparation, more than 20% of the epithelial cells are covered with bacteria (clue cells).[165] For the physician without a microscope a vaginal smear can be obtained and sent to the laboratory for Gram stain and microscopic examination.[166] The major problem with this Gram stain strategy is the delay until a diagnosis is made. When the diagnosis is established, either oral or vaginal treatment with clindamycin or metronidazole are effective. I favor vaginal therapy with either:

1. Clindamycin vaginal cream 2% at bedtime for 7 days. Recently, clindamycin vaginal suppositories have been introduced that can be used at bedtime for 5 days.
2. Metronidazole vaginal cream, one dose at bedtime for 5 days.

There is no evidence that treating the man improves the cure rates, but in women with recurrent bacterial vaginosis, I suggest the women, in addition to their local vaginal treatment, have their partners use a condom.

Trichomonas Vaginitis

Trichomonas vaginitis is less common than *Candida* vaginitis or bacterial vaginosis. It should be suspected in women with an excessive alkaline vaginal discharge and a vaginal smear loaded with white blood cells. The microscopic examination is not a sensitive mode of diagnosis,[167] and if *Trichomonas* is suspected and no trichomonads are seen, a culture or PCR test[168] for *Trichomonas* should be done. This infectious disease entity requires simultaneous treatment of the man and woman with metronidazole to prevent reinfection. I favor 2 g PO with one dose and appropriate warnings about no alcohol ingestion for at least 24 hours. Some women are infected with less susceptible strains of *trichomonas vaginalis*. The CDC has suggested an oral regimen of 2 g a day for 3 to 5 days.[2] In patients not cured with this regimen, I have used intravenous metronidazole 4 g a day for 4 to 5 days.

Other Causes of Vaginitis

Too little emphasis is placed on other causes of vaginitis by most gynecologists, but awareness of other possibilities can avoid therapeutic missteps by the physician. The error most frequently made by clinicians seeing a patient with persistent symptoms who does not have any of the three aforementioned infections is to get a vaginal culture and then treat one of the aerobic bacterial isolates with antibiotics. This is misguided, for the vagina is never sterile; bacteria will always be recovered from asymptomatic and symptomatic women; and antibiotics may cause other problems.

Allergic Vaginitis

The most common other cause of a persistent or recurrent vaginitis is an allergic vaginitis. This entity has been identified by the presence of IgE in vaginal secretions.[169] The three most common causes for this surface vaginal reaction are an allergy to the male ejaculate, to the non-oxynol 9 in the spermicide used with a diaphragm and condom, and to the chemical propylene glycol, a preservative present in most vaginal creams and suppositories. A hint of the type of allergy can be gained by a history of worsening symptoms when the woman is exposed to these entities. The patient's symptoms can be lessened by the male use of a condom or avoidance of patient contact with non-oxynol 9 or propylene glycol and the concomitant use of oral antihistamines.

Desquamative Vaginitis

Another chronic type of vaginitis, desquamative vaginitis, most commonly is seen in Ashkenazi Jewish women. Women with desquamative vaginitis have an excessive purulent vaginal discharge, an alkaline pH, and a smear loaded with white blood cells.[170] They have no mucopus when cervical mucus is examined and often have a vaginal culture with heavy growth of group B streptococcus. These women can often benefit from a 2-week course of intravaginal clindamycin cream 2%.

Vulvar Vestibulitis

Another often-missed diagnosis is vulvar vestibulitis (VV).[171] The chief complaint is pain at any attempts at coital entry, but 75% of patients also have an excessive vaginal discharge. Too commonly the physician following the rote of a rapid pelvic examination inserts a speculum to evaluate the discharge without examining the vulva. The cause of this syndrome is not known, but one recent study found that 40% of the women with VV had a gene polymorphism in which they did not produce interleukin-1-RA.[172]

Toxic Shock Syndrome

Toxic shock syndrome is a fearsome life-threatening clinical entity in which patients have multiple organ system insults. It was first described and named by Todd et al in 1978.[173] Subsequent studies have shown that it is caused by a particular strain of *Staphylococcus*, which produces a specific toxin, TSS-1, and this toxin wreaks havoc in susceptible women with no demonstrable antibodies to TSS-1.[174] An outbreak of cases in the early 1980s seemed linked to the introduction of a new superabsorbent tampon, which created a vaginal environment favorable to this bacterium's replication.[175] The withdrawal of this tampon from the commercial market was followed by a precipitous drop in the number of reported cases.[176] Seriously ill patients in shock, with a desquamative skin lesion and abnormal laboratory studies of such organ systems as the kidney and liver, however, are still being seen in gynecologic practices. In fact one study in Colorado using an enhanced passive reporting system showed a continuing frequency of the disease. The major difference has been that cases have been recognized and treated earlier.[177] The prerequisites are still there. A patient without TSS-1 antibodies with an infection of a *S. aureus* strain that produces TSS-1 can develop toxic shock syndrome. Examples include a postpartum or postoperative infection.[178] In addition a toxic shock–like syndrome has been reported in patients with a group A streptococcal infection.[179] Treatment should include drainage of an infected wound if present, appropriate intravenous hydration, and antibiotic treatment with clindamycin 900 mg IV every 8 hours.

Pelvic Inflammatory Disease

Pelvic inflammatory disease (PID) remains the biggest dichotomy between most house officers' urban training experience and their subsequent patient contacts in private practice. During residency, PID is the obvious diagnosis for the febrile patient seen in the emergency room with an exquisitely tender pelvis or the critically ill patient with pelvic masses who is admitted because of the suspicion of a pelvic abscess. In neither of these scenarios is the diagnosis in question; the only therapeutic quandries are the choice of antibiotics and the clinical decision of whether an operation is indicated.

In contrast the problem for the physician in private practice will be to make the diagnosis in patients with minimal or no symptoms. Patients can have few symptoms associated with PID early in the course of a *N. gonorrhoeae* infection. Instead the clinician should be alert to seemingly unrelated problems that could be early signs of a gonococcal infection. One study of sexually active women seen in an emergency room found a high incidence of positive *N. gonorrhoeae* cervical cultures in women with symptoms of urinary urgency and frequency and no significant bacterial growth on a urine culture, no abnormal vaginal bleeding, no evident pelvic abnormalities on pelvic examination, and no new vaginal discharge.[101] In such patients a test for *N. gonorrhoeae* should be done. Most asymptomatic or minimally symptomatic patients with a pelvic infection will be infected with *C. trachomatis*. The heat shock protein (HSP) of *C. trachomatis* elicits tubal and endometrial damage because of its similarity to the HSP of human pelvic epithelium.[180] The CDC has attempted to confront the problem of minimal symptomatology by easing the criteria needed by the physician to make the diagnosis of a pelvic infection.[2] There is merit to this, and physicians should be aware that a sensitive diagnostic test in an afebrile patient who has an active pelvic infection is an immediate examination of vaginal secretions in a saline wet preparation under the microscope. The presence of many white blood cells makes a strong case for the diagnosis of pelvic infection.[181] These are the patients who should be tested for *C. trachomatis*, and the standard in the United States should be the most sensitive and specific test, the PCR.[88] Increasing physician awareness of the paucity of symptoms in women with pelvic inflammatory disease is not enough. Women need to be educated about the dangers of unprotected intercourse with new sexual partners, and the United States needs the development of self-testing PCR kits to be made available to an educated public. Studies have shown that patient self-collection of an introital sample with PCR testing is every bit as sensitive as the same PCR testing when a physician gathers a sample using a speculum.[182]

In the past there has been much discussion about the best therapeutic approach to these patients, with the twin goals of an immediate response to antibiotic treatment and the long-term outcome of patient tubes so that a normal intrauterine pregnancy can be achieved in the future. I personally favor inpatient care, for with intravenous antibiotics, you can be assured that the patient will receive the antibiotics ordered. For the physician making this decision, various intravenous regimens are endorsed by the CDC (Table 27–8).[2] There are difficulties in making the decision for in-hospital treatment: There have been no prospective comparative studies reported that demonstrate either short-term or long-term benefit to hospitalization as compared to outpatient therapy, and in their office practices, nearly all physicians recognizing an asymptomatic or minimally symptomatic patient with this infection will opt for outpatient therapy. In their minds this woman is just not sick enough for admission. Again, various outpatient antibiotic regimens are endorsed by the CDC (Table 27–9),[2] and these have the same problems of analysis as noted for the inpatient treatment options. The CDC recommends a clinical assessment of the severity of infection in the decision to admit a patient; their criteria for admission are listed in Table 27–10. At least one obstetric-gynecologic infectious disease group has raised concerns about these admission guidelines. They believe patients to be admitted should include teenagers, who have a risk for subsequent tubal damage and who are not the most conscientious people about taking medication when they do not feel ill.[183]

TABLE 27–8 ■ **Intravenous Antibiotic Regimens Endorsed by the Centers for Disease Control and Prevention for the Treatment of Pelvic Inflammatory Disease**

A. Cefotetan 2 g IV q 12 h
   or
   Cefoxitin 2 g IV q 6 h plus Doxycyline 100 mg IV or PO q 12 h
B. Clindamycin 900 mg IV q 8 h
   plus
   Gentamicin loading dose IV 2 mg/kg followed by maintenance dose 1.5 mg/kg q 8 h. Single daily dosing may be substituted.
C. Alternative Regimens
   1. Ofloxacin 400 mg IV q 12 h plus metronidazole 500 mg IV q 8 h
   2. Ampicillin-Sulbactam 3 g IV q 6 h plus doxycycline 100 mg IV or PO q 12 h

TABLE 27–9 ■ **Outpatient Therapies Endorsed by the Centers for Disease Control and Prevention for the Treatment of Pelvic Inflammatory Disease**

A. Ofloxacin 400 mg PO bid × 14 d or levofloxacin 500 mg orally once daily with or without metronidazole 500 mg PO bid × 14 d
B. Ceftriazone 250 mg IM (one dose)
   or
   Cefoxitin 2 g IM plus probenecid 1 g PO (each, one dose) or other third generation cephalosporaid (ceftizoxime or cefotaxime)
   plus
   Doxycycline 100 mg PO bid × with or without metronidazole 500 mg PO bid for 14 d

Note: I do not favor regimen A or B if metronidazole is not given, because it gives too limited coverage of gram-negative anaerobes.

TABLE 27–10 ■ **Centers for Disease Control and Prevention Criteria for Hospitalization of Patients with Pelvic Inflammatory Disease**

1. Surgical emergencies such as appendicitis cannot be excluded.
2. The patient is pregnant.
3. The patient does not respond to oral antibiotic therapy.
4. The patient is unable to follow or tolerate an outpatient oral regimen.
5. The patient is thought to have severe illness, nausea and vomiting, or high fever.
6. The patient is thought to have a tubo-ovarian abscess.
7. The patient is immunodeficient.

Note: I believe all teenagers should also be admitted.

Infection After Abortion

The current heated political debate about a woman's right to terminate a pregnancy strays from an important fact of infection after abortion. Voices on one side sponsor the mother's choice, whereas their opponents want to stop the killing of the unborn. One reality that needs to be emphasized is that abortions will be done, whether they are legal or not. In the United States the major impact on maternal health with the legalization of abortion was the near elimination of maternal deaths, the majority of which were due to infection.[184] In contrast is the example of Brazil from 1978 to 1987, a society in which there was no national family planning program, and abortion was highly restricted. This resulted in heavy reliance upon illegal abortions to control excess fertility, and there was a 172% increase in abortion-related mortality in the 10-year time period studied.[185] Whatever the law, abortions will continue, and some women will develop an infection afterward.

Currently women who develop an infection after abortion are a population group that usually responds to antibiotic therapy.[152] Fortunately most pregnancy terminations are now done early in pregnancy. The more advanced the pregnancy, the higher the risk of infection, in part because of the higher risk of uterine perforation and retained tissue.[186] The care of these women is straightforward. They need to be carefully examined to determine the extent of the infection, including the use of vaginal ultrasound to see if there is any evidence of retained tissue or a uterine perforation. Endocervical cultures should be obtained as well as a PCR test for *C. trachomatis*. Most of these patients are not seriously ill and have no evidence of retained tissue or uterine damage. They can be treated as outpatients with oral ofloxacin 400 mg twice a day and oral metronidazole 500 mg twice a day for 5 days. The ofloxacin should be given for 14 days if this patient tests positive for *C. trachomatis*. More seriously ill patients should be admitted and blood cultures obtained. Criteria for admission include any of the following: a late abortion, i.e., beyond 12 weeks' gestation, an oral temperature above 38°C (100.4°F), and evidence of retained tissue or a uterine perforation. Intravenous antibiotics should be administered, clindamycin 900 mg every 8 hours and gentamicin 1.5 mg/kg every 8 hours. Any retained tissue should be removed by curettage as soon as possible after antibiotics are begun. If there is evidence of abscess formation, intravenous metronidazole 500 mg every 8 hours should be substituted for the clindamycin, and penicillin G 5 MU every 6 hours should be added to the regimen. Rarely, more extensive operative care will be needed including drainage or aspiration of a pelvic abscess or hysterectomy in the patient with extensive uterine damage and infection who is not responding to antibiotic treatment.

Postoperative Infections

The gynecologic patient with a postoperative infection presents a different set of diagnostic and therapeutic problems for the practitioner today. The widespread use of prophylactic antibiotics has reduced the incidence of postoperative site infections, but their prior use will influence subsequent antibiotic selection. The increasing use of laparoscopic operative procedures and early discharge policies means that most of these women will be first evaluated after hospital discharge in the physician's office or the emergency room. Because of personal and insurance pressures the physician will be inclined to treat all but the most seriously ill as outpatients.

The initial examination should be complete to determine the severity and the extent of the infection. Abdominal wound and pelvic operative sites should be examined for the presence of any collection that is amenable to drainage. Drainage alone is often sufficient for a cure, and the drainage fluid can be submitted for culture. If antibiotics are thought to be advisable because no drainage fluid is obtained, oral ciprofloxacin 500 mg twice a day and oral metronidazole 500 mg twice a day can be given for 5 days. More seriously ill patients should be hospitalized and treated with intravenous antibiotics.

There are three categories of patients with postoperative infections that need to be identified and treated with different strategies: The first and least common is the sick patient with an oral temperature above 39°C (102.2°F) and no physical or imaging findings of an abscess. My concern in this patient is a group A streptococcal infection.[158] Operative site and blood cultures should be obtained. Because of the unfavorable impact of the Eagle effect on the effectiveness of systemic penicillin therapy,[159] I favor intravenous antibiotics, clindamycin 900 mg every 8 hours and gentamicin 1.5 mg/kg every 8 hours. The second category is the most common, patients who will have marked induration of the operative sites and often infected fluid collections amenable to extraperitoneal drainage. These women can be effectively treated by simple drainage coupled with a variety of single intravenous antibiotic regimens including ampicillin-sulbactam 3 g every 6 hours, cefotaxime 1 g every 8 hours, cefotetan 2 g every 12 hours, cefoxitin 2 g every 6 hours, imipenem-cilastatin 500 mg every 8 hours, meropenem 500 mg every 8 hours, piperacillin 4 g every 6 hours, or piperacillin-tazobactam 3.375 g every 6 hours.[188] Again, physicians should not use the same family of antibiotics for treatment that was used for prophylaxis. Finally, there is a small group of women who have evidence of a pelvic abscess on imaging studies that is not amenable to extraperitoneal drainage. For these women I favor penicillin G 5 MU every 6 hours, gentamicin 1.5 mg/kg every 8 hours, and metronidazole 500 mg every 8 hours. In these sick women, peak and trough levels of gentamicin should be obtained to ensure therapeutic levels have been achieved.[189] If complete resolution of the infection is not achieved, needle aspiration of the abscess or laparoscopy or laporotomy to drain the abscess should be used.

REFERENCES

1. Centers for Disease Control: Congenital syphilis—United States, 1983–85. JAMA 1986;256:3206–3208.
2. Centers for Disease Control and Prevention: 1998 Guidelines for treatment of sexually transmitted diseases. MMWR Morb Mortal Wkly Rep 1998;47(RR-1):28–41.
3. Rolfs RT, Joesoef MR, Hendershot EF, et al: A randomized trial of enhanced therapy for early syphilis in patients with and without human immunodeficiency virus infection. N Engl J Med 1997;337:307–314.
4. Prenatal viral and parasitic infections: ACOG Pract Bull 2000;20:1–13.
5. Kimball AC, Kean BH, Fuchs F: Congenital toxoplasmosis: a prospective study of 4,048 obstetric patients. Am J Obstet Gynecol 1971;111:211–218.
6. Guerina NG, Hsu H-W, Meissner HC, et al: Neonatal serologic screening and early treatment for congenital *Toxoplasma gondii* infection. N Engl J Med 1999;3330:1858–1863.
7. Sever JL, Ellenberg JH, Ley AC, et al: Toxoplasmosis: Maternal and pediatric findings in 23,000 pregnancies. Pediatrics 1988;82:181–192.
8. Department of Health and Human Services: FDA Public Health Advisory: Limitations of *Toxoplasma* IgM commercial test kits. 25 July 1997.

9. Grover CM, Thulliez P, Remington JS, et al: Rapid prenatal diagnosis of congenital *Toxoplasma* infection by using polymerase chain reaction and amniotic fluid. J Clin Microbiol 1990;28:2297–2310.

10. Daffos F, Forestier F, Cupella-Pavlovsky M, et al: Prenatal management of 746 pregnancies at risk for congenital toxoplasmosis. N Engl J Med 1988;318:271–275.

11. Centers for Disease Control: US PHS/IDSA guidelines for the prevention of opportunistic infections in persons infected with human immunodeficiency virus: A summary. MMWR Morb Mortal Wkly Rep 1995;45:1–34.

12. Foulon W, Naessens A, Derde MP: Evaluation of the possibilities for preventing congenital toxoplasmosis. Am J Perinatol 1994;11:57–62.

13. Centers for Disease Control and Prevention: Tetanus surveillance—United States, 1991–1994. MMWR Morb Mortal Wkly Rep 1997;46:15–25.

14. Vitek CR, Bogatyreva EY, Wharton M: Diphtheria surveillance and control in the former Soviet Union and the newly independent states. J Infect Dis 2000;181:S23–S26.

15. Centers for Disease Control: Diphtheria acquired by US citizens in the Russian Federation and Ukraine—1994. MMWR 1995;44:237, 243–244.

16. Landsberger EJ, Hager WD, Grossman JH III: Successful management of varicella pneumonia complicating pregnancy. A report of three cases. J Reprod Med 1986;31:311–314.

17. Pastuszak AL, Levy M, Schick B, et al: Outcome of the maternal varicella infection in the first 20 weeks of pregnancy. N Engl J Med 1994;330:901–905.

18. Smegmo RA, Asperilla MO: Use of acyclovir for varicella pneumonia during pregnancy. Obstet Gynecol 1991;78:1112–1116.

19. Centers for Disease Control and Prevention: Prevention of varicella. MMWR Morb Mortal Wkly Rep 1999;48:(RR-6):1–5.

20. Smith WJ, Jackson LA, Walts DH, et al: Prevention of chicken pox in reproductive age women: Cost effectiveness of routine prenatal screening with post-partum vaccination of susceptibles. Obstet Gynecol 1998;92:535–545.

21. Harris JW: Influenza occurring in pregnant women: A statistical study of thirteen hundred and fifty cases. JAMA 1919;72:978–980.

22. Freeman DW, Barno A: Deaths from Asian influenza associated with pregnancy. Am J Obstet Gynecol 1959;78:1172–1175.

23. Centers for Disease Control and Prevention: Prevention and control of influenza. MMWR Morb Mortal Wkly Rep 1999;48:(RR-4):1–28.

24. Finland M, Dublin TD: Pneumococcal pneumonias complicating pregnancy and the puerperium. JAMA 1939;122:1027–1033.

25. Whitney CG, Farley MM, Hadler J, et al: Increasing prevalence of multidrug-resistant *Streptococcus pneumoniae* in the United States. N Engl J Med 2000;343:1917–1924.

26. Centers for Disease Control and Prevention: Prevention of pneumococcal disease. MMWR 1997;46:(RR-8):1–24.

27. Zangwill KM, Schuchat A, Wenger JD: Group B streptococcal disease in the United States, 1990: Report from a multistage active surveillance system. MMWR Morb Mortal Wkly Rep 1992;41:25–32.

28. Goodman JR, Berg RL, Gribble RK, et al: Longitudinal study of group B streptococcus carriage in pregnancy. Infect Dis Obstet Gynecol 1997;5:237–243.

29. Schuchat A, Whitney C, Zangwill K: Prevention of perinatal group B streptococcal disease: A public health perspective. MMWR Morb Mortal Wkly Rep 1996;45:1–24.

30. Hager WD, Schuchat A, Gibbs R, et al: Prevention of perinatal group B streptococcal infection: Current controversies. Obstet Gynecol 2000;96:141–145.

31. Yow MD, Mason EO, Leeds LF, et al: Ampicillin prevents intrapartum transmission of group B streptococcus. JAMA 1979;241:1245–1247.

32. Ledger WJ: CDC guidelines for prevention of perinatal group B streptococcal disease: Are they appropriate? Infect Dis Clin Pract 1998;7:188–193.

33. Towers CV, Carr MH, Padilla G, et al: Potential consequences of widespread antepartal use of ampicillin. Am J Obstet Gynecol 1998;179:879–883.

34. Rouse DJ, Andrews WW, Lin F-YC, et al: Antibiotic susceptibility profile of group B streptococcus acquired vertically. Obstet Gynecol 1998;92:931–934.

35. Burman LG, Christensen P, Christensen K, et al: Prevention of excess neonatal morbidity associated with group B streptococci by vaginal chlorhexidine coinfection during labour. The Swedish Chlorhexidine Study Group. Lancet 1992;340:65–69.

36. Linnan MJ, Moscola L, Lou XD, et al: Epidemic listeriosis associated with Mexican-style cheese. N Engl J Med 1988;319:823–828.

37. Lorber B: Listeriosis. Clin Infect Dis 1997;24:1–11.

38. Gregg NM: Congenital cataract following German measles in the mother. Trans Ophthalmol Soc Aust 1941;3:35–46.

39. Schluter WW, Reef SE, Redd SC, et al: Changing epidemiology of congenital rubella syndrome in the United States. J Infect Dis 1998;178:636–641.

40. Centers for Disease Control and Prevention: Congenital rubella syndrome among the Amish—Pennsylvania, 1991–1992. MMWR Morb Mortal Wkly Rep 1992;41:468–471.

41. Howson CP, Katz M, Johnston RB Jr, et al: Chronic arthritis after rubella vaccination. Clin Infect Dis 1992;15:307–312.

42. Demmier GJ: Summary of a workshop on surveillance for congenital cytomegalovirus disease. Rev Infect Dis 1991;13:315–329.

43. Fowler KB, Stagno S, Pass RF, et al: The outcome of congenital cytomegalovirus infection in relation to maternal antibody status. N Engl J Med 1992;326:663–667.

44. Breining MK, Kingsley LA, Armstrong JA, et al: Epidemiology of genital herpes in Pittsburgh: Serologic, sexual and racial correlates of apparent and inapparent herpes simplex infections. J Infect Dis 1990;162:299–305.

45. Brown ZA, Benedetti J, Ashley R, et al: Neonatal herpes simplex virus infection in relation to asymptomatic maternal infection at the time of labor. N Engl J Med 1991;324:1247–1252.

46. Mead PB, Amstey MS, Gall SA, et al: Letter to the editor. J Reprod Med 1991;36:831–833.

47. Scott LL, Sanchez PJ, Jackson GL, et al: Acyclovir suppression to prevent cesarean delivery after first episode of genital herpes. Obstet Gynecol 1996;87:67–73.

48. Brown ZA, Selek S, Zeh J, et al: The acquisition of herpes simplex virus during pregnancy. N Engl J Med 1997;337:509–515.

49. Centers for Disease Control and Prevention: Prevention of perinatal transmission of hepatitis B: Prenatal screening for all pregnant women with hepatitis B surface antigen. MMWR Morb Mortal Wkly Rep 1998;37:341–346.

50. Beasley RP, Wang LY, Lee GC: Prevention of perinatally transmitted hepatitis B virus infections with hepatitis B immune globulin and hepatitis B vaccine. Lancet 1983;2:1099–1102.

51. Hollinger FB: Comprehensive control (or elimination) of hepatitis B virus transmission in the United States. Gut 1996;38 (Suppl 2):S24–S30.

52. Ingardia CJ, Kelly L, Steinfeld JD, et al: Hepatitis B vaccination in pregnancy: Factors influencing efficacy. Obstet Gynecol 1999;93:983–986.

53. Jurema MW, Polaneczky M, Ledger WJ: Hepatitis B immunization in postpartum women. Am J Obstet Gynecol 2001;185:355–358.

54. Connor EM, Sperling RS, Gelbert R, et al: Reduction of maternal-infant transmission of human immunodeficiency virus types with zidovidine treatment. N Engl J Med 1994;331:1173–1180.

55. Centers for Disease Control and Prevention: Recommendations of the US Public Health Service Task Force on the use of zidovidine to reduce perinatal transmission of human immunodeficiency virus. MMWR Morb Mortal Wkly Rep 1994;43:1–20.

56. Minkoff H, Mofenson M: The role of obstetrical interventions in the prevention of pediatric human immunodeficiency virus infection. Am J Obstet Gynecol 1994;171:1167–1175.

57. The European Collaborative Study: Cesarean section and risk of vertical transmission of HIV-1 infection. Lancet 1994;343:1464–1467.

58. Centers for Disease Control and Prevention: Report of the NIH panel to define principles of therapy of HIV infection and guidelines for the use of antiretroviral agents in HIV infected adults and adolescents. MMWR Morb Mortal Wkly Rep 1998;77(RR-5):1–82.

59. Minkoff H, Augenbraun M: Anti-retroviral therapy for pregnant women. Am J Obstet Gynecol 1997;176:478–489.

60. Sperling RS, Shapiro DE, Coombs RW, et al: Maternal viral load, zidovudine treatment, and the risk of transmission of human immunodeficiency virus types from mother to infant. N Engl J Med 1996;335:1621–1629.

61. Shah K, Kashima H, Polk BF, et al: Rarity of cesarean delivery in cases of juvenile-onset respiratory papillomatosis. Obstet Gynecol 1986;68:795–799.

62. Bosch FX, Manos MN, Munoz N, et al: Prevalence of human papillomavirus in cervical cancer: A world wide perspective. J Natl Cancer Inst 1995;87:796–802.

63. Manos MM, Kinney WK, Hurley LB: Identifying women with cervical neoplasia using human papillomavirus DNA testing for equivocal Papanicolaou results. JAMA 1999;1605–1610.

64. Bauer HM, Ting Y, Greer CE, et al: Genital human papillomavirus infection in female university students as determined by a PCR-based method. JAMA;1991;265:472–477.

65. Lowe RS, Brown DR, Bryan JJ, et al: Human papillomavirus type II (HPV-II) neutralizing antibodies in the serum and genital mucosal secretions of African Green monkeys immunized with HPV II virus-like particles expressed in yeast. J Infect Dis 1997;176:1141–1145.

66. Ledger WJ, Jeremias J, Witkin SS: Testing for high risk human papillomavirus types will become a standard of clinical care. Am J Obstet Gynecol 2000;182:860–865.

67. Harger JH, Adler SP, Koch WC, et al: Prospective evaluation of 618 pregnant women exposed to parvovirus B19: Risks and symptoms. Obstet Gynecol 1998;91:413–420.

68. Esteban JI, Gonzales A, Hernandes JM, et al: Evaluation of antibodies to hepatitis C virus in a study of transfusion associated hepatitis. N Engl J Med 1990;323:1107–1112.

69. Iworson S, Norkraus G, Wejstål R: Hepatitis C: Natural history of a unique infection. Clin Infect Dis 1995;20:1361–1370.

70. Centers for Disease Control and Prevention: Recommendations for prevention and control of hepatitis C virus (HCV) infection and HCV-related chronic disease. MMWR Morb Mortal Wkly Rep 1998;47:(RR-19):1–39.

71. Vogt M, Lang T, Klinger C, et al: Prevalence and clinical outcome of hepatitis C in children who underwent cardiac surgery before the implementation of blood-donor screening. N Engl J Med 1999;341:866–870.

72. Thomas DL, Villano SA, Riester KA, et al: Perinatal transmission of hepatitis C virus from human immunodeficiency virus type-1-infected mothers. J Infect Dis 1998;177:1480–1488.

73. Hunt CM, Carson KL, Sharara AI: Hepatitis C in pregnancy. Obstet Gynecol 1997;89:883–890.

74. Harris RE: The significance of eradication of bacteriuria during pregnancy. Obstet Gynecol 1979;53:71–73.

75. Rouse DJ, Andrews WW, Goldberg RL, et al: Screening and treatment of asymptomatic bacteriuria in pregnancy to prevent pyelonephritis: A cost effectiveness and cost benefit analysis. Obstet Gynecol 1995;86:119–123.

76. Romero R, Oyarzun E, Mazor M, et al: Meta-analysis of the relationship between asymptomatic bacteriuria and preterm delivery/low birth weight. Obstet Gynecol 1989;73:576–582.

77. Mittendorf R, Williams MA, Kass EA: Prevention of preterm delivery and low birth weight associated with asymptomatic bacteriuria. Clin Infect Dis 1992;14:927–932.

78. Kundsin RB, Leviton A, Alfred EN, et al: *Ureaplasma urealyticum* infection of the placenta in pregnancies that ended prematurely. Obstet Gynecol 1996;87:122–127.

79. Regan JA, Chao S, James LS: Premature rupture of membranes, preterm delivery and Group B streptococcal colonization of mothers. Am J Obstet Gynecol 1981;141:184–186.

80. Hillier SL, Nugent RP, Eschenbach DA, et al: Association between bacterial vaginosis and preterm delivery of a low birth weight infant. N Engl J Med 1995;333:1737–1742.

81. Pastorek JG, Cotch MF, Martin DH, et al: Clinical and microbiological correlates of vaginal *Trichomonas* during pregnancy. Clin Infect Dis 1996;23:1075–1080.

82. Elliot B, Brunham RG, Laga M, et al: Maternal gonococcal disease as a preventable risk factor for low birth weight. J Infect Dis 1990;161:531–536.

83. Hauth JC, Goldenberg RL, Andrews WW, et al: Reduced incidence of preterm delivery with metronidazole and erythromycin in women with bacterial vaginosis. N Engl J Med 1995;333:1732–1736.

84. Carey JC, Klebanoff MA, Hauth JC, et al: Metronidazole to prevent preterm delivery in pregnant women with asymptomatic bacterial vaginosis. N Engl J Med 2000;342:534–540.

85. Ledger WJ, Gee C, Lewis WP: Guidelines of antibiotic prophylaxis in gynecology. Am J Obstet Gynecol 1975;121:1038–1045.

86. Burke JF: The effective period of preventive antibiotic action in experimental incisions and dermal lesions. Surgery 1961;50:161–168.

87. Hoyme UB, Möller U, Saling E: Results and potential consequences of the Thurinqia premature preventional campaign 2000. German Journal of Obstetrics and Gynecology. 2002;62:257–263.

88. Witkin SS, Jeremias J, Toth M, et al: Detection of *Chlamydia trachomatis* by the polymerase chain reaction in the cervices of women with acute salpingitis. Am J Obstet Gynecol 1993;168:1438–1442.

89. Hammerschlag MR, Cummings C, Roblin PM, et al: Efficacy of neonatal ocular prophylaxis for the prevention of chlamydial and gonococcal conjunctivitis. N Engl J Med 1989; 320:769–772.

90. Crombleholme WR, Schachter J, Grossman M, et al: Amoxicillin therapy for *Chlamydia trachomatis* in pregnancy. Obstet Gynecol 1990;75:752–756.

91. Sweet RL, Ledger WJ: Puerperal infectious morbidity. Am J Obstet Gynecol 1973;117:1093–1100.

92. Chow AW, Jewesson PJ: Pharmacokinetics and safety of antimicrobial agents during pregnancy. Rev Infect Dis 1985;7:287–313.

93. Gordon HR, Phelps D, Blanchard K: Prophylactic cesarean section antibiotics: Maternal and neonatal morbidity, before and after cord clamping. Obstet Gynecol 1979;53:151–156.

94. Wax JR, Hersey K, Philput C, et al: Single dose cefazolin prophylaxis for post cesarean infection: Before vs. after cord clamping. J Matern Fetal Med 1997;6:61–65.

95. Faro S, Martens MG, Hammill HA, et al: Antibiotic prophylaxis: Is there a difference? Am J Obstet Gynecol 1990;162:900–909.

96. Harwylshyn PA, Bernstein P, Papsin FR: Short term antibiotic prophylaxis in high risk patients following cesarean section. Am J Obstet Gynecol 1983;145:285–289.

97. Noyes N, Berkeley AS, Freedman K, et al: Incidence of postpartum endomyometritis following single-dose antibiotic prophylaxis with either ampicillin/sulbactam, cefazolin, or cefotetan in high risk cesarean section patients. Infect Dis Obstet Gynecol 1998;6:220–223.

98. Duff P, Gibbs RS, Jorgensen JH, et al: The pharmacokinetics of prophylactic antibiotics administered by intraoperative irrigation at the time of cesarean section. Obstet Gynecol 1982;60:409–412.

99. Berkeley AS, Hirsch JC, Freedman KS, et al: Cefotaxime for cesarean section in labor. Intravenous administration vs. lavage. J Reprod Med 1990;35:214–218.

100. Conover WB, Moore TR: Comparison of irrigation and intravenous antibiotic prophylaxis at cesarean section. Obstet Gynecol 1989;63:787–791.

101. Curran JW, Rendtorff RC, Chandler RW, et al: Female gonorrhea. Its relation to abnormal uterine bleeding, urinary tract symptoms, and cervicitis. Obstet Gynecol 1975;45:195–198.

102. Nichols RL: Surgical wound infection. Am J Med 1991;91(3B):54S–64S.

103. Cruse PJE, Foord R: A five-year prospective study of 23,649 surgical wounds. Arch Surg 1973;107:206–210.

104. Balthazar ER, Colt J, Nichols RL: Pre-operative hair removal: A random, prospective study. South Med J 1982;75:799–801.

105. Culver DH, Horan TC, Gaynes RP, et al: Surgical wound infection rates by wound class, operative procedure, and patient risk index. Am J Med 1991;91(3B):152S–157S.

106. Morrow CP, Hernandez WL, Townsend DE, et al: Pelvic celiotomy in the obese patient. Am J Obstet Gynecol 1977;127:335–339.

107. Karl RC, Mertz JJ, Veith FJ, et al: Prophylactic antimicrobial drugs in surgery. N Engl J Med 1966;275:305–308.

108. Price DJE, Sleigh JD: Control of infection due to *Klebsiella aerogenes* in a neurosurgical unit by withdrawal of all antibiotics. Lancet 1970;2:1213–1215.

109. Ledger WJ, Reite A, Headington JT: The surveillance of infection on an inpatient gynecology service. Am J Obstet Gynecol 1972;113:662–670.

110. Ledger WJ, Campbell C, Taylor D, et al: Adnexal abscess as a late complication of pelvic operations. Surg Gynecol Obstet 1969;129:973–978.

111. Sawin SW, Pilevsky ND, Berlin JA, et al: Comparability of perioperative morbidity between abdominal myomectomy and hysterectomy for woman with uterine myomas. Am J Obstet Gynecol 2000;183:1448–1455.

112. Sawaya GF, Grady D, Kerlikowske K, et al: Antibiotics at the time of induced abortion: The case for universal prophylaxis based on a meta-analysis. Obstet Gynecol 1996;87:884–890.

113. Pittaway DE, Winfield AC, Maxson W, et al: Prevention of acute pelvic inflammatory disease after hysterosalpingography: Efficacy of doxycycline prophylaxis. Am J Obstet Gynecol 1988;147:623–626.

114. Soper DE, Bump RC, Hurt WG: Bacterial vaginosis and trichomoniasis vaginitis are risk factors for cuff cellulitis after abdominal hysterectomy. Am J Obstet Gynecol 1990;163:1016–1023.

115. Shapiro M, Munoz A, Tager IB, et al: Risk factors for infection in the operative site after abdominal or vaginal hysterectomy. N Engl J Med 1982;307:1661–1666.

116. Hemsell DL, Martin JN Jr, Pastorek JG II, et al: Single dose antimicrobial prophylaxis at abdominal hysterectomy. J Reprod Med 1988;33:939–944.

117. Darj E, Stralin E-B, Nilsson S: The prophylactic effect of doxycycline on postoperative infection rate after first trimester abortion. Obstet Gynecol 1987;70:755–758.

118. Berkeley AS, Freedman KS, Ledger WJ, et al: Comparison of a cefotetan and cefoxitin prophylaxis for abdominal and vaginal hysterectomy. Am J Obstet Gynecol 1988;158:705–709.

119. Shapiro M, Townsend TR, Rosner B, et al: Use of antimicrobial drugs in general hospitals. Patterns of prophylaxis. N Engl J Med 1979;301:351–355.

120. Petersdorf RG, Curtin JA, Hoeprich PD, et al: A study of antibiotic prophylaxis in unconscious patients. N Engl J Med 1957;257:1001–1009.

121. Grossman JH III, Adams RL: Vaginal flora in women undergoing hysterectomy with antibiotic prophylaxis. Obstet Gynecol 1979;53:23–26.

122. Berkeley AS, Hayworth SD, Hirsch JC, et al: Controlled comparative study of moxalactam and cefazolin for prophylaxis of abdominal hysterectomy. Surg Gynecol Obstet 1985;161:457–461.

123. Spruill FG, Minette LJ, Sturner WQ: Two surgical deaths associated with cephalothin. JAMA 1974;229:440–441.

124. Bloomberg RJ: Cefotetan-induced anaphylaxis. Am J Obstet Gynecol 1988;159:125–126.

125. Ledger WJ, Puttler OL: Death from pseudomembranous enterocolitis. Obstet Gynecol 1975;45:609–613.

126. Pettet JD, Baggenstoss AH, Dearing WH, et al: Postoperative pseudomembranous enterocolitis. Surg Gynecol Obstet 1954;98:546–552.

127. Smith CV, Gallup D, Gibbs RL, et al: Oral doxycycline vs parenteral cefazolin: Prophylaxis for vaginal hysterectomy. Infect Surg 1989;8:64–67.

128. Livengood CH III, Addison WA: Adnexal abscess as a delayed complication of vaginal hysterectomy. Am J Obstet Gynecol 1982;143:596–597.

129. Benson WL, Brown RL, Schmidt PM: Comparison of short and long courses of ampicillin for vaginal hysterectomy. J Reprod Med 1985;30:874–878.

130. Burkman RT, Tonascia JA, Atienza MF, et al: Untreated endocervical gonorrhea and endometritis following effective abortion. Am J Obstet Gynecol 1976;126:648–651.

131. Moller BR, Ahrons S, Laurin J, et al: Pelvic infection after elective abortion associated with *Chlamydia trachomatis*. Obstet Gynecol 1982;59:210–213.

132. Pursley TJ, Blomquist IK, Abraham J, et al: Fluconazole-induced congenital anomalies in three infants. Clin Infect Dis 1996;22:336–340.

133. Watts DH, Krohn MA, Hillier SL, et al: Bacterial vaginosis as a risk factor for post cesarean endometritis. Obstet Gynecol 1990;75:52–58.

134. Klebanoff MA, Carey JC, Hauth JC, et al: Failure of metronidazole to prevent preterm delivery among pregnant women with asymptomatic *Trichomonas vaginalis* infection. N Engl J Med 2001;345:487–493.

135. Stamm WE, Counts GW, Running KR, et al: Diagnosis of coliform infection in acutely dysuric women. N Engl J Med 1982;307:463–468.

136. Hooper DC, Wolfson JS: Mode of action of the quinolone antimicrobial agents: Review of recent information. Rev Infect Dis 1989;11:S902–S911.

137. Graham JM, Oshiro BT, Blanco JD, et al: Uterine contractions after antibiotics for pyelonephritis in pregnancy. Am J Obstet Gynecol 1993;168:577–580.

138. Towers CV, Kaminskas CM, Garite TJ, et al: Pulmonary injury associated with antepartum pyelonephritis: Can patients at risk be identified? Am J Obstet Gynecol 1991;164:974–978.

139. Millar LK, Wing DA, Paul RH, et al: Outpatient treatment of pyelonephritis in pregnancy: A randomized controlled trial. Obstet Gynecol 1995;86:560–564.

140. Whalley PJ, Cunningham FG, Martin FG: Transient renal dysfunction associated with acute pyelonephritis of pregnancy. Obstet Gynecol 1975;46:174–177.

141. Stamm WE, Hooton TM, Johnson JR, et al: Urinary tract infections: From pathogens to treatment. J Infect Dis 1989;159:400–406.

142. Klostersky J, Daneau D, Swing G, et al: Antibacterial activity in serum and urine as a therapeutic guide in bacterial infections. J Infect Dis 1974;129:187–193.

143. Lorian V, Sabath LD: Effect of pH on the activity of erythromycin against 500 isolates of gram-negative bacilli. Appl Microbiol 1970;20:754–756.

144. Yost NP, Bloom SL, Richey SD, et al: An appraisal of treatment guidelines for antepartum community acquired pneumonia. Am J Obstet Gynecol 2000;183:131–135.

145. Bartlett JG, Powell SF, Mandell LA, et al: Practice guidelines for the management of community acquired pneumonia in adults. Clin Infect Dis 2000;31:347–382.

146. Bartlett JG, Mundy LM: Community acquired pneumonia. N Engl J Med 1995;333:1618–1624.

147. Koh KS, Chan FH, Monfared AH, et al: The changing perinatal and maternal outcome in chorioamnionitis. Obstet Gynecol 1979;53:730–734.

148. Grether JK, Nelson KB: Maternal infection and cerebral palsy in infants of normal birth weight. JAMA 1997;278:207–211.

149. Leitich H, Egarter C, Reisenberger K, et al: Concomitant use of glucocorticoids: A comparison of two meta-analyses on antibiotic treatment in preterm premature rupture of membranes. Am J Obstet Gynecol 1998;178:899–908.

150. Ledger WJ, Reite AM, Headington JT: A system for infectious disease surveillance on an obstetric service. Obstet Gynecol 1971;37:769–778.

151. Hager WD, Barton JR: Treatment of sporadic acute puerperal mastitis. Infect Dis Obstet Gynecol 1996;4:97–101.

152. Ledger WJ, Kriewall TJ, Gee C: The fever index. A technic for evaluating the clinical response to bacteremia. Obstet Gynecol 1975;45:603–608.

153. Dinsmoor MJ, Newton ER, Gibbs RS: A randomized double-blind, placebo-controlled trial of oral antibiotic therapy following intravenous antibiotic therapy for postpartum endometritis. Obstet Gynecol 1991;77:60–62.

154. Locksmith GJ, Duff P: Assessment of the value of routine blood cultures in the evaluation and treatment of patients with chorioamnionitis. Infect Dis Obstet Gynecol 1994;2:111–114.

155. DiZerega G, Yonekura L, Roy S, et al: A comparison of clindamycin-gentamicin and penicillin-gentamicin in the treatment of post-cesarean section endomyometritis. Am J Obstet Gynecol 1979;134:238–242.

156. DelPriore G, Jackson-Stone M, Shim EK, et al: A comparison of once daily and 8-hour gentamicin dosing in the treatment of post-partum endometritis. Obstet Gynecol 1996;87:994–1000.

157. Sweet RL, Ledger WJ: Cefoxitin: Single agent treatment of mixed aerobic-anaerobic pelvic infections. Obstet Gynecol 1979;54:193–198.

158. Ledger WJ, Headington JT: Group A beta-hemolytic streptococcus: An important cause of serious infections in obstetrics and gynecology. Obstet Gynecol 1972;39:474–482.

159. Stevens DL, Gibbons AE, Bergstrom R, Winn V: The Eagle effect revisited: Efficacy of clindamycin, erythromycin and penicillin in the treatment of streptococcal myositis. J Infect Dis 1988;158:23–28.

160. Soper DE, Brockwell NJ, Dalton HP: The importance of wound infection in antibiotic failures in the therapy of postpartum endometritis. Surg Gynecol Obstet 1992;174:265–269.

161. Gilbert DN, Dworkin RJ, Ruber SR, et al: Outpatient parenteral antimicrobial drug therapy. N Engl J Med 1997;337:829–838.

162. Abbott O: Clinical and microscopic diagnosis of vaginal yeast infection: A prospective analysis. Ann Emerg Med 1995;25:587–591.

163. Ledger WJ, Polaneczky MM, Yih MC, et al: Difficulties in the diagnosis of *Candida* vaginitis. Infect Dis Clin Pract 2000;9:66–69.

164. Redondo-Lopez V, Lynch M, Schmitt C, et al: *Torulopsis glabrata* vaginitis: Clinical aspects and susceptibility to antifungal agents. Obstet Gynecol 1990;76:651–655.

165. Amsel R, Totten PA, Spiegel, CA, et al: Non-specific vaginitis. Diagnostic criteria and microbial and epidemiologic association. Am J Med 1983;74:14–22.

166. Schwebke JR, Hillier SL, Sobel JD, et al: Validity of the vaginal Gram stain for the diagnosis of bacterial vaginosis. Obstet Gynecol 1996;88:573–576.

167. Krieger JN, Tan MR, Stevens CE, et al: Diagnosis of trichomoniasis: Comparison of conventional wet mount examination with cytologic studies, cultures and monoclonal antibody staining of direct specimens. JAMA 1988;259:1223–1227.

168. Jeremias J, Draper D, Ziegert M, et al: Detection of *Trichomonas vaginalis* using the polymerase chain reaction in pregnant and non-pregnant women. Infect Dis Obstet Gynecol 1994;2:16–19.

169. Witkin SS, Jeremias J, Ledger WJ: A localized vaginal allergic response in women with recurrent vaginitis. J Allergy Clin Immunol 1998;81:412–416.

170. Sobel JD: Desquamative inflammatory vaginitis: A new subgroup of purulent vaginitis responsive to topical 2% clindamycin therapy. Am J Obstet Gynecol 1994;171:1215–1220.

171. Ledger WJ, Kessler A, Leonard GH, et al: Vulvar vestibulitis: A complex clinical entity. Infect Dis Obstet Gynecol 1996;4:269–275.

172. Jeremias J, Ledger WJ, Witkin SS: Interleukin 1 receptor antagonist gene polymorphism in women with vulvar vestibulitis. Am J Obstet Gynecol 2000;182:283–285.

173. Todd J, Fishaut M, Kapral RF, et al: Toxic shock syndrome associated with phage-group-1 staphylococci. Lancet 1978;2:1116–1118.

174. Schlievert PM: Staphylococcal enterotoxin B and toxic-shock syndrome toxin–1 are significantly associated with non-menstrual TSS. Lancet 1986;1:1149–1150.

175. Centers for Disease Control: Follow-up on toxic shock. MMWR Morb Mortal Wkly Rep 1980;29:441–445.

176. Centers for Disease Control: Toxic shock syndrome—United States, 1970–1980. MMWR Morb Mortal Wkly Rep 1981;30:25–33.

177. Todd J, Kurtz B, Combs P, et al: Epidemiology of TSS in Colorado, 1970–96. European Conference on Toxic Shock Syndrome. London, Royal Society of Medicine Press Limited, 1998, pp 24–26.

178. Wager GP: Toxic shock syndrome: A review. Am J Obstet Gynecol 1983;146:93–102.

179. Nyirjesy P, Jones RS, Chatrvani A, et al: Streptococcal toxic shock–like syndrome as an unusual complication of laparoscopic tubal ligation. A case report. J Reprod Med 1994;39:649–651.

180. Witkin SS, Jeremias J, Toth M, et al: Proliferative response to conserved epitopes of the *Chlamydia trachomatis* and human 60 kilodalton heat shock proteins by lymphocytes from women with salpingitis. Am J Obstet Gynecol 1994;171:455–460.

181. Peipert JF, Boardman L, Hogan JW, et al: Laboratory evaluation of acute upper genital tract infection. Obstet Gynecol 1996;87:730–736.

182. Polaneczky MM, Witkin SS, Pollock L, et al: Self-testing for *Chlamydia trachomatis* infection in women. Obstet Gynecol 1998;91:375–378.

183. Hemsell DL, Ledger WJ, Martens M, et al: Concerns regarding the Centers for Disease Control: Published guidelines for pelvic inflammatory disease. Clin Infect Dis 2001;32:103–107.

184. Stubblefield PG, Grimes DA: Septic abortion. N Engl J Med 1994;331:310–314.

185. LaGuardia KD, Rotholz MV, Belfort P: A 10 year review of maternal mortality in a municipal hospital in Rio de Janeiro: A cause for concern. Obstet Gynecol 1990;75:27–32.

186. Grimes DA, Cates W Jr, Selik RM: Fatal septic abortion in the United States, 1975–1977. Obstet Gynecol 1981;57:739–744.

187. Garvey P, Ledger WJ: Group A streptococcus in the gynecologic patient. Infect Dis Obstet Gynecol 1997;5:391–394.

188. Hemsell DL: Infection after hysterectomy. Infect Dis Obstet Gynecol 1997;5:52–56.

189. Zaske DE, Cipolle RJ, Strate RG, et al: Increased gentamicin dosage requirements: Rapid elimination in 249 gynecology patients. Am J Obstet Gynecol 1981;139:896–900.

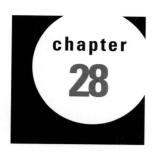

Urinary Tract Infections

THOMAS M. HOOTON, MD

EPIDEMIOLOGY

Urinary tract infection (UTI) in adults includes women with acute sporadic or recurrent uncomplicated cystitis, women with acute uncomplicated pyelonephritis, complicated UTI (a large heterogeneous group that includes all others with symptomatic UTI), and asymptomatic bacteriuria (Table 28–1). Complicated UTIs are by definition associated with conditions that increase the risk of serious complications or treatment failure. It is generally safe to assume that a premenopausal, sexually active, nonpregnant woman with recent onset of dysuria, frequency, or urgency who has not had urologic instrumentation recently and who has no history of a genitourinary tract abnormality has an uncomplicated lower (cystitis) or upper (pyelonephritis) UTI. It can be argued that many UTIs categorized as being complicated (Table 28–1), such as many episodes of acute cystitis in men, older women, and pregnant women with no history of genitourinary tract abnormalities, are really uncomplicated UTIs, but these groups are at greater risk for having occult renal or prostatic infection and should be managed accordingly. Recommendations for evaluation and treatment differ for uncomplicated and complicated urinary tract infections, and thus it is important to try to distinguish between the two. Complicating conditions are not always obvious, however, and may become obvious only after treatment has begun. The conditions shown in Table 28–1 only serve as guidelines for the clinician who must decide on the basis of limited clinical information whether to embark on a more extensive evaluation and treatment course when he or she is confronted with a patient with UTI.

Uncomplicated Urinary Tract Infection

Acute uncomplicated urinary tract infections are among the most common conditions causing people to seek outpatient medical care. One recent survey estimated that as many as 11 million women in the U.S. had at least one presumed UTI treated with antibiotics in 1995 and that the cost for evaluation and management of UTIs was $1.6 billion.[1] In this survey the self-reported cumulative lifetime risk of UTI in women was 60%.[1] In a recent large prospective study of young sexually active women the incidence of cystitis was approximately 0.5 per person-year.[2] Although there are few data on the incidence of pyelonephritis, which occurs about 28-fold less frequently than cystitis does,[3] a recent population-based study in Canada showed that the overall rate of hospitalization for pyelonephritis in women was about 1 case per 1000 population.[4] This rate is almost certainly an underestimate, since the study evaluated only patients with more severe disease who required hospitalization; in the United States up to 75% of patients presenting to emergency departments with acute pyelonephritis do not require hospitalization.[5,6]

TABLE 28–1 ■ **Categories of Urinary Tract Infection (UTI) in Adults**

Acute uncomplicated cystitis in young women
Recurrent acute uncomplicated cystitis in young women
Acute uncomplicated pyelonephritis in young women
Complicated UTI
  Acute cystitis in adult who has a condition suggesting possible occult renal or prostatic involvement but without other known complicating factors
    Male sex
    Elderly
    Pregnancy
    Recent urinary tract instrumentation
    Childhood UTI
    Symptoms for >7 d at presentation
    Diabetes mellitus well controlled
UTI in adult with potentially serious condition complicating management
  Obstruction or other structural abnormality
    Urolithiasis
    Malignancies
    Ureteral and urethral strictures
    Bladder diverticuli
    Renal cysts
    Fistulas
    Ileal conduits and other urinary diversions
  Functional abnormality
    Neurogenic bladder
    Vesicoureteral reflux
  Foreign bodies
    Indwelling catheter
    Ureteral stent
    Nephrostomy tube
  Other conditions
    Renal failure
    Renal transplantation
    Diabetes mellitus poorly controlled
    Immunosuppression
    Multi-drug-resistant uropathogens
    Hospital-acquired infection
    Prostatitis-related UTI
    Upper tract infection in adult other than young healthy woman
    Other functional or anatomic abnormality of the urinary tract
Asymptomatic bacteriuria

Uncomplicated UTIs, including episodes of acute cystitis, are associated with considerable morbidity. Foxman and Frerichs found that on average each episode of urinary tract infection in young women was associated with 6.1 days of symptoms, 2.4 days of restricted activity, 1.2 days in which they were not able to attend classes or work, and 0.4 bed days.[7]

Recurrent Acute Uncomplicated Urinary Tract Infection

A recurrent UTI is a symptomatic UTI that follows clinical resolution of a previous UTI, generally, but not necessarily, after treatment. Recurrent UTIs are common among young healthy women even though they generally have anatomically and physiologically normal urinary tracts. In a recent study of college women with their first urinary tract infection, 27% experienced at least one culture-confirmed recurrence within the 6 months following the initial infection,[8] and 2.7% had a second recurrence over this time period. In a Finnish study of women ages 17 to 82 years who had *Escherichia coli* cystitis, 44% had a recurrence within 1 year.[3] No large population-based studies have yet been performed to determine what proportion of women with UTI develop a pattern of high-frequency recurrences.

Although recurrent acute uncomplicated cystitis among young healthy women may occasionally be due to a persistent focus of infection (relapse), most are reinfections that in many cases are due to the persistence of the initially infecting strain in the fecal flora.[9] Thus the bacteria associated with recurrent cystitis and recurrent pyelonephritis often appear to be phenotypically or genotypically identical to the bacterial strain that caused the initial infection, suggesting that in women with recurrent UTI, selected *E. coli* strains become uniquely adapted for colonizing and infecting that particular host.[9] It is useful to try to distinguish clinically between relapse and reinfection because of therapeutic implications. Thus a recurrence is considered to be a reinfection if it is caused by a strain different from the one causing the original infection. Because it is generally not possible to distinguish between relapse and reinfection with the originally infecting strain, a recurrence often is defined clinically as a relapse if it is caused by the same species that caused the original UTI and if it occurs within 2 weeks after treatment, and it is considered a reinfection if it occurs more than 2 weeks after treatment of the original UTI. An exception would be the situation in which a post-treatment urine culture has been performed and has no growth of the uropathogen, in which case any subsequent recurrence is a reinfection. Most recurrences appear in the first 3 months after the initial urinary tract infection,[10,11] although clustering has not been found in some studies.[3]

There is no evidence that recurrent urinary tract infection in the absence of anatomic or functional abnormalities of the urinary tract leads to blood pressure elevation or renal disease.

Complicated Urinary Tract Infection

Complicated urinary tract infections encompass a heterogeneous group of infectious entities (Table 28–1) for which no population-based studies have been done and for which overall incidence data do not exist. The incidence of nosocomial UTI, one of the most common types of complicated UTI, is approximately 5 per 100 admissions in a university tertiary care hospital, with catheter-associated UTIs accounting for 88% of these infections.[12] Nosocomial UTIs account for up to 40% of hospital-acquired infections and for more than 1 million infections in U.S. hospitals each year. Although the rate of hospital-acquired UTI per 1000 patient days has not changed much over the past 20 years in the United States, the number of infections and the proportion of hospital-acquired infections contributed by UTIs has dropped considerably (42% in 1975 to 30% in 1995) as the average length of stay has dropped (National Nosocomial Infections Study [NNIS], unpublished data, 1995). Patients who develop hospital-acquired UTIs have their hospital stays extended by approximately 3 days and are nearly three times more likely to die during hospitalization than are patients without such infections. In 1995 in the United States it was estimated that 565,000 hospital-acquired UTIs contributed to the deaths of almost 9000 patients and caused $403 million in extra charges (NNIS, unpublished data, 1995). For those patients with significant anatomic abnormalities of the genitourinary tract, whether congenital or postsurgical, UTIs are a tremendous burden. Likewise among persons with spinal cord injury or diabetes, UTIs often cause considerable morbidity and occasionally death. Pregnant women who do not receive appropriate prenatal care may suffer significantly from the sequelae of UTI.

Asymptomatic Bacteriuria

Asymptomatic bacteriuria is defined as a uropathogen count of 10^5 cfu/ml or higher in a clean-voided urine specimen in the absence of symptoms. To reduce the chances that contamination with perineal flora is the source of bacteriuria, many authorities require that two or more consecutive urine cultures have counts of 10^5 cfu/ml or higher of the same species.[13] Approximately 5% of young, healthy sexually active women in a recent population-based study had a uropathogen count of 10^5 cfu/ml or higher in voided urine.[14] When these women were followed up with monthly urine cultures for 6 months, 21% had at least one urine culture with a uropathogen count of 10^5 cfu/ml or higher, and approximately 5% had two or more consecutive urine cultures with the same species of uropathogen. However, persistent asymptomatic bacteriuria with the same strain was rare.[14] In another recent population-based study of women ages 38 to 60 years in Sweden, bacteriuria was observed in 3% to 5% and increased with age.[15] The spectrum of organisms causing asymptomatic bacteriuria is similar to that seen in symptomatic UTI, with *E. coli* found in 80% of the cultures. Asymptomatic bacteriuria increases the short-term risk of subsequent symptomatic UTI, and the risk is higher among women with asymptomatic bacteriuria accompanied by pyuria. It is possible that such episodes of asymptomatic bacteriuria with pyuria represent the early stages of a symptomatic UTI. Risk factors for asymptomatic bacteriuria in young women appear to be similar to those for symptomatic UTI and include sexual intercourse and use of spermicidal products.

The prevalence of asymptomatic bacteriuria in women increases with age.[16] Thus, the prevalence in ambulatory noncatheterized women is reported to be approximately 6% to 10% among women over 60 years of age, 15% to 20% in women ages 65 to 90, and 22% to 43% in those 90 years of age and older. The incidence among institutionalized elderly women is even higher, 25% to 53%, varying with the underlying degree of disability.[16] Asymptomatic bacteriuria is found rarely in men less than 50 years of age, in 12% of ambulatory men older than 65, and in up to 37% of elderly men who are institutionalized.[16] Many episodes of asymptomatic bacteriuria in the elderly are transient, although bacteriuria tends to be more persistent than in younger women. Asymptomatic bacteriuria is more likely to be persistent in those with long-term indwelling catheters.

It is not clear whether age in and of itself predisposes to bacteriuria, although the high incidence in the elderly is most likely due to conditions frequently seen in this age group, including obstructive uropathy, loss of estrogen and the resulting adverse effects on vaginal microflora, loss of bactericidal activity of prostatic secretions, adverse effects on bladder emptying caused by uterine prolapse and cystocele in women, perineal soiling from fecal incontinence in demented persons, and frequent instrumentation and bladder catheter use.[16] As with younger populations, the risk of bacteriuria appears to be multifactorial and complex, and the relative importance of different factors is difficult to determine.

Asymptomatic bacteriuria generally is assumed to be a benign condition. No differences in mortality or incidence of severe kidney disease were found in a Swedish study during a 24-year follow-up between those with and those without bacteriuria at baseline.[15] Although early studies reported that asymptomatic bacteriuria in elderly men and women was associated with a higher mortality, this association has not been borne out in more recent studies in which underlying illness has been adjusted for.[17] Asymptomatic bacteriuria, however, may lead to serious complications in some clinical conditions such as pregnancy, genitourinary manipulation, and renal transplantation.[13]

PATHOGENESIS

Uncomplicated Urinary Tract Infection

Host Factors

Most uncomplicated UTIs in women appear to result from the interaction of infecting *E. coli* strains with the woman's epithelial cells in the absence of underlying functional or anatomic abnormalities of the urinary tract. In general, uropathogens originate in the person's rectal flora and enter the bladder via the urethra with an interim phase of periurethral and distal urethral colonization. Recurrently infecting strains, even those that are identical to the initially infecting strain, presumably persist or are reacquired in the gastrointestinal tract and cause recurrent UTI via the same mechanism. In men, colonizing uropathogens may also come from a sex partner's vagina or rectum. Hematogenous seeding of the urinary tract by potential uropathogens such as *Staphylococcus aureus* is the source of some urinary tract infections, but this is more likely to occur in the setting of persistent bloodstream infection or urinary tract obstruction. It is certainly possible, however, that some episodes of pyelonephritis are caused by transient bacteremia or lymphatic spread with uropathogens.

Recently another hypothesis has been proposed to explain the origin of urinary pathogens in some women with identical-strain recurrent UTI. Thus recent studies in mice have convincingly demonstrated that uropathogenic *E. coli* strains invade host epithelial cells, replicate, invade to deeper epithelial cell layers, where they can persist for several weeks in a quiescent state, and eventually re-emerge to cause recurrent bacteriuria.[18] The bladder persistence theory of recurrent UTI is supported by small studies of patients with a UTI history.[19] These animal and human studies suggest that in certain persons, uropathogens persist in the bladder epithelium and subsequently surface to produce asymptomatic bacteriuria or symptomatic UTI. This model of recurrent UTI is supported by the finding that bacteria associated with a recurrent UTI often appear to be identical to the bacterial strain that caused the initial infection.

Many host factors appear to predispose young healthy women to uncomplicated urinary tract infection. Sexual intercourse and spermicide use, especially in conjunction with diaphragm use, are factors most clearly demonstrated to predispose women to both sporadic[2] and recurrent UTI.[20] Recent antibiotic use also is associated with an increased risk of UTI, presumably because of the adverse effects of antibiotics on vaginal flora. Likewise a previous recurrent UTI is a strong risk factor for a subsequent UTI. In contrast, no associations have been demonstrated between recurrent UTI in young women and precoital and postcoital voiding patterns, frequency of urination, delayed voiding habits, wiping patterns, douching, bathing habits, or use of noncotton pantyhose or tights.[20] In healthy postmenopausal women, risk factors for recurrent UTI include incontinence, a cystocele, increased postvoid residual urine, being a nonsecretor of histo–blood group antigens, and having had a prior UTI.[21]

Recently published data suggest that genetic factors may be associated with an increased risk of recurrent UTI. In a case-control study of women with and without recurrent UTI, patients were more likely to have a mother with a history of recurrent UTI and to have had their first UTI at 15 years or younger.[20] These variables were the factors most strongly associated with recurrent UTI after frequency of sexual intercourse. Another case-control study demonstrated that female family members of women with recurrent UTI were significantly more likely to have a history of recurrent UTI than were female family members of controls.[22] A genetic predisposition to recurrent UTI is further suggested by the finding that nonsecretors of histo–blood group antigens have a threefold to fivefold greater risk of recurrent UTI than secretors have. This observation may explain why *E. coli* attaches to uroepithelial cells from young women with a history of recurrent UTI in greater numbers than it does to uroepithelial cells from controls. In this regard the vaginal epithelium of nonsecretors has been shown to express unique globoseries glycosphingolipids that bind uropathogenic *E. coli*.[23] Recently published data suggest that nonsecretor status is also associated with pyelonephritis in women.[24] In addition the P1 phenotype is overrepresented among girls and women with recurrent pyelonephritis.

In patients with cystitis or pyelonephritis, interleukin (IL)-6 and IL-8 are present in the urine, suggesting a potential role for these molecules in UTI pathogenesis.[25] IL-8 is a potent neutrophil chemotactic molecule, and induction of IL-8 after infection with uropathogenic *E. coli* correlates well with the appearance of neutrophils in the urine. The receptors for IL-8 on neutrophils are CXCR1 and CXCR2. Studies of the murine IL-8 receptor homologue (mIL-8Rh) in knockout mice suggest that the absence of mIL-8Rh leads to the accumulation of neutrophils in the subepithelial cell layers of the bladder or kidney.[26] This receptor defect prevents proper migration of the neutrophils into the bladder lumen. The resultant tissue neutrophilia may lead to more tissue damage and pyelonephritis. In addition a preliminary analysis of CXCR1 expression on the neutrophils of 12 children with a history of recurrent pyelonephritis, compared with age-matched controls, has demonstrated a consistently lower CXCR1 expression, which the authors suggest may explain their susceptibility to recurrent pyelonephritis.[26] In all eight of the children with recurrent pyelonephritis who were further tested, neutrophils contained lower CXCR1 mRNA levels than neutrophils in controls did. Thus alterations in these cytokine receptors may correlate with susceptibility to recurrent UTI or pyelonephritis because of an altered neutrophil response or an accumulation of neutrophils in the kidney tissue.

Antibacterial characteristics of urine, normal anatomy and function of the urinary tract, and other host defense mechanisms are thought to be important factors associated with UTI risk but have not been shown to be clearly associated with UTI in healthy persons. The host's inflammatory and immunologic responses help determine the clinical consequences of UTI.

The large difference in UTI incidence between men and women is thought to be due to a variety of factors, including the greater distance between the usual source of uropathogens, the anus, and the urethral meatus in men, the drier environment surrounding the male urethra, the greater length of the male urethra, and the antibacterial activity of prostatic fluid. Risk factors associated with urinary tract infections in healthy men include intercourse with an infected female partner, homosexuality, and lack of circumcision, although these factors are often not present in men with UTI. Uropathogenic strains infecting young men largely have been highly urovirulent, suggesting that UTIs in otherwise healthy men are most likely to occur when a highly urovirulent strain enters the urethra and progresses to infect the bladder or kidney.

Uropathogen Virulence Determinants

In addition to these and other host factors that modulate UTI risk, certain virulence determinants of uropathogens have been demonstrated to provide a selective advantage to those strains possessing them with regard to colonization and infection.[27,28] These virulence determinants provide uropathogens with a survival advantage as they compete with other bacteria for a niche in the genitourinary flora. Virulence factors are much more important in the normal host than in the host who has a functional or anatomic abnormality of the genitourinary tract. Several bacterial properties (including P fimbriae, type 1 fimbriae, hemolysin, aerobactin, serum resistance, and the K1 capsule) are fairly well established as virulence factors in acute symptomatic *E. coli* UTI.[28] It appears that whereas P-fimbriae are important in the development of pyelonephritis, type 1 fimbriae are important in the development of cystitis. Whether vaginal colonization and subsequent UTI occur is the result of a dynamic interaction between these host characteristics and uropathogen virulence determinants. Adhering bacteria stimulate epithelial and other cells to produce cytokines and other proinflammatory factors, which results in an inflammatory response, the magnitude and localization of which determines many features of UTI.[27] Asymptomatic bacteriuria may either be the consequence of bacterial attenuation by the host or a primary condition in which bacteria of low virulence chronically colonize the urinary tract without causing a symptomatic response. In a recent study of asymptomatic bacteriuria in young women, however, the proportions of strains with hemolysin and *papG*, the gene that encodes the G adhesin on P fimbriae, were almost identical among *E. coli* strains causing asymptomatic bacteriuria and symptomatic UTI.[14] In addition DNA typing data showed that identical *E. coli* strains caused episodes of asymptomatic and symptomatic UTI in the same woman. Thus the bacterial and host factors that result in asymptomatic bacteriuria vs. symptomatic UTI remain unknown.

Complicated Urinary Tract Infection

The initial steps leading to uncomplicated UTI probably also occur in most persons who develop a complicated UTI. Factors that predispose persons to complicated UTI generally do so by causing obstruction or stasis of urine flow, facilitating entry of uropathogens into the urinary tract by bypassing normal host defense mechanisms, pro-viding a nidus for infection that is not readily treatable with antimicrobials, or by compromising the host immune system (Table 28–1).[29,30] Uropathogen virulence determinants appear to be of much less importance in the pathogenesis of complicated UTIs than in the pathogenesis of uncomplicated UTIs. Infection with multiple-drug-resistant uropathogens is more likely than with uncomplicated UTI, especially in those infections that develop in institutional settings and in patients with frequent recurrences that require frequent antimicrobial administration.

Obstruction of urine flow, the chief factor contributing to complicated UTI, interferes with local mucosal defense mechanisms by overdistending the urinary tract, and the resulting residual urine pool provides a continuous media for bacterial growth. Urinary catheters allow easy access of uropathogens to the urinary tract either through or around the catheter. Fistulas provide direct access of uropathogens in the bowel to the urinary tract. Passage of uropathogens from the bladder to the renal pelvis and parenchyma is facilitated by vesicoureteral reflux or by alteration of the normal peristaltic effect of the ureter, as with pregnancy or obstruction. Biofilms on urinary catheters and other foreign bodies provide a nidus from which it is difficult or impossible to eradicate uropathogens with antimicrobials. The physiologic and anatomic changes in pregnancy, including hydroureter, decreased ureteral peristalsis, decreased bladder tone, and urine stasis, increase the risk of UTI, especially pyelonephritis, in pregnancy. Urinary tract infections are more likely to occur or to have serious consequences in certain conditions that impair host defenses, such as diabetes mellitus, neutropenia, renal transplantation, and possibly the acquired immunodeficiency syndrome. Diabetes in particular is associated with several syndromes of complicated UTI, including intrarenal and perirenal abscess, emphysematous pyelonephritis and cystitis, papillary necrosis, and xanthogranulomatous pyelonephritis, probably due to the combination of bladder dysfunction, glycosuria, and vascular disease that complicate diabetes.[31]

SPECTRUM OF ETIOLOGIC AGENTS

The spectrum of etiologic agents is similar in uncomplicated upper and lower urinary tract infection, with *E. coli* the causative pathogen in 70% to 95% and *Staphylococcus saprophyticus* in 5% to more than 20%[32] (Table 28–2). In a recent study of acute pyelonephritis, *S. saprophyticus* was isolated from only 2% of patients.[32] Occasionally other Enterobacteriaceae, such as *Proteus mirabilis*, *Klebsiella* spp, or Enterobacter spp or enterococci are isolated from such patients. Uncomplicated UTI is also caused on occasion by group B streptococococci and, rarely, *Pseudomonas aeruginosa*, *Citrobacter* spp, or other uropathogens.

TABLE 28–2 ■ **Bacteria That Cause Urinary Tract Infection**

	Uncomplicated (%)	Complicated* (%)
GRAM-NEGATIVE		
Escherichia coli	70–95	21–54
Proteus mirabilis	1–2	1–10
Klebsiella spp	1–2	2–17
Citrobacter spp	<1	5
Enterobacter spp	<1	2–10
Pseudomonas aeruginosa	<1	2–19
Other	<1	6–20
GRAM-POSITIVE		
Coagulase-negative staphylococci	5–>20[†]	1–4
Enterococci	1–2	1–23
Group B streptococci	<1	1–4
Staphylococcus aureus	<1	1–2
Other	<1	2

*Data from Nicolle.[30]

[†]*Staphylococcus saprophyticus.*

On the other hand a broad range of bacteria cause complicated infections, and such infections are often caused by strains resistant to multiple antimicrobial agents. Although *E. coli* is the predominant uropathogen in complicated UTI, uropathogens other than *E. coli*, including *Citrobacter* spp, *Enterobacter* spp, *P. aeruginosa*, enterococci, and *S. aureus* account for a relatively higher proportion of cases than in uncomplicated urinary tract infections (Table 28–2). The proportion of infections caused by fungi also appears to be increasing. *Candida* spp are especially common in patients with indwelling urinary catheters, especially those who have had previous antibiotic therapy. *S. saprophyticus* is rarely isolated in the elderly. Patients with chronic conditions, such as spinal cord injury and neurogenic bladder, are relatively more likely to have polymicrobial and multiple-drug-resistant infections. The diversity and antimicrobial resistance of uropathogens in complicated UTI reflect the fact that persons with such UTIs tend to acquire their infections in the hospital setting or to have frequent UTIs requiring multiple courses of antibiotics.[30]

DIAGNOSIS AND MANAGEMENT OF CLINICAL URINARY TRACT INFECTION SYNDROMES

Acute Uncomplicated Cystitis in Young Healthy Women

Women with acute uncomplicated cystitis generally present with acute onset of symptoms including dysuria, frequency, urgency, or suprapubic pain. Acute dysuria in a young sexually active woman is usually caused by acute cystitis, acute urethritis due to *Chlamydia trachomatis*,

Neisseria gonorrhoeae, or herpes simplex virus, or by vaginitis due to *Candida* or *Trichomonas vaginalis*.[33] A distinction between these three entities can usually, but not always, be made with data from the history and physical examination and simple laboratory tests. Pyuria is present in almost all women with acute cystitis, as well as in most women with urethritis caused by *N. gonorrhoeae* or *C. trachomatis*, and its absence strongly suggests an alternative diagnosis. Hematuria is common in women with UTI but not in women with urethritis or vaginitis. A history of vaginal symptoms, sexually transmitted diseases (STD), multiple sexual partners, or a sexual partner with symptoms of urethritis increases the likelihood of an STD as the cause for the urinary symptoms.

The definitive diagnosis of UTI is made in the presence of significant bacteriuria, the traditional standard for which is a uropathogen count of 10^5 cfu/ml or higher in voided midstream urine. This standard is based on previous studies of women with acute pyelonephritis and asymptomatic bacteriuria. Up to one-third of cystitis patients, however, have lower colony counts, which are missed by using the traditional definition. The Infectious Disease Society of America consensus definition of cystitis is a uropathogen count of 10^3 cfu/ml or higher (sensitivity 80% and specificity 90%).[34] Thus reliance on the traditional threshold of 10^5 cfu/ml or higher in voided midstream urine in the diagnosis of cystitis frequently will result in missed diagnoses.

Urine cultures generally are not necessary in women with uncomplicated cystitis, however, since the causative organisms and their antimicrobial susceptibility profiles are so predictable and since culture results become available only after therapeutic decisions have been made. This recommendation requires reassessment given the striking increases reported in the incidence of antimicrobial-resistant uropathogens causing uncomplicated UTIs.[35]

There appear to be no long-term adverse effects with respect to renal function or increased mortality associated with acute cystitis, even in women with frequent recurrences, and in the nonpregnant population, untreated cystitis appears to progress infrequently to symptomatic upper tract infection. Thus the significance of lower UTI in the nonpregnant woman appears to be limited to the morbidity of symptoms caused by the infection, which may be substantial. In fact most lower UTIs (50% to 70%) will clear spontaneously if untreated, although symptoms may persist for several months.[36] A more recent placebo-controlled cystitis treatment study showed that in 26% of women given placebo, bacteriuria spontaneously cleared by 2 weeks, but no data were provided on the status of symptoms or longer follow-up.[37]

Knowledge of the antimicrobial susceptibility profile of uropathogens causing uncomplicated UTI in the community should guide therapeutic decisions. *E. coli* in patients with uncomplicated UTI are often resistant to sulfonamides and amoxicillin, and *E. coli* is less often resistant to trimethoprim, TMP-SMX, nitrofurantoin, and the fluoroquinolones. However, there has been an increase in resistance to trimethoprim and TMP-SMX among urinary strains seen in outpatients in the United States and Europe, which is cause for concern.[33] In the United States the prevalence of resistance to TMP-SMX among *E. coli* strains causing uncomplicated cystitis is higher than 20% in some areas of the country.[38] A recently described disseminated *E. coli* clonal group (clonal group A) appears to contribute substantially to TMP-SMX resistance among strains causing uncomplicated cystitis and pyelonephritis in some areas in the United States, and the authors speculate that this strain may be entering new environments by one or more contaminated products ingested by community residents.[39] Although nitrofurantoin has maintained excellent activity against almost all *E. coli* causing uncomplicated UTI, it is not active against some strains of *Enterobacter* spp and *Klebsiella* spp, most strains of *Proteus* spp or *Serratia* spp, and no strains of *Pseudomonas* spp. In one recent large study, in vitro resistance to nitrofurantoin was reported for 6% to 9% of all uropathogens over the years 1992 to 1996 but for 41% of all non–*E. coli* isolates over these years.[40] Fluoroquinolones remain active against almost all *E. coli* causing uncomplicated cystitis in the United States, but fluoroquinolone-resistant strains in uncomplicated UTI are being reported in other countries. Moreover, in female outpatients older than 50 in the United States, resistance to nitrofurantoin and fluoroquinolones appears to be substantially higher in this group[38] than among younger women.

Antimicrobials used in the treatment of acute uncomplicated cystitis are shown in Table 28–3. Three-day regimens are generally recommended for the treatment of acute uncomplicated cystitis because of comparable efficacy, better adherence, lower cost, and lower frequency of adverse reactions than with longer regimens.[41] Single-dose regimens, while highly effective in most women

(especially TMP-SMX and fluoroquinolones), are somewhat less effective than multiday regimens.[41,42] Further, concern has been raised that single-dose regimens are less likely to be effective in treatment of infections in which an unrecognized complicating factor is present such as pregnancy, diabetes, or an anatomic or functional abnormality of the urinary tract. Single-dose therapy appears to be suboptimal in treatment of occult upper UTI, and in fact, relapse following single-dose treatment suggests the presence of upper UTI.

Higher cure rates generally have been observed with TMP-SMX and fluoroquinolones than with β-lactams regardless of the site of infection and duration of treatment.[41] In acute uncomplicated cystitis, one should expect eradication of the infecting pathogen after single-dose treatment with trimethoprim or TMP-SMX in 85% to 95% of cases and after single-dose treatment with β-lactams, with which cure rates have been more variable, in approximately 50% to 85%, depending on the site of infection. Factors possibly contributing to the poorer results seen with some of the β-lactam agents than with trimethoprim, TMP-SMX or fluoroquinolones are the much shorter time that β-lactams are present in high concentrations in urine and their inferior ability to effectively eradicate carriage of *E. coli* in the vaginal and fecal reservoirs.

Trimethoprim or TMP-SMX in a 3-day oral regimen should be considered the first-line agent for uncomplicated cystitis in women who can tolerate this agent and in areas where resistance is uncommon.[41] Trimethoprim achieves cure rates similar to those with TMP-SMX[41] and may have fewer side effects and therefore is the preferred first-line drug for some authorities. Although it is often believed that in vitro resistance to TMP-SMX may not predict whether treatment will fail in patients with cystitis because the drugs achieve high and prolonged urinary concentrations, this is not the case.[43] Most *E. coli* strains show high-level resistance (minimum inhibitory concentration 2000 μg/ml), and recent studies clearly demonstrate high failure rates when TMP-SMX is used to treat UTIs caused by strains that are resistant to TMP-SMX.[43,44] TMP-SMX can accelerate the metabolism and decrease the effectiveness of oral contraceptives,[45] and women should be counseled appropriately when this combination is used.

Fluoroquinolones are reasonable first-line agents in women who are known or are suspected of having antimicrobial-resistant organisms or who are allergic to or otherwise do not tolerate more conventional regimens, or in areas where resistance to TMP-SMX is over 10% to 20%.[41] Fluoroquinolones generally are not regarded as first-line therapy because of concerns regarding the promotion of quinolone resistance. Cost is a minor consideration in the setting of cystitis. Nitrofurantoin should be considered as an alternative to fluoroquinolones because it has no other uses than for uncomplicated UTI, and it does not select for resistance to other commonly used

TABLE 28–3 ■ Oral Regimens for Acute Uncomplicated Cystitis

Drug, dose	Interval
Amoxicillin, 250 mg	q8h
Amoxicillin, 500 mg	q12h
Amoxicillin-clavulanate, 500/125 mg	q12h
Cefixime, 400 mg	q24h
Cefpodoxime proxetil, 100 mg	q12h
Fluoroquinolones	
Ciprofloxacin, 250 mg	q12h
Gatifloxacin, 400 mg	q24h
Levofloxacin, 250 mg	q24h
Fosfomycin tromethamine	Single 3-g sachet
Nitrofurantoin monohydrate macrocystals	
(Macrobid), 100 mg	q12h
Nitrofurantoin macrocystals, 50 mg	q6h
Trimethoprim, 100 mg	q12h
TMP-SMX 160/800 mg	q12h

See text for additional information about these regimens.

antibiotics. Nitrofurantoin does not appear to be as effective in short-course regimens as TMP-SMX or fluoroquinolones are and therefore should be used in regimens of 7 days or longer. The short plasma half-life of nitrofurantoin, 20 minutes, may limit its usefulness with short-course regimens.

First- and second-generation cephalosporins have in vitro activity against most uropathogens causing uncomplicated UTI, but they appear to be less effective in the treatment of uncomplicated UTI, especially in short-course regimens, than TMP-SMX and fluoroquinolones.[46,47] Amoxicillin should be used only when the causative uropathogen is known to be susceptible, since over 30% of uropathogenic strains can be expected to be resistant to this drug. Amoxicillin-clavulanate provides broader empiric coverage but has a high rate of gastrointestinal side effects, which may be less common with use of the new twice-daily formulations, which contain less clavulanate. Cefixime and cefpodoxime proxetil are broad-spectrum third-generation oral cephalosporins that demonstrate in vitro activity against most uropathogens causing uncomplicated cystitis, but clinical data are sparse, especially with short-course regimens. Cefixime is less active against gram-positive organisms and therefore may not reliably eradicate S. saprophyticus. None of these agents should be used in short-course regimens for uncomplicated cystitis, especially in women with moderate-to-severe symptoms. Although fosfomycin tromethamine is approved for the single-dose treatment of uncomplicated cystitis, it appears to be less effective than multiday regimens of TMP-SMX or fluoroquinolones.[41]

Given the increasing prevalence of TMP-SMX resistance among uropathogens, it is useful to examine predictors of in vitro resistance. One recent study of UTIs in patients presenting to emergency departments showed that the most important independent risk factors for TMP-SMX resistance were recent antibiotic use and recent TMP-SMX use.[48] It is reasonable, therefore, to use trimethoprim or TMP-SMX for acute cystitis if the woman has no history of allergy to the drug and has not been taking antibiotics in the past 3 to 6 months (for any reason) and if the incidence of TMP-SMX resistance is not known to be more than 20%.[35] Interestingly, fecal colonization with drug-resistant uropathogens has been reported after travel to Mexico, among children attending day care centers, and among family member of patients with a UTI caused by a trimethoprim-resistant strain.[35] It is not clear whether such factors should be considered in choosing an empiric regimen for cystitis.

Routine post-treatment cultures in asymptomatic women are not indicated because of the considerable costs necessary to detect a single case of asymptomatic bacteriuria and because the benefit of detecting and treating asymptomatic bacteriuria in healthy women has been demonstrated only in pregnancy and prior to urologic instrumentation or surgery.[13] In women whose symptoms persist a urine culture and antimicrobial susceptibility testing should be performed, and a longer course of therapy, usually with a fluoroquinolone, should be used and modified according to culture and susceptibility results. In those women whose symptoms resolve but later recur, the approach should be the same as with sporadic infections except that a culture and susceptibility test should be considered if only a few weeks separate the recurrences.

Recurrent Acute Uncomplicated Cystitis in Young Healthy Women

Cystitis that recurs during or within the first week following treatment suggests possible relapse and should be managed with a pretreatment urine culture, antimicrobial susceptibility testing, and treatment with a fluoroquinolone for 7 days unless the culture results dictate otherwise. There is no reason outside of a research study to perform sophisticated typing of initial and recurrent cystitis strains, since one cannot eliminate the possibility of recurrence even if the strains are identical. Later recurrences of cystitis should be managed with short-course regimens of antimicrobials as described for sporadic infections.

Women with recurrent UTIs should be informed about the behavioral factors associated with such infections, so that they can modify such behavior as appropriate. Thus if the woman uses a spermicidal product (even spermicide-coated condoms), she should be counseled about the known association of such products with UTI and that her UTI risk will be reduced by changing to a nonspermicidal product. The effect of increasing fluid intake or changing voiding habits on the risk of urinary tract infection is not known. Although early postcoital micturition has not been confirmed as being protective, it is reasonable to encourage women to urinate soon after intercourse. Women with frequent recurrent urinary tract infections who do not wish to change their method of contraception and who do not benefit from behavioral modification suggestions should be offered antimicrobial management. Many women use cranberry juice to prevent UTIs. Although several small studies support its efficacy, there are as yet no definitive data supporting its use in the prevention of recurrent UTI.[49,50]

Antimicrobial prophylaxis has been demonstrated to be highly effective in reducing the risk of recurrent UTI in women.[51] One should consider antimicrobial prophylaxis for women who experience three or more infections over a 12-month period after successful treatment of any existing infection, although prophylaxis should be considered whenever the woman feels her life is being adversely impacted by frequent recurrences. There are several alternative approaches to choose from, and selection of the optimal method of antimicrobial prophylaxis is based on the frequency and pattern of recurrences. Continuous prophylaxis, postcoital prophylaxis, or intermittent self-treatment (which is not really a prophylaxis method) have all been demonstrated to be effective in the management of recurrent uncomplicated urinary tract infections.

Continuous prophylaxis (Table 28–4) has been demonstrated in numerous studies in different populations to decrease recurrences by 95% when compared with placebo or with patients' prior experience.[49,51] Most authorities advocate a 6-month trial of prophylaxis, with the dose administered at night, after which the regimen is discontinued and the patient observed for further infection. The rationale for the 6-month prophylaxis period is based on observations that urinary tract infections seem to cluster in some women.[10,11] It appears, however, that most women revert to the previous pattern of recurrent infections once prophylaxis is stopped unless other factors, such as sexual activity or spermicide use, are modified. Some authorities advocate a longer period of prophylaxis, such as 2 or more years, in women who continue to have symptomatic infections, and use of TMP-SMX or other agents for as long as 5 years has been reported to be effective and well tolerated.

Postcoital prophylaxis (Table 28–4) may be a more efficient and acceptable method of prevention than continuous prophylaxis in women whose urinary tract infections appear to be temporally related to sexual intercourse. In the only placebo-controlled trial done to date[52] the infection rate seen with postcoital TMP-SMX (40/200 mg) was 0.3 per patient-year compared with 3.6 per patient-year in placebo-treated women, and the regimen was effective for patients with both low and high

intercourse frequencies. These results compare favorably with those observed in other studies with continuous prophylaxis. Several other agents used after coitus have demonstrated comparable reduction in infection rates in uncontrolled studies (Table 28–4). Depending on the frequency of intercourse, postcoital prophylaxis usually requires considerably less consumption of antimicrobial than does continuous prophylaxis.

Some women do not want to take antimicrobials over an extended period. If such women are reliable, they may be candidates for self-treatment with a short-course antimicrobial regimen. In studies of educated women, UTI has been correctly self-diagnosed in at least 84% of documented UTIs (many of the rest have sterile pyuria), and self-therapy with TMP-SMX, norfloxacin, ofloxacin, or levofloxacin has been as effective as observed in clinical studies.[53,54] Use of this strategy should be restricted to those women who have clearly documented recurrent infections and who are motivated, comply with medical instructions, and have a good relationship with a medical provider. Such women should be reminded to call their provider if the symptoms are not completely resolved within 48 hours.

Intravaginal application of estriol has been demonstrated to dramatically reduce the risk of recurrent UTI in postmenopausal women with highly recurrent UTI.[55] The beneficial effect of topical estrogen presumably occurred through the normalization of the vaginal flora, which resulted in increased vaginal lactobacilli and reduced vaginal coliforms. This approach offers an alternative to the antimicrobial strategies discussed earlier for postmenopausal women.

Alternative approaches to prevention of recurrent uncomplicated UTI include the use of probiotics, such as vaginal lactobacillus suppositories, to normalize the vaginal flora and reduce the incidence of vaginal colonization with uropathogens and, thus, reduce the risk of UTI. This approach, although promising, has been studied little and as yet has not been demonstrated to be effective. Vaccination is another potentially useful approach to preventing recurrent UTIs. Whole cell vaccines, made from combinations of heat-killed uropathogenic strains delivered by injection or by a vaginal suppository, have to date had only partial success, with their protective effect diminishing over several weeks.[56] One promising approach is the development of a vaccine based on E. coli type 1 fimbriae components.[57] Virtually all uropathogenic strains of E. coli assemble type 1 pili that contain the FimH adhesin. Sera from animals vaccinated with candidate FimH vaccines inhibited binding of uropathogenic E. coli to human bladder cells in vitro. Immunization with FimH reduced in vivo colonization of the bladder mucosa by more than 99% in a murine cystitis model. Furthermore, passive systemic administration of immune sera to FimH also reduced bladder colonization by uropathogenic E. coli. This promising approach is currently undergoing human trials.

TABLE 28–4 ■ Antimicrobial Prophylaxis Regimens for Women with Recurrent Acute Uncomplicated Cystitis

Antimicrobial	Dose and frequency
CONTINUOUS PROPHYLAXIS	
Cefaclor	250 mg daily
Cephalexin	125–250 mg daily
Fluoroquinolone*†	
Ciprofloxacin	125 mg daily
Norfloxacin	200 mg daily
Nitrofurantoin	50–100 mg daily
Trimethoprim	100 mg daily
TMP-SMX†	40/200 mg daily
TMP-SMX†	40/200 mg thrice weekly
POSTCOITAL PROPHYLAXIS	
Cephalexin	250 mg
Fluoroquinolone*†	
Ciprofloxacin	125 mg
Norfloxacin	200 mg
Ofloxacin	100 mg
Nitrofurantoin	50 or 100 mg
TMP-SMX†	40/200 mg
TMP-SMX†	80/400 mg

*Women should be cautioned about pregnancy when fluoroquinolones are being used. Other fluoroquinolones are likely to be as effective for prophylaxis.

†TMP-SMX can induce the metabolism of oral contraceptives, and thereby decrease their effectiveness.[45]

Acute Uncomplicated Pyelonephritis in Young Healthy Women

Acute pyelonephritis is suggested by fever, chills, flank pain, nausea and vomiting, fever, and costovertebral angle tenderness. Cystitis symptoms are variably present, and some women experience acute onset of upper UTI signs and symptoms with no lower UTI symptoms at all. The presentation of acute pyelonephritis varies from mild to severe, which may involve a sepsis syndrome with or without shock and renal failure. Pyuria is almost always present, but leukocyte casts, specific for upper UTI, are seen infrequently. Women with acute uncomplicated pyelonephritis may be stratified into those who are ill enough to require hospitalization, generally for parenteral therapy, and those who can be managed in the outpatient setting with oral agents (the majority). Although approximately 12% of patients hospitalized with acute uncomplicated pyelonephritis have bacteremia, there is no evidence that bacteremia portends a worse prognosis or warrants longer therapy in an otherwise healthy person with pyelonephritis.

Microscopic evaluation of the urine may be useful in patients with suspected acute pyelonephritis in whom distinction of gram-positive and gram-negative infections can influence empiric therapy. A urine culture should be performed in all women with acute uncomplicated pyelonephritis. In contrast to cystitis, up to 95% of episodes of pyelonephritis are associated with a uropathogen count of 10^4 cfu/ml or higher.[34]

The availability of effective oral antimicrobials, especially the fluoroquinolones, allows for initial oral therapy in appropriate patients or, in those requiring parenteral therapy, the timely conversion from intravenous to oral therapy and the reduced need for hospitalization, resulting in great cost savings. Indications for admission to the hospital include inability to maintain oral hydration or take medications, uncertain social situation or concern about compliance, uncertainty about the diagnosis, and severe illness with high fevers, severe pain, and marked debility. Outpatient therapy, on the other hand, has been shown to be safe and effective for selected patients, even some who are febrile and vomiting, who can be stabilized with parenteral fluids and antibiotics in an urgent care facility and sent home on oral antibiotics under close supervision.

There are many effective oral (Table 28–5) and parenteral (Table 28–6) regimens for use in patients with acute uncomplicated pyelonephritis.[41] For those patients who can be managed in the outpatient setting, an oral fluoroquinolone, such as ciprofloxacin, gatifloxacin, or levofloxacin, should be used for initial empiric treatment of infection caused by gram-negative bacilli. Of note, moxifloxacin, a newer fluoroquinolone, achieves lower urinary levels than the others and should not be used for pyelonephritis. TMP-SMX or other agents can be used if the infecting strain is known to be susceptible. An initial

TABLE 28–5 ■ Oral Regimens for Acute Uncomplicated Pyelonephritis and Complicated Urinary Tract Infection

Drug, dose	Interval
Amoxicillin, 500 mg	q8h
Amoxicillin, 875 mg	q12h
Amoxicillin-clavulanate, 500/125 mg	q8h
Amoxicillin-clavulanate, 875/125 mg	q12h
Cefixime, 400 mg	q24h
Cefpodoxime proxetil, 200 mg	q12h
Fluoroquinolone	
Ciprofloxacin, 500 mg	q12h
Gatifloxacin, 400 mg	q24h
Levofloxacin, 250–500 mg	q24h
TMP-SMX, 160/800 mg	q12h

See text for additional information about these regimens. Nonfluoroquinolone regimens should be used only when susceptibility data support their use.

TABLE 28–6 ■ Parenteral Regimens for Acute Uncomplicated Pyelonephritis and Complicated Urinary Tract Infection

Drug, dose	Interval
Ampicillin, 1 g (+ gentamicin)	q6h
Aztreonam, 1 g	q8–12h
β-lactam or β-lactamase inhibitor	
Ampicillin-sulbactam, 1.5 g*	q6h
Piperacillin-tazobactam, 3.375 g*	q6–8h
Ticarcillin-clavulanate, 3.2 g*	q8h
Cefepime, 1 g	q12h
Ceftriaxone, 1–2 g	q24h
Fluoroquinolone	
Ciprofloxacin, 200–400 mg	q12h
Gatifloxacin, 400 mg	q24h
Levofloxacin, 250–500 mg	q24h
Gentamicin, 3–5 mg/kg (+/- ampicillin)	q24h
Gentamicin, 1 mg/kg (+/- ampicillin)	q8h
Imipenem-cilastatin, 250–500 mg*	q6–8h
TMP-SMX 160/800 mg	q12h

*Recommended if *Staphylococcus aureus* coverage desirable, as for treatment of a renal or perirenal abscess or when the Gram stain suggests *S. aureus* infection.

See text for additional information about these regimens.

intravenous dose of a fluoroquinolone, ceftriaxone, or aminoglycoside may be warranted in the woman who appears more ill. If enterococcus is suspected from the Gram stain, amoxicillin should be added to the treatment regimen until the causative organism(s) is identified. Cefixime and cefpodoxime proxetil also appear to be effective for the treatment of acute uncomplicated pyelonephritis, although published data are sparse. Cefixime may not perform as well against *S. saprophyticus* infections. Nitrofurantoin should not be used for the treatment of pyelonephritis, since it does not achieve reliable tissue levels.

For hospitalized patients, ceftriaxone is an effective and inexpensive (if given in a dosage of 1 g 24 hours) agent if the Gram stain does not suggest infection caused by gram-positive pathogens. Aminoglycosides given once daily are cost effective, associated with low toxicity (since a switch to oral therapy usually can be made in 1 to 3 days), and may provide a therapeutic advantage over TMP-SMX and β-lactams because of their marked concentration in renal tissue. Ciprofloxacin, gatifloxacin, and levofloxacin, which reach high concentrations in the infected kidney, are effective for the parenteral treatment of uncomplicated pyelonephritis. If enterococcus is suspected on the basis of the Gram stain, ampicillin plus gentamicin, ampicillin-sulbactam, or piperacillin-tazobactam are reasonable broad-spectrum empiric choices. TMP-SMX should not be used alone for empiric therapy for pyelonephritis in areas with a high incidence of resistance to this agent. Patients with acute uncomplicated pyelonephritis can often be switched to oral therapy at 24 to 48 hours, although longer intervals of parenteral therapy occasionally are indicated.

A recently published study in outpatient women with acute uncomplicated pyelonephritis demonstrated the superiority of a 7-day regimen of ciprofloxacin over a 14-day regimen of TMP-SMX.[32] The higher clinical and microbiologic failure rate observed in the TMP-SMX group was due to the high incidence of resistance to TMP-SMX among causative uropathogens. Eighteen percent of the strains were resistant to TMP-SMX, whereas only one isolate was resistant to ciprofloxacin. Among the women infected with TMP-SMX-resistant uropathogens who were treated with TMP-SMX, only 50% were cured microbiologically and 35% clinically at 4 to 11 days after treatment.

For those mildly to moderately ill patients who have a rapid response with resolution of fever and symptoms soon after treatment is initiated, treatment usually can be discontinued at 7 days. Treatment should be extended to 10 or 14 days for those who are sicker or who do not have a rapid response. Of note, β-lactam regimens shorter than 14 days have been associated with unacceptably high failure rates. Patients with severe pyelonephritis who require hospitalization may warrant longer therapy. However, 6-week regimens have been shown to be no more effective than 14-day regimens for uncomplicated pyelonephritis and cause more side effects.[58]

Routine post-treatment urine cultures in asymptomatic patients probably are not cost effective for the reasons given above for acute cystitis. In women whose pyelonephritis symptoms recur soon after discontinuation of treatment, a repeat urine culture and renal evaluation should be performed. In the patient with no urologic abnormality, retreatment with a 2-week regimen using another agent should be considered. For those patients whose infection persists with the same strain as the initially infecting strain, a 6-week regimen with an appropriate antibiotic is usually curative. In those women whose symptoms resolve but recur weeks or months later, the approach should be the same as with sporadic episodes of pyelonephritis.

Complicated Urinary Tract Infection

Acute Cystitis in Adult Who Has a Condition Suggesting Possible Occult Renal or Prostatic Involvement but Without Other Known Complicating Factors

This category includes men and women with acute cystitis who are more likely to have occult renal or prostatic infection and who may not respond as well to short-course therapy as young women with uncomplicated cystitis do (Table 28–1). Symptoms, signs, and laboratory findings in this group are the same as in acute uncomplicated cystitis. Episodes of cystitis in persons in this group generally are caused by uropathogens having the same antimicrobial susceptibility profile as those causing acute uncomplicated cystitis. Some patients in this category, such as those with diabetes or pregnancy, warrant special attention because of the serious complications that can occur if treatment is inadequate.

The management approach to patients in this category is similar to that for women with uncomplicated cystitis, generally including the same choice of antibiotic regimens (Table 28–3). Except in pregnancy a fluoroquinolone is the empiric antibiotic of choice, especially in someone who has recently been exposed to antimicrobials, because the consequences of treatment failure are greater than in women with uncomplicated cystitis. Fluoroquinolones should not be used in pregnant women. Nitrofurantoin generally should be avoided, since it does not achieve reliable tissue concentrations and would be ineffective for occult prostatitis or pyelonephritis. It is a safe alternative agent, however, for the treatment of mild cystitis in pregnancy. β-lactams are also considered safe in pregnancy. Amoxicillin should be used only when the causative uropathogen is known to be susceptible, however, or for empiric treatment of mild cystitis in pregnancy. Oral third-generation cephalosporins and amoxicillin-clavulanate provide broader coverage than amoxicillin and are preferable in pregnant women with more severe symptoms. A parenteral dose of ceftriaxone may be used for empiric coverage pending results of antimicrobial susceptibility testing in pregnant women with severe cystitis. Although it is likely that short-course treatment will be effective in many patients in this category, regimens of at least 7 days generally are recommended. A pretreatment urine culture should be obtained routinely in patients in this category, whereas the need for a post-treatment culture is less certain, except in pregnant women. In men, early recurrence of UTI with the same species suggests a prostatic source of infection and warrants evaluation for prostatitis.

Urinary Tract Infection in Adult with Potentially Serious Condition Complicating Management

Patients in this category may have, in addition to the classic symptoms and signs of uncomplicated cystitis and pyelonephritis, nonspecific symptoms such as fatigue, irritability, nausea, headache, and abdominal or back pain or other vague symptoms. This is especially true among patients at the extremes of age and those with neurologic disease. Signs and symptoms may occasionally be insidious and exist for weeks to months before diagnosis. Complicated urinary tract infection, like uncomplicated urinary tract infection, is generally associated with pyuria and bacteriuria, although these may be absent if the infection does not communicate with the collecting system. Because of the diverse spectrum of causative uropathogens and their unpredictable susceptibility profile, a urine culture with antimicrobial susceptibility testing should always be performed in patients with suspected complicated UTI. As with uncomplicated UTI, a colony count threshold of 10^3 cfu/ml or higher should be used to diagnose complicated UTI except when urine cultures are obtained through a catheter in which a level of 10^2 cfu/ml or higher is evidence of infection.[34]

It is difficult to generalize about antimicrobial therapy for complicated UTI given the wide variety of underlying conditions (Table 28–1), diverse spectrum of possible etiologic agents (Table 28–2), and high rates of drug resistance. Attempts must be made to correct any underlying anatomic, functional, or metabolic defect, since antibiotics alone often will not be successful otherwise.[30] Empiric therapy should be broad spectrum, especially for those with more severe disease. For empiric therapy in patients with mild-to-moderate illness who can be treated with oral medication, the fluoroquinolones provide the broadest spectrum of antimicrobial activity, covering most expected pathogens, and achieve high levels in the urine and urinary tract tissue. If the infecting pathogen is known to be susceptible, TMP-SMX or other agents are reasonable therapeutic choices. Thus it is not clear that any agent or class of agents has superior efficacy when the infecting organism is susceptible.

For initial treatment in more seriously ill, hospitalized patients, several parenteral antimicrobial agents, all having a broad spectrum of coverage, are available to choose from (Table 28–6). If enterococcus is suspected on the basis of the Gram stain, ampicillin plus gentamicin, piperacillin-tazobactam, or imipenem are reasonable broad spectrum empiric agents. *S. aureus* is relatively more likely to be found in complicated UTIs than in uncomplicated UTIs, and if it is suspected clinically or by Gram stain results, the therapeutic regimen should have activity against this pathogen.

The antimicrobial regimen can be modified when the infecting strain has been identified and antimicrobial susceptibilities are known. Patients given parenteral therapy can be switched to oral treatment after clinical improvement. Comparative trials to define optimal treatment length for complicated UTI are lacking, and long term success of antimicrobial treatment depends upon whether the underlying genitourinary abnormality, if present, can be corrected.[30] At least 7 to 14 days of therapy is generally recommended, but longer therapy is indicated in patients in whom an underlying complicating factor continues to compromise management.[33] On the other hand, some patients who have mild cystitis can be successfully treated with a 7-day regimen. A urine culture should be repeated 1 or 2 weeks after the completion of therapy.

Recurrent UTI, both relapse and reinfection, is common in persons with complicated UTIs in which the underlying genitourinary abnormality cannot be corrected. In populations with relatively uniform and well-characterized urologic abnormalities, at least 50% of patients experience recurrent UTI within 6 weeks of therapy.[30] Guidelines for conducting clinical trials suggest that the expected cure rates for complicated UTIs should be higher than 40% 4 to 6 weeks after treatment.[34] Thus the goals of antimicrobial therapy (cure, prophylaxis, or suppression) should be clearly elucidated when therapy is initiated, especially when definitive corrective action is not performed.[30]

Renal insufficiency is more common among patients with complicated UTI, and thus it is important to make appropriate dosage adjustments when one is treating such patients. Effective treatment of UTI has been associated with therapeutic antimicrobial concentrations in urine, but the extent to which tissue concentrations of antibiotics are important for cure has not been established. Renal perfusion of antimicrobials into infected renal tissue and urine is impaired, and some antimicrobials, such as aminoglycosides, may not achieve optimal concentrations in the urine.[59] A more prolonged course of therapy may be necessary to cure UTIs in patients with renal failure.[30]

Complicated Urinary Tract Infection in Special Populations
Pregnant Women

UTI in pregnant women presents a special problem because of the risk of perinatal complications. Although pregnant women appear to be at no greater risk of having asymptomatic bacteriuria than nonpregnant women are (prevalence approximately 4% to 7%), pregnant women with asymptomatic bacteriuria, compared to those without bacteriuria, are at much greater risk of symptomatic UTI later in pregnancy (20% to 40% vs. 2%, respectively).[60] Symptomatic UTI during pregnancy, especially pyelonephritis, is associated with an increased risk of premature delivery and possibly other maternal and fetal complications of pregnancy and should be treated aggressively with regimens considered to be safe in pregnancy. Treatment of asymptomatic bacteriuria decreases the risk of subsequent UTI by up to 90% and thus the morbidity associated with symptomatic UTI. Therefore, pregnant women should be screened early in pregnancy for asymptomatic bacteriuria. It should be noted, however, that most studies have not shown a decrease in prematurity with successful treatment of bacteriuria. Moreover only 40% to 70% of women who subsequently develop a symptomatic UTI are identified through routine screening.

Antimicrobials considered to be safe for use in pregnancy are shown in Table 28–7. Seven-day regimens should be considered for cystitis, although 3-day regimens also appear to be effective.[60] Longer regimens are indicated for pyelonephritis. Pregnant women with pyelonephritis should be hospitalized in most cases. Three-day regimens with several of these antibiotics have been shown to be effective in the treatment of asymptomatic bacteriuria and is the optimal duration when one considers both efficacy and reduced drug exposure to the fetus. A post-treatment culture should be obtained at 1 week to ensure bacteriologic cure and if negative should be followed with monthly cultures until delivery. If the post-treatment culture is positive, a longer course with an antibiotic to which the causative uropathogen is susceptible should be used. Prophylaxis may be indicated in some, after eradication of bacteriuria, who have frequent recurrences of bacteriuria. Prophylaxis may also be indicated in pregnant women who have a previous history of recurrent UTI.[9]

Young Healthy Men

It has been conventional to consider all UTIs in men as complicated, since most that occur in the newborn, the infant, or the elderly are associated with urologic abnormalities, bladder outlet obstruction (e.g., due to prostatic hyperplasia), or instrumentation. A small number of 15- to 50-year-old men, however, suffer acute cystitis with no known urologic abnormalities or instrumentation. The incidence of symptomatic UTI in such men ranges from 5 to 8 per 10,000 men annually. Risk factors associated with these infections include homosexuality, intercourse with an infected female partner, and lack of circumcision. It is reasonable to consider cystitis in these young men as being complicated, because they may have occult prostatitis. As in women, symptoms of dysuria, frequency, urgency, suprapubic pain, or hematuria and laboratory findings of pyuria are typical of cystitis in men. A midstream urine culture is recommended to confirm the diagnosis of UTI in men, using colony count criteria similar to that recommended for women.[61] Urethritis must be considered in sexually active men, and examination for penile ulcerations and urethral discharge, evaluation of a urethral swab specimen Gram stain, and diagnostic tests for *N. gonorrheae* and *C. trachomatis* are warranted. A urethral Gram stain demonstrating leukocytes and predominant gram-negative rods suggests *E. coli* urethritis, which may precede or accompany urinary tract infection. Chronic prostatitis should be considered, particularly in men who have had recurrent UTIs (see Patients with Prostatitis).

The microbial agents causing UTIs in young men are similar to those causing UTIs in young women, and the causative uropathogens also tend to have the same susceptibility patterns. Thus the antimicrobials recommended for the treatment of uncomplicated cystitis in women are appropriate for empiric use in men (Table 28–3), although 7-day regimens are recommended. Nitrofurantoin and β-lactams probably should not be used in men with cystitis, since they do not achieve reliable tissue concentrations and would be ineffective for occult prostatitis. Fosfomycin should also be avoided. Fluoroquinolones provide the best antimicrobial spectrum and prostatic penetration for treating these infections in men.

Catheterized Patients

Approximately 15% to 25% of patients in general hospitals have a catheter inserted at some time during their stay, and most are catheterized for 2 to 4 days.[62] Over 100,000 patients in nursing homes, on the other hand, are catheterized for months to years.[62] The incidence of bacteriuria associated with indwelling catheters is 3% to 10% per day, and the duration of catheterization is the most important risk factor for the development of catheter-associated bacteriuria. Most episodes of catheter-associated bacteriuria are asymptomatic. Although fewer than 5% of catheter-associated bacteriuria episodes are complicated by bacteremia, catheter-associated bacteriuria is the most common source of gram-negative bacteremia in hospitalized patients. The risk of UTI is lower if antimicrobials are given during the first few days of catheterization or within 48 hours of discontinuation of the catheter, but subsequent infections are more likely to be caused by antimicrobial-resistant organisms.[30] In hospitals and nursing homes, asymptomatic catheter-associated bacteriuria comprises a huge reservoir of resistant organisms, particularly on critical care units, and these bacteria are easily transmitted between patients. In fact, about 15% of episodes of hospital-acquired bacteriuria occur in clusters, and they often involve highly antibiotic-resistant organisms. Complications of long-term catheterization (more than 30 days) include almost universal bacteriuria, often with polymicrobic and antibiotic-resistant flora, and in addition to cystitis, pyelonephritis, and bacteremia as seen with short-term catheterization, frequent febrile episodes, catheter obstruction, stone formation associated with urease-producing uropathogens, local genitourinary infections, fistula formation, and bladder cancer.[62]

TABLE 28–7 ■ Antimicrobials Used for Urinary Tract Infection During Pregnancy

Amoxicillin
Amoxicillin-clavulanate
Cefixime
Cefpodoxime proxetil
Fosfomycin tromethamine
Nitrofurantoin
Trimethoprim
TMP-SMX

Trimethoprim and TMP-SMX should be avoided in the first trimester, and TMP-SMX should be avoided at term. See Table 28–3 for doses for cystitis.

Routine screening or treatment of asymptomatic catheterized patients is not indicated, since treatment does not reduce the complications of bacteriuria and can lead to antimicrobial resistance. Some authorities, however, recommend that women with bacteriuria acquired during short-term urethral catheterization should receive treatment after catheter removal to reduce the risk of subsequent symptomatic UTI.[63] Whether this approach has long-term benefits is still unknown. Symptomatic infections, often polymicrobial and caused by multiple-drug-resistant uropathogens, warrant broad-spectrum antimicrobial therapy. Patients with mild cystitis should be treated for 5 to 7 days to reduce the risk of drug resistance. Longer treatment regimens are indicated in patients with moderate-to-severe cystitis or pyelonephritis. However, the optimal duration of therapy for catheter-associated UTIs has not been determined. Since bacteria may be sequestered and protected from antibiotics in a biofilm on the catheter surface, it is reasonable to replace the catheter at the start of antibiotic therapy, especially those that have been in place for several days, although there are little data to support this recommendation.[33,64]

Preventive measures are indicated to reduce the morbidity, mortality, and costs of catheter-associated infection. Effective strategies include avoidance of the catheter when possible and, when the catheter is necessary, sterile insertion, prompt removal, and strict adherence to a closed collecting system.[33,62,65] Although randomized trials have not been performed, intermittent catheterization appears to result in lower rates of bacteriuria than long-term indwelling catheterization does, and in men, condom catheterization appears to have the lowest, although not negligible, risk. Suprapubic catheters also appear to be associated with a lower risk of UTI than urethral catheters are.[65] Other approaches that have been effective in some studies, but not others, include preconnected catheter-collecting tube units, disinfectants in collecting bags, silver oxide–coated catheters, and the regular periurethral application of antimicrobial creams. Silver alloy catheters, however, do appear to be effective in reducing the risk of UTI, although cost-effectiveness analysis is needed to assess whether these novel catheters should be used routinely.[65] Systemic antimicrobial agents (and, in intermittently catheterized patients, bladder irrigation with antibacterial agents) prevent or delay the onset of bacteriuria, but their routine use in catheterized persons is discouraged because of the cost and the potential for the development of antimicrobial resistance. Prophylactic systemic antimicrobial agents may be useful, however, in patients at high risk for serious complications if UTI occurs, such as pregnant women who are undergoing short-term catheterization or patients undergoing transurethral resection of the prostate or renal transplantation.[65] In addition, prophylaxis with TMP-SMX has been demonstrated to be beneficial in patients undergoing renal transplantation and requiring indwelling catheterization.[65]

Spinal Cord Injury Patients

Spinal cord injury (SCI) alters the dynamics of voiding and often requires bladder drainage with catheters. The use of catheters, elevated intravesicle pressures, and increased postvoid residuals heighten the risk for and severity of UTIs in persons with SCI. Eighty percent of persons with SCI have a UTI within 16 years of their injury.[66] Urinary tract infection and its complications of urosepsis, renal failure, and urolithiasis previously were associated with increased mortality in patients with SCI, but improved bladder management has markedly reduced the mortality in such patients.[67] The diagnosis of UTI in persons with SCI, often problematic, is based on the combination of symptoms and signs, which are often nonspecific, pyuria, and significant bacteriuria with uropathogens often present in quantities higher than 10^5 cfu/ml. Fluoroquinolones are the empiric oral agents of choice in patients with mild-to-moderate infection, although many uropathogens, even in the outpatient setting, are resistant to this class of antibiotics, and parenteral antibiotics may be needed. As with other types of complicated UTI, the optimal duration of therapy has not been established, but generally 7 to 14 days of therapy is recommended.[67]

Asymptomatic bacteriuria appears to have no long-term serious sequelae in the person with SCI who has low intravesicle pressure, but it is not known whether this low risk persists over the person's lifetime. Most authorities recommend against routine treatment of asymptomatic bacteriuria in persons with SCI because the long-term benefit is unclear and because treatment increases the selection pressure for antimicrobial-resistant uropathogens.[67] Likewise, antibiotic prophylaxis is generally not recommended because of its unproven benefit in several studies and the concern about emergence of antimicrobial resistance.[68] It is preferable instead to try to optimize the patient's bladder drainage method and to monitor patients closely for any evidence of symptoms or signs that may suggest UTI and to treat the UTI accordingly. For some patients, particularly outpatients with frequent symptomatic UTIs for whom there are no correctable risk factors, antimicrobial prophylaxis may be useful. A promising approach to prevention of UTI in persons with SCI is bacterial interference with an asymptomatic bacteriuria-causing *E. coli* strain. Long-term bladder colonization was achieved with a reduction in the number of symptomatic UTIs in a small number of patients tested with *E. coli* 83972.[69] Further study of this approach is warranted.

Patients with Prostatitis

The terminology used to describe prostatitis has long been confusing. In 1995 the National Institute of Diabetes and Digestive and Kidney Diseases Working Group on Prostatitis proposed a new classification for prostatitis disorders: I, acute bacterial prostatitis; II, chronic bacterial prostatitis; III, chronic prostatitis–chronic pelvic pain syndrome (CPPS) (IIIa, inflammatory [previously, chronic nonbacterial prostatitis], and IIIb, noninflammatory [previously, prostatodynia]); and IV, asymptomatic inflammatory prostatitis.[70] The new classification system recognizes that we have a limited understanding of the causes of the syndrome for most patients, that organs other than the prostate may be important in causing the symptoms, and that urologic pain complaints are a primary component of the syndromes.

In the United States there are approximately 2 million physician visits annually for prostatitis.[71] Prostatitis symptoms are experienced by approximately 50% of adult men, and prostatic symptoms account for 25% of office visits for men with genitourinary complaints.[72] Of men with genitourinary complaints attending a special prostatitis clinic, only 5% had chronic bacterial prostatitis, 64% had chronic nonbacterial prostatitis (inflammatory CPPS), and 31% had prostatodynia (noninflammatory CPPS).[73] The distinction between the various prostatitis syndromes is based on symptoms and signs and a quantitative evaluation of leukocytes and bacteria in urine and prostatic fluids.[74] The standard localization test, however, has never been properly validated and is inconvenient, time consuming, expensive, and difficult to perform.[75] As a result only a minority of physicians, including urologists, perform the diagnostic test as it was originally described,[74] and there appears to be little correlation between use of the test and the prescribing of antibiotics for symptoms.[76] Moreover, men classified as having chronic bacterial prostatitis may have physical findings, response to antibiotic therapy, and prognosis similar to those of other chronic pelvic pain syndromes previously described.[77]

The pathogenesis of prostatitis is believed to be related to ascending urethral infection or reflux of infected urine into the prostatic ducts. Prostatic calculi, commonly found in adult men, may provide a nidus for bacteria and protection from antimicrobial agents. The organisms most commonly causing bacterial prostatitis are gram-negative bacilli, including *E. coli*, *Proteus* spp, *Klebsiella* spp, and *P. aeruginosa*, and less commonly, enterococci. The role of staphylococci as pathogen or commensal in prostatitis continues to be debated.[75]

TMP-SMX and fluoroquinolones have been most successful in the treatment of prostatitis. Penicillins and cephalosporins do not penetrate the prostate well and generally are not recommended, although carbenicillin indanyl is approved for this condition. Among the fluoroquinolones, ciprofloxacin, levofloxacin, and gatifloxacin are all likely to be effective.

Acute bacterial prostatitis, which is rare, is manifested by typical UTI symptoms of dysuria, frequency, urgency, fever, and chills. Obstructive voiding symptoms and pain in the low back, rectum, or perineum are often present. The prostate is warm, tender, and swollen, but prostatic massage is contraindicated in men in whom the diagnosis of acute prostatitis is being considered because it is painful and may precipitate bacteremia. The patient will usually have pyuria and a positive urine culture. Patients who are severely ill require hospitalization and parenteral antibiotics, but many patients can be treated in the outpatient setting with oral fluoroquinolones. The recommended length of treatment is at least 30 days to help prevent the development of chronic bacterial prostatitis,[78] although many men with a diagnosis of chronic bacterial prostatitis have not had acute bacterial prostatitis. Abscess formation is rare.

Chronic bacterial prostatitis often is characterized by recurrent urinary tract infections with the same uropathogen with intervening asymptomatic periods. Between such UTIs, men may complain of dysuria, ejaculatory pain, hemospermia, or pelvic or genital pain. The prostate typically is normal to palpation during asymptomatic periods. Chronic bacterial prostatitis is characterized by 10 leukocytes or more per high-power field in expressed prostatic secretions or postmassage voided urine in the absence of significant pyuria in first-voided and midstream urine specimens and a uropathogen colony count that is at least 10-fold higher in the expressed prostatic secretions or postmassage voided urine than in the first-voided midstream urine. In addition, macrophage-laden fat droplets (oval fat bodies) are usually prominent in men with bacterial prostatitis. Cure rates historically have been low for this condition, 30% to 40% with TMP-SMX, but are up to 90% with the fluoroquinolones, which are the antibiotics of choice. The optimal duration of treatment is unknown, but most authorities recommend at least 1 to 3 months.[72,78] In some men with recalcitrant chronic bacterial prostatitis, surgical intervention should be considered, but morbidity is high. In men in whom surgery is not desired or feasible, long-term, low-dose suppressive therapy may be used to prevent symptomatic urinary tract infections. Effective regimens include daily low doses of a fluoroquinolone, TMP-SMX, or nitrofurantoin.[79]

Patients with Renal Abscess

Renal cortical and corticomedullary abscesses and perirenal abscesses occur in 1 to 10 per 10,000 hospital admissions.[80] Patients usually present with fever, chills, back or abdominal pain, and costovertebral angle tenderness but may have no urinary symptoms or findings if the abscess does not communicate with the collecting system, as is often the case with a cortical abscess. Bacteremia at the time of diagnosis is more common with corticomedullary and perirenal abscesses. The clinical presentation may be insidious and nonspecific, especially with perirenal abscess, and the diagnosis may not be made until hospital admission or at autopsy. Computed tomography (CT) is recommended to establish the diagnosis and location of a renal or perirenal abscess. Empiric antibiotic therapy should be broad and cover *S. aureus* and other uropathogens causing complicated UTI (Table 28–6) and modified as appropriate on the basis of urine culture results.

A renal cortical abscess (renal carbuncle) usually is caused by *S. aureus*, which reaches the kidney through the hematogenous route. Treatment with antibiotics is usually effective, and drainage ordinarily is not required unless the patient is slow to respond. A renal corticomedullary abscess, in contrast, usually results from ascending UTI in association with an underlying urinary tract abnormality such as obstructive uropathy or vesicoureteral reflux and is usually caused by common uropathogenic species such as *E. coli*. Such abscesses may extend deep into the renal parenchyma, perforate the renal capsule, and form a perinephric abscess. Treatment with antimicrobial agents without drainage is usually effective if the abscess is not large and if the underlying urinary tract abnormality can be corrected. Aspiration of the abscess may be necessary in some cases, and nephrectomy occasionally may be required in patients with diffuse renal involvement or with severe sepsis. Perinephric abscesses usually occur in the setting of obstruction or other complicating factor and result from ruptured intrarenal abscesses, hematogenous spread, or spread from a contiguous infection. Causative uropathogens are those commonly found in complicated UTIs (Table 28–2), including *S. aureus* and enterococci, and polymicrobic infections are common. A previously high mortality has been lowered with earlier diagnosis and therapy. In contrast to the other types of abscesses, drainage of pus is the cornerstone of therapy, and nephrectomy is sometimes indicated.

Patients with Papillary Necrosis

Most cases of papillary necrosis occur in diabetics, almost always in conjunction with a urinary tract infection, but the condition also complicates sickle cell disease, analgesic abuse, and obstruction.[81] Renal papillae are vulnerable to ischemia because of the sluggish blood flow in the vasa recta, and relatively modest ischemic insults may cause papillary necrosis. The clinical features are those typical of pyelonephritis, but passage of sloughed papillae into the ureter may also cause renal colic, renal insufficiency or failure, or obstruction with severe urosepsis. Papillary necrosis in the setting of pyelonephritis is associated with pyuria and bacteriuria. The microbial spectrum is typical of complicated UTI (Table 28–2). The retrograde pyelogram is the preferred diagnostic procedure. Radiologic findings include an irregular papillary tip, dilated calyceal fornix, extension of contrast material into the parenchyma, and a separated crescent-shaped papilla surrounded by contrast, called the "ring sign." Broad-spectrum antibiotics are indicated. Papillae obstructing the ureter may require removal with a cystoscopic ureteral basket or by insertion of a ureteral stent.

Patients with Emphysematous Pyelonephritis

Emphysematous pyelonephritis is a fulminant, necrotizing, life-threatening variant of acute pyelonephritis caused by gas-forming organisms including *E. coli, Klebsiella pneumoniae, P. aeruginosa,* and *P. mirabilis.*[82] Up to 90% of cases occur in diabetics, and obstruction may be present. Symptoms are suggestive of pyelonephritis, and a flank mass may be present. Dehydration and ketoacidosis are common. Pyuria and a positive urine culture are usually present. Gas usually is detected by a plain abdominal radiograph or ultrasound. CT is the diagnostic modality of choice, however, since it can better localize the gas than ultrasonography can. Accurate localization of gas is important, since gas may also form in an infected obstructed collecting system or renal abscess, which, although serious, do not carry the same grave prognosis and are managed differently. Emergent drainage or nephrectomy in conjunction with broad-spectrum antibiotics is the treatment of choice.[83] Medical treatment is associated with a mortality of 60% to 80%, which falls to 20% or less with surgical intervention.[31,83]

Asymptomatic Bacteriuria

Asymptomatic bacteriuria is a common and generally benign infection,[13,14] but is a predictor of subsequent symptomatic UTI in some settings. Pyuria is often present in asymptomatic bacteriuria but has no known prognostic significance except that it is a stronger predictor for symptomatic UTI in young women. Causative uropathogens are the same as those causing UTIs in the same population. Treatment for asymptomatic bacteriuria generally is not warranted, although recommendations vary according to the clinical setting.[13] Treatment considerations for patients who are catheterized, have spinal cord injury, or who are pregnant have been discussed. Patients with asymptomatic bacteriuria who may be at high risk for serious complications and thus who warrant a more aggressive approach to diagnosis and treatment include pregnant women, renal transplant patients, patients undergoing urologic surgery or surgery involving a prosthetic device, and neutropenic patients. Some authorities also advise treatment of asymptomatic bacteriuria found in patients who undergo clean intermittent catheterization, patients with anatomic or functional abnormalities of the urinary tract, diabetics, and patients with urea-splitting bacteria, such as *P. mirabilis, Klebsiella* spp, and others.[13] Evidence-based guidelines for screening and treatment of asymptomatic bacteriuria in these populations are needed.

UROLOGIC EVALUATION

Most women with recurrent uncomplicated cystitis have no anatomic or functional abnormality of the urinary tract and therefore do not need an evaluation of their urinary tract. Studies of the value of excretory urography and of cystoscopy in women with recurrent cystitis have demonstrated that significant abnormalities which influence subsequent management of urinary tract infections are uncommon.[33] Thus routine urologic evaluation of recurrent cystitis patients creates unnecessary expense and a potential for toxicity. Likewise, routine urologic investigation of young women with acute pyelonephritis is generally not cost effective and has a low diagnostic yield, although it is reasonable to obtain such an evaluation after two episodes of pyelonephritis or if any complicating factor is identified with any of the recurrences. A urologic evaluation is probably not necessary in a man who has had a single episode of cystitis with no obvious complicating factors and whose infection responds promptly to treatment. A complete urologic evaluation including cystoscopy and excretory urography should be performed in patients who have persistent hematuria after the UTI has been eradicated.

Urologic consultation and evaluation of the urinary tract should be considered in patients who present with symptoms or signs of obstruction, urolithiasis, flank mass, or urosepsis. A urologic evaluation should also be considered for those patients with any UTI who have not had a satisfactory clinical response after 72 hours of treatment with an appropriate antimicrobial to rule out a complicating factor. Contrast-enhanced CT scanning of the kidneys is the imaging modality with the highest yield in adult patients with renal infection because of its superior resolution and sensitivity in detecting renal abnormalities and perirenal fluid collections.[84] Spiral (helical) CT may be superior to conventional CT.[84,85] Noncontrast spiral CT appears to be a rapid, safe, and sensitive method for evaluating patients with suspected renal stones. Renal ultrasound is also a useful modality, especially for detection of stones and abscesses, and is often more readily accessible than CT. However, it is less sensitive than CT for detection of many of the conditions present in patients with complicated UTI. Excretory urography has assumed a less important role in evaluating acutely ill patients in the CT era, and the role of magnetic resonance imaging remains to be determined. A plain abdominal radiograph may be used to detect gas in the urinary tracts of diabetics with suspected pyelonephritis, but it is not as sensitive or specific as CT.

REFERENCES

1. Foxman B, Barlow R, D'Arcy H, et al: Urinary tract infection: Self-reported incidence and associated costs. Ann Epidemiol 2000;10:509–515.
2. Hooton TM, Scholes D, Hughes JP, et al: A prospective study of risk factors for symptomatic urinary tract infection in young women. N Engl J Med 1996;335:468–474.
3. Ikaheimo R, Siitonen A, Heiskanen T, et al: Recurrence of urinary tract infection in a primary care setting: Analysis of a 1-year follow-up of 179 women. Clin Infect Dis 1996;22:91–99.
4. Nicolle LE, Friesen D, Harding GK, Roos LL: Hospitalization for acute pyelonephritis in Manitoba, Canada, during the period from 1989 to 1992: Impact of diabetes, pregnancy, and aboriginal origin. Clin Infect Dis 1996;22:1051–1056.
5. Safrin S, Siegel D, Black D: Pyelonephritis in adult women: Inpatient versus outpatient therapy. Am J Med 1988;85:793–798.
6. Pinson AG, Philbrick JT, Lindbeck GH, Schorling JB: ED management of acute pyelonephritis in women: A cohort study. Am J Emerg Med 1994;12:271–278.
7. Foxman B, Frerichs RR: Epidemiology of urinary tract infection. I. Diaphragm use and sexual intercourse. Am J Public Health 1985;75:1308.
8. Foxman B: Recurring urinary tract infection: Incidence and risk factors. Am J Public Health 1990;80:331–333.
9. Stapleton A, Stamm WE: Prevention of urinary tract infection. Infect Dis Clin North Am 1997;11:719–733.
10. Kraft JK, Stamey TA: The natural history of symptomatic recurrent bacteriuria in women. Medicine 1977;56:55.
11. Stamm WE, McKevitt M, Roberts PL, White NJ: Natural history of recurrent urinary tract infections in women. Rev Infect Dis 1991;13:77.
12. Bronsema DA, Adams JR, Pallares R, et al: Secular trends in rates and etiology of nosocomial urinary tract infections at a university hospital. J Urol 1993;150:414–416.
13. Zhanel GG, Harding GKM, Guay DRP: Asymptomatic bacteriuria: Which patients should be treated? Arch Intern Med 1990;150:1389–1396.
14. Hooton TM, Scholes D, Stapleton AE, et al: A prospective study of asymptomatic bacteriuria in sexually active young women. N Engl J Med 2000;343:992–997.
15. Bengtsson C, Bengtsson U, Bjorkelund C, et al: Bacteriuria in a population sample of women: 24-year follow-up study: Results from the prospective population-based study of women in Gothenburg, Sweden. Scand J Urol Nephrol 1998;32:284–289.
16. Nicolle LE: Asymptomatic bacteriuria in elderly. Infect Dis Clin North Am 1997;11:647–662.
17. Yoshikawa TT, Nicolle LE, Norman DC: Management of complicated urinary tract infection in older patients. J Am Geriatr Soc 1996;44:1235–1241.
18. Mulvey MA, Schilling JD, Martinez JJ, Hultgren SJ: Bad bugs and beleaguered bladders: Interplay between uropathogenic Escherichia coli and innate host defenses. Proc Natl Acad Sci USA 2000;97:8829–8835.
19. Elliott TS, Reed L, Slack RC, Bishop MC: Bacteriology and ultrastructure of the bladder in patients with urinary tract infections. J Infect 1985;11:191–199.
20. Scholes D, Hooton TM, Roberts PL, et al: Risk factors for recurrent urinary tract infection in young women. J Infect Dis 2000;182:1177–1182.
21. Raz R, Gennesin Y, Wasser J, et al: Recurrent urinary tract infection in postmenopausal women. Clin Infect Dis 2000;30:152–156.
22. Hopkins WJ, Dillon CC, Uehling DT: Pedigree analysis demonstrates a familial predisposition to recurrent urinary tract infection. J Urol 2001;165(Suppl):7 (Abstract 32).
23. Stapleton A, Nudelman E, Clausen H, et al: Binding of uropathogenic Escherichia coli R45 to glycolipids extracted from vaginal epithelial cells is dependent on histo-blood group secretor status. J Clin Invest 1992;90:965–972.
24. Ishitoya S, Terai A, Yamamoto S, Ogawa O: Non-secretor status is associated with female acute uncomplicated pyelonephritis. J Urol 2001;165(Suppl):6 (Abstract 23).
25. Benson M, Jodal U, Agace W, et al: Interleukin (IL)-6 and IL-8 in children with febrile urinary tract infection and asymptomatic bacteriuria. J Infect Dis 1996;174:1080–1084.
26. Frendeus B, Godaly G, Hang L, et al: Interleukin 8 receptor deficiency confers susceptibility to acute experimental pyelonephritis and may have a human counterpart. J Exp Med 2000;192:881–890.
27. Svanborg C, Godaly G: Bacteral virulence in urinary tract infection. Infect Dis Clin North Am 1997;11:513–529.
28. Johnson JR: Virulence factors in Escherichia coli urinary tract infection. Clin Microbiol Rev 1991;4:80–128.

29. Ronald AR, Harding GKM: Complicated urinary tract infections. Infect Dis Clin North Am 1997;11:583–592.

30. Nicolle LE: A practical guide to the management of complicated urinary tract infection. Drugs 1997;53:583–592.

31. Patterson JE, Andriole VT: Bacterial urinary tract infections in diabetes. Infect Dis Clin North Am 1997;11:735–750.

32. Talan DA, Stamm WE, Hooton TM, et al: Comparison of ciprofloxacin (7 days) and trimethoprim-sulfamethoxazole (14 days) for acute uncomplicated pyelonephritis in women: A randomized trial. JAMA 2000;283:1583–1590.

33. Stamm WE, Hooton TM: Management of urinary tract infections in adults. N Engl J Med 1993;329:1328–1334.

34. Rubin UH, Shapiro ED, Andriole VT, et al: Evaluation of new anti-infective drugs for the treatment of urinary tract infection. Clin Infect Dis 1992;15:S216–S227.

35. Gupta K, Hooton TM, Stamm WE: Increasing antimicrobial resistance and the management of uncomplicated community-acquired urinary tract infections. Ann Intern Med 2001;135:41–50.

36. Hooton TM, Stamm WE. Diagnosis and treatment of uncomplicated urinary tract infection. Infect Dis Clin North Am 1997;11:551–581.

37. Asbach HW: Single dose oral administration of cefixime 400 mg in the treatment of acute uncomplicated cystitis and gonorrhoea. Drugs 1991;42(Suppl 4):10.

38. Gupta K, Sahm DF, Mayfield D, Stamm WE: Antimicrobial resistance among uropathogens that cause community-acquired urinary tract infections in women: A nationwide analysis. Clin Infect Dis 2001;33:89–94.

39. Manges AR, Johnson JR, Foxman B, et al: Widespread distribution of urinary tract infection caused by a multidrug-resistant *Escherichia coli* clonal group. N Engl J Med 2001;345:1055–1057.

40. Gupta K, Scholes D, Stamm WE: Increasing prevalence of antimicrobial resistance among uropathogens causing acute uncomplicated cystitis in women. JAMA 1999;281:736–738.

41. Warren JW, Abrutyn E, Hebel JR, et al: Guidelines for antimicrobial treatment of uncomplicated acute bacterial cystitis and acute pyelonephritis in women. Clin Infect Dis 1999;29:745–758.

42. Norrby SR: Short-term treatment of uncomplicated lower urinary tract infections in women. Rev Infect Dis 1990;12:458–467.

43. Stamm WE: An epidemic of urinary tract infection? N Engl J Med 2001;345:1055–1056.

44. McCarty JM, Richard G, Huck W, et al: A randomized trial of short-course ciprofloxacin, ofloxacin, or trimethoprim/sulfamethoxazole for the treatment of acute urinary tract infection in women. Am J Med 1999;106:292–299.

45. Oral contraceptives. Med Lett 2000;42:42–44.

46. Greenberg RN, Reilly PM, Luppen KL, et al: Randomized study of single-dose, three-day, and seven-day treatment of cystitis in women. Infect Dis 1986;153:277–282.

47. Hooton TM, Winter C, Tiu F, Stamm WE: Randomized comparative trial and cost analysis of 3-day antimicrobial regimens for treatment of acute cystitis in women. JAMA 1995;273:41.

48. Wright SW, Wrenn KD, Haynes ML: Trimethoprim-sulfamethoxazole resistance among urinary coliform isolates. J Gen Intern Med 1999;14:606–609.

49. Hooton TM: Recurrent urinary tract infection in women. Int J Antimicrob Agents 2001;17:259–268.

50. Kontiokari T, Sundqvist K, Nuutinen M, et al: Randomised trial of cranberry-lingonberry juice and *Lactobacillus* GG drink for the prevention of urinary tract infections in women. BMJ 2001;322:1–5.

51. Nicolle LE, Ronald AR: Recurrent urinary tract infection in adult women: Diagnosis and treatment. Infect Dis Clin North Am 1987;1:793–806.

52. Stapleton A, Latham RH, Johnson C, Stamm WE: Postcoital antimicrobial prophylaxis for recurrent urinary tract infection. JAMA 1990;264:703–706.

53. Schaeffer AJ, Stuppy BA: Efficacy and safety of self-start therapy in women with recurrent urinary tract infections. J Urol 1999;161:207–211.

54. Gupta K, Hooton TM, Roberts PL, Stamm WE: Patient-initiated treatment of uncomplicated recurrent urinary tract infections in young women. Ann Intern Med 2001;135:9–16.

55. Raz R, Stamm WE: A controlled trial of intravaginal estriol in postmenopausal women with recurrent urinary tract infections. N Engl J Med 1993;329:753–756.

56. Uehling DT, Hopkins WJ, Balish E, et al: Vaginal mucosal immunization for recurrent urinary tract infection: Phase II clinical trial. J Urol 1997;157:2049–2052.

57. Langermann S, Palaszynski S, Barnhart M, et al: Prevention of mucosal *Escherichia coli* infection by FimH-adhesin-based systemic vaccination. Science 1997;276:607–611.

58. Bergeron MG: Current concepts in the treatment of pyelonephritis. Intern Med 1989;10:65.

59. Craven R, Bennett W, Hartwell M, et al: Serum, urine and tissue antibiotic concentrations in patients with renal disease. Proc Am Soc Nephrol 1976;8:12.

60. Patterson TF, Andriole VT: Detection, significance, and therapy of bacteriuria in pregnancy. Infect Dis Clin North Am 1997;11:593–608.

61. Lipsky BA, Ireton RC, Fihn SD, et al: Diagnosis of bacteriuria in men: Specimen collection and culture interpretation. J Infect Dis 1987;155:847.

62. Warren JW: Catheter-associated urinary tract infections. Infect Dis Clin North Am 1997;11:609–622.

63. Harding GKM, Nicolle LE, Ronald AR, et al: How long should catheter-acquired urinary tract infection in women be treated? Ann Intern Med 1991;114:713–719.

64. Raz R, Schiller D, Nicolle LE: Chronic indwelling catheter replacement before antimicrobial therapy for symptomatic urinary tract infection. J Urol 2000;164:1254–1258.

65. Saint S, Lipsky BA: Preventing catheter-related bacteriuria: Should we? Can we? How? Arch Intern Med 1999;159:800–808.

66. DeVivo MJ, Black KJ, Stover S: Causes of death during the first 12 years after spinal cord injury. Arch Phys Med Rehabil 1993;74:248–254.

67. Cardenas DD, Hooton TM: Urinary tract infection in persons with spinal cord injury. Arch Phys Med Rehabil 1995;76:272–280.

68. The prevention and management of urinary tract infection among people with spinal cord injuries: National Institute on Disability and Rehabilitation Research Consensus Statement: January 27–29, 1992. J Am Paraplegia Soc 1992;15:194–204.

69. Hull R, Rudy D, Donovan W, et al: Urinary tract infection prophylaxis using *Escherichia coli* 83972 in spinal cord injured patients. J Urol 2000;163:872–877.

70. Krieger JN, Nyberg L Jr, Nickel JC: NIH consensus definition and classification of prostatitis. JAMA 1999;282:236–237.

71. Collins MM, Stafford RS, O'Leary MP, Barry MJ: How common is prostatitis? A national survey of physician visits. J Urol 1998;159:1224–1228.

72. Brannigan RE, Schaeffer AJ: Prostatitis syndromes. Curr Opin Infect Dis 1996;9:37–41.

73. Brunner H, Weidner W, Schiefer HG: Studies of the role of *Ureaplasma urealyticum* and *Mycoplasma hominis* in prostatitis. J Infect Dis 1983;147:807–813.

74. Meares EM Jr, Stamey TA: Bacteriologic localization patterns in bacterial prostatitis and urethritis. Invest Urol 1968; 5:492–518.

75. Lipsky BA: Prostatitis and urinary tract infection in men: What's new;what's true? Am J Med 1999;106:327–334.

76. Mc Naughton CM, Fowler FJ, Elliott DB, et al: Diagnosing and treating chronic prostatitis: Do urologists use the four-glass test? Urology 2000;55:403–407.

77. Pavone-Macaluso M, Di Trapani D, Pavone C: Prostatitis, prostatosis and prostalgia. Psychogenic or organic disease? Scand J Urol Nephrol 1991;138(Suppl):77–82.

78. Meares EM: Prostatitis. Med Clin North Am 1991;75:405–424.

79. Falagas ME, Gorbach SL: Practice guidelines: Prostatitis, epididymitis, and urethritis. Infect Dis Clin Pract 1995;4:325–333.

80. Dembry LM, Andriole VT: Renal and perirenal abscesses. Infect Dis Clin North Am 1997;11:663–680.

81. Mandel EE: Renal medullary necrosis. Am J Med 1952; 13:322–327.

82. McHugh TP, Albanna SE, Stewart NJ: Bilateral emphysematous pyelonephritis. Am J Emerg Med 1998;16:166–169.

83. Tang HJ, Yen MY, Chen YS, et al: Clinical characteristics of emphysematous pyelonephritis. J Microbiol Immunol Infect 2001;34:125–130.

84. Pewitt EB, Schaeffer AJ: Urinary tract infection in urology, including acute and chronic prostatitis. Infect Dis Clin North Am 1997;11:623–646.

85. Wyatt SH, Urban BA, Fishman EK: Spiral CT of the kidneys: Role in characterization of renal disease. Part I: Nonneoplastic disease. Crit Rev Diagn Imag 1995;36:1–37.

JOHN F. TONEY, MD

Sexually Transmitted Diseases

The term sexually transmitted diseases (STDs) refers to the more than 25 infectious organisms noted to be spread primarily through sexual activity. Despite the burdens, costs, complications, and preventable nature of STDs, they remain a significant public health problem. The extent of the problem has been largely unrecognized by the public, legislative policymakers, and public health and health care professionals in the United States.[1] STDs are associated with significant national morbidity and many harmful and costly clinical complications involving reproductive health, fetal and perinatal health, and cancer. Infection with some STDs significantly increases the risk of acquiring human immunodeficiency virus (HIV) infection.[2,3]

The magnitude of the STD problem our nation faces is significant. In 1995, STDs were the most common reportable diseases in the United States and accounted for 87% of the top 10 infections most frequently reported to the Centers for Disease Control and Prevention (CDC).[4] Every year an estimated 15 million new STD infections are acquired in the United States, and nearly 4 million adolescents are infected with an STD.[5] An estimated $17 billion annually is spent in direct and indirect costs on the treatment of the major STDs and their complications, including sexually transmitted HIV infection.[1]

Recognizing STD infections has been problematic for both health care providers and persons at risk. Because most STDs are asymptomatic or produce symptoms so mild that they often are ignored, a low index of suspicion that they are infected is held by infected persons who should (but may not) seek medical attention and by their health care providers (if they do seek medical evaluation). This becomes extremely important with infections such as HIV, chlamydial infection, gonorrhea, human papillomavirus (HPV) infection, hepatitis B virus (HBV) infection, and others that may cause prolonged subclinical infection. There can be a significant delay between the initial infection and the recognition of a clinically significant health problem with these agents, as noted with cervical cancer caused by HPV, liver cancer caused by HBV infection,[6] and infertility or ectopic pregnancy resulting from unrecognized or undiagnosed chlamydial infection or gonorrhea.[7]

The risk of acquiring an STD depends on many factors. There are gender differences encountered with most STDs, with women having a higher risk than men for most STDs and young women being more susceptible to certain STDs than are older women. Certain racial and ethnic groups (currently African American and Hispanic populations) have higher rates of STDs. Other factors influencing a person's risk for exposure and acquisition of STDs include social and behavioral factors (including poverty, access to health care, substance abuse, sexual coercion, and secrecy in discussing sexuality).

Information available to the public regarding STD prevention has been sparse. Although sexually oriented messages and images created by the media have increased significantly, little information regarding contraception, sexuality, or the risks of early, unprotected sexual behavior as STD prevention messages has been publicized.[8] With other health problems (such as smoking), mass media campaigns have been effective in bringing about significant changes in awareness, attitude, knowledge, and behavior[9] and could be created for STDs as well.

This chapter focuses primarily on the therapy and prevention of many of the prominent STDs encountered in the United States, with a brief review of clinical identification of these infections.

CLINICAL APPROACH TO THE EVALUATION FOR STDS

Taking a Sexual History

One of the medical interview components that is problematic for health care providers is the discussion of sex and sexual activity. Asking sensitive questions about a patient's current and distant sexual activity and past STD experience and ascertaining the likelihood of exposure to STDs (especially HIV) can be troubling.[10] As providers acquire additional STD interview skills, however, they will note increased comfort with asking these personal questions. Reviewing some of the general considerations that can facilitate provider and patient comfort during the STD portion of an examination is important.

A focused sexual history should include the four Ps: sexual *practices*, *past* STDs, sexual *partners*, and *protection* from STDs. Table 29–1 lists many general areas of consideration clinicians should be aware of and incorporate into their examination when they are taking a sexual

TABLE 29–1 ■ Taking a Sexual History—General Considerations

- Obtain the history with the patient fully clothed.
- Interview the patient alone or with an unrelated translator.
- Assure the patient of the confidential nature of the information he or she gives.
- Discuss the medical necessity of an accurate, complete, specific sexual behavioral history.
- Make no assumptions regarding gender, gender role, or specific sexual behaviors; always use gender-neutral terminology.
- Be nonjudgmental and objective.
- Use active listening and open-ended inquiry to ascertain whether the patient understands the questions posed.
- Use active listening for informational content, emotional content, comprehension, omitted information, and so forth.
- Begin with the least sensitive questions (e.g., general health history); then progress to sexual behaviors, substance use, and so forth.
- Discuss specific sexual and substance use behavior; do not use labels (e.g., straight, bisexual, gay, funny, sissy, punk, shooter).
- Become comfortable with the use of a broad range of sexual terms but do not assume patients know the meaning of them (e.g., fellatio, anal sex).

TABLE 29–2 ■ Sexually Transmitted Disease (STD) Risk Indicators (Risk Dependent on Specific STD)

- High number of lifetime sex partners
- Adolescence
- Residence in high-incidence area
- History of prior STD diagnosis and treatment
- Sex partner with a known STD diagnosis
- More than one recent sex partner (past 1–4 mo)
- Sex partner with other recent sex partners (past 1–4 mo)
- Inconsistent use of barrier contraceptive methods with casual or multiple partners
- New partner in the last 2 or 3 mo
- Commercial sex or exchange of sex for drugs
- A recent or past history of sexual assault or abuse
- Current use or a history of injection drug use or substance abuse by patient or sex partners

history. The discovery of STD risk indicators (Table 29–2) during the interview is crucial, with the risk of STD acquisition dependent on the specific STD of potential or known exposure.

The STD history is similar to the medical interview most clinicians use, with the addition of the specific areas noted above. When inquiring about the current visit, the clinician should elicit the reason for the visit, characterize all signs and symptoms noted by the patient, determine the past medical and STD history, determine current and recent medications taken, and note any prior drug allergies or adverse effects known to the patient. In women, information regarding their last menstrual period (LMP), parity, hygiene practices, and use of contraception, and a history of Pap smear examinations should be delineated as well. In both genders, HIV risk assessment should be determined.

Although many clinicians are knowledgeable about which questions to ask patients in a sexual history, they may be uncertain how to ask them. Introducing the topic of sexual activity has become somewhat easier recently, as medications used to treat sexual dysfunction in men (erectile dysfunction) are well known and widely advertised. However, some important questions remain difficult to ask. Table 29–3 reviews examples of introducing the topic of sex during an examination (including both adolescents and adults), asking about the number of sexual partners, STD and pregnancy prevention, sexual activity and practices, history of past STDs, and risk of exposure to HIV or hepatitis viruses that may be sexually transmitted.

Physical Examination

A complete physical examination, including the genital and rectal area, should be completed in any routine medical assessment and is especially necessary when the chance of infection with STDs is possible. A complete review of performing a male and female genital examination is available in several reference books.[11–15]

TABLE 29–3 ■ Brief Guide to Taking a Sexual History

INTRODUCTORY STATEMENTS AND QUESTIONS

ADOLESCENTS

Now I am going to take a few minutes to ask you some sensitive questions. Your answers are important. They will help me to help you be healthy. Anything we discuss will be completely confidential. I won't discuss this with anyone, not even your parents, without your permission.

OR

Some of my patients your age have started having sex. Have you had sex?

ADULTS

Now I am going to take a few minutes to ask you some direct questions about your sexual practices. These questions are very personal, but your answers are important for me to know so I can help you be healthy. I ask these questions to all my patients regardless of age or marital status. Like the rest of this visit, this information is strictly confidential.

PARTNER IDENTIFICATION

Do you have sex with men, women, or both?
In the past 2 months, how many partners have you had sex with?
In the past 12 months, how many partners have you had sex with?

PREGNANCY PREVENTION

Are you or your partner trying to get pregnant? If no, What are you doing to prevent pregnancy?

SEXUALLY TRANSMITTED DISEASE (STD) PROTECTION

What do you do to protect yourself from STDs and HIV?

SEXUAL PRACTICES

To understand your risks for STDs, I need explicit information about the kind of sex you have had over the last year:
Have you had vaginal sex, meaning "penis in vagina sex"?
Have you had anal sex, meaning "penis in rectum/anus sex"?
Have you had oral sex, meaning "mouth on penis/vagina"?
If the answer to any of the above is yes, Do you use condoms: never, sometimes, or always?
For condom answers:
  If answer is never. Why don't you use condoms?
  If answer is sometimes: In what situations, or with whom, do you not use condoms?

PAST HISTORY OF STDS

Have you ever had an STD?
Have any of your partners had an STD?

QUESTIONS TO IDENTIFY HIV AND HEPATITIS RISK

Have you or any of your partners injected drugs?
Have any of your partners exchanged money or drugs for sex?

CLOSING STATEMENTS

Is there anything else about your sexual practices that I need to know about?

DISEASES ASSOCIATED WITH GENITAL ULCERATION

Most young, sexually active persons in the United States who have genital ulcers have genital herpes, syphilis, or chancroid, with genital herpes being the most prevalent of these diseases. Less common ulcerative diseases in the United States, although endemic in many parts of the world, include lymphogranuloma venereum and granuloma inguinale. A patient who has genital ulcers may have more than one of these diseases. Each of these diseases has been associated with an increased risk for HIV infection. Pain, or the lack thereof, may be useful in differentiating these diseases (Fig. 29–1). Several representative photographs are included for reference (Fig. 29–2).

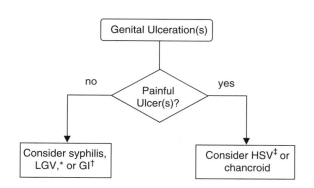

*LGV = lymphogranuloma venereum
†GI = granuloma inguinale
‡HSV = herpes simplex

FIGURE 29–1. General guide in the differentiation of genital ulcerations.

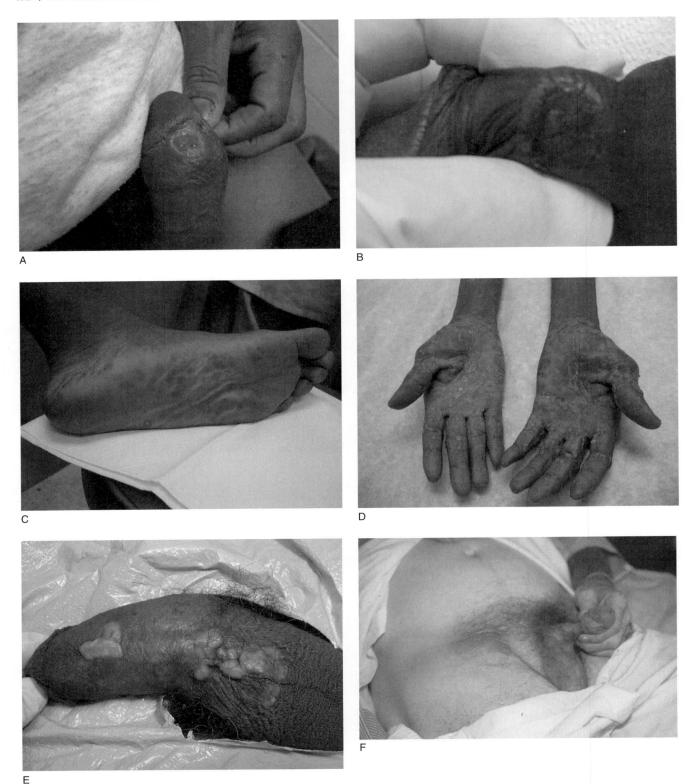

FIGURE 29–2. *A,* Syphilitic chancre. *B,* Syphilitic chancre showing induration. *C,* Secondary syphilitic rash of the foot. *D,* Secondary syphilitic rash involving the hands. *E,* Condylomata lata of secondary syphilis. *F,* Chancroid with penile ulcer and bubo that was aspirated.

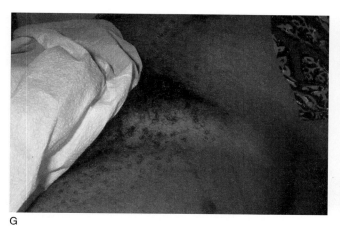

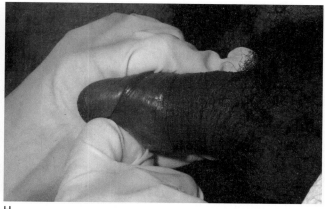

G   H

FIGURE 29–2. *Continued G*, Lymphogranuloma venereum with inguinal adenopathy. *H*, Lymphogranuloma venereum with ulcer of the prepuce.

Syphilis

Syphilis is a systemic disease that results from infection by the spirochete *Treponema pallidum*, which cannot be cultured in vitro. It is slightly longer than the diameter of a white blood cell (10 to 20 μm) and thin (0.1 μm in diameter). Initial inoculation occurs via visible or microscopic abrasions of the skin or mucous membranes that can result from sexual contact, with the risk of infection after a sexual exposure approximating 30%.[16] Other routes of transmission are vertical (in utero from an infected pregnant woman via hematogenous spread to her fetus) or, uncommonly, by direct contact with a nongenital skin area. The average incubation period of syphilis is 3 weeks but may be up to 3 months, with a smaller inoculum prolonging the time until symptom development[16] as the doubling time of the organism is approximately 30 to 33 hours.[17] The disease is characterized by episodes of active disease interrupted by periods of latent infection. Patients who have syphilis may seek treatment for signs or symptoms of primary infection (i.e., an ulcer or chancre at the infection site that typically remains painless), secondary infection (i.e., manifestations that include but are not limited to skin rash, mucocutaneous lesions, and lymphadenopathy), or tertiary infection (e.g., cardiac, ophthalmic, auditory abnormalities and gummatous lesions). Primary (1°) and secondary (2°) stages are considered to be new or incident infections; other stages are considered as distant infections. Early clinical manifestations (1° and 2° stages) primarily involve the skin and mucosal surfaces; latent disease has no clinical signs or symptoms and is detected by serologic testing; late manifestations may affect virtually any organ system.

Primary Syphilis

The hallmark of primary syphilis is the development of a chancre, a dermatologic lesion that progresses from a macule to papule to ulcer, typically remaining painless,

and demonstrates induration with a nonpurulent ulcer base. Multiple chancres are noted in up to 25% of primary syphilis cases.[18] The chancre heals spontaneously, usually without scarring, within 1 to 6 weeks, heralding the end of the primary stage. Chancres may appear on any moist mucosal area infected, including external male and female genitalia, the cervix, and the oral cavity. Atypical chancres may occur and can mimic herpes or chancroid.

Secondary Syphilis

The secondary lesions of syphilis generally are seen 3 to 6 weeks after the primary chancre appears; primary and secondary stages therefore may overlap. In the secondary stage, generalized or localized skin eruptions with mucosal lesions can occur. These eruptions or rashes may be mild or florid, depending on the patient's immune response. The lesions may persist for weeks to months. The secondary stage results from multiplication of the bacteria at multiple organ sites after hematogenous spread. Because the organism grows better at lower temperatures, the most common clinical findings are mucocutaneous. This stage is often accompanied by generalized lymphadenopathy and constitutional symptoms, most commonly malaise.[16,19]

Syphilis Rash

The appearance of secondary syphilis rash is nonspecific (i.e., macular, papular, pustules, or any combination), with usually nonpruritic lesions scattered on the trunk and extremities; it involves the palms and soles (discrete, scaly, oval lesions) in more than half of cases. Any new onset macular, papular, or squamous rash should be evaluated to rule out secondary syphilis.

Mucocutaneous Lesions

Other findings of secondary syphilis include mucous patches (flat silver-gray erosions involving the mouth, pharynx, larynx, genitals, or anus) and condylomata lata (moist, gray-white wartlike growths appearing on the genitals, perianal area, and perineum, in gluteal folds, nasolabial folds, axillae, between toes, and under breasts). Secondary syphilis (especially condylomata lata) should be included in the differential diagnosis of any lesion with the appearance of condylomata acuminata (i.e., HPV infection), and syphilis serology should be performed. Symptoms of secondary syphilis may persist for weeks to months before spontaneously remitting even without treatment. In serologic tests the syphilis antibody titers usually are highest during this stage, and despite the presence of antibodies, the patient cannot clear the infection. Sometimes secondary signs and symptoms recur, usually during the first year of infection.

Other Manifestations

Patients with secondary syphilis may exhibit additional clinical manifestations. Alopecia, or patchy hair loss, may occur in the occipital and bitemporal areas or as a loss of lateral eyebrows. Generalized lymphadenopathy is a common manifestation that may be confused with HIV infection or other infections or malignancies. Hepatic and renal involvement with syphilis may occur, but usually it is not clinically significant.

Latent Syphilis

Latent syphilis infection indicates infection without noticeable clinical manifestations. In this stage the host immune response suppresses infection enough to eliminate any signs or symptoms of disease but does not eradicate the infection completely and is detected by serologic testing. Latent syphilis acquired within the preceding year is referred to as *early latent* syphilis; all other cases of latent syphilis are either *late latent* syphilis or *latent syphilis* of *unknown duration*. Treatment for both late latent syphilis and tertiary syphilis theoretically may require a longer duration of therapy because organisms are dividing more slowly; however, the validity of this concept has not been assessed. The natural history of late latent syphilis generally follows the rule of thirds: one-third of patients will serorevert back to a nonreactive rapid plasma reagin (RPR) with no recurrence of disease; one-third will remain reactive by RPR but remain free of symptoms or signs of disease; and the remaining one-third will go on to develop tertiary syphilis, sometimes after decades of chronic, persistent asymptomatic infection.

Tertiary (Late) Syphilis

Patients with tertiary syphilis may develop granulomatous lesions (gummas) in the skin or viscera, cardiovascular disease (including aortic aneurysm, aortic valve insufficiency, coronary stenosis, and myocarditis), or neurologic disease (acute meningitis, hearing loss, meningovascular disease, general paresis, tabes dorsalis, and gummatous disease of the brain and spinal cord).

Untreated syphilis ultimately can have potentially devastating sequellae, which include the complications of neurosyphilis and tertiary syphilis. Late benign (gummatous) syphilis is noted by the granulomatous or gummatous lesions that may occur in eyes, viscera (lung, stomach, liver, genitals, breast, eyes, brain, and heart), and skeletal, spinal, and mucosal areas. The average onset of these lesions is 10 to 15 years after the initial infection. These destructive lesions clinically can mimic carcinoma or other noninfectious diseases.

Cardiovascular syphilis involves predominantly the ascending aorta. The pathologic process is an endarteritis obiterans of aortic vasa vasorum, which over time results in the loss of elasticity of the aorta. This clinically presents as an ascending aortic aneurysm, aortic insufficiency, or coronary ostial stenosis. On average, cardiovascular syphilis appears 20 to 30 years after infection and has been noted in 10% of untreated infected individuals. Central nervous system invasion with *T. pallidum* occurs early in syphilis infection in 30% to 40% of patients. Most patients, however, eventually clear this site of infection with conventional therapy. Asymptomatic neurosyphilis can occur at any stage. Early forms of neurosyphilis usually appear a few months to a few years after infection if it goes untreated. Clinical manifestations include acute syphilitic meningitis, basilar meningitis (that typically involves cranial nerves VI, VII, and VIII), or meningovascular syphilis (an endarteritis that presents as a strokelike syndrome or seizures). Late forms of neurosyphilis usually occur decades after infection and rarely are seen. Clinical manifestations of parenchymatous involvement include general paresis and tabes dorsalis. Ocular involvement can also be manifested in early or late disease. Uveitis may be the most common early presentation, but the most discussed ocular manifestation is an Argyll Robertson pupillary response.

Congenital Syphilis

Untreated syphilis infection in a pregnant woman can have tragic repercussions for a developing fetus. Syphilis can be transmitted from mother to fetus at any stage of maternal infection, although risk of fetal infection is greatest in more recently acquired maternal infection (i.e., primary and secondary > early latent > late latent). Syphilis can be transmitted at any point during the pregnancy, although the risk of fetal infection is greatest during late pregnancy. The optimal diagnosis and management of congenital syphilis requires the following:

- A complete physical examination of both mother and child
- Laboratory evaluation of any abnormal newborn fluids (e.g., nasal discharge) or lesions
- Consideration of the timing of any treatment received by the mother (e.g., before becoming pregnant, during pregnancy and > 4 weeks prior to delivery, or within the final 4 weeks of the pregnancy)

- Type of maternal treatment (e.g., penicillin vs. non-penicillin regimen)
- Serologic maternal response to therapy (i.e., rule out "treatment failure" in mother)
- In communities and populations where the incidence of syphilis is high or for patients at high risk, serologic testing should be performed twice during the third trimester (at 28 weeks' gestation and at delivery) in addition to routine early screening

Seropositive pregnant women should be considered infected unless an adequate treatment history is documented in the medical records and sequential serologic antibody titers have declined.[20]

Syphilis Serology

Serologic tests for syphilis include a variety of assays that fall into two general categories: nontreponemal and treponeme specific.

Nontreponemal Assays

Nontreponemal assays, such as the RPR and VDRL, are useful to screen for syphilis infection (past or present), to evaluate the effectiveness of therapy for a syphilis infection, and in patients with a history of previous treatment for syphilis, to determine the likelihood of reinfection. The quantitative result of nontreponemal tests typically will rise in early infection, peak during the secondary stage, and decline over time even without treatment. The RPR and VDRL are, for clinical purposes, equivalent tests, although when an individual's titers are assessed over time the same test should be used to avoid quantitative variations between tests (i.e., RPR titers often are slightly higher than VDRL titers for the same specimen).

Treponeme-Specific Assays

Treponeme-specific assays most often are used to confirm a syphilis diagnosis in a patient with a reactive RPR or VDRL and, in so doing, rule out a biologic false-positive nontreponemal result. Treponeme-specific assays should only be used as a qualitative test (i.e., reactive vs. nonreactive). Although quantitative results are often reported by laboratories, these do not correlate well with disease activity and should not be used to guide clinical management. A host of treponeme-specific assays are available clinically and include fluorescent treponemal antibody—absorption (FTA-ABS), *T. pallidum* particle agglutination (TP-PA) (which has replaced the microhemagglutination assay for *T. pallidum* (MHA-TP)), and IgG enzyme immunoassay (EIA). Treponeme-specific tests most often remain reactive for life in patients infected with syphilis even following adequate therapy.

The diagnosis of syphilis must take into consideration the results of both a nontreponemal test (NTT) and a treponemal test (TT).[21] Table 29–4 summarizes the interpretation of each of the four possible serologic scenarios: (1) NTT nonreactive, TT nonreactive; (2) NTT

TABLE 29–4 ■ Syphilis Serology Interpretation

Test results	Interpretation
NTT (–) TT (–)	Primary syphilis, very early (incubating)
	Primary syphilis after treatment
	Never had syphilis
	HIV:
	Delayed seroconversion (Hicks)
	Spontaneous TT antibody loss (Hass)
NTT (+) TT (–)	Biologic false positive
	Autoimmune: antiphospholipids (15%–20%)
	Age
	Addiction
	Miscellaneous (infectious, noninfectious)
NTT (–) TT (+)	Primary syphilis, early
	Secondary syphilis with prozone phenomenon
	Late syphilis, untreated
	Syphilis successfully treated
	HIV, advanced
	False-positive TT
NTT (+) TT (+)	Untreated syphilis
	Infections with other *Treponema* or close relatives
	Successfully treated syphilis with coincidental biologic false positives
	Both NTT and TT false positives
	Systemic lupus erythematosus and others

NTT, nontreponemal test; TT, treponemal test.
From Jurado RL: Syphilis serology: A practical approach. Infect Dis Clin Pract 1996;5:351–358.

nonreactive, TT reactive; (3) NTT reactive, TT nonreactive; and (4) NTT reactive, TT reactive. Rarely, a phenomenon called the prozone effect causes a false-negative reaction. In the prozone effect the reaction is overwhelmed by antibody excess, which may occur in late primary or in secondary syphilis. If clinical suspicion of secondary syphilis is high, the laboratory should dilute the serum to at least a 1/16 dilution to rule out the prozone effect. Figure 29–3 is a proposed algorithm for NTT and TT testing.

No test can be used alone to diagnose neurosyphilis. The VDRL cerebrospinal fluid (CSF) test is highly specific, but it is insensitive, as are other tests for neurosyphilis, and must be interpreted in relation to other test results and the clinical assessment. With this in mind the diagnosis of neurosyphilis usually depends on various combinations of reactive serologic test results, abnormalities of CSF cell count or protein, or a reactive VDRL-CSF with or without clinical manifestations.

The sensitivity of serologic tests in untreated syphilis is reviewed in Table 29–5. Sequential serologic tests in individual patients should be performed by the same testing method (e.g., VDRL or RPR), preferably by the same laboratory. After treatment, nontreponemal tests usually become nonreactive with time; in some patients, however, nontreponemal antibodies can persist at a low titer for a long time (sometimes lifelong). This response is referred

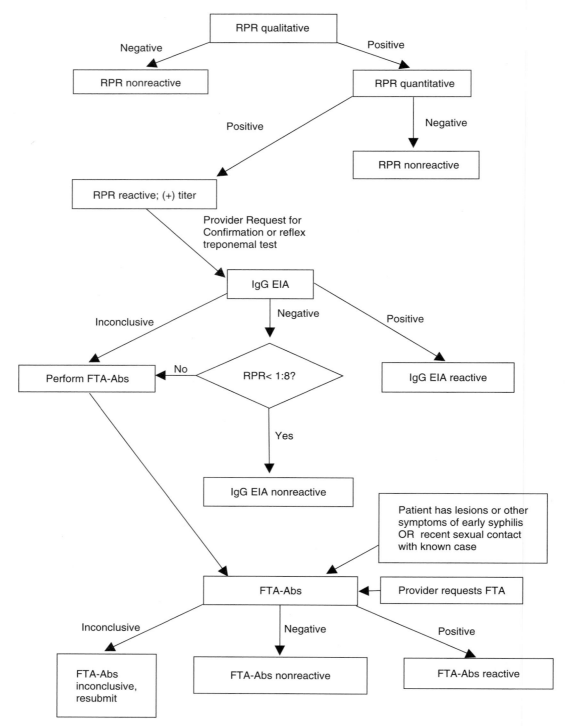

FIGURE 29–3. Proposed syphilis test algorithm using IgG EIA.

to as being "serofast." Most patients with reactive treponemal tests will have lifelong reactive tests, regardless of disease activity or amount of effective treatment, but 15% to 25% of patients treated during the primary stage revert to being serologically nonreactive after 2 to 3 years.

Some HIV-infected patients can have atypical serologic test results (i.e., unusually high, unusually low, or fluctuating titers). When serologic tests and clinical syndromes suggestive of early syphilis do not correspond with one another in these patients, other tests for syphilis (e.g., darkfield microscopy, biopsy) should be considered. Serologic tests are accurate and reliable for the diagnosis of syphilis for most HIV-infected patients and useful for following the response to treatment.

TABLE 29–5 ■ **Sensitivity of Serologic Tests in Untreated Syphilis**

Test	Percent positive (range)			
	Primary	Secondary	Latent	Tertiary
VDRL or rapid plasma reagin (RPR)	78 (74–87)	100	95 (88–100)	71 (37–94)
Fluorescent treponemal antibody absorption (FTA-ABS)	84 (70–100)	100	100	96
TREPONEMAL AGGLUTINATION				
T. pallidum particle agglutination (TP-PA)* (Microhemagglutination assay for T. pallidum [MHA-TP] no longer available†)	84 (84–100)	100	100	Unknown (TP-PA has not been tested for known late syphilis)

*FTA-ABS and TP-PA generally are considered equally sensitive in the primary stage of disease.
†The MHA-TP has been replaced by the TP-PA.

Management of Syphilis

General Management

Central nervous system involvement is common in many stages of syphilis. In most patients with primary, secondary, and latent syphilis the prognostic significance is unknown. Conventional therapy is effective for most immunocompetent patients with asymptomatic central nervous system involvement in primary and secondary syphilis.

Penicillin G is the preferred drug for treatment of all stages of syphilis when given intravenously or intramuscularly. The preparation(s) used (i.e., benzathine, aqueous procaine, or aqueous crystalline), the dosage, and the length of treatment depend on the stage and clinical manifestations of disease. Almost all the recommendations for the treatment of syphilis are based on the opinions of STD experts and are reinforced by case series, clinical trials, and 50 years of clinical experience, as randomized, controlled clinical trials generally have not been performed.

Management of Sex Partners

Sexual transmission of T. pallidum occurs only in the presence of mucocutaneous syphilitic lesions, which are uncommon after the first year of infection. Persons exposed sexually to a patient who has syphilis in any stage, however, should be evaluated clinically and serologically according to the following recommendations[20]:

- Persons sexually exposed (even if the partner is seronegative) within 90 days preceding the diagnosis of primary, secondary, or early latent syphilis should be treated presumptively.
- Persons exposed more than 90 days before the diagnosis of primary, secondary, or early latent syphilis in a sex partner should be treated presumptively if serologic test results are not available immediately and their follow-up is uncertain.
- Patients with syphilis of unknown duration who have high nontreponemal serologic test titers (i.e., >1:32) can be assumed to have early syphilis. Serologic titers should not be used, however, to differentiate early from late latent syphilis for the purpose of determining treatment.
- Long-term sex partners of patients who have latent syphilis should be evaluated clinically and serologically for syphilis and treated on the basis of the findings. Partners are at risk if the time period from sexual contact until treatment is (1) 3 months plus duration of symptoms for primary syphilis, (2) 6 months plus duration of symptoms for secondary syphilis, and (3) 1 year for early latent syphilis.

Treatment of Syphilis

The treatment of early, latent, and late syphilis is listed in Table 29–6. Treatment of syphilis in pregnancy should be appropriate for the stage of syphilis encountered. No alternatives to penicillin have been proved consistently effective for treatment of syphilis during pregnancy. Pregnant women who have a history of penicillin allergy should be desensitized and treated with penicillin if possible. Tetracycline and doxycycline should not be used during pregnancy. Erythromycin should not be used because it does not reliably cure an infected fetus. Data currently are insufficient to recommend azithromycin or ceftriaxone to treat syphilis in pregnancy. Treatment for congenital syphilis depends on the clinical evaluation of both the newborn and the mother and is outlined in Table 29–7. In the treatment of early syphilis, an HIV-infected person may be at greater risk than HIV-negative patients for neurologic complications and may have higher rates of treatment failure with currently recommended regimens.[22] These risks are not precisely defined and are probably minimal. No treatment regimens for syphilis have been demonstrated to be more effective in preventing neurosyphilis in HIV-infected patients than the syphilis regimens recommended for HIV-negative patients.[23] Careful follow-up after therapy is essential.

Jarisch-Herxheimer Reaction

Patients treated for syphilis should be warned that a Jarisch-Herxheimer reaction may occur within the first

TABLE 29–6 ▪ **Recommended Treatment of Syphilis by Stage**

Stage	Recommended treatment	Alternative treatment
Incubating (10–90 d after exposure, negative serology, no clinical lesions)	2.4 MU benzathine penicillin IM	Penicillin allergic: Doxycycline 100 mg PO bid × 14 d
Primary (chancre)	2.4 MU benzathine penicillin IM	Penicillin allergic: Doxycycline 100 mg PO bid × 14 d
Secondary (e.g., mucocutaneous manifestations, rash)	2.4 MU benzathine penicillin IM	Penicillin allergic: Doxycycline 100 mg PO bid × 14 d
Latent		Penicillin allergic
Early (<1 y duration)	2.4 MU benzathine penicillin IM	Doxycycline 100 mg PO bid × 14 d
Late (>1 y duration or unknown duration)	7.2 MU benzathine penicillin IM given as 2.4 MU qwk × 3 wk	Doxycycline 100 mg PO bid × 28 d
Tertiary (gummatous, cardiovascular)	7.2 MU benzathine penicillin IM given as 2.4 MU qwk × 3 wk	Penicillin allergic Doxycycline 100 mg PO bid × 28 d
Neurosyphilis	Aqueous crystalline penicillin G 18–24 MU/d administered as 3–4 MU IV q4h or as continuous infusion × 10–14 d OR Procaine penicillin 2.4 MU IM qd PLUS probenecid 500 mg PO qid, both × 10–14 d (some specialists give 2.4 MU of benzathine penicillin IM qwk for up to 3 wk after IV or IM treatment completed)	Ceftriaxone 2 g/d IM or IV for 10–14 d OR desensitize to penicillin

From CDC: Sexually Transmitted Diseases Treatment Guidelines 2002. MMWR Morb Mortal Wkly Rep 2002;51(RR-6):26–28.

TABLE 29–7 ▪ **Syphilis Treatment of Infants in the First Month of Life**

Setting	Treatment
Proven or highly probable disease	Aqueous crystalline penicillin G 100,000–150,000 U/kg/d, given as 50,000 U/kg IV q12h for the first 7 d of life and q8h thereafter × 3 d for a total of 10 d OR Procaine penicillin G 50,000 U/kg IM qd × 10 d
Normal physical examination and a serum rapid plasma reagin (RPR) VDRL titer the same or less than fourfold the maternal titer and Mother was not treated, inadequately treated, or has no documentation of having received treatment Mother was treated with erythromycin or other nonpenicillin regimen Mother received treatment <4 wk before delivery Mother has early syphilis and a nontreponemal titer that has either not decreased fourfold or has increased fourfold	Aqueous crystalline penicillin G 100,000–150,000 U/kg/d given as 50,000 U/kg IV q12h for the first 7 d of life and q8h thereafter × 3 d for a total of 10 days OR Procaine penicillin G 50,000 U/kg IM qd × 10 d OR Benzathine penicillin G 50,000 U/kg IM in a single dose
Normal physical examination and a serum quantitative nontreponemal serologic titer the same or less than fourfold the maternal titer and Mother was treated during pregnancy; treatment was appropriate for the stage of infection; treatment was administered >4 wk before delivery Mother's nontreponemal titers decreased fourfold after appropriate therapy for early syphilis or remained stable and low for late syphilis Mother has no evidence of reinfection or relapse	Benzathine penicillin G 50,000 U/kg IM in a single dose (some experts would not treat but follow serology closely)
Normal physical examination and a serum quantitative nontreponemal serologic titer the same or less than fourfold the maternal titer and Mother's treatment was adequate before pregnancy Mother's nontreponemal serologic titer remained low and stable before and during pregnancy and at delivery (VDRL <1:2; RPR <1:4)	No treatment is required (some experts would treat with benzathine penicillin G 50,000 U/kg IM as a single injection, particularly if follow-up is uncertain)

From CDC: Sexually Transmitted Diseases Treatment Guidelines 2002. MMWR Morb Mortal Wkly Rep 2002;51(RR-6):26–28.

24 hours after treatment (usually 2 to 8 hours after treatment). Symptoms include local and systemic exacerbation of existing, or unrecognized, manifestations of primary or secondary syphilis in the face of malaise, myalgias, headache, nausea or vomiting, tender adenopathy, pharyngitis, or fever. Treatment is supportive utilizing antipyretics and analgesics, and symptoms usually resolve within 24 hours. Patients should be counseled that the reaction does not represent an allergic reaction to penicillin. During pregnancy this reaction has been associated with fetal distress and preterm labor (the greatest risk occurring during the first 48 hours after treatment).

Prevention

The major effective prevention measures persons can practice include sexual abstinence, monogamy, and reduction in the number of sexual contacts. Barriers such as condoms do not protect against all body secretions and skin lesions. Nevertheless they should be used as part of an overall educational program stressing sex with uninfected partners and monogamy. Screening for syphilis should include high-risk populations (patients with other STDs, detention and corrections populations, pregnant women). Pregnant women should have syphilis screening at least at first prenatal visit and in high-incidence areas, rescreening in third trimester and at delivery.

Genital Herpes Simplex Virus Infections

Genital herpes is a recurrent, life-long viral infection. Two serotypes of herpes simplex virus (HSV) have been identified: HSV-1 and HSV-2; most cases of recurrent genital herpes are caused by HSV-2. The prevalence of genital HSV is significant; at least 50 million people in the United States have active genital HSV infection, and at least 1 million new cases occur each year.[5] Most persons infected with HSV-2 have not been diagnosed. Many such persons have mild or unrecognized infections but shed virus intermittently in the genital tract. On any given day, HSV-2 causes subclinical reactivation in about 1% of infected persons.[24] Most genital herpes infections are transmitted by persons unaware that they have the infection or who are asymptomatic when transmission occurs. Rarely, first-episode genital herpes manifests as severe genital ulcerative disease that requires hospitalization. Most persons with clinical genital HSV have lesions characterized by painful grouped vesicles in the anogenital region that rapidly ulcerate and form shallow tender lesions. The initial episode may be associated with inguinal adenopathy, fever, headache, myalgias, and aseptic meningitis; recurrences usually are less severe than the initial episode. Routes of transmission are sexual (genital to genital and oral to genital) and perinatal (mother to child).

Diagnosis of HSV Infection

The clinical diagnosis of genital herpes is both insensitive and nonspecific. The typical painful multiple vesicular or ulcerative lesions are absent in many infected persons. Up to 30% of first-episode cases of genital herpes are caused by HSV-1, but recurrences are much less frequent for genital HSV-1 infection than genital HSV-2 infection. Therefore the distinction between HSV serotypes influences prognosis and counseling. For these reasons the clinical diagnosis of genital herpes should be confirmed by laboratory testing. Cell culture isolation of HSV is the preferred virologic test in patients who present with genital ulcers or other mucocutaneous lesions. The sensitivity of culture declines rapidly as lesions begin to heal, usually within a few days of onset. Polymerase chain reaction (PCR) assays for HSV DNA are available, but their role in the diagnosis of genital ulcer disease has not been well defined. Detection of type-specific HSV-2 antibody indicates anogenital infection, as almost all HSV-2 infections are sexually acquired, but the presence of HSV-1 antibody does not distinguish anogenital from orolabial infection. Accurate type-specific assays for HSV antibodies based on the HSV-specific glycoprotein G2 are available for the diagnosis of infection with HSV-2, and glycoprotein G1 is available for diagnosis of infection with HSV-1. Because false-negative HSV cultures are common, especially in patients with recurrent infection or with healing lesions, type-specific serologic tests are useful in confirming a clinical diagnosis of genital herpes. Additionally such tests can be used to diagnose persons with unrecognized infection and to manage sex partners of persons with genital herpes.

Therapy of Genital Herpes

The mainstay in the management of genital herpes is antiviral chemotherapy. Systemic antiviral medications partially control the symptoms and signs of herpes episodes when used to treat first clinical episodes and recurrent episodes or when used as daily suppressive therapy. These medications, however, neither eradicate latent virus nor reduce the risk, frequency, and severity of recurrences after drug discontinuation. Topical therapy with antiviral drugs is not recommended, since it offers minimal clinical benefit. Intravenous therapy mainly is used for severe primary infection and complications such as urinary retention secondary to sacral radiculitis, aseptic meningitis, or progressive or invasive mucocutaneous HSV. Table 29–8 reviews current recommendations for the management of genital herpes. Immunocompromised patients may have prolonged or severe episodes of genital, perianal, or oral herpes. Lesions caused by HSV are common among HIV-infected patients and may be severe, painful, and atypical. Episodic or suppressive therapy with oral antiviral agents often is used. Some persons may have acyclovir-resistant HSV infections; for them, sodium phosphonoformate (Foscarnet) intravenously is considered the therapy of choice. Cidofovir gel is currently under investigation and is not available for use.

TABLE 29–8 ■ Management of Genital Herpes Infection

Manifestation	Treatment
First clinical episode of genital herpes	Acyclovir 400 mg PO tid × 7–10 d OR Acyclovir 200 mg PO five times a day × 7–10 d OR Famciclovir 250 mg PO tid × 7–10 d OR Valacyclovir 1 g PO bid × 7–10 d
Episodic therapy for recurrent genital herpes	Acyclovir 400 mg PO tid × 5 d OR Acyclovir 200 mg PO five times a day × 5 d OR Acyclovir 800 mg PO bid × 5 d OR Famciclovir 125 mg PO bid × 5 d OR Valacyclovir 500 mg PO bid × 3–5 d OR Valacyclovir 1 g PO qd × 5 d
Suppressive therapy for recurrent genital herpes	Acyclovir 400 mg PO bid OR Famciclovir 250 mg PO bid OR Valacyclovir 500 mg PO qd OR Valacyclovir 1 g PO qd
Severe genital herpes	Acyclovir 5–10 mg/kg IV q8h × 2–7 d or until clinical improvement, followed by oral antiviral therapy to complete at least 10 d total therapy
Episodic infection in persons infected with HIV	Acyclovir 400 mg PO tid × 5–10 d OR Acyclovir 200 mg PO five times a day × 5–10 d OR Famciclovir 500 mg PO bid × 5–10 d OR Valacyclovir 1 g PO bid × 5–10 d
Daily suppressive therapy in persons infected with HIV	Acyclovir 400–800 mg PO bid or tid OR Famciclovir 500 mg PO bid OR Valacyclovir 500 mg PO bid

From CDC: Sexually Transmitted Diseases Treatment Guidelines 2002. MMWR Morb Mortal Wkly Rep 2002;51(RR-6):26–28.

Management of Sex Partners

Sex partners of patients with genital herpes can benefit from evaluation and counseling. Sex partners with symptoms should be evaluated and treated like patients who have known genital lesions. Asymptomatic sex partners of patients who have genital herpes should be questioned regarding any history of genital lesions, educated to recognize potential symptoms of herpes, and offered type-specific serologic testing for HSV infection.

Prevention

Condoms reduce the risk of HSV transmission to uninfected partners, especially from men to women when the infected areas are covered or protected by the condom. Susceptible pregnant women whose partners have known oral or genital HSV or whose status is unknown should be counseled to avoid unprotected genital and oral sexual contact in late pregnancy to prevent neonatal HSV, which is associated with initial maternal infection near the time of delivery.

Chancroid

Chancroid is an acute infection manifested by deep genital ulceration and by the frequent occurrence of inguinal adenopathy and bubo formation. The responsible agent is *Haemophilus ducreyi*, a gram-negative coccobacillus. In the United States, chancroid usually occurs in discrete outbreaks, although the disease is endemic in some areas. Chancroid frequently coexists with other STDs; about 10% of persons who have chancroid acquired in the United States are coinfected with *T. pallidum* or HSV. The diagnosis of chancroid requires the identification of *H. ducreyi* on special culture media that is not widely available; even when selective media is used, the culture sensitivity is less than 80%. A probable diagnosis can be made if all the following criteria are met:

1. The patient has one or more painful genital ulcers.
2. The patient has no evidence of *T. pallidum* infection by darkfield examination of ulcer exudate or by a serologic test for syphilis performed at least 7 days after onset of ulcers.
3. The clinical presentation, appearance of genital ulcers, and regional lymphadenopathy, if present, are typical of chancroid.
4. A test for HSV performed on the ulcer exudate is negative.[20]

The combination of a painful ulcer and tender inguinal adenopathy, symptoms occurring in one-third of patients, suggests a diagnosis of chancroid. These signs accompanied by suppurative inguinal adenopathy are almost pathognomonic for chancroid.

Treatment of Chancroid

The treatment of chancroid, when effective, cures the infection, resolves the clinical symptoms, and prevents transmission to others. Buboes may require drainage by aspiration if they are large or painful or for diagnostic purposes. Buboes may appear to worsen in the 1 to 2 days following therapy, and patients may need additional antibiotic therapy for resolution. The antibiotics recommended for the treatment of chancroid include azithromycin 1 g orally in a single dose, ceftriaxone 250 mg intramuscularly in a single dose, ciprofloxacin 500 mg orally twice a day for 3 days, or erythromycin base 500 mg orally three times a day for 7 days. Patients should be reexamined in 3 to 5 days for evidence of symptomatic improvement, in 7 to 10 days for evidence of clinical improvement, and then weekly until healed. Uncircumcised patients or those who have HIV infection do not respond as well to treatment as do those who are circumcised or HIV-negative. Patients should be tested for HIV infection at the time chancroid is diagnosed and be retested for syphilis and HIV 3 months after the diagnosis of chancroid if the initial test results were negative.

Sex partners of patients who have chancroid should be examined and treated regardless of whether they have symptoms of the disease if they had sexual contact with the patient during the 10 days preceding the patient's onset of symptoms

Granuloma Inguinale (Donovanosis)

Granuloma inguinale is a genital ulcerative disease caused by the intracellular gram-negative bacterium *Calymmatobacterium granulomatis*. The bacteria can be seen in infected tissue as intracellular bacterial inclusions known as Donovan bodies[25] but cannot be cultured on artificial media. This is an uncommon disease in the United States, although it is endemic in certain tropical and developing areas, including India, Papua New Guinea, central Australia, and southern Africa. The disease commonly presents as painless, progressive ulcerative lesions without regional lymphadenopathy. The lesions are highly vascular (beefy red appearance) and bleed easily on contact. The clinical presentation, however, can also include hypertrophic, necrotic, or sclerotic variants. The diagnosis requires visualization of intracellular Donovan bodies on tissue crush preparation or biopsy. The lesions may develop secondary bacterial infection or may be coinfected with another sexually transmitted pathogen.

Treatment of Granuloma Inguinale

Antibiotic treatment of granuloma inguinale halts progression of the lesions, although prolonged therapy may be required to allow granulation and reepithelialization of the ulcers. Relapse can occur 6 to 18 months after apparently effective therapy is discontinued. Several antimicrobial regimens have been effective, but few controlled trials have been published. Recommended agents used to treat granuloma inguinale include doxycycline 100 mg orally twice a day for at least 3 weeks or TMP-SMZ one double-strength (800 mg/160 mg) tablet orally twice a day for at least 3 weeks. Alternatively, ciprofloxacin 750 mg orally twice a day for at least 3 weeks, or erythromycin base 500 mg orally four times a day for at least 3 weeks, or azithromycin 1 g orally once per week for at least 3 weeks may be used. Patients should be followed clinically until signs and symptoms have resolved.

Management of Sex Partners

Persons who have had sexual contact with a patient who has granuloma inguinale within the 60 days before onset of the patient's symptoms should be examined and offered therapy. However, the value of empiric therapy in the absence of clinical signs and symptoms has not been established.

Lymphogranuloma Venereum

Lymphogranuloma venereum (LGV) is caused by *Chlamydia trachomatis* serovars L1, L2, or L3. The disease occurs rarely in the United States but is endemic in many areas of the world. The most common clinical manifestation of LGV among heterosexuals is tender inguinal or femoral lymphadenopathy that is most commonly unilateral. Women and homosexually active men may have proctocolitis or inflammatory involvement of perirectal or perianal lymphatic tissues resulting in fistulas and strictures. A self-limited genital ulcer sometimes occurs at the site of inoculation. By the time patients seek care, however, the ulcer commonly has disappeared. The diagnosis of LGV usually is made serologically and by exclusion of other causes of inguinal lymphadenopathy or genital ulcers. Complement fixation titers higher than 1:64 are consistent with the diagnosis of LGV, and some experts suggest using a titer of higher than 1:128. The diagnostic utility of serologic methods other than complement fixation is unknown.

Treatment of Lymphogranuloma Venereum

Treatment cures infection and prevents ongoing tissue damage, although tissue reaction can result in scarring. Buboes may require aspiration through intact skin or incision and drainage to prevent the formation of inguinal and femoral ulcerations. Doxycycline is the preferred treatment. A dose of 100 mg orally twice a day for 21 days is the standard therapy. Erythromycin base 500 mg orally four times a day for 21 days may be used alternatively, and some experts believe azithromycin 1 g orally once weekly for 3 weeks is likely effective for LGV, although azithromycin clinical data are lacking.

DISEASES CHARACTERIZED BY GENITAL DISCHARGES

Gonococcal Infections

An estimated 600,000 new *Neisseria gonorrhoeae* infections occur each year in the United States. Most infections among men produce symptoms that cause them to seek curative treatment soon enough to prevent serious sequelae, but this may not be soon enough to prevent transmission to others. Men commonly are symptomatic with a purulent urethral discharge often accompanied by dysuria. Epididymitis is an infrequent local complication in men, and other uncommon complications include inguinal lymphadenitis, penile edema, periurethral abscess or fistula, accessory (Tyson's) gland infection, balanitis, urethral stricture, and perhaps prostatitis.

Among women, many gonococcal infections do not produce recognizable symptoms until there are complications (e.g., pelvic inflammatory disease [PID]). Both symptomatic and asymptomatic cases of PID can result in tubal scarring that causes infertility or ectopic pregnancy. Accessory gland infection (Skene's, Bartholin's gland infections) can result from gonococcal infection and often is unilateral; if the duct becomes occluded, an abscess may form. In women, gonococcal perihepatitis (Fitz-Hugh–Curtis syndrome) and inflammation of the liver capsule can develop: spillage of infected material from the fallopian tubes into the peritoneum involves the liver capsule, causing the inflammation. Gonococcal infection during pregnancy can be associated with premature rupture of membranes, preterm delivery, and postpartum endometritis.

Both men and women can acquire gonococcal infection in the anorectal area. In 35% to 50% of women with gonococcal cervicitis who do not acknowledge rectal sexual contact, the rectal mucosa has been reported to be infected with gonococcus, presumably from perineal contamination with infected cervical secretions. Both sexes may also develop gonococcal pharyngeal infection, conjunctivitis, and disseminated gonococcal disease. Perinatal gonococcal infection can involve the eyes and respiratory tract of the newborn.

Diagnosis of Gonorrhea

The diagnosis of gonorrhea is usually made by one of several laboratory methods: (1) Gram stain on a smear of a characteristic genital discharge, (2) culture on selective median, (3) nonamplified tests such as EIA, DNA probe, or direct fluorescent antibody (DFA), or (4) amplified tests such as PCR, ligase chain reaction (LCR), or transcription mediated amplification (TMA). For a detailed review of these tests the reader is referred to the chapter on gonorrhea in the companion text.

Treatment of Gonorrhea

The treatments for gonococcal infections are outlined in Table 29–9. Patients infected with *N. gonorrhoeae* often are coinfected with *C. trachomatis*; this finding led to the recommendation that patients treated for gonococcal infection also be treated routinely with a regimen effective against uncomplicated genital *C. trachomatis* infection. Some experts feel that the routine use of dual therapy has significantly decreased the incidence of chlamydial infection. Routine cotreatment may hinder the development of antimicrobial-resistant *N. gonorrhoeae*, as most gonococci in the United States are susceptible to doxycycline and azithromycin. However, one or more types of resistance is present in 20% to 30% of gonococcal infections in the United States. Quinolone-resistant *N. gonorrhoeae* (QRNG), common in parts of

TABLE 29–9 ■ Treatment of Gonorrhea

Site of infection	Recommended therapy
Uncomplicated cervical, urethral, and rectal gonorrhea	Cefixime 400 mg PO in a single dose OR Ceftriaxone 125 mg IM in a single dose OR Ciprofloxacin 500 mg PO in a single dose OR Ofloxacin 400 mg PO in a single dose OR Levofloxacin 250 mg PO in a single dose PLUS, if chlamydial infection is not ruled out, Azithromycin 1 g PO in a single dose OR Doxycycline 100 mg PO bid × 7 d Alternate for the above: Spectinomycin 2 g IM
Pharyngeal gonorrhea	Ceftriaxone 125 mg IM in a single dose OR Ciprofloxacin 500 mg PO in a single dose PLUS, if chlamydial infection is not ruled out, Azithromycin 1 g PO in a single dose OR Doxycycline 100 mg PO bid × 7 d
Gonococcal conjunctivitis (adult)	Ceftriaxone 1 g IM in a single dose
Ophthalmia neonatorum (infant)	Ceftriaxone 25–50 mg/kg IV or IM in a single dose, not to exceed 125 mg
Disseminated gonococcal infection (DGI)	Initial therapy (hospitalized): Ceftriaxone 1 g IM or IV q 24h Alternative regimens: Cefotaxime 1 g IV q 8h OR Ceftizoxime 1 g IV q 8h OR Ciprofloxacin 400 mg IV q 12h OR Ofloxacin 400 mg IV q 12h OR Levofloxacin 250 mg/d IV OR Spectinomycin 2 g IM q 12h Continue the above for 24–48 h after improvement begins; then switch to one of the following regimens to complete at least 1 wk of antimicrobial therapy: Cefixime 400 mg PO bid OR Ciprofloxacin 500 mg PO bid OR Ofloxacin 400 mg PO bid OR Levofloxacin 500 mg PO qd

From CDC: Sexually Transmitted Diseases Treatment Guidelines 2002. MMWR Morb Mortal Wkly Rep 2002;51(RR-6):26–28.

Asia and the Pacific, continues to spread, making the treatment of gonorrhea with quinolones inadvisable in many areas of the United States. QRNG is becoming more common in areas on the West Coast. Quinolones are no longer recommended for the treatment of gonorrhea in Hawaii and should not be used to treat infections that may have been acquired in Asia or the Pacific (including Hawaii). Recent data from California demonstrate an increased incidence of QRNG; therefore the use of fluoroquinolones in California is probably inadvisable. Clinicians should obtain a recent travel history, including histories from sex partners, in those persons with gonorrhea to ensure appropriate antibiotic therapy.

Chlamydial Infections

Chlamydial genital infection occurs frequently among sexually active adolescents and young adults in the United States, with an estimated 3 million or more new infections per year.[5] Asymptomatic infection is common among both men and women. Sexually active adolescent women should be screened for chlamydial infection at least annually, even if symptoms are not present. Annual screening of all sexually active women between the ages of 20 and 25 years is also recommended, as is screening of older women with risk factors (e.g., those who have a new sex partner and those with multiple sex partners).[26] Several important sequelae can result from C. trachomatis infection in women; the most serious of these include PID, ectopic pregnancy, and infertility. Some women who have apparently uncomplicated cervical infection already have subclinical upper reproductive tract infection. Chlamydial perihepatitis is also a possibility with untreated disease.

Chlamydial infection in men commonly manifests as urethritis, although more than 50% are asymptomatic. The incubation period is unknown (probably about 5 to 10 days in symptomatic infection). Some of the symptoms and signs noted on examination include discharge, dysuria, and urethral discharge. Complications of chlamydial infection in men include epididymitis and Reiter's syndrome; the risk of chlamydial prostatitis is unknown.

Chlamydia Testing

A brief review of current testing for *Chlamydia* is included in Table 29–10. Detection of *Chlamydia* usually is done by cell culture, EIA, DFA, nonamplified genetic probe, or more recently by nucleic acid amplification testing (NAAT). The reader is referred to the chapter on *Chlamydia* in the companion text for specifics regarding *Chlamydia* testing.

Treatment of Chlamydial Infection

The following recommended treatment and alternative regimens cure chlamydial infection and usually relieve symptoms. Uncomplicated chlamydial infection can be treated with azithromycin 1 g orally in a single dose or doxycycline 100 mg orally twice a day for 7 days. Alternative regimens include erythromycin base 500 mg orally four times a day for 7 days, erythromycin ethylsuccinate 800 mg orally four times a day for 7 days, ofloxacin 300 mg orally twice a day for 7 days, or levofloxacin 500 mg orally for 7 days.

Patients do not need to be retested for *Chlamydia* after completing treatment with doxycycline or azithromycin unless symptoms persist or reinfection is suspected. A test of cure may be considered 3 weeks after completion of treatment with erythromycin.

A chlamydial cause should be considered for all infants under 30 days of age who have conjunctivitis. Ocular exudate from infants being evaluated for chlamydial conjunctivitis should also be tested for *N. gonorrhoeae*. Erythromycin base or ethylsuccinate 50 mg/kg/d orally divided into four doses daily for 14 days is recommended. Topical antibiotic therapy alone is inadequate for treatment of chlamydial infection and is unnecessary when systemic treatment is administered.

TABLE 29–10 ■ *Chlamydia* Test Performance Characteristics

Test	Sensitivity*	Specificity	Detectability level (elementary bodies)
Enzyme immunoassay (EIA)	40%–60%	99.5%[†]	1000–10,000
Nonamplified genetic probe	40%–65%	99.0%	1000–10,000
Direct fluorescent antibody (DFA)	50%–70%	99.8%	1000–10,000
Cell culture	50%–90%	99.9%	10–100
Nucleic acid amplification tests (NAATs)			
Ligase chain reaction (LCR)	Over 90% for cervical, urethral, and urine testing	99.7%	1–10
Polymerase chain reaction (PCR)			
Transcriptase mediated amplification (TMA)			
Strand displacement amplification (SDA)			

*Defined using a combination of different test methods, including culture, DFA, and PCR or LCR directed against a target sequence distinct from that used in the routine PCR or LCR assays.
†Specificity using confirmatory assays.

Management of Sex Partners

Patients should be instructed to refer their sex partners for evaluation, testing, and treatment. The following recommendations on exposure intervals are based on limited evaluation. Sex partners should be evaluated, tested, and treated if they had sexual contact with the patient during the 60 days preceding the onset of the patient's symptoms or diagnosis of chlamydial infection. The most recent sex partner should be evaluated and treated even if the time of the last sexual contact was more than 60 days before symptom onset or diagnosis. Patients should be instructed to abstain from sexual intercourse until they and their sex partners have completed treatment. Abstinence should be continued until 7 days after a single-dose regimen or after completion of a 7-day regimen.

DISEASES CHARACTERIZED BY URETHRITIS AND CERVICITIS

Management of Men with Urethritis

Urethritis that is due to an infection is characterized by urethral discharge of mucopurulent or purulent material and sometimes by dysuria or urethral pruritus. Asymptomatic infections are common. The principal bacterial pathogens of proven clinical importance in men who have urethritis are *N. gonorrhoeae* and *C. trachomatis*. Testing to determine the specific cause is recommended because both chlamydial infection and gonorrhea must be reported to state health departments, and a specific diagnosis may enhance partner notification and improve compliance with treatment, especially in the exposed partner. Nongonococcal urethritis (NGU) is diagnosed when gram-negative intracellular diplococci cannot be identified on urethral smears. *C. trachomatis* is a frequent cause (i.e., 15% to 55% of cases); however, the incidence differs by age group, with a lower incidence of this organism in older men. The proportion of NGU cases caused by *Chlamydia* has been declining gradually. Complications of NGU among men infected with *C. trachomatis* include epididymitis and Reiter's syndrome. The cause of most cases of nonchlamydial NGU is unknown. *Ureaplasma urealyticum* and *Mycoplasma genitalium* have been implicated as causes of NGU in some studies.[27] *Trichomonas vaginalis* and HSV sometimes cause NGU.

Clinicians should document the presence of urethritis. Urethritis can be documented on the basis of any of the following signs:

1. Mucopurulent or purulent discharge.
2. Gram stain of urethral secretions demonstrating more than 5 white blood cells (WBCs) per oil immersion field. The Gram stain is the preferred rapid diagnostic test for evaluating urethritis. It is highly sensitive and specific for documenting both urethritis and the presence or absence of gonococcal infection.

Gonococcal infection is confirmed by documenting the presence of WBCs containing intracellular gram-negative diplococci.

3. Positive WBC esterase test on first-void urine or microscopic examination of first-void urine demonstrating more than 10 WBCs per high power field.

If none of these criteria is present, treatment should be deferred, and the patient should be tested for *N. gonorrhoeae* and *C. trachomatis* and followed closely if test results are negative. Empiric treatment of symptoms without documentation of urethritis is recommended only for patients at high risk for infection who are unlikely to return for a follow-up evaluation. Such patients should be treated for gonorrhea and chlamydial infection. Partners of patients treated empirically should be evaluated and treated.

Treatment of Nongonococcal Urethritis

Treatment should be initiated as soon as possible after diagnosis. Single-dose regimens have the advantage of improved compliance. Recommended regimens include either azithromycin 1 g orally in a single dose or doxycycline 100 mg orally twice a day for 7 days. Alternatively, erythromycin base 500 mg orally four times a day for 7 days, erythromycin ethylsuccinate 800 mg orally four times a day for 7 days, ofloxacin 300 mg twice a day for 7 days, or levofloxacin 500 mg once daily for 7 days may be given. Patients should be instructed to return for evaluation if symptoms persist or recur after completion of therapy. Symptoms alone, without documentation of signs or laboratory evidence of urethral inflammation, are not a sufficient basis for re-treatment. Patients should be instructed to abstain from sexual intercourse until 7 days after therapy is initiated. Patients should refer for evaluation and treatment all sex partners they have had within the preceding 60 days.

Patients who have persistent or recurrent urethritis should be re-treated with the initial regimen if they did not comply with the treatment regimen or if they were re-exposed to an untreated sex partner. Otherwise a culture of an intraurethral swab specimen and a first-void urine specimen for *T. vaginalis* should be performed. Some cases of recurrent urethritis following doxycycline treatment may be caused by tetracycline-resistant *U. urealyticum*. In this situation, treatment with metronidazole 2 g orally in a single dose plus erythromycin base 500 mg orally four times a day for 7 days or erythromycin ethylsuccinate 800 mg orally four times a day for 7 days may be curative.

Management of Mucopurulent Cervicitis

Mucopurulent cervicitis is an inflammatory process of the cervical epithelium and stroma caused by certain infectious agents that can result in an ascending infection of the upper genital tract. Clinically, mucopurulent cervicitis (MPC) is characterized by a yellow or green endocervical exudate visible in the endocervical canal or on an endocervical swab specimen. Some specialists also diagnose MPC on the basis of easily induced cervical bleeding. Although some experts consider an increased number of polymorphonuclear leukocytes on endocervical Gram stain as being useful in the diagnosis of MPC, this criterion has not been standardized, has a low positive-predictive value (PPV), and is not available in some settings. MPC often is asymptomatic, but some women have an abnormal vaginal discharge and vaginal bleeding (e.g., after sexual intercourse). MPC can be caused by *C. trachomatis* or *N. gonorrhoeae*; however, in most cases neither organism can be isolated. MPC can persist despite repeated courses of antimicrobial therapy. Because relapse or reinfection with *C. trachomatis* or *N. gonorrhoeae* usually does not occur in persons with persistent cases of MPC, other nonmicrobiologic determinants (e.g., inflammation in the zone of ectopy) might be involved. Patients who have MPC should be tested for *C. trachomatis* and for *N. gonorrhoeae* with the most sensitive and specific test available.

Treatment of MPC

The results of sensitive tests for *C. trachomatis* or *N. gonorrhoeae* (e.g., culture or nucleic acid amplification tests) should determine the need for treatment unless the likelihood of infection with either organism is high or the patient is unlikely to return for treatment. Empiric treatment should be considered for a patient who is suspected of having gonorrhea or a chlamydial infection if (1) the incidence of these infections is high in the patient population (2) the patient might be difficult to locate for treatment. If the decision to provide empiric treatment is made, the regimen should include coverage for *Chlamydia* and *N. gonorrhoeae*. Single-dose regimens have the important advantage of improved compliance through directly observed therapy.

PELVIC INFLAMMATORY DISEASE

PID comprises a spectrum of inflammatory disorders of the upper female genital tract, including any combination of endometritis, salpingitis, tubo-ovarian abscess, and pelvic peritonitis. Sexually transmitted organisms, especially *N. gonorrhoeae* and *C. trachomatis*, are implicated in many cases; however, microorganisms that comprise the vaginal flora (e.g., anaerobes, *Gardnerella vaginalis*, *Haemophilus influenzae*, enteric gram-negative rods, and *Streptococcus agalactiae*) also have been associated with PID. In addition, cytomegalovirus (CMV), *Mycoplasma hominis*, or *U. urealyticum* may be the responsible agent in some cases of PID.

Many women with PID have subtle or mild symptoms; thus acute PID is difficult to diagnose. Delay in diagnosis and effective treatment probably contributes to inflammatory sequelae in the upper reproductive tract. Laparoscopy can be used to obtain a more accurate diagnosis of salpingitis and a more complete bacteriologic diagnosis but cannot be used if PID is indicated by mild symptoms. Consequently a diagnosis of PID usually is based on clinical findings. The clinical diagnosis of acute PID is imprecise. No single historical, physical, or laboratory finding is both sensitive and specific for the diagnosis of acute PID. Because of the difficulty of diagnosis and the potential for damage to the reproductive health of women even from apparently mild or atypical PID, health care providers should maintain a low threshold for the diagnosis of PID. Diagnosis and management of other common causes of lower abdominal pain (e.g., ectopic pregnancy, acute appendicitis, and functional pain) are unlikely to be impaired by initiating empiric antimicrobial therapy for PID. Empiric treatment of PID should be initiated in sexually active young women and other women at risk for STDs if uterine or adnexal tenderness or cervical motion tenderness is present and no other cause(s) for the illness can be identified.

Most women with PID have either mucopurulent cervical discharge or evidence of WBCs on a microscopic evaluation of a saline preparation of vaginal fluid. If the cervical discharge appears normal and no white blood cells are found on the saline preparation, the diagnosis of PID is unlikely, and alternative causes of pain should be investigated.

Approximately 25% of women with a single episode of symptomatic PID will experience sequelae, including ectopic pregnancy, infertility, or chronic pelvic pain. Tubal infertility occurs in 8% of women after one episode of PID, in 20% after two episodes, and in 40% after three episodes.

Treatment of Pelvic Inflammatory Disease

PID treatment regimens must provide empiric, broad-spectrum coverage of likely pathogens. Antimicrobial coverage should include *N. gonorrhoeae*, *C. trachomatis*, anaerobes, gram-negative facultative bacteria, and streptococci. Although PID frequently is treated on an outpatient basis, there are no long-term studies comparing the efficacy of outpatient and parenteral regimens in preventing sequelae. The need to eradicate anaerobes from women who have PID has not been determined definitively; however, many women who have PID also have bacterial vaginosis. The decision to hospitalize should be left to the discretion of the health care provider. Many randomized trials have demonstrated the efficacy of both parenteral and oral regimens.[28] The time to switch from intravenous to oral therapy (in those patients started on IV therapy) classically has been after at least 48 hours of substantial clinical improvement, but this time designation is arbitrary. Therapy initiated with cefotetan 2 g intravenously every 12 hours or cefoxitin 2 g intravenously every 6 hours plus doxycycline 100 mg orally or intravenously every 12 hours is effective and can be switched to oral therapy. Alternatively, clindamycin 900 mg intravenously every 8 hours plus gentamicin with a loading dose of 2 mg/kg followed by a maintenance dose of 1.5 mg/kg every 8 hours can be used, with once-daily gentamicin dosing also a consideration. Additional parenteral therapy for PID has been described but with little clinical trial data. Oral therapy for PID includes ofloxacin 400 mg orally twice a day for 14 days or levofloxacin 500 mg orally once daily for 14 days with or without metronidazole 500 mg orally twice a day for 14 days. The following could also be used: ceftriaxone 250 mg intramuscularly in a single dose or cefoxitin 2 g intramuscularly in a single dose plus probenecid 1 g orally administered concurrently in a single dose, another parenteral third-generation cephalosporin (e.g., ceftizoxime or cefotaxime) plus doxycycline 100 mg orally twice a day for 14 days could be given with or without metronidazole 500 mg orally twice a day for 14 days (metronidazole if bacterial vaginosis is a concern).

Patients should exhibit significant clinical improvement within 3 days after initiation of therapy. Patients who do not improve within this period usually require hospitalization, additional diagnostic tests, and possible surgical intervention.

Management of Sex Partners

Male sex partners of women with PID should be examined and treated if they had sexual contact with the patient during the 60 days preceding the patient's onset of symptoms. Male partners of women who have PID caused by *C. trachomatis* or *N. gonorrhoeae* often are asymptomatic. Sex partners should be treated empirically with regimens effective against both of these infections, regardless of the cause of the PID or pathogens isolated from the infected woman.

BACTERIAL VAGINOSIS

Bacterial vaginosis (BV) is a clinical syndrome resulting from replacement of the normal hydrogen peroxide–producing *Lactobacillus* spp. in the vagina with high concentrations of anaerobic bacteria (e.g., *Prevotella* spp and *Mobiluncus* spp), *G. vaginalis*, *M. hominis*, and streptococci. BV is the most common cause of vaginal discharge or malodor; however, up to 50% of women with BV may not report symptoms. The cause of the microbial alteration is not fully understood. BV is associated with having multiple sex partners, douching, and lack of vaginal lactobacilli; it is unclear whether BV results from acquisition of a sexually transmitted pathogen. Women who have never been sexually active are rarely affected. Treatment of the male sex partner has not been beneficial in preventing the recurrence of BV.

BV can be diagnosed by clinical or Gram stain criteria. Clinical criteria require three of the following symptoms or signs (Amsel's criteria)[29]:

1. Homogeneous, white, noninflammatory discharge that smoothly coats the vaginal walls
2. Clue cells on microscopic examination
3. pH of vaginal fluid higher than 4.5
4. Fishy odor of vaginal discharge before or after the addition of 10% KOH (i.e., the whiff test)

Another test for BV is to apply the Nugent criteria: the relative proportions of bacterial morphotypes on a gram-stained slide are estimated to give a score between 0 and 10. A score of less than 4 is normal, 4 to 6 is intermediate, and over 6 is BV.

Treatment of Bacterial Vaginosis

For nonpregnant women with BV, first-line treatment with metronidazole or clindamycin offers the following benefits: (1) relief of vaginal symptoms and signs of infection and (2) reduction of the risk for infectious complications after abortion or hysterectomy. Other potential benefits include the reduction of other infectious complications (e.g., HIV and other STDs). All women who have symptomatic disease require treatment. BV during pregnancy is associated with adverse pregnancy outcomes, including premature rupture of the membranes, preterm labor, preterm birth, and postpartum endometritis. Because of the increased risk for postoperative infectious complications associated with BV, some specialists recommend that before performing surgical abortion or hysterectomy, providers screen for and treat women with BV in addition to providing routine prophylaxis,[30,31] but data here are sparse.

BV can be treated with metronidazole 500 mg orally twice a day for 7 days, metronidazole gel 0.75% one full applicator (5 g) intravaginally once a day for 5 days or clindamycin cream 2% one full applicator (5 g) intravaginally at bedtime for 7 days. Other options for treatment, but somewhat less effective, include metronidazole 2 g orally in a single dose, clindamycin 300 mg orally twice a day for 7 days, or clindamycin ovules 100 g intravaginally once at bedtime for 3 days. Patients should be advised to abstain from alcohol during treatment with metronidazole and for 24 hours afterward. Trials are currently underway to evaluate the efficacy of vaginal lactobacilli suppositories in addition to oral metronidazole for the treatment of BV. Clindamycin cream and ovules are oil based and might weaken latex condoms and diaphragms. Routine treatment of sex partners is not recommended.

Treatment of BV during pregnancy is indicated, since it is associated with adverse pregnancy outcomes (e.g., premature rupture of the membranes, chorioamnionitis, preterm labor, preterm birth, postpartum endometritis, and post–cesarean wound infection). Metronidazole 250 mg orally three times a day for 7 days or clindamycin 300 mg orally twice a day for 7 days is recommended, as existing data do not support the use of topical agents during pregnancy. Evidence from three trials suggests an increase in adverse events (e.g., prematurity and neonatal infections) after use of clindamycin cream.[32–34] Multiple studies and meta-analyses have not demonstrated a consistent association between metronidazole use during pregnancy and teratogenic or mutagenic effects in newborns.[35–37]

TRICHOMONAS VAGINITIS

Trichomoniasis is caused by the protozoan *T. vaginalis*. There are an estimated 5 million cases annually in the United States, which cost an estimated $375 million dollars to diagnose and treat. Trichomoniasis is almost always sexually transmitted; fomite transmission is rare. Because *T. vaginalis* may persist for months to years in epithelial crypts and periglandular areas, distinguishing between persistent, subclinical infection and remote sexual acquisition is not always possible. Transmission between female sex partners has been documented.

Most men who are infected with *T. vaginalis* do not have symptoms; others have NGU. Many infected women have symptoms characterized by a diffuse, malodorous, yellow-green discharge with vulvar irritation. Some women, however, have minimal or no symptoms. Vaginal trichomoniasis has been associated with adverse pregnancy outcomes, particularly premature rupture of the membranes, preterm delivery, and low birth weight. Diagnosis of vaginal trichomoniasis usually is made by microscopic examination of vaginal secretions, but this method has a sensitivity of only about 60% to 70%. Culture is the most sensitive commercially available method of diagnosis.

Treatment of Trichomoniasis

Treatment of patients and sex partners with trichomoniasis relieves symptoms, effects microbiologic cure, and reduces transmission. Recommended treatment of trichomoniasis includes either metronidazole 2 g orally in a single dose or metronidazole 500 mg twice a day for 7 days. Metronidazole gel has been approved for treatment of BV. As is the case with other topically applied antimicrobials that are unlikely to achieve therapeutic levels in the urethra or perivaginal glands, metronidazole gel is considerably less efficacious for the treatment of trichomoniasis (<50%) than oral preparations of metronidazole are and is not recommended for use.

Follow-up is unnecessary for men and women who become asymptomatic after treatment or who are initially asymptomatic. If treatment fails with either regimen, the patient should be re-treated with metronidazole 500 mg twice a day for 7 days. If treatment fails again, the patient should be treated with a single, 2-g dose of metronidazole once a day for 3 to 5 days.

Management of Sex Partners

Sex partners of patients with *T. vaginalis* should be treated. Patients should be instructed to avoid sex until they and their sex partners are cured (i.e., when therapy has been completed and patient and partner[s] are asymptomatic).

VULVOVAGINAL CANDIDIASIS

Vulvovaginal candidiasis (VVC) usually is caused by *Candida albicans* but occasionally is caused by other *Candida* spp or yeasts. Typical symptoms of VVC include pruritus and vaginal discharge. Other symptoms include vaginal soreness, vulvar burning, dyspareunia, and external dysuria. None of these symptoms is specific for VVC. An estimated 75% of women will have at least one episode of VVC, and 40% to 45% will have two or more episodes. On the basis of clinical presentation, microbiology, host factors, and response to therapy, VVC can be classified as either uncomplicated or complicated (usually implying either a non-*albicans Candida* infection, recurrent or severe disease, or infection in women who have uncontrolled diabetes, debilitation, or immunosuppression or who are pregnant). A diagnosis of *Candida* vaginitis is suggested clinically by pruritus and erythema in the vulvovaginal area; a white discharge may also be present. The diagnosis can be made in a woman who has signs and symptoms of vaginitis when either (1) a wet preparation (saline, 10% KOH) or Gram stain of vaginal discharge demonstrates yeasts or pseudohyphae or (2) a culture or other test is positive for a yeast species. Recurrent VVC (RVVC), usually defined as four or more episodes of symptomatic VVC each year, affects a small percentage of women (<5%). The pathogenesis of RVVC is poorly understood, and most women who have RVVC have no apparent predisposing or underlying conditions. Vaginal cultures should be obtained from patients with RVVC to confirm the clinical diagnosis and to identify unusual species, including non-*albicans* species, particularly *Candida glabrata*. Severe vulvovaginitis (i.e., extensive vulvar erythema, edema, excoriation, and fissure formation) has lower clinical response rates in patients treated with short courses of topical or oral therapy.

Treatment of Vulvovaginal Candidiasis

Short-course topical formulations (i.e., single dose and regimens of 1 to 3 days) effectively treat uncomplicated VVC. The topically applied azole drugs are more effective than nystatin. Treatment with azoles relieves symptoms, and cultures are negative in 80% to 90% of patients who complete therapy. A number of topical agents are available for treatment (Table 29–11). Alternatively, fluconazole 150-mg oral tablet taken as a single dose can also be used. The creams and suppositories in this regimen are oil based and may weaken latex condoms and diaphragms. VVC usually is not acquired through sexual intercourse; treatment of sex partners is not recommended but may be considered in women who have

TABLE 29–11 ■ Topical Agents for Treatment of Vulvovaginal Candidiasis (VVC)

Butoconazole 2% cream 5 g intravaginally × 3 d*

OR

Butoconazole 2% cream 5 g (Butaconazole 1—sustained release) single intravaginal application

OR

Clotrimazole 1% cream 5 g intravaginally × 7–14 d*

OR

Clotrimazole 100-mg vaginal tablet × 7 d*

OR

Clotrimazole 100-mg vaginal tablet, 2 tablets × 3 d*

OR

Clotrimazole 500-mg vaginal tablet, 1 tablet in a single application

OR

Miconazole 2% cream 5 g intravaginally × 7 d*

OR

Miconazole 100 mg vaginal suppository, one suppository × 7 d*

OR

Miconazole 200 mg vaginal suppository, one suppository × 3 d*

OR

Nystatin 100,000-U vaginal tablet, one tablet × 14 d

OR

Tioconazole 6.5% ointment 5 g intravaginally in a single application

OR

Terconazole 0.4% cream 5 g intravaginally × 7 d

OR

Terconazole 0.8% cream 5 g intravaginally × 3 d

OR

Terconazole 80 mg vaginal suppository, 1 suppository × 3 d

*Over-the-counter (OTC) preparations.

From CDC: Sexually Transmitted Diseases Treatment Guidelines 2002. MMWR Morb Mortal Wkly Rep 2002; 51(RR-6):26–28.

recurrent infection. A minority of male sex partners may have balanitis, which is characterized by erythematous areas on the glans of the penis in conjunction with pruritus or irritation. These men benefit from treatment with topical antifungal agents to relieve symptoms.

RVVC therapy revolves around the use of short-duration oral or topical azole therapy as well. To maintain clinical and mycologic control, however, specialists recommend a longer duration of initial therapy (e.g., 7 to 14 days of topical therapy or a 150-mg oral dose of fluconazole repeated 3 days later) to achieve fungal remission before a maintenance antifungal regimen is initiated. Suppressive maintenance antifungal therapies are effective in reducing RVVC. However, 30% to 40% of women will have recurrent disease once maintenance therapy is discontinued. Maintenance antifungals are selected on the basis of pharmacologic characteristics of individual agents and route of administration. Recommended regimens include clotrimazole (500-mg vaginal suppository once weekly), ketoconazole (100-mg dose once daily), fluconazole (100- to 150-mg dose once weekly), and itraconazole (400-mg dose once monthly or 100-mg dose once daily). Although all maintenance regimens should be continued for 6 months, an estimated 1 in 10,000 to 15,000 people exposed to ketoconazole may develop hepatotoxicity. Patients receiving long-term ketoconazole should be monitored for toxicity. Routine treatment of sex partners is controversial.

Severe vulvovaginitis has lower clinical response rates in patients treated with short courses of topical or oral therapy. Either 7 to 14 days of topical azole or 150 mg of fluconazole in two sequential doses (second dose 72 hours after initial dose) is recommended.

Vulvovaginal Candidiasis in the Compromised Host

Women with underlying debilitating medical conditions (e.g., those with uncontrolled diabetes or those receiving corticosteroid treatment) do not respond well to short-term therapies. Efforts to correct modifiable conditions should be made, and more prolonged (i.e., 7 to 14 days) conventional antifungal treatment is necessary.

VVC often occurs during pregnancy. Only topical azole therapies, applied for 7 days, are recommended for use in pregnant women.

The attack rate of VVC in HIV-infected women is unknown. Vaginal *Candida* colonization rates in HIV-infected women are higher than among seronegative women with similar demographic characteristics and high-risk behaviors, and the colonization rates correlate with increasing severity of immunosuppression. Symptomatic VVC is more common in seropositive women and similarly correlates with severity of immunodeficiency. In addition, among HIV-infected women, systemic azole exposure is associated with the isolation of non-*albicans Candida* spp from the vagina. On the basis of available data, therapy for VVC in HIV-infected women should not differ from that for seronegative women. Although long-term prophylactic therapy with fluconazole at a dose of 200 mg weekly has been effective in reducing *C. albicans* colonization and symptomatic VVC, it is not recommended for routine primary prophylaxis in HIV-infected women in the absence of recurrent VVC. Given the frequency of RVVC in the immunocompetent healthy population, RVVC should not be considered a sentinel sign to justify HIV testing.

GENITAL HUMAN PAPILLOMAVIRUS INFECTION (GENITAL WARTS)

Genital HPV infection is common, with exact numbers of infection unknown but estimated to be approximately 20 million new infections in the United States each year. Many clinic-based studies suggest a genital HPV prevalence of 50% or more, with the highest occurrence in the 20- to 24-year age group. More than 30 types of HPV can infect the genital tract. Most HPV infections are asymptomatic, unrecognized, or subclinical. Visible genital warts usually are caused by HPV types 6 or 11. Other HPV types in the anogenital region (e.g., types 16, 18, 31, 33, and 35) have been strongly associated with cervical neoplasia. In addition to their presence an the external genitalia (i.e., the penis, vulva, scrotum, perineum, and perianal skin), genital warts also can be present on the uterine cervix and in the vagina, urethra, anus, and mouth; these warts are sometimes symptomatic. Intra-anal warts are seen predominantly in patients who have had receptive anal intercourse; these warts are distinct from perianal warts, which can occur in men and women who do not have a history of anal sex. In addition to the genital area, HPV types 6 and 11 have been associated with conjunctival, nasal, oral, and laryngeal warts. Patients who have visible genital warts can be infected simultaneously with multiple HPV types.

Treatment of Genital Human Papillomavirus Infection

The primary goal of treating visible genital warts is the removal of symptomatic warts. In most patients, treatment can induce wart-free periods. If left untreated, visible genital warts may resolve on their own, remain unchanged, or increase in size or number. Determining whether treatment of genital warts will reduce transmission is difficult, because no laboratory marker of infectivity has been established and because clinical studies evaluating the persistence of HPV DNA in genital tissue after treatment have had variable findings. Existing data indicate that currently available therapies for genital warts may reduce, but probably not eradicate, infectivity. Treatment of genital warts should be guided by the preference of the patient, the available resources, and the experience of the health care provider. No definitive

evidence suggests that any of the available treatments is superior to the others, and no single treatment is ideal for all patients or all warts. Locally developed and monitored treatment algorithms have been associated with improved clinical outcomes and should be encouraged. Because of uncertainty regarding the effect of treatment on future transmission and the possibility for spontaneous resolution, an acceptable alternative for some patients is to forgo treatment and await spontaneous resolution.

In general, warts located on moist surfaces or in intertriginous areas respond better to topical treatment than do warts on drier surfaces. The treatment modality should be changed if a patient has not improved substantially after three provider-administered treatments or if warts have not completely cleared after six treatments. Complications are rare if treatments for warts are used properly. Patients should be warned that persistent hypopigmentation or hyperpigmentation are common with ablative modalities. Depressed or hypertrophic scars are uncommon but can occur, especially if the patient has had insufficient time to heal between treatments. Rarely, treatment can result in disabling chronic pain syndromes (e.g., vulvodynia or hyperesthesia of the treatment site).

Treatment regimens for genital HPV can be divided into two treatment settings: patient applied and provider administered. For patient-applied treatments, patients must be able to identify and reach warts to be treated. Patient-applied therapy includes podofilox 0.5% solution or gel; the patient should apply podofilox solution with a cotton swab or podofilox gel with a finger to visible genital warts twice a day for 3 days, followed by 4 days of no therapy. This cycle may be repeated, as necessary, for up to four cycles. The total wart area treated should not exceed 10 cm², and the total volume of podofilox should be limited to 0.5 ml per day. Most patients experience mild-to-moderate pain or local irritation after treatment. The safety of podofilox during pregnancy has not been established. A newer form of therapy is to use an immune-response modifier such as imiquimod 5% cream. Patients should apply imiquimod cream once daily at bedtime three times a week for up to 16 weeks. The treatment area should be washed with soap and water 6 to 10 hours after the application. Local inflammatory reactions are common with imiquimod; these reactions usually are mild to moderate. The safety of imiquimod during pregnancy has not been established.

Many provider-applied therapies are available to the clinician: cryotherapy with liquid nitrogen or a cryoprobe, topical podophyllin resin 10% to 25% in a compound tincture of benzoin, topical trichloroacetic acid (TCA) or bichloroacetic acid (BCA) 80% to 90% solution, and surgical removal. Less commonly, intralesional interferon or laser surgery has been used. Cryotherapy destroys warts by thermal-induced cytolysis. Health care providers must be trained in the proper use of this therapy, because overtreatment or undertreatment may result in poor efficacy or complications. Pain after application of the liquid nitrogen, followed by necrosis and sometimes blistering, is common. Podophyllin resin, which contains several compounds including antimitotic podophyllin lignans, is another treatment option. The resin is most frequently compounded at 10% to 25% in a tincture of benzoin. However, podophyllin resin preparations differ in the concentration of active components and contaminants. The shelf life and stability of podophyllin preparations are unknown. A thin layer of podophyllin resin must be applied to the warts and allowed to air dry before the treated area comes into contact with clothing; overapplication or failure to air dry can result in local irritation caused by spread of the compound to adjacent areas. Both TCA and BCA are caustic agents that destroy warts by chemical coagulation of the proteins. Although these preparations are widely used, they have not been investigated thoroughly. TCA solutions have a low viscosity comparable to that of water and can spread rapidly if applied excessively; thus they can damage adjacent tissues. Both TCA and BCA should be applied sparingly and allowed to dry before the patient sits or stands. If pain is intense, the acid can be neutralized with soap or sodium bicarbonate. Surgical therapy is a treatment option that has the advantage of usually eliminating warts at a single visit. Such therapy, however, requires substantial clinical training, additional equipment, and a longer office visit. Once local anesthesia is applied, the visible genital warts can be physically destroyed by electrocautery, in which case no additional hemostasis is required. Care must be taken to control the depth of electrocautery to prevent scarring. Alternatively the warts can be removed either by tangential excision with a pair of fine scissors or a scalpel or by curettage. Carbon dioxide laser surgery may be useful in the management of extensive warts or intraurethral warts, particularly for those patients who have not responded to other treatments. Interferons, either natural or recombinant, used for the treatment of genital warts have been administered systemically (i.e., subcutaneously at a distant site or intramuscularly) and intralesionally (i.e., injected into the warts). Systemic interferon is not effective. The efficacy and recurrence rates of intralesional interferon are comparable to other treatment modalities. Interferon is likely effective because of its antiviral or immunostimulating effects. Interferon therapy, however, is not recommended for routine use because of inconvenient routes of administration, frequent office visits, and the association between its use and a high frequency of systemic adverse effects. Site-specific treatment regimens are listed in Table 29–12.

Follow-up

After visible genital warts have cleared, a follow-up evaluation is not mandatory but may be helpful. Patients should be cautioned to watch for recurrences, especially during the first 3 months after treatment. Women should be counseled to undergo regular Pap screening as

TABLE 29–12 ■ Treatment of Genital Herpesvirus (HPV) Infection by Site

Site	Recommended therapy
External genital warts (EGW)	Patient applied: Podofilox 0.5% solution or gel OR Imiquimod 5% cream Provider applied: Cryotherapy OR Podophyllin resin 10%–25% OR Trichloroacetic acid (TCA) or bichloroacetic acid (BCA) 80%–90% OR Surgical removal *Alternatives*: Intralesional interferon or laser surgery
Cervical warts	Treatment by a specialist
Vaginal warts	Cryotherapy or TCA or BCA 80%–90%
Urethral meatus warts	Cryotherapy or podophyllin 10%–25%
Anal warts	Cryotherapy, TCA or BCA 80%–90%, or surgical removal
Oral warts	Cryotherapy or surgical removal

From CDC: Sexually Transmitted Diseases Treatment Guidelines 2002. MMWR Morb Mortal Wkly Rep 2002;51(RR-6):26–28.

recommended for women without genital warts. The presence of genital warts is not an indication for a change in the frequency of Pap tests or for cervical colposcopy.

Management of Sex Partners

Examination of sex partners is not necessary for the management of genital warts because no data indicate that reinfection plays a role in recurrences. Additionally, providing treatment solely for the purpose of preventing future transmission cannot be recommended because the value of treatment in reducing infectivity is not known. The counseling of sex partners provides an opportunity for these partners to (1) learn about implications of having a partner who has genital warts and about their potential for future disease transmission and (2) receive STD and Pap screening. Female sex partners of patients who have genital warts should be reminded that cytologic screening for cervical cancer is recommended for all sexually active women.

The management and treatment of subclinical genital HPV infection is complex and is discussed at length in the complementary text, to which readers are referred for a detailed discussion of this condition.

REFERENCES

1. Institute of Medicine (IOM). Eng TR, Butler WT (eds): The Hidden Epidemic: Confronting Sexually Transmitted Diseases. Washington, DC, National Academy Press, 1997.

2. St. Louis ME, Wasserheit JN, Gayle HD: Janus considers the HIV pandemic—Harnessing recent advances to enhance AIDS prevention [Editorial]. Am J Pub Health 1997;87:10–12.

3. Centers for Disease Control and Prevention (CDC): HIV Prevention through Early Detection and Treatment of Other Sexually Transmitted Diseases — United States Recommendations of the Advisory Committee for HIV and STD Prevention. MMWR Morb Mortal Wkly Rep 1998;47(RR-12):1–31.

4. Centers for Disease Control and Prevention (CDC): Ten leading national notifiable infectious diseases—United States, 1995. MMWR Morb Mortal Wkly Rep 1996;45:883–884.

5. American Social Health Association: Sexually Transmitted Diseases in America: How Many Cases and at What Cost? Menlo Park, Calif, Kaiser Family Foundation, 1998.

6. Beasley RP, Hwang LY, Lin CC, et al: Hepatocellular carcinoma and hepatitis B virus. A prospective study of 22,707 men in Taiwan. Lancet 1981;2(8256):1129–1133.

7. Marchbanks P, Annegers J, Coulam C, et al: Risk factors for ectopic pregnancy: A population-based study. JAMA 1988;259:1823–1827.

8. Lowry D, Schindler J: Prime time TV portrayals of sex, "Safe sex and AIDS: A longitudinal analysis." Journalism Q 1993;70:628–637.

9. Flay B: Mass media and smoking cessation: A critical review. Am J Public Health 1987;77:153–160.

10. Curtis JR, Holmes KK: Individual-level risk assessment for STD/HIV infections. In Holmes KK, Mårdh PA, Sparling PF, Weisner PJ, (eds): Sexually Transmitted Diseases, 3rd ed. New York, McGraw-Hill, 1999, pp 669–683.

11. Seidel HM: Mosby's Guide to Physical Examination. 3rd ed. St. Louis, Mosby Inc, 1995.

12. MacLaren A: Primary care for women: Comprehensive sexual health assessment. J Nurse-Midwifery 1995;40:104–119.

13. Bates B: A Guide to Physical Examination and History Taking. 5th ed. Philadelphia, JB Lippincott, 1991, pp 369–385.

14. Hacker N, Moore J: Essentials of Obstetrics and Gynecology. 2nd ed. Philadelphia, WB Saunders, 1992, pp 12–21.

15. Tanagho E, McAninch J: Smith's General Urology, 14th ed. Stamford, Conn, Appleton & Lange, 1995, pp 43–44.

16. Magnuson HJ, Thomas EW, Olansky S, et al: Inoculation syphilis in human volunteers. Medicine (Baltimore) 1956; 35:33–42.

17. Chapel TA: The variability of syphilitic chancres. Sex Trans Dis 1978;5:68.

18. Chapel TA: Physician recognition of the signs and symptoms of secondary syphilis. JAMA 1981;246:250–251.

19. Mindel A, Tovey SJ, Timmins DJ, Williams P: Primary and secondary syphilis, 20 years experience. 2. Clinical features. Genitourin Med 1989;65:1–3.

20. Centers for Disease Control and Prevention (CDC): Sexually transmitted diseases treatment guidelines 2002. MMWR Morb Mortal Wkly Rep 2002;51(RR-6):26–28.

21. Jurado RL: Syphilis serology: A practical approach. Infect Dis Clin Pract 1996;5:351–358.

22. Bolan G. Management of syphilis in HIV-infected persons. In Sande MA, Volberding PA (eds): Medical Management of AIDS, 5th ed. Philadelphia, WB Saunders, 1997, pp 399–411.

23. Rolfs RT, Joesoef MR, Hendershot EF, et al: A randomized trial of enhanced therapy for early syphilis inpatients with and without human immunodeficiency virus infection. N Engl J Med 1997;337:307–314.

24. Prober CG, Corey L, Brown ZA, et al: The management of pregnancies complicated by genital infections with herpes simplex virus. Clin Infect Dis 1992;15:1031–1038.

25. Joseph AK, Rosen T: Laboratory techniques used in the diagnosis of chancroid, granuloma inguinale, and lymphogranuloma venereum. Dermatol Clin 1994;12:1–8.

26. Recommendations for the prevention and management of Chlamydia trachomatis infection. MMWR Morb Mortal Wkly Rep 1993;42:1–39.

27. Horner P, Thomas B, Gilroy CB, et al: Role of Mycoplasma genitalium and Ureaplasma urealyticum in acute and chronic nongonococcal urethritis. Clin Infect Dis 2001;32:995–1003.

28. Walker CK, Kahn JG, Washington AE, et al: Pelvic Inflammatory disease: Meta-analysis of antimicrobial regimen efficacy. J Infect Dis 1993;168:969–978.

29. Amsel R, Totten PA, Spiegel CA, et al: Nonspecific vaginitis: Diagnostic criteria and microbial and epidemiologic associations. Am J Med 1983;74:14–22.

30. Soper DE, Bump RC, Hurt WG: Bacterial vaginosis and trichomoniasis vaginitis are risk factors for cuff cellulitis after abdominal hysterectomy. Am J Obstet Gynecol 1990; 163:1016–1021.

31. Watts DH, Krohn MA, Hillier SL, Eschenbach DA: Bacterial vaginosis as a risk factor for postcesarean endometritis. Obstet Gynecol 1990;75:52–58.

32. McGregor JA, French JI, Jones W, et al: Bacterial vaginosis is associated with prematurity and vaginal fluid mucinase and sialidase: Results of a controlled trial of topical clindamycin cream. Am J Obstet Gynecol 1994;170:1048–1059.

33. Joesoef MR, Hillier SL, Wiknjosastro G, et al: Intravaginal clindamycin treatment for bacterial vaginosis: Effects on preterm delivery and low birth weight. Am J Obstet Gynecol 1995;173:1527–1531.

34. Vermeulen GM, Bruinse HW: Prophylactic administration of clindamycin 2% vaginal cream to reduce the incidence of spontaneous preterm birth in women with an increased recurrence risk: A randomised placebo-controlled double-blind trial. Br J Obstet Gynaecol 1999;106:652–657.

35. Piper JM, Mitchel EF, Ray WA: Prenatal use of metronidazole and birth defects: No association. Obstet Gynecol 1993; 82:348–352.

36. Caro-Paton T, Carvajal A, Martin de Diego I, et al: Is metronidazole teratogenic? A meta-analysis. Br J Clin Pharmacol 1997;44:179–182.

37. Burtin P, Taddio A, Ariburnu O, et al: Safety of metronidazole in pregnancy: A meta-analysis. Am J Obstet Gynecol 1995; 172:525–529.

Therapy and Prophylaxis for Infectious Complications of Human Immunodeficiency Virus

RAY Y. CHEN, MD
J. MICHAEL KILBY, MD

The outlook for HIV-1-infected patients in the developed world has brightened considerably over the past 5 years, as reflected by declines in AIDS-related mortality and in severe complications of immunodeficiency in the United States. These improvements have been attributed to the availability of more antiretroviral treatment options and the administration of more potent combination regimens (highly active antiretroviral therapy or HAART). It is important to recognize, however, that improving trends in AIDS-related morbidity and mortality were apparent before the widespread use of HAART. This observation suggests more successful prevention and treatment of opportunistic infections has also played a significant role in prolonging survival and improving quality of life for HIV-1-infected patients.

The care of HIV-1-infected patients is a rapidly moving field, particularly because of the dramatic benefits of HAART, and any attempt to provide detailed guidelines on opportunistic infection prevention and treatment is at risk of becoming obsolete within a relatively short time. In this chapter we address the diversity of potential infectious complications of HIV-1 infection by using an outline based on broad categories of organisms (bacteria, fungi, viruses, and parasites and protozoa). Each category is further broken down into commonly encountered specific organisms. These discussions begin with brief reviews regarding the treatment of infections caused by each organism in the context of HIV-1 or AIDS. Because certain infections (e.g., herpes simplex virus, syphilis, hepatitis B and C, and *Mycobacterium tuberculosis*) are covered more fully elsewhere in this textbook, they are mentioned only briefly here. Thus, greater emphasis is placed on AIDS-defining conditions and treatment principles relatively unique to the setting of HIV-1 infection. Each overview of treatment is followed by recommendations regarding the use of primary or secondary prophylaxis or both to decrease the risk of infection or active disease. For the most common and severe opportunistic infections, these recommendations are often based on conclusive clinical trials. For less frequently encountered infections, recommendations about the need for prophylaxis or prevention measures—and the specific agents and dosages to be used—are sometimes extrapolated from treatment experience or are based on anecdotal clinical observations. Importantly, we will also discuss currently evolving recommendations about the potential for discontinuation of primary prevention or maintenance therapy for specific opportunistic infections among previously immunocompromised patients who have favorably responded to HAART. Finally, we summarize in tables the overall opportunistic infection prophylaxis recommendations compiled from these categories of potential pathogens, organizing this information from the standpoint of the degree of immunosuppression and other special considerations related to risk (e.g., gender, geography, serologic status).

BACTERIA

"Typical" Pyogenic Bacterial Infections

Most of the infections incorporated by the Centers for Disease Control and Prevention (CDC) into the clinical definition of AIDS are conditions not commonly encountered in the care of immunocompetent persons. Thus this chapter primarily focuses on opportunistic infections normally defended against by pathogen-specific T lymphocyte immune responses. HIV infection is primarily a disorder of cell-mediated immunity; however, deficits in T cell help are also associated with dysfunction of humoral immune responses. These combined deficits also predispose patients to infections caused by more "typical" bacterial pathogens, particularly intracellular (*Salmonella*) and encapsulated (pneumococcus) bacteria that require efficient antibody responses or opsonization for clearance.

In general, HIV-infected patients with relatively high absolute CD4+ T cell counts (>>200 cells/μl) are not at substantially higher risk for routine, community-acquired infections than the general population is. However, in a subset of otherwise healthy HIV-infected patients, recurrent bacterial pneumonia or sinusitis develops. HIV-infected patients with CD4 counts less than 200/μl are at greater risk for chronic or refractory bacterial sinusitis, sometimes involving the posterior sinuses and requiring surgical drainage in addition to antibiotic therapy.[1] Community-acquired sinusitis in this setting may be associated with organisms such as *Pseudomonas aeruginosa*, normally encountered only in nosocomial respiratory infections.[2] It is also important to remember that refractory or rapidly progressive sinus disease in highly immunocompromised patients must be evaluated aggressively; sinusitis symptoms in persons with advanced AIDS may be due to fungal disease, particularly *Aspergillus* and other molds, or to atypical presentations of lymphoma or other neoplastic diseases.

The risk of bacterial pneumonia among HIV-infected persons increases as the absolute CD4 cell count declines, with over two-thirds of reported cases occurring when the absolute CD4 count is less than 200/μl.[3] Patients with AIDS are at substantial risk for disease due to *Streptococcus pneumoniae*. In a San Francisco study, the crude rate ratio for developing invasive pneumococcal disease in persons with AIDS was 51.3 (confidence internal 40.3 to 65.3).[4] Patients with AIDS were much more likely to have pneumococcal bacteremia concurrent with lung infiltrates than were HIV-negative patients with pneumococcal pneumonia, so blood cultures are essential for febrile HIV-infected patients with pneumonia. *Haemophilus influenzae* pneumonia, again with a high risk of concurrent bacteremia, has also been well described among patients with advanced HIV infection.[5] Community-acquired pneumonia due to organisms such as

Staphylococcus aureus and *P. aeruginosa*, which normally are associated only with hospital-acquired infections, also develops in patients with advanced HIV disease.[3] Atypical or unusual bacterial pathogens, for example, *Rhodococcus equi*, *Nocardia asteroides,* and *Legionella* spp, should also be considered when patients with advanced immunosuppression develop severe or refractory pneumonia, and bronchoscopy is frequently needed to confirm the responsible organism. Although these considerations are crucial for choosing initial empiric antibacterial therapy for HIV-infected patients, once specific pathogens are identified, general treatment principles of pneumonia and sinusitis are the same for HIV-infected patients as for other persons with underlying medical conditions.

Patients with advanced AIDS are at higher risk for bacteremia and invasive infections due to *S. aureus* than the general population is, although this may largely be attributable to the use of long-term in-dwelling intravenous lines rather than deficits in cellular immune responses.[6] Patients with advanced AIDS may be at higher risk than the general population for methicillin-resistant staphylococcal disease, which is not surprising because of the selection pressure from long-term or recurring courses of antibacterial treatments. In general there is not an extremely high risk of bacterial skin and soft tissue infections among HIV-infected patients, although pyomyositis (deep muscle infection similar to "tropical pyomyositis") due to *S. aureus* is occasionally reported in HIV-infected patients.[7]

There are no data to support long-term antibacterial therapy administered to HIV-infected patients solely to prevent "typical" bacterial pathogens. A portion of the benefits derived from prophylaxis with TMP-SMX (the primary prevention strategy for *Pneumocystis* pneumonia), however may relate to a decreased overall risk for bacterial infections. For example, in one study prophylaxis with TMP-SMX was associated with protection from salmonellosis, infection with *Haemophilus* spp and *Staphylococcus* spp, but not from pneumococcal or pseudomonal disease.[8] Prophylaxis with macrolides (clarithromycin or azithromycin administered to advanced AIDS patients to prevent mycobacteremia), with or without TMP-SMX, had a significant protective effect against bacterial infections (i.e., respiratory tract infections, skin and soft tissue infections, abscesses, and bacteremias).[9] Another study, however, suggested that antiretroviral therapy had a significant influence on the incidence of bacterial pneumonia and that administration of TMP-SMX or macrolide prophylaxis did not.[10] Another important preventive measure is to promote smoking cessation, which should help to diminish the increased risk of bacterial respiratory infections and increased susceptibility to emphysema observed in HIV-infected patients.[11,12]

Salmonella and Other Enteric Bacteria

HIV-infected patients are at increased risk for bacterial diarrhea, including infections due to *Shigella*,

Salmonella, and Campylobacter species. Disease recurrences following initial resolution are observed much more commonly in patients with AIDS than in HIV-negative patients.[13] This is particularly well described with nontyphoidal Salmonella, which may cause frequent relapses in some HIV-infected patients unless prolonged suppressive therapy is given. Recurrent salmonellosis has long been recognized as an AIDS-defining condition.[14] As with the bacterial respiratory infections described above, enteric bacterial infections are much more likely to be complicated by bacteremia in HIV-infected patients than are diarrheal syndromes in the general population. Although antimicrobial therapy is not generally indicated for uncomplicated salmonellosis in immunocompetent patients, HIV-infected patients should receive therapy to ameliorate the symptoms of acute diarrheal illness and to help prevent bacteremia and extraintestinal spread. Antibacterial treatment is also indicated for HIV-infected patients with Shigella infections, and the choice of specific therapy must be based on in vitro susceptibilities. Fluoroquinolones are generally the drugs of choice for salmonellosis and other enteric syndromes, and ciprofloxacin 500 to 750 mg twice daily has been used successfully for diarrhea or complications including bacteremia.[15] Although there are no definitive guidelines based on large clinical trials regarding duration of therapy, patients with advanced HIV disease may require life-long therapy as a protection against Salmonella (and less commonly Shigella) disease recurrences.

Campylobacter spp are among the chief bacterial causes of diarrhea worldwide and typically are transmitted following ingestion of contaminated food or water. HIV-infected men who have sex with men are at particularly high risk for Campylobacter infections, probably because of fecal contact during sexual activities. Uncomplicated diarrheal syndromes frequently resolve with rehydration and conservative measures. As with other enteric infections, however, HIV-infected patients with Campylobacter diarrhea are much more likely to become bacteremic than immunocompetent hosts are.[16] Since the earliest recognition of the epidemic, homosexual men were noted to be at significantly increased risk for infections due to Campylobacter jejuni, Campylobacter coli, and several organisms initially referred to as CLO (Campylobacter-like organisms) because of their morphology.[17] The CLO organisms have been reclassified as Helicobacter spp. Helicobacter cinaedi is an example of a CLO that has been well described as a cause of bacteremia in men with AIDS.[18] The treatment of choice for Campylobacter enteric infections has been erythromycin. Although ciprofloxacin has also been used successfully, Campylobacter isolates with fluoroquinolone resistance have been recognized increasingly.

Even though risk factors unique to HIV infection have not been identified for listeriosis, Listeria monocytogenes infections have been reported at higher frequencies in HIV-infected populations.[19] Patients with CD4 counts below 50/µl are at particular risk, often presenting with bacteremia or meningitis.[20] Treatment with standard antimicrobial therapy (e.g., intravenous ampicillin with or without gentamicin for 2 to 4 weeks) is often effective. Although recurrent disease following initial treatment is a potential concern, this phenomenon has not been reported to be a common problem among HIV-infected patients, in contrast to infections with other enteric bacteria.

It is particularly important for HIV-infected patients to adhere closely to proper handwashing and food preparation techniques to avoid enteric infections. Most of these bacterial pathogens can be transmitted via unwashed raw produce, contaminated water or unpasteurized milk, undercooked meats, or dishes containing eggs or dairy products. Shigella and Campylobacter are frequently transmitted from human to human, because of inadequate handwashing or fecal-oral contact. Immunocompromised patients should avoid direct contact with the feces of pets, including cats and dogs (particularly those less than 6 months old with diarrhea, which may shed Salmonella or Campylobacter species) or reptiles. (Pet turtles or iguanas have been associated with the transmission of unusual Salmonella species pathogenic to humans.) Although primary prophylaxis against Salmonella and other enteric infections is not recommended, TMP-SMX prophylaxis for Pneumocystis may secondarily decrease enteric bacterial infections among patients with absolute CD4 counts below 200/µl. In addition, it should be noted that the antiretroviral drug zidovudine has significant anti-Salmonella effects and may provide a protective effect for patients at risk for recurrent Salmonella bacteremia.[21]

Clostridium difficile

Although not specifically designated an HIV-associated pathogen, C. difficile is a relatively common infection in HIV-infected patients, likely as a consequence of frequent hospitalizations and courses of antibacterial therapies. The presentation of C. difficile colitis and the responses to standard therapies are generally comparable to the experience in the general population.[22,23]

Treponema pallidum

The treatment of syphilis is described in detail in Chapter 29. It is important to recognize that presentations of syphilis may be atypical among HIV-infected patients.[24] Occasionally patients are described who appear to develop "late stage" sequelae of syphilis at an accelerated pace. HIV-infected patients may be at higher risk for central nervous system manifestations, and some experts recommend a lower threshold for a diagnostic lumbar puncture when patients present with signs of secondary syphilis. Although routine treatment guidelines can generally be used, some HIV-infected patients may have atypical responses to therapy or relapses after a prolonged period, and careful clinical follow-up is indicated.[25]

Mycobacterium tuberculosis

The treatment of tuberculosis is covered extensively in Chapter 31. HIV-infected patients are at much higher risk for tuberculosis than the general population, even when the absolute CD4 count is not substantially suppressed. The diagnostic cutoff for the purified protein derivative (PPD) skin test for HIV-infected patients is 5 mm rather than the 10 or 15 mm used to define a positive response in other persons at risk. Often when persons with early HIV infection present, they have positive skin tests and cavitary apical lung infiltrates easily recognizable as pulmonary tuberculosis. Patients with more advanced HIV or AIDS, however, have a high rate of atypical presentations of lung disease—diffuse infiltrates, deceptively normal chest radiographs, pleural effusions, thoracic adenopathy—and a high rate of extrapulmonary disease of all descriptions. In most cases, following the general guidelines for tuberculosis therapy is also effective for HIV-infected patients, but patients with extrapulmonary disease may require more prolonged courses of therapy and consultation with experienced clinicians. In some (particularly urban) areas HIV-infected patients are at substantially higher risk for multidrug-resistant tuberculosis relative to the overall local community. Directly observed therapy and close involvement of local health department officials are strongly recommended for optimal care in HIV-infected tuberculosis cases. Careful attention to potential drug interactions with antimycobacterial agents is important, particularly rifampin or rifabutin, which can lower levels of certain antiretroviral drugs (particularly non-nucleoside reverse transcriptase and protease inhibitors).[26,27]

Mycobacterium avium Complex and Other Nontuberculous Mycobacteria

The most common mycobacterial infection among HIV-infected patients in the United States is due to *Mycobacterium avium* complex (MAC, also called *M. avium-intracellulare* or MAI). MAC infection typically manifests as disseminated bacteremia in the setting of advanced AIDS, often presenting with hectic subacute fevers, weight loss, nonspecific abdominal pain, anemia, and an elevated alkaline phosphatase level. There may be hepatic and splenic enlargement and superficial and deep lymphadenopathy.[28] MAC is not a common respiratory pathogen in AIDS patients, except perhaps for patients who have concurrent pulmonary disease (emphysema or bronchiectasis). Isolation of MAC from stool or respiratory secretions in the absence of convincing evidence of infection may represent colonization and does not necessarily require systemic therapy.

Before the development of the second-generation macrolide antibiotics the treatment of MAC infection was relatively complex (often four or more agents in combination), poorly tolerated, and not very effective.[29–32] With the advent of clarithromycin and azithromycin, however, treatment efficacy and tolerability improved considerably.[33,34] Because monotherapy with clarithromycin led to the development of resistance,[35] current recommendations for the treatment of MAC infection are to use at least two agents.[36] The macrolides, especially clarithromycin, have been established as the backbone of any MAC regimen.[37] The standard dose is 500 mg PO twice daily; higher doses have been associated with *shorter* survival.[35] Although azithromycin is likely as efficacious as clarithromycin, there are fewer data from clinical trials regarding azithromycin-based regimens for the treatment of MAC. Ethambutol is recommended as the second agent on the basis of studies that demonstrated a significantly reduced rate of relapse when ethambutol was added to clarithromycin-based regimens.[38,39]

For patients with more extensive disease, rifabutin has been recommended as a third agent. Rifabutin has demonstrated efficacy against MAC in non-macrolide-based regimens.[40] Its impact as a third agent in addition to clarithromycin and ethambutol, however, seems to be limited to preventing the development of clarithromycin resistance, with no effect on bacteriologic response or survival.[41] Rifabutin has many potential adverse effects, the most common of which is an orange-brown discoloration of body secretions. Uveitis, although relatively uncommon, has also been described[42] and is primarily dose related[43] for example, when rifabutin is taken in combination with other drugs, such as fluconazole, which may elevate rifabutin levels above the therapeutic range.[26] Rifabutin has significant drug interactions with many medications taken by HIV-infected patients, although it is a less potent inducer of hepatic enzymes than rifampin. Clofazimine, once a common component of multidrug MAC treatment regimens, is no longer recommended, as studies have shown negligible antimycobacterial activity[44] and an association with increased mortality.[45] Antibiotics commonly used against MAC along with their dosages, pregnancy categories, common adverse effects, and drug interactions are listed in Table 30–1.

Patients who initially respond to effective multidrug therapy but subsequently relapse may fail for multiple reasons, including poor adherence, drug intolerance, or poor absorption.[46,47] The development of drug resistance is also a possibility. MAC resistance to macrolides is well described and involves a point mutation in the central loop of domain V of the 23S rRNA, conferring resistance to both clarithromycin and azithromycin.[48–50] In patients for whom therapy fails, susceptibility testing might be considered to evaluate for macrolide-resistant strains, which can help in determining patient adherence and in guiding therapy. In vitro susceptibility testing for other

TABLE 30–1 ■ Drugs Commonly Used to Treat MAC Infection

Drug	Adult dosage	Pregnancy category*	Adverse effects	Drug interactions
Clarithromycin	500 mg bid	C	Diarrhea, nausea, abnormal taste, dyspepsia, abdominal pain, headache, ↑LFT, ↑PT, ↑BUN	↑es rifabutin levels; ↓ed by fluconazole; arrhythmias with terfenadine, astemizole, cisapride
Azithromycin	500–600 mg qd	B	Same	
Rifabutin	300 mg qd	B	Neutropenia, anemia, thrombocytopenia, rash, nausea, abdominal pain, diarrhea, discolored body fluids, uveitis, myalgias, arthritis, ↑LFT	↓es clarithromycin; ↓ dosage with protease inhibitors; ↑ dosage with efavirenz; no data with nevirapine or delavirdine; ↑ed by clarithromycin and fluconazole
Ethambutol	15 mg/kg/d	C	Optic neuritis, abdominal pain, nausea, confusion, headache, gout, peripheral neuropathy	↓ed absorption with Al³⁺ antacids
Ciprofloxacin	500–750 mg bid	C	Nausea, diarrhea, abdominal pain, headache, restlessness	↓ed absorption with Al³⁺, Ca²⁺, Mg²⁺, antacids, ↑es theophylline level
Amikacin	10–15 mg/kg/d	D	Nephrotoxicity, ototoxicity	

*Pregnancy categories: A, safety has been established in human studies; B, safety is presumed on the basis of animal studies; C, uncertain safety—animal studies show an adverse effect but no human studies; D, unsafe—evidence of risk that may in certain clinical circumstances be justifiable.
BUN, blood urea nitrogen; LFT, liver function tests; PT, prothrombin time.

MAC treatment drugs, however, has not been shown to correlate well with response to treatment in vivo and therefore cannot be recommended to guide therapy.[51,52] The appropriate therapy in patients who develop macrolide resistance is not clear but probably should continue to include a macrolide, as both drug-resistant and drug-susceptible species may be present.[53]

Infections with other nontuberculous mycobacteria, although much less common than disseminated MAC, have also been well described in HIV-infected patients. *Mycobacterium genavense* causes disseminated disease in AIDS patients; the clinical presentation and responses to treatment appear to be similar to those of MAC infection.[54] *Mycobacterium haemophilum* causes disseminated cutaneous skin and bone lesions in patients with low CD4 counts; although treatment regimens have not been established in clinical trials, clarithromycin and rifabutin have shown promise in animal models and have been anecdotally successful in humans.[55] *Mycobacterium kansasii* is endemic in certain U.S. states (Florida, Louisiana, Texas, Illinois) and can cause symptomatic pulmonary infections in patients with AIDS. Only about 20% of HIV-infected patients with *M. kansasii* infection have mycobacteremia, so lysis-centrifugation blood cultures are not so helpful diagnostically compared to disseminated MAC cases.[56] *M. kansasii* often responds to a conventional antituberculosis regimen such as isoniazid, ethambutol, and rifampin, but this organism also has in vitro sensitivity to macrolides or sulfamethoxazole in many cases. For patients receiving drugs that may interact adversely with rifampin, clarithromycin, or rifabutin have been tried in place of rifampin. Treatment for a minimum of 15 months following culture-negativity is recommended. Other "atypical" mycobacteria—including *M. fortuitum*, *M. xenopi*, and *M. gordonae*—may

represent laboratory contaminants or avirulent colonizers when they are isolated from nonsterile sites (i.e., sputum) in the setting of early HIV infection but may cause respiratory disease or disseminated infections in patients with advanced immunosuppression.[57–59] Treatment regimens for these infections are not well defined. *M. gordonae* is often sensitive to antituberculosis drugs and clarithromycin, *M. xenopi* has variable in vitro sensitivities, and *M. fortuitum* is generally not susceptible to conventional tuberculosis drugs. Amikacin, cefoxitin, and probenecid have been used as "induction" therapy, followed by TMP-SMX or doxycycline for a total of at least 6 months.

The use of adjuvant agents in treating patients with refractory mycobacterial disease is still under study. Interferon (IFN)-γ and granulocyte-macrophage colony-stimulating factor (GM-CSF) have both had positive results initially.[60,61] Oral dexamethasone has been shown to reduce refractory symptoms in patients on combination therapy, but the long-term effects on survival are not clear and may be associated with the development of new opportunistic infections.[62,63]

The use of antibiotics for primary prophylaxis of MAC infection has been well established. Although some of the MAC prophylaxis studies included patients with higher CD4 counts (50 to 150/μl), the bulk of disease in these studies occurred in patients within the lowest CD4 count range. Therefore, current U.S. Public Health Service–Infectious Diseases Society of America (USPHS/IDSA) guidelines recommend prophylaxis for patients with CD4 counts below 50/μl (Table 30–2). (USPHS/IDSA Prevention of Opportunistic Infections Working Group: 2001 USPHS/IDSA Guidelines for the Prevention of Opportunistic Infections in Persons Infected with Human Immunodeficiency Virus. Found at

TABLE 30–2 ■ Primary Prophylaxis and Vaccination Regimens[*]

Pathogen	Indication	Prophylactic regimen[†]
Pneumocystis carinii	CD4 count <200/μl or oropharyngeal candidiasis	**Trimethoprim-sulfamethoxazole TMP-SMX 1 DS or SS PO qd** Dapsone 50 mg PO bid or 100 mg PO qd Dapsone 50 mg PO qd + pyrimethamine 50 mg PO qwk + leucovorin 25 mg PO qwk Dapsone 200 mg PO qwk + pyrimethamine 75 mg PO qwk + leucovorin 25 mg PO qwk Aerosolized pentamidine 300 mg qmo Atovaquone 1500 mg PO qd TMP-SMX 1 DS PO 3×/wk
Toxoplasma gondii	CD4 count <100/μl and *Toxoplasma* IgG antibody positive	**TMP-SMX 1 DS PO qd** TMP-SMX 1 SS PO qd Dapsone 50 mg PO qd + pyrimethamine 50 mg PO qwk + leucovorin 25 mg PO qwk Atovaquone 1500 mg PO qd ± pyrimethamine 25 mg PO qd or leucovorin 10 mg PO qd
Mycobacterium avium complex	CD4 count <50/μl	**Azithromycin 1200 mg PO qwk** **Clarithromycin 500 mg PO bid** Rifabutin 300 mg PO qd Azithromycin 1200 mg PO qwk + rifabutin 300 mg PO qd
Streptococcus pneumoniae	CD4 count >200/μl; may be given at CD4 count <200/μl, but efficacy likely diminished	**23 valent polysaccharide vaccine**
Hepatitis B virus	Anti-HBc-negative patients	**Hepatitis B vaccination** (3 doses)
Influenza virus	All patients annually	**Inactivated trivalent influenza virus**
Hepatitis A virus	Anti-HAV-negative patients who are intravenous drug users, men who have sex with men, hemophiliacs, have chronic liver disease (hepatitis B or C)	**Hepatitis A vaccination** (2 doses)

[*]Based on the 2001 USPHS/IDSA Guidelines for the Prevention of Opportunistic Infections in Persons Infected with Human Immunodeficiency Virus, found at *www.hivatis.org*.
[†]Bold-face regimens are first line.
DS, double strength; SS, single strength.

www.hivatis.org.) Recommended prophylactic regimens include clarithromycin 500 mg twice daily or azithromycin 1200 mg once weekly, both of which were associated with a 65% to 70% relative risk reduction of MAC infection.[64,65] MAC prophylaxis is associated with reductions in febrile illnesses, hospitalization, and mortality. In patients who cannot tolerate macrolides, rifabutin 300 mg once daily has been shown to be efficacious but is only about half as effective as macrolide prophylaxis.[66,67] Pregnant patients should receive prophylaxis under the same guidelines as other patients, but withholding prophylaxis in the first trimester is also acceptable (2001 Guidelines). Clarithromycin should not be used in pregnancy, as it is teratogenic in animals. Azithromycin seems to be safe in pregnancy[68] and is the drug of choice for MAC prevention in this setting. Secondary prophylaxis regimens are listed in Table 30–3.

For patients whose CD4 counts increase to over 100/μl in response to antiretroviral therapy, current data indicate that primary MAC prophylaxis may be safely discontinued.[69–72] The current guidelines recommend discontinuing primary MAC prophylaxis for patients who have sustained a CD4 count above 100/μl for longer than three months. Primary prophylaxis should be reinstituted if the patient's CD4 count falls below 50/μl. Discontinuation of secondary prophylaxis has been less well studied. On the basis of current data,[73–75] however, the 2001 Guidelines state that the discontinuation of secondary prophylaxis in patients who have completed 12 months of MAC therapy, have no signs or symptoms of MAC infection, and have sustained a CD4 count above 100/μl for 6 months or longer is reasonable to consider. Secondary prophylaxis should be restarted if the patient's CD4 count falls below 100/μl.

Bartonella Infections

Bartonella spp cause several syndromes in HIV-infected patients, including cat-scratch disease, bacillary angiomatosis, peliosis hepatis, and low-grade bacteremia or endocarditis.[76] These infections usually are treated with macrolides (erythromycin 500 mg PO or IV every 6 hours) although doxycycline (100 mg PO or IV every 12 hours) may also be effective. Following initial treatment,

TABLE 30–3 ■ Secondary Prophylaxis Regimens*

Pneumocystis carinii	**Trimethoprim-sulfamethoxazole (TMP-SMX) 1 DS or SS PO qd**[†]
	Dapsone 50 mg PO bid or 100 mg PO qd
	Dapsone 50 mg PO qd + pyrimethamine 50 mg PO qwk + leucovorin 25 mg PO qwk
	Dapsone 200 mg PO qwk + pyrimethamine 75 mg PO qwk + leucovorin 25 mg PO qwk
	Aerosolized pentamidine 300 mg qmo
	Atovaquone 1500 mg PO qd
	TMP-SMX 1 DS PO 3×/wk
Toxoplasma gondii	**Sulfadiazine 500–1000 mg PO qid + pyrimethamine 25–50 mg PO qd + leucovorin 10–25 mg PO qd**
	Clindamycin 300–450 mg PO q6–8h + pyrimethamine 25–50 mg PO qd + leucovorin 10–25 mg PO qd
	Atovaquone 750 mg PO q6–12h ± pyrimethamine 25 mg PO qd or leucovorin 10 mg PO qd
Mycobacterium avium complex	**Clarithromycin 500 mg PO bid + ethambutol 15 mg/kg PO qd ± rifabutin 300 mg PO qd**
	Azithromycin 500 mg PO qd + ethambutol 15 mg/kg PO qd ± rifabutin 300 mg PO qd
Cytomegalovirus	**Ganciclovir 5–6 mg/kg IV 5–7 d/wk or 1000 mg PO tid**
	Foscarnet 90–120 mg/kg IV qd
	Ganciclovir retinal implant q6–9mo + ganciclovir 1000–1500 mg PO tid (for retinitis)
	Cidofovir 5 mg/kg IV fowk + probenecid 2 g PO 3 h before, then 1 g PO 2 h after, then 1 g PO 8 h after dose
	Valganciclovir 900 mg PO qd
Cryptococcus neoformans	**Fluconazole 200 mg PO qd**
	Amphotericin B 0.6–1 mg/kg IV qwk to 3×/wk
	Itraconazole capsule 200 mg PO qd
Histoplasma capsulatum	**Itraconazole capsule 200 mg PO bid**
	Amphotericin B 1 mg/kg IV qwk
Coccidioides immitis	**Fluconazole 400 mg PO qd**
	Amphotericin B 1 mg/kg IV qwk
	Itraconazole capsule 200 mg PO bid

*Based on the 2001 USPHS/IDSA Guidelines for the Prevention of Opportunistic Infections in Persons Infected with Human Immunodeficiency Virus, found at *www.hivatis.org.*

[†]Bold-face regimens are first line.

DS, double strength; SS, single strength.

life-long suppression may be necessary. Treatment for these syndromes is described in further detail in Chapter 37. Bartonellosis may be best avoided by taking precautions regarding cat exposures. Keeping pet cats should not be prohibited for HIV-infected patients, but certain considerations are worth noting. These infections are spread particularly via bites or scratches from flea-infested young cats, which often have asymptomatic chronic bacteremia. Choosing adult cats as pets, emphasizing flea control strategies, declawing pets, and avoiding rough play may help to decrease the incidence of *Bartonella* infections.[77]

FUNGI

*Pneumocystis carinii**

Many drugs have been evaluated for the treatment of *P. carinii* pneumonia (PCP); the most extensive clinical experience over the years has been with TMP-SMX and pentamidine. Although both are efficacious, TMP-SMX

*Although *Pneumocystis carinii* was previously categorized as a protozoan infection, most experts now contend it is more closely related to the fungi.

has been established as the drug of choice[78–80] on the basis of studies showing either that these agents are equivalent or that TMP-SMX is associated with increased survival.[81–83] TMP-SMX works by inhibiting the biosynthesis of tetrahydrofolic acid; trimethoprim inhibits dihydrofolate reductase, and sulfamethoxazole inhibits dihydropteroate synthase. Recent reports have suggested that *P. carinii* may develop sulfa resistance in response to drug-selective pressure, but the clinical significance of this is still uncertain, and thus no change in therapy is recommended at this time.[84] The convenience of TMP-SMX includes its oral and intravenous formulations and its low cost. For patients with mild disease (Pao_2 >80 mm Hg) and no gastrointestinal difficulties, oral TMP-SMX at a dose of two double strength tablets every 8 hours may be used for a total of 21 days. For patients with more serious disease, intravenous TMP-SMX should be administered at a dose of 15 to 20 mg/kg/d of trimethoprim divided every 6 hours. This may be switched to the oral formulation after the patient has improved to finish the 21 days of therapy.

The difficulty with TMP-SMX is the high rate of intolerance to it, especially among HIV-infected patients.[85,86] The most common adverse effect of TMP-SMX is skin rash.[79] The rash is characteristically generalized, maculopapular, and pruritic, occurring 8 to

12 days after initiation of therapy. Mild rashes have been successfully treated with antihistamines or antipyretics during therapy. Severe rashes, for example, when there is mucous membrane involvement, bullae formation, or intolerable pruritus, require discontinuation of therapy. Fever, if present, usually coincides with the cutaneous eruptions.[87] The next most common adverse effect is bone marrow suppression, especially neutropenia and thrombocytopenia, which often leads to discontinuation of the drug.[79] In an attempt to ameliorate this effect, folinic acid (leucovorin) has been studied in conjunction with TMP-SMX to see if folate replacement would reduce the incidence of bone marrow suppression. Although folinic acid was associated with a decreased incidence of neutropenia, it was also associated with a higher rate of therapeutic failure and death and thus is not recommended.[88] Other commonly seen adverse effects of TMP-SMX include nausea, vomiting, and hepatotoxicity. Less commonly seen adverse reactions include hyperkalemia with metabolic acidosis, hypersensitivity reactions, and tremor.[89–92] A number of studies have reported success with oral desensitization of HIV-infected patients to sulfonamides.[93–96]

Patients with PCP often are noted to have a decline in oxygenation during the first 3 to 5 days of therapy; the decline is believed to be due to an increase in inflammation from anti-*Pneumocystis* therapy, analogous to the Jarisch-Herxheimer reaction.[97] Because of this, the patient should not be presumed to have "treatment failure" until treated for at least 1 week. Patients who have mild disease still retain a pulmonary reserve and can tolerate an initial decline in oxygenation. In patients who have more severe disease, however, any decline in oxygenation can lead to respiratory failure. Corticosteroids administered early in treatment have been shown to reduce this early deterioration and improve survival.[98–101] As a result, corticosteroids are now recommended as adjunctive therapy (whether the primary therapy is TMP-SMX or an alternative regimen) in adults and adolescents (children >13 years of age) with PaO_2 below 70 mm Hg or an alveolar-arterial oxygen gradient higher than 35 mm Hg. Oral prednisone should be started within 72 hours of the initiation of anti-*Pneumocystis* therapy; the following regimen should be used: days 1 to 5: prednisone 40 mg twice a day; days 6 to 10: prednisone 40 mg once a day; days 11 to 21: prednisone 20 mg once a day. If the intravenous route is required, methylprednisolone is recommended at 75% of the prednisone dose.[102] The adverse effects of short-term corticosteroids are well described and include oral candidiasis, hyperglycemia, and mucocutaneous herpes simplex virus infection.[103] There has been concern that steroids may increase the incidence of more serious opportunistic infections as well, such as reactivated tuberculosis or cytomegalovirus.[104] To date, however, there has been no conclusive evidence to this effect.[105–107]

For patients who cannot tolerate TMP-SMX, several alternatives are available. For patients with moderate-to-severe disease the intravenous options include pentamidine, trimetrexate, and clindamycin. Although pentamidine's mechanism of action is not clearly defined, it has been shown to have efficacy similar to that of TMP-SMX in certain studies[81,83] but decreased efficacy in another.[82] Pentamidine traditionally has been dosed at 4 mg/kg/d, but some studies have used 3 mg/kg/d.[108,109] The dose should not be adjusted for renal impairment because the amount of renal clearance is minimal.[110] The main problem with intravenous pentamidine, as with TMP-SMX, is its high incidence of severe adverse effects, often requiring discontinuation of the drug. Hypoglycemia, generally mild but sometimes fatal, occurs in up to 35% of patients,[111,112] because of pancreatic islet cell damage. If enough of the pancreas is damaged, frank diabetes mellitus and pancreatitis can subsequently result.[113,114] The development of hypoglycemia strongly correlates with the duration and dosage of pentamidine, prior pentamidine use within the last 3 weeks, and the development of nephrotoxicity, which can also occur independently from hypoglycemia.[112,115–118] Hypoglycemia can occur more than 3 weeks after initiation of therapy, so serum glucose levels should be monitored closely during the entire treatment time.[112] Other well-described adverse effects include cardiac arrhythmias that may be fatal, hyperkalemia, and elevated liver transaminase levels.[112,116,119–121] Hypotension, more prevalent in the past, is less of an issue when the duration of administration is increased to at least 1 hour.[122] Several trials have compared the efficacy of inhaled pentamidine with intravenous pentamidine for the treatment of PCP. Although inhaled pentamidine is better tolerated and potentially useful in patients with mild disease who cannot tolerate many of the systemic treatment options, it is associated with a high rate of relapse and is therefore generally not recommended for the treatment of PCP.[123–125] After patients have improved clinically, pentamidine may be changed to an oral regimen (discussed below) to complete 21 days of therapy.

Trimetrexate, a derivative of methotrexate, is an inhibitor of protozoan dihydrofolate reductase and is 1500 times more potent than trimethoprim.[126] Because of its bone marrow suppressive effects, trimetrexate is administered concurrently with folinic acid, which "rescues" mammalian bone marrow but does not enter eukaryotic cells such as *P. carinii* to protect them. Trimetrexate was studied in small trials to establish its efficacy and optimal dose[127,128] and had higher rates of failure and mortality than TMP-SMX but was better tolerated.[129] Its use is therefore limited to a second-line status, for patients who fail or do not tolerate TMP-SMX. The primary adverse effect of trimetrexate is bone marrow suppression, with rash, hepatic toxicity, and peripheral neuropathy also occasionally reported. The recommended dose of trimetrexate is 45 mg/m^2/d IV with leucovorin 20 mg/m^2 PO or IV every 6 hours.

Clindamycin-primaquine was first demonstrated to have activity against *P. carinii* in the rat model in 1987,[130] yet its mechanism of action still remains unknown. Since then, several small noncomparative trials have demonstrated the safety and efficacy of this combination.[131–135] There have been three double-blind, randomized trials comparing clindamycin-primaquine with TMP-SMX.[136–138] The difficulty with comparing these three trials to each other is that all used differing doses of clindamycin and primaquine, with two using intravenous and oral clindamycin and one using only oral. Another limitation is that all of these trials were small. What is similar, however, is that all patients had relatively mild disease (Pao$_2$ >50 mm Hg or Pao$_2$-Pao$_2$ gradient ≤45 mm Hg). With these limitations in mind, all three trials found that clindamycin-primaquine has efficacy similar to that of TMP-SMX, possibly with fewer adverse effects. Common side effects of clindamycin are rash, diarrhea (including *C. difficile* associated), nausea, vomiting, abdominal pain, and neutropenia. Primaquine is associated with hemolytic anemia in patients with glucose-6-phosphate dehydrogenase (G-6-PD) deficiency, and patients of African, Asian, or Mediterranean descent should be screened before treatment. Primaquine is also associated with nausea, vomiting, abdominal pain, and methemoglobinemia.[139] Clindamycin-primaquine therefore is recommended for patients with relatively mild disease who can tolerate an oral regimen, as primaquine only has an oral formulation. The recommended dose is clindamycin 600 mg IV every 8 hours or 300 to 450 mg PO every 6 hours, with primaquine 30 mg base PO once daily for 21 days.

For patients with milder disease who do not tolerate sulfa drugs, there are several alternative oral regimens. Clindamycin-primaquine, discussed above, is one option. Trimethoprim-dapsone is another, although both agents in this combination have similarities to the sulfa drugs. Dapsone, also known as diaminodiphenylsulfone, is a sulfone antibiotic related to the sulfonamides. Dapsone initially was found to be effective against *P. carinii* in rats,[140] and similar to sulfamethoxazole, dapsone inhibits dihydropteroate synthase in the folate synthesis pathway.[141] A substantial proportion of patients who do not tolerate sulfamethoxazole, however, are able to take dapsone. The exact amount of cross-reactivity between the two drugs is unclear, but studies have estimated from 0 to 55%.[142] These studies examined rates of all adverse effects of the two drugs. Another study, looking specifically at the cross-reactivity rates of hypersensitivity reactions (rash, pruritus, hives, anaphylactic reaction, or drug fever), found that 21.7% of patients who developed a hypersensitivity reaction to TMP-SMX also reacted to dapsone.[142] Although none of the three patients with anaphylactic reactions to TMP-SMX had a cross-reaction with dapsone, one should consider the use of dapsone in

this situation carefully. Trimethoprim-dapsone has the same mechanism of action as TMP-SMX. Dapsone by itself is less efficacious than TMP-SMX.[143] TMP-dapsone, however, has efficacy similar to that of TMP-SMX but with fewer side effects.[137,144,145] When used together, trimethoprim and dapsone have a bidirectional clearance interaction such that serum levels of both drugs are boosted.[146] Dapsone is associated with a number of side effects, the most significant of which is a dose-dependent hemolytic anemia, generally seen at higher doses (≥200 mg/d).[147] Hemolysis can be seen with or without G-6-PD deficiency, but patients with this deficiency are at greatest risk. G-6-PD screening should be considered before dapsone treatment is initiated, especially among patients of African, Asian, or Mediterranean descent. A spectrum of methemoglobinemia can also occur, from asymptomatic to life-threatening disease.[139] More common adverse effects include rash, nausea, vomiting, bone marrow suppression, and hepatic enzyme abnormalities. For patients who develop a hypersensitivity reaction (e.g., fever and rash) to dapsone, a desensitization scheme has been proposed.[148] A "sulfone syndrome," composed of fever, exfoliative dermatitis, jaundice, lymphadenopathy, hemolytic anemia, and methemoglobinemia and thought to be a hypersensitivity reaction, has been reported to occur after 6 to 8 weeks of treatment.[147] Dapsone is dosed at 100 mg/d and TMP as 15 to 20 mg/d PO or IV divided every 8 hours, for 21 days.

Atovaquone is an oral antimalarial agent that initially was found to have activity against *P. carinii* in the rat model.[149] Its mechanism of action is thought to be as a selective and potent inhibitor of the protozoal mitochondrial electron transport chain, preventing pyrimidine biosynthesis.[150] After demonstrating efficacy in HIV-infected patients,[151] atovaquone was compared head-to-head in two separate trials, one with TMP-SMZ and the other with pentamidine.[152,153] The patients included in these trials had relatively mild episodes of PCP with Pao$_2$–Pao$_2$ 45 mm Hg or lower or Pao$_2$ 60 mm Hg or higher. Atovaquone's efficacy was less than that of TMP-SMX and similar to that of pentamidine. Atovaquone was better tolerated, however, than both TMP-SMX and pentamidine, as it had fewer side effects. These side effects include rash, hepatic transaminase abnormalities, nausea, vomiting, diarrhea, and fever. The tablet formulation of atovaquone is poorly absorbed with significant individual variation.[79] Atovaquone tablets have now been replaced by atovaquone liquid suspension, which is much better absorbed. The recommended dose is 750 mg (5 ml) twice daily with food for 21 days; it is supplied in a 210 ml bottle (21-day supply).

There is strong evidence to support primary PCP prophylaxis for all patients with CD4 cell counts lower than 200/μl or a history of oropharyngeal candidiasis.[154–156] Other considerations for PCP prophylaxis are a CD4 percentage under 14% or a history of any AIDS-defining illness. As with the discussion of PCP treatment options, there are many possible prophylactic regimens. TMP-SMX has again been established as the prophylactic regimen of choice through many randomized trials comparing it with aerosolized pentamidine,[157] dapsone, or dapsone-pyrimethamine[158,159] or in trials comparing all three regimens.[160–163] The superiority of TMP-SMX over other regimens is most apparent at lower CD4 count ranges.[160,164] TMP-SMX has the added benefit of affording protection against toxoplasmosis[165] and likely a diversity of other infectious complications of AIDS as well.[8] Daily TMP-SMX is slightly more efficacious than thrice weekly TMP-SMX,[166] but TMP-SMX single strength (SS) and double strength (DS) as daily doses are equivalent.[167] Studies comparing dapsone or dapsone-pyrimethamine with aerosolized pentamidine show either equivalent PCP prevention[168–170] or better protection with dapsone-based regimens,[162,163] with this protective effect being more pronounced at lower CD4 counts.[160] Dapsone-based regimens also protect against toxoplasmosis, whereas pentamidine does not.[158,162,168,170,171] Atovaquone 1500 mg once daily has efficacy similar to that of daily dapsone therapy[172] or monthly aerosolized pentamidine[173] but is more expensive. See Table 30–2 for suggested dosing guidelines. Secondary prophylaxis regimens are listed in Table 30–3. TMP-SMX (first-line) or dapsone (second-line) prophylaxis is recommended in pregnancy. Because of the theoretical risk of teratogenicity in the first trimester, aerosolized pentamidine with its lack of systemic absorption may be an acceptable alternative during this period (2001 Guidelines).

Of all the opportunistic infections in HIV-infected persons, the discontinuation of primary and secondary prophylaxis for PCP after immune reconstitution has been the most studied. Based on multiple observational studies and randomized trials,[69,174–180] the 2001 Guidelines recommend discontinuing primary and secondary prophylaxis for patients who respond to HAART with an increase in CD4 count to higher than 200 cells/μl for more than 3 months. The only exception is in patients who developed PCP at a CD4 count higher than 200/μl. These guidelines suggest that these patients should continue secondary prophylaxis for life regardless of CD4 count rise. For the other patients, prophylaxis should be restarted if the CD4 count falls below 200/μl.

Candida albicans and Other Yeasts

Many agents are available for the treatment of candidiasis, depending on the location of infection, the extent of infection, and the degree of immunosuppression of the patient. The three main classes currently available are (1) the polyenes, including nystatin and amphotericin B, (2) the azoles, including the imidazoles (clotrimazole) and the triazoles (fluconazole), and (3) the echinocandins (caspofungin—the only drug available in this class at present). Suggested dosing guidelines are listed in Table 30–4.

TABLE 30–4 ■ Treatment Options for Mucosal Candidiasis

Medication	Dosage
OROPHARYNGEAL	**TREAT FOR 7–14 D**
Nystatin suspension	5 ml (100,000 U/ml) swish and swallow 4–5×/d
Clotrimazole oral troche	10 mg 5×/d
Fluconazole	100 mg PO qd
Itraconazole oral suspension	100 mg PO qd on empty stomach
Ketoconazole	200 mg PO qd
ESOPHAGEAL	**TREAT FOR 14–21 D**
Fluconazole	200–400 mg PO qd
Itraconazole	200 mg PO qd as oral suspension
Amphotericin B	0.3–0.6 mg/kg/d IV × 10–14 d
Caspofungin*	70 mg IV × 1, then 50 mg IV qd
VULVOVAGINAL	
Fluconazole	150 mg PO × 1
Miconazole intravaginal	100 mg suppository† qhs × 7 d
	200 mg suppository qhs × 3 d
	2% cream† qhs × 7 d
Clotrimazole intravaginal	100 mg suppository† qhs × 7 d
	200 mg suppository† qhs × 3 d
	500 mg suppository × 1
	1% cream† qhs × 7 d

*Not an FDA approved indication.
†Available over the counter.

Oropharyngeal candidiasis (OPC) can often be treated topically. When compared with oral fluconazole, nystatin is less effective, has a bitter taste, and must be taken multiple times each day.[181,182] Clotrimazole troches, however, have cure rates comparable to those of fluconazole, but associated relapse rates may be higher[183–185] and adherence may be lower because of frequent dosing (five times per day). Fluconazole has the simplest and most effective regimen currently available.[186] The problem with fluconazole is the potential development of resistance.[187] Several reports have identified OPC refractory to fluconazole in HIV patients with recurrent candidiasis.[188–193] A number of studies have identified the extent of prior fluconazole exposure and degree of immunosuppression (CD4 <50/μl) as significant risk factors.[185,194–198] Prolonged itraconazole use also is associated with the development of resistance to itraconazole and cross-resistance to fluconazole.[199] Despite the effectiveness of fluconazole prophylaxis against mucosal candidiasis,[200–203] prolonged prophylaxis is not recommended because of the potential development of resistance (2001 Guidelines).[204,205] In addition, acute candidiasis is relatively easy to treat and is not life threatening, while primary prophylaxis is expensive and has the potential for drug interactions (2001 Guidelines). In patients who have frequent or severe recurrences of mucosal candidiasis, an oral azole may be considered for long-term suppression with the recognition that these persons will be at higher risk for thrush that is refractory to therapy in the future (2001 Guidelines).

Esophageal candidiasis requires systemic therapy (Table 30–4), with fluconazole being the recommended first-line agent. Patients should be treated for 14 to 21 days, longer than for OPC. In patients who develop candidiasis refractory to fluconazole, itraconazole oral suspension has been shown to be effective in most cases[206-208] and more effective than itraconazole capsules.[206,209] Relatively low doses of amphotericin B IV may also be considered. Itraconazole and ketoconazole capsules both have limited oral bioavailability, requiring an acidic gastric environment for optimal absorption.[210,211] They are as efficacious[212,213] but not as well absorbed as fluconazole and therefore are less clinically effective.[214-216] Caspofungin, although not approved by the U.S. Food and Drug Administration (FDA) for the treatment of *Candida* species, has in vitro activity against *Candida* and may be a reasonable option in cases refractory to all other treatments. Voriconazole showed efficacy in one small study and may be a viable future option.[217]

The treatment of vulvovaginal candidiasis is largely based on studies in HIV-negative women.[218] A number of over-the-counter preparations are available (Table 30–4). A single oral dose of fluconazole has been shown to be just as efficacious as 7-day topical clotrimazole[219] with likely better compliance. Fluconazole has been associated with congenital anomalies when given to pregnant patients[220,221] and therefore should be avoided in pregnancy. Topical therapy appears to be safe in pregnancy.

Resistant candidal mucosal infections can occur at all these mucosal sites and may be difficult to treat. The National Committee for Clinical Laboratory Standards has proposed interpretive breakpoints for antifungal susceptibility testing of *Candida* spp.[222] These in vitro results seem to correlate well with in vivo responses[223,224] and may be useful in deciding which agent to use. The mechanism of resistance is likely a combination of the development of *Candida albicans* strains resistant to fluconazole[225] and the selection of non-*albicans* strains that are inherently resistant to fluconazole.[226] The most effective long-term therapy of resistant infections is immune recovery,[227,228] and declining rates of OPC have been seen in the HAART era.[229]

Cryptococcus neoformans

C. neoformans may cause disseminated disease, pneumonitis, and other localized organ disease in patients with or without immune dysfunction but is most commonly associated with meningoencephalitis in patients with advanced AIDS (often those with absolute CD4 counts <50/mm^3). Although there is a suggestion of geographic variation (more commonly diagnosed on the East Coast of the United States; more common in Africa than in the Americas), cryptococcal meningitis occurs virtually worldwide. Previously the outlook for immunocompromised patients with cryptococcal meningitis was poor, but treatment options have improved on the basis of results of randomized clinical trials and the introduction of orally bioavailable azole compounds.

Low-dose amphotericin B deoxycholate (0.3 to 0.4 mg/kg/d) with flucytosine for 4 to 6 weeks was established as the treatment regimen of choice for cryptococcal meningitis before the era of AIDS, with cure rates ranging from 75% to 85%.[230,231] The efficacy of this regimen in HIV-infected patients, however, was lower in one retrospective study showing survival rates ranging from 45% to 55%,[232] and the relapse rate was high, suggesting the importance of long-term suppression. With the advent of the azole antifungal agents, fluconazole with or without flucytosine was compared with low-dose amphotericin B as a primary treatment regimen and achieved similar to slightly better results.[233-236] Itraconazole also demonstrated efficacy against cryptococcal meningitis[237] but is inferior to low-dose amphotericin B with flucytosine.[238] Overall cure rates improved significantly, however, with higher dose amphotericin B (0.7 to 1 mg/kg/d) as initial treatment.[239] Subsequent studies established the current recommendation of induction therapy in HIV-infected patients, that higher dose amphotericin B be used with flucytosine (100 mg/kg/d) for 14 days (60% to 93% cerebrospinal fluid [CSF] sterilization).[240,241] This dose of flucytosine, lower than previously used in HIV-negative hosts, is associated with less risk of anemia than the previous "full" dose. The flucytosine dose must also be further adjusted on the basis of renal function. Flucytosine alone is not acceptable therapy for meningitis. The combination of flucytosine and amphotericin B initially appears to be associated with fewer relapses following induction than amphotericin B alone is, but amphotericin B alone is acceptable for those who do not tolerate flucytosine.[233] Although previously used for milder presentations of cryptococcal meningitis, oral fluconazole is generally no longer recommended for induction therapy.

Amphotericin B, although basically the "gold standard" for treating a variety of life-threatening fungal infections, is notoriously difficult to administer and can have diverse and severe adverse effects.[242,243] The drug does not achieve significant tissue levels when administered orally and therefore must be given intravenously. Amphotericin B metabolism is complex, and many of its metabolites are virtually inert, with traces remaining in the tissues many weeks or months after administration. For this reason, day-to-day dose variations do not have short-term impact comparable to that of drugs with predictable clearance rates; the most important factor regarding toxicity may be the total cumulative dose rather than the daily dosage administered. Formerly some experts recommended an initial test dose (~1 mg) to assess for the potential of rare anaphylactic reactions. This is generally not necessary with current preparations of amphotericin B. If a test dose is given, however, it should not be at the expense of delaying a therapeutic dose. Premedication with acetaminophen, diphenhydramine, antiemetics, or meperidine may forestall febrile reactions, rigors, headaches, myalgias, nausea, vomiting, and general malaise. It appears most prudent, however, to individualize predose adjunctive regimens on the basis of the experience with the first dose.[244] Amphotericin B must be suspended in 5% dextrose in water, and the rate of infusion may need to be adjusted on the basis of the intensity of adverse effects; however, if infusion-related events are not life threatening, slowing the rate of infusion in some cases merely extends the duration of adverse symptoms. The most common non-infusion-related complication of ampotericin B is nephrotoxicity; in most patients receiving higher doses of amphotericin B the serum creatinine rises and electrolyte abnormalities (hypokalemia, hypomagnesemia, renal tubular acidosis) develop, requiring careful replacement. Hydration with normal saline during and after infusions appears to lower the risk of renal toxicity. Considerable caution must be used when patients require contrast dye for radiologic studies or need to receive other nephrotoxic agents (aminoglycosides or cidofovir) in addition to amphotericin B. Although decisions must be based on the risks and benefits of continuing therapy for life-threatening disease, clinicians often choose to give alternate day doses or to withhold dosing all together when the creatinine rises to significant levels (>3 mg/dl). Amphotericin B typically causes a mild normocytic anemia, which is important to recognize when there is pre-existing anemia related to HIV infection or concurrently administered myelosuppressive compounds such as zidovudine or 5-flucytosine. For those patients who do not tolerate amphotericin B the lipid formulations of amphotericin (liposomal amphotericin and amphotericin B lipid complex) have been shown in preliminary studies to have equal clinical efficacy for cryptococcal meningitis with significantly less nephrotoxicity and fewer infusion-related complications.[245–247] Amphotericin B emulsified in lipid suspension (Intralipid) has also been shown to have similar efficacy while reducing infusion-related toxicity but does not reduce the risk of nephrotoxicity.[248] In addition, a precipitate forms with this formulation that must be removed by in-line filters. These filters also remove an unknown amount of amphotericin B. For these reasons, amphotericin B emulsified in lipid suspension is not recommended. Under extreme circumstances, in refractory cases in which systemic antifungal therapy has failed, intraventricular amphotericin B has been used.[249]

The primary recommendation for consolidation therapy following induction is fluconazole 400 mg PO daily for 8 weeks or until CSF cultures are sterile.[241] Itraconazole 400 mg PO daily is less effective but is an acceptable alternative for those who cannot tolerate fluconazole; overall, however, fluconazole tends to be better tolerated than itraconazole by most patients. Consolidation therapy must be followed by lifelong maintenance therapy to prevent relapse[250–252] unless immune reconstitution occurs as a result of HAART. The current recommendations suggest that the discontinuation of secondary prophylaxis against cryptococcal meningitis may be safe in patients who have successfully completed induction therapy, remain asymptomatic, and have a sustained level (>6 months) of CD4 counts above 100 to 200/μl (2001 Guidelines). Maintenance therapy should be reinstituted should the CD4 count fall below this level again. Fluconazole 200 mg PO daily has demonstrated efficacy in preventing relapse[250,253] and is superior to itraconazole.[254] Thus the current recommendation for the treatment of cryptococcal meningitis in AIDS patients is induction therapy with amphotericin B 0.7 to 1 mg/kg/d IV and flucytosine 25 mg/kg every 6 hours PO for 14 days, consolidation therapy with fluconazole 400 mg PO once daily for 8 weeks, and then maintenance therapy with fluconazole 200 mg PO once daily.[255] Serial monitoring of serum cryptococcal antigen has no proven prognostic value, but following CSF cryptococcal antigen levels may have some prognostic value, particularly in patients with persistent symptoms or only marginal improvement. Unchanging or increasing CSF cryptococcal antigen levels during acute therapy is associated with lack of response, and rising titers during suppressive therapy is associated with relapse. Falling titers, however, are not always associated with treatment success.[256]

One of the most important therapeutic goals in cryptococcal meningitis is the management of elevated intracranial pressure (ICP).[257] Elevated ICP in cryptococcal meningitis has been associated with increased morbidity and imminent death.[258] Thus patients with a baseline opening pressure higher than 250 mm H_2O should undergo lumbar CSF drainage to achieve a closing pressure 50% of the initial opening pressure or 200 mm H_2O or lower. This should be repeated daily until the opening pressure stabilizes. In patients with a normal baseline opening pressure, a second lumbar puncture should be done after induction therapy (2 weeks after starting therapy) to exclude elevated opening pressure and to evaluate CSF culture status. In selected cases, neurosurgical consultation for consideration of a CSF shunt may be necessary when pressure cannot be normalized through antifungal therapy and conservative measures alone.[255]

Primary prevention of cryptococcal meningitis using oral fluconazole has been shown to be effective in AIDS patients.[201,203,259,260] Despite this, primary prevention is not recommended routinely because of the relative infrequency of cryptococcal disease, the lack of survival benefit with prophylaxis, the possibility of drug interactions, the potential for antifungal drug resistance, and the high cost of prolonged therapy (2001 Guidelines). Particularly important from the resistance standpoint is the potential development of fluconazole-resistant mucosal *Candida* infections following long-term azole prophylaxis.[187,196]

Histoplasma capsulatum

Unlike *Cryptococcus* and *Pneumocystis*, which are prevalent throughout the United States, *Histoplasma* is more restricted geographically. It is particularly common in midwestern and central U.S. river valley regions, and in certain high-risk cities (Kansas City, Indianapolis, Memphis, Nashville) up to 25% of AIDS patients eventually develop disseminated infection. Histoplasmosis may present as isolated pulmonary disease (often mimicking tuberculosis) in patients with higher CD4 counts, but the most common disease manifestation is disseminated infection (fever, weight loss, lymphadenopathy, organomegaly) in the setting of advanced AIDS.[261]

The choice of induction therapy for histoplasmosis depends on the severity of disease presentation. Patients presenting with severe illness, such as "sepsis syndrome" or marked cytopenia or organ failure, should be admitted to the hospital and treated with amphotericin B or an amphotericin lipid preparation (especially if renal insufficiency is present). Except for severe sepsis presentations the initial response rate to amphotericin B preparations typically approaches 90%.[261] Liposomal amphotericin B clears fungemia more rapidly than itraconazole does,[262] and this may be an important consideration when patients present with severe or rapidly progressive disease. For patients with milder disease, however, itraconazole 400 mg/d is highly effective for induction therapy.[263] Although published experience with this approach is limited, itraconazole 200 mg three times a day is sometimes used for the initial 2 to 3 days of induction therapy to achieve higher levels more quickly in AIDS patients with significant disease and the potential for suboptimal drug absorption, and 200 mg twice daily is given thereafter.[264]

It is important to consider drug interactions between itraconazole and inducers of cytochrome P450 enzymes (ritonavir, rifampin, anticonvulsants, which commonly are given to HIV-infected patients), because these medications may significantly lower itraconazole levels. In addition, itraconazole inhibits P450 enzymes and therefore can increase the toxicity of concurrently administered drugs (phenytoin, coumadin, digoxin, many others) metabolized by these enzymes.[26] Itraconazole requires an acidic environment for gastric absorption, so it is not effective when administered to patients with achlorhydria or when given at the same time or in close proximity to antacids or blockers of acid secretion. The drug is generally well tolerated, with less than 10% incidence of discontinuation for toxicity, usually gastrointestinal upset or rash. Fluconazole is less potent than itraconazole against histoplasmosis, but reasonable response rates may be seen when high doses (800 mg/d) are used, for example, for patients intolerant of itraconazole or unable to discontinue drugs they are taking that are contraindicated with itraconazole.[265] Because fluconazole penetrates CSF better than itraconazole does, high-dose fluconazole may be a better choice for patients with meningitis due to *H. capsulatum*. However, clinical evidence of resistance to fluconazole has recently been described in patients receiving the drug for treatment of histoplasmosis.[266] Ketoconazole is ineffective for induction therapy.[261]

The duration of induction therapy must be based on the rapidity of the treatment response but typically lasts between 3 and 14 days. In most patients fever and severe symptoms resolve within 1 week of beginning itraconazole therapy.[263] The rate of relapse for patients with AIDS, however, is high—up to 80%—if therapy is discontinued following induction.[261] Maintenance therapy with intermittent amphotericin B infusions (50 to 100 mg given weekly or every 2 weeks) was over 90% effective in preventing relapses following amphotericin B induction therapy.[261,267] Daily oral itraconazole (200 to 400 mg/d), however, is also highly effective[268] and is now more commonly used for "secondary prophylaxis" because of its convenience and toxicity profile. Itraconazole 200 mg once daily or twice daily may be used for maintenance therapy. Some experts recommend checking an itraconazole serum concentration 2 hours after drug administration, especially among patients with the potential for limited drug absorption or drug-drug interactions, in order to choose a dosing regimen that will achieve itraconazole blood levels higher than 1 μg/ml.[264] Fluconazole is less successful than itraconazole for maintenance therapy also, with relapse rates of 10% to 30% depending on the doses used.[265,269] Although published data are limited at present, it may be possible to discontinue long-term maintenance histoplasmosis therapy for patients who have had significant, persistent (greater than a year) immunologic improvements on antiretroviral combination therapy.

In general, primary prevention for disseminated histoplasmosis is not recommended for widespread use because of the risk-to-benefit ratio projections, which take into account the relative infrequency of these infections and the high cost of antifungal therapies. Itraconazole solution, however, should be strongly considered for patients living in high-risk areas, particularly those patients with CD4 counts lower than 100/μl who may have significant exposures to contaminated soil.[270]

Coccidioides immitis

Coccidioidomycosis is another example of a dimorphic fungus complicating HIV infection only among patients who have been exposed to the geographic area endemic for this pathogen. Exposures are most common in hot, dry, dusty areas, particularly the San Joaquin Valley area in California and parts of Arizona. As is true for many HIV-associated opportunistic infections, the epidemiologic clues are not limited to recent exposures, as patients may have had primary infection years before, and reactivation disease developed once they became immunosuppressed. Most immunocompetent hosts have subclinical primary infection, whereas about one-third have a self-limited respiratory illness. Patients with HIV infection and relatively high absolute CD4 cell counts tend to present with focal pneumonia or pulmonary nodules; the prognosis is generally quite good, and these patients often respond to therapy much like HIV-negative hosts do. When patients have advanced AIDS, for example, absolute CD4 cell counts lower than 50/µl, they more often present with diffuse reticulonodular pneumonitis. This presentation may be rapidly progressive and even fatal despite aggressive therapy. Disseminated disease, particularly meningitis, arthritis, and skin disease, has also been well described in the setting of AIDS.[271,272]

Patients with focal pneumonia often can be treated on an outpatient basis with oral azole therapy. Although it has significant activity, ketoconazole is no longer frequently used in HIV-infected patients because it is poorly absorbed and drug interactions are common. Therefore oral fluconazole or itraconazole at doses of at least 400 mg a day are the best choices, although neither is currently FDA approved for this indication. The efficacy of fluconazole and itraconazole for coccidioidomycosis appears to be generally comparable.[273] Because of the greater frequency of poor drug absorption and undesirable drug interactions with itraconazole (described in the discussions of *Cryptococcus* and *Histoplasma* infections), fluconazole may be a better choice overall. Patients presenting with more severe manifestations of pneumonitis or disseminated disease require treatment with amphotericin B 1 mg/kg/d, which can be gradually tapered to two to three times per week and eventually to oral azole therapy if there is a favorable initial response.[274]

Meningitis previously required intrathecal amphotericin B administration, but there is a growing experience with high-dose fluconazole (800 mg/d),[275] which penetrates CSF more reliably than itraconazole does. Patients who do not respond to this therapy should be referred to experienced clinicians for consideration of intrathecal amphotericin B. Although there are theoretical concerns about antagonism between amphotericin B and azole therapy, combination therapy is sometimes attempted as a last resort for severe coccidioidomycosis. This consideration is particularly pertinent for a patient with AIDS and concurrent meningeal and pulmonary manifestations of coccidioidomycosis, where high-dose fluconazole plus intravenous amphotericin B may be warranted (however, this strategy is not proven to be effective and must be approached with caution).

Although antibody titers may still rise during the course of treatment of acute disease, in general serum anticoccidioidal antibody titers provide a useful assay for monitoring long-term treatment responses. Generally, high-dose therapy for coccidioidomycosis has been recommended for life following induction therapy for HIV-infected patients. Some experts, however, have slowly tapered the "maintenance" azole dose over time,

monitoring antibody titers every few months for evidence of breakthrough. Relapse rates among HIV-infected patients are likely to be high if no therapy is continued, although clinicians might consider discontinuation of therapy for patients who presented with focal pneumonia and afterward had significant, sustained immunologic responses to combination antiretroviral therapy. Because of the refractory, potentially life-threatening recurrences seen with meningitis, however, these patients should receive at least 400 mg daily of fluconazole for life.[274,276]

Primary prophylaxis, as with the other invasive mycoses, generally is not recommended for HIV-infected patients because of the cost and potential adverse effects involved. Prophylactic azole therapy might be a consideration for patients with advanced AIDS living in high-risk areas, particularly those who have high-risk occupations or avocations involving frequent exposures to contaminated soils. Another approach for these selected patients is to periodically screen with antibody titers, so that one can intervene with therapy at the first signs of seroconversion. HIV-infected patients who undergo subclinical seroconversion (or whose pre-existing positive titers demonstrate a rising trend) should begin fluconazole 400 mg daily even if there is no radiographic or symptomatic evidence of disease.[274]

Penicillium marneffei

P. marneffei is a fungal pathogen increasingly recognized as a cause of disseminated disease in HIV-infected patients in Southeast Asia. Common manifestations include fever and wasting, respiratory disease, joint disease, and a characteristic umbilicated papular rash. Itraconazole (400 mg/d) is effective for mild-to-moderate disease, although amphotericin B (0.6 mg/kg/d) may be required initially for severely ill patients.[277,278] Fluconazole is less effective than itraconazole, with initial antifungal failure rates of greater than 60% vs. approximately 25% for these two agents, respectively.[277] The relapse rate is high (~50%) regardless of initial therapy, and therefore long-term maintenance therapy is generally indicated. A randomized clinical trial of itraconazole 200 mg daily vs. placebo as secondary prophylaxis demonstrated no relapses in the itraconazole group vs. higher than 50% relapses in the placebo group (relapses occurring a median of 24 weeks after discontinuation of induction therapy).[279] Because the incidence of penicilliosis and cryptococcosis are both high among AIDS patients in Thailand, a trial of itraconazole 200 mg daily as primary prophylaxis has also been carried out. This study showed a significant reduction in the incidence of cryptococcosis and penicilliosis combined from 16.7% to 16% when itraconazole was given, although a survival advantage was not demonstrated.[280]

Other Dimorphic Fungi: *Blastomyces dermatitidis, Paracoccidioides brasiliensis,* and *Sporothrix schenckii*

Other dimorphic fungi occasionally are seen in the setting of HIV infection but are not as strongly associated with AIDS as cryptococcosis, histoplasmosis, and penicilliosis. Blastomycosis rarely complicates advanced AIDS, but when it does occur, severe disseminated and rapidly progressive central nervous system involvement has been reported.[281] Similarly, paracoccidioidomycosis rarely is seen in AIDS patients, even in highly endemic areas of South America, but when it does occur, atypically rapid progression and meningeal involvement may be seen.[282] Sporotrichosis is uncommon in HIV-infected patients, but unusual presentations including meningitis have been reported in this setting.[283] For all of these endemic mycoses the general recommendation (extrapolated in large part from the experience with HIV-negative hosts) has been for induction (for severe or disseminated disease) with amphotericin B followed by consolidation with itraconazole 400 mg daily. Subsequently itraconazole may be reduced to 200 mg daily as maintenance, but frequent relapses are common if patients discontinue antifungal therapy completely. Careful attention to drug absorption (although the newer itraconazole solution formulation partially overcomes this concern) and potential drug interactions is critical when itraconazole is administered to HIV-infected patients.

Aspergillus and Other Molds

Although less common than mucosal yeast infections and dimorphic fungal infections, a variety of "mold" or mycelial opportunistic infection has also been reported in the setting of advanced AIDS. Often these infections occur when additional immunosuppressive risk factors, such as high-dose steroid administration, prolonged drug-associated neutropenia, or neoplastic disease, are present in addition to HIV infection. These mold infections can cause a spectrum of disease from localized sinus, skin, or other soft tissue infections to disseminated disease. Both local and disseminated disease can be rapidly progressive and fatal. For example, devastating local sinus or periorbital infections can be due to *Aspergillus, Pseudallescheria,* or the agents of zygomycosis, such as *Rhizopus* and *Mucor. Aspergillus fumigatus* causes skin infections, pulmonary disease including invasive tracheobronchitis, and disseminated disease in severely immunocompromised patients. Previously unusual pathogens such as the agents of phaeohyphomycosis (*Alternaria* and others) have been reported to cause localized abscesses or disseminated disease in AIDS patients.[284,285]

Treatment of invasive mold infections in AIDS patients is largely based on anecdotal cases and extrapolation from the limited literature regarding management of these infections in other types of immunocompromised hosts. Traditionally, high-dose intravenous amphotericin B (0.7 to 1.5 mg/kg/d) has been the gold standard for severe invasive fungal disease. Response rates generally are limited (complete cure occurs in a small minority; roughly 60% have at least a partial response), and data are further limited because these patients are often dying of advanced underlying conditions in addition to the mold infection.[286,287] Surgical débridement is indicated in many cases in addition to aggressive antifungal therapy if there is any hope for cure or sustained palliation. Newer lipid formulations of amphotericin may allow higher dose exposures with less renal toxicity. Itraconazole shows some activity against the invasive molds, particularly when used at high doses (600 mg/d), and may be an alternative to amphotericin preparations or a way to consolidate therapy following induction with intravenous amphotericin.[286,288] The newer oral itraconazole solution may provide some pharmacokinetic advantages over capsules in this setting. Caspofungin was recently approved for *Aspergillus* disease that has been refractory to azole or amphotericin treatment; experience with this agent in HIV-infected patients is limited.[289] Other classes of antifungal therapy currently are under investigation. Life-long therapy often is needed for any invasive mold infection because of the high risk of relapses and inexorable disease progression.[284,290]

Because hyphal elements are widespread in the environment, primary prevention of these infections is generally not feasible. There is no evidence to support continuous antifungal therapy to prevent these infections in the setting of advanced AIDS. Obviously the potential for occurrence of these infections provides additional impetus to avoid prolonged neutropenia and long-term high-dose corticosteroids or other immunosuppressive compounds whenever possible in the care of HIV-infected patients.

VIRUSES

Cytomegalovirus

Infection with cytomegalovirus (CMV) is endemic throughout the U.S. population; most sexually active adults in the United States are seropositive for the virus but have no attributable signs or symptoms of disease. In the setting of severely depressed cellular immunity, however, CMV can reactivate to cause disseminated disease or end-organ damage.[291] The most common manifestation among patients with AIDS is CMV retinitis, the leading cause of blindness in HIV-infected persons. The next most common end-organ damage is gastrointestinal disease, particularly esophagitis and colitis.[292] For reasons that are poorly understood, CMV only occasionally is implicated as the sole pathogen in HIV-infected patients with pneumonitis,[293] whereas CMV pnuemonitis is quite common in the setting of organ or bone marrow transplantation. When *Pneumocystis* pneumonitis or pneumococcal pneumonia is diagnosed but CMV inclusion cells are also seen in bronchoscopy specimens, it is not usually necessary to give anti-CMV therapy in addition to targeting these more virulent HIV-associated pulmonary pathogens.[294] Finally, CMV may cause central nervous system disease,[295] including encephalitis and polyradiculopathy, in HIV-infected patients (this is discussed further in Chapter 12). All these manifestations tend to occur at low absolute CD4 counts (<50/μl), and all are encountered much less frequently in the HAART era.

Most of the treatment data in this section refers to the CMV retinitis experience. In general, treatment principles for HIV-related CMV disease are assumed to be similar for ophthalmologic, gastrointestinal, pulmonary, and neurologic disease, but there are few large clinical trials involving extraocular disease. The overall therapeutic strategy (e.g., local instillation of drug or systemic therapy) and the aggressiveness of therapy (e.g., all intravenous therapy, intravenous followed by oral maintenance therapy, or all oral therapy) for CMV retinitis need to be based on the pattern of retinal involvement. Experienced ophthalmologists should to be involved in the decision-making process, since the therapeutic plan is so dependent on the location and extent (e.g., bilateral vs. unilateral, peripheral vs. central sight-threatening lesions) of retinal damage. Ongoing retinal damage may cause irreversible blindness and necessitates prompt and aggressive therapy, but the results may be less devastating for other CMV end-organ disease. For nonsevere gastrointestinal disease, such as a single esophageal ulcer, it may be possible to administer a trial of oral valganciclovir, with the knowledge that one could escalate to parenteral forms of therapy if there were an insufficient early disease response. For similar reasons, maintenance therapy has not been consistently recommended following initial treatment for typical gastrointestinal CMV disease; the consequences of intermittent "reinduction" are generally less dire in this setting than in retinal or central nervous system involvement.

Typically induction therapy for CMV disease is given for 2 to 6 weeks or until a significant response is observed, and then long-term maintenance therapy is required to prevent relapses (unless sustained and significant immune reconstitution can be achieved with HAART). Investigational assays are available that quantify plasma CMV antigen or DNA viral load, and these appear to correlate with disease progression or treatment response.[296] There has been no consensus regarding the clinical use of these tests, however, and generally treatment decisions are based on clinically detectable responses to therapy (such as serial dilated retinal examinations, chest radiograph changes, or endoscopic or neurologic examinations). For retinitis, dilated retinal examinations typically are carried out every 4 weeks during the early stages of treatment to monitor progress. In addition patients are instructed to report any new visual changes ("floaters" or blind spots) promptly so that immediate evaluations can be performed.

In recent years three parenteral agents have been available for CMV induction therapy: ganciclovir, foscarnet, and cidofovir. Ganciclovir, a nucleoside analog, was the first approved therapy for CMV retinitis. Induction therapy is administered intravenously at 5 mg/kg twice daily for 14 to 21 days, followed by maintenance therapy (assuming a favorable initial response) at 5 mg/kg once daily.[297] The most common adverse events due to ganciclovir are catheter-related and hematologic complications. The incidence of neutropenia and thrombocytopenia are approximately 25% and 5%, respectively. Less commonly associated problems include nausea, vomiting, and rash.

Foscarnet, a pyrophosphate analog, is an alternative agent. Because it works by an entirely different mechanism than ganciclovir does, these drugs can be used strategically when concerns about drug-resistant virus arise. Foscarnet is begun at an induction dose of 90 to 120 mg/kg intravenously twice daily (typically for 14 to 21 days) and then continued at 90 mg/kg daily as maintenance therapy, with adjustment (and readjustments during therapy, if necessary) for renal function. Normal saline boluses should be given prior to each infusion to help avoid renal toxicity. The most common adverse effects are catheter-related events and nephrotoxicity, including the wasting of cations (leading to low magnesium, potassium, and calcium). Nausea and gastrointestinal upset sometimes occur. Genital ulcerations and periurethral pain are sometimes reported; these symptoms likely are caused by crystallization of drug metabolites in the urine.

Ganciclovir and foscarnet appear to be equally efficacious against CMV retinitis.[298] Although data are limited, either agent appears to have high initial response rates for gastrointestinal, pulmonary, or neurologic disease.[295,299–301] The choice of therapy therefore often centers on side-effect profiles and convenience, both of which may slightly favor ganciclovir in many scenarios. In the pre-HAART era, foscarnet was associated with a slightly better overall mortality than ganciclovir was, despite similar effects on retinitis progression, and it was speculated that this might reflect favorable antiretroviral effects of foscarnet in addition to anti-CMV effects.[302] Although initial response rates are favorable with either of these drugs, the median time to retinitis progression on ganciclovir or foscarnet therapy in the pre-HAART era was in the range of 2 to 4 months (compared with 2 to 3 weeks if therapy was deferred all together).[297,303] Therefore the long-term outcome following monotherapy with an intravenous agent against CMV retinitis was often disappointing in the pre-HAART era.

A third systemic agent, cidofovir, has also been shown to be efficacious for primary treatment of CMV retinitis. Cidofovir is a nucleotide analog that does not require phosphorylation by viral enzymes to achieve its active form. It has potent in vitro anti-CMV activity and a prolonged intracellular half-life allowing infrequent dosing. When intravenous cidofovir was given 5 mg/kg weekly for 2 weeks and then every other week thereafter to patients with peripheral CMV retinitis, the median time to disease progression was extended to approximately 4 months compared with less than 1 month in patients who had therapy deferred.[304,305] Thus this approach to induction was at least comparable to, and perhaps better than, the success rates with foscarnet or ganciclovir. Another significant advantage that cidofovir has over foscarnet or ganciclovir was that its administration does not require prolonged intravenous access, and patients could come into clinic for intermittent infusions. On the other hand, cidofovir requires a rather complex infusion protocol to diminish the risks of nephrotoxicity. Urinalysis and serum creatinine should be evaluated prior to each infusion. Patients must take probenecid around the time of infusion (2 g PO 3 hours prior to cidofovir, followed by 1 g at 1 hour and 6 hours after cidofovir), and this agent is associated with toxicities of its own including rash and vomiting. Normal saline should be administered before and during the cidofovir infusion. Cidofovir doses need to be adjusted or discontinued if serum creatinine rises or significant proteinuria is documented. The most common adverse event is nephrotoxicity, manifest as renal insufficiency or proteinuria, which may require discontinuation in up to 25% of patients. Other associated adverse events include neutropenia (15%), nausea, and headaches. Although not observed in all cidofovir trials, iritis and loss of pressure in the globe (hypotony, a condition that can lead to irreversible blindness) have also been reported in association with cidofovir.[306] Although the complex infusion protocol and the potentially irreversible toxicities involved are serious limitations, cidofovir is still a valid consideration for many patients because of the convenience of biweekly rather than daily infusions (which may circumvent the need for long-standing intravenous catheters).

A logical strategy for overcoming the inconvenience and line-related toxicities of these parenteral agents was to strive for orally bioavailable alternatives. Oral ganciclovir has been used for maintenance therapy following induction with intravenous ganciclovir with some success,[307] and this approach may be particularly effective when patients have partial immune reconstitution on HAART and are therefore less likely to require high-dose CMV suppression. Although oral ganciclovir's bioavailability is limited compared with that of the intravenous formulation, preliminary studies of high-dose oral therapy appear promising.[308] Valganciclovir is a newly available prodrug of ganciclovir that achieves drug concentrations similar to those seen with intravenous ganciclovir induction therapy. In preliminary reports from a nonblinded, randomized clinical trial involving 160 HIV-infected patients with CMV retinitis, oral valganciclovir

appeared to be as effective as intravenous ganciclovir for induction therapy.[309] Oral valganciclovir has recently been approved for CMV retinitis induction therapy at a dose of 900 mg twice daily for 21 days, followed by 900 mg once daily for maintenance. The most common adverse events reported include neutropenia, anemia, thrombocytopenia, and gastrointestinal upset.

Drug-resistant CMV can be a significant problem among patients who have received long-term monotherapy with ganciclovir or foscarnet.[310,311] Cidofovir may be effective when CMV retinitis is clinically refractory to ganciclovir or foscarnet,[312] although some isolates have cross-resistance to ganciclovir and cidofovir. Because of concerns about resistance and the high rate of relapse, therapeutic combinations also have been evaluated for refractory CMV retinitis. The combination of intravenous ganciclovir and foscarnet, although inconvenient, does appear to produce more prolonged disease-free intervals than either drug alone.[303] Some experts have recommended combined foscarnet and ganciclovir for severe CMV central nervous system disease, but this has not been studied in randomized trials. Some form of combination therapy may be indicated for patients with refractory disease or frequent relapses despite intravenous therapy. A phase I study of combined biweekly cidofovir and oral ganciclovir (3 g/d) for CMV retinitis demonstrated no disease progression over a median of 5 to 6 months of follow-up, but several persons developed anterior uveitis and hypotony of the globe.[313]

Another approach to improvement of treatment options for CMV retinitis involves strategies for local intraocular therapy. Administering ganciclovir directly into the vitreous body is effective but requires weekly injections.[314] Therefore a surgically implanted sustained-release delivery system was developed. In a multicenter clinical trial, patients with newly diagnosed CMV retinitis were randomized to receive intravenous ganciclovir or one of two implant delivery strategies (1 μg/h or 2 μg/h of ganciclovir). The median time to disease progression was 71 days for the intravenous group vs. 221 and 191 days with the 1 μg/h and 2 μg/h implants, respectively.[315] Visual impairment was common in the first few weeks after the surgery, but this was temporary in all cases. Although endophthalmitis, retinal detachment, and other surgical complications are potential concerns, such adverse events have been seen only occasionally with this approach. On a more limited basis, intraocular approaches have been attempted using foscarnet[316] and cidofovir[317] as well.

The primary limitation of the local treatment approaches is that intraocular therapy does not provide protection from disease in the contralateral eye or from extraocular CMV manifestations. One approach to consider for overcoming this problem is the combination of an intraocular implant, to achieve high local drug levels at the site of infection, and daily oral therapy, to provide at least moderate drug levels to suppress disease at sites other than the affected eye. In a recent clinical trial, 377 patients with unilateral retinitis were randomized to groups receiving intravenous ganciclovir, a ganciclovir implant plus high-dose oral ganciclovir (4.5 g/d), or the implant plus placebo. The incidence of new CMV disease was significantly higher in the placebo plus implant group (44%) than in the implant plus oral ganciclovir and the intravenous ganciclovir groups (24% and 20%, respectively).[318] In another recent study involving 61 subjects the combination of a ganciclovir implant and oral ganciclovir was comparable to intravenous cidofovir alone in terms of disease progression.[319]

There is no firm consensus on, or standardized approach to, CMV retinitis treatment at the present time because of so many rapidly evolving treatment choices and because HAART has so drastically affected the incidence, presentation, and management of this opportunistic infection. Although the clinical experience with newer therapies is somewhat limited, there appear to be promising alternatives to life-long parenteral therapy, including oral valganciclovir alone or a ganciclovir implant plus oral therapy, which will make long-term treatment of CMV disease much more feasible in the HAART era.[320] There is increasing evidence that CMV retinitis maintenance therapy may be safely discontinued if CD4 counts above 100 or 150/µl are achieved on HAART.[321–325] Current guidelines therefore recommend that the discontinuation of secondary prophylaxis be considered in patients with CD4 counts >100–150 cells/µl[326] (2001 Guidelines) for ≥6 months. The extent of the retinal lesion, the vision in the contralateral eye, and the availability of regular ophthalmologic follow-up must also be considered. Patients who discontinue maintenance therapy should continue regular ophthalmologic examinations to monitor for relapse. Maintenance therapy should be restarted should the patient's CD4 cell count fall below 100–150 cells/µl (2001 Guidelines).

Primary prophylaxis against CMV disease has been a matter of some controversy but is not commonly used at present. In one study, oral ganciclovir reduced the risk of CMV retinitis by half when administered to patients with CD4 counts below 50/µl (or <100/µl for those with a history of other AIDS-defining illnesses), although without a statistically significant improvement in overall survival.[327] Renal insufficiency and cytopenias requiring cell growth factors (erythropoietin and G-CSF) were significantly more common in the ganciclovir group than in the placebo group. Another similar study, enrolling subjects with CD4 counts below 100/µl to compare 3 g of oral ganciclovir with placebo as primary CMV prophylaxis, had different results.[328] There was no difference in CMV disease rates seen, but there was a trend toward improved survival in the treated group. Generally the emphasis in prevention of CMV disease should be on maintaining absolute CD4 counts at higher levels with HAART. It is possible that emerging assays to quantify CMV viremia will help to identify patients at highest risk

for CMV end-organ disease, so that targeted pre-emptive therapy will be possible for patients unable to benefit from HAART.

Herpes Simplex Virus

Herpes simplex virus (HSV) treatment is discussed in detail elsewhere. HIV-infected patients are at risk for severe presentations of mucosal HSV disease[329] and appear to shed more HSV than immunocompetent hosts do.[330] Other HSV manifestations occasionally seen in HIV-infected patients include proctitis in men who have sex with men and esophagitis. Interestingly there is no evidence to suggest that HSV encephalitis is more common in HIV-infected patients than in the general population.

Mucosal HSV lesions may be typical crops of vesicles but in more advanced HIV infection may become confluent, leading to extensive ulceration, and have been mistaken for bacterial cellulitis or neoplastic disease by clinicians unfamiliar with HSV manifestations in immunocompromised hosts. Treatment for HSV generally is similar to that recommended for normal hosts. Patients with advanced HIV may require parenteral therapy for severe presentations (acyclovir 5 mg/kg IV every 8 hours for 10–14 days), whereas most cases can be treated with acyclovir (200 to 400 mg five times daily), valacyclovir (500 mg twice daily), or famciclovir (125 to 250 mg twice daily). Oral therapy with acyclovir (400 mg twice daily), valacyclovir (500 mg daily or twice daily), or famciclovir (125 mg twice daily) also appears to be effective for suppressive therapy. Valacyclovir was associated with hemolytic uremic syndrome when administered at high doses (>3 g/d) to HIV-infected patients in a CMV prevention trial, but this complication has not been commonly reported at routine HSV treatment doses. The treatment of recurrent disease can be individualized following recommendations for HIV-negative patients, although patients with HIV infection more often require ongoing suppressive therapy to avoid frequent relapses. HIV-infected patients who have received continuous therapy, however, are at risk for acyclovir-unresponsive HSV disease. Acyclovir-unresponsive HSV lesions may be deeply ulcerating and fail to heal for many months.[331] Higher doses of oral therapy (such as acyclovir 800 mg five times a day) are sometimes effective, but the recommended therapy for true acyclovir-resistant HSV disease is foscarnet (40 mg/kg IV every 8 hours).[332] Cidofovir and various investigational topical therapies have also been used successfully in anecdotal reports and small case series.

Primary prophylaxis for HSV disease is not recommended for HIV-infected patients. Condoms are useful in reducing the risk of HSV transmission, and patients should avoid sexual contact when either partner has active genital lesions, although genital shedding may occur with or without active lesions.

Varicella-Zoster Virus

Many adults have been previously infected with varicella-zoster virus (chickenpox). HIV-infected children with chickenpox may have more severe manifestations than immunocompetent hosts have.[333] "Shingles," the cutaneous rash associated with relapses of varicella-zoster disease, has been recognized as a common complication of HIV infection since early in the epidemic. Most outbreaks occur in the classic dermatomal distribution, but patients with advanced HIV disease are at higher risk for multidermatomal involvement or disseminated disease. Central nervous system complications including meningitis, encephalitis, myelitis, and rapidly progressive retinal necrosis have been reported in patients with AIDS.[334] AIDS patients are uniquely at risk for recurrences of herpes zoster, either in the same dermatomal distribution or in different anatomic locations.[334]

Traditional therapy for uncomplicated herpes zoster in immunocompromised patients has been acyclovir (800 mg PO five times a day). Famciclovir (500 mg three times daily) or valacyclovir (1 g three times daily) are often used now because of convenience; the possibility of a link between high-dose valacyclovir and thrombotic thrombocytopenic purpura/hemolytic uremic syndrome in HIV-infected patients should be kept in mind, although again this has not been encountered with routine episodic use. As with HSV, acyclovir-resistant varicella-zoster virus has been reported in the setting of advanced HIV infection among patients who previously have received long-term acyclovir.[335,336] Foscarnet (40 mg/kg every 8 hours or 60 mg/kg every 12 hours) is the treatment of choice for treatment-refractory disease.[337]

Long-term administration of therapy to prevent outbreaks of varicella-zoster is generally not recommended, although occasionally suppressive therapy has been attempted in AIDS patients with multiple recurrences. For children and adult HIV-infected patients with no history of exposure to chickenpox, avoidance of exposure is the only way to prevent infection. Susceptible household members should be vaccinated against varicella-zoster virus. If HIV-infected patients are exposed, varicella-zoster immune globulin should be given as soon as possible but within 96 hours after contact. Varicella vaccine might be a consideration in the future for adults who have never had primary varicella infection, but this is not currently recommended because of the potential risk for disseminated infection with the vaccine strain live virus.

Other Human Herpesviruses

Epstein-Barr virus (EBV) is associated with several HIV-related manifestations: oral hairy leukoplakia (a generally benign mucosal finding that is a marker for cellular immunosuppression), primary central nervous system lymphoma, and a variety of other lymphomas. There are no definitive studies of treatment for oral hairy leukoplakia, and the condition sometimes regresses spontaneously, but case reports suggest that acyclovir may have a favorable response when treatment is desired for cosmetic purposes.[338] Although antiviral treatment has been attempted investigationally for EBV-related malignancies, there has been no evidence to support the hypothesis that antiviral therapy has any effect once neoplastic transformation has already taken place.

Human herpesvirus-6 and -7 (HHV-6 and HHV-7) are recently characterized viruses, the causes of the childhood exanthem subitum (roseola, sixth disease) and febrile seizures, and have been studied as potential cofactors in HIV progression. Although these viruses are under investigation as contributors to HIV disease, there is no definitive HIV-related disease association at this time and certainly no proven indication for targeted antiviral treatment.[339,340]

Human herpesvirus-8 (HHV-8) has been strongly linked with Kaposi's sarcoma, a common neoplastic complication of advanced HIV-related immunosuppression. Although early anecdotal evidence suggested that antiviral therapy such as foscarnet might lead to Kaposi's sarcoma remission,[341] antiherpetic therapy is not currently a routine part of tumor management. As with EBV-related malignancies, it seems unlikely that antiherpes therapy will play an important therapeutic role after neoplastic transformation has taken place. Potent antiretroviral therapy, on the other hand, appears to slow progression of Kaposi's sarcoma and may even bring about persistent remission in some cases.[342]

Human Papillomavirus

Human papillomaviruses (HPV) cause common warts and genital warts, and certain subtypes are strongly linked with squamous cell carcinoma, including cervical and anal cancer. Cutaneous, genital, and perirectal warts in HIV-infected patients may be treated with a variety of local therapies including cryosurgery, laser surgery, podophyllin-podofilox, bichloracetic and trichloracetic acids, immune-modulating local therapies such as α-IFN injections and imiquimod cream. These treatments are described in more detail in Chapter 31. Occasionally immunocompromised patients may have more extensive warts (giant condylomata acuminata) requiring more aggressive therapy. No targeted, systemic antiviral therapies have been shown to benefit patients after HPV-related malignancies have developed.

Screening for HPV-related malignancies is an important part of HIV clinical care. Pelvic examination with regular Papanicolaou (Pap) smears to screen for early signs of dysplasia or neoplasia is a well-established prevention effort indicated for all sexually active females and is particularly important in immunocompromised hosts, in whom cervical cancer may develop more often and more rapidly (invasive cervical cancer is categorized as an AIDS-defining illness among HIV-infected women). Pap smears appear to have sensitivity and specificity in HIV-infected women similar to that in uninfected hosts, and HIV-infected women have a high incidence of the papillomavirus subtypes linked with neoplasia.[343-345] Evidence to support routine perianal Pap smears for men who have rectal intercourse is growing so that one can intervene as quickly as possible if premalignant changes or malignancy is detected.[346,347]

Pharmacologic therapy for primary HPV prevention is not available at this time. As with other sexually transmitted diseases, appropriate counseling regarding safer sex practices and condom use should lower rates of HPV transmission.

Hepatitis Viruses

Because of common routes of transmission, HIV-infected patients may be coinfected with viral hepatitis. There is no known therapy for hepatitis A, typically a benign and self-limited infection. Treatment options for hepatitis B and C are evolving, although published experience with treating HIV-coinfected patients is limited. These treatments are discussed in more detail in Chapter 10. Lamivudine (3TC) is an antiretroviral drug that also has significant activity against hepatitis B,[348] so this should be considered when an antiretroviral regimen is chosen for dually infected patients. Conversely, when dually infected patients discontinue lamivudine as part of an antiretroviral regimen, there may be a "flare" of hepatitis signs and symptoms.[349] Other antiretroviral agents, including adefovir, tenofovir, and emtricitabine (FTC), also have antiviral activity against hepatitis B and are under study for coinfected patients. Overall, long-term remission rates and adverse event profiles generally were disappointing in the past when α-IFN alone was administered for hepatitis B or C infection. However, recent improvements involving pegylated interferon and combination therapies (ribavirin and interferon formulations) for immunocompetent hosts raise expectations that such therapies will also prove effective among HIV-infected patients (particularly with hepatitis C coinfection). Indeed preliminary experience suggests response rates of immunocompetent HCV-infected hosts are comparable to those of patients co-infected with hepatitis C and HIV when treatment with IFN-alfa2b plus ribavirin is administered.[350]

No pharmacologic strategies have proven to be effective for the prevention of hepatitis infections. Highly effective vaccines are available, however, against hepatitis A and hepatitis B (including a formulation containing vaccines against both viruses). Vaccination against hepatitis B is strongly recommended for HIV-infected patients at risk for sexual or blood-borne transmission; vaccination in childhood is approaching nearly universal acceptance in the United States. Hepatitis A vaccination has been recommended for HIV-infected patients not known to be immune, particularly men who have sex with men, patients traveling to developing countries, and during community outbreaks. There is no approved hepatitis C vaccine.

JC Virus

JC virus (which should not be confused with Jakob-Creutzfeldt virus, the cause of another enigmatic central nervous system disorder) is a polyomavirus associated with progressive multifocal leukoencephalopathy (PML). PML occurs rarely in immunocompetent hosts. It is more often diagnosed among patients with severe cellular immunodeficiency, especially due to AIDS. There are no known symptoms related to the initial (respiratory?) infection, but patients with immunodeficiency experience an insidious but rapidly progressive onset of diverse neurologic signs and symptoms (e.g., hemiparesis, gait difficulty, mental status changes, seizures) corresponding with white matter disease on magnetic resonance imaging. Currently no therapy is approved for PML. A large trial involving cytosine arabinoside (ara-C) was stopped prematurely because of lack of evidence of efficacy.[351] There are anecdotal reports about potential anti-PML activity of other compounds, but controlled clinical trials are lacking. Cidofovir, the nucleoside analog approved for anti-CMV therapy, has in vitro activity against polyomaviruses, and case reports suggest the possibility of clinical effectiveness[352,353]; however, preliminary reports from recent open label studies have been disappointing. Although benefit is not universal,[354] some patients with PML appear to have significant improvement or even complete remission when effective HAART is initiated.[355,356] There are no known primary prevention strategies against PML.

PROTOZOA AND PARASITES

Toxoplasma gondii

Definitive diagnosis of toxoplasmic encephalitis requires the demonstration of the tachyzoite form of *T. gondii* in a tissue specimen. Because of the morbidity associated with brain biopsies, the standard of care is empiric treatment of the patient with suspected *Toxoplasma* infection and assessment for clinical response after 7 to 14 days[357] (Fig. 30–1). Those without clinical or radiographic improvement after a trial of empiric therapy require definitive diagnosis with a brain biopsy. Pyrimethamine (a dihydrofolate reductase inhibitor) and sulfadiazine (a dihydrofolate synthetase inhibitor) block sequential steps in the metabolism of folic acid and are well established as the first-line treatment of toxoplasmic encephalitis.[358,359] Leucovorin (folinic acid) is added to reduce the bone marrow suppressive effects of pyrimethamine. Retrospective analyses of pyrimethamine, sulfadiazine, and leucovorin in combination have shown success rates of

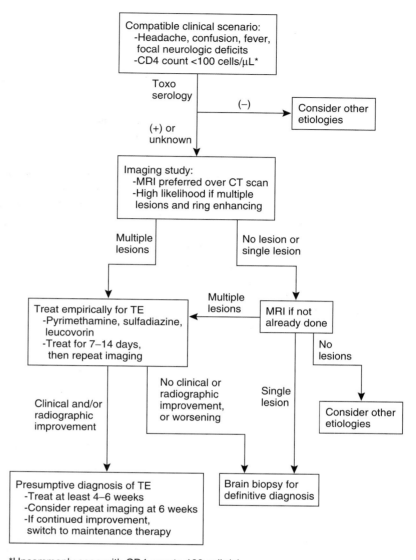

FIGURE 30–1. Algorithm for the management of suspected toxoplasmic encephalitis (TE). CT, computed tomography; MRI, magnetic resonance imaging.

*Uncommonly seen with CD4 count >100 cells/μL

up to 95%.[360] Unfortunately, adverse effects of this therapy have also been reported in up to 62% of patients, with rash, leukopenia, nausea, thrombocytopenia, and fever being the most common.[360,361] Up to 44% of patients have a reaction severe enough to require a change in therapy.[360] Less common side effects include encephalopathy, psychosis, and crystalluria, which have been attributed to sulfadiazine.[362–365] A number of studies have reported success with oral desensitization of HIV-infected patients to sulfonamides.[93–95]

For patients who do not tolerate pyrimethamine-sulfadiazine, second-line therapy is pyrimethamine-clindamycin. Several studies have shown this regimen to be either as efficacious or only slightly less efficacious than pyrimethamine-sulfadiazine but somewhat better tolerated.[359,366–368] Data on the management of patients who do not tolerate sulfadiazine or clindamycin are limited. The macrolide class, including azalides and ketolides, have excellent efficacy in vitro and in murine models,[369–372] but experience in human trials is limited.[373–376] Similarly, atovaquone has shown good efficacy in vitro and in mice[370,377] and reasonable activity as a salvage regimen in small human trials.[378–380] These agents are reasonable third-line alternatives when used in combination with pyrimethamine and leucovorin. A number of other agents have been evaluated either in vitro or in small, noncomparative human trials, including dapsone, trimetrexate, pentamidine, and doxycycline.[381–385] Although they cannot be recommended for treatment now, these agents may prove to be effective treatment alternatives in the future.

The use of corticosteroids in the treatment of *Toxoplasma* encephalitis (TE) has not been well evaluated but one study noted no difference in outcome between patients who received corticosteroids and patients who did not.[386] In this trial, however, only patients with evidence of elevated ICP received steroids. Thus it may be that those patients who did receive steroids would have done worse had they not received steroids. The difficulty with using corticosteroids, especially when empirically treating, is that other processes, most notably lymphoma, may respond to steroids and thereby obfuscate the diagnosis. If patients have biopsy-proven TE and cerebral edema, corticosteroids likely will not cause harm and may be beneficial. If there is no evidence of increased ICP, steroids are not indicated. For those patients without a proven diagnosis and with cerebral edema, steroids should be considered with the caveat that if these patients improve, the improvement may be due to the steroids and not the primary therapy. These patients should be followed closely after steroids are discontinued.

Standard dosing regimens for TE are listed in Table 30–5. Treatment should be given for 4 to 6 weeks, followed by repeat imaging. If the patient does well with clinical and radiologic improvement, lifelong maintenance therapy should be given unless immune reconstitution occurs with HAART. Secondary prophylaxis regimens for TE are listed in Table 33–3. Current guidelines allow the discontinuation of secondary prophylaxis in those patients who successfully complete induction therapy, remain asymptomatic, and have a CD4 cell count above 200/μl for 6 months or longer (2001

Guidelines).[74,75,387,388] Secondary prophylaxis should be restarted if the CD4 count falls below 200/μl.

Primary prophylaxis for TE is well established and is achieved concomitantly with PCP prophylaxis using TMP-SMX.[165,389] For patients who do not tolerate sulfa medications, the combination of pyrimethamine and dapsone has similar efficacy[389,390] and is better than pyrimethamine alone[391,392] and aerosolized pentamidine.[170,171,389] Dapsone alone has an efficacy similar to that of aerosolized pentamidine.[168] The toxicity profile of pyrimethamine-dapsone is similar to that of TMP-SMX with rash, fever, nausea, and bone marrow suppression.[170,171,390] The bone marrow suppression can be ameliorated with leucovorin. Atovaquone, which has demonstrated activity as a salvage regimen,[378–380] may be a reasonable third-line agent. Clindamycin alone is inadequate,[393] and the clindamycin-pyrimethamine combination demonstrates too much toxicity to be recommended as primary prophylaxis.[394] Suggested prophylactic regimens and their dosages are listed in Table 30–2. Similar to the discontinuation of secondary prophylaxis, the discontinuation of primary prophylaxis for TE has been well studied in observational and randomized trials.[69,74,178,387,395] On the basis of these results, the current guidelines recommend discontinuing primary prophylaxis in patients who have a rise in CD4 count to above 200/μl for 3 months or longer (2001 Guidelines). In pregnant patients, primary prophylaxis with TMP-SMX may be given. Pyrimethamine should not be used because of its potential for teratogenicity and the low incidence of toxoplasmosis during pregnancy. Secondary prophylaxis with regimens including pyrimethamine, however, should be maintained during pregnancy for those patients still requiring continued therapy (Table 33–3). HIV-infected pregnant patients who develop primary toxoplasmosis during pregnancy should be managed closely for the possibility of congenital toxoplasmosis (2001 Guidelines).

Spore-Forming Protozoa

Microsporidium, Cryptosporidium, Isospora, and *Cyclospora* are all spore-forming protozoa that can infect the gastrointestinal tract of HIV-infected patients. In general these pathogens have been characterized relatively recently, and treatment guidelines have not been firmly established. All of these enteric protozoan infections appear to be much less commonly encountered in the HAART era.

The order Microsporidia contains organisms from a variety of genera (*Encephalitozoon, Enterocytozoon*, and others) that likely can exist in asymptomatic carriers or can cause self-limited enteritis in normal hosts, whereas they have been implicated in chronic diarrhea and wasting among AIDS patients. Less commonly, these organisms have been identified at the sites of local infections such as sinusitis, conjunctivitis, and hepatitis in the

TABLE 30–5 ■ Treatment Regimens for Toxoplasmic Encephalitis

Drug	Dosage
ACUTE TREATMENT	
First line	
Pyrimethamine	200 mg PO ×1, then 75–100 mg PO qd
Leucovorin (folinic acid)	10–15 mg PO qd
Sulfadiazine	1–1.5 g PO q6h
Second line	
Pyrimethamine and leucovorin	As above
Clindamycin	600 mg PO/IV q6h
Third line	
Pyrimethamine and leucovorin	As above
With one of the following:	
Clarithromycin	1000 mg PO bid
Azithromycin	1200–1500 mg PO qd
Atovaquone	750 mg PO q6h with food
SUPPRESSIVE TREATMENT	
First line	
Pyrimethamine	25–50 mg PO qd
Leucovorin	10–25 mg PO qd
Sulfadiazine*	500–1000 mg PO qid
Second line	
Pyrimethamine and leucovorin	As above
Clindamycin*	300–450 mg PO q6–8h
Third line	
Atovaquone, with or without	750 mg PO q6–12h
Pyrimethamine	25 mg PO qd
Leucovorin	10 mg PO qd

*Sulfadiazine-pyrimethamine protects against both toxoplasmosis and *Pneumocystis carinii* pneumonia. Clindamycin-pyrimethamine only protects against toxoplasmosis.

setting of advanced HIV infection. Although several investigational agents are currently being evaluated, there is no established treatment for microsporidiosis beyond supportive care.[396] The antiparasitic drug albendazole (400 mg twice daily) showed promise in a small pilot study, improving clearance and delaying relapse compared with no treatment.[397] Many cases of microsporidiosis dramatically improve once patients have partial immune reconstitution on effective antiretroviral therapy.[398,399]

In HIV-infected patients with only mild or moderate immunosuppression, *Cryptosporidium parvum* causes self-limited enteritis indistinguishable from the subacute diarrheal illness seen in immunocompetent hosts. In this situation, supportive care and rehydration are often sufficient. Among patients with advanced AIDS, however, *Cryptosporidium* infection often leads to chronic, severe diarrhea, malabsorption, and wasting. In some patients with low CD4 counts, the biliary tract also becomes involved.[400] No antibiotic therapy has proven effective for *Cryptosporidium* infection, although various agents have been studied. Paromomycin is an aminoglycoside agent with in vitro activity against the protozoan, but clinical trial experience has demonstrated inconsistent or limited effectiveness.[401,402] Similarly, azithromycin had anecdotal success, but clinical trials have not clearly demonstrated meaningful activity.[403] Nitazoxanide is an antiparasitic drug that has shown potential in a randomized clinical trial involving HIV-infected hosts with *Cryptosporidium* infection.[404] Bovine hyperimmune colostrum (as a means to deliver polyclonal antibodies to the gut) has also shown preliminary evidence of activity, both as a pre-"experimental challenge" prophylaxis[405] and as a therapy.[406] Outside of these investigational approaches the primary treatment focus has been on aggressive fluid and electrolyte management. In the past this approach sometimes meant life-long intravenous fluids and hyperalimentation in severe cases. Agents to slow gut motility are sometimes effective; there is no evidence that the somatostatin analog octreotide provides significant advantages over much less expensive over-the-counter agents such as loperamide.[407] As with microsporidiosis, many cases are greatly ameliorated once patients have experienced immunologic improvements on antiretroviral treatment,[398,399] and improving HIV suppression may be the most important treatment consideration.

Isospora belli and the more recently identified *Cyclospora* spp are larger protozoa that share some clinical characteristics with microsporidial and cryptosporidial infections, causing self-limited diarrhea in normal hosts but chronic diarrhea and wasting in advanced HIV cases. *Isospora* appears to be much less common in the United States than in HIV-infected patients in Africa and the developing world.[400] *Cyclospora* may be more likely to cause nausea and upper gastrointestinal upset than other enteric protozoa. These protozoa differ from *Microsporidium* and *Cryptosporidium*, however, in that treatment is much more straightforward.

TMP-SMX is effective for treatment of both *Isospora*[408,409] and *Cyclospora*[410] infections. One double strength tablet twice daily for 7 to 10 days has been shown to be effective for either infection in HIV-negative hosts and for *Isospora* in HIV-infected hosts, and higher doses (one double strength tablet four times a day) were used successfully in HIV-infected patients with *Cyclospora* infection in Peru. Both infections tend to relapse without maintenance therapy, and one double strength tablet daily of TMP-SMX is recommended for patients with AIDS as prophylaxis against *Pneumocystis* infection anyway.

Other Enteric Parasites

Other parasites, although not specific to HIV infection, are sometimes diagnosed in the HIV clinic setting.[410,411] *Giardia lamblia* tends to present in the same manner as in normal hosts, sometimes causing crampy abdominal pain and mild diarrhea. *Giardia* infection usually responds to treatment with metronidazole 500 mg twice daily for 5 to 7 days. Stool colonization with *Entamoeba* spp that are typically nonvirulent has been reported in gay men who are at risk for fecal-oral contact, but in general, invasive amebic infections are not more common in the HIV setting than in the general population.[411–413] In the event of invasive *Entamoeba histolytica* infection, standard therapy is generally effective (metronidazole 750 mg three times daily for 14 days plus a "luminally active agent" such as iodoquinol 650 mg three times daily for 20 days to eradicate colonization).

SUMMARY AND CONCLUSIONS

Preventing and Treating Opportunistic Infections in the HAART Era

There is growing evidence to support the safety of discontinuing primary prophylaxis against some common HIV-associated opportunistic infections (particularly, *Pneumocystis*, toxoplasmosis, and MAC) when patients have sustained, significant immunologic improvements on HAART. Generally, less data is available on whether it is prudent to discontinue secondary prophylaxis (or maintenance therapy) for these infections following administration of effective HAART. However, there is encouraging early data about the safety of stopping therapy in these settings as well. Persons who have had potentially life-threatening infections, such as fungal meningitis or disseminated infections slow to respond to conventional therapy, clearly warrant cautious consideration about the potential risks and benefits of withholding therapy. On the other hand, a downside of continuing multiple prophylactic drugs once the absolute CD4 count has significantly improved is the resulting "polypharmacy" and the inherent risks of drug-drug interactions.

Another layer of complexity in the HAART era is the relatively uncommon phenomenon of "immune reconstitution syndromes."[414,415] Although many opportunistic infections become more responsive to therapy or even remit spontaneously following HAART-induced immunologic improvements, occasionally patients experience transient immune-mediated flares of disease activity soon after beginning effective antiretroviral therapy. This has been particularly reported in cases of granulomatous disease (e.g., MAC adenitis), CMV retinitis (inflammatory uveitis), and viral hepatitis. Often these post-HAART phenomena involve local tissue inflammatory symptoms (e.g., tender fluctuant adenopathy related to MAC or leukocyte infiltrates in the anterior chamber of the eye related to CMV) as opposed to the nonspecific signs and symptoms attributed to widespread dissemination unchecked by organized immune responses. Case reports suggest that most of these reconstitution events resolve spontaneously without intervention, although occasionally clinicians have attempted temporary cessation of HAART or even corticosteroid therapy[416] to improve febrile manifestations.

Prophylaxis and Vaccination Recommendations

Recommendations regarding treatment and prevention of opportunistic infection are evolving over time, particularly in light of the overall improvements in, and greater complexity of, antiretroviral treatment options. With this caveat in mind, however, we summarized recommendations about primary prophylaxis and vaccination recommendations for HIV-infected patients in Tables 30–2 and 30–3 on the basis of the literature cited throughout this chapter and in particular the recently available USPHS/IDSA guidelines on this subject.

REFERENCES

1. Godofsky EW, Zinreich J, Armstrong M, et al: Sinusitis in HIV-infected patients: A clinical and radiographic review. Am J Med 1992;93:163–170.
2. O'Donnell JG, Sorbello AF, Condoluci DV, Barnish MJ: Sinusitis due to *Pseudomonas aeruginosa* in patients with human immunodeficiency virus infection. Clin Infect Dis 1993;16:404–406.
3. Hirschtick RE, Glassroth J, Jordan MC, et al: Bacterial pneumonia in persons infected with the human immunodeficiency virus. Pulmonary Complications of HIV Infection Study Group. N Engl J Med 1995;333:845–851.
4. Nuorti JP, Butler JC, Gelling L, et al: Epidemiologic relation between HIV and invasive pneumococcal disease in San Francisco County, California. Ann Intern Med 2000;132:182–190.
5. Cordero E, Pachon J, Rivero A, et al: *Haemophilus influenzae* pneumonia in human immunodeficiency virus–infected patients. The Grupo Andaluz para el Estudio de las Enfermedades Infecciosas. Clin Infect Dis 2000;30:461–465.
6. Senthilkumar A, Kumar S, Sheagren JN: Increased incidence of *Staphylococcus aureus* bacteremia in hospitalized patients with acquired immunodeficiency syndrome. Clin Infect Dis 2001;33:1412–1416.
7. Al Tawfiq JA, Sarosi GA, Cushing HE: Pyomyositis in the acquired immunodeficiency syndrome. South Med J 2000;93:330–334.
8. Dworkin MS, Williamson J, Jones JL, Kaplan JE: Prophylaxis with trimethoprim-sulfamethoxazole for human immunodeficiency virus–infected patients: Impact on risk for infectious diseases. Clin Infect Dis 2001;33:393–398.
9. Currier JS, Williams P, Feinberg J, et al: Impact of prophylaxis for *Mycobacterium avium* complex on bacterial infections in patients with advanced human immunodeficiency virus disease. Clin Infect Dis 2001;32:1615–1622.
10. Sullivan JH, Moore RD, Keruly JC, Chaisson RE: Effect of antiretroviral therapy on the incidence of bacterial pneumonia in patients with advanced HIV infection. Am J Respir Crit Care Med 2000;162:64–67.
11. Diaz PT, King MA, Pacht ER, et al: Increased susceptibility to pulmonary emphysema among HIV-seropositive smokers. Ann Intern Med 2000;132:369–372.
12. Niaura R, Shadel WG, Morrow K, et al: Human immunodeficiency virus infection, AIDS, and smoking cessation: The time is now. Clin Infect Dis 2000;31:808–812.
13. Kartalija M, Sande MA: Diarrhea and AIDS in the era of highly active antiretroviral therapy. Clin Infect Dis 1999;28:701–705.
14. Smith PD, Macher AM, Bookman MA, et al: *Salmonella typhimurium* enteritis and bacteremia in the acquired immunodeficiency syndrome. Ann Intern Med 1985;102:207–209.
15. Jacobson MA, Hahn SM, Gerberding JL, et al: Ciprofloxacin for *Salmonella* bacteremia in the acquired immunodeficiency syndrome (AIDS). Ann Intern Med 1989;110:1027–1029.
16. Molina J, Casin I, Hausfater P, et al: *Campylobacter* infections in HIV-infected patients: Clinical and bacteriological features. AIDS 1995;9:881–885.
17. Quinn TC: Diversity of *Campylobacter* species and its impact on patients infected with human immunodeficiency virus. Clin Infect Dis 1997;24:1114–1117.
18. Kiehlbauch JA, Tauxe RV, Baker CN, Wachsmuth IK: *Helicobacter cinaedi*-associated bacteremia and cellulitis in immunocompromised patients. Ann Intern Med 1994;121:90–93.
19. Angulo FJ, Swerdlow DL: Bacterial enteric infections in persons infected with human immunodeficiency virus. Clin Infect Dis 1995;21(Suppl 1):S84–S93.
20. Berenguer J, Solera J, Diaz MD, et al: Listeriosis in patients infected with human immunodeficiency virus. Rev Infect Dis 1991;13:115–119.
21. Casado JL, Valdezate S, Calderon C, et al: Zidovudine therapy protects against *Salmonella* bacteremia recurrence in human immunodeficiency virus–infected patients. J Infect Dis 1999;179:1553–1556.
22. Lu SS, Schwartz JM, Simon DM, Brandt LJ: *Clostridium difficile*-associated diarrhea in patients with HIV positivity and AIDS: A prospective controlled study. Am J Gastroenterol 1994;89:1226–1229.
23. Hutin Y, Molina JM, Casin I, et al: Risk factors for *Clostridium difficile*-associated diarrhoea in HIV-infected patients. AIDS 1993;7:1441–1447.
24. Hutchinson CM, Hook EW III, Shepherd M, et al: Altered clinical presentation of early syphilis in patients with human immunodeficiency virus infection. Ann Intern Med 1994;121:94–100.
25. Malone JL, Wallace MR, Hendrick BB, et al: Syphilis and neurosyphilis in a human immunodeficiency virus type-1 seropositive population: Evidence for frequent serologic relapse after therapy. Am J Med 1995;99:55–63.
26. Piscitelli SC, Gallicano KD: Interactions among drugs for HIV and opportunistic infections. N Engl J Med 2001;344:984–996.
27. Kuper JI, D'Aprile M: Drug-Drug interactions of clinical significance in the treatment of patients with *Mycobacterium avium* complex disease. Clin Pharmacokinet 2000;39:203–214.

28. Horsburgh CR Jr: The pathophysiology of disseminated *Mycobacterium avium* complex disease in AIDS. J Infect Dis 1999;179(Suppl 3):S461–S465.

29. Agins BD, Berman DS, Spicehandler D, et al: Effect of combined therapy with ansamycin, clofazimine, ethambutol, and isoniazid for *Mycobacterium avium* infection in patients with AIDS. J Infect Dis 1989;159:784–787.

30. Hoy J, Mijch A, Sandland M, et al: Quadruple-drug therapy for *Mycobacterium avium-intracellulare* bacteremia in AIDS patients. J Infect Dis 1990;161:801–805.

31. Chiu J, Nussbaum J, Bozzette S, et al: Treatment of disseminated *Mycobacterium avium* complex infection in AIDS with amikacin, ethambutol, rifampin, and ciprofloxacin. California Collaborative Treatment Group. Ann Intern Med 1990; 113:358–361.

32. Kemper CA, Meng TC, Nussbaum J, et al: Treatment of *Mycobacterium avium* complex bacteremia in AIDS with a four-drug oral regimen. Rifampin, ethambutol, clofazimine, and ciprofloxacin. The California Collaborative Treatment Group. Ann Intern Med 1992;116:466–472.

33. Dautzenberg B, Truffot C, Legris S, et al: Activity of clarithromycin against *Mycobacterium avium* infection in patients with the acquired immune deficiency syndrome. A controlled clinical trial. Am Rev Respir Dis 1991;144(3 Pt 1):564–569.

34. Young LS: Treatment and prophylaxis of *Mycobacterium avium* complex. Int J STD AIDS 1996;7(Suppl 1):23–27.

35. Chaisson RE, Benson CA, Dube MP, et al: Clarithromycin therapy for bacteremic *Mycobacterium avium* complex disease. A randomized, double-blind, dose-ranging study in patients with AIDS. AIDS Clinical Trials Group Protocol 157 Study Team. Ann Intern Med 1994;121:905–911.

36. Masur H: Recommendations on prophylaxis and therapy for disseminated *Mycobacterium avium* complex disease in patients infected with the human immunodeficiency virus. Public Health Service Task Force on Prophylaxis and Therapy for *Mycobacterium avium* Complex. N Engl J Med 1993;329:898–904.

37. Shafran SD, Singer J, Zarowny DP, et al: A comparison of two regimens for the treatment of *Mycobacterium avium* complex bacteremia in AIDS: Rifabutin, ethambutol, and clarithromycin versus rifampin, ethambutol, clofazimine, and ciprofloxacin. Canadian HIV Trials Network Protocol 010 Study Group. N Engl J Med 1996;335:377–383.

38. May T, Brel F, Beuscart C, et al: Comparison of combination therapy regimens for treatment of human immunodeficiency virus–infected patients with disseminated bacteremia due to *Mycobacterium avium*. ANRS Trial 033 Curavium Group. Agence Nationale de Recherche sur le Sida. Clin Infect Dis 1997;25:621–629.

39. Dube MP, Sattler FR, Torriani FJ, et al: A randomized evaluation of ethambutol for prevention of relapse and drug resistance during treatment of *Mycobacterium avium* complex bacteremia with clarithromycin-based combination therapy. California Collaborative Treatment Group. J Infect Dis 1997;176:1225–1232.

40. Sullam PM, Gordin FM, Wynne BA: Efficacy of rifabutin in the treatment of disseminated infection due to *Mycobacterium avium* complex. The Rifabutin Treatment Group. Clin Infect Dis 1994;19:84–86.

41. Gordin FM, Sullam PM, Shafran SD, et al: A randomized, placebo-controlled study of rifabutin added to a regimen of clarithromycin and ethambutol for treatment of disseminated infection with *Mycobacterium avium* complex. Clin Infect Dis 1999;28:1080–1085.

42. Markowitz M, Vesanen M, Tenner-Racz K, et al: The effect of commencing combination antiretroviral therapy soon after HIV-1 infection on viral replication and antiviral immune responses. J Infect Dis 1999;179:527–537.

43. Shafran SD, Singer J, Zarowny DP, et al: Determinants of rifabutin-associated uveitis in patients treated with rifabutin, clarithromycin, and ethambutol for *Mycobacterium avium* complex bacteremia: A multivariate analysis. Canadian HIV Trials Network Protocol 010 Study Group. J Infect Dis 1998;177:252–255.

44. Kemper CA, Havlir D, Haghighat D, et al: The individual microbiologic effect of three antimycobacterial agents, clofazimine, ethambutol, and rifampin, on *Mycobacterium avium* complex bacteremia in patients with AIDS. J Infect Dis 1994;170:157–164.

45. Chaisson RE, Keiser P, Pierce M, et al: Clarithromycin and ethambutol with or without clofazimine for the treatment of bacteremic *Mycobacterium avium* complex disease in patients with HIV infection. AIDS 1997;11:311–317.

46. Gordon SM, Horsburgh CR Jr, Peloquin CA, et al: Low serum levels of oral antimycobacterial agents in patients with disseminated *Mycobacterium avium* complex disease. J Infect Dis 1993;168:1559–1562.

47. Wallace RJ Jr, Brown BA, Griffith DE, et al: Reduced serum levels of clarithromycin in patients treated with multidrug regimens including rifampin or rifabutin for *Mycobacterium avium–M. intracellulare* infection. J Infect Dis 1995; 171:747–750.

48. Nash KA, Inderlied CB: Genetic basis of macrolide resistance in *Mycobacterium avium* isolated from patients with disseminated disease. Antimicrob Agents Chemother 1995; 39:2625–2630.

49. Meier A, Heifets L, Wallace RJ Jr, et al: Molecular mechanisms of clarithromycin resistance in *Mycobacterium avium*: Observation of multiple 23S rDNA mutations in a clonal population. J Infect Dis 1996;174:354–360.

50. Picardeau M, Varnerot A, Lecompte T, et al: Use of different molecular typing techniques for bacteriological follow-up in a clinical trial with AIDS patients with *Mycobacterium avium* bacteremia. J Clin Microbiol 1997;35:2503–2510.

51. Sison JP, Yao Y, Kemper CA, et al: Treatment of *Mycobacterium avium* complex infection: Do the results of in vitro susceptibility tests predict therapeutic outcome in humans? J Infect Dis 1996;173:677–683.

52. Shafran SD, Talbot JA, Chomyc S, et al: Does in vitro susceptibility to rifabutin and ethambutol predict the response to treatment of *Mycobacterium avium* complex bacteremia with rifabutin, ethambutol, and clarithromycin? Canadian HIV Trials Network Protocol 010 Study Group. Clin Infect Dis 1998;27:1401–1405.

53. Dube MP, Torriani FJ, See D, et al: Successful short-term suppression of clarithromycin-resistant *Mycobacterium avium* complex bacteremia in AIDS. California Collaborative Treatment Group. Clin Infect Dis 1999;28:136–138.

54. Pechere M, Opravil M, Wald A, et al: Clinical and epidemiologic features of infection with *Mycobacterium genavense*. Swiss HIV Cohort Study. Arch Intern Med 1995; 155:400–404.

55. Straus WL, Ostroff SM, Jernigan DB, et al: Clinical and epidemiologic characteristics of *Mycobacterium haemophilum*, an emerging pathogen in immunocompromised patients. Ann Intern Med 1994;120:118–125.

56. Campo RE, Campo CE: *Mycobacterium kansasii* disease in patients infected with human immunodeficiency virus. Clin Infect Dis 1997;24:1233–1238.

57. Shafer RW, Sierra MF: *Mycobacterium xenopi, Mycobacterium fortuitum, Mycobacterium kansasii*, and other nontuberculous mycobacteria in an area of endemicity for AIDS. Clin Infect Dis 1992;15:161–162.

58. El Helou P, Rachlis A, Fong I, et al: *Mycobacterium xenopi* infection in patients with human immunodeficiency virus infection. Clin Infect Dis 1997;25:206–210.

59. Lessnau KD, Milanese S, Talavera W: *Mycobacterium gordonae*: A treatable disease in HIV-positive patients. Chest 1993;104:1779–1785.

60. Zegans ME, Walton RC, Holland GN, et al: Transient vitreous inflammatory reactions associated with combination antiretroviral therapy in patients with AIDS and CMV retinitis. Am J Ophthalmol 1998;125:292–300.

61. Kemper CA, Bermudez LE, Deresinski SC: Immunomodulatory treatment of *Mycobacterium avium* complex bacteremia in patients with AIDS by use of recombinant granulocyte-macrophage colony-stimulating factor. J Infect Dis 1998;177:914–920.

62. Dorman SE, Heller HM, Basgoz NO, Sax PE: Adjunctive corticosteroid therapy for patients whose treatment for disseminated *Mycobacterium avium* complex infection has failed. Clin Infect Dis 1998;26:682–686.

63. Wormser GP, Horowitz H, Dworkin B: Low-dose dexamethasone as adjunctive therapy for disseminated *Mycobacterium avium* complex infections in AIDS patients. Antimicrob Agents Chemother 1994;38:2215–2217.

64. Pierce M, Crampton S, Henry D, et al: A randomized trial of clarithromycin as prophylaxis against disseminated *Mycobacterium avium* complex infection in patients with advanced acquired immunodeficiency syndrome. N Engl J Med 1996;335:384–391.

65. Oldfield EC III, Fessel WJ, Dunne MW, et al: Once weekly azithromycin therapy for prevention of *Mycobacterium avium* complex infection in patients with AIDS: A randomized, double-blind, placebo-controlled multicenter trial. Clin Infect Dis 1998;26:611–619.

66. Havlir DV, Dube MP, Sattler FR, et al: Prophylaxis against disseminated *Mycobacterium avium* complex with weekly azithromycin, daily rifabutin, or both. California Collaborative Treatment Group. N Engl J Med 1996;335:392–398.

67. Benson CA, Williams PL, Cohn DL, et al: Clarithromycin or rifabutin alone or in combination for primary prophylaxis of *Mycobacterium avium* complex disease in patients with AIDS: A randomized, double-blind, placebo-controlled trial. The AIDS Clinical Trials Group 196/Terry Beirn Community Programs for Clinical Research on AIDS 009 Protocol Team. J Infect Dis 2000;181:1289–1297.

68. Adair CD, Gunter M, Stovall TG, et al: *Chlamydia* in pregnancy: A randomized trial of azithromycin and erythromycin. Obstet Gynecol 1998;91:165–168.

69. Dworkin MS, Hanson DL, Kaplan JE, et al: Risk for preventable opportunistic infections in persons with AIDS after antiretroviral therapy increases CD4+ T lymphocyte counts above prophylaxis thresholds. J Infect Dis 2000;182:611–615.

70. El Sadr WM, Burman WJ, Grant LB, et al: Discontinuation of prophylaxis for *Mycobacterium avium* complex disease in HIV-infected patients who have a response to antiretroviral therapy. Terry Beirn Community Programs for Clinical Research on AIDS. N Engl J Med 2000;342:1085–1092.

71. Furrer H, Telenti A, Rossi M, Ledergerber B: Discontinuing or withholding primary prophylaxis against *Mycobacterium avium* in patients on successful antiretroviral combination therapy. The Swiss HIV Cohort Study. AIDS 2000;14:1409–1412.

72. Currier JS, Williams PL, Koletar SL, et al: Discontinuation of *Mycobacterium avium* complex prophylaxis in patients with antiretroviral therapy–induced increases in CD4+ cell count. A randomized, double-blind, placebo-controlled trial. AIDS Clinical Trials Group 362 Study Team. Ann Intern Med 2000;133:493–503.

73. Aberg JA, Yajko DM, Jacobson MA: Eradication of AIDS-related disseminated *Mycobacterium avium* complex infection after 12 months of antimycobacterial therapy combined with highly active antiretroviral therapy. J Infect Dis 1998;178:1446–1449.

74. Kirk O, Lundgren JD, Pedersen C, et al: Can chemoprophylaxis against opportunistic infections be discontinued after an increase in CD4 cells induced by highly active antiretroviral therapy? AIDS 1999;13:1647–1651.

75. Soriano V, Dona C, Rodriguez-Rosado R, et al: Discontinuation of secondary prophylaxis for opportunistic infections in HIV-infected patients receiving highly active antiretroviral therapy. AIDS 2000;14:383–386.

76. Koehler JE, Tappero JW: Bacillary angiomatosis and bacillary peliosis in patients infected with human immunodeficiency virus. Clin Infect Dis 1993;17:612–624.

77. Mohle-Boetani JC, Koehler JE, Berger TG, et al: Bacillary angiomatosis and bacillary peliosis in patients infected with human immunodeficiency virus: clinical characteristics in a case-control study. Clin Infect Dis 1996;22:794–800.

78. Masur H: Prevention and treatment of *Pneumocystis* pneumonia. N Engl J Med 1992;327:1853–1860.

79. Warren E, George S, You J, Kazanjian P. Advances in the treatment and prophylaxis of *Pneumocystis carinii* pneumonia. Pharmacotherapy 1997;17:900–916.

80. Drugs for parasitic infections. Med Lett 1998;17:900–916.

81. Wharton JM, Coleman DL, Wofsy CB, et al: Trimethoprim-sulfamethoxazole or pentamidine for *Pneumocystis carinii* pneumonia in the acquired immunodeficiency syndrome. A prospective randomized trial. Ann Intern Med 1986;105:37–44.

82. Sattler FR, Cowan R, Nielsen DM, Ruskin J: Trimethoprim-sulfamethoxazole compared with pentamidine for treatment of *Pneumocystis carinii* pneumonia in the acquired immunodeficiency syndrome. A prospective, noncrossover study. Ann Intern Med 1988;109:280–287.

83. Klein NC, Duncanson FP, Lenox TH, et al: Trimethoprim-sulfamethoxazole versus pentamidine for *Pneumocystis carinii* pneumonia in AIDS patients: Results of a large prospective randomized treatment trial. AIDS 1992;6:301–305.

84. Kovacs JA, Gill VJ, Meshnick S, Masur H: New insights into transmission, diagnosis, and drug treatment of *Pneumocystis carinii* pneumonia. JAMA 2001;286:2450–2460.

85. Gordin FM, Simon GL, Wofsy CB, Mills J: Adverse reactions to trimethoprim-sulfamethoxazole in patients with the acquired immunodeficiency syndrome. Ann Intern Med 1984;100:495–499.

86. Kovacs JA, Hiemenz JW, Macher AM, et al: *Pneumocystis carinii* pneumonia: A comparison between patients with the acquired immunodeficiency syndrome and patients with other immunodeficiencies. Ann Intern Med 1984;100:663–671.

87. Jung AC, Paauw DS: Management of adverse reactions to trimethoprim-sulfamethoxazole in human immunodeficiency virus-infected patients. Arch Intern Med 1994;154:2402–2406.

88. Safrin S, Lee BL, Sande MA: Adjunctive folinic acid with trimethoprim-sulfamethoxazole for *Pneumocystis carinii* pneumonia in AIDS patients is associated with an increased risk of therapeutic failure and death. J Infect Dis 1994;170:912–917.

89. Greenberg S, Reiser IW, Chou SY, Porush JG: Trimethoprim-sulfamethoxazole induces reversible hyperkalemia. Ann Intern Med 1993;119:291–295.

90. Kelly JW, Dooley DP, Lattuada CP, Smith CE: A severe, unusual reaction to trimethoprim-sulfamethoxazole in patients infected with human immunodeficiency virus. Clin Infect Dis 1992;14:1034–1039.

91. Porras MC, Lecumberri JN, Castrillon JL: Trimethoprim/sulfamethoxazole and metabolic acidosis in HIV-infected patients. Ann Pharmacother 1998;32:185–189.

92. Slavik RS, Rybak MJ, Lerner SA: Trimethoprim/sulfamethoxazole-induced tremor in a patient with AIDS. Ann Pharmacother 1998;32:189–192.

93. Torgovnick J, Arsura E: Desensitization to sulfonamides in patients with HIV infection. Am J Med 1990;88:548–549.

94. Tenant-Flowers M, Boyle MJ, Carey D, et al: Sulphadiazine desensitization in patients with AIDS and cerebral toxoplasmosis. AIDS 1991;5:311–315.

95. Gluckstein D, Ruskin J: Rapid oral desensitization to trimethoprim-sulfamethoxazole (TMP-SMZ): Use in prophylaxis for *Pneumocystis carinii* pneumonia in patients with AIDS who were previously intolerant to TMP-SMZ. Clin Infect Dis 1995;20:849–853.

96. Leoung GS, Stanford JF, Giordano MF, et al: Trimethoprim-sulfamethoxazole (TMP-SMZ) dose escalation versus direct rechallenge for *Pneumocystis carinii* pneumonia prophylaxis in human immunodeficiency virus–infected patients with previous adverse reaction to TMP-SMZ. J Infect Dis 2001;184:992–997.

97. Bozzette SA: The use of corticosteroids in *Pneumocystis carinii* pneumonia. J Infect Dis 1990;162:1365–1369.

98. Montaner JS, Lawson LM, Levitt N, et al: Corticosteroids prevent early deterioration in patients with moderately severe *Pneumocystis carinii* pneumonia and the acquired immunodeficiency syndrome (AIDS). Ann Intern Med 1990;113:14–20.

99. Gagnon S, Boota AM, Fischl MA, et al: Corticosteroids as adjunctive therapy for severe *Pneumocystis carinii* pneumonia in the acquired immunodeficiency syndrome. A double-blind, placebo-controlled trial. N Engl J Med 1990;323:1444–1450.

100. Bozzette SA, Sattler FR, Chiu J, et al: A controlled trial of early adjunctive treatment with corticosteroids for *Pneumocystis carinii* pneumonia in the acquired immunodeficiency syndrome. California Collaborative Treatment Group. N Engl J Med 1990;323:1451–1457.

101. Nielsen TL, Eeftinck Schattenkerk JK, Jensen BN, et al: Adjunctive corticosteroid therapy for *Pneumocystis carinii* pneumonia in AIDS: A randomized European multicenter open label study. J Acquir Immune Defic Syndr 1992;5:726–731.

102. Consensus statement on the use of corticosteroids as adjunctive therapy for *Pneumocystis* pneumonia in the acquired immunodeficiency syndrome. The National Institutes of Health–University of California Expert Panel for Corticosteroids as Adjunctive Therapy for *Pneumocystis* Pneumonia. N Engl J Med 1990;323:1500–1504.

103. Caumes E, Roudier C, Rogeaux O, et al: Effect of corticosteroids on the incidence of adverse cutaneous reactions to trimethoprim-sulfamethoxazole during treatment of AIDS-associated *Pneumocystis carinii* pneumonia. Clin Infect Dis 1994;18:319–323.

104. Jensen AM, Lundgren JD, Benfield T, et al: Does cytomegalovirus predict a poor prognosis in *Pneumocystis carinii* pneumonia treated with corticosteroids? A note for caution. Chest 1995;108:411–414.

105. Bozzette SA, Morton SC: Reconsidering the use of adjunctive corticosteroids in *Pneumocystis* pneumonia? J Acquir Immune Defic Syndr Hum Retrovirol 1995;8:345–347.

106. Jones BE, Taikwel EK, Mercado AL, et al: Tuberculosis in patients with HIV infection who receive corticosteroids for presumed *Pneumocystis carinii* pneumonia. Am J Respir Crit Care Med 1994;149:1686–1688.

107. Martos A, Podzamczer D, Martinez-Lacasa J, et al: Steroids do not enhance the risk of developing tuberculosis or other AIDS-related diseases in HIV-infected patients treated for *Pneumocystis carinii* pneumonia. AIDS 1995;9:1037–1041.

108. Conte JE Jr, Chernoff D, Feigal DW Jr, et al: Intravenous or inhaled pentamidine for treating *Pneumocystis carinii* pneumonia in AIDS. A randomized trial. Ann Intern Med 1990;113:203–209.

109. Conte JE Jr, Hollander H, Golden JA: Inhaled or reduced-dose intravenous pentamidine for *Pneumocystis carinii* pneumonia. A pilot study. Ann Intern Med 1987;107:495–498.

110. Conte JE Jr: Pharmacokinetics of intravenous pentamidine in patients with normal renal function or receiving hemodialysis. J Infect Dis 1991;163:169–175.

111. Sattler FR, Waskin H: Pentamidine and fatal hypoglycemia. Ann Intern Med 1987;107:789–790.

112. Waskin H, Stehr-Green JK, Helmick CG, Sattler FR: Risk factors for hypoglycemia associated with pentamidine therapy for *Pneumocystis* pneumonia. JAMA 1988;260:345–347.

113. Salmeron S, Petitpretz P, Katlama C, et al: Pentamidine and pancreatitis. Ann Intern Med 1986;105:140–141.

114. Zuger A, Wolf BZ, el Sadr W, et al: Pentamidine-associated fatal acute pancreatitis. JAMA 1986;256:2383–2385.

115. Stahl-Bayliss CM, Kalman CM, Laskin OL: Pentamidine-induced hypoglycemia in patients with the acquired immune deficiency syndrome. Clin Pharmacol Ther 1986;39:271–275.

116. O'Brien JG, Dong BJ, Coleman RL, et al: A 5-year retrospective review of adverse drug reactions and their risk factors in human immunodeficiency virus–infected patients who were receiving intravenous pentamidine therapy for *Pneumocystis carinii* pneumonia. Clin Infect Dis 1997;24:854–859.

117. Comtois R, Pouliot J, Vinet B, et al: Higher pentamidine levels in AIDS patients with hypoglycemia and azotemia during treatment of *Pneumocystis carinii* pneumonia. Am Rev Respir Dis 1992;146:740–744.

118. Stehr-Green JK, Helmick CG: Pentamidine and renal toxicity. N Engl J Med 1985;313:694–695.

119. Bibler MR, Chou TC, Toltzis RJ, Wade PA: Recurrent ventricular tachycardia due to pentamidine-induced cardiotoxicity. Chest 1988;94:1303–1306.

120. Taylor AJ, Hull RW, Coyne PE, et al: Pentamidine-induced torsades de pointes: Safe completion of therapy with inhaled pentamidine. Clin Pharmacol Ther 1991;49:698–700.

121. Kleyman TR, Roberts C, Ling BN: A mechanism for pentamidine-induced hyperkalemia: Inhibition of distal nephron sodium transport. Ann Intern Med 1995;122:103–106.

122. Helmick CG, Green JK: Pentamidine-associated hypotension and route of administration. Ann Intern Med 1985;103:480.

123. Conte JE Jr, Chernoff D, Feigal DW Jr, et al: Intravenous or inhaled pentamidine for treating *Pneumocystis carinii* pneumonia in AIDS. A randomized trial. Ann Intern Med 1990;113:203–209.

124. Soo Hoo GW, Mohsenifar Z, Meyer RD: Inhaled or intravenous pentamidine therapy for *Pneumocystis carinii* pneumonia in AIDS. A randomized trial. Ann Intern Med 1990;113:195–202.

125. Montgomery AB, Feigal DW Jr, Sattler F, et al: Pentamidine aerosol versus trimethoprim-sulfamethoxazole for *Pneumocystis carinii* in acquired immune deficiency syndrome. Am J Respir Crit Care Med 1995;151:1068–1074.

126. Allegra CJ, Kovacs JA, Drake JC, et al: Activity of antifolates against *Pneumocystis carinii* dihydrofolate reductase and identification of a potent new agent. J Exp Med 1987;165:926–931.

127. Allegra CJ, Chabner BA, Tuazon CU, et al: Trimetrexate for the treatment of *Pneumocystis carinii* pneumonia in patients with the acquired immunodeficiency syndrome. N Engl J Med 1987;317:978–985.

128. Sattler FR, Allegra CJ, Verdegem TD, et al: Trimetrexate-leucovorin dosage evaluation study for treatment of *Pneumocystis carinii* pneumonia. J Infect Dis 1990;161:91–96.

129. Sattler FR, Frame P, Davis R, et al: Trimetrexate with leucovorin versus trimethoprim-sulfamethoxazole for moderate to severe episodes of *Pneumocystis carinii* pneumonia in patients with AIDS: A prospective, controlled multicenter investigation of the AIDS Clinical Trials Group Protocol 029/031. J Infect Dis 1994;170:165–172.

130. Queener SF, Bartlett MS, Richardson JD, et al: Activity of clindamycin with primaquine against *Pneumocystis carinii* in vitro and in vivo. Antimicrob Agents Chemother 1988;32:807–813.

131. Toma E, Fournier S, Poisson M, et al: Clindamycin with primaquine for *Pneumocystis carinii* pneumonia. Lancet 1989; 1(8646):1046–1048.
132. Black JR, Feinberg J, Murphy RL, et al: Clindamycin and primaquine as primary treatment for mild and moderately severe *Pneumocystis carinii* pneumonia in patients with AIDS. Eur J Clin Microbiol Infect Dis 1991;10:204–207.
133. Ruf B, Rohde I, Pohle HD: Efficacy of clindamycin/primaquine versus trimethoprim/sulfamethoxazole in primary treatment of *Pneumocystis carinii* pneumonia. Eur J Clin Microbiol Infect Dis 1991;10:207–210.
134. Toma E: Clindamycin/primaquine for treatment of *Pneumocystis carinii* pneumonia in AIDS. Eur J Clin Microbiol Infect Dis 1991;10:210–213.
135. Noskin GA, Murphy RL, Black JR, Phair JP: Salvage therapy with clindamycin/primaquine for *Pneumocystis carinii* pneumonia. Clin Infect Dis 1992;14:183–188.
136. Toma E, Fournier S, Dumont M, et al: Clindamycin/primaquine versus trimethoprim-sulfamethoxazole as primary therapy for *Pneumocystis carinii* pneumonia in AIDS: A randomized, double-blind pilot trial. Clin Infect Dis 1993; 17:178–184.
137. Safrin S, Finkelstein DM, Feinberg J, et al: Comparison of three regimens for treatment of mild to moderate *Pneumocystis carinii* pneumonia in patients with AIDS. A double-blind, randomized, trial of oral trimethoprim-sulfamethoxazole, dapsone-trimethoprim, and clindamycin-primaquine. ACTG 108 Study Group. Ann Intern Med 1996;124:792–802.
138. Toma E, Thorne A, Singer J, et al. Clindamycin with primaquine vs. trimethoprim-sulfamethoxazole therapy for mild and moderately severe *Pneumocystis carinii* pneumonia in patients with AIDS: A multicenter, double-blind, randomized trial (CTN 004). CTN-PCP Study Group. Clin Infect Dis 1998;27:524–530.
139. Sin DD, Shafran SD: Dap. J Acquir Immune Defic Syndr Hum Retrovirol 1996;12:477–481.
140. Hughes WT, Smith BL: Efficacy of diaminodiphenylsulfone and other drugs in murine *Pneumocystis carinii* pneumonitis. Antimicrob Agents Chemother 1984;26:436–440.
141. Voeller D, Kovacs J, Andrawis V, et al: Interaction of *Pneumocystis carinii* dihydropteroate synthase with sulfonamides and diaminodiphenyl sulfone (dapsone). J Infect Dis 1994;169:456–459.
142. Holtzer CD, Flaherty JF Jr, Coleman RL: Cross-reactivity in HIV-infected patients switched from trimethoprim-sulfamethoxazole to dapsone. Pharmacotherapy 1998; 18:831–835.
143. Mills J, Leoung G, Medina I, et al: Dapsone treatment of *Pneumocystis carinii* pneumonia in the acquired immunodeficiency syndrome. Antimicrob Agents Chemother 1988; 32:1057–1060.
144. Leoung GS, Mills J, Hopewell PC, et al: Dapsone- trimethoprim for *Pneumocystis carinii* pneumonia in the acquired immunodeficiency syndrome. Ann Intern Med 1986; 105:45–48.
145. Medina I, Mills J, Leoung G, et al: Oral therapy for *Pneumocystis carinii* pneumonia in the acquired immunodeficiency syndrome. A controlled trial of trimethoprim-sulfamethoxazole versus trimethoprim-dapsone. N Engl J Med 1990;323:776–782.
146. Lee BL, Medina I, Benowitz NL, et al: Dapsone, trimethoprim, and sulfamethoxazole plasma levels during treatment of *Pneumocystis* pneumonia in patients with the acquired immunodeficiency syndrome (AIDS). Evidence of drug interactions. Ann Intern Med 1989;110:606–611.
147. Hughes WT: Use of dapsone in the prevention and treatment of *Pneumocystis carinii* pneumonia: A review. Clin Infect Dis 1998;27:191–204.
148. Metroka CE, Lewis NJ, Jacobus DP: Desensitization to dapsone in HIV-positive patients. JAMA 1992;267:512.
149. Hughes WT, Gray VL, Gutteridge WE, et al: Efficacy of a hydroxynaphthoquinone, 566C80, in experimental *Pneumocystis carinii* pneumonitis. Antimicrob Agents Chemother 1990;34:225–228.
150. Hughes WT, Kennedy W, Shenep JL, et al: Safety and pharmacokinetics of 566C80, a hydroxynaphthoquinone with anti–*Pneumocystis carinii* activity: A phase I study in human immunodeficiency virus (HIV)–infected men. J Infect Dis 1991;163:843–848.
151. Falloon J, Kovacs J, Hughes W, et al: A preliminary evaluation of 566C80 for the treatment of *Pneumocystis* pneumonia in patients with the acquired immunodeficiency syndrome. N Engl J Med 1991;325:1534–1538.
152. Hughes W, Leoung G, Kramer F, et al: Comparison of atovaquone (566C80) with trimethoprim-sulfamethoxazole to treat *Pneumocystis carinii* pneumonia in patients with AIDS. N Engl J Med 1993;328:1521–1527.
153. Dohn MN, Weinberg WG, Torres RA, et al: Oral atovaquone compared with intravenous pentamidine for *Pneumocystis carinii* pneumonia in patients with AIDS. Atovaquone Study Group. Ann Intern Med 1994;121:174–180.
154. Phair J, Munoz A, Detels R, et al: The risk of *Pneumocystis carinii* pneumonia among men infected with human immunodeficiency virus type 1. Multicenter AIDS Cohort Study Group. N Engl J Med 1990;322:161–165.
155. Kaplan JE, Hanson DL, Navin TR, Jones JL: Risk factors for primary *Pneumocystis carinii* pneumonia in human immunodeficiency virus–infected adolescents and adults in the United States: Reassessment of indications for chemoprophylaxis. J Infect Dis 1998;178:1126–1132.
156. Kovacs JA, Masur H: Prophylaxis against opportunistic infections in patients with human immunodeficiency virus infection. N Engl J Med 2000;342:1416–1429.
157. Schneider MM, Hoepelman AI, Eeftinck Schattenkerk JK, et al: A controlled trial of aerosolized pentamidine or trimethoprim-sulfamethoxazole as primary prophylaxis against *Pneumocystis carinii* pneumonia in patients with human immunodeficiency virus infection. The Dutch AIDS Treatment Group. N Engl J Med 1992;327:1836–1841.
158. Podzamczer D, Salazar A, Jimenez J, et al: Intermittent trimethoprim-sulfamethoxazole compared with dapsone-pyrimethamine for the simultaneous primary prophylaxis of *Pneumocystis* pneumonia and toxoplasmosis in patients infected with HIV. Ann Intern Med 1995;122:755–761.
159. Hughes WT: Use of dapsone in the prevention and treatment of *Pneumocystis carinii* pneumonia: A review. Clin Infect Dis 1998;27:191–204.
160. Bozzette SA, Finkelstein DM, Spector SA, et al: A randomized trial of three anti-*Pneumocystis* agents in patients with advanced human immunodeficiency virus infection. NIAID AIDS Clinical Trials Group. N Engl J Med 1995;332:693–699.
161. Ioannidis JP, Cappelleri JC, Skolnik PR, et al: A meta-analysis of the relative efficacy and toxicity of *Pneumocystis carinii* prophylactic regimens. Arch Intern Med 1996;156:177–188.
162. Bucher HC, Griffith L, Guyatt GH, Opravil M: Meta-analysis of prophylactic treatments against *Pneumocystis carinii* pneumonia and *Toxoplasma* encephalitis in HIV-infected patients. J Acquir Immune Defic Syndr Hum Retrovirol 1997;15:104–114.
163. Mallolas J, Zamora L, Gatell JM, et al: Primary prophylaxis for *Pneumocystis carinii* pneumonia: A randomized trial comparing cotrimoxazole, aerosolized pentamidine and dapsone plus pyrimethamine. AIDS 1993;7:59–64.
164. Saah AJ, Hoover DR, Peng Y, et al: Predictors for failure of *Pneumocystis carinii* pneumonia prophylaxis. Multicenter AIDS Cohort Study. JAMA 1995;273:1197–1202.

165. Carr A, Tindall B, Brew BJ, et al: Low-dose trimethoprim-sulfamethoxazole prophylaxis for toxoplasmic encephalitis in patients with AIDS. Ann Intern Med 1992;117:106–111.

166. El Sadr WM, Luskin-Hawk R, Yurik TM, et al: A randomized trial of daily and thrice-weekly trimethoprim-sulfamethoxazole for the prevention of *Pneumocystis carinii* pneumonia in human immunodeficiency virus–infected persons. Terry Beirn Community Programs for Clinical Research on AIDS (CPCRA). Clin Infect Dis 1999;29:775–783.

167. Schneider MM, Nielsen TL, Nelsing S, et al: Efficacy and toxicity of two doses of trimethoprim-sulfamethoxazole as primary prophylaxis against *Pneumocystis carinii* pneumonia in patients with human immunodeficiency virus. Dutch AIDS Treatment Group. J Infect Dis 1995;171:1632–1636.

168. Torres RA, Barr M, Thorn M, et al: Randomized trial of dapsone and aerosolized pentamidine for the prophylaxis of *Pneumocystis carinii* pneumonia and toxoplasmic encephalitis. Am J Med 1993;95:573–583.

169. Girard PM, Landman R, Gaudebout C, et al: Dapsone-pyrimethamine compared with aerosolized pentamidine as primary prophylaxis against *Pneumocystis carinii* pneumonia and toxoplasmosis in HIV infection. The PRIO Study Group. N Engl J Med 1993;328:1514–1520.

170. Opravil M, Hirschel B, Lazzarin A, et al: Once-weekly administration of dapsone/pyrimethamine vs. aerosolized pentamidine as combined prophylaxis for *Pneumocystis carinii* pneumonia and toxoplasmic encephalitis in human immunodeficiency virus–infected patients. Clin Infect Dis 1995;20:531–541.

171. Girard PM, Landman R, Gaudebout C, et al: Dapsone-pyrimethamine compared with aerosolized pentamidine as primary prophylaxis against *Pneumocystis carinii* pneumonia and toxoplasmosis in HIV infection. The PRIO Study Group. N Engl J Med 1993;328:1514–1520.

172. El Sadr WM, Murphy RL, Yurik TM, et al: Atovaquone compared with dapsone for the prevention of *Pneumocystis carinii* pneumonia in patients with HIV infection who cannot tolerate trimethoprim, sulfonamides, or both. Community Program for Clinical Research on AIDS and the AIDS Clinical Trials Group. N Engl J Med 1998;339:1889–1895.

173. Chan C, Montaner J, Lefebvre EA, et al: Atovaquone suspension compared with aerosolized pentamidine for prevention of *Pneumocystis carinii* pneumonia in human immunodeficiency virus–infected subjects intolerant of trimethoprim or sulfonamides. J Infect Dis 1999;180:369–376.

174. Furrer H, Egger M, Opravil M, et al: Discontinuation of primary prophylaxis against *Pneumocystis carinii* pneumonia in HIV-1 infected adults treated with combination antiretroviral therapy. N Engl J Med 1999;340:1301–1306.

175. Weverling GJ, Mocroft A, Ledergerber B, et al: Discontinuation of *Pneumocystis carinii* pneumonia prophylaxis after start of highly active antiretroviral therapy. Lancet 1999;353:1293–1298.

176. Yangco BG, Von Bargen JC, Moorman AC, Holmberg SD: Discontinuation of chemoprophylaxis against *Pneumocystis carinii* pneumonia in patients with HIV infection. HIV Outpatient Study (HOPS) Investigators. Ann Intern Med 2000;132:201–205.

177. Schneider MM, Borleffs JC, Stolk RP, et al: Discontinuation of prophylaxis for *Pneumocystis carinii* pneumonia in HIV-1-infected patients treated with highly active antiretroviral therapy. Lancet 1999;353:201–203.

178. Mussini C, Pezzotti P, Govoni A, et al: Discontinuation of primary prophylaxis for *Pneumocystis carinii* pneumonia and toxoplasmic encephalitis in human immunodeficiency virus type I–infected patients: The changes in opportunistic prophylaxis study. J Infect Dis 2000;181:1635–1642.

179. Furrer H, Opravil M, Rossi M, et al: Discontinuation of primary prophylaxis in HIV-infected patients at high risk of *Pneumocystis carinii* pneumonia: Prospective multicentre study. AIDS 2001;15:501–507.

180. Trikalinos TA, Ioannidis JP: Discontinuation of *Pneumocystis carinii* prophylaxis in patients infected with human immunodeficiency virus: A meta-analysis and decision analysis. Clin Infect Dis 2001;33:1901–1909.

181. Pons V, Greenspan D, Lozada-Nur F, et al: Oropharyngeal candidiasis in patients with AIDS: Randomized comparison of fluconazole versus nystatin oral suspensions. Clin Infect Dis 1997;24:1204–1207.

182. Flynn PM, Cunningham CK, Kerkering T, et al: Oropharyngeal candidiasis in immunocompromised children: A randomized, multicenter study of orally administered fluconazole suspension versus nystatin. The Multicenter Fluconazole Study Group. J Pediatr 1995;127:322–328.

183. Koletar SL, Russell JA, Fass RJ, Plouffe JF: Comparison of oral fluconazole and clotrimazole troches as treatment for oral candidiasis in patients infected with human immunodeficiency virus. Antimicrob Agents Chemother 1990;34:2267–2268.

184. Pons V, Greenspan D, Debruin M: Therapy for oropharyngeal candidiasis in HIV-infected patients: A randomized, prospective multicenter study of oral fluconazole versus clotrimazole troches. The Multicenter Study Group. J Acquir Immune Defic Syndr 1993;6:1311–1316.

185. Sangeorzan JA, Bradley SF, He X, et al: Epidemiology of oral candidiasis in HIV-infected patients: Colonization, infection, treatment, and emergence of fluconazole resistance. Am J Med 1994;97:339–346.

186. Vazquez JA: Options for the management of mucosal candidiasis in patients with AIDS and HIV infection. Pharmacotherapy 1999;19:76–87.

187. Fichtenbaum CJ, Powderly WG: Refractory mucosal candidiasis in patients with human immunodeficiency virus infection. Clin Infect Dis 1998;26:556–565.

188. Boken DJ, Swindells S, Rinaldi MG: Fluconazole-resistant *Candida albicans*. Clin Infect Dis 1993;17:1018–1021.

189. Sanguineti A, Carmichael JK, Campbell K: Fluconazole-resistant *Candida albicans* after long-term suppressive therapy. Arch Intern Med 1993;153:1122–1124.

190. Newman SL, Flanigan TP, Fisher A, et al: Clinically significant mucosal candidiasis resistant to fluconazole treatment in patients with AIDS. Clin Infect Dis 1994;19:684–686.

191. White A, Goetz MB: Azole-resistant *Candida albicans*: Report of two cases of resistance to fluconazole and review. Clin Infect Dis 1994;19:687–692.

192. Horn CA, Washburn RG, Givner LB, et al: Azole-resistant oropharyngeal and esophageal candidiasis in patients with AIDS. AIDS 1995;9:533–534.

193. Revankar SG, Kirkpatrick WR, McAtee RK, et al: A randomized trial of continuous or intermittent therapy with fluconazole for oropharyngeal candidiasis in HIV-infected patients: Clinical outcomes and development of fluconazole resistance. Am J Med 1998;105:7–11.

194. Baily GG, Perry FM, Denning DW, Mandal BK: Fluconazole-resistant candidosis in an HIV cohort. AIDS 1994;8:787–792.

195. Maenza JR, Keruly JC, Moore RD, et al: Risk factors for fluconazole-resistant candidiasis in human immunodeficiency virus–infected patients. J Infect Dis 1996;173:219–225.

196. Maenza JR, Merz WG, Romagnoli MJ, et al: Infection due to fluconazole-resistant *Candida* in patients with AIDS: Prevalence and microbiology. Clin Infect Dis 1997;24:28–34.

197. Johnson EM, Davey KG, Szekely A, Warnock DW: Itraconazole susceptibilities of fluconazole susceptible and resistant isolates of five *Candida* species. J Antimicrob Chemother 1995;36:787–793.

198. Fichtenbaum CJ, Koletar S, Yiannoutsos C, et al: Refractory mucosal candidiasis in advanced human immunodeficiency virus infection. Clin Infect Dis 2000;30:749–756.

199. Goldman M, Cloud GA, Smedema M, et al: Does long-term itraconazole prophylaxis result in in vitro azole resistance in mucosal *Candida albicans* isolates from persons with advanced human immunodeficiency virus infection? The National Institute of Allergy and Infectious Diseases Mycoses study group. Antimicrob Agents Chemother 2000;44:1585–1587.

200. Stevens DA, Greene SI, Lang OS: Thrush can be prevented in patients with acquired immunodeficiency syndrome and the acquired immunodeficiency syndrome–related complex. Randomized, double-blind, placebo-controlled study of 100-mg oral fluconazole daily. Arch Intern Med 1991;151:2458–2464.

201. Powderly WG, Finkelstein D, Feinberg J, et al: A randomized trial comparing fluconazole with clotrimazole troches for the prevention of fungal infections in patients with advanced human immunodeficiency virus infection. NIAID AIDS Clinical Trials Group. N Engl J Med 1995;332:700–705.

202. Schuman P, Capps L, Peng G, et al: Weekly fluconazole for the prevention of mucosal candidiasis in women with HIV infection. A randomized, double-blind, placebo-controlled trial. Terry Beirn Community Programs for Clinical Research on AIDS. Ann Intern Med 1997;126:689–696.

203. Havlir DV, Dube MP, McCutchan JA, et al: Prophylaxis with weekly versus daily fluconazole for fungal infections in patients with AIDS. Clin Infect Dis 1998;27:1369–1375.

204. Powderly WG, Mayer KH, Perfect JR: Diagnosis and treatment of oropharyngeal candidiasis in patients infected with HIV: A critical reassessment. AIDS Res Hum Retroviruses 1999;15:1405–1412.

205. Powderly WG, Gallant JE, Ghannoum MA, et al: Oropharyngeal candidiasis in patients with HIV: suggested guidelines for therapy. AIDS Res Hum Retroviruses 1999;15:1619–1623.

206. Cartledge JD, Midgley J, Youle M, Gazzard BG: Itraconazole cyclodextrin solution—effective treatment for HIV-related candidosis unresponsive to other azole therapy. J Antimicrob Chemother 1994;33:1071–1073.

207. Phillips P, De Beule K, Frechette G, et al: A double-blind comparison of itraconazole oral solution and fluconazole capsules for the treatment of oropharyngeal candidiasis in patients with AIDS. Clin Infect Dis 1998;26:1368–1373.

208. Saag MS, Fessel WJ, Kaufman CA, et al: Treatment of fluconazole-refractory oropharyngeal candidiasis with itraconazole oral solution in HIV-positive patients. AIDS Res Hum Retroviruses 1999;15:1413–1417.

209. Wilcox CM, Darouiche RO, Laine L, et al: A randomized, double-blind comparison of itraconazole oral solution and fluconazole tablets in the treatment of esophageal candidiasis. J Infect Dis 1997;176:227–232.

210. Lake-Bakaar G, Tom W, Lake-Bakaar D, et al: Gastropathy and ketoconazole malabsorption in the acquired immunodeficiency syndrome (AIDS). Ann Intern Med 1988; 109:471–473.

211. Blum RA, D'Andrea DT, Florentino BM, et al: Increased gastric pH and the bioavailability of fluconazole and ketoconazole. Ann Intern Med 1991;114:755–757.

212. Smith DE, Midgley J, Allan M, et al: Itraconazole versus ketaconazole in the treatment of oral and oesophageal candidosis in patients infected with HIV. AIDS 1991;5:1367–1371.

213. de Repentigny L, Ratelle J: Comparison of itraconazole and ketoconazole in HIV-positive patients with oropharyngeal or esophageal candidiasis. Human Immunodeficiency Virus Itraconazole Ketoconazole Project Group. Chemotherapy 1996;42:374–383.

214. De Wit S, Weerts D, Goossens H, Clumeck N: Comparison of fluconazole and ketoconazole for oropharyngeal candidiasis in AIDS. Lancet 1989;1(8641):746–748.

215. Laine L, Dretler RH, Conteas CN, et al: Fluconazole compared with ketoconazole for the treatment of *Candida* esophagitis in AIDS. A randomized trial. Ann Intern Med 1992;117:655–660.

216. Barbaro G, Barbarini G, Di Lorenzo G. Fluconazole compared with itraconazole in the treatment of esophageal candidiasis in AIDS patients: A double-blind, randomized, controlled clinical study. Scand J Infect Dis 1995;27:613–617.

217. Hegener P, Troke PF, Fatkenheuer G, et al: Treatment of fluconazole-resistant candidiasis with voriconazole in patients with AIDS. AIDS 1998;12:2227–2228.

218. Reef SE, Levine WC, McNeil MM, et al: Treatment options for vulvovaginal candidiasis, 1993. Clin Infect Dis 1995;20(Suppl 1):S80–S90.

219. Sobel JD, Brooker D, Stein GE, et al: Single oral dose fluconazole compared with conventional clotrimazole topical therapy of *Candida* vaginitis. Fluconazole Vaginitis Study Group. Am J Obstet Gynecol 1995;172(4 Pt 1):1263–1268.

220. Pursley TJ, Blomquist IK, Abraham J, et al: Fluconazole-induced congenital anomalies in three infants. Clin Infect Dis 1996;22:336–340.

221. Aleck KA, Bartley DL: Multiple malformation syndrome following fluconazole use in pregnancy: Report of an additional patient. Am J Med Genet 1997;72:253–256.

222. Rex JH, Pfaller MA, Galgiani JN, et al: Development of interpretive breakpoints for antifungal susceptibility testing: Conceptual framework and analysis of in vitro–in vivo correlation data for fluconazole, itraconazole, and *Candida* infections. Subcommittee on Antifungal Susceptibility Testing of the National Committee for Clinical Laboratory Standards. Clin Infect Dis 1997;24:235–247.

223. Walsh TJ, Gonzalez CE, Piscitelli S, et al: Correlation between in vitro and in vivo antifungal activities in experimental fluconazole-resistant oropharyngeal and esophageal candidiasis. J Clin Microbiol 2000;38:2369–2373.

224. Walmsley S, King S, McGeer A, et al: Oropharyngeal candidiasis in patients with human immunodeficiency virus: Correlation of clinical outcome with in vitro resistance, serum azole levels, and immunosuppression. Clin Infect Dis 2001;32:1554–1561.

225. Redding S, Smith J, Farinacci G, et al: Resistance of *Candida albicans* to fluconazole during treatment of oropharyngeal candidiasis in a patient with AIDS: Documentation by in vitro susceptibility testing and DNA subtype analysis. Clin Infect Dis 1994;18:240–242.

226. Sobel JD, Ohmit SE, Schuman P, et al: The evolution of *Candida* species and fluconazole susceptibility among oral and vaginal isolates recovered from human immunodeficiency virus (HIV)–seropositive and at-risk HIV-seronegative women. J Infect Dis 2001;183:286–293.

227. Zingman BS: Resolution of refractory AIDS-related mucosal candidiasis after initiation of didanosine plus saquinavir. N Engl J Med 1996;334:1674–1675.

228. Arribas JR, Hernandez-Albujar S, Gonzalez-Garcia JJ, et al: Impact of protease inhibitor therapy on HIV-related oropharyngeal candidiasis. AIDS 2000;14:979–985.

229. Martins MD, Lozano-Chiu M, Rex JH: Declining rates of oropharyngeal candidiasis and carriage of *Candida albicans* associated with trends toward reduced rates of carriage of fluconazole-resistant *C. albicans* in human immunodeficiency virus–infected patients. Clin Infect Dis 1998;27:1291–1294.

230. Bennett JE, Dismukes WE, Duma RJ, et al: A comparison of amphotericin B alone and combined with flucytosine in the treatment of cryptoccal meningitis. N Engl J Med 1979;301:126–131.

231. Dismukes WE, Cloud G, Gallis HA, et al: Treatment of cryptococcal meningitis with combination amphotericin B and flucytosine for four as compared with six weeks. N Engl J Med 1987;317:334–341.

232. Chuck SL, Sande MA: Infections with *Cryptococcus neoformans* in the acquired immunodeficiency syndrome. N Engl J Med 1989;321:794–799.

233. Saag MS, Powderly WG, Cloud GA, et al: Comparison of amphotericin B with fluconazole in the treatment of acute AIDS-associated cryptococcal meningitis. The NIAID Mycoses Study Group and the AIDS Clinical Trials Group. N Engl J Med 1992;326:83–89.

234. Larsen RA, Bozzette SA, Jones BE, et al: Fluconazole combined with flucytosine for treatment of cryptococcal meningitis in patients with AIDS. Clin Infect Dis 1994;19:741–745.

235. Menichetti F, Fiorio M, Tosti A, et al: High-dose fluconazole therapy for cryptococcal meningitis in patients with AIDS. Clin Infect Dis 1996;22:838–840.

236. Mayanja-Kizza H, Oishi K, Mitarai S, et al: Combination therapy with fluconazole and flucytosine for cryptococcal meningitis in Ugandan patients with AIDS. Clin Infect Dis 1998;26:1362–1366.

237. Denning DW, Tucker RM, Hanson LH, et al: Itraconazole therapy for cryptococcal meningitis and cryptococcosis. Arch Intern Med 1989;149:2301–2308.

238. de Gans J, Portegies P, Tiessens G, et al: Itraconazole compared with amphotericin B plus flucytosine in AIDS patients with cryptococcal meningitis. AIDS 1992;6:185–190.

239. Larsen RA, Leal MA, Chan LS: Fluconazole compared with amphotericin B plus flucytosine for cryptococcal meningitis in AIDS. A randomized trial. Ann Intern Med 1990;113:183–187.

240. de Lalla F, Pellizzer G, Vaglia A, et al: Amphotericin B as primary therapy for cryptococcosis in patients with AIDS: Reliability of relatively high doses administered over a relatively short period. Clin Infect Dis 1995;20:263–266.

241. van der Horst CM, Saag MS, Cloud GA, et al: Treatment of cryptococcal meningitis associated with the acquired immunodeficiency syndrome. National Institute of Allergy and Infectious Diseases Mycoses Study Group and AIDS Clinical Trials Group [see comments]. N Engl J Med 1997;337:15–21.

242. Gallis HA, Drew RH, Pickard WW: Amphotericin B: 30 years of clinical experience. Rev Infect Dis 1990;12:308–329.

243. Medoff G, Kobayashi GS: Strategies in the treatment of systemic fungal infections. N Engl J Med 1980;302:145–155.

244. Goodwin SD, Cleary JD, Walawander CA, et al: Pretreatment regimens for adverse events related to infusion of amphotericin B. Clin Infect Dis 1995;20:755–761.

245. Coker RJ, Viviani M, Gazzard BG, et al: Treatment of cryptococcosis with liposomal amphotericin B (AmBisome) in 23 patients with AIDS. AIDS 1993;7:829–835.

246. Sharkey PK, Graybill JR, Johnson ES, et al: Amphotericin B lipid complex compared with amphotericin B in the treatment of cryptococcal meningitis in patients with AIDS. Clin Infect Dis 1996;22:315–321.

247. Leenders AC, Reiss P, Portegies P, et al: Liposomal amphotericin B (AmBisome) compared with amphotericin B both followed by oral fluconazole in the treatment of AIDS-associated cryptococcal meningitis. AIDS 1997;11:1463–1471.

248. Joly V, Aubry P, Ndayiragide A, et al: Randomized comparison of amphotericin B deoxycholate dissolved in dextrose or Intralipid for the treatment of AIDS-associated cryptococcal meningitis. Clin Infect Dis 1996;23:556–562.

249. Polsky B, Depman MR, Gold JW, et al: Intraventricular therapy of cryptococcal meningitis via a subcutaneous reservoir. Am J Med 1986;81:24–28.

250. Bozzette SA, Larsen RA, Chiu J, et al: A placebo-controlled trial of maintenance therapy with fluconazole after treatment of cryptococcal meningitis in the acquired immunodeficiency syndrome. California Collaborative Treatment Group. N Engl J Med 1991;324:580–584.

251. Spitzer ED, Spitzer SG, Freundlich LF, Casadevall A: Persistence of initial infection in recurrent *Cryptococcus neoformans* meningitis. Lancet 1993;341:595–596.

252. Brandt ME, Pfaller MA, Hajjeh RA, et al: Molecular subtypes and antifungal susceptibilities of serial *Cryptococcus neoformans* isolates in human immunodeficiency virus–associated cryptococcosis. Cryptococcal Disease Active Surveillance Group. J Infect Dis 1996;174:812–820.

253. Powderly WG, Saag MS, Cloud GA, et al: A controlled trial of fluconazole or amphotericin B to prevent relapse of cryptococcal meningitis in patients with the acquired immunodeficiency syndrome. The NIAID AIDS Clinical Trials Group and Mycoses Study Group. N Engl J Med 1992;326:793–798.

254. Saag MS, Cloud GA, Graybill JR, et al: A comparison of itraconazole versus fluconazole as maintenance therapy for AIDS-associated cryptococcal meningitis. National Institute of Allergy and Infectious Diseases Mycoses Study Group. Clin Infect Dis 1999;28:291–296.

255. Saag MS, Graybill RJ, Larsen RA, et al: Practice guidelines for the management of cryptococcal disease. Infectious Diseases Society of America. Clin Infect Dis 2000;30:710–718.

256. Powderly WG, Cloud GA, Dismukes WE, Saag MS: Measurement of cryptococcal antigen in serum and cerebrospinal fluid: Value in the management of AIDS-associated cryptococcal meningitis. Clin Infect Dis 1994;18:789–792.

257. Denning DW, Armstrong RW, Lewis BH, Stevens DA: Elevated cerebrospinal fluid pressures in patients with cryptococcal meningitis and acquired immunodeficiency syndrome. Am J Med 1991;91:267–272.

258. Graybill JR, Sobel J, Saag M, et al: Diagnosis and management of increased intracranial pressure in patients with AIDS and cryptococcal meningitis. The NIAID Mycoses Study Group and AIDS Cooperative Treatment Groups. Clin Infect Dis 2000;30:47–54.

259. Quagliarello VJ, Viscoli C, Horwitz RI: Primary prevention of cryptococcal meningitis by fluconazole in HIV-infected patients. Lancet 1995;345:548–552.

260. Singh N, Barnish MJ, Berman S, et al: Low-dose fluconazole as primary prophylaxis for cryptococcal infection in AIDS patients with CD4 cell counts of ≤ 100/mm3: Demonstration of efficacy in a positive, multicenter trial. Clin Infect Dis 1996;23:1282–1286.

261. Wheat LJ, Connolly-Stringfield PA, Baker RL, et al: Disseminated histoplasmosis in the acquired immune deficiency syndrome: Clinical findings, diagnosis and treatment, and review of the literature. Medicine (Baltimore) 1990;69:361–374.

262. Wheat LJ, Cloud G, Johnson PC, et al: Clearance of fungal burden during treatment of disseminated histoplasmosis with liposomal amphotericin B versus itraconazole. Antimicrob Agents Chemother 2001;45:2354–2357.

263. Wheat J, Hafner R, Korzun AH, et al: Itraconazole treatment of disseminated histoplasmosis in patients with the acquired immunodeficiency syndrome. AIDS Clinical Trial Group. Am J Med 1995;98:336–342.

264. Wheat J, Sarosi G, McKinsey D, et al: Practice guidelines for the management of patients with histoplasmosis. Infectious Diseases Society of America. Clin Infect Dis 2000;30:688–695.

265. Wheat J, MaWhinney S, Hafner R, et al: Treatment of histoplasmosis with fluconazole in patients with acquired immunodeficiency syndrome. National Institute of Allergy and Infectious Diseases Acquired Immunodeficiency Syndrome

Clinical Trials Group and Mycoses Study Group. Am J Med 1997;103:223–232.

266. Wheat LJ, Connolly P, Smedema M, et al: Emergence of resistance to fluconazole as a cause of failure during treatment of histoplasmosis in patients with acquired immunodeficiency disease syndrome. Clin Infect Dis 2001;33:1910–1913.

267. McKinsey DS, Gupta MR, Driks MR, et al: Histoplasmosis in patients with AIDS: Efficacy of maintenance amphotericin B therapy. Am J Med 1992;92:225–227.

268. Wheat J, Hafner R, Wulfsohn M, et al: Prevention of relapse of histoplasmosis with itraconazole in patients with the acquired immunodeficiency syndrome. The National Institute of Allergy and Infectious Diseases Clinical Trials and Mycoses Study Group Collaborators. Ann Intern Med 1993;118:610–616.

269. Norris S, Wheat J, McKinsey D, et al: Prevention of relapse of histoplasmosis with fluconazole in patients with the acquired immunodeficiency syndrome. Am J Med 1994;96:504–508.

270. Hajjeh RA, Pappas PG, Henderson H, et al: Multicenter case-control study of risk factors for histoplasmosis in human immunodeficiency virus–infected persons. Clin Infect Dis 2001;32:1215–1220.

271. Stevens DA. Coccidioidomycosis. N Engl J Med 1995;332:1077–1082.

272. Singh VR, Smith DK, Lawerence J, et al: Coccidioidomycosis in patients infected with human immunodeficiency virus: Review of 91 cases at a single institution. Clin Infect Dis 1996;23:563–568.

273. Galgiani JN, Catanzaro A, Cloud GA, et al: Comparison of oral fluconazole and itraconazole for progressive, nonmeningeal coccidioidomycosis. A randomized, double-blind trial. Mycoses Study Group. Ann Intern Med 2000;133:676–686.

274. Galgiani JN, Ampel NM, Catanzaro A, et al: Practice guideline for the treatment of coccidioidomycosis. Infectious Diseases Society of America. Clin Infect Dis 2000;30:658–661.

275. Galgiani JN, Catanzaro A, Cloud GA, et al: Fluconazole therapy for coccidioidal meningitis. The NIAID-Mycoses Study Group. Ann Intern Med 1993;119:28–35.

276. Dewsnup DH, Galgiani JN, Graybill JR, et al: Is it ever safe to stop azole therapy for *Coccidioides immitis* meningitis? Ann Intern Med 1996;124:305–310.

277. Supparatpinyo K, Nelson KE, Merz WG, et al: Response to antifungal therapy by human immunodeficiency virus–infected patients with disseminated *Penicillium marneffei* infections and in vitro susceptibilities of isolates from clinical specimens. Antimicrob Agents Chemother 1993;37:2407–2411.

278. Sirisanthana T, Supparatpinyo K, Perriens J, Nelson KE: Amphotericin B and itraconazole for treatment of disseminated *Penicillium marneffei* infection in human immunodeficiency virus–infected patients. Clin Infect Dis 1998;26:1107–1110.

279. Supparatpinyo K, Perriens J, Nelson KE, Sirisanthana T: A controlled trial of itraconazole to prevent relapse of *Penicillium marneffei* infection in patients infected with the human immunodeficiency virus. N Engl J Med 1998;339:1739–1743.

280. Chariyalertsak S, Supparatpinyo K, Sirisanthana T, Nelson KE: A controlled trial of itraconazole as primary prophylaxis for systemic fungal infections in patients with advanced human immunodeficiency virus infection in Thailand. Clin Infect Dis 2002;34:277–284.

281. Pappas PG, Pottage JC, Powderly WG, et al: Blastomycosis in patients with the acquired immunodeficiency syndrome. Ann Intern Med 1992;116:847–853.

282. Goldani LZ, Sugar AM: Paracoccidioidomycosis and AIDS: An overview. Clin Infect Dis 1995;21:1275–1281.

283. Penn CC, Goldstein E, Bartholomew WR: *Sporothrix schenckii* meningitis in a patient with AIDS. Clin Infect Dis 1992;15:741–743.

284. Cunliffe NA, Denning DW: Uncommon invasive mycoses in AIDS. AIDS 1995;9:411–420.

285. Perfect JR, Schell WA: The new fungal opportunists are coming. Clin Infect Dis 1996;22(Suppl 2):S112–S118.

286. Denning DW, Lee JY, Hostetler JS, et al: NIAID Mycoses Study Group Multicenter Trial of Oral Itraconazole Therapy for Invasive Aspergillosis. Am J Med 1994;97:135–144.

287. Khoo SH, Denning DW: Invasive aspergillosis in patients with AIDS. Clin Infect Dis 1994;19(Suppl 1):S41–S48.

288. Caillot D, Bassaris H, McGeer A, et al: Intravenous itraconazole followed by oral itraconazole in the treatment of invasive pulmonary aspergillosis in patients with hematologic malignancies, chronic granulomatous disease, or AIDS. Clin Infect Dis 2001;33:E83–E90.

289. Keating GM, Jarvis B: Caspofungin. Drugs 2001;61:1121–1129.

290. Patterson TF, Kirkpatrick WR, White M, et al: Invasive aspergillosis. Disease spectrum, treatment practices, and outcomes. I3 Aspergillus Study Group. Medicine (Baltimore) 2000;79:250–260.

291. Gallant JE, Moore RD, Richman DD, et al: Incidence and natural history of cytomegalovirus disease in patients with advanced human immunodeficiency virus disease treated with zidovudine. The Zidovudine Epidemiology Study Group. J Infect Dis 1992;166:1223–1227.

292. Goodgame RW: Gastrointestinal cytomegalovirus disease. Ann Intern Med 1993;119:924–935.

293. Salomon N, Gomez T, Perlman DC, et al: Clinical features and outcomes of HIV-related cytomegalovirus pneumonia. AIDS 1997;11:319–324.

294. Bozzette SA, Arcia J, Bartok AE, et al: Impact of *Pneumocystis carinii* and cytomegalovirus on the course and outcome of atypical pneumonia in advanced human immunodeficiency virus disease. J Infect Dis 1992;165:93–98.

295. McCutchan JA: Cytomegalovirus infections of the nervous system in patients with AIDS. Clin Infect Dis 1995;20:747–754.

296. Spector SA, Wong R, Hsia K, et al: Plasma cytomegalovirus (CMV) DNA load predicts CMV disease and survival in AIDS patients. J Clin Invest 1998;101:497–502.

297. Spector SA, Weingeist T, Pollard RB, et al: A randomized, controlled study of intravenous ganciclovir therapy for cytomegalovirus peripheral retinitis in patients with AIDS. AIDS Clinical Trials Group and Cytomegalovirus Cooperative Study Group. J Infect Dis 1993;168:557–563.

298. Combination foscarnet and ganciclovir therapy vs monotherapy for the treatment of relapsed cytomegalovirus retinitis in patients with AIDS. The Cytomegalovirus Retreatment Trial. The Studies of Ocular Complications of AIDS Research Group in Collaboration with the AIDS Clinical Trials Group. Arch Ophthalmol 1996;114:23–33.

299. Dieterich DT, Kotler DP, Busch DF, et al: Ganciclovir treatment of cytomegalovirus colitis in AIDS: A randomized, double-blind, placebo-controlled multicenter study. J Infect Dis 1993;167:278–282.

300. Blanshard C, Benhamou Y, Dohin E, et al: Treatment of AIDS-associated gastrointestinal cytomegalovirus infection with foscarnet and ganciclovir: A randomized comparison. J Infect Dis 1995;172:622–628.

301. Rodriguez-Barradas MC, Stool E, Musher DM, et al: Diagnosing and treating cytomegalovirus pneumonia in patients with AIDS. Clin Infect Dis 1996;23:76–81.

302. Mortality in patients with the acquired immunodeficiency syndrome treated with either foscarnet or ganciclovir for cytomegalovirus retinitis. Studies of Ocular Complications of AIDS Research Group, in collaboration with the AIDS Clinical Trials Group. N Engl J Med 1992;326:213–220.

303. Foscarnet-Ganciclovir Cytomegalovirus Retinitis Trial. 4. Visual outcomes. Studies of Ocular Complications of AIDS Research Group in collaboration with the AIDS Clinical Trials Group. Ophthalmology 1994;101:1250–1261.

304. Lalezari JP, Stagg RJ, Kuppermann BD, et al: Intravenous cidofovir for peripheral cytomegalovirus retinitis in patients with AIDS. A randomized, controlled trial. Ann Intern Med 1997;126:257–263.

305. Parenteral cidofovir for cytomegalovirus retinitis in patients with AIDS: The HPMPC peripheral cytomegalovirus retinitis trial. A randomized, controlled trial. Studies of Ocular Complications of AIDS Research Group in Collaboration with the AIDS Clinical Trials Group. Ann Intern Med 1997;126:264–274.

306. Davis JL, Taskintuna I, Freeman WR, et al: Iritis and hypotony after treatment with intravenous cidofovir for cytomegalovirus retinitis. Arch Ophthalmol 1997;115:733–737.

307. Drew WL, Ives D, Lalezari JP, et al: Oral ganciclovir as maintenance treatment for cytomegalovirus retinitis in patients with AIDS. Syntex Cooperative Oral Ganciclovir Study Group. N Engl J Med 1995;333:615–620.

308. Lalezari JP, Friedberg DN, Bissett J, et al: High dose oral ganciclovir treatment for cytomegalovirus retinitis. J Clin Virol 2002;24:67–77.

309. Curran M, Noble S. Valganciclovir. Drugs 2001;61:1145–1150.

310. Erice A, Chou S, Biron KK, et al: Progressive disease due to ganciclovir-resistant cytomegalovirus in immunocompromised patients. N Engl J Med 1989;320:289–293.

311. Erice A, Gil-Roda C, Perez JL, et al: Antiviral susceptibilities and analysis of UL97 and DNA polymerase sequences of clinical cytomegalovirus isolates from immunocompromised patients. J Infect Dis 1997;175:1087–1092.

312. Lalezari JP, Holland GN, Kramer F, et al: Randomized, controlled study of the safety and efficacy of intravenous cidofovir for the treatment of relapsing cytomegalovirus retinitis in patients with AIDS. J Acquir Immune Defic Syndr Hum Retrovirol 1998;17:339–344.

313. Jacobson MA, Wilson S, Stanley H, et al: Phase I study of combination therapy with intravenous cidofovir and oral ganciclovir for cytomegalovirus retinitis in patients with AIDS. Clin Infect Dis 1999;28:528–533.

314. Cochereau-Massin I, LeHoang P, Lautier-Frau M, et al: Efficacy and tolerance of intravitreal ganciclovir in cytomegalovirus retinitis in acquired immune deficiency syndrome. Ophthalmology 1991;98:1348–1353.

315. Musch DC, Martin DF, Gordon JF, et al: Treatment of cytomegalovirus retinitis with a sustained-release ganciclovir implant. The Ganciclovir Implant Study Group. N Engl J Med 1997;337:83–90.

316. Diaz-Llopis M, Espana E, Munoz G, et al: High dose intravitreal foscarnet in the treatment of cytomegalovirus retinitis in AIDS. Br J Ophthalmol 1994;78:120–124.

317. Rahhal FM, Arevalo JF, Chavez dlP, et al: Treatment of cytomegalovirus retinitis with intravitreous cidofovir in patients with AIDS. A preliminary report. Ann Intern Med 1996;125:98–103.

318. Martin DF, Kuppermann BD, Wolitz RA, et al: Oral ganciclovir for patients with cytomegalovirus retinitis treated with a ganciclovir implant. Roche Ganciclovir Study Group. N Engl J Med 1999;340:1063–1070.

319. The ganciclovir implant plus oral ganciclovir versus parenteral cidofovir for the treatment of cytomegalovirus retinitis in patients with acquired immunodeficiency syndrome: The Ganciclovir Cidofovir Cytomegalovirus Retinitis Trial. Am J Ophthalmol 2001;131:457–467.

320. Martin DF, Dunn JP, Davis JL, et al: Use of the ganciclovir implant for the treatment of cytomegalovirus retinitis in the era of potent antiretroviral therapy: Recommendations of the International AIDS Society–USA panel. Am J Ophthalmol 1999;127:329–339.

321. Whitcup SM, Fortin E, Lindblad AS, et al: Discontinuation of anticytomegalovirus therapy in patients with HIV infection and cytomegalovirus retinitis. JAMA 1999;282:1633–1637.

322. Macdonald JC, Torriani FJ, Morse LS, et al: Lack of reactivation of cytomegalovirus (CMV) retinitis after stopping CMV maintenance therapy in AIDS patients with sustained elevations in CD4 T cells in response to highly active antiretroviral therapy. J Infect Dis 1998;177:1182–1187.

323. Jabs DA, Bolton SG, Dunn JP, Palestine AG: Discontinuing anticytomegalovirus therapy in patients with immune reconstitution after combination antiretroviral therapy. Am J Ophthalmol 1998;126:817–822.

324. Jouan M, Saves M, Tubiana R, et al: Discontinuation of maintenance therapy for cytomegalovirus retinitis in HIV-infected patients receiving highly active antiretroviral therapy. AIDS 2001;15:23–31.

325. Berenguer J, Gonzalez J, Pulido F, et al: Discontinuation of secondary prophylaxis in patients with cytomegalovirus retinitis who have responded to highly active antiretroviral therapy. Clin Infect Dis 2002;34:394–397.

326. Whitcup SM: Cytomegalovirus retinitis in the era of highly active antiretroviral therapy. JAMA 2000;283:653–657.

327. Spector SA, McKinley GF, Lalezari JP, et al: Oral ganciclovir for the prevention of cytomegalovirus disease in persons with AIDS. Roche Cooperative Oral Ganciclovir Study Group. N Engl J Med 1996;334:1491–1497.

328. Brosgart CL, Louis TA, Hillman DW, et al: A randomized, placebo-controlled trial of the safety and efficacy of oral ganciclovir for prophylaxis of cytomegalovirus disease in HIV-infected individuals. Terry Beirn Community Programs for Clinical Research on AIDS. AIDS 1998;12:269–277.

329. Safrin S, Ashley R, Houlihan C, et al: Clinical and serologic features of herpes simplex virus infection in patients with AIDS. AIDS 1991;5:1107–1110.

330. Augenbraun M, Feldman J, Chirgwin K, et al: Increased genital shedding of herpes simplex virus type 2 in HIV-seropositive women. Ann Intern Med 1995;123:845–847.

331. Erlich KS, Mills J, Chatis P, et al: Acyclovir-resistant herpes simplex virus infections in patients with the acquired immunodeficiency syndrome. N Engl J Med 1989;320:293–296.

332. Safrin S, Crumpacker C, Chatis P, et al: A controlled trial comparing foscarnet with vidarabine for acyclovir-resistant mucocutaneous herpes simplex in the acquired immunodeficiency syndrome. The AIDS Clinical Trials Group. N Engl J Med 1991;325:551–555.

333. Leibovitz E, Cooper D, Giurgiutiu D, et al: Varicella-zoster virus infection in Romanian children infected with the human immunodeficiency virus. Pediatrics 1993;92:838–842.

334. Glesby MJ, Moore RD, Chaisson RE: Clinical spectrum of herpes zoster in adults infected with human immunodeficiency virus. Clin Infect Dis 1995;21:370–375.

335. Jacobson MA, Berger TG, Fikrig S, et al: Acyclovir-resistant varicella zoster virus infection after chronic oral acyclovir therapy in patients with the acquired immunodeficiency syndrome (AIDS). Ann Intern Med 1990;112:187–191.

336. Linnemann CC Jr, Biron KK, Hoppenjans WG, Solinger AM: Emergence of acyclovir-resistant varicella zoster virus in an AIDS patient on prolonged acyclovir therapy. AIDS 1990;4:577–579.

337. Safrin S, Berger TG, Gilson I, et al: Foscarnet therapy in five patients with AIDS and acyclovir-resistant varicella-zoster virus infection. Ann Intern Med 1991;115:19–21.

338. Resnick L, Herbst JS, Ablashi DV, et al: Regression of oral hairy leukoplakia after orally administered acyclovir therapy. JAMA 1988;259:384–388.

339. Spira TJ, Bozeman LH, Sanderlin KC, et al: Lack of correlation between human herpesvirus-6 infection and the course of human immunodeficiency virus infection. J Infect Dis 1990;161:567–570.

340. Di Luca D, Mirandola P, Ravaioli T, et al: Human herpesviruses 6 and 7 in salivary glands and shedding in saliva of healthy and human immunodeficiency virus positive individuals. J Med Virol 1995;45:462–468.

341. Morfeldt L, Torssander J: Long-term remission of Kaposi's sarcoma following foscarnet treatment in HIV-infected patients. Scand J Infect Dis 1994;26:749–752.

342. Dupont C, Vasseur E, Beauchet A, et al: Long-term efficacy on Kaposi's sarcoma of highly active antiretroviral therapy in a cohort of HIV-positive patients. CISIH 92. Centre d'information et de soins de l'immunodeficience humaine. AIDS 2000;14:987–993.

343. Wright TC Jr, Ellerbrock TV, Chiasson MA, et al: Cervical intraepithelial neoplasia in women infected with human immunodeficiency virus: Prevalence, risk factors, and validity of Papanicolaou smears. New York Cervical Disease Study. Obstet Gynecol 1994;84:591–597.

344. Sun XW, Kuhn L, Ellerbrock TV, et al: Human papillomavirus infection in women infected with the human immunodeficiency virus. N Engl J Med 1997;337:1343–1349.

345. Ellerbrock TV, Chiasson MA, Bush TJ, et al: Incidence of cervical squamous intraepithelial lesions in HIV-infected women. JAMA 2000;283:1031–1037.

346. Goldie SJ, Kuntz KM, Weinstein MC, et al: The clinical effectiveness and cost-effectiveness of screening for anal squamous intraepithelial lesions in homosexual and bisexual HIV-positive men. JAMA 1999;281:1822–1829.

347. Palefsky JM, Holly EA, Hogeboom CJ, et al: Anal cytology as a screening tool for anal squamous intraepithelial lesions. J Acquir Immune Defic Syndr Hum Retrovirol 1997;14:415–422.

348. Dienstag JL, Schiff ER, Wright TL, et al: Lamivudine as initial treatment for chronic hepatitis B in the United States. N Engl J Med 1999;341:1256–1263.

349. Bessesen M, Ives D, Condreay L, et al: Chronic active hepatitis B exacerbations in human immunodeficiency virus–infected patients following development of resistance to or withdrawal of lamivudine. Clin Infect Dis 1999;28:1032–1035.

350. Landau A, Batisse D, Piketty C, et al: Long-term efficacy of combination therapy with interferon-alpha2b and ribavirin for severe chronic hepatitis C in HIV-infected patients. AIDS 2001;15:2149–2155.

351. Hall CD, Dafni U, Simpson D, et al: Failure of cytarabine in progressive multifocal leukoencephalopathy associated with human immunodeficiency virus infection. AIDS Clinical Trials Group 243 Team. N Engl J Med 1998;338:1345–1351.

352. De Luca A, Giancola ML, Ammassari A, et al: Cidofovir added to HAART improves virological and clinical outcome in AIDS-associated progressive multifocal leukoencephalopathy. AIDS 2000;14:F117–F121.

353. De Luca A, Giancola ML, Ammassari A, et al: Potent antiretroviral therapy with or without cidofovir for AIDS-associated progressive multifocal leukoencephalopathy: Extended follow-up of an observational study. J Neurovirol 2001;7:364–368.

354. Tantisiriwat W, Tebas P, Clifford DB, et al: Progressive multifocal leukoencephalopathy in patients with AIDS receiving highly active antiretroviral therapy. Clin Infect Dis 1999;28:1152–1154.

355. Clifford DB, Yiannoutsos C, Glicksman M, et al: HAART improves prognosis in HIV-associated progressive multifocal leukoencephalopathy. Neurology 1999;52:623–625.

356. Albrecht H, Hoffmann C, Degen O, et al: Highly active antiretroviral therapy significantly improves the prognosis of patients with HIV-associated progressive multifocal leukoencephalopathy. AIDS 1998;12:1149–1154.

357. Cohn JA, McMeeking A, Cohen W, et al: Evaluation of the policy of empiric treatment of suspected *Toxoplasma* encephalitis in patients with the acquired immunodeficiency syndrome. Am J Med 1989;86:521–527.

358. Leport C, Raffi F, Matheron S, et al: Treatment of central nervous system toxoplasmosis with pyrimethamine/sulfadiazine combination in 35 patients with the acquired immunodeficiency syndrome. Efficacy of long-term continuous therapy. Am J Med 1988;84:94–100.

359. Luft BJ, Brooks RG, Conley FK, et al: Toxoplasmic encephalitis in patients with acquired immune deficiency syndrome. JAMA 1984;252:913–917.

360. Porter SB, Sande MA: Toxoplasmosis of the central nervous system in the acquired immunodeficiency syndrome. N Engl J Med 1992;327:1643–1648.

361. Haverkos HW. Assessment of therapy for *Toxoplasma* encephalitis. The TE Study Group. Am J Med 1987;82:907–914.

362. Sahai J, Heimberger T, Collins K, et al: Sulfadiazine-induced crystalluria in a patient with the acquired immunodeficiency syndrome: A reminder. Am J Med 1988;84:791–792.

363. Reboli AC, Mandler HD: Encephalopathy and psychoses associated with sulfadiazine in two patients with AIDS and CNS toxoplasmosis. Clin Infect Dis 1992;15:556–557.

364. Simon DI, Brosius FC III, Rothstein DM: Sulfadiazine crystalluria revisited. The treatment of *Toxoplasma* encephalitis in patients with acquired immunodeficiency syndrome. Arch Intern Med 1990;150:2379–2384.

365. Molina JM, Belenfant X, Doco-Lecompte T, et al: Sulfadiazine-induced crystalluria in AIDS patients with *Toxoplasma* encephalitis. AIDS 1991;5:587–589.

366. Foppa CU, Bini T, Gregis G, et al: A retrospective study of primary and maintenance therapy of toxoplasmic encephalitis with oral clindamycin and pyrimethamine. Eur J Clin Microbiol Infect Dis 1991;10:187–189.

367. Dannemann BR, Israelski DM, Remington JS: Treatment of toxoplasmic encephalitis with intravenous clindamycin. Arch Intern Med 1988;148:2477–2482.

368. Katlama C, De Wit S, O'Doherty E, et al: Pyrimethamine-clindamycin vs. pyrimethamine-sulfadiazine as acute and long-term therapy for toxoplasmic encephalitis in patients with AIDS. Clin Infect Dis 1996;22:268–275.

369. Araujo FG, Guptill DR, Remington JS: Azithromycin, a macrolide antibiotic with potent activity against *Toxoplasma gondii*. Antimicrob Agents Chemother 1988;32:755–757.

370. Huskinson-Mark J, Araujo FG, Remington JS: Evaluation of the effect of drugs on the cyst form of *Toxoplasma gondii*. J Infect Dis 1991;164:170–171.

371. Araujo FG, Khan AA, Slifer TL, et al: The ketolide antibiotics HMR 3647 and HMR 3004 are active against *Toxoplasma gondii* in vitro and in murine models of infection. Antimicrob Agents Chemother 1997;41:2137–2140.

372. Luft BJ: In vivo and in vitro activity of roxithromycin against *Toxoplasma gondii* in mice. Eur J Clin Microbiol 1987;6:479–481.

373. Fernandez-Martin J, Leport C, Morlat P, et al: Pyrimethamine-clarithromycin combination for therapy of acute *Toxoplasma* encephalitis in patients with AIDS. Antimicrob Agents Chemother 1991;35:2049–2052.

374. Raffi F, Struillou L, Ninin E, et al: Breakthrough cerebral toxoplasmosis in patients with AIDS who are being treated with clarithromycin. Clin Infect Dis 1995;20:1076–1077.

375. Farthing C, Rendel M, Currie B, Seidlin M: Azithromycin for cerebral toxoplasmosis. Lancet 1992;339:437–438.

376. Jacobson JM, Hafner R, Remington J, et al: Dose-escalation, phase I/II study of azithromycin and pyrimethamine for the treatment of toxoplasmic encephalitis in AIDS. AIDS 2001;15:583–589.

377. Araujo FG, Huskinson J, Remington JS: Remarkable in vitro and in vivo activities of the hydroxynaphthoquinone 566C80 against tachyzoites and tissue cysts of *Toxoplasma gondii*. Antimicrob Agents Chemother 1991;35:293–299.

378. Kovacs JA: Efficacy of atovaquone in treatment of toxoplasmosis in patients with AIDS. The NIAID-Clinical Center Intramural AIDS Program. Lancet 1992;340:637–638.

379. Torres RA, Weinberg W, Stansell J, et al: Atovaquone for salvage treatment and suppression of toxoplasmic encephalitis in patients with AIDS. Atovaquone/Toxoplasmic Encephalitis Study Group. Clin Infect Dis 1997;24:422–429.

380. Katlama C, Mouthon B, Gourdon D, et al: Atovaquone as long-term suppressive therapy for toxoplasmic encephalitis in patients with AIDS and multiple drug intolerance. Atovaquone Expanded Access Group. AIDS 1996;10:1107–1112.

381. Allegra CJ, Boarman D, Kovacs JA, et al: Interaction of sulfonamide and sulfone compounds with *Toxoplasma gondii* dihydropteroate synthase. J Clin Invest 1990;85:371–379.

382. Derouin F, Piketty C, Chastang C, et al: Anti-*Toxoplasma* effects of dapsone alone and combined with pyrimethamine. Antimicrob Agents Chemother 1991;35:252–255.

383. Morris JT, Kelly JW: Effective treatment of cerebral toxoplasmosis with doxycycline. Am J Med 1992;93:107–108.

384. Masur H, Polis MA, Tuazon CU, et al: Salvage trial of trimetrexate-leucovorin for the treatment of cerebral toxoplasmosis in patients with AIDS. J Infect Dis 1993;167:1422–1426.

385. Lindsay DS, Blagburn BL, Hall JE, Tidwell RR: Activity of pentamidine and pentamidine analogs against *Toxoplasma gondii* in cell cultures. Antimicrob Agents Chemother 1991;35:1914–1916.

386. Luft BJ, Hafner R, Korzun AH, et al: Toxoplasmic encephalitis in patients with the acquired immunodeficiency syndrome. Members of the ACTG 077p/ANRS 009 Study Team. N Engl J Med 1993;329:995–1000.

387. Miro JM, Lopez JC, Podzamczer D, et al: Discontinuation of toxoplasmic encephalitis prophylaxis is safe in HIV-1- and *T. gondii*-coinfected patients after immunologic recovery with HAART. 7th Conference on Retroviruses and Opportunistic Infections. Abstract 230. 2000.

388. Guex AC, Radziwill AJ, Bucher HC. Discontinuation of secondary prophylaxis for toxoplasmic encephalitis in human immunodeficiency virus infection after immune restoration with highly active antiretroviral therapy. Clin Infect Dis 2000;30:602–603.

389. Antinori A, Murri R, Ammassari A, et al: Aerosolized pentamidine, cotrimoxazole and dapsone-pyrimethamine for primary prophylaxis of *Pneumocystis carinii* pneumonia and toxoplasmic encephalitis. AIDS 1995;9:1343–1350.

390. Podzamczer D, Salazar A, Jimenez J, et al: Intermittent trimethoprim-sulfamethoxazole compared with dapsone-pyrimethamine for the simultaneous primary prophylaxis of *Pneumocystis* pneumonia and toxoplasmosis in patients infected with HIV. Ann Intern Med 1995;122:755–761.

391. Jacobson MA, Besch CL, Child C, et al: Primary prophylaxis with pyrimethamine for toxoplasmic encephalitis in patients with advanced human immunodeficiency virus disease: Results of a randomized trial. Terry Beirn Community Programs for Clinical Research on AIDS. J Infect Dis 1994;169:384–394.

392. Leport C, Chene G, Morlat P, et al: Pyrimethamine for primary prophylaxis of toxoplasmic encephalitis in patients with human immunodeficiency virus infection: A double-blind, randomized trial. ANRS 005-ACTG 154 Group Members. Agence Nationale de Recherche sur le SIDA. AIDS Clinical Trial Group. J Infect Dis 1996;173:91–97.

393. Remington JS, Vilde JL: Clindamycin for toxoplasma encephalitis in AIDS. Lancet 1991;338:1142–1143.

394. Jacobson MA, Besch CL, Child C, et al: Toxicity of clindamycin as prophylaxis for AIDS-associated toxoplasmic encephalitis. Community Programs for Clinical Research on AIDS. Lancet 1992;339:333–334.

395. Furrer H, Opravil M, Bernasconi E, et al: Stopping primary prophylaxis in HIV-1-infected patients at high risk of *Toxoplasma* encephalitis. Swiss HIV Cohort Study. Lancet 2000;355:2217–2218.

396. Conteas CN, Berlin OG, Ash LR, Pruthi JS: Therapy for human gastrointestinal microsporidiosis. Am J Trop Med Hyg 2000;63:121–127.

397. Molina JM, Chastang C, Goguel J, et al: Albendazole for treatment and prophylaxis of microsporidiosis due to *Encephalitozoon intestinalis* in patients with AIDS: A randomized double-blind controlled trial. J Infect Dis 1998;177:1373–1377.

398. Carr A, Marriott D, Field A, et al: Treatment of HIV-1-associated microsporidiosis and cryptosporidiosis with combination antiretroviral therapy. Lancet 1998;351:256–261.

399. Maggi P, Larocca AM, Quarto M, et al: Effect of antiretroviral therapy on cryptosporidiosis and microsporidiosis in patients infected with human immunodeficiency virus type 1. Eur J Clin Microbiol Infect Dis 2000;19:213–217.

400. Goodgame RW: Understanding intestinal spore-forming protozoa: Cryptosporidia, microsporidia, isospora, and cyclospora. Ann Intern Med 1996;124:429–441.

401. Hewitt RG, Yiannoutsos CT, Higgs ES, et al: Paromomycin: No more effective than placebo for treatment of cryptosporidiosis in patients with advanced human immunodeficiency virus infection. AIDS Clinical Trial Group. Clin Infect Dis 2000;31:1084–1092.

402. White AC Jr, Chappell CL, Hayat CS, et al: Paromomycin for cryptosporidiosis in AIDS: A prospective, double-blind trial. J Infect Dis 1994;170:419–424.

403. Flanigan TP, Soave R: Cryptosporidiosis. Prog Clin Parasitol 1993;3:1–20.

404. Rossignol JF, Ayoub A, Ayers MS: Treatment of diarrhea caused by *Cryptosporidium parvum*: A prospective randomized, double-blind, placebo-controlled study of nitazoxanide. J Infect Dis 2001;184:103–106.

405. Okhuysen PC, Chappell CL, Crabb J, et al: Prophylactic effect of bovine anti-*Cryptosporidium* hyperimmune colostrum immunoglobulin in healthy volunteers challenged with *Cryptosporidium parvum*. Clin Infect Dis 1998;26:1324–1329.

406. Greenberg PD, Cello JP: Treatment of severe diarrhea caused by *Cryptosporidium parvum* with oral bovine immunoglobulin concentrate in patients with AIDS. J Acquir Immune Defic Syndr Hum Retrovirol 1996;13:348–354.

407. Simon DM, Cello JP, Valenzuela J, et al: Multicenter trial of octreotide in patients with refractory acquired immunodeficiency syndrome–associated diarrhea. Gastroenterology 1995;108:1753–1760.

408. DeHovitz JA, Pape JW, Boncy M, et al: Clinical manifestations and therapy of *Isospora belli* infection in patients with the acquired immunodeficiency syndrome. N Engl J Med 1986;315:87–90.

409. Pape JW, Verdier RI, Johnson WD Jr: Treatment and prophylaxis of *Isospora belli* infection in patients with the acquired immunodeficiency syndrome. N Engl J Med 1989;320:1044–1047.

410. Pape JW, Verdier RI, Boncy M, et al: *Cyclospora* infection in adults infected with HIV. Clinical manifestations, treatment, and prophylaxis. Ann Intern Med 1994;121:654–657.

411. Cotte L, Rabodonirina M, Piens MA, et al: Prevalence of intestinal protozoans in French patients infected with HIV. J Acquir Immune Defic Syndr 1993;6:1024–1029.

412. Jessurun J, Barron-Rodriguez LP, Fernandez-Tinoco G, Hernandez-Avila M: The prevalence of invasive amebiasis is not increased in patients with AIDS. AIDS 1992;6:307–309.

413. Allason-Jones E, Mindel A, Sargeaunt P, Williams P: *Entamoeba histolytica* as a commensal intestinal parasite in homosexual men. N Engl J Med 1986;315:353–356.

414. DeSimone JA, Pomerantz RJ, Babinchack TJ: Inflammatory reactions in HIV-1-infected persons after initiation of highly active antiretroviral therapy. Ann Intern Med 2000; 133:447–454.

415. Ledergerber B, Egger M, Erard V, et al: AIDS-related opportunistic illnesses occurring after initiation of potent antiretroviral therapy: The Swiss HIV Cohort Study. J Infect Dis 1999;282:2220–2226.

416. Furrer H, Malinverni R: Systemic inflammatory reaction after starting HAART in AIDS patients treated for extrapulmonary tuberculosis. Am J Med 1999;106:371–372.

chapter
31

Tuberculosis Treatment: Theory and Practice

C. ROBERT HORSBURGH JR., MD

WILLIAM J. BURMAN, MD

GENERAL PRINCIPLES

Active Tuberculosis Disease and Latent Tuberculosis Infection

After exposure to *Mycobacterium tuberculosis*, a person either escapes infection or becomes infected. This primary infection may progress to symptomatic tuberculosis (active TB), or the host immune response may control the infection, leading to a condition known as latent tuberculosis infection (LTBI).

TB that becomes active soon after the organism is acquired is called *primary* (active) *TB*. Primary TB usually begins as a pulmonary process and then undergoes a brief period of hematogenous dissemination. The initial site (most commonly the lung) may heal spontaneously, with subsequent appearance of disease anywhere else in the body and occasionally in multiple sites. If primary active TB is controlled by the host and progresses to the latent state, the host continues to harbor viable tubercle bacilli but is not ill. It is estimated that roughly 95% of persons with normal immunity who become infected with *M. tuberculosis* do not become ill but progress asymptomatically to the latent state. Over a period of months to decades the latent state may reactivate, with the appearance of clinical disease; this condition is called *reactivation* (active) *TB*. The factors that lead to reactivation tuberculosis are not completely understood, but any condition that depresses cellular immunity, such as human immunodeficiency virus (HIV) infection, cancer, therapy with immunosuppressive agents, or malnutrition increases the risk of reactivation. Most patients in whom reactivation TB develops do not have recognized immunologic deficits; nonetheless among patients with reactivation TB who have recognized immunologic deficits, HIV infection is by far the most common cause. Immunocompetent persons with latent TB have a 10% lifetime risk that the reactivation TB will develop. HIV-infected persons who have latent TB have a *yearly* risk of reactivation of 5% to 10%, however, without effective antiretroviral therapy.

Most cases of active TB in the United States occur within 1 to 2 years after exposure to *M. tuberculosis*. From a diagnostic and therapeutic perspective the distinction between primary and reactivation TB is not so important, as primary and reactivation TB are for the most part clinically indistinguishable.

Diagnosis of Active Tuberculosis

Most patients are symptomatic, but some may be minimally so. Symptoms may be protean and localize to any part of the body. Thus it is essential to obtain cultures from any suspected site. Roughly 80% of patients with active TB in the United States have TB pneumonia.[1] Other less commonly involved sites include lymph node (7.4%), pleura (4.1%), bone and joint (2.1%), genitourinary (1.2%), and central nervous system (1%). *M. tuberculosis* does not colonize man and is not found in the environment. Therefore a culture from any site that reveals *M. tuberculosis* indicates active TB (the only exception being laboratory cross-contamination, see Diagnosis of Active Tuberculosis). Disseminated disease is defined as active TB in more than one discrete location or organ system. This condition is more common among HIV-infected persons with TB, and all HIV-infected persons with localized disease should have a blood culture for *M. tuberculosis* performed in addition to other diagnostic tests.

Obtaining cultures and susceptibility testing are essential for adequate management of the tuberculosis patient.[2,3] The Centers for Disease Control and Prevention (CDC) recommend that all patient isolates be tested for susceptibility to the first-line TB drugs (see antimycobacterial agents and Toxicities). A qualified laboratory should be able to perform such testing and return results to the clinician within 6 weeks of obtaining the culture. The clinician should ensure that specimens are sent to a laboratory with adequate experience and quality control in culturing and identifying *M. tuberculosis*.

Obtaining susceptibility testing results and adjusting the regimen on the basis of the findings are essential to adequate management of the TB patient. Ideally, susceptibilities are ordered on the initial isolate. Since cultures may remain positive for the first several weeks of therapy, however, additional cultures should be obtained for susceptibility testing during this period if such testing was not obtained initially. Because *M. tuberculosis* remains viable on laboratory plates for many weeks to months and most laboratories keep these plates for several months, previous cultures may also be retrieved for susceptibility testing if this was not performed.

When TB is diagnosed in children who are unable to produce a sputum sample, the susceptibility testing of samples from associated adult cases should be used as a guide to therapy. It is not necessary with follow-up cultures to have susceptibility testing performed unless there is clinical or laboratory evidence of failure or relapse. In the event of either of these the laboratory should be informed and a request made for repeat susceptibility testing of the new isolate.

When cultures have not been obtained or isolates fail to grow, the diagnosis of active TB may be made on clinical grounds, but this is less reliable. An algorithm for making such a diagnosis is shown in Table 31–1. The following should be obtained: chest radiograph, smears for acid-fast bacilli, tuberculin skin test, and history of exposure to a person with active TB.[2] It should be noted that the tuberculin skin test is useful if positive, but a negative skin test does not exclude the possibility of

TABLE 31–1 ■ Criteria for Definitive Diagnosis of Active Tuberculosis

1. Signs, symptoms, and chest radiograph (for pulmonary site)
   AND
   Culture or nucleic acid amplification test of *Mycobacterium tuberculosis*
   OR
2. Signs, symptoms and chest radiograph (for pulmonary site)
   AND
   Smear positive for acid-fast bacilli, or histologic evidence of granuloma, or positive purified protein derivative (PPD) skin test
   AND
   Clinical improvement with antituberculosis treatment

active TB; up to 25% of persons with active TB do not respond to a tuberculin skin test when they are first seen (although most become positive after being placed on therapy).

Even when TB is suspected on clinical grounds, a diagnosis in the absence of culture confirmation requires that other potential causes of the clinical syndrome be excluded and the response to a course of antituberculosis therapy be evaluated. Thus when culture confirmation is not available, a patient may be a suspected case of TB for as long as 3 months. Even when these criteria are applied, persons with nontuberculous mycobacterial disease may mistakenly be considered to have tuberculosis when cultures are not available.

In addition, evaluation of previous chest radiographs is required to determine if apparent disease in the absence of culture is active and requires treatment or is old healed disease. Old healed disease that has received a full course of treatment does not need further attention, but old healed disease that has not been treated is a form of latent TB and requires treatment for latent TB (see Treatment of Latent Tuberculosis).

A positive culture for *M. tuberculosis* in a patient without clinical signs and symptoms of TB or for whom there is another explanation for the clinical presentation (e.g., bacterial pneumonia) should be carefully evaluated for the possibility of laboratory cross-contamination. Even in laboratories with reasonable experience in processing and identifying *M. tuberculosis*, contamination occurs in 3% to 5% of positive cultures; in less experienced laboratories the rate of false-positive cultures can be as high as 30%.[4] When the clinical situation raises doubt that a positive culture represents active TB, several steps can be taken to help identify a false-positive culture for *M. tuberculosis*: obtain additional cultures (these may be positive even if the patient has been on therapy for several weeks), consult with the laboratory to determine the rate of growth on culture plates (growth of only a few colonies further raises suspicion of contamination), and order molecular typing of *M. tuberculosis* isolates processed at the same laboratory on the same day as the suspect isolate (isolates matching those from a confirmed TB case are diagnostic of cross-contamination). Investing energy in determining whether a suspect culture result represents contamination can prevent unnecessary diagnostic tests, treatment costs, toxicity of antituberculosis agents, and public health evaluation of persons exposed to the index case.

Diagnosis of Latent Tuberculosis Infection

Persons with latent TB are asymptomatic, and latent TB can only be detected by evidence of immune sensitization to *M. tuberculosis*. This is established by tuberculin skin testing with *M. tuberculosis* purified protein derivative (PPD). Other immunologic tests, such as testing for lymphocyte activation to antigens from *M. tuberculosis*, are being evaluated and may prove to be useful in the future. Diagnosis of latent TB also requires that active TB be excluded. In practice this usually requires obtaining a chest radiograph that shows no abnormalities. In circumstances in which the radiograph is ambiguous, however, sputum cultures should be obtained and treatment for latent TB delayed until cultures are shown to be negative and it has been conclusively established that the patient does not have active TB.

Criteria for diagnosis of latent TB by skin testing depend on the probability of infection with *M. tuberculosis* and the potential for reactivation in a person with such infection. Thus a 5 mm PPD skin test reaction indicates latent TB in a person with HIV infection or in a person who has had close contact with a person with active TB; a 15 mm reaction is required for the diagnosis in a person with no known risks for TB infection (see Table 31–2).[2] As a general rule, PPD skin testing is not recommended for persons who do not fall into one of the risk groups (e.g., persons in whom latent TB would only be diagnosed with a skin test result of 15 mm or greater). Although it is possible that a person who has received Bacille Calmette-Guérin (BCG) vaccine may have a false-positive PPD skin test reaction, this possibility becomes less likely as the time from BCG vaccination lengthens, so that in most cases BCG vaccination status has little impact on the interpretation of the PPD reaction. In the United States it is recommended that the PPD skin test reaction be interpreted without regard to BCG vaccination status.[2]

Diagnosis of latent TB is difficult in persons who are so immunologically impaired that they cannot respond to

TABLE 31–2 ■ Criteria for Diagnosis of Latent Tuberculosis Infection (LTBI)

PPD Skin Test		
Reaction: 5 mm of induration	**Reaction: 10 mm of induration**	**Reaction: 15 mm of induration**
Human immunodeficiency virus (HIV)–positive persons	Recent immigrants (i.e., within the last 5 y) from high-prevalence countries	Persons with no risk factors for TB
Recent contacts of tuberculosis (TB) patients	Injection drug users	
Fibrotic changes on chest radiograph consistent with prior TB	Residents and employees[†] of the following high-risk congregate settings: prisons and jails, nursing homes and other long-term care facilities for the elderly, hospitals and other health care facilities, residential facilities for patients with acquired immunodeficiency syndrome (AIDS), and homeless shelters	
Patients with organ transplants and other immunosuppressed patients (receiving the equivalent of 15 mg/d of prednisone for 1 mo or more)*	Mycobacteriology laboratory personnel	
	Persons with the following clinical conditions that place them at high risk: silicosis, diabetes mellitus, chronic renal failure, some hematologic disorders (e.g., leukemias and lymphomas), other specific malignancies (e.g., carcinoma of the head or neck and lung), weight loss of 10% of ideal body weight, gastrectomy, and jejunoileal bypass	
	Children younger than 4 y of age or infants, children, and adolescents exposed to adults at high risk	

PPD, purified protein derivative.

*Risk of TB in patients treated with corticosteroids increases with higher dose and longer treatment.

†For persons who are otherwise at low risk and are tested at the start of employment, a 15-mm induration is considered positive.

Adapted from American Thoracic Society, Centers for Disease Control and Prevention: Diagnostic standards and classification of tuberculosis in adults and children. Am J Respir Crit Care Med 2000;161:1376–1395.

a PPD skin test (anergic persons). Anergy occurs primarily among persons with advanced HIV infection, and as many as 80% of them may not be able to respond to such testing. If such a person is exposed to *M. tuberculosis* but has no evidence of active TB, treatment of presumed latent TB may be warranted, despite a negative tuberculin skin test. Anergy skin test panels do not contribute additional useful information and are not recommended.

PPD skin test–negative HIV-infected persons who are not contacts of persons with active TB should not receive treatment for latent TB but should be tested with PPD after responding to combination antiretroviral therapy. In persons whose CD4 cell count has risen to $100/mm^3$ or higher, PPD skin testing should be performed to assure that latent TB is not present.

Children are more likely than adults to progress to active disease upon initial infection. Therefore children who have substantial exposure to an adult with TB but who are skin test negative on initial testing should also receive presumptive treatment for latent TB until repeat skin tests (6 to 12 weeks later) confirm that they have not become infected.

Theoretical Basis for TB Therapy

As shown in Figure 31–1 the number of organisms in a person with active TB falls rapidly over the first phase of therapy with active agents. This phase usually lasts about 2 months and is termed the *induction phase* of therapy. After this point the number of organisms falls more slowly. Addition of more drugs cannot prevent this slowing in the rate of elimination of the organisms. Rather it is believed that the organisms alter their metabolism (or a subpopulation of organisms emerges) in such a way that a prolonged second phase of therapy is needed to eliminate them. These organisms are called *persisters*, and the second phase of therapy is called the *continuation phase*.

Because the number of organisms is large during the induction phase, the multiple drug regimen is continued throughout this phase to prevent the emergence of drug resistance. Once the number of organisms decreases, the number of drugs can be reduced, but never to a single agent. The actual number of organisms cannot be measured, so induction phase is usually defined as the first 2 months of therapy, and the continuation phase is defined as months 3 through 6. Clinical studies of the treatment of active TB have established that this approach can achieve high success rates (over 95% cures), whereas shorter regimens have substantially lower cure rates. Thus the overall course of therapy for active TB must be at least 6 months.

In a patient with latent TB, the total body burden of organisms is much smaller, probably on the order of 10^2 to 10^3/organisms. In addition these organisms probably are not replicating. In such cases, treatment with a single agent is adequate and does not pose a risk for the emergence of drug resistance. Latent TB treatment regimens may therefore include only a single drug. Combination therapy with rifampin and pyrazinamide allows treatment for a shorter duration with no loss of efficacy.

Antimycobacterial Agents and Toxicities

Many common antibiotics are not active against *M. tuberculosis*. Those that are active against *M. tuberculosis* can be divided into two groups: the most active, best tolerated, and most commonly used agents, known as first-line agents (Table 31–3), and those less active, more toxic, or less commonly used, known as second-line agents (Table 31–4). Second-line agents generally should

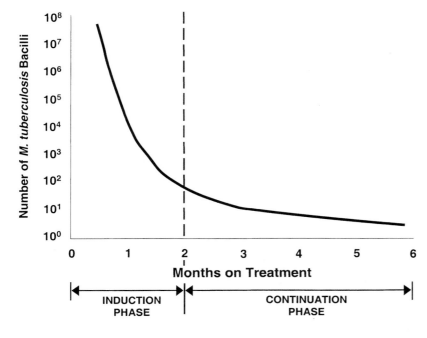

FIGURE 31–1. Time course of mycobacterial burden in a patient with pulmonary tuberculosis (TB) during treatment. Mycobacterial burden decreases dramatically during the first 2 months (induction phase) and slowly during the next 4 months (continuation phase).

TABLE 31–3 ■ First-Line Antituberculosis Agents: Dosages

Drug	Route	Dose in mg/kg* [Maximum dose]						
		Children daily	Adults daily	Children 2/wk†	Adults 2/wk†	Children 3/wk†	Adults 3/wk†	Adults weekly
Isoniazid	PO	10–20 [300 mg]	5 [300 mg]	20–40 [900 mg]	15 [900 mg]	20–40 [900 mg]	15 [900 mg]	15 [900 mg]
Rifampin	PO	10–20 [600 mg]	10 [600 mg]	10–20 [600 mg]	10 [600 mg]	10–20 [600 mg]	10 [600 mg]	—
Rifabutin	PO	—	5 [300 mg]	—	5 [300 mg]	—	5 [300 mg]	—
Rifapentine	PO	—	—	—	—	—	—	10 [600 mg]
Pyrazinamide	PO	15–30 [2 g]	15–30 [2 g]	50–70 [4 g]	50–70 [4 g]	50–70 [3 g]	50–70 [3 g]	—
Ethambutol	PO	15–25	15–25	50	50	25–30	25–30	—
Streptomycin	IM or IV	20–40 [1 g]	15 [1 g]	25–30 [1.5 g]	25–30 [1.5 g]	25–30 [1.5 g]	25–30 [1.5 g]	—

*Maximum dose is given in brackets. Doses are for children under 12 y. Adjust weight-based doses as weight changes.
†All regimens administered two or three times a week should be used with directly observed therapy.
Adapted from Simone PM, Horsburgh CR, Castro KG: Antimycobacterial drugs. Gorbach SL, Bartlett JG, Blacklow NR (eds): Infections Diseases, 2nd ed. Philadelphia, WB Saunders, 1997, pp 359–376.

TABLE 31–4 ■ Second-Line Antituberculosis Drug Dosages

Drug*	Daily dose† [Maximum dose] (Usual dose)
Cycloserine	15–20 mg/kg PO in divided doses [1 g] (250–500 mg bid)
Ethionamide	15–20 mg/kg PO in divided doses [1 g] (250–500 mg bid)
p-Aminosalicylic acid	150 mg/kg PO in divided doses [12 g] (4 g tid)
Capreomycin	15–30 mg/kg IM or IV qd [1 g]
Kanamycin and amikacin	15–30 mg/kg IM or IV qd [1 g]
Ofloxacin	600–800 mg/d PO (400 mg bid)
Levofloxacin	750 mg/d PO

*Use these drugs only in consultation with a clinician experienced in the management of drug-resistant tuberculosis. Adjust weight-based dosages as weight changes.
†Doses for children are the same as those for adults.

not be used for treatment of tuberculosis without consultation with a specialist in this area.

As can be seen from the dosing schedules, dosing more than once daily generally is not required and is only used when such dosing improves tolerance. The slow growth of *M. tuberculosis* and the postantibiotic effect of the first-line agents allow effective intermittent dosing schedules, in which drugs can be given twice or thrice weekly with excellent clinical results. Such intermittent treatment schedules also facilitate direct supervision of medication administration, or directly observed therapy

(DOT), which can greatly improve adherence and lead to substantially higher cure rates.[6] Intermittent dosing without DOT is not recommended.

Serious toxicities are uncommon, but side effects that are not dose limiting are frequent (Table 31–5). Clinicians should be reticent about discontinuing the first-line drugs in the absence of severe toxicity. The rifamycins are particularly important in shortening the duration of therapy and decreasing relapse, yet inexperienced clinicians may inappropriately discontinue rifampin.[7] Isoniazid (INH), rifamycins (rifampin, rifabutin, and rifapentine), and pyrazinamide can cause drug-induced hepatitis that may be fatal. This rare complication can be avoided with early recognition of hepatitis and discontinuation of the offending drug. Specific guidelines for monitoring such toxicity are given under Treatment of Active Tuberculosis, Monitoring the Patient. INH may also cause peripheral neuropathy; neuropathy is more common among certain patient groups, such as patients with alcoholism, malnutrition, diabetes, uremia, seizure disorders, or pregnancy. Supplemental pyridoxine (50 mg/d) is recommended when INH is given to such patients. Rifampin, INH, and pyrazinamide can each cause skin rash, but discontinuation of the offending agent usually is not necessary. Administration of pyrazinamide may be accompanied by hyperuricemia, but usually this is clinically insignificant. Accompanying arthralgias may be treated symptomatically. Ethambutol may cause retrobulbar neuritis, but this is rare when the lower dose range is employed (15 mg/kg). Streptomycin can cause ototoxicity and neurotoxicity, particularly among older patients. Some authorities recommend against the use of aminoglycosides in persons over 60 years of age, particularly when toxicity monitoring cannot be assured.

TABLE 31–5 ■ Antituberculosis Drugs: Adverse Reactions

Drug	Adverse reactions	Monitoring	Comments

Isoniazid	Hepatic enzyme elevation
	Hepatitis
	Peripheral neuropathy
	Mild effects on central nervous system
	Drug interactions
	Rash
		Baseline measurements of hepatic enzymes for adults
		Repeat measurements
		  If baseline results are abnormal
		  If patient is at high risk for adverse reactions
		  If patient has symptoms of adverse reactions
			Hepatitis risk increases with age and alcohol consumption
			Pyridoxine can prevent peripheral neuropathy

Rifampin	Gastrointestinal upset
	Drug interactions
	Hepatitis
	Thrombocytopenia
	Influenza-like symptoms
	Rash
	Interstitial nephritis
		Baseline measurements for adults
		  Complete blood count and platelets
		  Hepatic enzymes
		Repeat measurements
		  If baseline results are abnormal
		  If patient has symptoms of adverse reactions
			See Table 31–6 for drug interactions
			Colors body fluids orange
			
			May permanently discolor soft contact lenses

Rifabutin	Rash
	Gastrointestinal upset
	Drug interactions
	Hepatitis
	Neutropenia
	Joint pain
		Baseline measurements for adults
		  Complete blood count and platelets
		  Hepatic enzymes
		Repeat measurements
		  If baseline results are abnormal
		  If patient has symptoms of adverse reactions
			See Table 31–6 for drug interactions
			Colors body fluids orange
			May permanently discolor soft contact lenses

Rifapentine	Rash
	Gastrointestinal upset
	Drug interactions
	Hepatitis
	Neutropenia
	Joint pain
		Baseline measurements for adults
		  Complete blood count and platelets
		  Hepatic enzymes
		Repeat measurements
		  If baseline results are abnormal
		  If patient has symptoms of adverse reactions
			See Table 31–6 for drug interactions
			Colors body fluids orange
			May permanently discolor soft contact lenses

Pyrazinamide	Hepatitis
	Rash
	Gastrointestinal upset
	Joint aches
	Hyperuricemia
	Gout (rare)
		Baseline measurements for adults
		  Uric acid
		  Hepatic enzymes
		Repeat measurements
		  If baseline results are abnormal
		  If patient has symptoms of adverse reactions
			Treat hyperuricemia only if patient has symptoms

Ethambutol	Optic neuritis	Baseline and monthly tests
		  Visual activity
		  Color vision
			Not recommended for children too young to be monitored for changes in vision unless tuberculosis is drug resistant

Streptomycin	Ototoxicity (hearing loss or vestibular dysfunction)
	Renal toxicity
		Baseline and repeated tests as needed
		  Hearing
		  Kidney function
			Avoid or reduce dose in adults older than 60 y

Cycloserine	Psychosis Convulsions Depression Headaches Rash	Assess mental status Measure serum drug levels	Start with low dosage and increase as tolerated Pyridoxine may decrease central nervous system effects
Ethionamide	Gastrointestinal irritation Hepatotoxicity Hypersensitivity Metallic taste Bloating	Measure hapatic enzyme levels	Start with low dosage and increase as tolerated May cause hypothyroid condition, especially if used with p-amino-salicylic acid
p-Aminosalicylic acid	Gastrointestinal irritation Hypersensitivity	Measure hepatic enzyme levels Assess volume status	Start with low dosage and increase as tolerated

TABLE 31–5 ■ Antituberculosis Drugs: Adverse Reactions *(Continued)*

Drug	Adverse reactions	Monitoring	Comments

Capreomycin	Hepatotoxicity
	Sodium load
	Toxicity
	  Auditory
	  Vestibular
	  Renal
		Assess
		  Vestibular function
		  Hearing function
		Measure
		  Blood urea nitrogen
		  Creatinine level
			Monitor cardiac patients for sodium load
			After bacteriologic conversion, dosage may be reduced to 2 or 3 times/wk

Kanamycin and amikacin	Toxicity
	  Auditory
	  Vestibular
	  Renal
		Assess
		  Vestibular function
		  Hearing function
		Measure
		  Blood urea nitrogen
		  Creatinine level
			After bacteriologic conversion, dosage may be reduced to 2 or 3 times/wk

Ofloxacin and levofloxacin	Gastrointestinal upset
	Dizziness
	Hypersensitivity
	Drug interactions
	Headaches
	Restlessness
		Drug interactions	Should not be used in children
			Avoid
			  Antacids
			  Iron
			  Zinc
			  Sucralfate

Adapted from Simone PM, Horsburgh CR, Castro KG: Antimycobacterial drugs. In Gorbach SL, Bartlett JG, Blacklow NR (eds): Infectious Diseases, 2nd ed. Philadelphia, WB Saunders, 1997, pp 359–376.

Drug Interactions

INH may increase phenytoin and carbamazepine levels, which should be monitored when the two drugs are coadministered. All the rifamycins can decrease clearance of other drugs, as they induce hepatic microsomal enzymes. Many drugs can potentially be affected, including methadone, coumadin, estrogens, theophylline, and several classes of antiretroviral agents (Table 31–6).[8] When rifamycins are coadministered with other pharmacologic agents, the package insert should always be consulted for potential interactions, and where possible, there should be therapeutic drug monitoring or dose adjustment or both. Rifampin, rifabutin, and rifapentine have similar levels of activity against *M. tuberculosis* and identical mechanisms of action. Thus they are not useful when rifampin resistance is present. Rifampin and rifabutin, however, have different hepatic microsomal enzyme induction profiles, and thus rifabutin may offer advantages over rifampin in individual cases when rifampin resistance is not present.

Preventing Emergence of Resistance

Drug-resistant *M. tuberculosis* organisms occur spontaneously and are present in any population of *M. tuberculosis* that is sufficiently large (10^5 to 10^6 organisms). If single-drug treatment is used in the presence of such a resistant subpopulation, a completely resistant population of organisms will emerge in 2 to 4 months, and clinical treatment will fail concurrently. Since the average number of organisms in a person with active pulmonary tuberculosis is 10^8 to 10^{11}, resistance can be reliably predicted if active TB is treated with a single drug. Therefore to prevent failure of therapy caused by the emergence of drug resistance, treatment of active TB is initiated with a minimum of three drugs. In situations in which there is a reasonable probability of complete initial resistance to a single drug, four drugs are recommended for initiation so that there will be three active drugs in the regimen. When the susceptibility results are known at the outset of therapy (as in a close contact of a person whose isolate has known susceptibility), the appropriate three drugs may be used. In the United States, over 84% of the population lives in an area in which there is resistance to at least one first-line agent in more than 4% of isolates.[3] Therefore the recommended initial regimen for the United States is four-drug therapy. Since susceptibility results may take 6 weeks (or in some cases, longer) a prolonged period of treatment with four drugs is often required.

Despite therapy with several drugs, emergence of drug resistance during therapy is still the most common situation in which drug resistance occurs. This is nearly always the result of failure to adhere to the regimen. Thus ensuring adherence to the regimen and identifying failure to do so are essential to the management of patients with tuberculosis. Physicians and other care providers are not good judges of a patient's likelihood of adhering to a TB treatment regimen and also are not easily able to determine when patients are not compliant.[9] Adherence to prolonged courses of medication is difficult, and physicians themselves are poor at adhering to regimens with many medications. For this reason DOT is recommended for all patients with TB. In a DOT program a health care provider (physician, nurse, or outreach worker) administers and observes ingestion of each medication dose by the patient. The CDC recommends DOT for all patients, and this strategy is associated

TABLE 31–6 ■ Clinically Significant Drug-Drug Interactions Involving the Rifamycins

Drug class	Drugs whose concentrations are substantially decreased by the rifamycins	Comments
Anti-infectives	HIV-1 protease inhibitors	Can be used with rifabutin
	Non-nucleoside reverse transcriptase inhibitors	Delavirdine should not be used with any rifamycin
	Macrolide antibiotics	Azithromycin has no significant interaction with rifamycins
	Doxycycline	May require use of an alternative drug or drug combination
	Azole antifungal agents	Itraconazole and ketoconazole concentrations may be subtherapeutic with any of the rifamycins
		Fluconazole can be used with rifamycins, but the dose may have to be increased
	Atovaquone	Consider alternate form of *Pneumocystis carinii* treatment or prophylaxis
	Chloramphenicol	Consider use of an alternative antibiotic
Hormone therapy	Ethinylestradiol, norethindrone	Women of reproductive potential on oral contraceptives should be advised to add a barrier method of contraception when on a rifamycin
	Tamoxifen	May require alternative therapy
	Levothyroxine	Monitoring of serum thyroid-stimulating hormone recommended; may require higher dose of levothyroxine
Narcotics	Methadone	Rifampin may require methadone dose increase
		Rifabutin infrequently causes methadone withdrawal
Anticoagulants	Warfarin	Monitor prothrombin time; may require 2- or 3-fold dose increase
Immunosuppressive agents	Cyclosporine, tacrolimus, corticosteroids	Rifabutin may allow concomitant use of cyclosporine and a rifamycin
Anticonvulsants	Phenytoin, carbamazepine	Therapeutic drug monitoring recommended; may require dose increase
Cardiovascular agents	Calcium-channel blockers	Clinical monitoring recommended; may require change to an alternate drug
	Beta-blockers	Clinical monitoring recommended; may require dose increase or change to an alternate drug
	Angiotensin-converting enzyme inhibitors and angiotensin receptor antagonists	Monitor clinically; may require a dose increase or use of an alternate drug
	Digitalis preparations	Therapeutic drug monitoring recommended; may require dose increase
	Quinidine	Therapeutic drug monitoring recommended; may require dose increase
	Antiarrhythmics	Clinical monitoring recommended; may require change to an alternative drug
Theophylline	Theophylline	Therapeutic drug monitoring recommended; may require dose increase
Hypoglycemics	Sulfonylurea agents	Monitor blood glucose; may require dose increase or change to an alternative drug
Psychotropic drugs	Tricyclic antidepressants	Therapeutic drug monitoring recommended; may require dose increase or change to alternative drug
	Antipsychotics	Monitor clinically; may require a dose increase or use of an alternative drug
	Benzodiazepines	Monitor clinically; may require a dose increase or use of an alternative drug

with substantially higher cure rates and less emergence of drug resistance than self-administered therapy is.[6,10]

Failure to adhere to the treatment regimen is of particular importance in TB, since patients feel greatly improved after 4 to 8 weeks of therapy and yet need to continue treatment for 4 more months, a time when they are asymptomatic. Failure to take one or two agents in a multidrug regimen is more serious than failing to take all the medications because this behavior facilitates the emergence of drug resistance. Ensuring adherence for the full course of therapy is the most difficult challenge of TB therapy, and failure to adhere is one of the most difficult conditions to diagnose and treat.

If treatment is with self-administered therapy, a particularly useful strategy for prevention of selective nonadherence is the use of fixed-dose combination capsules. These are available as INH + rifampin (Rifamate: 300 mg rifampin and 150 mg INH) and INH + rifampin + pyrazinamide (Rifater: 120 mg rifampin, 50 mg INH, and 300 mg pyrazinamide). Using such fixed dose combinations ensures that if one drug is discontinued, the other will be as well. This greatly decreases the risk of emergence of drug resistance. In addition, since the large number of pills in many antituberculosis regimens is likely to contribute to nonadherence, combination pills may increase adherence by decreasing the number of pills that have to be taken.

The public health cost of failure due to nonadherence is also great; in a recent study in San Francisco, 44% of new tuberculosis cases were attributable to three patients who did not adhere to the treatment regimen.[11] These three patients remained infectious and transmitted *M. tuberculosis* to 65 additional patients. Few if any of these secondary cases would have occurred if adherence had been assured.

Practice Guidelines for Tuberculosis

The Infectious Disease Society of America has developed practice guidelines for the treatment of active and latent tuberculosis (Table 31–7).[3] These guidelines are meant to be the minimum standards that will allow care providers and programs to monitor their proficiency in meeting basic standards of care for patients with tuberculosis.

The Health Department: A Partner in Patient Management

Cases of active TB must be reported to the local health department in all areas of the United States. Reporting cases of TB to public health authorities serves several functions:

1. It allows public health investigators to perform contact and source-case investigations to determine if other cases of untreated, infectious TB are present in the community.

2. It allows monitoring of adherence to therapy by TB patients, who might otherwise continue to spread TB in the community.
3. It allows identification of infected contacts and administration of treatment for latent TB infection (TLTBI) to eligible candidates.
4. It permits record keeping and surveillance to determine if public health TB control efforts are achieving their goal of prevention of spread of TB.[3]

To allow the health department to perform these functions adequately, prompt notification of cases of active TB by clinicians and hospitals is essential. It is preferable to report suspected cases (based on clinical diagnosis or the presence of acid-fast bacilli in clinical specimens) rather than wait for definitive culture confirmation. In many areas the health department also offers diagnostic tests and medications at no cost, consultation in selecting and monitoring the regimen, and access to statutory intervention when patients pose a continuing risk of transmitting TB to others.

TREATMENT OF ACTIVE TUBERCULOSIS

Induction Phase Regimen

Recommended regimens for induction phase therapy in the United States are shown in Table 31–8.[12,13] The efficacy of these regimens has been established in randomized, prospective clinical trials.[14–16] The susceptibility of the organism causing disease usually is not known at the initiation of therapy, and imputation by epidemiologic circumstances is highly inaccurate. In most areas of the United States there is a greater than 4% chance of at least monoresistant active TB. Therefore each of the three recommended options for TB treatment in the United States includes four drugs. In a case in which the infecting isolate is known to be susceptible to INH, rifampin, and pyrazinamide before the initiation of therapy, the regimens can be used without the addition of ethambutol or streptomycin. In some situations in which drug interactions preclude the use of rifampin, rifabutin may be substituted.

Regimen 2 is the regimen most commonly used in the United States and is most appropriate for patients diagnosed in hospital. Hospitalized patients can receive daily therapy for 2 weeks while in hospital, changing to twice-weekly therapy after clinical improvement has been established and the patient is ready for discharge. Many health departments favor this regimen because it facilitates DOT. Intermittent regimens should always be used with DOT, as there is less tolerance for missed doses than with daily therapy. Persons receiving one of the INH-containing regimens who are at increased risk for the development of peripheral neuropathy, such as patients with alcoholism, malnutrition, diabetes, uremia, seizure disorders, and pregnancy, should receive supplemental pyridoxine (50 mg/d). When the patient fails to adhere to

TABLE 31–7 ■ Infectious Disease Society of America Tuberculosis (TB) Practice Guidelines

Guideline	Performance indicator
1. Obtain bacteriologic confirmation and susceptibility testing for patients with TB or suspected of having TB	90% of adults with or suspected of having TB have 3 cultures for mycobacteria obtained before initiation of antituberculosis therapy (50% of children 0–12 y)
2. Place persons with suspected or confirmed smear-positive pulmonary or laryngeal tuberculosis in respiratory isolation until noninfectious	90% of persons with sputum smear positive for TB remain in respiratory isolation until smear converts to negative
3. Begin treatment of patients with confirmed or suspected TB with HRZ or HRZE(S), depending on local resistance patterns	90% of all TB patients are started on HRZE or HRZS in geographic areas where >4% of TB isolates are resistant to isoniazid
4. Report each case of TB promptly to the local public health department	100% of persons with active TB are reported to the local public health department within 1 wk of diagnosis
5. Perform HIV testing for all TB patients	80% of all TB patients have HIV status determined within 2 mo of a diagnosis of TB
6. Treat patients with TB caused by a susceptible organism for 6 mo using an ATS/CDC-approved regimen	90% of all TB patients complete 6 mo of therapy within 12 mo of beginning treatment
7. Re-evaluate TB patients who are smear positive at 3 mo for possible nonadherence or drug resistance	90% of all TB patients who are smear positive at 3 mo have sputum culture and susceptibility testing performed within 1 mo of the 3 mo visit
8. Add 2 or more new antituberculosis agents when TB treatment failure is suspected	100% of TB patients with suspected treatment failure are prescribed 2 or more new antituberculosis agents
9. Perform tuberculin skin testing on all patients with HIV infection, a history of injecting drug use, homelessness, incarceration, or contact with a person with pulmonary TB	80% of persons in the indicated population groups receive tuberculin skin test and return for reading
10. Administer treatment for latent tuberculosis infection (TLTBI) to all persons with latent TB infection unless prior TLTBI can be documented.	75% of patients with positive tuberculin skin tests who are candidates for TLTBI complete a course of therapy within 12 mo of initiation

Adapted from Horsburgh CR Jr, Feldman S, Ridzon R: Practice guidelines for the treatment of tuberculosis. Clin Infect Dis 2000;31:633–639.
ATS, American Thoracic Society; CDC, Centers for Disease Control and Prevention; HRZ, isoniazid, rifampin, and pyrazinamide; HRZE, HRZ and ethambutol; HRZS, HRZ and streptomycin.

TABLE 31–8 ■ Induction Regimen Options for Treatment of Pulmonary and Extrapulmonary Tuberculosis*

Option	Total duration (wk)	Drugs	Interval and duration of induction
1		Isoniazid Rifampin Pyrazinamide Ethambutol or Streptomycin	Daily × 8 wk
2		Isoniazid Rifampin Pyrazinamide Ethambutol or streptomycin	Daily × 2 wk; then 2/wk[†] × 6 wk
3		Isoniazid Rifampin Pyrazinamide Ethambutol or streptomycin	3/wk[†] × 8 wk

*Note: for all patients, if susceptibility results show resistance to any of the first-line drugs or if the patient remains symptomatic or smear or culture positive after 3 mo, consult a tuberculosis medical expert.
[†]Directly observed therapy should be used with all regimens administered two or three times weekly.
Adapted from Simone PM, Horsburgh CR, Castro KG: antimycobacterial drugs. In Gorbach SL, Bartlett JG, Blacklow NR (eds): Infectious Diseases, 2nd ed. Philadelphia, WB Saunders, 1997, pp 359–376.

the dosing schedule for induction, it can be difficult to determine when induction phase therapy has been completed. However, completion of the required number of doses within 10 weeks is adequate.

Continuation Phase Regimen: Drug-Susceptible Disease

Overall duration of therapy (induction plus continuation phases) is 6 months. Recommended continuation phase regimens for active TB caused by organisms susceptible to the first-line agents are shown in Table 31–9. Because the number of organisms is still substantial, two drugs are essential to prevent the emergence of drug resistance. Any of the three continuation regimens may be used following any of the induction regimens, but none of these continuation phase regimens should be initiated without confirmation that the organism is susceptible to INH and rifampin. Patients with poor clinical responses to induction phase therapy should be considered for an extension of continuation phase therapy; those with cavitary lung disease whose sputum cultures are positive at the end of induction should receive continuation phase therapy for 7 months (31 weeks) rather than 4 months.

The once-weekly rifapentine regimen should only be used in persons who have non-cavitary pulmonary disease (even if the cavity has subsequently closed).[17] This once-weekly regimen has the distinct advantage of reducing the number of doses by 50 percent. The rifapentine regimen also substantially reduces the effort and expense of direct observation. When the patient fails to adhere to the dosing schedule for continuation, it can difficult to determine when therapy has been completed. However, completion of the required number of doses for both induction and continuation within 9 months of initiating induction is considered adequate.

Drug-Resistant Disease

Resistance or Intolerance to Isoniazid Alone

Persons with active TB caused by organisms resistant to INH alone or persons who are unable to tolerate INH should not be treated with one of the standard three-drug induction regimens but can receive one of the standard four-drug regimens, omitting the INH when resistance or intolerance is recognized. Because pyrazinamide is not as effective at preventing emergence of resistance as other first-line agents, there can be no simplification of the regimen after induction, and the pyrazinamide is also given for the full 6 months. Persons with disease due to INH-resistant organisms should receive a 6-month course of therapy with (1) rifampin, pyrazinamide, and ethambutol or (2) rifampin, pyrazinamide, and streptomycin, given either daily or intermittently.

Resistance or Intolerance to Rifampin Alone

Persons with active TB caused by organisms resistant to rifamycins alone or persons who are unable to tolerate rifamycins should not be treated with one of the standard three-drug induction regimens. Substitution of one rifamycin for another is not useful for rifampin-resistant isolates, since there is nearly complete cross-resistance between these agents. Intolerance to rifamycins is also likely to be shared by these agents, although there is less experience in this area. Because regimens lacking rifampin are not as effective at reducing the burden of organisms during the first 2 months of therapy, there can be no simplification of the regimen after induction, and the same regimen is used for the full course of therapy. Moreover, unlike the situation with INH monoresistance, TB treatment regimens lacking rifampin must be given for a longer time to ensure acceptable response rates. Persons with disease due to INH-resistant organisms should receive 9 months of therapy with INH, pyrazinamide, and streptomycin. This regimen may be given daily or twice weekly, but such intermittent therapy must be directly observed. Practically, 9 months of injectable therapy can only be given intermittently, and even this may be difficult for patients to tolerate because of pain at the site of repeated injections. If this regimen is intolerable, INH, pyrazinamide, and ethambutol may be given, but the duration of treatment must be 18 months (Pyrazinamide may be discontinued after 4 to 6 months).

TABLE 31–9 ■ Continuation Regimens for Treatment of Pulmonary and Extrapulmonary Tuberculosis

Option	Drugs	Interval and duration	Comments
1	Isoniazid Rifampin	Daily or 2/wk* × 18 wk*	Ethambutol or streptomycin should be continued until susceptibility to isoniazid and rifampin is demonstrated
2	Isoniazid Rifampin	2/wk × 18 wk*	Regimen should be directly observed; After the initial phase, continue ethambutol or streptomycin until susceptibility to isoniazid and rifampin is demonstrated, unless drug resistance is unlikely
3	Isoniazid Rifapentine	Weekly × 18 wk*	Regimen should be used for patients without cavitary lung disease and should be directly observed

Adapted from Simone PM, Horsburgh CR, Castro KG: Antimycobacterial drugs. In Gorbach SL, Bartlett JG, Blacklow NR (eds): Infectious Diseases, 2nd ed. Philadelphia, WB Saunders, 1997, pp 359–376.

*Duration should be extended to 31 weeks if patient has cavitary lung disease and cultures are positive at the completion of induction phase therapy.

Resistance or Intolerance to Pyrazinamide Alone

Persons with active TB caused by organisms resistant to pyrazinamide or persons who are unable to tolerate pyrazinamide should not be treated with one of the standard three-drug induction regimens. Such patients should receive 2-month induction phase therapy with (1) INH, rifampin, and ethambutol or (2) INH, rifampin, and streptomycin. The regimen may be simplified after 6 to 8 weeks when susceptibility to INH and rifampin have been demonstrated. Inability to provide pyrazinamide during induction, however, results in longer overall therapy, and these regimens should be given for 9 months.

Resistance or Intolerance to Ethambutol Alone or Streptomycin Alone

Patients with active TB caused by such organisms are uncommon, but they may be safely and effectively treated with any of the three standard induction regimens shown in Table 31–8 (using a fourth drug to which the isolate is susceptible). Continuation phase therapy is then instituted with one of the standard regimens shown in Table 31–9. Duration and dosing are the same as for drug-susceptible disease.

Resistance or Intolerance to Both Isoniazid and Rifampin

Isolates resistant to INH and rifampin are multiple-drug resistant organisms (MDR-TB). Since these organisms are usually resistant to other agents in addition to INH and rifampin, regimens must be tailored to the susceptibility pattern of the individual isolate. Consultation with a specialist in the treatment of patients with MDR-TB is the standard of care.[18]

Resistance or Intolerance to Both Isoniazid and Streptomycin

Treatment of active TB in patients with these resistant organisms or with intolerance to these agents can be accomplished with a regimen containing rifampin, pyrazinamide, ethambutol, and amikacin or kanamycin, as there is no cross-resistance between amikacin or kanamycin and streptomycin. It is preferable to give the oral agents daily and the amikacin intermittently, although data from clinical trials are lacking. Duration of the therapy may vary from 6 to 9 months: patients who continue to be culture positive at 2 months (or who have an otherwise unacceptable clinical response) should receive 9 months of treatment.

Resistance or Intolerance to Both Isoniazid and Ethambutol

Treatment of active TB in patients with these organisms or with intolerance to these agents can be accomplished with a regimen containing rifampin, pyrazinamide, a flouroquinolone, and streptomycin. It is preferable to give the oral agents daily and the streptomycin intermittently, although data from clinical trials are lacking. Duration of the therapy may vary from 6 to 9 months:

patients who continue to be culture positive at 2 months (or who have an otherwise unacceptable clinical response) should receive 9 months of treatment.

Role of Corticosteroids

Administration of corticosteroids in addition to antimycobacterial agents in the treatment of tuberculosis disease has been advocated as a means of blunting the immune response to the mycobacteria and decreasing immune-mediated tissue damage. In patients with mild-to-moderate disease this does not appear to be necessary, but steroids may be used when there is extensive pulmonary disease as an aid to maintaining adequate tissue oxygenation. In addition, when there is potentially life-threatening closed space infection such as in TB meningitis or TB pericarditis, administration of a several week course of high-dose steroids is recommended to reduce inflammation and scarring.[19] Despite concerns that such treatment might impair protective host responses, if does not appear that there are adverse consequences to its use.

Expected Outcome

With any of the standard courses of treatment outlined above, over 95% of patients should be cured of their disease and have no residual organisms. The remaining 5% may experience either treatment failure (failure to convert cultures to negative or breakthrough while on therapy) or relapse (recurrence of disease after completion of treatment). Such relapses are usually the result of failure to eliminate the disease, with gradual recrudescence and clinical reappearance of symptoms and signs of active disease. Most cases of relapse occur within 1 year of completion of a course of treatment.[17] Tissue damage, if extensive, may be permanent, and impaired pulmonary function is not uncommon after extensive pulmonary TB. Similarly, neurologic sequelae after TB meningitis can be substantial. Drug resistance should always be a concern in a patient with failure or relapse, but the risk is greatest in cases in which therapy has failed. A specialist in the treatment of tuberculosis should be consulted when either failure or relapse is suspected.

Monitoring the Patient

Patients should be seen biweekly during induction phase therapy and monthly during continuation phase therapy. These visits are important both to monitor the response of the disease and to identify medication side effects. For patients with pulmonary TB, three sputum samples should be obtained (preferably first morning samples on three consecutive days prior to inception of therapy) for smear, culture, and susceptibility testing, along with a chest radiograph (including apical lordotic view for better visualization of lung apices if upper lobe disease is present). Hematocrit, complete blood count, and liver function tests are adequate laboratory studies. These tests are also useful for establishing baseline values for monitoring toxicity of antimycobacterial agents. For patients with extrapulmonary TB, samples and schedules for clinical and laboratory follow-up must be individualized.

Smears and Cultures

For patients with pulmonary disease a sputum sample should be obtained monthly for smear and culture; this should be performed until three successive specimens have negative culture results. Failure to convert cultures to negative may indicate the need for prolongation of the course of therapy or alteration of the regimen and are an important indicator of likely nonadherence. If this occurs, patients not on DOT must be placed on DOT, and the DOT records of patients on DOT must be reviewed to assure that direct observation is occurring and that patients are not spitting out pills after the outreach worker departs. Smear conversion may lag behind culture conversion, as some patients continue to excrete nonviable bacilli, and this phenomenon can be diagnostically confusing.

Chest Radiographs

Follow-up chest radiographs are not necessary at each visit but should be obtained at month 2 and at the conclusion of therapy. Progressive worsening of the radiograph at 2 months may indicate problems with the regimen (such as unsuspected drug resistance or malabsorption of medications) or nonadherence. It is important, however, to look at the initial and 2-month films together, as written reports alone may not allow adequate comparison. The film obtained at the conclusion of therapy is important as a baseline for evaluation of possible relapse.

Liver Enzymes

Active TB, even that apparently confined to the lung, may involve the liver, and mild elevation of liver enzymes is common in patients with TB. This is not an impediment to initiation of therapy with INH, rifampin, and pyrazinamide despite their known potential for hepatotoxicity. Since the initial elevations are often the result of active TB, therapy improves of hepatic parameters in many cases. When initial transaminases are elevated, they should be monitored at least monthly until they return to the normal range. If clinical symptoms later suggest hepatitis, the transaminases should be repeated, as drug-induced hepatitis can occur at any time during a course of therapy and may require discontinuation of the hepatotoxic agent. Patients should be cautioned to note the symptoms of hepatitis, including nausea, fatigue, abdominal pain, jaundice, and dark urine, but in practice these symptoms are frequently associated with the underlying disease and may be less helpful. Occurrence of these symptoms at a time when clinical disease is improving, however, should initiate an investigation for drug-induced hepatitis. Since early cessation of the offending agent can lead to resolution of the hepatitis and continued ingestion may be fatal, prompt attention to the possibility of drug-induced hepatitis is essential.

Clinical Monitoring

Weight and temperature should be obtained at each visit. Fever usually resolves within 4 weeks but can persist longer; however, a search for possible failure of the treatment and other causes of fever should be initiated should this occur. Continued weight loss should also be investigated, as most patients gain weight with successful treatment. Specific abnormalities related to the site of involvement of TB in the individual case should, of course, also be monitored. Patients who will be taking ethambutol at the 25 mg/kg dose for a prolonged period should have a color vision test performed at baseline and at monthly follow-up visits.

Adherence

Patients not receiving DOT should be questioned at each visit about their regularity of medication ingestion. For those suspected of failing to take at least 80% of any of their medication, a DOT program should be instituted. For patients on DOT the records of DOT visits should be reviewed at each visit. Patients who do not present for follow-up appointments must be located and evaluated. State laws governing detention of infectious TB patients vary, but all states have some mechanism for ensuring adherence of such patients.[20] Although enforcement of these statutes is rarely necessary, patients and health care providers should be aware that adherence to treatment of infectious pulmonary TB can be legally enforced.[21,22] The local health department can provide valuable assistance in locating such patients and ensuring adherence.

Managing Drug Toxicities

When a drug side effect is noted, one of two strategies can be employed: (1) stopping all medications with readministration of each, one by one, over subsequent 3 to 4-day intervals or (2) discontinuation of the most likely offending agent, followed by resumption of that agent with discontinuation of a second candidate if the symptom or sign fails to resolve. As a general rule the first strategy is preferred for more serious side effects, and the latter is used when side effects are less severe. Mild side effects may be treated symptomatically without discontinuation of the antibacterial agent, as in the case of mild skin rashes or arthralgias. There is an important caveat with either of the two strategies, however: the patient should not be treated with a regimen that contains a single drug for more than 1 week in induction phase or 2 weeks in continuation phase to avoid the emergence of drug resistance. Thus it is important to identify the causal agent promptly and, if the regimen needs to be changed, to substitute an alternative regimen within 1 or 2 weeks. Except in cases in which the active TB is life threatening, patients with extensive toxicity (such as markedly elevated liver enzymes) may have all antituberculosis medications discontinued for 2 to 3 weeks before therapy is restarted. Consultation with a specialist with experience in managing such reactions is recommended.

Pharmacokinetic Monitoring

Serum drug levels of most of the antimycobacterial agents can be obtained by sending specimens to one of several commercial laboratories. However, there is little role for such monitoring in most TB case management. Patients failing therapy without a clear explanation for failure may benefit from pharmacologic monitoring, as problems with drug absorption and drug interactions have been reported, leading to low serum drug levels and clinical failure. Other causes of failure, however, such as nonadherence and drug resistance, are much more common and should first be excluded.[23]

Identifying a Failing Regimen

Failure is difficult to identify before the end of induction, since the clinical response to treatment is variable and some patients who will be cured may take 2 months to manifest a clinical response. However, improvement of signs or symptoms followed by recrudescence of these signs or symptoms should prompt a re-evaluation of both the patient and the regimen. Similarly, at the end of the 2-month induction period, sputum cultures should be negative in 80% of patients. Patients whose cultures are not negative at 2 months are at increased risk of failure and relapse.[24] When failure or relapse is suspected, consultation with a specialist in tuberculosis treatment should be sought. The patient should be interviewed and examined to assess adherence to the regimen; culture and susceptibility results should be reviewed; and repeat cultures (with susceptibility testing) and radiograph should be obtained.

Other possible causes of recurrent signs and symptoms should be investigated and excluded. In patients with HIV infection who are receiving combination antiretroviral therapy along with therapy for active TB, immune reconstitution reactions should be considered when one is evaluating new or recrudescent signs or symptoms, particularly fevers, swollen lymph nodes, headache, and pulmonary infiltrates; these may occur in up to one-third of patients with HIV and TB who are receiving combination antiretroviral therapy.[25] Immune reconstitution reactions can also occur in persons with TB who do not have HIV infection, but they are unusual (they occur in up to 25% of immunocompetent patients with nodal TB) and are usually manifested as enlarging lymph nodes.

If susceptibility is unchanged and adherence is assured (i.e., DOT), then it may be advisable to extend the duration of the continuation phase therapy for persons in specific high-risk groups, such as patients with a positive sputum culture at 2 months.[24] If drug resistance or substantial nonadherence is confirmed or suspected, a single drug should never be added to the regimen, since

resistance to all currently employed agents may be present, and effective monotherapy is being introduced.[26,27] Inevitably this will lead to resistance to the newly introduced agent and will greatly complicate future management. At least two drugs that can be expected to be active should be added. This nearly always leads to administration of one or more of the second-line agents, and consultation with a specialist in the treatment of drug-resistant TB is advised.

Special Situations

Human Immunodeficiency Virus Coinfection

Persons with HIV infection are uniquely susceptible to infection with *M. tuberculosis*, and progression to active disease is common. Among those who initially contain the disease, reactivation disease is common. Therefore active TB is a common clinical condition among persons with HIV, and in many locales a substantial proportion of TB patients have HIV coinfection. For this reason it is recommended that all TB patients have HIV serologic testing performed at the time of TB diagnosis. Persons with early HIV infection have the usual clinical manifestations of active TB and respond well to standard treatment regimens.[28] Thus specifically tailored TB treatment regimens are not required to control the TB. Such persons, however, are also likely to benefit from treatment of the HIV infection with combination antiretroviral therapy, particularly those patients with advanced HIV disease (CD4 cell count less than 200/mm^3), and a number of the medications that comprise combination antiretroviral therapy have serious drug interactions with antituberculous medications, thus requiring modification of the TB regimen, the antiretroviral regimen, or both.

Most authorities recommend that patients with TB and HIV receive combination antiretroviral therapy along with TB therapy, since TB can accelerate the course of HIV disease. Antiretroviral therapy for HIV infection is a repidly changing field of medicine. Furthermore, there are complex drug-drug interactions between the rifamycins and two commonly exployed classes of antiretroviral drugs, HIV-1 protease inhibitors and nonnucleoside reverse-transcriptase inhibitors. Therefore, it is difficult to make general recommendations regarding the most appropriate antiretroviral regimen for an HIV-infected patient with active TB. The first priority in the co-infected patient is always appropriate treatment of TB; untreated or inappropriately treated TB is a severe disease in an immunocompromised patient. Antiretroviral therapy is recommended during TB therapy, but it should not be started until there is initial control of TB, mangement of initial adverse reactions to TB therapy, and the patient is ready for the adherence challenge of multidrug antiretroviral therapy. Doses of both TB drugs and antiretroviral drugs may need to be adjusted when treating TB in a patient concurrently receiving antiretroviral therapy. Because of these complexities, management of patients with HIV-related TB should always involve a care provider with experience in such treatment.[8,28]

Tuberculosis in the Pregnant Patient

Untreated Active TB in a pregnant woman can have poor outcomes for the patient and fetus, and TB treatment is indicated. Pyrazinamide is not routinely recommended for use in pregnancy in the United States because of insufficient safety data, so the regimen recommended above for pyrazinamide-resistant or intolerant patients should be given. Aminoglycosides should also be avoided in pregnancy because of potential fetal ototoxicity, so the regimen containing INH, rifampin, and ethambutol is preferred. Antituberculosis medications are not excreted in any great degree in breast milk, and TB therapy is not a contraindication to breast feeding.

Disseminated Tuberculosis or Tuberculosis Meningitis

All forms of active tuberculosis respond well to the standard 6-month treatment regimens. In cases in which clinical response is suboptimal, the clinician may opt to extend the duration of TB treatment. In such situations, however, it is imperative that failure of the initial regimen and other diseases be excluded as possible explanations for the suboptimal clinical response. Neither ethambutol nor streptomycin penetrate cerebrospinal fluid well, and these agents should not be relied upon for treatment of TB meningitis. Consultation with a specialist is advised when managing such patients.

Therapy of Active Tuberculosis in Persons with Impaired Renal Function

Neither INH nor rifampin is excreted by the kidney, so that adjustment of dosing of these agents in patients with impaired renal function is not necessary. Ethambutol and pyrazinamide can be used at normal doses with mild-to-moderate renal impairment, but in complete renal failure, doses should be reduced by half. INH, rifampin, and ethambutol are not removed by dialysis, but pyrazinamide is removed and should be replaced after dialysis.[29] Aminoglycosides can be used in patients with renal impairment when serum drug levels are carefully monitored, but in general, use of these agents to treat TB in persons with renal impairment can be avoided.

Treatment of Active Tuberculosis in Children

For most forms of active TB in children, recommendations for regimens and management of TB parallel those for TB in adults (with adjustment of dosing for the weight of the patient). Because of the difficulty in obtaining sputum samples from children, however, the diagnosis more often is based on clinical criteria, and monitoring the success of treatment relies more heavily on chest radiographs. In the selection of a treatment regimen, the inability to monitor color vision in very young children makes ethambutol less desirable, and quinolones generally are avoided because of their potential for interference with bone and joint development.

TREATMENT OF LATENT TUBERCULOSIS

Latent Tuberculosis Regimens

Recommended regimens for treatment of presumed drug-susceptible latent TB are shown in Table 31–10. The efficacy of each of the first four of these regimens has been established in randomized, prospective clinical trials.[30] Because persons with latent TB are culture negative, it is not possible to know the susceptibility of the

TABLE 31–10 ■ Recommended Drug Regimens for Treatment of Latent Tuberculosis Infection (TLTBI)

Preferred regimens	Interval and duration	Comments
Isoniazid	Daily × 9 mo	In human immunodeficiency virus (HIV)-infected patients, isoniazid may be administered concurrently with nucleoside reverse transcriptase inhibitors (NRTIs), protease inhibitors, or non-nucleoside reverse transcriptase inhibitors (NNRTIs)
Isoniazid	2/wk × 9 mo	Directly observed therapy (DOT) must be used with twice-weekly dosing
ALTERNATIVE REGIMENS		
Rifampin plus pyrazinamide	Daily × 2 mo	May also be offered to persons who are contacts of patients with isoniazid-resistant, rifampin-susceptible TB In HIV-infected patients, protease inhibitors or NNRTIs generally should not be administered concurrently with rifampin; rifabutin may be used as an alternative
Isoniazid	Daily × 6 mo	Not indicated for HIV-infected persons, those with fibrotic lesions on chest radiographs, or children
Rifampin	Daily × 4 mo	For persons who are contacts of patients with isoniazid-resistant, rifampin-susceptible TB

Adapted from Centers for Disease Control and Prevention: Targeted tuberculin testing and treatment of latent tuberculosis infection. MMWR Morb Mortal Wkly Rep 2000;49(RR-6):1–51.

isolate with which they are infected. However, as over 90% of *M. tuberculosis* isolates in the United States are susceptible to INH, rifampin, and pyrazamide, it is assumed that this will be the case unless the source case is known to have drug resistance. The preferred regimen is 9 months of INH. The 9-month INH regimen can be given daily or twice weekly. If one of these preferred regimens cannot be tolerated, rifampin and pyraminamine for 2 months or rifampin alone for 4 months can be used. Cost-benefit concerns may lead health departments to employ the second-line regimen of INH (daily or twice weekly) for 6 months, but this regimen is not as effective as the 9-month INH regimen. When INH is given twice weekly, DOT should be employed. Persons receiving one of the INH-containing regimens who are at increased risk for the development of peripheral neuropathy, such as patients with alcoholism, malnutrition, diabetes, uremia, or seizure disorders or who are pregnant, should receive supplemental pyridoxine (50 mg/d).

Previous recommendations from the CDC suggested that INH not be given to persons over the age of 35 unless they were in a group at high risk for reactivation of their latent TB. This recommendation attempted to balance the risk for a false-positive PPD skin test with the increasing potential for INH hepatotoxicity in older persons. The most recent recommendations increase the cutoff for a positive PPD skin test among such persons from 10 mm to 15 mm.[2] By doing this the risk of reactivation TB among skin-test-positive persons is increased because most of the false-positive results were in the 10- to 14-mm group. Therefore the risk of INH hepatitis is outweighed by the benefit of protection from reactivation TB in all age groups, and the 35-year age cutoff no longer applies.

When a patient with latent TB is a recent PPD skin test converter (an increase of 10 mm in PPD size within 2 years) and the source case has active TB that is resistant to INH or when the patient cannot tolerate INH, one of the rifampin-based regimens should be used; the 2-month rifampin-pyrazinamide regimen is preferred. Persons intolerant to pyrazinamide can receive rifampin alone for 4 months. When the person with latent TB is a recent PPD skin test converter and the source case has active TB that is resistant to rifampin alone, the 9-month INH regimen should be given.

If there is a high likelihood that the patient with latent TB has acquired disease that is multidrug resistant, treatment of the latent TB must be individualized and based on the susceptibility pattern of the source case from whom the patient acquired the *M. tuberculosis* infection. There are no data on the efficacy of such individualized latent TB treatment regimens, however, and many are difficult to tolerate. Moreover, when it is unclear whether the person with latent TB has acquired drug-susceptible or drug-resistant infection, one of the standard regimens should be given, since these are known to be effective when the isolate is susceptible.

Expected Outcome

Treatment of latent TB with one of the preferred regimens in Table 31–10 reduces the risk of reactivation TB by as much as 90%.[30] The 6-month INH regimen reduces the risk by 50% to 60%. Although this is substantial and statistically significant, it is less than the reduction achieved by the preferred regimens. The 4-month rifampin regimen has not been evaluated in a clinical trial, although a 3-month regimen of rifampin achieved a 50% reduction in reactivation TB among persons with silicosis.[31]

Monitoring Treatment for Latent Tuberculosis

Adherence

Latent TB treatment regimens are largely self-administered, and care providers should monitor adherence carefully. Considerable encouragement and reiteration of the benefit of adhering to treatment may be needed. Many clinics give a single month of medicine per visit and see patients monthly (every 2 weeks for patients taking the 2-month regimen), thus providing regular opportunities to monitor adherence and reinforce the patient's resolve to complete the course of therapy. DOT (using intermittent regimens) is used mostly in treating latent TB in children and is infrequently recommended for adults.

Drug Toxicity

Since patients with latent TB are asymptomatic, they may be less willing to tolerate the adverse effects of medications. The potential toxicities are the same whether the drugs are given for latent or active TB and include hepatitis and rash from INH, rifampin, and pyrazinamide, peripheral neuritis from INH, and arthralgias and hyperuriciemia from pyrazinamide. Gastrointestinal intolerance related to any of the three drugs is possible but is less likely to be caused by pyrazinamide when a dose of only 20 mg/kg is used.

For patients with a history or physical examination suggestive of hepatitis or risk factors for hepatitis, such as alcoholism or intravenous drug use, and for pregnant, postpartum, and HIV-infected persons, baseline liver function tests should be obtained. When initial liver function test results show elevated levels, they should be monitored at each visit until they return to the normal range. In persons not receiving follow-up testing, and in whom clinical symptoms suggesting hepatitis develop, liver function tests should be obtained, as drug-induced hepatitis may occur at any time during a course of therapy. Patients should be cautioned to note the symptoms of hepatitis, such as nausea, fatigue, abdominal pain, jaundice, and dark urine. Since early cessation of the offending agent can lead to resolution and since continued ingestion of the offending agent may be fatal, prompt attention to the possibility of drug-induced hepatitis is essential.

Patients with intolerance to INH, rifampin, or pyrazinamide theoretically may be rechallenged after the toxicity has subsided, but this is not recommended for patients receiving these drugs in latent TB treatment regimens. Gaining patient adherence to treatment of latent TB is difficult enough without risking recurrence of an adverse reaction, however minor. Discoloration of urine and other secretions (such as tears) in persons taking rifampin may be problematic for some patients (particularly those who wear contact lenses), and patients should be advised about this phenomenon before they start a rifampin-based regimen.

Special Situations

Latent Tuberculosis Treatment in Persons Coinfected with HIV

HIV coinfection greatly increases the risk of reactivation TB in a person with latent TB; therefore assuring completion of latent TB treatment assumes even greater importance in such patients. Latent TB treatment is a "standard of care" recommendation in this population.[32] The regimens are the same as those recommended for treatment of latent TB in HIV-negative persons. When an INH regimen is selected, the 9-month regimen should be used. When a rifamycin-containing regimen is given to persons also taking combination antiretroviral therapy, regimens will require substitution of rifabutin for rifampin and the antiretroviral dosing adjustments needed for treatment active TB.[8] Patients on antiretroviral regimens containing multiple protease inhibitors or protease inhibitors and non-nucleoside reverse transcriptase inhibitors should be treated with the INH regimen, as pharmacokinetic interactions with rifamycin are complex and not easily predictable.

Latent Tuberculosis Treatment in the Pregnant Patient

As pyrazinamide is not recommended in pregnancy, the INH regimen is preferred. Anecdotal evidence suggests that the risk of INH hepatotoxicity may be increased in pregnancy, however, particularly in Hispanic women. Thus the risk of hepatotoxicity must be balanced with the potential benefit from treatment. On the other hand, patients who only seek medical care when pregnant may not return for latent TB treatment after delivery; thus delaying treatment may mean not treating. Cost benefit studies have shown that latent TB treatment with INH during pregnancy is beneficial in some populations. Any pregnant woman who has additional risk factors for progression of latent TB (such as recent infection, HIV infection, or injection drug use) should receive treatment without delay.

Treatment of Latent Tuberculosis in Children

Children under the age of 5 years are likely to have recent TB infection and are considered at increased risk for reactivation on this basis. The 9-month INH regimen is the only recommended regimen for children. Pyridoxine is not routinely recommended for coadministration,

except in breast-feeding infants and children with potential dietary deficiency of this vitamin.

ACKNOWLEDGMENT We thank John Bernardo, MD, for his thoughtful review of this chapter.

REFERENCES

1. Centers for Disease Control and Prevention: Reported tuberculosis in the United States, 1999. August 2000.
2. American Thoracic Society, Centers for Disease Control and Prevention: Diagnostic standards and classification of tuberculosis in adults and children. Am J Respir Crit Care Med 2000;161:1376–1395.
3. Horsburgh CR Jr, Feldman S, Ridzon R: Practice guidelines for the treatment of tuberculosis. Clin Infect Dis 2000;31:633–639.
4. Burman WJ, Reves RR: Review of false-positive cultures for *Mycobacterium tuberculosis* and recommendations for avoiding unnecessary treatment. Clin Infect Dis 2000;31:1390–1395.
5. Simone PM, Horsburgh CR Jr, Castro KG: Antimycobacterial drugs. In Gorbach SL, Bartlett JG, Blacklow NR (eds): Infectious Diseases, 2nd ed. Philadelphia, WB Saunders, 1997, pp 359–376.
6. Davidson BL: A controlled comparison of directly observed therapy vs self-administered therapy for active tuberculosis in the urban United States. Chest 1998;114:1239–1243.
7. Cook SV, Fujiwara PI, Frieden TR: Rates and risk factors for discontinuation of rifampicin. Int J Tuberc Lung Dis 2000; 4:118–122.
8. Burman WJ, Gallicano K, Peloquin C: Therapeutic implications of drug interactions in the treatment of human immunodeficiency virus-related tuberculosis. Clin Infect Dis 1999;28:419–429.
9. Sumartojo E: When tuberculosis treatment fails. A social behavioral account of patient adherence. Am Rev Respir Dis 1993;147:1311–1320.
10. Weis SE, Slocum PC, Blais FX, et al: The effect of directly observed therapy on the rates of drug resistance and relapse in tuberculosis. N Engl J Med 1994;330:1179–1184.
11. Small PM, Hopewell PC, Singh SP, et al: The epidemiology of tuberculosis in San Francisco. A population-based study using conventional and molecular methods. N Engl J Med 1994;330:1703–1709.
12. American Thoracic Society, Centers for Disease Control and Prevention, Infectious Disease Society of America: Treatment of tuberculosis. Am J Resp Crit Care Med 2002 (in press).
13. Centers for Disease Control and Prevention: Core Curriculum on Tuberculosis. What the Clinician Should Know, 4th ed. Atlanta, US Department of Health and Human Services, 2000.
14. Fox W, Ellard GA, Mitchison DA: Studies on the treatment of tuberculosis undertaken by the British Medical Research Council Tuberculosis Units, 1946–86, with subsequent publications. Int J Tuberc Lung Dis 1999;3:S231–S279.
15. Combs DL, O'Brien RJ, Geiter LJ: USPHS tuberculosis short-course chemotherapy trial 21: Effectiveness, toxicity and acceptability. The report of final results. Ann Intern Med 1990;112:397–406.
16. Cohn DL, Catlin BBJ, Petersen KL, et al: A 62-dose, 6 month therapy for pulmonary and extrapulmonary tuberculosis. Ann Intern Med 1990;112:407–415.
17. Tuberculosis Trials Consortium: Rifapentine and isoniazid once a week versus rifampicin and isoniazid twice a week for treatment of drug-susceptible pulmonary tuberculosis in HIV-negative patients: A randomised clinical trial. Lancet 2002;360:528–34.
18. Iseman MD: Treatment of multidrug-resistant tuberculosis. N Eng J Med 1993;329:784–791.

19. Dooley DP, Carpenter JL, Rademacher S: Adjunctive corticosteroid therapy for tuberculosis: A critical reappraisal of the literature. Clin Infect Dis 1997;25:872–887.

20. Centers for Disease Control: Tuberculosis Control Laws—United States, 1993. MMWR Morb Mortal Wkly Rep 1993;42(RR-15):1–26.

21. Singleton L, Turner M, Haskal R, et al: Long-term hospitalization for tuberculosis control. JAMA 1997;278:838–842.

22. Oscherwitz T, Tulsky JP, Roger S, et al: Detention of persistently nonadherent patients with tuberculosis. JAMA 1997;278:843–846.

23. Peloquin CA: Using therapeutic drug monitoring to dose antimycobacterial drugs. Clin Chest Med 1997;18:79–87.

24. Gordin F, Chaisson R, TB Trials Consortium: TBTC study 22: Risk factors for relapse in HIV-negative patients. Am J Respir Crit Care Med 2000;161:A252.

25. Narita M, Ashkin D, Hollender ES, Pitchenik AE: Paradoxical worsening of tuberculosis following antiretroviral therapy in patients with AIDS. Am J Respir Crit Care Med 1998; 158:157–161.

26. Mahmoudi A, Iseman MD: Pitfalls in the care of patients with tuberculosis. JAMA 1993;270:65–68.

27. Rao SN, Mookerjee AL, Obasanjo OO, Chaisson RE: Errors in the treatment of tuberculosis in Baltimore. Chest 2000;117: 734–737.

28. Centers for Disease Control and Prevention: Prevention and treatment of tuberculosis among patients infected with human immunodeficiency virus: Principles of therapy and revised recommendations. MMWR Morb Mortal Wkly Rep 1998; 47(RR-20):1–58.

29. Malone RS, Fish DN, Spiegel DM, et al: The effect of hemodialysis on isoniazid, rifampin, pyrazinamide, and ethambutol. Am J Respir Crit Care Med 1999;159:1580–1584.

30. Centers for Disease Control and Prevention: Targeted tuberculin testing and treatment of latent tuberculosis infection. MMWR Morb Mortal Wkly Rep 2000;49(RR-6):1–51.

31. A double-blind placebo-controlled clinical trial of three antituberculosis chemoprophylaxis regimens in patients with silicosis in Hong Kong. Am Rev Respir Dis 1992;145:36–41.

32. USPHS/IDSA Prevention of Opportunistic Infections Working Group. 1999 USPHS/IDSA guidelines for the prevention of opportunistic infections in persons infected with human immunodeficiency virus. Clin Infect Dis 2000;30:S29–S65.

chapter
32

Nontuberculous Mycobacterial Infections

JAMES L. COOK, MD

Nontuberculous mycobacteria (NTM) are environmental pathogens[1] that are relatively uncommon causes of noncontagious disease in humans. NTM have been recognized as human pathogens since the late 1940s.[2] The true incidence and prevalence of NTM infections in the United States is uncertain, however, since there has been no well-organized national reporting or data gathering system. Limited data are available from the Public Health Laboratory Information System (PHLIS) at the Centers for Disease Control and Prevention (CDC) for the period 1993 through 1996, when laboratory reports were collected from state public health laboratories across the United States. These data provide a laboratory-based estimate of the number of NTM-positive cultures, by species, state, region, and body site reported during that period. These data can be viewed at http://www.cdc.gov/ncidod/dastlr/TB/ntmfinal.pdf.

NTM disease initially was recognized as a tuberculosis (TB)-like illness, presenting as upper lobe cavitary disease in men with underlying pulmonary disease. Because of the low incidence of these infections compared with that of TB and the associated lack of experience that most clinicians have with NTM disease, there was little change in this perception in the general medical community until the middle 1980s. With the onset of the AIDS epidemic, it rapidly became apparent that infections with *Mycobacterium avium* complex (MAC)—the most common of the NTM infections in the United States—were also the most common opportunistic bacterial infections in these highly immunosuppressed patients. The increased national awareness of the importance of MAC infections in the context of human immunodeficiency virus (HIV) disease stimulated a collateral increase in the recognition of the prevalence of these infections in the general population. Over the past two decades there has been a growing appreciation of the problems of NTM disease in a variety of HIV-negative patient populations, including older women with underlying bronchiectasis, others with structural lung abnormalities, and those with a variety of environmental exposures to these pathogens. The increased frequency of diagnosis of NTM infections is likely the consequence of both increased clinical and laboratory diagnostic acumen and a true increase in infection incidence.

Treatment for NTM infections initially was modeled after the treatment of TB, especially multidrug-resistant tuberculosis (MDR-TB). This was a result of both the absence of clinical studies of optimal NTM disease treatment and the observation that like MDR-TB, most NTM are resistant to a variety of antibiotics. With the onset of the HIV epidemic there was an intensive study of NTM treatment regimens. These efforts further advanced understanding of the key elements of NTM treatment strategies and development of effective prophylactic regimens for HIV-infected patients.

The primary goal of this chapter will be to focus on general principles of the treatment of NTM disease. General guidelines will also be provided for disease caused by specific NTM species. In keeping with the theme of this text, discussions of epidemiology, microbiology, and NTM pathogenesis will be limited to considerations of regional differences in diagnosis, empiric treatment, and antibiotic regimen design.

HOW TO PROCEED UNTIL MYCOBACTERIAL IDENTIFICATION IS AVAILABLE

A not uncommon clinical question is how to treat a patient with an acid-fast bacilli (AFB)-positive sputum smear who is suspected of having NTM-induced disease. Public health concerns mandate consideration of TB for questions of respiratory isolation and initiation of empiric therapy. Standard TB regimens, however, are not highly effective against NTM infections. It can be helpful under these circumstances to consider the regional epidemiology of NTM infections and the site of NTM infection in the design of an empiric treatment plan pending mycobacterial identification. The Runyon Classification of NTM was based on both growth rates and pigmentation characteristics of mycobacterial colonies.[3] Even though this scheme is used less frequently in the era of biochemical and molecular diagnostics, it does provide a means to represent the relationships among the most clinically relevant NTM (Fig. 32–1).

A few NTM species cause most of the disease. Observations from the PHLIS NTM database provide regional epidemiologic information that can be used to guide empiric anti-NTM therapy. These data show that *Mycobacterium avium-intracellulare* (MAI) causes more infections than any other NTM species in all regions of the United States (Fig. 32–2A). The second most com-

monly reported laboratory isolates nationwide were rapidly growing mycobacteria (RGM: *Mycobacterium fortuitum*, *Mycobacterium abscessus*, and *Mycobacterium chelonae*). Reporting rates for other species of NTM varied by geographic region. Two examples illustrate this point. *Mycobacterium kansasii* isolates were reported more commonly in the South Central, North Central, and South Eastern regions of the United States (78% of 2784 isolates; Fig. 32–2B). In contrast, *Mycobacterium simiae* isolates were relatively more common in the Mountain and South Central regions of the United States (72% of 760 isolates; Fig. 32–2C). Variations in the regional incidence of NTM disease are also observed in other countries and regions outside of the United States. *Mycobacterium malmoense* infection is one example. This NTM species was first identified as a cause of pulmonary disease in the late 1970s and is recognized as a major NTM pathogen in England and northern Europe.

Final laboratory identification of an NTM isolate from a clinical specimen may require many weeks. Epidemiologic data on NTM incidence can be used to develop a strategy for empiric therapy pending mycobacterial species identification. In addition to regional epidemiology several questions can be used to formulate this strategy (Table 32–1). The first is whether TB can be excluded as the diagnosis. A nuclear acid amplification assay using sputum specimens can be used to confirm or exclude the diagnosis of TB with reasonable certainty in a patient with an AFB smear-positive specimen.[4] Another question is whether the patient's clinical status warrants initiation of empiric therapy before identification of the mycobacterial pathogen. Whether the patient is AFB smear-positive or smear-negative, the absence of clinical

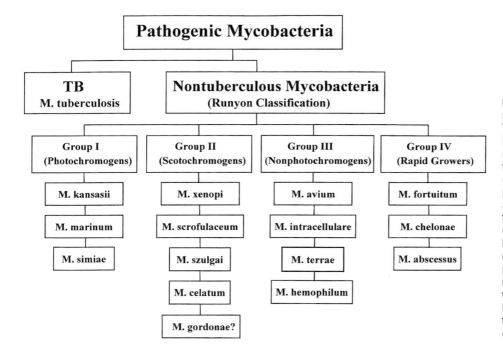

FIGURE 32–1. Runyon Classification of nontuberculous mycobacteria (NTM). The three categories of slowly growing NTM (groups I, II, and III) are based upon usual pigmentation characteristics of mycobacterial colonies. Photochromogens produce yellow-orange pigmentation on exposure to light but are mostly nonpigmented when cultured in the dark. Scotochromogens exhibit pigmentation irrespective of light exposure. Nonchromogenic mycobacterial colonies are usually nonpigmented or weakly pigmented and do not change their pigmentation characteristics with light exposure. Group IV NTM are distinguished from species in the other categories by rapid growth in culture (usually within 1 week).

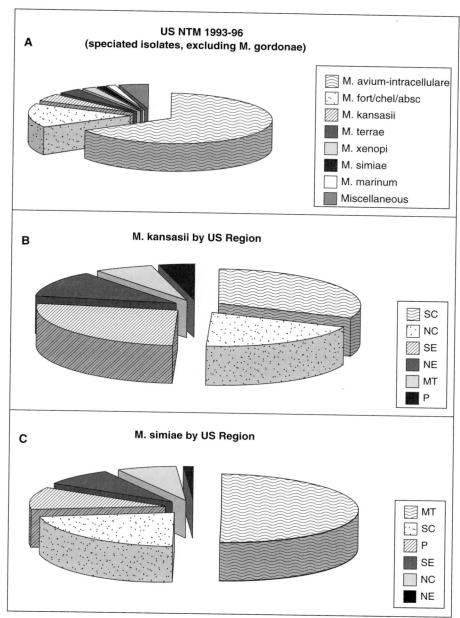

FIGURE 32–2. Nontuberculous mycobacteria (NTM) reporting patterns from state public health laboratories in the United States between 1993 and 1996 recorded on the Public Health Laboratory Information Service (PHLIS) database. **A,** NTM isolates that were speciated, other than *Mycobacterium gordonae*; 66% (714/54, 120) were *Mycobacterium avium-intracellulare*. **B,** *Mycobacterium kansasii* isolates reported by U.S. geographic region; 78% of isolates were reported from three U.S. regions: South Central (SC) (856/2784, 31%), South East (SE) (784/2784, 27%), and North Central (NC) (549/2784, 20%). **C,** *Mycobacterium simiae* isolates reported by U.S. geographic region; 72% of isolates were reported from two U.S. regions: Mountain (MT) (383/760, 50%) and South Central (SC) (169/760, 22%). NE, North East; P, Pacific. Figure legends are represented clockwise in pie figures.

signs and symptoms or of evidence of severe disease allows time to complete microbiologic studies and to consider the best approach to therapy. Rapid growth of NTM from sputum or other specimens (culture often positive within 1 week for rapid growers) raises suspicion about RGM as the pathogens and can be used to guide empiric therapy. If RGM are suspected and if the clinical circumstance dictates initiation of therapy before mycobacterial identification and antibiotic susceptibility testing are completed, a different empiric treatment strategy from that for MAI or other NTM infections is appropriate (Tables 32–2 to 32–4). In uncommon cases it is possible to use the site of an NTM infection to plan empiric therapy. Finding an AFB-positive smear from a

TABLE 32–1 ■ Questions to Guide Initiation of Empiric Therapy for Suspected Nontuberculosis Mycobacterial (NTM) Disease

1. What are the most prevalent NTM in the region?
2. Can TB be excluded with a rapid diagnostic test?
3. Does the patient's clinical status warrant starting therapy before mycobacterial identification?
4. Is the mycobacterium a rapid grower?
5. Does the site of infection suggest infection caused by a rapidly growing mycobacterium?

soft tissue infection associated with trauma and soil contamination suggests an RGM. RGM are also more common than slowly growing NTM as pathogens in hospital-acquired infections associated with sternal wound infections, augmentation mammoplasties, contaminated suture material, or peritoneal dialysis.[5]

WHETHER TO TREAT? WHEN TO TREAT? WHEN NOT TO TREAT?

A common dilemma is what to do about the first positive NTM culture result. This is usually a sputum culture but can also be a culture from another site that should be sterile. If only a single specimen has been tested, several questions arise about the clinical significance of the culture result and the approach to therapy.

False-Positive Cultures for *Mycobacterium gordonae*

Mycobacteria can contaminate laboratory buffers and other water sources and therefore can produce false-positive culture results. The most noteworthy problem of this type results from contamination with *M. gordonae*.[6–11] For this reason it is common practice among physicians experienced in treating NTM infections to assume that a *M. gordonae* isolate associated with a clinical specimen is a contaminant until proven otherwise. It is therefore usually appropriate to seek an alternative diagnosis for a patient with a culture positive for *M. gordonae* unless there is extensive supporting clinical information and multiple positive cultures for the same species. Other mycobacteria are less likely to cause a false-positive culture result. Even TB, however, can be the source of laboratory cross-contamination.[12]

The Single Positive Culture

It is also possible that the first positive culture is a true positive but that only a single positive will be obtained after testing multiple clinical specimens. If it is only possible to obtain a single positive sputum culture (or culture from another site), the decision must be made about whether the diagnosis of NTM-induced disease is worth pursuing. After multiple negative follow-up cultures, it may be necessary to proceed with bronchoscopy, lung

biopsy, or repeat culture of another site to confirm the diagnosis if warranted by the clinical situation. The issue of a single positive culture can be more problematic with clinical specimens from normally sterile sites (e.g., joint or spinal fluid) because of the difficulty of repeated sampling. The summary point about the first positive NTM culture from any site is that confirmation should be sought through repeated cultures, and corroborating clinical and radiographic evidence should be obtained to complement the culture data.

"Colonization" with NTM?

A finding of more than one positive mycobacterial culture can raise the question of mycobacterial colonization vs. true infection and disease. For example, patients with bronchiectasis can present with minimal symptoms and repeated sputum cultures positive for NTM. Physicians who have followed such patients are increasingly impressed that the concept of NTM "colonization" of the airways is probably incorrect. Conversely, most of these patients appear to have slowly progressive, invasive disease. The availability of high-resolution computed tomography (CT) scans has made it possible to see a variety of pulmonary prenchymal changes caused by NTM infection[13] despite no definitive changes in routine chest radiography. It is unlikely that the use of pulmonary hygiene, in the absence of antimicrobial therapy, will eliminate these infections.

Decision to Treat Based on Mycobacterial Species Isolated

It is also appropriate to consider the species of mycobacterium identified in a clinical specimen when one is deciding whether to start therapy for a patient with a culture positive for NTM. Pulmonary NTM disease will be used as the model for this point. Detection of *M. kansasii*, *M. xenopi*, or *M. simiae* in patients with a clinical presentation compatible with pulmonary disease usually indicates the presence of mycobacterial disease that should be treated with antimicrobial therapy. It is appropriate to start treatment with a multidrug antimycobacterial regimen when the culture positive status for these species is confirmed. In contrast, patients with sputum cultures that are positive for MAI, RGM, or other NTM may or may not require prompt

TABLE 32-2 ■ Guidelines for Treatment of Disease Caused by Slowly Growing Nontuberculous Mycobacteria: *Mycobacterium avium-intracellulare* (MAI) and *Mycobacterium kansasii*

DISEASE	SUSCEPTIBILITY PATTERN	CORE REGIMEN (ALTERNATIVE DRUG)	CORE DRUG DOSAGES	CORE DRUG DOSING STRATEGIES	ANCILLARY THERAPY (ALTERNATIVE DRUG)	COMMENTS
*M. avium-intracellulare*						
Pulmonary (bronchiectasis + nodular, patchy infiltrates; cavitary disease)	Clarithromycin susceptible (MIC ≤ 8.0)	Clarithromycin (Azithromycin) Ethambutol Rifampin (Rifabutin)	500–1000 mg (250–500) mg 25 (2 mo) → 15 mg/kg 450–600 mg (150–300) mg	3×/wk or qd	Aminoglycoside Amikacin (Streptomycin) IM, 15 mg/kg IV, 12 mg/kg 2–3/wk or 5 d/wk ?Inhaled Tobramycin 300 mg qd (Amikacin) (500) mg qd	Thrice weekly oral therapy for mild disease; highest tolerated macrolide dose up to max shown; ?daily therapy for more severe disease; add aminoglycoside therapy for 1–3 mo for moderate-to-severe disease ?Use of inhaled aminoglycoside for continuation after parenteral treatment or for salvage regimen or palliative therapy
Pulmonary (bronchiectasis + nodular, patchy infiltrates; cavitary disease)	Clarithromycin-resistant (MIC > 8.0)	Ethambutol Rifampin (Rifabutin) Added drugs, e.g., Fluoroquinolone Clofazimine	Same as above Same as above Standard dose 100–200 mg	qd	Same	Base retreatment on susceptibility testing data; seek at least 3 effective drugs; more likely to use initial aminoglycoside therapy in retreatment of moderate-to-severe disease unless limited by previous toxicity
Soft tissue, bone, or joint infection	Same as for pulmonary disease	Same as above	Same as above	qd	Same	Excision, débridement, foreign body removal are important
Lymphadenitis	Assume Clarithromycin susceptibility	Clarithromycin-based regimen with two effective drugs is conservative approach ??Clarithromycin monotherapy for minimal disease	Same as above	qd	NA	Only use antibiotic therapy for disease that is refractory to excision, nonresectable, or recurrent; avoid incision and drainage if possible
Disseminated in immunosuppressed patient	Same as for pulmonary disease	Same as for pulmonary disease, except rifabutin instead of rifampin	Same as above, except consider reduced rifabutin dose	qd	Same as for pulmonary disease	Consider macrolide and rifabutin interactions with antiretroviral drugs[66,67]
Prophylaxis in HIV-positive patient	Assume Clarithromycin susceptibility	Azithromycin (Rifabutin)	1200 mg (300 mg)	Weekly qd	NA	Exclude active TB when rifabutin is used

Continued

TABLE 32-2 ■ Guidelines for Treatment of Disease Caused by Slowly Growing Nontuberculous Mycobacteria: Mycobacterium avium-intracellulare (MAI) and Mycobacterium kansasii (Continued)

DISEASE	SUSCEPTIBILITY PATTERN	CORE REGIMEN (ALTERNATIVE DRUG)	CORE DRUG DOSAGES	CORE DRUG DOSING STRATEGIES	ANCILLARY THERAPY (ALTERNATIVE DRUG)	COMMENTS
			*Mycobacterium kansasii*			
Pulmonary (nodular and cavitary disease)	Rifampin-susceptible	Rifampin (Rifabutin) / Ethambutol / Isoniazid	450–600 (150–300) mg / 25(2 mo) → 15 mg/kg / 300 mg	qd	Aminoglycoside, Amikacin (Streptomycin) IM, 15 mg/kg IV, 12 mg/kg 2–3x/wk or 5 d/wk	Clarithromycin or fluoroquinolone alternative if isoniazid-intolerant or hepatotoxicity
Pulmonary (nodular and cavitary disease)	Rifampin-resistant	Ethambutol / Isoniazid / Added drugs, e.g., Clarithromycin / Fluoroquinolone / Ethionamide / Cycloserine	25(2 mo) → 15 mg/kg / 300 mg / 500–1000 mg / Standard qd dose / 250–750 mg / 250–750 mg	qd / qd / May need divided daily dose	Same as above	Base treatment on susceptibility testing data; seek at least 3 effective drugs, not previously used; more likely to use initial aminoglycoside therapy in retreatment of moderate-to-severe disease unless limited by previous toxicity; *not* Pyrazinamide or Para-aminosalicylic acid ("always" resistant); Ethionamide and Cycloserine more toxic that other options
Soft tissue, bone, joint infection	Same as for pulmonary disease	Same as above	Same as above	qd	Same	Excision, débridement, foreign body removal are important
Disseminated in immuno-suppressed patient	Same as for pulmonary disease	Same as for pulmonary disease, except use rifabutin instead of rifampin	Same as above, except consider reduced rifabutin dose	qd	Same as for pulmonary disease	Consider macrolide and rifabutin interactions with antiretroviral drugs[66,67]

MIC, minimum inhibitory concentration; NA, not applicable.

TABLE 32–3 ■ Slowly Growing Nontuberculous Mycobacteria (NTM) other than *M. avium-intracellulare* (MAI) and *M. kansasii*

Mycobacterial species	Empiric regimen until susceptibility testing data available; doses as for MAI (Table 32–2) (alternative drug)	Alternative or additional drugs (see MAI recommendations [Table 32–2] for doses and comments; otherwise standard doses)	Ancillary therapy for moderate-to-severe disease (alternative drug)	Comments
M. xenopi (and less common NTM—e.g., szulgai, terrae, malmoense, genavense, gordonae, hemophilum, celatum)	Rifampin (Rifabutin) Ethambutol Clarithromycin (Azithromycin)	Fluoroquinolone Others based on susceptibility data	Aminoglycoside, Amikacin (Streptomycin) IM, 15 mg/kg IV, 12 mg/kg 2–3×/wk or 5 d/wk	*M. xenopi* susceptibility testing data are variable but may show a relatively high degree of susceptibility despite a limited response to therapy; *M. terrae*: tenosynovitis is most common presentation; débridement can be important[*]; *M. gordonae*: usually a contaminant, rarely a pathogen; *M. celatum*: limited data on resistance to rifamycins and benefit of ethambutol-clarithromycin-fluoroquinolone regimen[91]; *M. ulcerans*: débridement and skin grafting important; multidrug antibiotic therapy may be useful[†]
M. simiae	Ethambutol Clarithromycin (Azithromycin) Fluoroquinolone	Ethionamide Cycloserine	Same as above	Usually resistant to most standard TB drugs; limited clinical data in AIDS patients and mouse model data on ethambutol-clarithromycin-fluoroquinolone regimen[83,86]
M. marinum	Rifampin (Rifabutin) Ethambutol Clarithromycin (Azithromycin)	Fluoroquinolone Doxycycline TMP-SMX	Amikacin IV, 12 mg/kg qd	Aminoglycoside therapy rarely necessary unless severe disease requires complementary parenteral therapy during débridement

NOTES: Limited data on the optimal therapy for slowly growing NTM other than MAI and *M. kansasii*—American Thoracic Society guidelines.[38] Advisable to start therapy with an empiric, 3-drug regimen and then to base treatment on the results of antibiotic susceptibility testing of the clinical isolate. For severe illness, initial empiric aminoglycoside therapy can be started and then reviewed as soon as susceptibility data are available. Same empiric guidelines can be used for pulmonary diseases or for soft tissue, bone, joint, or disseminated infection, considering the same comments as for MAI in Table 32–2.

[*]Data from Smith DS, Lindholm-Levy P, Huitt GA, et al: *Mycobacterium terrae*: Case reports, literature review, and in vitro antibiotic susceptibility testing. Clin Infect Dis 2000;30:444–453.

[†]Data from Portaels F, Traore H, De Ridder K, Meyers WM: In vitro susceptibility of *Mycobacterium ulcerans* to clarithromycin. Antimicrob Agents Chemother 1998;42:2070–2073.

TABLE 32–4 ■ Guidelines for Treatment of Disease Caused by Rapidly Growing Nontuberculous Mycobacteria (RGM)

Mycobacterial species	Oral agents	Parenteral β-lactam dose	Parenteral aminoglycoside dose	Comments
M. fortuitum	Clarithromycin Fluoroquinolone Doxycycline Sulfonamide ?Oxazalidinones	Cefoxitin 2 g IV q8–12h OR Imipenem-cilastatin 500 mg IV q8–12h	Amikacin 12 mg/kg IV qd	*M. fortuitum* isolates are usually more susceptible in vitro and more responsive to therapy than the other two major RGM species are; *M. fortuitum* may be susceptible to linezolid[93]
M. abscessus	Clarithromycin Fluoroquinolone ?Oxazalidinones	Same as above	Same as above ?Inhaled Tobramycin (Amikacin) 300 (500) mg qd	Linezolid can be active in vitro against *M. abscessus*[93] and can be effective in vivo[94] ?Use of inhaled aminoglycoside for continuation after parenteral treatment in patients for whom parenteral aminoglycoside therapy is contraindicated or for patients for whom an added drug is needed for long-term disease suppression
M. chelonae	Clarithromycin Fluoroquinolone ?Oxazalidinones	Same as above	Same as above ?Inhaled Tobramycin (Amikacin) 300 (500) mg qd	*M. chelonae* is more likely than *M. fortuitum* or *M. abscessus* to be resistant to cefoxitin; linezolid may be less active in vitro against *M. chelonae* than *M. abscessus* or *M. fortuitum*[93] ?Use of inhaled aminoglycoside for continuation after parenteral treatment in patients for whom parenteral aminoglycoside therapy is contraindicated or for patients for whom an added drug is needed for long-term disease suppression

NOTES: Limited data on the optimal therapy for rapidly growing nontuberculous mycobacteria—American Thoracic Society guidelines.[38] Advisable to start therapy with an empiric 2- or 3-drug regimen and then to base treatment upon the results of antibiotic susceptibility testing of the clinical isolate. *For limited soft tissue infection,* oral antibiotic therapy may be sufficient. *For moderate to severe pulmonary disease or other infection,* advisable to start therapy with two effective i.v. antibiotics (i.e., β-lactam + aminoglycoside) with or without oral agents and then to make a transition to a 2-drug oral regimen for long-term therapy after initial clinical response. *For soft tissue, bone, joint, or disseminated infection,* same comments apply as for *M. avium intracellulare* (Table 32–2).
Fluoroquinolone, e.g., ciprofloxacin, levofloxacin, gatifloxacin, moxifloxacin.

initiation of treatment. In these cases it is reasonable to consider the answers to several questions before starting therapy.

Consideration of Symptoms in Decision to Start Therapy

The first question is whether the patient is ill or has minimal or no symptoms. Occasionally patients will be referred for the question of the clinical significance of positive cultures for MAI in the absence of any clinical symptoms or in the setting of minimal symptoms. In this situation there is no rush to start antibiotic therapy. It is appropriate to consider the likelihood of clinical benefit as a result of therapy and to balance this against factors such as anticipated drug-related side effects, patient age, and the cost of medications.

Consideration of Disease Severity in Decision to Start Therapy

A second question regarding the decision of whether to start therapy is the extent of disease and the prospect for disease progression and loss of lung function as a consequence of withholding therapy. Evidence from previous serial radiographic and pulmonary function studies can often be used to plot the course of disease. Patients with progressive disease resulting in parenchymal abnormalities (including fibronodular, bronchiectatic, and cavitary changes) are usually sufficiently symptomatic to justify starting a multidrug antimycobacterial regimen. At the other end of the spectrum are patients who have few or no pulmonary parenchymal abnormalities that can be directly attributed to NTM infection. For example, patients may present with long-standing bronchiectasis but no evidence of nodular changes, patchy infiltrates, cavities, or other abnormalities outside of the areas of bronchiectasis. Such patients can have serial AFB smears and cultures to confirm the bacteriologic diagnosis, can be observed at regular intervals (e.g., every 3 to 6 months) and can have serial chest CT scans (e.g., every 6 to 12 months) to watch for any evidence of NTM disease progression. If these patients have progressive symptoms or other clinical signs of deterioration, they should be treated. There is a spectrum of clinical presentations between these extremes of minimal symptoms and radiographic abnormalities to severe symptoms and progressive parenchymal damage that requires clinical judgment about the timing of the initiation of antimycobacterial therapy. The treatment starting point usually is marked by a pivotal change in the clinical course that triggers action, such as more frequent fevers, cough, or fatigue, episodes of hemoptysis, or progressive pulmonary lesions observed radiographically. Deterioration of pulmonary function in cystic fibrosis patients with NTM infections can also justify antimycobacterial therapy.

Circumstances in Which Therapy Might Be Withheld

In some patients who have clear-cut progressive NTM disease, antimycobacterial therapy can be inappropriate. This situation usually involves either elderly patients who experience intractable treatment-related side effects or patients with end-stage mycobacterial disease. Even a two-drug suppressive antibiotic regimen can cause unacceptable gastrointestinal or other side effects in some elderly patients. It is appropriate to counsel such patients about the anticipated course of untreated NTM disease and to consider alternative forms of symptomatic therapy and support. It might be possible to reconsider an antibiotic treatment plan at a later date, after improvement in nutritional status or resolution of other factors that contributed to drug intolerance. In patients with far-advanced pulmonary NTM infection, a time may come when multidrug antibiotic therapy is inappropriate. The cachexia, anorexia, and malaise associated with end-stage mycobacterial disease can make it difficult for patients to tolerate an otherwise appropriate antibiotic regimen. A "drug treatment holiday" of 1 to 2 weeks off of therapy to allow patients to recover from antibiotic-related side effects (usually gastrointestinal) can provide a timeout for both the patient and the physician to consider the value and acceptability of resuming treatment. As with elderly patients, it might be possible and necessary to restart a suppressive, palliative regimen if patients begin to experience fevers and other unacceptable systemic symptoms off of therapy. Alternatively it may be decided that further antibiotic therapy is inappropriate and that the patient should be considered for hospice care or other forms of supportive therapy during the terminal phase of their illness.

The advisability of starting or continuing treatment can also be questioned for patients who have failed multiple rounds of antibiotic therapy for persistent or progressive NTM disease. The physician must decide whether to stop therapy or to treat with a minimal, hopefully suppressive, regimen. A decision to stop therapy requires patient education regarding anticipated consequences of the decision and mandates follow-up for signs of clinical deterioration. Some patients who appear to have gained no benefit from antibiotic therapy and who then stop treatment can experience rapid disease progression. A more conservative approach in this situation is reduction in the antibiotic dose or frequency of administration. Since thrice weekly dosing can be effective during initial treatment of NTM infection caused by MAI,[14,15] intermittent therapy might also be useful for palliation. All of these decisions about "fine-tuning" treatment in patients with complex or inadequate responses to therapy may be best done in collaboration with a consultant with experience in the management of patients with refractory NTM infections.

GENERAL PRINCIPLES OF ANTIBIOTIC THERAPY FOR NTM DISEASE

Some concepts about the approach to treatment of NTM disease are generally applicable to most infections, irrespective of the mycobacterial species or site of infection. These general concepts will be reviewed using the model of pulmonary infection with MAI. Specific points will be added for other mycobacterial species and for NTM infections involving other organ systems or body sites.

Considering the Long-Term Plan

It is useful to think through the long-term goals and consequences of therapy when planning treatment for each new patient. Consideration of the duration and complexity of therapy, the side effects and costs of the treatment regimen, and the chronicity of NTM disease and underlying disease processes requires planning and continuity of care that are unusual when contrasted with many other infectious processes.

Matching Intensity of Therapy with Severity of Disease

It is usually appropriate to attempt to match the intensity of therapy with the severity of NTM disease. For example, patients with minimal symptoms and minimal-to-moderate pulmonary involvement can tolerate and respond well to an intermittent oral antibiotic regimen.[14] In contrast, patients who are severely ill with cavitary pulmonary disease may require parenteral antibiotic therapy that complements the oral antibiotic regimen and, in some cases, is timed to provide optimum preoperative disease control and postoperative coverage for resection or débridement. Consideration should also be given to the role of ancillary measures such as pulmonary hygiene, nutritional support, management of drug-related side effects, psychosocial support for chronic illness, and the financial impact of the treatment plan on the patient. Patients with moderate-to-severe disease often require the support of other consultants and ancillary services. Coordination of these efforts requires an additional time commitment from the primary treating physician and support staff.

Points to Assist in Formulating NTM Treatment Plan

Several questions can be used to formulate the specific antibiotic regimen and plan for drug management. What antibiotics should be used? How will the response to therapy be evaluated? How should the patient be monitored for drug-induced side effects? What is the appropriate duration of therapy?

Antibiotic Monotherapy—"Never" (Rarely) Used

Guidelines for empiric antibiotic selection are provided in Tables 32–2 to 32–4 and will be discussed when infections with specific mycobacterial species are considered. Some general concepts can be considered here. It is important to treat most NTM infections with multiple effective antibiotics, and it is usually inappropriate to use single antibiotic therapy, so-called monotherapy. The lesson of avoidance of monotherapy for mycobacterial disease was learned during the early history of the treatment of tuberculosis, where such practices resulted in treatment-induced emergence of drug-resistance.

Clarithromycin monotherapy of *M. avium* infection in AIDS patients exemplifies this problem. Initial trials were designed to determine whether clarithromycin was effective as a single drug in the context of *M. avium* bacteremia in AIDS. Monotherapy was effective in reducing or eliminating MAC bacteremia but also resulted in the evolution of clarithromycin resistance in the MAI population during the relapse phase of infection.[16] This pattern recapitulates the so-called fall-and-rise phenomenon that was described in TB, that is, initial reduction in bacterial burden followed by relapse of infection associated with emergence of drug resistance. The problem of monotherapy-induced NTM resistance results from initial elimination of the drug-susceptible subpopulations of mycobacteria followed by the emergence of drug-resistant subpopulations during relapse. The advantage of using multiple drugs against such a heterogeneous mycobacterial population is that organisms resistant to drug A will usually be susceptible to drug B. Therefore, the likelihood of emergence of a resistant population to a given treatment regimen becomes the multiple of the incidences of resistance to each drug. For example, if the incidence of drug A resistance $= 10^{-6}$ and the incidence of drug B resistance $= 10^{-4}$, the combined likelihood of drug resistance to a treatment regimen of drug A + B $= 10^{-6} \times 10^{-4} = 10^{-10}$. This theoretical problem is clinically relevant in circumstances of high bacterial burden, such as mycobacterial bacteremia in AIDS patients or cavitary NTM-induced lung disease, in which antibiotic monotherapy can result in evolution of drug resistance, subsequent loss of the effectiveness of the antibiotic, and long-term treatment failure. In contrast, in circumstances of low bacterial burden, as can be observed in mycobacterial skin infections, this problem might not be of practical concern, and monotherapy has been reported to result in a good clinical response with a low incidence of disease relapse.[17] As a general practice, however, it is appropriate to start antimycobacterial therapy with at least two, and usually three, effective antibiotics and if possible to continue this therapy throughout the course of treatment.

Monitoring Response to Therapy

Three types of parameters usually are followed to assess the efficacy of antimycobacterial therapy in NTM disease: symptomatic, bacteriologic, and radiographic responses. Although it is convenient to think of the response to therapy as following a linear course of improvement, this is sometimes not the case. Even during successful treatment of NTM-induced pulmonary disease there is usually an initial delay prior to any noticeable response, which can be followed by a somewhat hectic course of gradual improvement in all three parameters (Fig. 32–3). Since many patients have underlying pulmonary disease (e.g., bronchiectasis), it is also common for patients to have chronic symptoms that persist, despite conversion to mycobacteria negative culture status and improvement in radiographic changes.

Symptomatic response is manifested as a reduction in cough, fatigue, malaise, and fever, and for more chronically ill patients, as a reversal of a pattern of weight loss. Drug-related side effects such as anorexia and nausea can complicate assessment of the clinical response but can usually be dissected from symptoms caused by NTM infection. It is useful to follow serial bacteriology studies to determine whether the bacterial burden is reduced and the culture status has converted to negative. In the context of pulmonary NTM disease, monthly or bimonthly studies of sputum AFB smear positivity and semiquantitative mycobacterial culture positivity can be useful. Since a desired symptomatic response to therapy is reduction in cough and sputum production, it can be difficult to follow bacteriology results very far in to the course of successful therapy.

For pulmonary disease, periodic chest CT scans are the most informative radiographic studies. Chest radiographs have limited value for the assessment of NTM-induced

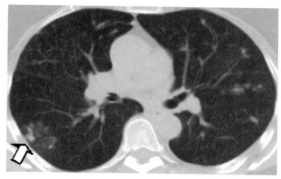

FIGURE 32–4. Peripheral clusters of nodules characteristic of nontuberculous mycobacteria–induced pulmonary disease.

lesions, other than large cavities, because of the common background problem of pulmonary changes from underlying disease and the insensitivity of plain films for mild-to-moderate bronchiectasis and associated nodular and parenchymal infiltrates. Pulmonary NTM cause CT changes that are different from those observed with TB. For example, clusters of nodules and patchy midlung field infiltrates associated with bronchiectasis are more common in pulmonary disease caused by NTM than in TB[13,18–20] (Fig. 32–4). Side-by-side comparisons of CT scans taken at 6- to 9-month intervals provide a radiographic correlation with symptomatic and bacteriologic parameters. Chest CT scans done at less than 4- to 6-month intervals may not show much change because of the relatively slow rate of improvement or progression of pulmonary NTM disease. Because of the frequency of underlying pulmonary abnormalities (especially bronchiectasis), it can be difficult to determine whether some changes seen on chest CT scan are associated with active NTM infection or with the underlying process, especially toward the end of a course of anti-NTM therapy when changes can be subtle.

Monitoring Drug-Induced Side Effects

Monitoring drug-related side effects during NTM therapy requires a combination of patient education, collaboration between the treating physician and ancillary support services, and assurance of longitudinal laboratory data analysis (Table 32–5).

Most patients tolerate a standard course of multidrug anti-NTM therapy with minor modifications in drug dosage. The most common long-term management problem follows initiation of therapy and the early symptomatic response. After a reduction in cough, malaise, and other systemic symptoms caused by NTM infection, patients usually report that their primary symptoms relate to medication-induced side effects, especially gastrointestinal symptoms associated with macrolide or fluoroquinolone therapy. Therefore most of the symptom management during a prolonged course of anti-NTM therapy involves attempts to support patients through drug-related side effects during a course of therapy sufficient to provide the best opportunity for cure or optimal bacteriologic response.

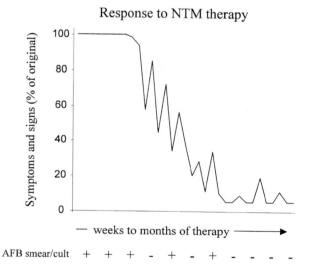

Response to NTM therapy

AFB smear/cult   +   +   +   -   +   -   +   -   -   -   -

FIGURE 32–3. Representation of the slow waxing and waning course of clinical response to anti-nontuberculous mycobacteria (NTM) therapy that is observed in some patients. Acid-fast bacilli (AFB) smears and cultures that are consistently positive prior to therapy can become intermittently positive during the transition toward the culture-negative status. Similarly, chest radiograph and chest computed tomography scan abnormalities may fluctuate over the course of therapy, with a general trend toward improvement.

TABLE 32–5 ■ Symptom, Laboratory, and Ancillary Test Monitoring During Therapy with Selected Anti-Nontuberculous Mycobacteria Antibiotics

Drug	Symptoms/patient education	Laboratory and ancillary test monitoring*
Clarithromycin or Azithromycin	Gastrointestinal symptoms; changes in hearing (usually late)	Baseline audiometry (repeat every 3 mo) and biochemistry panel with liver enzyme studies (repeat monthly)
Ethambutol	Gastrointestinal symptoms; numbness and tingling of the toes, feet, and fingers; visual changes	Baseline ophthalmologic examination (repeat eye chart and color vision testing monthly)
Rifampin or Rifabutin	Red-orange discoloration of urine and body secretions; flulike symptoms; nausea; ecchymoses (rarely); myalgias and arthralgias (rifabutin); visual changes (rifabutin)	Baseline complete blood count with differential and platelet counts; biochemical panel with liver enzyme studies; visual acuity testing (rifabutin) (repeat monthly)
Fluoroquinolone	Gastrointestinal symptoms; anxiety, insomnia, other central nervous system symptoms; symptoms of tendinitis (rare)	Baseline biochemical panel, including renal function and liver enzyme studies (repeat monthly)
Aminoglycoside IV access IM injection	Changes in hearing (acuity and tinnitus); changes in gait or balance; changes in renal function uncommon with daily or intermittent dosing; tenderness, exudation, or redness at the site of IV access or IM injection	Baseline audiometry and vestibular function testing; baseline biochemical panel including renal function studies (repeat every 2 wk)
Clofazimine	Anticipate skin pigmentation, photosensitivity; use sunblocks and protective clothing; gastrointestinal symptoms (relatively late in therapy); symptoms may persist for weeks to months because of long drug half-life	Routine laboratory studies of little value

*Monitoring studies should be repeated more frequently, as clinically indicated, for patients with changing symptoms or predisposition to increased risk (e.g., altered renal or hepatic function or visual or auditory acuity at baseline).

Because of the requirement for long-term therapy of NTM disease, drug-related side effects can be observed that are uncommon with shorter courses of therapy with the same medications. Examples include macrolide-induced changes in hearing, ethambutol-induced peripheral neuropathy, rifabutin-induced myalgias and arthralgias in patients on combined rifabutin and clarithromycin therapy, aminoglycoside-induced hearing changes, and clofazimine-induced gastrointestinal symptoms.

Patient Education Regarding Antibiotics

There are two advantages of patient education about the antibiotic regimen. First, improved patient understanding of anticipated drug-related effects and toxicity helps patients understand their treatment program and adhere to the regimen. Second, patient awareness of drug-related side effects provides early warning for needed laboratory testing and dosage modification or discontinuation of therapy.

MACROLIDE ANTIBIOTICS. The primary side effects noticed by patients taking macrolide antibiotics are gastrointestinal symptoms, including an unpleasant taste in the mouth, anorexia, and nausea. Most of these symptoms are dose related and therefore are less of a problem in patients using lower drug doses or intermittent dosing schedules. Other than the unpleasant taste, the side effects are partly related to the promotility effects of this

class of drugs on the gastrointestinal tract.[21] Nausea can also be a nonspecific component of the uncommon problem of clarithromycin-induced hepatotoxicity.[22] This dose-related problem is usually diagnosed through routine laboratory monitoring of liver enzyme levels. It is usually possible for patients with this problem to restart treatment at a lower drug dose after a period off of therapy to allow serum liver enzyme levels to return to normal. However, follow-up monitoring is required to check for recurrence.

A less common macrolide-induced side effect is reduced auditory acuity.[23,24] This problem is related to both dose and duration of therapy and can occur with either clarithromycin or azithromycin. Patients usually first notice problems with conversational hearing. Education about this possible problem and periodic audiometry testing (e.g., approximately every 3 months during therapy) may be helpful for early detection. With discontinuation of the offending drug, usually normal or near-normal hearing, slowly returns, although irreversible hearing loss has been reported.[24] Assessment of this problem is frequently confounded by treatment of patients of advanced age who have age-related hearing limitations.

ETHAMBUTOL. Although some patients experience gastrointestinal symptoms related to ethambutol therapy, this is usually difficult to distinguish from the more common problem of macrolide-induced symptoms. Otherwise, ethambutol rarely causes symptoms that are specifically attributable to this agent. One uncommon symptom is ethambutol-induced peripheral neuropathy.[25,26] This usually presents as numbness or tingling of the toes, feet, or fingers after months of therapy. These symptoms are usually slowly reversible but may not completely disappear after therapy is discontinued. The least common but most feared consequence of ethambutol therapy is optic neuritis and associated vision loss. Patients can experience a gradual reduction in visual acuity or photosensitivity. However, the symptoms can be subtle and, in retrospect, are often missed until they are well established. It is for this reason that visual acuity and red-green color vision are monitored monthly during therapy. It is important to stop ethambutol therapy promptly at the first symptoms or signs of reduction in visual acuity, since the symptoms of optic neuritis and the associated vision loss rarely are severe. Vision loss can be reversible. However, recovery of vision may require months to years. It is unclear whether monitoring using complete ophthalmologic examination vs. eye chart and color vision (Ishihara chart) testing affects the ability to detect ethambutol-induced optic neuritis, although ophthalmologic monitoring using visual evoked potential studies has been advocated by some.[26-28]

RIFAMPIN OR RIFABUTIN. A red-orange discoloration of the urine and other body secretions is predictable with rifampin or rifabutin therapy. It is important to alert patients to this, so that they are not alarmed. Occasional patients will experience rifamycin-induced flulike symptoms that can be difficult to distinguish from the systemic response to infection. Rifamycins can also cause hepatotoxicity, resulting in either no symptoms or nonspecific symptoms such as nausea at the time of detected serum enzyme level abnormalities. Treatment with rifabutin, especially in high doses or in combination with clarithromycin, can be associated with rheumatologic symptoms, including myalgias and arthralgias.[29-31] These symptoms are uncommon with rifampin therapy. Rifabutin therapy is also more likely than rifampin therapy to cause leukopenia and thrombocytopenia.

FLUOROQUINOLONES. Fluoroquinolone antibiotics can cause gastrointestinal symptoms, especially in elderly patients. Patients can also experience central nervous system symptoms, including anxiety, insomnia, and rarely seizures. Other agents, such as caffeine, chocolates, and bronchodilator medications, can increase fluoroquinolone-related neurologic symptoms. Fluoroquinolone therapy has also been associated with tendinitis, most notably of the Achilles tendon. Most of this information derives from case reports; therefore the incidence of this apparently uncommon complication is poorly understood.[32]

AMINOGLYCOSIDES. Aminoglycoside antibiotics can be used to complement oral antibiotics in the treatment of patients with severe systemic symptoms and moderate-to-severe pulmonary or extrapulmonary disease. Aminoglycoside doses are administered either once daily or on an intermittent schedule two or three times a week. With these dosing schedules, drug-induced nephrotoxicity is uncommon. The major problem encountered with these dosing strategies is aminoglycoside-induced ototoxicity and hearing loss. Vestibular toxicity, usually manifested by unsteady gait, occurs less commonly but should also be evaluated during patient follow-up visits. The other problem with aminoglycoside therapy is related to the parenteral route of administration. Ideally, when these drugs are needed, they can be given by intravenous infusion rather than by intramuscular injection. The intravenous route of administration can reduce the long-term morbidity of multiple injections and also achieves greater peak serum concentrations that may increase antibiotic tissue penetration. Intravenous infusion is usually best done through a peripherally inserted central venous catheter (PICC line) when possible but can require a surgically implanted central venous catheter for certain patients. Patient education about catheter-related problems of inflammation, exudation, and clotting can help provide early warning for catheter-related problems. Inhaled aminoglycoside therapy for disease suppression or palliation has been used in highly selected patients, although its benefit remains uncertain. There are usually few or no systemic side effects from inhaled aminoglycoside therapy because serum drug levels are low or undetectable.[33,34] Rarely, patients who have developed tinnitus as a result of previous parenteral aminoglycoside therapy will notice intermittent, mild tinnitus following inhaled aminoglycoside treatments. Patients can also experience hoarseness, bronchospasm, and a bad taste in the mouth as result of this route of therapy.

CLOFAZIMINE. Clofazimine usually is well tolerated early in the course of therapy. The major change noted by patients is dose- and time-related increasing skin pigmentation, resulting from drug deposition. This pigmentation is intensified by sun exposure. Therefore it is recommended that patients should use sunblocks and wear protective hats and clothing. Courses of clofazimine lasting for many months can be associated with nonspecific gastrointestinal symptoms, including nausea and abdominal discomfort and bloating. The symptoms are usually subtle but can be severe. Patients may have difficulty discerning the slow onset of clofazimine-related gastrointestinal symptoms from those associated with macrolide antibiotic therapy. If gastrointestinal symptoms worsen on a stable macrolide antibiotic dose several months into the treatment course, however, it is reasonable to reduce either the dose or dosing frequency of clofazimine. If the symptoms are moderate to severe, the drug should be stopped. Unfortunately this drug clears slowly because of its long half-life, and these gastrointestinal symptoms can take many months to resolve. The symptoms usually do lessen, however, within weeks after stopping the drug. Patients should also be aware that clofazimine deposition can occur at body sites other than the skin, lungs, and gastrointestinal tract. For example, during routine eye examinations, patients may be told that they have scleral discolorations. These can be related to clofazimine deposition.

Monitoring Laboratory Studies and Tests for Drug-Induced Abnormalities

Monitoring laboratory studies and ancillary tests complements, but does not replace, periodic clinical evaluation of drug-related side effects. As noted in Table 32–5, studies can be done periodically during patient follow-up to monitor for side effects of various antimycobacterial drugs used in NTM therapy. All studies should be done at baseline in most patients. The frequency of periodic reevaluation of these parameters is arbitrary and based on the average experience of serial evaluation of such patients. Customization of the frequency of the studies should be based upon changes in reported symptoms and individual patient risk factors. For example, patients with baseline liver enzyme abnormalities or evidence of renal dysfunction should be followed more carefully for drug-related, organ-specific abnormalities. A common baseline evaluation could include a complete blood count (CBC) with differential and platelet count and biochemical panel with renal function and liver enzyme studies plus a formal ophthalmologic evaluation and audiometry. Most of the studies, with the exception of ophthalmologic examination and audiometry, usually will have been done during the course of routine patient evaluation.

Planning Duration of Therapy

The proper duration of therapy for most NTM infections is unknown. Recommendations for NTM treatment are, in most cases, not based on the results of clinical trials but instead are derived from a general extrapolation from experience treating drug-resistant TB. TB treatment in the prerifampin era required at least 18 months of therapy for acceptable cure rates. TB cure rates with rifampin-containing regimens have been excellent with much shorter durations of therapy. The only NTM infection in which there is sufficient experience to expect that rifampin can shorten the duration of therapy is pulmonary disease caused by *M. kansasii*. Limited clinical experience suggests that *M. kansasii*–induced pulmonary disease can be treated with a rifampin-containing regimen for 12 months with a high cure and low relapse rate.[35,36] Initial observations indicated that this ability to shorten *M. kansasii* therapy to 12 months from the previous standard of 18 to 24 months might be related to the use of rifampin in the regimen. The results of one study, however, suggest that *M. kansasii* infections can respond to 12 months of therapy despite resistance of the mycobacterial population to rifampin.[37]

Treatment of pulmonary MAI infection in HIV-negative patients usually is started with at least three effective drugs (e.g., rifampin or rifabutin, ethambutol, and a macrolide) and continued for at least 12 months following sputum culture conversion to negative.[38] From 1 to 4 months of treatment usually are required to achieve culture conversion, depending on the severity of the disease.[39] Therefore on average the use of the guideline to treat for 12 months after culture conversion will require therapy for over 1 year and often as long as 18 months. For patients who have severe, cavitary pulmonary disease the addition of a parenteral aminoglycoside (or other antimycobacterial drug) may be necessary to obtain initial control of the disease and symptoms. In summary, it is most appropriate to consider discussions about the duration of therapy as an initial estimate of an average response that must be custom tailored to the individual patient when one is considering the severity of disease, the drug-responsiveness of the mycobacterial population, and other factors that complicate treatment.

This complexity in determining the duration of therapy is further confounded by the tendency for relapse of infections with RGM, especially *M. abscessus* and *M. chelonae*. Pulmonary or soft tissue infections with these mycobacteria can respond promptly to aggressive, multidrug therapy. However, sustaining a clinical and bacteriologic response is more difficult with pulmonary disease caused by RGM than by other NTM. The course can be one of treatment-induced remissions punctuated by periodic bacteriologic and clinical relapses that extends over many years. Therefore it is difficult to define specific recommendations for duration of therapy for these infections.

Setting Realistic Goals for Therapy

The spectrum of treatment-induced responses among different NTM infections probably reflects the balance between the inherent antibiotic resistance of the species and the availability of effective drugs. If one takes this broad perspective, drug-susceptible TB is the most easily cured of all mycobacterial infections. *M. kansasii* may be next in line. Then follows an ill-defined sequence of responses of other nontuberculous mycobacteria, ending with moderate-to-severe disease caused by RGM, which in general are the most difficult to treat. It is often helpful to consider this spectrum of anticipated treatment responses when setting realistic goals for therapy and discussing the long-term treatment plan with patients. Although there may be initial disappointment with the vagueness of the prognosis, patients usually understand the need to periodically reevaluate their individual response to therapy and to reevaluate goals and objectives as treatment proceeds.

In Vitro Antibiotic Susceptibility Testing

A question that commonly arises during plans to initiate anti-NTM therapy is, What is the proper use of in vitro susceptibility testing data in the design of the treatment regimen? There have been major improvements in the past decade in susceptibility testing assays. As would be predicted, the rate of development of these methods has exceeded the ability to test the clinical utility of the data. The use of susceptibility testing data will be considered for four groups of infections: *M. kansasii*, MAI, RGM, and other NTM.

Susceptibility Testing of *M. kansasii*

Historically this testing has been done on agar plates designed for testing of TB using the so-called proportion method.[40] In these studies the growth of a standard inoculum of mycobacteria in a control quadrant of a plate is compared with growth in quadrants with agar containing drug doses that originally were designed to test TB susceptibility. Relative inhibition of growth in the drug quadrants compared with the control quadrant is used to assess antibiotic susceptibility or resistance. On the basis of the results of proportion studies, *M. kansasii* strains from patients who have not been treated previously can be predicted to be consistently susceptible to rifampin and resistant to pyrazinamide and variably susceptible to isoniazid (INH). Susceptibility testing results with the BACTEC or broth microdilution methods have confirmed the consistent susceptibility to rifampin of *M. kansasii* isolates from previously untreated patients and have extended the results of proportion method studies to indicate that clarithromycin and newer generation fluoroquinolone antibiotics can also be effective in vitro.[41,42] In the BACTEC method a [^{14}C]-labeled fatty acid substrate (palmitic acid) that is metabolized by growing mycobacteria is included in liquid media. Measurement of the release of [$^{14}CO_2$] from the culture is used to develop a growth index for the antibiotic-free control culture and for cultures containing different antibiotic concentrations. The presence or absence of detectable growth and the relative differences in growth rates are used to define antibiotic susceptibility. Clinical studies of rifampin-containing regimens indicate that they are highly effective in achieving cure of *M. kansasii* disease.[35,36] The value of susceptibility testing of other antibiotics for first-round therapy is uncertain. It is appropriate, however, to use in vitro testing results with other drugs to design re-treatment plans for previously treated patients with rifampin-resistant *M. kansasii* disease.

Susceptibility Testing of *Mycobacterium avium-intracellulare*

MAI testing against a variety of antimycobacterial drugs commonly is done using minimum inhibitory concentration (MIC) determinations with liquid culture methods such as BACTEC.[40] Clarithromycin testing for MAI is currently the only in vitro susceptibility data supported by clinical trials. Initial trials were done with clarithromycin monotherapy to establish its independent effectiveness in disseminated *M. avium* infection, mostly

MAC bacteremia in AIDS patients.[16] Most isolates from patients not previously treated with macrolide antibiotics had MICs below 2 µg/ml (considered to be highly susceptible). In contrast, isolates recovered from clarithromycin-treated patients who had initial clinical and bacteriologic responses followed by relapses of infection had MICs that were usually greater than 32 µg/ml (considered to be highly resistant). The accepted breakpoint for clarithromycin susceptibility is 8 µg/ml. There are no such extensive correlations between susceptibility testing data and clinical trials for other antimycobacterial drugs used in MAI regimens. The conservative recommendation for MAI susceptibility testing is to determine whether the clinical isolate is or is not susceptible to clarithromycin and to base initial treatment (or revision of empiric treatment) on these data (see Table 32–2).

Other MAI susceptibility testing data can be reserved for use in patients who either fail to respond to the initial clarithromycin-based regimen or who have a relapse of infection after an initial response. The key question is whether clarithromycin resistance has emerged. The secondary question is whether other antibiotics that might be used to design a re-treatment regimen show in vitro activity against a recently acquired mycobacterial isolate. It is desirable to try to select multiple, previously unused drugs with high-level in vitro activity. Because of the short list of possibly useful antibiotics, however, it is usually necessary to use a combination of previously used antibiotics with the best possible added agents, based on susceptibility testing data.

Susceptibility Testing of Other Slowly Growing Nontuberculous Mycobacteria

Other slowly growing, pathogenic NTM continue to be tested with the proportion method, in a manner similar to that done for TB or *M. kansasii*.[40] There have not been enough studies of broth culture MIC determinations to validate the use of this approach for routine susceptibility testing of NTM other than MAI. Insufficient clinical trial information is available to test correlations between in vitro susceptibility results and clinical outcome for organisms such as *M. xenopi*, *M. simiae*, *M. szulgai*, *M. marinum*, *M. malmoense*, or other uncommon NTM pathogens. Recent clinical studies suggest that some of these species are susceptible to a combination of rifampin and ethambutol, but they do not resolve the issue of the correlation between drug susceptibility testing and clinical outcome.[43]

Susceptibility Testing of Rapidly Growing Mycobacteria

Testing of RGM has been done with a variety of laboratory methods, including agar dilution, disk diffusion, and agar disk elution. The antibiotic broth microdilution method is increasingly used for MIC determinations.[44] Since RGM are resistant to conventional TB drugs, there is no role for agar plate proportion method testing of these organisms. A different panel of drugs is tested against RGM compared with either TB or MAI, including cefoxitin, amikacin, clarithromycin, fluoroquinolones, doxycycline, TMP-SMX, imipenem, and sulfonamides.

Because of their relatively rapid growth, results of antibiotic testing of RGM are often available during initiation of antibiotic therapy. Since there are notable variations in the patterns of susceptibility to specific drugs among these species, it is useful to know both the identity of the mycobacterial species and the susceptibility data before initiating therapy. For example, M. fortuitum and M. abscessus isolates are usually susceptible to cefoxitin, whereas M. chelonae isolates can be resistant.[38] Antibiotic testing panels for RGM contain both oral and parenteral agents. Therefore these data can be used to define both highly aggressive parenteral regimens and suppressive oral regimens, depending on the clinical situation.

There are no controlled clinical trials comparing different antimycobacterial treatment regimens for RGM. Anecdotal information suggests that treatment with drugs determined to be effective in vitro can result in a favorable clinical outcome. There are, however, also occasional observations that patients whose RGM isolates are judged to be resistant by in vitro testing do have positive clinical responses. For example, patients whose M. abscessus or M. chelonae isolates show in vitro resistance to both clarithromycin and fluoroquinolone antibiotics can experience clinical improvement or stabilization when treated with a two-drug suppressive regimen using these drug classes. This apparent discrepancy could result from the relatively stringent criteria for laboratory "susceptibility." In vitro susceptibility is defined as greater than 99% growth inhibition at a given antibiotic concentration compared with the antibiotic-free control culture. There may be circumstances in which less effective antibiotic-induced growth inhibition as measured in vitro could result in clinical improvement. The final analysis of the proper role of RGM susceptibility testing awaits comparative clinical studies. In the meantime, it is reasonable to test all isolates for antibiotic susceptibility using the microtiter dilution method of MIC determination and to use combinations of at least two effective drugs to treat most RGM infections.

ANTIBIOTICS USED IN THERAPY OF DISEASE CAUSED BY NONTUBERCULOUS MYCOBACTERIA

Macrolide Antibiotics

The primary use of the newer macrolide antibiotics—clarithromycin and azithromycin—in NTM therapy is to treat disease caused by MAI. Prior to the availability of this new class of drugs the clinical response to treatment of pulmonary MAI infection was inconsistent and associated with an unacceptable rate of treatment failures. In the premacrolide era there was some hope that fluoroquinolone antibiotics would dramatically change the results of multidrug therapy of MAI disease. It was not until the inclusion of clarithromycin and azithromycin in multidrug protocols, however, that a major change in clinical response was noted.

Most data on the efficacy of clarithromycin and azithromycin against MAI infection have been generated through intensive investigation of the optimal treatment regimen for disseminated M. avium infection in AIDS patients. Extensive in vitro testing, studies in macrophages, animal model experiments, and clinical trials produced the current understanding of the importance of these drugs in treating M. avium infection.[16,45–53] Initial studies have also been done of the use of these macrolide antibiotics to treat HIV-negative patients with pulmonary MAI disease.[14,15,23,54–56] The available data indicate that macrolide antibiotics are the keystone in the treatment regimen for MAI infection in both clinical settings.

Following are some questions that have evolved regarding the optimal use of these macrolide antibiotics for NTM disease. What are the relative advantages of clarithromycin vs. azithromycin? What doses and dosing intervals should be used? What problems are encountered during macrolide therapy?

Most clinical studies of macrolide efficacy have tested the role of clarithromycin in MAI therapy. Dose range studies indicate that 500 mg of clarithromycin may be the best twice daily dose for treatment of disseminated M. avium infection in HIV-infected patients. By extrapolation from these studies, a 500-mg twice daily dose of clarithromycin commonly is used to treat HIV-negative patients with pulmonary MAI infection and NTM infections at other sites. There are data, however, suggesting that clarithromycin or azithromycin given either as a single daily dose or intermittently in a thrice weekly schedule can be equally effective.[14,56] Reduced cost and better drug tolerance make these intermittent regimens attractive. It is likely that macrolide treatment protocols involving multiple daily doses will be phased out as acceptance is gained for single daily dosing and intermittent therapy. Studies to date have not stratified patients on the basis of NTM disease severity. Therefore it remains to be determined whether daily dosing offers any advantage over intermittent therapy for patients with more severe disease.

Results of studies comparing the relative benefits of clarithromycin vs. azithromycin in treating M. avium infection in either HIV-positive or HIV-negative patients are varied. Some data suggest an advantage for clarithromycin-containing regimens, whereas other studies have not confirmed this difference.[14,50,57] Some patients who experience unacceptable gastrointestinal toxicity from clarithromycin find azithromycin more tolerable. Furthermore azithromycin does not block hepatic cytochrome function and therefore causes fewer problems with drug-drug interactions than clarithromycin does. One approach to a macrolide-based regimen for treatment of MAI (or other NTM) infection is to attempt to use clarithromycin as the macrolide component and to reserve azithromycin as an alternative agent for patients who are clarithromycin-intolerant or for situations in which drug-drug interactions caused by clarithromycin create a management problem. There are two uncommon situations in which azithromycin might have an advantage over clarithromycin in the treatment of NTM-induced disease. Patients with bronchiectasis can have coinfections with other bacteria. Studies of the relative activities of azithromycin and clarithromycin in vitro against *Haemophilus influenzae* have shown that azithromycin is a more active agent.[58] Therefore azithromycin is the preferred agent in patients with bronchiectasis who have a demonstrated coinfection with *H. influenzae*. Another uncommon situation in which azithromycin might have an advantage over clarithromycin is the circumstance of a pregnant patient who has NTM disease that requires therapy. Azithromycin is rated as a category B drug; thus the chance of fetal harm is considered to be remote but possible. Clarithromycin is rated as a category C drug, which generally is contraindicated in pregnancy.

There are few laboratory and clinical data regarding the value of these macrolide antibiotics for treatment of NTM other than MAI. Both in vitro and animal model data suggest the efficacy of clarithromycin and azithromycin against *M. kansasii*,[41,59-61] although one in vitro report suggested slightly reduced activity of azithromycin vs. clarithromycin.[62] Other NTM, including *M. marinum, M. xenopi, M. szulgai,* and *M. malmoense*, are best considered to be similar to MAI in their response to macrolide antibiotics until susceptibility testing can be completed. The one possible exception may be *M. simiae*, which has been reported to be relatively resistant to clarithromycin.[59]

Early studies with macrolide antibiotic monotherapy suggested that other than drug-related side effects the most important problem for the long-term treatment of patients with MAI infection is emergence of macrolide resistance.[45,46,54,63] This is a problem of antibiotic-induced selection of drug-resistant subpopulations of mycobacteria. The incidence of clarithromycin-resistant organisms within a MAI population has been estimated at 10^{-7} to 10^{-8}.[47] Therefore the problem of selection for drug resistance is greater in patients with high bacterial burdens, such as AIDS patients with *M. avium* bacteremia and HIV-negative patients with MAI-induced cavitary pulmonary disease. Several studies were done early in the AIDS epidemic to attempt to identify the best agent (or agents) to add in a multidrug NTM regimen to protect against emergence of macrolide resistance. The consensus from these studies was that ethambutol was the best second drug to add to the regimen.[64] Results of studies seeking to identify the next best drug to add to a clarithromycin + ethambutol regimen have been vari-

able.[48,51,65] The results of these and other studies have led to a consensus that a rifamycin may be the best third agent.

Ethambutol

Ethambutol dosing strategies for NTM therapy are borrowed from information developed for TB treatment. When daily dosing is used, patients usually are started on a dose of approximately 25 mg/kg for the first 2 months of therapy, and then the dose is reduced to approximately 15 mg/kg for the duration of treatment. One concern that arises in managing long-term ethambutol dosing is the problem of ensuring that the reduction of the 25 mg/kg dose to 15 mg/kg occurs at 2 months. This dose change is done to minimize the likelihood of ethambutol-induced optic neuritis and other neurotoxicity. If patient follow-up or other factors make the assurance of ethambutol dose reduction a problem, it is reasonable to start with the maintenance dose of 15 mg/kg. Ethambutol also has been used successfully in a rifampin (or rifabutin) + clarithromycin (or azithromycin) regimen in an intermittent dosing schedule administered in a dose of 25 mg/kg three times per week to treat pulmonary MAI infection in HIV-negative patients.[14,15]

The use of ethambutol to treat NTM infections other than MAI or *M. kansasii* is based on anecdotal observations and small numbers of patients. Ethambutol commonly is added to a rifamycin as the core of a regimen to which a third drug is added, such as a macrolide, a fluoroquinolone, or an aminoglycoside. This rifampin + ethambutol + X strategy provides a reasonable empiric basis for treatment of most unusual NTM infections (other than RGM infections) until data can be obtained about susceptibility of the clinical isolate, and, if needed, expert consultation can be sought to optimize treatment design (Table 32–3).

Rifamycins

Rifampin and rifabutin have been used interchangeably to treat NTM infections with the exception of treatment of AIDS patients, in whom rifabutin is the drug of choice. The advantage of rifabutin in this setting is that it is less active at inducing hepatic metabolism of other drugs, including clarithromycin and several antiretroviral drugs. A relative disadvantage of rifabutin compared with rifampin is that rifabutin tends to cause a greater incidence of drug-related side-effects, including leukopenia, thrombocytopenia, uveitis, and rheumatologic symptoms. These are rifabutin dose-related side effects that can be made worse by clarithromycin + rifabutin therapy, since clarithromycin increases rifabutin blood levels.

One approach that can be used for decision making in the choice of rifampin vs. rifabutin is to separate considerations of treatment of HIV-positive and HIV-negative patients. For HIV-positive patients who will likely be treated with multiple antiretroviral drugs, rifabutin is the drug of choice. Even then, rifabutin dosing and drug-drug interactions must be considered carefully, depending on the design of the antiretroviral regimen.[66,67] For HIV-negative patients with NTM-induced pulmonary disease (or localized disease at another site), rifampin can be used as the first choice for the rifamycin component of the regimen and replaced with rifabutin if patients are rifampin intolerant or if there is a problem with rifampin interactions with other components of the patient's drug treatment regimen.

Rifampin reduces serum clarithromycin concentrations more than rifabutin does.[68] The clinical significance of this observation is uncertain, since excellent clinical and bacteriologic responses have been obtained with regimens containing clarithromycin plus either of these two rifamycins. It is possible that intracellular concentrations of these antibiotics and other factors at the site of infection have effects on therapy that cannot be predicted from serum drug level measurements.

Fluoroquinolones

For infections caused by MAI and most other NTM, fluoroquinolone antibiotics play a supporting role but are not one of the core drugs in primary therapy. Ciprofloxacin, levofloxacin, and newer fluoroquinolones, such as gatifloxacin and moxifloxacin, can have excellent in vitro activity against MAI, *M. kansasii*, RGM, and other NTM. This antibiotic class, however, is generally less active against mycobacteria than against other more susceptible bacterial species, possibly because of genetic differences in the targeted bacterial DNA gyrase.[42] Studies of ciprofloxacin in the treatment of disseminated *M. avium* infections in AIDS patients indicate that its results are inferior to those obtained with macrolide antibiotics.[69]

For most NTM infections other than MAI, fluoroquinolone antibiotics are probably best considered as a candidate X agent in the rifampin + ethambutol + X strategy described in the Ethambutol discussion. In a clinical situation in which rifampin cannot be used, a fluoroquinolone antibiotic can be used as a third drug in a clarithromycin + ethambutol regimen. It is useful to have evidence of fluoroquinolone susceptibility of the clinical isolate when one is making these decisions. Furthermore, if possible, there should be at least one other highly active agent in the multidrug regimen. When a fluoroquinolone is the only active agent in the treatment protocol, fluoroquinolone resistance can emerge, just as when fluoroquinolones are used in monotherapy.

The relative clinical role of newer fluoroquinolone antibiotics vs. ciprofloxacin is based upon anecdotal experience and not comparison trials. In vitro data suggest that the newer agents can have lower MIC values for selected mycobacterial isolates.[70–74] Whether this in vitro advantage will translate into better clinical outcomes than

are achieved with ciprofloxacin-containing regimens remains to be tested.

One clinical situation in which fluoroquinolone antibiotics can assume a more prominent role is treatment of certain patients with purulent bronchiectasis and superimposed NTM infection. Such patients can have infections with multiple bacteria, including *Pseudomonas aeruginosa* and other gram-negative pathogens. Addition of a fluoroquinolone antibiotic to the anti-NTM regimen in such cases can have a dual advantage. The drug can add intensity to the anti-NTM regimen (assuming that the mycobacterial isolate is sensitive to the fluoroquinolone) and also can provide activity against the gram-negative pathogen(s). This circumstance can be observed in patients with cystic fibrosis who have NTM disease or in non–cystic fibrosis bronchiectasis patients who have been treated previously with repeated courses of other antibiotics and are colonized and infected with these gram-negative pathogens.

Dosing (and especially the timing of dosing) of fluoroquinolone antibiotics must be done with consideration of substances that interfere with their absorption, such as those that contain divalent or trivalent cations (e.g., calcium, magnesium, and iron), which include antacids and multivitamins. This adds to the complexity of patient adherence to a multidrug anti-NTM regimen.

Aminoglycosides

Either streptomycin or amikacin is commonly recommended for use as an added agent to multidrug oral anti-NTM regimens during the first few months of therapy for patients with moderate-to-severe disease.[38] When such therapy is required, it has been common to use intramuscular injections of the aminoglycoside once daily, 5 days per week as the dosing schedule. An alternative that can have comparable clinical results is intermittent intramuscular injections given two or three times a week. The reduced frequency of injections decreases morbidity but can still be difficult for some patients to tolerate over a prolonged course of therapy. Some physicians increasingly favor the use of intravenous aminoglycoside therapy over intramuscular injections for two reasons: First, intravenous therapy has the theoretical advantage of achieving higher peak serum drug concentrations than intramuscular therapy does. Whether this translates into improved clinical outcome has not been studied. Second, intravenous therapy is usually better tolerated by patients than repeated intramuscular injections. The primary disadvantage of intravenous aminoglycoside therapy is the cost of drug administration. This requires initial placement of a central venous line and arrangement for periodic intravenous drug administration in either a health care setting or the home. A secondary disadvantage is that intravenous therapy is associated with an incidence (albeit fairly small) of serious line-related complications.

Laboratory and clinical data are mixed regarding the advantages of adding aminoglycoside therapy to a multidrug oral NTM regimen. There are currently no clinical studies showing that aminoglycoside therapy is preferable to a clarithromycin-based, multidrug regimen. There are anecdotal cases, however, of patients with pulmonary NTM disease who have failed to respond to the best available oral antibiotic regimen but who have had clinical and bacteriologic responses to the addition of aminoglycoside therapy. Aminoglycoside therapy may also be useful as a component of a re-treatment regimen for patients with relapsing NTM infection associated with the evolution of resistance to other drugs.

A third route of aminoglycoside administration that has been used in highly selected patients with pulmonary NTM infections is nebulization, primarily of tobramycin or amikacin. This is usually done in a setting in which previous parenteral aminoglycoside therapy was effective but had to be discontinued because of its ototoxicity. There are no clinical trial data to support the use of aerosolized aminoglycosides to treat NTM-induced pulmonary disease. A case series, however, has indicated that mycobacterial disease can respond to nebulized aminoglycoside therapy, as evidenced by repression of pulmonary TB.[75] Even if in vitro susceptibility testing data show only marginal susceptibility or resistance of the mycobacterial isolate to the aminoglycoside (using standard breakpoints for intravenous therapy), it is possible that the high drug concentrations achieved in respiratory secretions following inhaled therapy might be effective in inhibiting mycobacterial growth in lung areas reached by the nebulized drug. One approach to consider if inhaled aminoglycoside therapy is used is to set an arbitrary period of treatment of approximately 2 to 4 months and to define criteria of improvement including symptomatic response and reduced mycobacterial colony counts in the sputum. These parameters can be used to evaluate the utility of continuing and to justify the expense and inconvenience of this therapy.

Clofazimine

This antileprosy medication was found to have in vitro activity against many isolates of MAI and occasional strains of TB. It has a variable reputation, however, in the treatment of NTM disease. Studies have evaluated clofazimine as a companion drug to macrolide antibiotics in the treatment of disseminated *M. avium* disease in AIDS patients. Among the results are data showing that clofazimine + ciprofloxacin are inferior to clarithromycin when they are added to a core regimen of rifabutin + ethambutol.[69] Clofazimine is also inferior to the combination of rifabutin + ethambutol in preventing the emergence of resistance to clarithromycin.[48]

In a multicenter study of the value of adding clofazimine to a core regimen of clarithromycin + ethambutol the mortality was increased in the clofazimine-treated group (61% vs. 38%).[65] However, there was also a higher level of baseline bacteremia in patients in the clofazimine arm. Other studies have not reported a clofazimine-related increase in mortality in this patient population, but they usually were not designed to test this question. Clofazimine has been used for many years as a component of treatment regimens for MAI pulmonary disease in HIV-negative patients, and there are no known reports of increased mortality associated with clofazimine therapy in this patient population. Therefore the reasons for the apparently increased mortality in AIDS patients treated with clofazimine in addition to clarithromycin + ethambutol are unknown. Clofazimine has well-known immunosuppressive effects that have been used therapeutically in autoimmune skin disorders and chronic graft-vs.-host rejection.[76] It is possible that such an immunosuppressive effect could be critical in patients already suppressed by HIV infection but would not be clinically significant in immunocompetent patients with mycobacterial infections. Another possibility is that changes in gastrointestinal tract function as a result of clofazimine deposition, could adversely affect antiretroviral therapy. Whether these speculations or other explanations explain the increased mortality reported in one study in AIDS patients with *M. avium* bacteremia treated with a clofazimine-containing antimycobacterial regimen is unknown.

Clofazimine has a prolonged half-life that is variably cited to be from 10 days to over 70 days.[77,78] Skin pigmentation related to drug deposition appears slowly during the initiation of therapy and disappears slowly over several weeks after therapy is discontinued. Symptoms of clofazimine-induced gastrointestinal and dermatologic side effects can persist for many months. Furthermore, in some patients, nearly therapeutic serum drug levels can be detected for at least 4 to 6 months after clofazimine therapy is discontinued. A beginning dosage of 100 to 200 mg daily is well tolerated. After prolonged courses of therapy, some patients will notice vague gastrointestinal symptoms that can only be distinguished from macrolide-induced symptoms by the late onset of clofazimine-related symptoms. The symptoms are usually mild and can be controlled by either reducing the clofazimine dose to 50 mg daily or reducing the dose and dosing frequency to a twice weekly schedule. In some cases the gastrointestinal symptoms can be more severe, and the drug must be discontinued. It is occasionally possible to restart therapy at a lower dose after several weeks off of treatment.

The role of clofazimine in treating NTM infections remains uncertain. Other than for treatment of leprosy, it is best considered as an alternative to complement core regimens based on macrolide + ethambutol therapy for MAI-induced disease or rifampin + ethambutol + X regimens for other NTM infections. For example, in HIV-negative patients with pulmonary MAI disease who are intolerant of rifamycins, clofazimine can be added to clarithromycin + ethambutol as a third agent. A minor advantage of clofazimine is its extremely low cost compared with the cost of other anti-NTM drugs.

Other Drugs Used in Treatment of Nontuberculous Mycobacteria Disease

Several other drugs, some of which are used to treat TB and some of which are conventional antibiotics, can also be used to treat selected types of NTM infections. These include INH, ethionamide, cycloserine, TMP-SMX and other sulfonamides, tetracyclines, cefoxitin, and imipenem. These drugs are referred to in Table 32–3 and will be discussed with the treatments for infections caused by specific NTM species.

TREATMENT OF DISEASE CAUSED BY SPECIFIC NTM SPECIES

Management of NTM infections can be divided into considerations of therapy for slowly growing NTM and therapy for rapidly growing NTM (RGM). In this discussion, pulmonary disease will be used as the model for considerations of these two groups of NTM infections. Differences in the approaches to therapy for mycobacterial disease at other sites will be contrasted with the approach to pulmonary infection and are referred to in Table 32–2.

Mycobacterium avium-intracellulare

Studies of optimal therapy for disseminated *M. avium* infections in AIDS patients demonstrated the importance of macrolides in the treatment regimens for this class of slowly growing mycobacteria. Almost all MAI isolates are initially susceptible to clarithromycin (and azithromycin) if patients have not been treated with repeated courses of these antibiotics for other reasons. These drugs and fluoroquinolone antibiotics, however, are increasingly used as empiric therapy for recurrent flares of bronchiectasis (and other chronic pulmonary problems). Therefore it is anticipated that there will be a slowly increasing number of patients presenting with a first diagnosis of macrolide-resistant MAI infection. Since this is still an uncommon problem, it is reasonable to start empiric therapy for patients with a first diagnosis of pulmonary MAI disease with a macrolide-containing regimen and then to do follow-up testing to confirm macrolide susceptibility of the clinical isolate.

Clarithromycin, ethambutol, and rifampin used on a three times weekly or daily basis is an appropriate initial regimen for such patients[14] (Table 32–2). Whether daily therapy has an advantage over thrice weekly therapy for patients with severe disease has not been studied. If tolerated, daily therapy might be appropriate under such circumstances, at least until clinical improvement is achieved. If patients are intolerant of clarithromycin, azithromycin can be used as an alternative macrolide that may be less likely to cause gastrointestinal problems. Rifabutin can be used as an alternative to rifampin for patients in whom drug-drug interactions limit rifampin use. Some practitioners prefer to start the multidrug regimen with rifabutin rather than rifampin because of reports that rifabutin has greater antimycobacterial activity in vitro. Rifabutin, however, is more likely than rifampin to cause side effects over the course of therapy—an observation that limits its therapeutic advantage in practice.

The decision about adding a parenteral aminoglycoside to a multidrug oral antimycobacterial regimen usually depends on the severity of disease and clinical illness as balanced against the increased risk for drug-induced toxicity. For patients with progressive cavitary disease with fevers, diaphoresis, and cachexia from MAI infection, the addition of an aminoglycoside to a three-drug oral antibiotic regimen has been observed to improve the rate of symptomatic improvement and disease control. One study in AIDS patients with *M. avium* bacteremia who were treated with rifampin, ethambutol, ciprofloxacin, and clofazimine as the oral regimen, with or without the addition of amikacin for the first month of therapy, failed to show that amikacin improved clinical response or reduced bacteremia.[79] No such comparative study is available for HIV-negative patients with pulmonary MAI disease or in patients treated with a macrolide-containing regimen. In one case series, however, patients with severe pulmonary disease more often failed a rifampin + ethambutol + clarithromycin regimen than did patients treated with the same regimen but with kanamycin added during the initial phase of therapy.[39] At present there appears to be a consensus among physicians experienced in the treatment of patients with moderate-to-severe NTM disease that aminoglycoside therapy for the first few weeks to months of treatment can be beneficial.

Parenteral aminoglycoside therapy is often most conveniently administered through a PICC line. These lines do not require an operating room setting for placement and if cared for properly usually are well tolerated for weeks to months of therapy. Intravenous aminoglycoside therapy can be effective when given either once daily (usually 5 days per week) or 2 or 3 times a week. Whether daily therapy is any more effective than intermittent therapy in controlling severe disease is unknown. A combination of disease severity, cost, patient convenience, and other factors usually determines the decision about frequency of administration. In cases in which the oral antibiotic regimen is marginal and in which it might be desirable to use aminoglycoside therapy for a longer time, it is reasonable to choose the intermittent dosing schedule to attempt to slow the appearance of dose-related ototoxicity and prolong the availability of the drug. If daily therapy is thought to be needed initially because of disease severity, it is also possible to change to an intermittent dosing schedule once clinical improvement is achieved.

Defining the best treatment regimen for patients with clarithromycin-resistant MAI infections is a problem. In the premacrolide era, clinical and bacteriologic responses were obtained with rifampin, ethambutol, and two or three additional drugs. Some of these regimens (e.g., those including ethionamide or cycloserine) were associated with a high rate of drug-induced side effects and in addition were probably less effective than current clarithromycin-containing regimens. If clarithromycin resistance has been defined, other drug susceptibility testing data are also often available. In that case, drugs can be selected for the retreatment regimen based on antibiotic susceptibility data. For example, one approach is to retreat with a rifampin + ethambutol–based regimen with the addition of at least two other effective drugs to which the mycobacterial isolate has been shown to be susceptible. For moderate-to-severe disease caused by a clarithromycin-resistant mycobacterial population, addition of a parenteral aminoglycoside may assume greater importance in the regimen. Newer fluoroquinolone antibiotics can have lower MIC values against MAI isolates than ciprofloxacin has and therefore might offer a clinical advantage. This possibility remains to be tested. In contrast to clarithromycin-susceptible MAI disease, there are no data demonstrating the utility of intermittent antibiotic treatment regimens for patients with clarithromycin-resistant disease.

Treatment of MAI (or other slowly growing NTM) infections of soft tissue, bone, or joints can present challenges different from those of pulmonary disease treatment. Decisions about the initial antibiotic regimen are similar. A problem that arises more commonly with infections at these other sites is definition of the role of surgery, in addition to antibiotic therapy, in the treatment plan. Drainage of pus and débridement of devitalized tissue are essential. It is also important to remove foreign bodies or sequestra and to consider healing by second intention rather than by primary closure for débrided spaces.

MAI has become the most common cause of mycobacterial lymphadenitis, currently outnumbering cases caused by TB and *Mycobacterium scrofulaceum* in most populations outside of areas of high TB incidence. Where the anatomy permits, complete surgical excision is usually curative for MAI-induced lymphadenitis and has often been completed during the diagnostic procedure. In circumstances in which complete excision of the involved lymph nodes is not possible (e.g., with involvement near the facial nerve), only limited excision may be done, or antibiotic therapy may be used instead of surgical excision. Nonexcisional incision and drainage of infected nodes and related masses should be discouraged because of the possibility of persistent draining sinus tracts in areas of mycobacterial infection. When antibiotic therapy is needed to treat lymphadenitis, the conservative approach is to use a macrolide-based regimen containing at least two effective drugs. This avoids the theoretical problem of emergence of macrolide resistance during therapy. There are, however, no clinical trials

showing that macrolide monotherapy results in treatment failure and emergence of resistance in the setting of MAI lymphadenitis. Therefore, since the bacterial burden is relatively low in most of these infections, it is possible that monotherapy could have a high cure rate, as has been observed with MAI-induced cutaneous diseases.[17] The correct length of antibiotic treatment for NTM-induced lymphadenitis is unknown, but treatment for 4 to 6 months beyond resolution of clinical disease is probably appropriate. Longer therapy may be required for more extensive disease.

Treatment of AIDS patients with disseminated *M. avium* infections and low CD4 lymphocyte counts is based on the same general concepts used in treating MAI infections in immunocompetent patients, with one important exception—the role of rifamycin antibiotics. Rifampin is more active than rifabutin at inducing the hepatic cytochrome P450 enzyme class, CYP3A. Furthermore many of the currently used antiretroviral drugs are heavily metabolized by these hepatic enzymes and are themselves also often inhibitors or inducers of these enzymes. Therefore the use of rifamycins to treat *M. avium* infections in AIDS patients can be problematic. If a rifamycin is used, rifabutin is the drug of choice. Furthermore, if rifabutin is used, its dose or dosing frequency may have to be altered, depending on the drug composition of the antiretroviral regimen. A collaborative interaction between the treating physician and the pharmacist can be useful for ongoing review of the potential drug-related complications of therapy. It is also useful to refer to reviews of the problems of drug-drug interactions between rifamycins, macrolides, and antiretroviral drugs.[66,67]

Some general observations about drug-drug interactions between antimycobacterial and antiretroviral agents that have been reviewed previously[66] will be listed. There are three general observations about the effects of rifabutin on antiretroviral drugs that can be related to the class of the antiviral agent. For protease inhibitors, antiretroviral activity is proportionate to the serum concentration of the drug. Therefore rifabutin-induced reductions in the serum concentration of protease inhibitors can be critical. The nucleoside analogue reverse transcriptase inhibitors (NRTIs) are not metabolized by CYP3A. Furthermore the antiretroviral activity of NRTIs (e.g., zidovudine) is less dependent on serum concentration and more dependent on intracellular triphosphate levels.[80] Therefore rifabutin therapy probably has little clinically relevant effect on these agents. The rifabutin effect on the third major class of antiretrovirals, the non-nucleoside reverse transcriptase inhibitors (NNRTIs), varies with the drug and must be considered on a case by case basis.

The antiretrovirals can affect rifabutin levels, since antiviral agents can alter (both decrease and increase) CYP3A activity. The general guidelines that have been proposed for management of these drug-drug interactions[66] are as follows:

1. Do not give rifabutin with ritonavir, since the antiviral agent is such a potent inhibitor of rifabutin metabolism.
2. Reduce the rifabutin dose from 300 to 150 mg daily when it is being used with nelfinavir, indinavir, or amprenavir.
3. Increase the rifabutin dose to 600 mg daily when it is used with nevirapine or efavirenz (Table 32–6).

A major question that remains unanswered is whether the clinical significance of the drug-drug interactions between rifabutin and antiretroviral drugs would be lessened or eliminated by using rifabutin in a two or three times weekly intermittent dosing schedule.[66]

Mycobacterium kansasii

Isolation of *M. kansasii* from sputum or other body sites associated with a compatible clinical presentation should be interpreted as disease that should be treated and not as colonization. The general principles of decision making about treatment of MAI disease also apply to treating *M. kansasii* disease. The difference is the expected cure rate. For MAI-induced disease, clinical responses and cure rates are improving with the use of newer macrolide antibiotics. These responses, however, are still not at the high level that can be expected when treating *M. kansasii*–induced disease. Previously untreated patients receiving rifampin-containing multidrug regimens for *M. kansasii* disease can be expected to have cure rates in excess of 95%.[35,36,81,82]

The current recommendation for treatment of rifampin-susceptible *M. kansasii* disease is to use a three-drug regimen including rifampin, ethambutol, and INH[38] (Table 32–2). Previously treated patients with rifampin-resistant *M. kansasii* isolates or patients who are intolerant of one of these three agents should receive the best possible three-drug regimen based upon the results of in vitro susceptibility testing. Macrolide and fluoroquinolone antibiotics offer potentially excellent options to add to *M. kansasii* re-treatment regimens. There are insufficient clinical data available, however, to know whether these alternative regimens will have cure rates similar to those achieved with rifampin-containing regimens. Ethionamide and cycloserine can be highly active in vitro against *M. kansasii*.[40] These drugs have a much higher incidence of side effects and therefore should be relegated to third-line status unless other less toxic antibiotics are ineffective in vitro. Pyrazinamide and para-aminosalicylic acid are almost always ineffective when tested in vitro against *M. kansasii* and should not be used for treatment. The decision to use aminoglycoside therapy for either rifampin-susceptible or rifampin-resistant disease is best based on the same considerations on which the decision for MAI disease is based (Table 32–2).

Slowly Growing NTM Other Than MAI or *M. Kansasii*

There are even fewer data upon which to base the design of treatment regimens for other NTM than there are for MAI or *M. kansasii* disease. For most of these other NTM infections it is reasonable to start with an empiric rifampin + ethambutol + clarithromycin treatment regimen until susceptibility testing data are available. Previous comments about the relative advantages and disadvantages of rifampin vs rifabutin, clarithromycin vs azithromycin, and about the use of aminoglycoside therapy are also applicable here. Limited species-specific information is available that can be used for modifications to this empiric treatment approach for some species (Table 32–3).

For *M. simiae* infections it has been observed in small clinical studies and in animal model investigations that the combination of ethambutol + macrolide + fluoroquinolone can be effective.[83–86] This provides a reasonable alternative strategy for starting therapy for *M. simiae*–induced disease until susceptibility testing data are completed. This mycobacterial species has also been observed to be susceptible to ethionamide and cycloserine in vitro.[87] The use of these drugs must be considered carefully, however, since they are more likely than most other medications to induce treatment-limiting side effects.

The spectrum of antibiotics active against *M. marinum*, based on susceptibility testing data, can usually be broadened from the core rifampin + ethambutol + macrolide regimen to include conventional antibiotics including doxycycline, minocycline, sulfonamides, and selected newer fluoroquinolones, such as moxifloxacin.[88–90] Most often aminoglycoside therapy is unnecessary for *M. marinum* infections restricted to cutaneous or subcutaneous sites unless severe disease requires temporary intensification of therapy during surgical débridement.

Mycobacterium celatum is an uncommon pathogen that causes *M. avium*–like illness in AIDS patients and resembles *M. xenopi* in the laboratory but can be distinguished by high-performance liquid chromatograpy analysis. Limited data indicate that this species is resistant to rifamycins but may respond clinically to the combination of clarithromycin, ethambutol, and a fluoroquinolone.[91]

TABLE 32–6 ■ **Guidelines for Managing Interactions Between Rifabutin and Antiretroviral Drugs in AIDS Patients***

1. Do not use rifabutin with ritonavir.
2. Reduce the rifabutin dose from 300 mg to 150 mg/d when it is used with nelfinavir, indinavir, or amprenavir.
3. Increase the rifabutin dose to 600 mg/d when it is used with neviripine or efavirenz.

*Reviewed in Burman et al.[66]

Rapidly Growing Mycobacteria

Three species—*M. fortuitum, M. abscessus,* and *M. chelonae*—are responsible for most RGM infections. *M. fortuitum* clinical isolates tend to be susceptible in vitro to a broader spectrum of antibiotics than *M. abscessus* and *M. chelonae* are, including tetracyclines and sulfonamides. Infections caused by *M. fortuitum* also appear to respond better to antibiotic therapy[92] and to have a lower relapse rate than infections caused by the other two species.

For treatment of moderate-to-severe pulmonary disease caused by RGM, empiric therapy can be started with a parenteral β-lactam agent, such as cefoxitin, combined with parenteral aminoglycoside therapy with amikacin (Table 32–4). If the clinical isolate has already been found to be resistant to cefoxitin in vitro, imipenem can often be used as an alternative β-lactam antibiotic to complement amikacin therapy. Available clinical experience suggests that treatment with multiple daily doses of the β-lactam agent can be combined with once daily therapy with amikacin for the first few weeks of therapy until a clinical response is observed. Both clinical and bacteriologic responses can be prompt with such a parenteral treatment protocol. However, relapses are common upon discontinuation of this therapy. Prior to the availability of the newer macrolide and fluoroquinolone antibiotics, clinical and bacteriologic relapses were the rule when parenteral therapy was discontinued for patients with moderate-to-severe pulmonary RGM disease. Addition of a two-drug continuation regimen including a macrolide and fluoroquinolone, started during a 1-week overlap period at the end of intravenous β-lactam + aminoglycoside therapy, has maintained clinical improvement in some cases. Persistence of sputum culture positivity continues to be observed in most patients with moderate-to-severe pulmonary disease. There are uncommon cases, usually involving mild pulmonary disease or soft tissue infection, in which multidrug therapy has effected clinical and bacteriologic cure of RGM infections. The prognosis in most cases of pulmonary disease is that treatment-induced clinical remissions will be interrupted by periodic exacerbations over a long course of disease management.

Recent studies have tested the efficacy of linezolid, an oxazolidinone agent, in the search for drugs that are more effective against RGM.[93] The results of one in vitro study indicate that *M. fortuitum* is the most susceptible of the three common RGM. *M. chelonae* was intermediately susceptible, and *M. abscessus* isolates were relatively resistant to this drug. Clinical trial data are not yet available to determine whether disease caused by linezolid-susceptible RGM will respond to this drug as a component of a multidrug regimen. Case report information suggests this possibility, however.[94]

Because of the limitations of antibiotic therapy for cure of pulmonary disease caused by RGM, it is appropriate to consider surgical options for patients with localized infection. For example, if the patient has a localized area of bronchiectasis or a cavitary lesion with no disease or minimal disease involving other areas of the lung, a combined approach of antibiotic therapy and lobectomy may be appropriate. Ideally, patients should be treated for 1 to 2 months before surgery with an effective parenteral antibiotic regimen to reduce the mycobacterial burden to its nadir prior to lung resection. The best outcome is achieved with patients who have converted their sputum AFB smears and cultures to negative before surgery. Continued multidrug therapy for 6 to 12 months after surgery may be required if there is evidence of residual RGM disease. Unfortunately the clinical presentation of these patients usually involves diffuse lung involvement and multilobar bronchiectasis, in which case surgery usually is not an option.

Localized extrapulmonary disease caused by RGM can be associated with trauma and soil contamination, foreign bodies, and immunosuppression. In these settings the mycobacterial burden is usually lower than for diffuse pulmonary disease, especially cavitary lung disease. Therefore it is more likely that extrapulmonary disease can be cured. Thorough débridement and removal of foreign bodies is an essential component of the management of these infections. Pretreatment with a 1- or 2-week course of effective parenteral antimycobacterial therapy following the guidelines defined for pulmonary disease is appropriate prior to surgery. The optimal length of therapy after débridement or foreign body removal is unknown but should probably be extended at least 4 to 6 months after the disappearance of any signs of infection. For cases in which débridement or foreign body removal is incomplete, longer courses of suppressive therapy and repeated attempts at débridement may be required.

Disseminated disease caused by RGM fortunately is less common than disseminated disease caused by *M. avium.* Disseminated infections with RGM usually occur in the context of immunosuppression, either therapeutically induced or HIV-related. Successful treatment of these disseminated infections usually involves aggressive, multidrug therapy similar to that defined for pulmonary disease (Table 32–2) combined with efforts to reduce the immunosuppression. As with other NTM infections, controlling the immunosuppression may be as important as antibiotic therapy in the outcome of treatment.[95]

UNUSUAL PRESENTATIONS OF NONTUBERCULOUS MYCOBACTERIAL DISEASE

Pulmonary and Thoracic Disease

Patients can present with at least three unusual variations of thoracic NTM disease: hypersensitivity pneumonitis, empyema, and prominent mediastinal adenopathy.

Hypersensitivity Pneumonitis

NTM-induced hypersensitivity pneumonitis usually has been associated with infection through NTM-contaminated water bioaerosols. Patients with exposure to hot tubs or indoor swimming pools or with work-related exposures to contaminated fluid baths have presented with this syndrome[96-99] (Fig. 32–5).

Anecdotal reports indicate that patients can respond to multidrug antimycobacterial regimens. Some patients have been treated with a combination of antibiotics and oral corticosteroid therapy. It is appropriate to treat patients with a macrolide-based protocol as suggested for MAI infection (Table 32–2) until the mycobacterial species is known. After identification and susceptibility testing are completed, the antibiotic regimen should be modified to fit the responsible agent. If the deterioration in pulmonary function is extreme, oral corticosteroid therapy may be indicated. Although there have been concerns about even short-term immunosuppression in patients with NTM pulmonary disease, clinical experience indicates that corticosteroid therapy can be used to treat such patients who are on appropriate, multidrug, anti-NTM regimens.

Serial pulmonary function testing, measurement of oxygen saturation at rest and with exercise, and high-resolution chest CT scans can be used to monitor the response to therapy of NTM-induce hypersensitivity pneumonitis. Because of the low bacterial burden and the rapid disappearance of cough and sputum production with therapy, it is usually difficult to obtain follow-up sputum cultures to confirm the bacteriologic response to therapy. Normalization of pulmonary function, resolution of chest CT scan abnormalities, and completion of at least a 6-month course of antimycobacterial antibiotic therapy after resolution of clinical signs and symptoms is usually effective. When corticosteroid therapy is necessary, the dose can be tapered over weeks to months as allowed by improvement in pulmonary function and oxygenation. It is essential to attempt to eliminate the environmental source of NTM infection in these cases because relapses or reinfections with severe hypersensitivity pneumonitis can occur upon re-exposure to NTM bioaerosols.

Empyema

Pleural involvement with empyema is a rare complication of pulmonary NTM disease. There are few case reports of this complication.[100-102] In some cases, NTM-induced empyema can be related to rupture of a pleural-based mycobacterial cavity or infected pulmonary cystic structure. In patients with TB-induced empyema, chest tube drainage is rarely necessary because of the effectiveness of antibiotic therapy. In contrast, there is little data to suggest the proper course of action for NTM-induced empyema. Limited experience suggests that a combination of a multidrug anti-NTM regimen and chest tube drainage for large NTM-induced empyemas is appropriate. If the empyema is small and the infection is caused by a macrolide-susceptible NTM population, it may be possible to avoid chest tube drainage.

Prominent Mediastinal Adenopathy (Fig. 32–6)

Patients with prominent mediastinal adenopathy usually come to medical attention because of a differential diagnosis of malignancy associated with a mediastinal mass. They therefore have often already undergone an invasive procedure for biopsy of the lymph node or mass to establish the diagnosis of NTM infection. If complete surgical excision has been accomplished and there is no associated pulmonary disease (negative CT scan), no further NTM therapy may be necessary, similar to the observations for patients with NTM-induced cervical lymphadenitis. Conversely, if the mediastinal adenopathy is large and impinging on adjacent airways, an antimycobacterial regimen can be used to attempt to speed resolution. In some cases such lesions can result in a postobstructive right middle lobe syndrome. Whether antibiotic therapy reduces the likelihood of long-term problems with airway compression by scarred, and often calcified mediastinal lymph nodes is uncertain.

Postinjection Soft Tissue Abscess

NTM infections of the skin and soft tissues have been associated with injections with drugs or other agents contaminated with NTM.[103,104] RGM are most likely the responsible species. Therefore empiric antibiotic therapy should be targeted at these species (Table 32–4) until mycobacterial identification is available. These infections are relatively resistant to treatment with antibiotics alone. It is usually necessary to combine antibiotic therapy with débridement and, if possible, excision of the infected site. In cases in which complete excision is not possible, it is often necessary to allow these wounds to

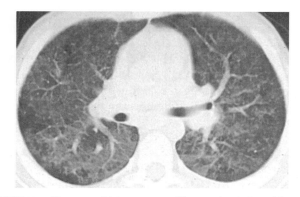

FIGURE 32–5. Hypersensitivity pneumonitis reaction induced by pulmonary infection with *Mycobacterium avium-intracellulare*. Mid-lung chest computed tomography image from a 12-year-old patient exposed to a decorative home fountain contaminated with mycobacteria. Radiographic abnormalities and oxygen desaturation completely disappeared over a several month course of therapy with oral antimycobacterial antibiotics and a tapering course of corticosteroids.

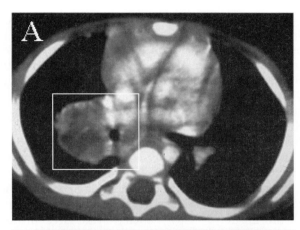

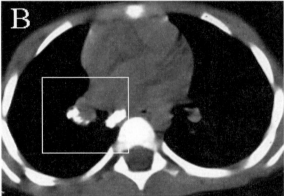

FIGURE 32–6. Prominent mediastinal adenopathy caused by *Mycobacterium avium-intracellulare* infection. **A,** Large, right-sided mediastinal mass in a 1-year-old. Biopsy revealed granuloma on histopathology, was positive for acid-fast bacilli on special staining, and grew *Mycobacterium avium-intracellulare*. **B,** Evolution of the mediastinal mass after 32 months of follow-up and treatment with a three-drug antimycobacterial regimen. Note the reduction in size and dense calcification of the lesions around the airway.

heal secondarily during continued antibiotic therapy. Limited experience suggests that continuation of the multidrug antimycobacterial regimen for 3 to 6 months after a surgical excision may be necessary for cure.[103] Attention should be paid to removal of all foreign bodies during débridement. If the infection can be linked with a therapeutic injection, it may be useful to do an epidemiologic investigation to determine whether other symptomatic patients might have been exposed to a common source.[104]

Head and Neck Infections

NTM infections of the head and neck, other than cervical lymphadenitis, are uncommon. RGM have been implicated in mycobacterial keratitis associated with corneal trauma, contact lens use, and injuries with residual foreign bodies.[105,106] Topical therapy with aminoglycoside-containing solutions and systemic antimycobacterial drug therapy have been used. In selected cases, however, a keratectomy plus antibiotic therapy may be needed.

Limited evidence from treatment of other infections suggests that systemic macrolide therapy can be effective for treatment of ocular infections.[107] NTM-induced otitis media is an uncommon problem, mostly of childhood. In one case series this problem was associated with placement of tympanostomy tubes and was caused by RGM.[108] Tube removal and prolonged antibiotic therapy were necessary. This is consistent with the general theme of foreign body removal, débridement, and antibiotic therapy for NTM infections at other sites.

NONTUBERCULOUS MYCOBACTERIAL DISEASE REFRACTORY TO THERAPY

In some cases, symptomatic improvement can require 1 or 2 months (or more) of continued antibiotic therapy despite good adherence to the treatment regimen and full susceptibility of the mycobacterial population to the drugs selected. Because of this lag time for improvement, questions often arise about the appropriateness of the treatment regimen (Table 32–7). After the first few weeks of therapy it is appropriate to review the medical regimen with the patient to be sure that treatment is being tolerated and that the patient is adhering to the dosing schedule. At this point anticipated drug-related side effects, timing of drug dosages, and other problems can be reviewed with the patient. This is also a good time to reassure patients that the response to treatment of NTM disease may require many weeks. Patient frustration with the appearance of drug-related side effects in the absence of any perceived clinical benefit can lead to problems with adherence to the treatment program. When patients have either failed to respond to therapy for several months or have shown evidence of disease progression despite appropriate treatment, it is reasonable to review the diagnosis, the possibility of another cause of the clinical problem, and alternative approaches to therapy.

TABLE 32–7 ■ **Questions to Guide the Approach to the Patient with an Unresponsive NTM Infection**

1. Adequacy of drug dosing?
2. Drug side effects and adherence to therapy?
3. Drug-drug interactions or other problems that affect drug absorption?
4. Mixed infection: multiple NTM (e.g., *M. avium-intracellulare* + rapidly growing NTM) or NTM + another pathogen (e.g., NTM + *Pseudomonas aeruginosa*)?
5. Changes in underlying pulmonary (or other) condition that complicate interpretation of the response to therapy (e.g., bronchiectasis, interstitial pulmonary fibrosis, immunosuppression, malignancy)?
6. Appearance of a new medical problem that confounds interpretation of the response to NTM therapy?
7. Requirement for excision or débridement (devitalized or poorly vascularized tissue; foreign bodies)?

Medications being used either for an underlying illness or for other medical problems should be reviewed to be sure they are not interfering with the efficacy of the antimycobacterial agents. It can also be useful to review options for reducing treatment-related immunosuppression that might improve the response to antimycobacterial therapy. Patients being treated with corticosteroids for underlying lung disease or with chemotherapy for a malignancy may benefit from an attempt to reduce immunosuppression during treatment of the mycobacterial infection.

Another question to consider is whether the NTM isolated from the sputum or other site is the only pathogen. Occasionally patients will have coinfection with two NTM species, for example, MAI and a RGM. These mixed mycobacterial infections usually are detected in the laboratory. Not all specimens, however, are positive for both pathogens. Therefore it is reasonable to submit repeated sputums or other clinical specimens for repeated cultures for mycobacteria to be sure that the pathogen that is the focus of antibiotic therapy is the only one detected. Patients can also have other infectious agents as copathogens with NTM. The problem of *P. aeruginosa* coinfection in patients with bronchiectasis or cystic fibrosis has been mentioned. Patients with bronchiectasis and cavitary lung disease can also have coinfection with other bacterial or fungal pathogens. The spectrum of possible copathogens is, of course, much broader for immunosuppressed patients, including those with AIDS.

Many patients with pulmonary NTM infections have another, underlying noninfectious process. When patients fail to respond clinically to apparently appropriate antimycobacterial therapy, it is appropriate to review the status of the underlying disease to determine whether its treatment is optimal. It can be difficult to distinguish between symptoms and radiographic manifestations of some underlying pulmonary problems and superimposed NTM infections. For example, patients with idiopathic pulmonary fibrosis, pulmonary malignancies, or severe underlying bronchiectasis can experience intervening exacerbations that can be difficult to distinguish from NTM-induced lung pathology. In these situations it is helpful to have serial semiquantitative bacteriology studies to support the decision making process. If sputums have converted from AFB smear and culture positive to negative on antimycobacterial therapy and if increasing lung pathology is detected, consideration must be given to another explanation for the process. Histopathologic diagnosis can be required in these circumstances.

In summary, there can be multiple explanations for an apparently inadequate response to treatment of NTM-induced pulmonary disease. Development of a checklist to review drug dosing, adherence to therapy, drug-drug interactions, possible evidence for alternative or coinfecting pathogens, and exacerbations of underlying illnesses or appearance of intervening illnesses can be useful when approaching this problem (Table 32–5).

Failure of NTM infections at extrapulmonary sites to respond to therapy suggests additional questions. The most common problem is inadequate response of a soft tissue NTM infection. Assuming that NTM susceptibility, drug dosing, and treatment adherence have been reviewed and are optimal, the most likely problem is inadequate débridement, foreign body removal, or vascularization of the site of NTM disease. These situations usually occur when complete excision of the infected site is difficult or impossible because of structural or functional limitations. Consideration of the persistence of devitalized or poorly vascularized tissue or foreign bodies is appropriate in this setting.

Unfortunately, many patients who have diffuse, severe pulmonary involvement with NTM infection have persistent symptoms despite the best available multidrug antimycobacterial therapy. In these cases it is often not possible to improve the clinical response by modifying the antibiotic treatment protocol to include new antimycobacterial drugs. Instead it may be necessary to revise the goals of therapy from cure to disease suppression or palliation. Reconsideration of the objectives can help reorient the focus of therapy and to educate the patient about changes in realistic treatment options.

Limited studies have evaluated the possible benefits of immunotherapy to complement antibiotic treatment of NTM disease.[109–111] The results of these and other preliminary studies indicate that some patients might respond to cytokine-induced enhancement of cellular immunity as a complement to antibiotic therapy. These investigations are still in the clinical trial stage.

In patients with NTM infections and severe immunosuppression associated with HIV infection, interpretation of a failure to respond to NTM therapy can be more complicated. Many of the questions listed above regarding appropriateness of the treatment regimen, adherence to the treatment protocol, possible drug-drug interactions, and coinfection with other pathogens apply in this circumstance. Because patients with AIDS can have nonspecific symptoms in response to NTM infection and other complicating illnesses, it can be difficult to distinguish NTM treatment failure from symptoms caused by another medical problem. Use of objective parameters, such as the level of *M. avium* bacteremia and, where available, quantitative changes in NTM-induced lesions, either in the lung or elsewhere, may help discriminate between failure of NTM therapy and the complication of a coinfection or another intervening illness.

REFERENCES

1. Falkinham JO III: Epidemiology of infection by nontuberculous mycobacteria. Clin Microbiol Rev 1996;9:177–215.
2. Feldman WH, Davie R, Moses HE: An unusual *Mycobacterium* isolated from sputum of a man suffering from pulmonary disease of long duration. Am Rev Tuberculosis 1943;48:82–93.
3. Runyon EH: Anonymous mycobacteria in pulmonary disease. Med Clin North Am 1959;43:273.

4. Centers for Disease Control and Prevention: Nucleic acid amplification tests for tuberculosis. MMWR Morb Mortal Wkly Rep 1996;45(43):950–952.

5. Wallace RJ Jr: The clinical presentation, diagnosis, and therapy of cutaneous and pulmonary infections due to the rapidly growing mycobacteria, *M. fortuitum* and *M. chelonae*. Clin Chest Med 1989;10:419–429.

6. Steere AC, Corrales J, von Graevenitz A: A cluster of *Mycobacterium gordonae* isolates from bronchoscopy specimens. Am Rev Respir Dis 1979;120:214–216.

7. Panwalker AP, Fuhse E: Nosocomial *Mycobacterium gordonae* pseudoinfection from contaminated ice machines. Infect Control 1986;7:67–70.

8. Stine TM, Harris AA, Levin S, et al: A pseudoepidemic due to atypical mycobacteria in a hospital water supply. JAMA 1987;258:809–811.

9. Cox R, deBorja K, Bach MC: A pseudo-outbreak of *Mycobacterium chelonae* infections related to bronchoscopy. Infect Control Hosp Epidemiol 1997;18:136–137.

10. Arnow PM, Bakir M, Thompson K, Bova JL: Endemic contamination of clinical specimens by *Mycobacterium gordonae*. Clin Infect Dis 2000;31:472–476.

11. Lalande V, Barbut F, Varnerot A, et al: Pseudo-outbreak of *Mycobacterium gordonae* associated with water from refrigerated fountains. J Hosp Infect 2001;48:76–79.

12. Centers for Disease Control and Prevention: Misdiagnoses of tuberculosis resulting from laboratory cross-contamination of *Mycobacterium tuberculosis* cultures—New Jersey, 1998. MMWR Morb Mortal Wkly Rep 2000;46:413–416.

13. Lynch DA, Simone PM, Fox MA, et al: CT features of pulmonary *Mycobacterium avium* complex infection. J Comput Assist Tomogr 1995;19:353–360.

14. Griffith DE, Brown BA, Cegielski P, et al: Early results (at 6 months) with intermittent clarithromycin-including regimens for lung disease due to *Mycobacterium avium* complex. Clin Infect Dis 2000;30:288–292.

15. Griffith DE, Brown BA, Girard WM, et al: Azithromycin-containing regimens for treatment of *Mycobacterium avium* complex lung disease. Clin Infect Dis 2001;32:1547–1553.

16. Dautzenberg B, Truffot C, Legris S, et al: Activity of clarithromycin against *Mycobacterium avium* infection in patients with the acquired immune deficiency syndrome. A controlled clinical trial. Am Rev Respir Dis 1991;144(3 Pt 1):564–569.

17. Wallace RJ Jr, Tanner D, Brennan PJ, Brown BA: Clinical trial of clarithromycin for cutaneous (disseminated) infection due to *Mycobacterium chelonae*. Ann Intern Med 1993;119:482–486.

18. Primack SL, Logan PM, Hartman TE, et al: Pulmonary tuberculosis and *Mycobacterium avium-intracellulare*: A comparison of CT findings. Radiology 1995;194:413–417.

19. Kasahara T, Nakajima Y, Niimi H, et al: [HRCT findings of pulmonary *Mycobacterium avium* complex: A comparison with tuberculosis]. Nihon Kokyuki Gakkai Zasshi 1998;36:122–127.

20. Hazelton TR, Newell JD Jr, Cook JL, et al: CT findings in 14 patients with *Mycobacterium chelonae* pulmonary infection. AJR Am J Roentgenol 2000;175:413–416.

21. Bortolotti M, Annese V, Mari C, et al: Dose-related stimulatory effect of clarithromycin on interdigestive gastroduodenal motility. Digestion 2000;62:31–37.

22. Brown BA, Wallace RJ Jr, Griffith DE, Girard W: Clarithromycin-induced hepatotoxicity. Clin Infect Dis 1995;20:1073–1074.

23. Dautzenberg B, Piperno D, Diot P, et al: Clarithromycin in the treatment of *Mycobacterium avium* lung infections in patients without AIDS. Clarithromycin Study Group of France. Chest 1995;107:1035–1040.

24. Ress BD, Gross EM: Irreversible sensorineural hearing loss as a result of azithromycin ototoxicity. A case report. Ann Otol Rhinol Laryngol 2000;109:435–437.

25. Argov Z, Mastaglia FL: Drug-induced peripheral neuropathies. BMJ 1979;1(6164):663–666.

26. Nair VS, LeBrun M, Kass I: Peripheral neuropathy associated with ethambutol. Chest 1980;77:98–100.

27. Kumar A, Sandramouli S, Verma L, et al: Ocular ethambutol toxicity: Is it reversible? J Clin Neuroophthalmol 1993;13:15–17.

28. Srivastava AK, Goel UC, Bajaj S, et al: Visual evoked responses in ethambutol induced optic neuritis. J Assoc Physicians India 1997;45:847–849.

29. Siegal FP, Eilbott D, Burger H, et al: Dose-limiting toxicity of rifabutin in AIDS-related complex: Syndrome of arthralgia/arthritis. AIDS 1990;4:433–441.

30. Griffith DE, Brown BA, Girard WM, Wallace RJ Jr: Adverse events associated with high-dose rifabutin in macrolide-containing regimens for the treatment of *Mycobacterium avium* complex lung disease. Clin Infect Dis 1995;21:594–598.

31. Le Gars L, Collon T, Picard O, et al: Polyarthralgia-arthritis syndrome induced by low doses of rifabutin. J Rheumatol 1999; 26:1201–1202.

32. Harrell RM: Fluoroquinolone-induced tendinopathy: What do we know? South Med J 1999;92:622–625.

33. Smith AL, Ramsey BW, Hedges DL, et al: Safety of aerosol tobramycin administration for 3 months to patients with cystic fibrosis. Pediatr Pulmonol 1989;7:265–271.

34. Ramsey BW, Pepe MS, Quan JM, et al: Intermittent administration of inhaled tobramycin in patients with cystic fibrosis. Cystic Fibrosis Inhaled Tobramycin Study Group. N Engl J Med 1999;340:23–30.

35. Ahn CH, Lowell JR, Ahn SS, et al: Short-course chemotherapy for pulmonary disease caused by *Mycobacterium kansasii*. Am Rev Respir Dis 1983;128:1048–1050.

36. Schraufnagel DE, Leech JA, Schraufnagel MN, Pollak B: Short-course chemotherapy for mycobacteriosis kansasii? CMAJ 1984;130:34–38.

37. Wallace RJ Jr, Dunbar D, Brown BA, et al: Rifampin-resistant *Mycobacterium kansasii*. Clin Infect Dis 1994;18:736–743.

38. Wallace RJ, Glassroth J, Olivier K, et al: Diagnosis and treatment of disease caused by nontuberculous mycobacteria. This official statement of the American Thoracic Society was approved by the Board of Directors, March 1997. Medical Section of the American Lung Association. Am J Respir Crit Care Med 1997;156(2 Pt 2):S1–S25.

39. Tanaka E, Kimoto T, Tsuyuguchi K, et al: Effect of clarithromycin regimen for *Mycobacterium avium* complex pulmonary disease. Am J Respir Crit Care Med 1999; 160:866–872.

40. Heifets L: Dilemmas and realities in drug susceptibility testing of *M. avium-intracellulare* and other slowly growing nontuberculous mycobacteria. In Heifets L (ed): Drug Susceptibility in the Chemotherapy of Mycobacterial Diseases. Boca Raton; Fla, CRC Press, 1991, pp 123–146.

41. Biehle J, Cavalieri SJ: In vitro susceptibility of *Mycobacterium kansasii* to clarithromycin. Antimicrob Agents Chemother 1992; 36:2039–2041.

42. Guillemin I, Jarlier V, Cambau E: Correlation between quinolone susceptibility patterns and sequences in the A and B subunits of DNA gyrase in mycobacteria. Antimicrob Agents Chemother 1998;42:2084–2088.

43. Research Committee of the British Thoracic Society. First randomised trial of treatments for pulmonary disease caused by *M. avium intracellulare, M. malmoense,* and *M. xenopi* in HIV negative patients: Rifampicin, ethambutol and isoniazid versus rifampicin and ethambutol. Thorax 2001;56:167–172.

44. Swenson JM, Thornsberry C, Silcox VA: Rapidly growing mycobacteria: Testing of susceptibility to 34 antimicrobial agents by broth microdilution. Antimicrob Agents Chemother 1982;22:186–192.

45. Dautzenberg B, Saint Marc T, Meyohas MC, et al: Clarithromycin and other antimicrobial agents in the treatment of disseminated *Mycobacterium avium* infections in patients with acquired immunodeficiency syndrome. Arch Intern Med 1993;153:368–372.

46. Chaisson RE, Benson CA, Dube MP, et al: Clarithromycin therapy for bacteremic *Mycobacterium avium* complex disease. A randomized, double-blind, dose-ranging study in patients with AIDS. AIDS Clinical Trials Group Protocol 157 Study Team. Ann Intern Med 1994; 121:905–911.

47. Grosset J, Ji B: Prevention of the selection of clarithromycin-resistant *Mycobacterium avium-intracellulare* complex. Drugs 1997; 54(Suppl 2):23–27.

48. May T, Brel F, Beuscart C, et al: Comparison of combination therapy regimens for treatment of human immunodeficiency virus–infected patients with disseminated bacteremia due to *Mycobacterium avium*. ANRS Trial 033 Curavium Group. Agence Nationale de Recherche sur le Sida. Clin Infect Dis 1997;25:621–629.

49. Roussel G, Igual J: Clarithromycin with minocycline and clofazimine for *Mycobacterium avium intracellulare* complex lung disease in patients without the acquired immune deficiency syndrome. GETIM. Groupe d'Etude et de Traitement des Infections a Mycobacteries. Int J Tuberc Lung Dis 1998;2:462–470.

50. Ward TT, Rimland D, Kauffman C, et al: Randomized, open-label trial of azithromycin plus ethambutol vs. clarithromycin plus ethambutol as therapy for *Mycobacterium avium* complex bacteremia in patients with human immunodeficiency virus infection. Veterans Affairs HIV Research Consortium. Clin Infect Dis 1998;27:1278–1285.

51. Cohn DL, Fisher EJ, Peng GT, et al: A prospective randomized trial of four three-drug regimens in the treatment of disseminated *Mycobacterium avium* complex disease in AIDS patients: Excess mortality associated with high-dose clarithromycin. Terry Beirn Community Programs for Clinical Research on AIDS. Clin Infect Dis 1999;29:125–133.

52. Gordin FM, Sullam PM, Shafran SD, et al: A randomized, placebo-controlled study of rifabutin added to a regimen of clarithromycin and ethambutol for treatment of disseminated infection with *Mycobacterium avium* complex. Clin Infect Dis 1999;28:1080–1085.

53. Benson CA, Williams PL, Cohn DL, et al: Clarithromycin or rifabutin alone or in combination for primary prophylaxis of *Mycobacterium avium* complex disease in patients with AIDS: A randomized, double-blind, placebo-controlled trial. The AIDS Clinical Trials Group 196/Terry Beirn Community Programs for Clinical Research on AIDS 009 Protocol Team. J Infect Dis 2000;181:1289–1297.

54. Wallace RJ Jr, Brown BA, Griffith DE, et al: Initial clarithromycin monotherapy for *Mycobacterium avium-intracellulare* complex lung disease. Am J Respir Crit Care Med 1994;149:1335–1341.

55. Wallace RJ Jr, Brown BA, Griffith DE, et al: Clarithromycin regimens for pulmonary *Mycobacterium avium* complex. The first 50 patients. Am J Respir Crit Care Med 1996;153(6 Pt 1):1766–1772.

56. Griffith DE, Brown BA, Murphy DT, et al: Initial (6-month) results of three-times-weekly azithromycin in treatment regimens for *Mycobacterium avium* complex lung disease in human immunodeficiency virus–negative patients. J Infect Dis 1998;178:121–126.

57. Dunne M, Fessel J, Kumar P, et al: A randomized, double-blind trial comparing azithromycin and clarithromycin in the treatment of disseminated *Mycobacterium avium* infection in patients with human immunodeficiency virus. Clin Infect Dis 2000;31:1245–1252.

58. Barry AL, Fuchs PC, Brown SD: Relative potencies of azithromycin, clarithromycin and five other orally administered antibiotics. J Antimicrob Chemother 1995;35:552–555.

59. Brown BA, Wallace RJ Jr, Onyi GO: Activities of clarithromycin against eight slowly growing species of nontuberculous mycobacteria, determined by using a broth microdilution MIC system. Antimicrob Agents Chemother 1992;36:1987–1990.

60. Yew WW, Piddock LJ, Li MS, et al: In-vitro activity of quinolones and macrolides against mycobacteria. J Antimicrob Chemother 1994;34:343–351.

61. Klemens SP, Cynamon MH: Activities of azithromycin and clarithromycin against nontuberculous mycobacteria in beige mice. Antimicrob Agents Chemother 1994;38:1455–1459.

62. Witzig RS, Franzblau SG: Susceptibility of *Mycobacterium kansasii* to ofloxacin, sparfloxacin, clarithromycin, azithromycin, and fusidic acid. Antimicrob Agents Chemother 1993;37:1997–1999.

63. Heifets L: Susceptibility testing of *Mycobacterium avium* complex isolates. Antimicrob Agents Chemother 1996;40:1759–1767.

64. Benson C: Disseminated *Mycobacterium avium* complex disease in patients with AIDS. AIDS Res Hum Retroviruses 1994;10:913–916.

65. Chaisson RE, Keiser P, Pierce M, et al: Clarithromycin and ethambutol with or without clofazimine for the treatment of bacteremic *Mycobacterium avium* complex disease in patients with HIV infection. AIDS 1997;11:311–317.

66. Burman WJ, Gallicano K, Peloquin C: Therapeutic implications of drug interactions in the treatment of human immunodeficiency virus–related tuberculosis. Clin Infect Dis 1999;28:419–429.

67. Kuper JI, D'Aprile M: Drug-drug interactions of clinical significance in the treatment of patients with *Mycobacterium avium* complex disease. Clin Pharmacokinet 2000;39:203–214.

68. Wallace RJ Jr, Brown BA, Griffith DE, et al: Reduced serum levels of clarithromycin in patients treated with multidrug regimens including rifampin or rifabutin for *Mycobacterium avium-M. intracellulare* infection. J Infect Dis 1995;171:747–750.

69. Shafran SD, Singer J, Zarowny DP, et al: A comparison of two regimens for the treatment of *Mycobacterium avium* complex bacteremia in AIDS: Rifabutin, ethambutol, and clarithromycin versus rifampin, ethambutol, clofazimine, and ciprofloxacin. Canadian HIV Trials Network Protocol 010 Study Group. N Engl J Med 1996; 335:377–383.

70. Gillespie SH, Billington O: Activity of moxifloxacin against mycobacteria. J Antimicrob Chemother 1999;44:393–395.

71. Tomioka H, Sato K, Akaki T, et al: Comparative in vitro antimicrobial activities of the newly synthesized quinolone HSR-903, sitafloxacin (DU-6859a), gatifloxacin (AM-1155), and levofloxacin against *Mycobacterium tuberculosis* and *Mycobacterium avium* complex. Antimicrob Agents Chemother 1999;43:3001–3004.

72. Fung-Tomc J, Minassian B, Kolek B, et al: In vitro antibacterial spectrum of a new broad-spectrum 8-methoxy fluoroquinolone, gatifloxacin. J Antimicrob Chemother 2000; 45:437–446.

73. Gozalbes R, Brun-Pascaud M, Garcia-Domenech R, et al: Prediction of quinolone activity against *Mycobacterium avium* by molecular topology and virtual computational screening. Antimicrob Agents Chemother 2000;44:2764–2770.

74. Kawakami K, Namba K, Tanaka M, et al: Antimycobacterial activities of novel levofloxacin analogues. Antimicrob Agents Chemother 2000;44:2126–2129.

75. Sacks LV, Pendle S, Orlovic D, et al: Adjunctive salvage therapy with inhaled aminoglycosides for patients with persistent smear-positive pulmonary tuberculosis. Clin Infect Dis 2001;32:44–49.

76. Lee SJ, Wegner SA, McGarigle CJ, et al: Treatment of chronic graft-versus-host disease with clofazimine. Blood 1997; 89:2298–2302.

77. Schaad-Lanyi Z, Dieterle W, Dubois JP, et al: Pharmacokinetics of clofazimine in healthy volunteers. Int J Lepr Other Mycobact Dis 1987;55:9–15.

78. Holdiness MR: Clinical pharmacokinetics of clofazimine. A review. Clin Pharmacokinet 1989;16:74–85.

79. Parenti DM, Williams PL, Hafner R, et al: A phase II/III trial of antimicrobial therapy with or without amikacin in the treatment of disseminated *Mycobacterium avium* infection in HIV-infected individuals. AIDS Clinical Trials Group Protocol 135 Study Team. AIDS 1998;12:2439–2446.

80. Barry MG, Khoo SH, Veal GJ, et al: The effect of zidovudine dose on the formation of intracellular phosphorylated metabolites. AIDS 1996;10:1361–1367.

81. Pezzia W, Raleigh JW, Bailey MC, et al: Treatment of pulmonary disease due to *Mycobacterium kansasii*: Recent experience with rifampin. Rev Infect Dis 1981;3:1035–1039.

82. Ahn CH, Lowell JR, Ahn SS, et al: Chemotherapy for pulmonary disease due to *Mycobacterium kansasii*: Efficacies of some individual drugs. Rev Infect Dis 1981;3:1028–1034.

83. Valero G, Moreno F, Graybill JR: Activities of clarithromycin, ofloxacin, and clarithromycin plus ethambutol against *Mycobacterium simiae* in murine model of disseminated infection. Antimicrob Agents Chemother 1994;38:2676–2677.

84. Valero G, Peters J, Jorgensen JH, Graybill JR: Clinical isolates of *Mycobacterium simiae* in San Antonio, Texas. An 11-yr review. Am J Respir Crit Care Med 1995;152(5 Pt 1):1555–1557.

85. Barzilai A, Rubinovich B, Blank-Porat D, et al: Successful treatment of disseminated *Mycobacterium simiae* infection in AIDS patients. Scand J Infect Dis 1998;30:143–146.

86. Al-Abdely HM, Revankar SG, Graybill JR: Disseminated *Mycobacterium simiae* infection in patients with AIDS. J Infect 2000;41:143–147.

87. Woods GL, Washington JA II: Mycobacteria other than *Mycobacterium tuberculosis*: Review of microbiologic and clinical aspects. Rev Infect Dis 1987;9:275–294.

88. Stone MS, Wallace RJ Jr, Swenson JM, et al: Agar disk elution method for susceptibility testing of *Mycobacterium marinum* and *Mycobacterium fortuitum* complex to sulfonamides and antibiotics. Antimicrob Agents Chemother 1983;24:486–493.

89. Forsgren A: Antibiotic susceptibility of *Mycobacterium marinum*. Scand J Infect Dis 1993;25:779–782.

90. Aubry A, Jarlier V, Escolano S, et al: Antibiotic susceptibility pattern of *Mycobacterium marinum*. Antimicrob Agents Chemother 2000;44:3133–3136.

91. Bonomo RA, Briggs JM, Gross W, et al: *Mycobacterium celatum* infection in a patient with AIDS. Clin Infect Dis 1998; 26:243–245.

92. Griffith DE, Girard WM, Wallace RJ Jr: Clinical features of pulmonary disease caused by rapidly growing mycobacteria. An analysis of 154 patients. Am Rev Respir Dis 1993; 147:1271–1278.

93. Wallace RJ Jr, Brown-Elliott BA, Ward SC, et al: Activities of linezolid against rapidly growing mycobacteria. Antimicrob Agents Chemother 2001;45:764–767.

94. Brown-Elliott BA, Wallace RJ Jr, Blinkhorn R, et al: Successful treatment of disseminated *Mycobacterium chelonae* infection with linezolid. Clin Infect Dis 2001;33:1433–1434.

95. Hadad DJ, Lewi DS, Pignatari AC, et al: Resolution of *Mycobacterium avium* complex bacteremia following highly active antiretroviral therapy. Clin Infect Dis 1998;26:758–759.

96. Embil J, Warren P, Yakrus M, et al: Pulmonary illness associated with exposure to *Mycobacterium avium* complex in hot tub water. Hypersensitivity pneumonitis or infection? Chest 1997;111:813–816.

97. Kreiss K, Cox-Ganser J: Metalworking fluid-associated hypersensitivity pneumonitis: A workshop summary. Am J Ind Med 1997;32:423–432.

98. Shelton BG, Flanders WD, Morris GK: *Mycobacterium* sp. as a possible cause of hypersensitivity pneumonitis in machine workers. Emerg Infect Dis 1999;5:270–273.

99. Moore JS, Christensen M, Wilson RW, et al: Mycobacterial contamination of metalworking fluids: Involvement of a possible new taxon of rapidly growing mycobacteria. Aihaj 2000;61:205–213.

100. Zvetina JR, Difilippo NM, Ali MM, Vandrunen M: *Mycobacterium kansasii* empyema. Tubercle 1981;62:135–138.

101. Haynes J Jr, Bass JB Jr, Maisel D: Thoracic empyema necessitatis with recovery of *Mycobacterium avium-intracellulare*. Ala J Med Sci 1987;24:138–139.

102. Kawamoto H, Yamagata M, Nakashima H, et al: Development of a case of *Mycobacterium avium* complex disease from right pleural effusion. Nihon Kokyuki Gakkai Zasshi 2000;38:706–709.

103. Villanueva A, Calderon RV, Vargas BA, et al: Report on an outbreak of postinjection abscesses due to *Mycobacterium abscessus*, including management with surgery and clarithromycin therapy and comparison of strains by random amplified polymorphic DNA polymerase chain reaction. Clin Infect Dis 1997;24:1147–1153.

104. Galil K, Miller LA, Yakrus MA, et al: Abscesses due to *Mycobacterium abscessus* linked to injection of unapproved alternative medication. Emerg Infect Dis 1999; 5:681–687.

105. Dugel PU, Holland GN, Brown HH, et al: *Mycobacterium fortuitum* keratitis. Am J Ophthalmol 1988;105:661–669.

106. Huang SC, Soong HK, Chang JS, Liang YS: Nontuberculous mycobacterial keratitis: A study of 22 cases. Br J Ophthalmol 1996;80:962–968.

107. Langtry HD, Balfour JA: Azithromycin. A review of its use in paediatric infectious diseases. Drugs 1998;56:273–297.

108. Franklin DJ, Starke JR, Brady MT, et al: Chronic otitis media after tympanostomy tube placement caused by *Mycobacterium abscessus*: A new clinical entity? Am J Otol 1994; 15:313–320.

109. Holland SM, Eisenstein EM, Kuhns DB, et al: Treatment of refractory disseminated nontuberculous mycobacterial infection with interferon gamma. A preliminary report. N Engl J Med 1994;330:1348–1355.

110. Kemper CA, Bermudez LE, Deresinski SC: Immunomodulatory treatment of *Mycobacterium avium* complex bacteremia in patients with AIDS by use of recombinant granulocyte-macrophage colony-stimulating factor. J Infect Dis 1998;177:914–920.

111. Lauw FN, van Der Meer JT, de Metz J, et al: No beneficial effect of interferon-gamma treatment in 2 human immunodeficiency virus-infected patients with *Mycobacterium avium* complex infection. Clin Infect Dis 2001;32:e81–e82.

section

10

Tropical Diseases

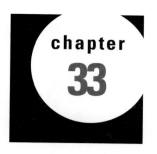

Leishmaniasis and Trypanosomiasis

LÍGIA CAMERA PIERROTTI, MD

LEISHMANIASIS

Leishmaniasis is a serious infectious disease worldwide, and its incidence is increasing, with endemic areas reporting a 500% increase over the past 7 years.[1] The World Health Organization (WHO) has estimated that 2 million new cases occur each year and that a 10th of the world's population is at risk of infection. Leishmaniasis is endemic in areas of the tropics, subtropics, and southern Europe and is seen on all continents except Australia and Antarctica; epidemic areas are also recognized. Cases seen within the United States are almost exclusively imported.

Leishmaniasis refers to several clinical syndromes, including cutaneous leishmaniasis (CL), mucosal leishmaniasis (ML), visceral leishmaniasis or kala-azar (VL), and post-kala-azar dermal leishmaniasis (PKDL). These syndromes are caused by protozoa belonging to the genus *Leishmania*, which are transmitted by different species of phebotomine sandflies. With some exceptions (e.g., VL in India and CL caused by *Leishmania tropica*), humans are usually incidental hosts of infection; natural hosts include a variety of rodents, small mammals, and dogs. Congenital and parenteral transmission can occur but are rare.

Case Definitions

Cutaneous Leishmaniasis

Over 90% of worldwide cases of CL occur in Afghanistan, Algeria, Iran, Iraq, Saudi Arabia, and Syria (Old World) and in Brazil and Peru (New World). Localized cutaneous leishmaniasis (LCL) is caused primarily by the organisms *L. major*, *L. tropica*, and *L. aethiopica* in the Old World. In the New World LCL is caused primarily by two independent complexes: *Viannia* subgenus (including *L. braziliensis, L. panamensis, L. guyanensis,* and *L. peruviana*) and *L. mexicana* species complex (especially *L. mexicana mexicana, L. mexicana amazonensis,* and *L. mexicana venezuelensis*).

LCL usually presents as skin ulcers involving exposed parts of the body bitten by the sand fly vector following a variable incubation period that averages several weeks (Fig. 33–1 and Color Plate 2). After approximately 6 to 12 months, ulcers spontaneously regress, leaving atrophic scars. Nodular lesions also can occur in exposed areas (Fig. 33–2 and Color Plate 2).

Diffuse cutaneous leishmaniasis (DCL) is a variant of CL that develops in the context of *Leishmania*-specific anergy and manifests as disseminated skin involvement.

Mucosal Leishmaniasis

ML is most commonly reported in the New World, although it has been found in the Mediterranean caused by *L. donovani infantum* and *L. major*. In the New World,

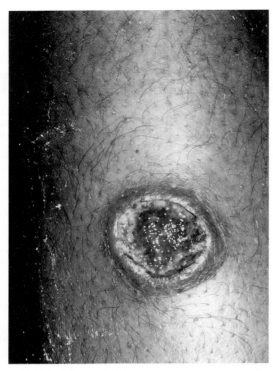

FIGURE 33–1. Localized cutaneous leishmaniasis in a Brazilian patient. An ulcer of the upper extremity caused by *Leishmania vianna brazilienses*. (Courtesy of Dr. Valdir Sabbaga Amato.) (See Color Plate 2.)

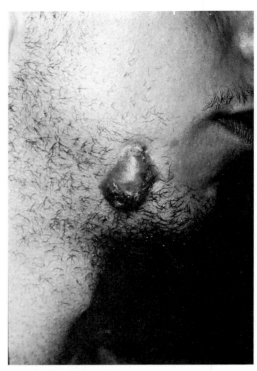

FIGURE 33–2. Localized cutaneous leishmaniasis in a Brazilian patient. A nodular lesion mimicking tumor that was caused by *Leishmania* sp. (Courtesy of Dr. Valdir Sabbaga Amato.) (See Color Plate 2.)

parasites of the *Viannia* subgenus (particularly *L. viannia braziliensis*) are the most common causes of ML, although cases caused by other parasites of the *Viannia* subgenus and *L. mexicana* complex have been reported. Typically, mucosal disease results in disfiguring and progressive ulceration at the nasal mucocutaneous junction and oropharyngeal area (Fig. 33–3 and Color Plate 2).

Only a small percentage (about 3%) of persons infected by *L. braziliensis* subspecies will have ML; it results from hematogenous or lymphatic dissemination of amastigotes from the skin to the naso-oropharyngeal mucosa. ML usually occurs years after the initial skin ulcer has healed, and some factors are associated with the risk of development of ML, including male sex, large or multiple primary lesions, lesions lasting longer than 1 year, and inadequate treatment of primary skin lesions. It is unclear if specific chemotherapy of primary *L. braziliensis* lesions decreases the risk of subsequent mucosal disease.

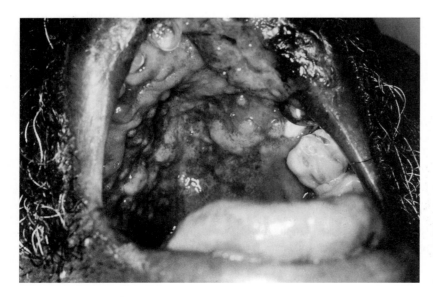

FIGURE 33–3. Mucocutaneous leishmaniasis in a Brazilian patient. A chronic lesion of the oropharyngeal mucosa caused by *Leishmania vianna brazilienses*. (Courtesy of Dr. Valdir Sabbaga Amato.) (See Color Plate 2.)

Visceral Leishmaniasis

Visceral leishmaniasis is a systemic disease caused primarily by parasites belonging to the *L. donovani* complex (*L. donovani donovani*, *L. donovani infantum*, *L. donovani chagasi*) that spread throughout the reticuloendothelial system. Parasites usually associated with LCL and ML can cause VL in rare cases, including *L. mexicana* complex, *L. tropica*, and *L. major*.

Infection remains asymptomatic or subclinical in many cases or can follow an acute, subacute, or chronic course. The classic patient with VL who is heavily infected throughout the mononuclear phagocyte system develops life-threatening disease after an incubation period of weeks to months and presents with fever, severe cachexia, hepatosplenomegaly (splenomegaly usually predominates), and pancytopenia.

In immunosuppressed hosts, such as transplant recipients and patients who are infected with human immunodeficiency virus (HIV), there is a potential either for reactivation of a previously asymptomatic infection or the acquisition of a new infection; unusual localization of the disease in these patients, including the gut, lungs, and central nervous system, have been reported.[2,3]

In HIV-infected patients, VL has emerged as a common opportunistic infection, particularly in southern Europe, where it is caused by *L. donovani infantum* and where 25% to 70% of adults with VL are coinfected with HIV.[2] In endemic regions of southern Europe, 1% to 5% of acquired immunodeficiency syndrome (AIDS) patients develop symptomatic VL, and VL transmission may be related to needle sharing.[2]

Post–Kala-Azar Dermal Leishmaniasis

PKDL develops at variable times after apparent cure of VL. The syndrome primarily is caused by *L. donovani donovani* and is endemic in East Africa and India. The skin lesions are often hypopigmented macules, papules, or nodules and usually are seen first on the face and later involve the limbs and trunk.

Laboratory Procedures

Leishmaniasis is diagnosed by microscopic visualization of amastigotes in smears of tissue aspirates or biopsy samples. Culture of the parasite from infected tissue can increase the diagnostic yield. Although skin testing, antibody detection, and most recently polymerase chain reaction (PCR) analysis have been evaluated for their usefulness in the diagnosis of leishmaniasis, each of these diagnostic methods has limitations.

In immunosuppressed patients, particularly in HIV-infected patients, massive parasitemia is common, which facilitates parasitologic diagnosis, both by conventional methods and unconventional means, such as examination of gastrointestinal tissue, peripheral blood smear, or culture of a buffy-coat preparation.

Pathogenesis

The resolution of leishmania infection in humans and animals depends on a cell-mediated immune response associated with an expansion of *Leishmania*-specific CD4$^+$ T cells of the T_H1 type, which secrete interferon (IFN)-γ and interleukin (IL)-2.[4] The spectrum of disease ranges from the absence of *Leishmania*-specific T_H1 responses and numerous organisms (VL, DCL) to protective T_H1 responses with few organisms (ML, PKDL), and the immune cells may be the cause of pathologic changes.[5,6]

The clinically polar forms of leishmaniasis associated with T_H1 and T_H2 cytokines have been considered in choices of therapy. IFN-γ, IL-2, anti-IL-10, or anti-IL-12 (which increases the number of T_H1-producing cells) could be effective in the treatment of diseases associated with the absence of a cellular immune response.

Treatment

Despite its toxicity and the need for prolonged parenteral therapy, pentavalent antimony (Sb^V)-containing compounds have been standard recommended therapy for leishmaniasis since their introduction in the 1930s. Two compounds are available: sodium stibogluconate (SSG; Pentostam; GlaxoWellcome, London) is used in Asia, much of Europe, and English-speaking parts of Africa; and meglumine antimoniate (SbV; Glucantime; Rhône-Poulenc, Paris), is used in Latin America and French-speaking parts of Africa and Europe. Their therapeutic efficacy is directly related to their content of Sb^V. Sodium stibogluconate solution contains about 10% (100 mg/ml) Sb^V, whereas meglumine antimoniate solution contains approximately 8.5% (85 mg/ml) Sb^V. These compounds have similar efficacy and side effects and both can be administered intramuscularly or intravenously. In the United States, Pentostam is available from the Centers for Disease Control and Prevention (CDC).

Pentavalent antimonials frequently are associated with adverse effects. Intramuscular injection is moderately painful. For intravenous infusion, dilution of the daily dose at least 1:10 with 5% dextrose in water is desirable to reduce the incidence of local thrombosis. Nausea, anorexia, abdominal pain, headache, myalgias, arthralgias, lethargy, and peripheral neuropathy are common, beginning about 7 to 10 days into therapy and resolving shortly after therapy is completed. In general, VL patients tolerate Sb^V better than CL or ML patients do. Hepatotoxicity, nephropathy, acute pancreatitis, and pancytopenia have been reported.[7] Cardiotoxicity is the most serious toxic effect; up to 40% of patients develop electrocardiogram (ECG) abnormalities including premature ventricular contractions, primary atrioventricular nodal block, prolonged PR interval, abnormal T waves, concave ST segments, and abnormal axis. Most often these changes develop gradually over the duration of therapy. Nevertheless, sudden death during antimony treatment has been reported in a few patients receiving the drug in high-dosage regimens.[8]

All patients receiving 20 mg/kg daily of antimony should have an ECG, serum chemistry tests (amylase, lipase, creatinine, liver enzyme tests), and complete blood cell count before treatment and weekly during treatment. Elderly patients with underlying cardiac, hepatic, or renal disease should be monitored more frequently. Therapy should be discontinued if significant elevations of serum amylase (fivefold) or lipase (15-fold), severe hypoplasia of the bone marrow, or elevations in serum transaminases (fivefold) develop. Usually the drug should be withheld for a few days until side effects resolve and re-treatment can be resumed at the same dose. Therapy should be interrupted if specific ECG changes occur during antimony treatment. These ECG changes include concave ST segments, prolongation of QT interval to more than 0.5 second, or significant arrhythmia.[9] T-wave flattening or inversion, the most common ECG abnormalities seen during antimony administration, are not criteria on which to base discontinuation of treatment.

Intramuscular or intravenous injections of pentamidine isethionate are an option for treatment of leishmaniasis, but their use is limited by toxic effects, particularly with higher doses and longer courses of treatment for VL.

Aminosidine (paromomycin sulfate) is an injectable aminoglycoside used either intravenously or intramuscularly with broad antiparasitic activity not shared by the other aminoglycosides. Pentamidine 2 to 4 mg/kg daily for up to 15 days is an effective but potentially toxic alternative, including renal and eighth cranial nerve toxicities, especially when used for periods longer than 10 days or in combination with other agents.

Conventional amphotericin B deoxycholate, 0.5 mg/kg given daily or 1 mg/kg every other day for up to 8 weeks, has also been used successfully to treat *Leishmania* infections. The widespread use of amphotericin B deoxycholate has been limited, however, because of its well-known infusion-related side effects (fever, chills, and thrombophlebitis), its poor tolerability, and the associated long-term problems of nephropathy, anemia, and hypokalemia. Also, amphotericin B should be used with caution in patients who previously received Sb[V] and in whom therapy failed. Amphotericin B should be started only after a rest period of at least 10 days for the patient who has ECG evidence of myocardial damage caused by Sb[V] (ST elevation or ST depression and T inversion) to avoid ventricular arrhythmia and cardiac arrest.[10]

Lipid forms of amphotericin B are thought to be highly effective against *Leishmania* and are associated with less renal toxicity than non-lipid-associated amphotericin B, because of excellent distribution into the intracellular compartment, where parasites reside in the human host, and is poorly cleared by the kidney.

Currently three lipid formulations of amphotericin B are available: liposomal amphotericin B (L-AmB [AmBisome], Gilend Sciences, San Dimas, California); amphotericin B cholesteryl sulfate dispersion (ABCD [Amphocil], Sequus Pharmaceuticals, Menlo Park, California); and amphotericin B lipid complex (ABLC [Abelcet], Liposome Company, Princeton, New Jersey).

Several studies have demonstrated the efficacy and safety of AmBisome for the treatment of VL in Brazil, India, Kenya, and the Mediterranean,[11-14] and it is the only drug currently approved by the U.S. Food and Drug Administration (FDA) for the treatment of VL in the United States.[15]

Although both amphotericin B cholesteryl sulfate dispersion and amphotericin B lipid complex have been used to treat patients with leishmaniasis, there is less experience with these drugs than with AmBisome. These two compounds have higher infusion-related side effects, including fever, chills, and increased respiratory rate.[16,17] These adverse events can be ameliorated by pretreatment with nonsteroidal anti-inflammatory drugs.

Lipid-associated amphotericin B formulations are taken up by the reticuloendothelial system, where the parasites reside in VL. How effective it is for other forms of leishmaniasis has not yet been assessed.

Despite the advantages of liposomal formulations of amphotericin B—being less toxic than amphotericin B deoxycholate and requiring shorter treatment courses (5 to 10 days)—in the absence of randomized, comparative trials it is not clear whether lipid-associated amphotericin B is more effective than amphotericin B deoxycholate in the treatment of VL. It is also difficult to determine which liposomal product should be used if a liposomal formulation is indicated. On the basis of the comparative frequency of infusion-related side effects, AmBisome appears to be the best option for VL therapy. Its high cost, however, is a major obstacle to its use in developing countries.

Although several oral agents have been tested, none has produced consistent results. Ketoconazole and itraconazole have been used for the treatment of leishmaniasis with variable results.

Theoretically *Leishmania* should be susceptible to allopurinol. However, its role as monotherapy and in combination therapy for leishmaniasis has not been clearly elucidated. If shown effective against *Leishmania*, allopurinol has the advantages of low cost and good oral bioavailability and tolerance.

Sitamaquine (WR 6026; Glaxo Smithkline) is an orally administered primaquine analogue that is extremely active against VL in animal models and has shown effectiveness in one phase II trial with VL patients treated for 28 days; 50% of these patients were cured.[18]

Another oral agent has been used in recent studies in Indian patients with kala-azar. The synthetic phospholipid derivative hexadecylphosphocholine, miltefosine, has been an effective drug for treating leishmaniasis, even in patients with antimony-unresponsive infection.[19–22] The primary adverse reactions to miltefosine are gastrointestinal, primarily vomiting and diarrhea. These side effects usually occur during the first 7 to 14 days of therapy, and in most patients the side effects subside as the drug is continued. Side effects have been largely graded as mild with a 100 mg/d dose.[21] Less frequently, asymptomatic increases in serum hepatic transaminases and serum levels of blood urea nitrogen and creatinine can develop. Pregnancy is a contraindication to the use of the drug because miltefosine is a teratogen in animals. Although retinopathy has developed in rats receiving long-term miltefosine treatment, retinal damage has not been found in humans.

Because cure of VL requires an effective cellular immune response to the organism, agents that stimulate cellular immunity have been considered to have an important role in the antileishmanial therapy. Previous work has demonstrated that therapy with three vaccinations of bacille Calmette-Guérin (BCG) plus killed *Leishmania* had the same cure rate that conventional antimony had in CL patients.[23] Although BCG vaccination has not been examined in the treatment of VL, this treatment option should be investigated.

IFN-γ, a T cell–derived cytokine that activates macrophages to kill intracellular *Leishmania*, has been used in humans with promising results as a supplement to Sb[V] therapy in patients who have failed to respond to conventional therapy with antimony and pentamidine.

With all treatment modalities usually a test of cure is not recommended, and repeat parasitologic testing is needed only if there is apparent clinical relapse. The presence of some residual parasites does not necessarily portend a poor outcome, whereas the apparent absence of parasites does not preclude relapse.

Treatment of Cutaneous Leishmaniasis

Lesions of LCL heal spontaneously over 1 month to 3 years even without treatment. Nevertheless, patients with lesions on the face or other cosmetically important area should be treated. Also, LCL caused by *L. braziliensis* and *L. panamensis* should be treated to reduce the risk of mucosal disease.

Antimony is the recommended drug for CL therapy for large or disfiguring lesions. The recommended dose is 10 to 20 mg of Sb[V]/kg daily for 2 to 4 weeks or longer if needed for Old World cases and 20 mg of Sb[V]/kg daily for 20 days for New World cases. The improvement of the skin lesions should begin during antileishmanial therapy, but re-epithelialization of large ulcers may continue after treatment. Thus the need for additional therapy should be assessed 4 to 6 weeks after therapy, and for patients who fail to respond, a second or even third course of Sb[V] may be successful, or an alternative drug may be necessary.[9]

A well-tolerated low-dose short-course of pentamidine is an acceptable alternative for CL unresponsive to antimonials. Previous trials have show that a relatively short course of pentamidine 2 mg/kg intramuscularly every other day for 7 days[24] or 3 mg/kg administered in four every-other-day injections[25] was effective (cure rate of 96%) for cutaneous disease. The same dose was tried every other day for only 4 days, but the cure rate was lower (84%).[25] Recently Hellier et al[26] included 11 patients in an open pilot study with Old World CL treated with three intramuscular injections of 4 mg/kg every other day and demonstrated a 73% cure rate with good drug tolerance.

The cure rate with aminosidine is inferior to that obtained with antimony compounds or pentamidine for CL. Even a higher daily dose (18 mg/kg daily) given for 14 days cured only 50% of patients in Colombia,[27] and similar results were seen in Belize.[28]

Amphotericin B deoxycholate is an alternative therapy for patients who fail to respond to pentavalent antimony. Prolonged treatment with a total of 2 to 3 g is generally required. The efficacy of liposomal formulations for cutaneous diseases has not yet been assessed.

Therapy with alternative agents can be considered for some relatively benign cosmetically unimportant lesions, particularly if caused by *L. major* (Old World) or *L. mexicana* (New World), which cause lesions that tend to self-heal without complications.[7,9]

Ketoconazole, given 600 mg daily for 4 weeks, was more effective than antimony against *L. mexicana* (cure rate of 89%) but less effective than antimony against *L. braziliensis* infections (cure rate of 30%).[29] Ketoconazole was also effective in approximately 70% of persons with *L. major* or *L. panamensis* lesions but is not as effective against *L. tropica*, *L. aethiopica*, or *L. braziliensis*.[30] Singh et al[31] failed to demonstrate efficacy of ketoconazole for *L. tropica* infections, with no cure obtained among 14 patients who received 400 mg daily of the drug for 10 weeks.

Several uncontrolled trials with itraconazole in Old World CL have shown good results,[32,33] but in a small double-blinded study with Old World CL cases, itraconazole 200 mg daily for 4 weeks was slightly less active than placebo.[34]

Allopurinol as monotherapy cannot be recommended for the treatment of CL. Although Ghanem et al[35] administered 1200 mg daily of allopurinol for 1 month and achieved a cure rate of 80% in 20 patients from Egypt, Velez et al[36] demonstrated no effect with a similar dose of allopurinol in Colombian patients. However, allopurinol apparently has been useful when used in combination with pentavalent antimonials to treat CL. In a randomized trial with CL patients the combination of allopurinol and Sb[V] was significantly superior to Sb[V] alone (cure rate of 71% vs. 39%, $P = .005$).[37] In addition the combination of allopurinol and Sb[V] seems effective for recurrent CL.[38]

Patients with CL unresponsive to conventional therapy have been cured with antimony in combination with systemic IFN-γ.[39] In contrast, Arana et al[40] demonstrated no benefit from treatment with Glucantime alone or in combination with IFN-γ in 66 CL patients.

Local therapies have been tried with variable results. Local heat therapy may be useful in treating an unresponsive lesion, but mechanical excision can pose a substantial risk of relapse.

Intralesional antimony therapy has been used extensively for Old World CL, with efficacy similar to that of intramuscular administration,[41] but this therapy has not been widely used in New World CL, and no large comparative trials have been conducted to support its recommendation.

A topical formulation of aminosidine commercially available in Israel has been used to successfully treat 23 of 27 patients with Old World CL.[42] In an uncontrolled trial that included New World CL patients, topical application of aminosidine achieved 70% cure,[43] but the true efficacy in a controlled trial remains to be assessed. Different topical formulations have caused significant local reactions. The best formulation and optimal dose regimen have yet to be determined. The role of topical aminosidine in combination with other drugs deserves further study. In one open, randomized trial, topical aminosidine combined with parenteral Glucantime at 20 mg/kg daily for 7 days cured 58% of patients, compared to an 84% cure rate in the group that received Sb^V alone for 20 days.[44]

Topical application of S-nitro-N-acetylpenicillamine, a nitric oxide donor, is a promising new treatment based on the leishmanicidal effects on macrophage-derived nitric oxide.[45]

In the Old World, DCL usually responds poorly to treatment with Sb^V but the combination of antimony compound and aminosidine has led to long-lasting clinical and parasitologic cures.[46] In the New World the DCL lesion usually improves after initial treatment with Sb^V, but the drug should be administered for several months after apparent clinical and parasitologic cure to limit relapse. The combination of allopurinol plus pentamidine has been unsuccessful in the treatment of DCL.[47]

Treatment of Mucosal Leishmaniasis

All patients with ML should be medically treated, and complementary surgery may be required after parasitologic cure for patients with extensive tissue destruction by leishmaniasis. In general, ML is more difficult to treat than CL is, and the response of ML to therapy is frequently unsatisfactory.

In one study, antimony 20 mg/kg daily for 28 days achieved complete clinical and parasitologic cure in approximately 60% of all lesions, and relapse occurred in 70% of patients.[48] The addition of allopurinol to Sb^V in a randomized trial showed no benefit in the treatment of ML.[49]

Amphotericin B deoxycholate is a treatment option in ML, and liposomal amphotericin formulations are also available for patients who fail to respond to antimony compounds. Long-term cure with AmBisome (2 to 5 g

total dose) in 83% of patients was reported in a small trial in Brazil that included six patients with antimony-unresponsive ML.[50]

As with CL, the combined therapy of Sb^V plus IFN-γ may provide a novel therapeutic approach for the treatment of antimony-resistant CL or ML.[39]

Treatment of Visceral Leishmaniasis

In light of the high case fatality rate of the disease (close to 100% in untreated patients) and given the relatively low sensitivity of most of the parasitologic tests, suspect cases should be treated promptly.

Although less than 10% of VL infections worldwide are resistant to pentavalent antimonials, reports of resistance to these drugs are increasing in parts of Europe, India, and East Africa. Currently, 35% to 64% of previously untreated cases in the state of Bihar, the epicenter of the Indian VL epidemic, are unresponsive to, or relapse after, conventional antimony therapy.[51–53] Resistance is also increasing in Sudan,[13] the other major epidemic area for kala-azar.

Where Sb^V has maintained a high level of efficacy in the treatment of kala-azar, it should be the first-line therapy. For areas where there is high-level resistance to Sb^V, alternative treatments are recommended. One alternative includes a prolonged (40 days or longer) initial treatment with Sb^V.[54] Another option is conventional amphotericin B. Several studies have shown the efficacy of conventional amphotericin B to be as high as 100% in untreated[55] and multidrug-refractory Indian VL patients.[56–58] A traditional regimen using doses of 1 mg/kg daily (total dose, 16 to 20 mg/kg)[57,58] or a regimen of 14 doses of 0.5 mg/kg given every other day for 28 to 30 days (total dose, 7 mg/kg)[55,56] have similar efficacy. In addition the drug can be safely given intravenously over 2 hours rather than 6 hours.[57]

The current FDA-approved regimen of AmBisome for VL is based on trials conducted in Europe and Brazil.[11,12,14] For immunocompetent patients the recommended dosage is 3 mg/kg daily on days 1 to 5, 13, and 21 (total 21 mg/kg), and the course of therapy may be repeated in those in whom parasite clearance is not achieved.[15] An alternative recommendation for immunocompetent patients is treatment on days 1 to 5 and 10 with 3 to 4 mg/kg daily for cases in Europe or Brazil, 3 mg/kg daily for Africa, and 2 to 4 mg/kg daily for India.[59] In one study of treatment of kala-azar under field conditions in Sudan, including severe and complicated cases in patients who were malnourished and had coexisting infections, a total dose of 24 mg/kg of AmBisome was given in six divided doses and found to be more effective (88% cure) than a regimen of 12 mg/kg given in three divided doses (50% cure).[13]

Amphocil has been used successfully in Brazilian patients with kala-azar. A regimen of 2 mg/kg for 5 to 10 days cured 29 of 30 patients.[16,17] In another study, low-dose therapy with Abelcet for VL patients in India who had had poor responses to Sb^V was studied; the long-term efficacy rate was 84% to 100%.[60]

For treatment of VL the recommended dose of pentamidine is 4 mg/kg intravenously given three times per week until initial parasitologic cure was achieved. With this recommended regimen the pentamidine was relatively effective but toxic. In a study of 312 antimony-resistant patients, treatment with pentamidine cured 75% of patients after 5 weeks of therapy (15 injections), and 94% were cured after 9 weeks of treatment (27 injections), but 21% of these patients had a relapse.[61] The addition of 3 weeks of antimony compound to a 5-week course of pentamidine did not raise the rate of parasitologic cure above that observed with pentamidine alone. After 6 months the rate of parasitologic cure was significantly higher in the group who received pentamidine followed by Sb[V] than in the groups who received pentamidine alone or the two drugs together.

Minor side effects with pentamidine include an uneasy feeling during intravenous injection, intestinal disturbances, cellulite, abscess formation, and allergic manifestations. Major reactions are associated with the high-dose and prolonged pentamidine regimens used for VL. Tachycardia or hypotension or both were reported in 20% of VL patients.[62] Hyperglycemia and hypoglycemia occurred in 10% and 8%, respectively, and four deaths were associated with the administration of pentamidine in another study.[61] Considering that pentamidine regimens for VL cases are not superior to regimens of antimonials and that it is more toxic, pentamidine should be used only in regions where treatment failure with antimony is common and in individual cases of antimony treatment failure.

Injectable aminosidine has been used as monotherapy for VL with activity superior to that of Sb[V] in India,[51] a region with a high level of antimony resistance.[51–53] In addition, aminosidine has been shown to act synergistically with antimony drugs.[63,64]

Reports are conflicting on whether ketoconazole is effective in the treatment of VL patients, and its use in these cases is not recommended. Ketoconazole 15 mg/kg/d was used for 21 days to treat Kenyan patients with VL and decreased the splenic parasite load in seven patients.[65] Also, in an Indian center, ketoconazole 200 mg three times a day for 4 weeks cured four of five patients in one study[66] and seven of nine patients' unresponsiveness to Sb[V] or pentamidine or both[67] in another study. However, an average drug dosage of 300 mg twice daily for 30 days failed to reduce the parasitic load in six patients described in another report.[68]

A more recent study with fluconazole for 30 days to treat patients with VL in India achieved less effective results (about 50% cure) and a high relapse rate.[69]

A large number of uncontrolled trials have shown allopurinol successfully used in combination with azoles[70–72] or antimony[73] for the treatment of VL in immunosuppressed patients. However, a controlled trial of Sb[V] alone (20 mg of Sb[V]/kg/d) vs Sb[V] plus allopurinol (20 mg/kg/d), each given for 30 days, demonstrated no advantage to the combination in 128 untreated cases of kala-azar.[74] Allopurinol apparently has been useful in combination with pentavalent antimonials in a few patients whose disease relapsed. Evidence on whether allopurinol in combination with other agents has a role in the treatment of leishmaniasis is not yet conclusive.

Recent studies have shown good results with miltefosine in the treatment of VL patients. Initial studies determined the safety, tolerance, and efficacy of 28 days of miltefosine therapy in a total of 75 VL patients who received drug doses that ranged from 50 to 100 mg on alternate days to 100 to 250 mg daily.[19,20] At day 28, 73 patients were considered to have clinical and parasitologic cure. Subsequently, in another study, 120 Indian patients were treated daily with various doses of miltefosine for a total of 28 to 42 days, and 95% of these subjects had long-term cure.[22] In one recently completed study, Sundar et al[21] treated 54 Indian VL patients with 100 mg daily of oral miltefosine in three randomized groups for 14 days (group A), 21 days (group B), and 28 days (group C), and cure was achieved in 89% of group A and 100% of groups B and C.

IFN-γ as monotherapy to treat VL has shown a measurable but incomplete antileishmanial effect,[75] indicating its limited efficacy in the treatment of these patients. Additional trials suggest that a subgroup of patients with VL who exhibit primary drug resistance or who fail to respond to repeated courses of conventional therapy with both antimony and pentamidine may benefit from treatment with IFN-γ plus Sb[V].[76,77] This approach may offer at best marginal benefit in settings with high-level resistance to antimony compounds[78] and seldom has been used since the lipid formulations of amphotericin B became available. IFN-γ may also play an important adjunctive role in accelerating responsiveness to conventional therapy in previously untreated patients with VL.[79,80]

After starting therapy for kala-azar, most patients feel better and become afebrile during the first week of treatment. Splenomegaly and biochemical abnormalities do not resolve for weeks to months in some cases. The recommended period for follow-up is 6 months. Parasites can persist in sterile sites such as the spleen after therapy even if clinical disease does not recur, and it may be that total eradication of the organism is not achievable.

Treatment of Post–Kala-Azar Dermal Leishmaniasis

Long-term therapy (up to 120 days) with Sb[V] has been successful in the treatment of PKDL in India.[81]

Treatment of Leishmaniasis in Immunosuppressed Patients

The management of Leishmania in HIV-coinfected patients should be individualized and based on an assessment of the clinical importance and evolution of the leishmanial infection and the stage of HIV infection. When treatment is indicated, more aggressive therapeutic regimens are warranted to induce a longer relapse-free period. Secondary prophylaxis should be given after initial treatment is completed.

Therapy of leishmaniasis in HIV-infected patients with antimonial pentavalent compounds is unsuccessful in more than 50% of patients. Furthermore conventional amphotericin B seems to provide no additional benefit in the treatment of leishmaniasis. Laguna et al[82] in an open, multicenter, randomized trial compared treatment with an antimony compound and conventional amphotericin B in HIV-infected patients with VL in Spain. These authors found no difference between the two drugs in an intention-to-treat analysis (cure rates of 66% vs. 62%) or an on-treatment analysis (85% vs. 93%); also no difference was found with respect to the probability of not having a relapse by 12 months after therapy (30% vs. 40%) and in survival after the diagnosis of leishmaniasis. None of the patients received highly active antiretroviral therapy.

AmBisome, in higher doses than those used to treat immunocompetent patients with kala-azar, is currently approved by the FDA to treat immunosuppressed patients with leishmaniasis. The recommended dose is 4 mg/kg daily on days 1 to 5, 10, 17, 24, 31, and 38 (total 40 mg/kg).[15] Unfortunately, although clinical trials including immunosuppressed patients have shown a high level of efficacy in these patients with doses ranging from 100 mg/d for 21 days to 4 mg/kg/d on days 1 to 5, 10, 17, 24, 31, and 38, with a cure rate of 94.7% at the end of treatment, the relapse rate was as high as 80% to 100%.[11,12,14]

Secondary prophylaxis with different schemes has been administered with no effectiveness measurable in the prevention of recurrence. Monthly administered antimonials, pentamidine every 3 to 4 weeks, AmBisome, allopurinol, and itraconazole have been used.[2]

Relapse is not rare and pancreatitis is common when pentavalent antimonials are used to treat VL in transplant recipients.[3] Alternative therapies in these patients are limited; pentamidine and amphotericin B may be highly toxic for renal transplant recipients. AmBisome should be considered as an alternative therapy because of its reduced nephrotoxicity and high efficacy.[83]

Prevention

Despite recent advances in immunoprophylaxis of leishmaniasis, no vaccine is available. Thus the control of leishmaniasis consists in control of vectors, detection and elimination of animal reservoirs, and treatment of infected patients. Control of this zoonosis is more difficult in areas where the natural cycle of the parasite involves sylvatic mammals, where the control of reservoir is obviously impossible.

TRYPANOSOMIASIS

Members of the family Trypanosomatidae, genus *Trypanosoma*, include the etiologic agents of American trypanosomiasis (Chagas' disease), endemic in Central and South America, and of human African trypanosomiasis (sleeping sickness), endemic in sub-Saharan Africa. Despite recent advances in the control of the transmission of trypanosomiasis, these diseases continue to be a serious health problem in regions where they are endemic.

American Trypanosomiasis

American trypanosomiasis is a zoonosis caused by *Trypanosoma cruzi*, a protozoan parasite found only in the Americas. *T. cruzi* is distributed among humans, many non-human mammalian species, and a large number of insects in all South and Central American countries and Mexico. The sylvatic cycle of *T. cruzi* has also been documented in southwestern and southern United States, but autochthonous *T. cruzi* infection in the United States is rare.

Most infected persons acquire the parasite through contact with various species of bloodsucking *Triatoma* insects harboring *T. cruzi*. Transmission of *T. cruzi* also occurs through blood transfusion, and this mode of transmission has become a major source of new infections in some regions. Rarely, transmission is through congenital exposure, oral contact, or laboratory exposure.

Case Definitions
Immunocompetent Patients
In humans, *T. cruzi* infection induces an acute phase with high levels of parasitemia characterized by a mild, self-limited systemic illness involving fever, malaise, anorexia, and headache. Edema of the face and lower extremities, generalized lymphadenopathy, and hepatosplenomegaly are often present. In immunocompetent patients the disease usually resolves spontaneously in 4 to 8 weeks without diagnosis or treatment. Next the patient enters the indeterminate phase of *T. cruzi* infection, a lifelong phase with no clinical manifestations of chronic Chagas' disease, low levels of parasitemia, and the presence of antibodies to many *T. cruzi* antigens.

Symptomatic chronic Chagas' disease typically appears years or even decades after the initial infection. Approximately 20% to 30% of the seroreactors develop chronic cardiomyopathy, and less than 10% develop gastrointestinal megaorgan syndromes.

Chronic chagasic cardiomyopathy is a panmyocarditis manifested by symptoms reflecting heart failure, arrhythmias, and thromboembolic events.

Gastrointestinal involvement is the second most common manifestation of chronic Chagas' disease. Although the most frequent findings are megaesophagus and megacolon, any hollow viscera can be affected, including stomach and small intestine.

Megaesophagus is the most common problem in chronic gastrointestinal Chagas' disease, causing dysphagia, pain, and regurgitation. Recurrent pulmonary infections and malnutrition are commonly reported in patients with recurrent regurgitation, and it can be fatal in untreated patients.

Patients with chagasic megacolon present with motility disturbances, colonic enlargement, the principal symptom of which is chronic constipation that increases in frequency and duration over months and years, and abdominal pain. Because of prolonged periods without bowel movements, these patients can develop toxic megacolon, volvulus, and acute obstruction, which can cause perforation, septicemia, and death.

Immunosuppressed Patients

T. cruzi can cause severe infection, frequently fatal, in immunosuppressed patients. Cases of severe reactivated chagasic infections, particularly meningoencephalitis and myocarditis, occur in patients with suppressed cellular immunity, including transplant recipients and AIDS patients.

The clinical manifestations in kidney transplant recipients can be indistinguishable from the acute phase of Chagas' disease and occasionally involve the CNS.[84,85] Because of the risk of reactivation of chagasic infection in patients following transplant, evaluation for signs and symptoms of Chagas' disease should be done periodically, and a search for *T. cruzi* infection should be performed when acute illness occurs.

The risk of Chagas' disease reactivation after heart transplantation is higher than after kidney transplantation because of the more intensive postoperative immunosuppression used in heart transplantation.[86,87] Since 1991, however, its incidence in heart transplant recipients has decreased because reduced doses of cyclosporine have been used.[88,89] In those who have undergone heart transplantation and suffered reactivated Chagas' disease, meningoencephalitis is rare; the disease is manifested as severe myocarditis and subcutaneous lesions.[86]

In AIDS patients, reactivation of Chagas' disease is manifested as a febrile syndrome accompanied by meningoencephalitis or acute myocarditis or both.[90,91] Most *T. cruzi* infection reactivations are in persons in advanced stages of AIDS with CD4 lymphocyte counts less than 200/mm³.

Laboratory Procedures

The diagnosis of acute Chagas' disease is made by direct microscopy, xenodiagnosis, and hemoculture. Serologic tests for anti–*T. cruzi* immunoglobulin (Ig) M play a limited role in the diagnosis of acute disease.

In immunosuppressed persons suspected of having reactivation of *T. cruzi* infection, specimens other than blood such as lymph node aspirates, bone marrow, cerebrospinal fluid, and pericardial fluid should be examined for parasites. The diagnosis of *T. cruzi* infection in immunosuppressed patients is usually difficult because the parasitologic approaches used to detect *T. cruzi* in acute infections are not sensitive enough to diagnose reactivation.

Chronic Chagas' disease usually is diagnosed by detecting IgG antibodies specific to *T. cruzi* antigens, and demonstration of the parasite is not necessary. The most common conventional tests for detecting IgG are complement fixation, indirect immunofluorescence, indirect hemagglutination, and enzyme-linked immunosorbent assays (ELISA). A persistent problem with these serodiagnostic assays has been the number of false-positive reactions, and improved tests for diagnosis of chronic Chagas' disease are needed. Most authorities recommend that sera be tested in different assays before being considered positive.

In recent years efforts have focused on the development of serologic assays using recombinant *T. cruzi* proteins or synthetic peptides for the diagnosis of both acute and chronic disease. PCR-based assays for Chagas' disease diagnosis have also been investigated. However, additional evaluation of these serologic and PCR-methods is needed.

Evaluation of all *T. cruzi*–infected patients should include serial ECGs repeated at periodic intervals. Minor ECG abnormalities are associated with an increased risk of disease progression, and persons with these findings should be followed closely.

Investigation for megaorgans should be done in *T. cruzi*–infected patients with symptoms suggesting esophageal or colon disease. For patients with megaesophagus, chest radiography, fluoroscopic barium studies, cine-esophagram, and endoscopy can be useful in the evaluation. For patients with megacolon a radiograph of the abdomen often discloses large amounts of feces, and after evacuation of the colon with enemas, the diagnosis can be confirmed with an air-contrast barium enema, which shows a characteristic lack of haustral markings and an enlarged colon diameter.

Pathogenesis

The pathogenesis of the gastrointestinal and cardiac lesions of chronic Chagas' disease is not well understood. There is evidence supporting an autoimmune process.[92,93] It is possible, however, that tissue injury could be caused by *T. cruzi* parasites during the acute and chronic phases of the infection, resulting in inflammatory lesions that develop over time.[94,95]

Treatment

Treatment of American trypanosomiasis is problematic because of the limited number of active drugs available, the necessity of taking them for extended periods, the high risk of toxicity, and the low efficacy. In addition the known variations in virulence and drug sensitivity of parasites from different geographic areas do not permit comparisons among therapy trials from different areas.

The only two drugs currently available specifically for treatment of *T. cruzi* are a nitroimidazole, Benznidazole (Rochagan, Roche 07–1051, Radanil), and a nitrofuran, nifurtimox (Lampit, Bayer 2502).[96,97] The efficacy of both drugs is similar, although *T. cruzi* strains have different drug susceptibilities.[98] Both drugs can have several adverse effects. In most cases, side effects do not justify cessation of treatment. Neither of these drugs is licensed in the United States or Europe, but they can be obtained from the Parasitic Disease Drug Service of the CDC, Atlanta, Georgia.

Benznidazole is given orally at 5 mg/kg daily in two or three doses for 30 to 60 days. Children tolerate the drug better than adults do and can tolerate doses of 5 to 10 mg/kg/d. Therapy should be administered under strict medical supervision. Peripheral neuritis, anorexia, weight loss, rash, and hematologic alterations (neutropenia, agranulocytosis, thrombocytopenia) are common adverse effects. In South America, especially Brazil, benznidazole is the drug of choice for specific therapy.

Nifurtimox is administered to adults in an oral dosage of 8 to 10 mg/kg/d in three divided doses after meals. Adolescents should receive 12.5 to 15 mg/kg/d and for children 1 to 10 years of age a higher dose of 15 to 20 mg/kg/d is needed. Recommended duration of treatment varies from a minimum of 30 days up to 120 days. Therapy with nifurtimox must be given under strict medical supervision because of the high incidence of side effects. Tremors, excitation, insomnia, seizures, anorexia, nausea, vomiting, abdominal pain, and weight loss are common. These symptoms usually disappear when the dosage is reduced or therapy is discontinued. Hemolytic anemia associated with glucose-6-phosphate dehydrogenase deficiency is dose dependent and appears near the end of treatment.

Ketoconazole and itraconazole have been used in animal and human therapy for *T. cruzi* infection without success,[99,100] although a recent report showed parasitologic cures in over 50% of chronically infected patients treated with itraconazole.[101] Allopurinol has also been used in clinical studies with varying efficacy.[101-103] Additional study is needed to assess its role in the therapy of Chagas' disease.

The use of recombinant IFN-γ with nifurtimox in one immunosuppressed patient with acute Chagas' disease was reported.[104] Although the use of immunomodulating agents, particularly in immunosuppressed patients, may be of benefit, its role in the treatment of chagasic disease needs further investigation.

A fourth generation of triazole derivatives, including posaconazole (SCH 56592) (Schering-Plough), has shown high efficacy in murine models of acute and chronic Chagas' disease, and clinical trials with this and other triazole derivatives are currently underway.

Positive parasitologic tests prove the presence of the parasite, but because of its low sensitivity, negative test results cannot prove the elimination of *T. cruzi* after specific therapy. Positive conventional serologic tests offer indirect but sensitive proof of parasite presence, especially when two or three consecutive tests are positive. Criteria of cure are serologic tests previously positive that become completely and consistently negative after specific therapy. In acute disease this seroconversion occurs approximately 12 months after the initiation of treatment, whereas in chronic forms, negative seroconversion is slow, taking years to occur, and requires a long follow-up to prove cure.

New promising perspectives have been studied to assess cure, especially in patients with chronic chagasic disease; they include serologic methods to detect lytic antibodies, other antigens substituting for live parasites in ELISA and Western blot tests, and PCR, but more studies are needed before they are used in clinical practical.

Treatment of Acute Chagas' Disease

Both benznidazole and nifurtimox reduce the duration and severity of acute Chagas' disease. Parasitologic cure is achieved in about 50% to 70% of treated patients with acute disease.[105]

In cases of acute and congenital disease, therapy should be initiated as early as possible. In cases due to laboratory exposure, therapy should be initiated before clinical or parasitologic indications of infection are seen. In these situations the recommended dose of benznidazole is 7 to 10 mg/kg daily for 10 days.

Treatment of Indeterminate and Asymptomatic Chronic Chagas' Disease

Specific treatment of the indeterminate or chronic phase of Chagas' disease is controversial because of the difficulty in assessing therapeutic efficacy in these infection phases. Some studies have demonstrated no benefits from treatments.[106,107] In others, parasitologic cure has been about 35%.[105] Braga et al[108] found no parasitologic cure among 34 treated patients with chronic chagasic disease by using improved laboratory methods to detect cure after treatment.

Recent studies implicate the parasite in the pathogenesis of chronic disease,[94,95] and some trials show benefits of specific therapy in the natural course of chronic disease in patients with or without parasitologic cure.[109,110] These findings have changed the previously accepted recommendation that therapy was not indicated in patients with chronic disease. Viotti et al[110] followed 131 patients with chronic chagasic disease treated with benznidazole and 70 patients with untreated chronic chagasic disease for an average of 8 years. The treated patients had a lower incidence of ECG changes (4% vs. 30%) and a lower rate of clinical deterioration (2% vs. 17%) that was independent of negative serologic or parasitologic results.

Additional studies have shown a good chance of cure when therapy is given during the first decade of life. In one study, 58% of 64 asymptomatic Brazilian school-age children treated with benznidazole became seronegative vs. 3(5%) of 65 untreated children (56% efficacy) over a 3-year follow-up period.[109]

Treatment of these patients may improve the prognosis by minimizing parasite invasion of tissues and diminishing inflammatory responses that damage the heart muscle and the peripheral autonomic nervous system, thus decreasing the risk of the development of chronic chagasic disease. In view of these new findings, authorities in the field who have been supported by WHO admit that the administration of antiparasitic drugs to chronically infected patients, particularly for infected children and adults up to a few years after infection, is a valid option, but each case should be considered individually.

Treatment of Symptomatic Chronic Chagas' Disease

Therapy of chronic chagasic cardiomyopathy is directed at ameliorating symptoms though the use of cardiotropic and antiarrhythmic drugs, and pacemakers for patients with severe arrhythmia. Prophylaxis of thromboembolic phenomena with anticoagulant therapy should be considered. Several studies have confirmed the important role of heart transplantation in the treatment of end-stage chagasic cardiomyopathy.[88,89,111] Although reactivation of *T. cruzi* parasitemia and Chagas' disease is possible, both can be successfully treated and allograft function preserved.[88] Long-term use of benznidazole for suppression of parasitemia is not justified.[88]

The best treatment choice for chagasic megaesophagus is balloon dilatation of the lower esophageal sphincter. Patients who fail to respond to repeated dilatation procedures should have surgical intervention. In general, dietary measures and anticholinergic drugs are of little use for these patients. The local injection of botulinum toxin to reduce lower esophageal sphincter pressure is an alternative still under study. Periodic esophagoscopy is recommended to monitor for esophageal carcinoma.

Chagasic patients in the early stages of colonic dysfunction can be managed with a diet high in fiber and increased fluid intake. More advanced disease requires regular use of laxatives and enemas. Severe disease may be complicated by toxic megacolon and volvulus. Volvulus without ischemic complications can be reduced with nonsurgical means, but complicated cases should be treated with urgent bowel resection. Even without complications, patients with advanced chagasic megacolon are best managed surgically with resection of the involved colon.

Treatment of Immunosuppressed Patients with Chagas' Disease

Benznidazole and nifurtimox are both effective in the treatment of disease reactivation in immunosuppressed patients. The dosage of benznidazole is the same as that recommended for immunocompetent patients and is given for a minimum of 60 days. If the diagnosis is made early and therapy is initiated immediately, resolution of symptoms has been seen after a few days of therapy, and parasitologic tests become negative within the first weeks of therapy. Otherwise the prognosis is poor, and most die within 20 days after the initial diagnosis.

Secondary prophylaxis is indicated for patients who achieve complete clinical remission. A committee of experts meeting in Uruguay in 1996 under the sponsorship of the Pan American Health Organization recommended benznidazole 5 mg/kg/d three times a week indefinitely as secondary prophylaxis.[112] Consensus has not been achieved for primary prophylaxis in chagasic HIV-infected patients.[112] Antiretroviral therapy in AIDS patients can decrease the number of cases of Chagas' disease reactivation because of the capacity of these drugs to maintain CD4 lymphocyte counts above 200/mm^3 for longer periods.[113]

The prolonged use of corticosteroids in patients with chronic chagasic disease has been associated with increased parasitemia,[114] although reactivation of the disease in these patients is rare, with only one case described in the literature.[115] Some studies have shown the efficacy of benznidazole and nifurtimox in preventing an increase in parasitemia.[116,117] The real risk-to-benefit ratio needs to be better defined, however, before the routine use of antiparasitic drugs associated with potentially serious side effects can be recommended for patients with chronic chagasic disease who have been taking corticosteroids for a prolonged period.

Although *T. cruzi* infection can reactivate in patients eligible for transplantation, American trypanosomiasis is not a contraindication to organ transplantation.

Prevention

In the absence of a vaccine or therapy free of side effects, control of Chagas' disease is to prevent its transmission. The strategies to eliminate vector and transfusion transmission—using insecticides to eliminate insects in homes and screening blood products—have achieved considerable success in reducing the transmission of *T. cruzi*.

African Trypanosomiasis

Human African trypanosomiasis (HAT) is an old disease restricted to sub-Saharan Africa. The agents responsible for HAT are two morphologically identical trypanosome subspecies, *Trypanosoma brucei gambiense* in West and Central Africa and *Trypanosoma brucei rhodesiense* in East Africa. They are transmitted to humans most often by bites from infected tsetse flies that are found uniquely in sub-Saharan Africa. Transmission is also possible through contamination with infected blood or congenital exposure. Humans are the primary reservoir in Gambian HAT, and antelope and cattle are the primary reservoirs in Rhodesian HAT with humans infected only incidentally.

Sleeping sickness has resurged as a major public health problem in endemic areas in recent years, in part related to fewer control programs. A severe epidemic began in the 1970s and continues today.[118] During the past 25 years, approximately 25 cases of imported

African trypanosomiasis have been reported to the CDC.[119–121]

Case Definitions

T. b. gambiense has a chronic, protracted course that may last for several years, whereas *T. b. rhodesiense* is an acute illness, that can cause death within weeks or months. However, both diseases are fatal if untreated. HAT is characterized by an early stage in which trypanosomes multiply in the bloodstream and lymphatic system over weeks (*T. b. rhodesiense*) or months (*T. b. gambiense*), and patients manifest nonspecific symptoms (hemolymphatic stage). After this nonspecific syndrome, patients develop the late-stage disease with central nervous system (CNS) involvement. Parasites reach the brain and meninges via the bloodstream and cause meningoencephalitis or meningomyelitis or both. During the CNS stage, which can last weeks (*T. b. rhodesiense*) to months (*T. b. gambiense*), trypanosomes are found in the cerebrospinal fluid (CSF) of patients with neurologic symptoms that include alteration of the circadian sleep-wake cycle, mental status changes, tone and sensory disorders, and coordination problems. Other complications include endocrinologic, cardiovascular, and renal disorders. The natural course of the disease includes body wasting, somnolence, coma, and death in untreated patients.

HAT is no more common or more severe in patients with HIV infection or AIDS despite both infections being endemic in sub-Saharan Africa.[122]

Laboratory Procedures

Definitive diagnosis of HAT requires demonstration of the parasite in at least one specimen, which can be found in the aspirate of lymph nodes and in peripheral blood during the first stage of the disease and in the CSF during the CNS stage. Bone marrow aspirate is an additional specimen that can be a source of parasites in cases in which they are not found in usual specimens.

As the disease progresses, trypanosomes are more difficult to find in the blood or lymph nodes and are easier to find in the CSF. Examination of CSF, however, is mandatory in all patients suspected of having HAT.[123] In any patient with trypanosomes in the CSF or a pleocytosis above 6/mm³, even without neurologic symptoms, CNS involvement is indicated, which has treatment implications.

Several serologic assays are available to aid in the diagnosis of HAT, but their results are not reliable, limiting their use in treatment decisions. Currently there are no PCR-based assays to assist in the diagnosis of HAT.

Treatment

The treatment of HAT is difficult, particularly after the parasite has crossed the blood-brain barrier. The medicines available are few and difficult to administer because of severe toxicity that can cause death. It has been estimated that between 3% and 5% of those treated in the last stage of illness die from the treatment.[124] In addition, parasite resistance to currently used drugs is a problem.[124]

This discussion will address the most important aspects of HAT treatment. A more complete review of treatment is available.[125]

Therapy of HAT depends on the infecting parasite (*T. b. gambiense* or *T. b. rhodesiense* trypanosomiases) and on whether there is CNS involvement. Because the separate geographic distributions of *T. b. gambiense* and *T. b. rhodesiense* have little overlap, it is not necessary to identify which subspecies is causing the disease. If there is doubt about the subspecies involved and laboratory analysis is not available, treatment decisions should be based on clinical presentation.

The drugs used include suramin, pentamidine, organic arsenicals, and more recently, eflornithine. Melarsoprol and suramin are not licensed for use in the United States but can be obtained from the Parasitic Disease Drug Service of the CDC in Atlanta, Georgia. Eflornithine can also be obtained from the Division of Control of Tropical Diseases of WHO.

Suramin (Bayer 205, naphuride, Antrypol) is effective for treatment of patients with HAT without CNS involvement. Although suramin is effective for both *T. b. gambiense* and *T. b. rhodesiense* infections, several studies have reported a high frequency of treatment failure (about 25% to 35%) with suramin monotherapy for Gambian HAT.[126,127] Thus, suramin rarely is used for early-stage Gambian disease. For early-stage Rhodesian disease, suramin is more effective than pentamidine.

Suramin is administered as five intramuscular or intravenous injections. The dosage for adults is 1 g and is given on days 1, 3, 7, 14, and 21. The dosage for children is 20 mg/kg intravenously by the same schedule. Although anaphylaxis is rare (approximately 1 of 20,000 treated patients), a 100- to 200-mg test dose should be given before start of therapy. Less severe side effects include fever, nausea, vomiting, urticaria, photophobia, arthralgias, and skin eruption. A transient proteinuria can occur, and a urinalysis should be done before giving each dose. If proteinuria increases or casts and red blood cells appear in the urine sediment, the drug should be discontinued. Suramin should not be used in patients with preexisting renal insufficiency.

Eflornithine (difluoromethylornithine, DFMO, Ornidyl) is active against both hemolymphatic and CNS stages of *T. b. gambiense* trypanosomiasis. Although highly effective for *T. b. gambiense* infection and relatively safe, the drug is expensive and should be reserved for late-stage illness of *T. b. gambiense* trypanosomiasis or for patients not responding to melarsoprol. Eflornithine is not recommended for *T. b. rhodesiense* infections because it is variably effective in these cases.[128] Limited data suggest that HIV-infected patients with HAT do not respond well to eflornithine, probably because the drug is trypanostatic and not trypanocidal; HIV-infected patients should be treated with melarsoprol.

The recommended dosage of eflornithine is 400 mg/kg/d intravenously in four divided doses for 7 to 14 days, followed by oral treatment with 300 mg/kg/d, also in four divided doses, for 3 to 4 weeks. Intravenous administration for 14 days followed by oral therapy for another 21 days was superior to 14 days of intravenous therapy alone in one study.[129] Seven days of intravenous eflornithine is recommended for patients who failed to respond to melarsoprol.

Side effects are usually mild and reversible and include fever, vomiting, diarrhea, anemia, and thrombocytopenia. Seizures and hearing loss have been reported rarely. Currently this drug is not commercially available in the United States and Canada. (In the United States, this drug may be obtained from Parasitic Disease Drug Service, CDC.)

For patients with *T. b. gambiense* CNS disease who cannot tolerate eflornithine, the alternative therapeutic approach is a combination of the arsenical tryparsamide (Tryparsone, Novatoxyl) and suramin. Tryparsamide is not effective against *T. b. rhodesiense*. The dosage of tryparsamide is one injection of 30 mg/kg (max. 2 g) intravenously every 5 days for a total of 12 injections. The dosage of suramin is 10 mg/kg intravenously every 5 days, also for a total of 12 injections. The course of both drugs may be repeated after 1 month. Tryparsamide can cause encephalopathy, fever, abdominal pain, vomiting, rash, tinnitus, and a variety of ocular symptoms.

Pentamidine isoethionate is an alternative treatment recommended for patients with *T. b. gambiense* hemolymphatic trypanosomiasis without CNS involvement.[130] *T. b. rhodesiense* infections usually do not respond to this drug. It is administered to both adults and children daily or every other day intramuscularly at a dose of 4 mg/kg/d for 7 to 10 injections. The most common adverse reactions of pentamidine are nausea, vomiting, abdominal pain, hypotension, and tachycardia, but these reactions generally are transient and usually do not warrant discontinuation of therapy. Other side effects include nephrotoxicity, abnormal liver function test results, neutropenia, rashes, hypoglycemia, and hyperglycemia.

Some authors recommend the combination of pentamidine and suramin to treat Gambian HAT. In one study, Neujean and Evens[127] reported better efficacy with this combination than with pentamidine alone (failure rate of 3% and 16%, respectively) in patients with *T. b. gambiense* infection and normal CSF.

The arsenical melarsoprol (Mel B, Arsobal) is the primary choice for HAT patients with CNS involvement due to either *T. b. gambiense* or *T. b. rhodesiense* infections. Also it is an alternative for hemolymphatic stage of *T. b. rhodesiense* infection in patients in whom suramin or pentamidine or both have failed or were not tolerated. However, it should never be the treatment choice for early-stage trypanosomiasis because of its high toxicity.

The recommended dosage of the arsenical melarsoprol is 2 to 3.6 mg/kg/d intravenously for 3 days for the first course, followed by two subsequent courses of 3.6 mg/kg/d for 3 days each, with a 7- to 10-day rest period between each series. In frail patients an initial dose of 18 mg followed by progressive drug increases has been recommended. Pretreatment with suramin for 2 to 4 days before melarsoprol therapy is started in debilitated patients has been advocated. Pediatric patients should be treated with 18 to 25 mg/kg intravenously given over 1 month; initial dose of 0.36 mg/kg should be increased gradually to a maximum of 3.6 mg/kg at intervals of 1 to 5 days for a total of 9 to 10 doses.

Reactive encephalopathy, the most important side effect, has been reported in 5% to 10% of patients, and 10% to 50% of these patients die. It is thought to result from the interaction of the drug with diseased brain tissue and trypanosomes, and it is rare in patients with minimal CNS involvement. Reactive encephalopathy generally occurs during the first course, and its onset may be sudden or insidious. Clinical manifestations include high fever, headache, tremor, impaired speech, seizures, and finally coma. The reaction may be fatal, but death rates have been reduced as experience with the drug has accumulated. Melarsoprol should be discontinued at the first sign of encephalopathy. It may be restarted cautiously using small doses a few days after signs of toxicity have resolved. Corticosteroids have been used to prevent arsenical encephalopathy.[131]

A number of other side effects with melarsoprol therapy, including local reactions with the extravasation of the drug, abdominal pain, vomiting, Jarisch-Herxheimer-type reactions, nephrotoxicity, abnormal liver function tests, and myocardial damage, have been reported.

Melarsoprol treatment failures have increased over the past 3 to 5 years. Some treatment centers in endemic countries for HAT including Angola, Democratic Republic of Congo, Sudan, and Uganda, have reported treatment failure rates over 20%.[118]

Relapses

After treatment of Gambian HAT, patients should be followed for at least 2 years, and a lumbar puncture should be done every 6 months to evaluate for relapse. Patients treated for Rhodesian HAT should have a more frequent lumbar puncture (every 3 months), at least during the first year. Frequently the patient is asymptomatic during relapses; in that case the diagnosis should be based on the presence of trypanosomes in the CSF or pleocytosis.

Prevention

Control programs include eradication of vectors and drug treatment of all infected humans and animals. Individuals can reduce their risk of acquiring infection with trypanosomes by avoiding areas known to harbor infected insects, by wearing clothing that reduces the biting of flies, and by using insect repellent. Chemoprophylaxis is not recommended because of the marked toxicity of the drugs active against HAT. No vaccine is currently available to prevent transmission of parasites.

ACKNOWLEDGMENTS: I thank Dr. Valdir Sabbaga Amato of the University of São Paulo, Brazil, who provided patient photographs and Dr. Larry M. Baddour for helpful suggestions in chapter development.

REFERENCES

1. World Health Organization, Division of Control of Tropical Diseases: Leishmaniasis control home page *www.who.int/health-topics/leishmaniasis.htm* (updated 2000).
2. Alvar J, Cavanate C, Gutierrez-Solar B, et al: *Leishmania* and human immunodefiency virus coinfection: The first 10 years. Clin Microbiol Rev 1997;10:298–319.
3. Berenguer J, Gomez-Campdera F, Padilla B, et al: Visceral leishmaniasis (kala-azar) in transplant recipients: Case report and review. Transplantation 1998;65:1401–1404.
4. Reiner SL, Locksley RM: Cytokines in the differentiation of Th1/Th2 CD4+ subsets in leishmaniasis. J Cell Biochem 1993;53:323–8.
5. Holaday BJ, Pompeu MM, Evans T, et al: Correlates of *Leishmania*-specific immunity in the clinical spectrum of infection with *Leishmania chagasi*. J Infect Dis 1993; 167(2):411–417.
6. Castes M, Cabrera M, Trujillo D, et al: T-cell subpopulations, expression of interleukin-2 receptor, and production of interleukin-2 and gamma interferon in human American cutaneous leishmaniasis. J Clin Microbiol 1988;26:1207–1213.
7. Berman JD: Human leishmaniasis: Clinical, diagnostic, and chemotherapeutic development in the last 10 years. Clin Infect Dis 1997;24:684–703.
8. Thakur CP: Harmful effect of high stibogluconate treatment of kala-azar in India. Trans R Soc Trop Med Hyg 1986; 80:672–673.
9. Herwaldt BL, Berman JD: Recommendations for treating leishmaniasis with sodium stibogluconate (Pentostam) and review of pertinent clinical studies. Am J Trop Med Hyg 1992;46:296–306.
10. Thakur CP: Sodium antimony gluconate, amphotericin, and myocardial damage. Lancet 1998;351(9120):1928–1929.
11. Davidson RN, Di Martino L, Gradoni L, et al: Liposomal amphotericin B (AmBisome) in Mediterranean visceral leishmaniasis: A multi-centre trial. Q. J. Med 1994;87:75–81.
12. Davidson RN, Di Martino L, Gradoni L, et al: Short-course treatment of visceral leishmaniasis with liposomal amphotericin B (AmBisome). Clin Infect Dis 1996;22:938–943.
13. Seaman J, Boer C, Wilkinson R, et al: Liposomal amphotericin B (AmBisome) in the treatment of complicated kala-azar under field conditions. Clin Infect Dis 1995;21:188–193.
14. Russo R, Nigro LC, Minniti S, et al: Visceral leishmaniasis in HIV-infected patients: Treatment with high dose liposomal amphotericin B (AmBisome). J Infect 1996;32:133–137.
15. Meyerhoff A: U.S. Food and Drug Administration: Approval of AmBisome (liposomal amphotericin B) for treatment of visceral leishmaniasis. Clin Infect Dis 1999;28:42–48.
16. Dietze R, Milan EP, Berman JD, et al: Treatment of Brazilian kala-azar with a short course of Amphocil (amphotericin B cholesterol dispersion). Clin Infect Dis 1993;17:981–986.
17. Dietze R, Fagundes SM, Brito EF, et al: Treatment of kala-azar in Brazil with Amphocil (amphotericin B cholesterol dispersion) for 5 days. Trans R Soc Trop Med Hyg 1995;89:309–311.
18. Sherwood JA, Gachihi GS, Muigai RK, et al: Phase 2 efficacy trial of an oral 8-aminoquinolone (WR6026) for treatment of visceral leishmaniasis. Clin Infect Dis 1994;19:1034–1039.
19. Sundar S, Rosenkaimer F, Makharia MK, et al: Trial of oral miltefosine for visceral leishmaniasis. Lancet 1998;352:1821–1823.
20. Sundar S, Gupta LB, Makharia MK, et al: Oral treatment of visceral leishmaniasis with miltefosine. Ann Trop Med Parasitol 1999;93:589–597.
21. Sundar S, Makharia A, More DK, et al: Short-course of oral miltefosine for treatment of visceral leishmaniasis. Clin Infect Dis 2000;31(4):1110–1113.
22. Jha TK, Sundar S, Thakur CP, et al: Miltefosine, an oral agent, for the treatment of Indian visceral leishmaniasis. N Engl J Med 1999;341:1795–1800.
23. Convit J, Castellanos PL, Rondon A, et al: Immunotherapy versus chemotherapy in localized cutaneous leishmaniasis. Lancet 1987;1(8530):401–405.
24. Soto-Mancipe J, Grogl M, Berman JD: Evaluation of pentamidine for the treatment of cutaneous leishmaniasis in Colombia. Clin Infect Dis 1993;16:417–425.
25. Soto J, Buffet P, Grol M, et al: Successful treatment of Colombian cutaneous leishmaniasis with four injections of pentamidine. Am J Trop Med Hyg 1994;50:107–111.
26. Hellier I, Dereure O, Tournillac I, et al: Treatment of Old World cutaneous leishmaniasis by pentamidine isethionate. An open study of 11 patients. Dermatology 2000;200:120–123.
27. Soto J, Grogl M, Berman J, et al: Limited efficacy of injectable aminosidine as single-agent therapy for Colombian cutaneous leishmaniasis. Trans R Soc Trop Med Hyg 1994;88:695–698.
28. Hepburn NC, Tidman MJ, Hunter JAA: Aminosidine [paromomycin] versus sodium stibogluconate for the treatment of American cutaneous leishmaniasis. Trans R Soc Trop Med Hyg 1994;88:700–703.
29. Navin TR, Arana BA, Arana FE, et al: Placebo-controlled clinical trial of sodium stibogluconate (Pentostam) versus ketoconazole for treating cutaneous leishmaniasis in Guatemala. J Infect Dis 1992;165:528–534.
30. Weinrauch L, Livshin R, el-On J: Ketoconazole in cutaneous leishmaniasis. Br J Dermatol 1987;117:666–668.
31. Singh S, Singh R, Sundar S: Failure of ketoconazole treatment in cutaneous leishmaniasis. Int J Dermatol 1995;34:120–121.
32. Dogra J, Aneja N, Lal BB, et al: Cutaneous leishmaniasis in India: Clinical experience with itraconazole (R51 211 Janssen). Ind J Dermatol 1990;29:661–662.
33. Van den Enden E, Van Gompel A, Stevens A, et al: Treatment of cutaneous leishmaniasis with oral itraconazole. Int J Dermatol 1994;33:285–286.
34. Akuffo H, Dietz M, Teklemariam S, et al: The use of itraconazole in the treatment of leishmaniasis caused by *Leishmania aethiopica*. Trans R Soc Trop Med Hyg 1990;84:532–534.
35. Ghanem BM, el-Shazly AM, Fawzy M, et al: Allopurinol in the treatment of zoonotic cutaneous leishmaniasis. J Egypt Soc Parasitol 1996;26:619–628.
36. Velez I, Agudelo S, Hendrickx E, et al: Inefficacy of allopurinol as monotherapy for Colombian cutaneous leishmaniasis. A randomized, controlled trial. Ann Intern Med 1997;126:232–236.
37. Martinez S, Gonzalez M, Vernaza ME: Treatment of cutaneous leishmaniasis with allopurinol and stibogluconate. Clin Infect Dis 1997;24:165–169.
38. Momeni AZ, Aminjavaheri M: Treatment of recurrent cutaneous leishmaniasis. Int J Dermatol 1995;34:129–133.
39. Falcoff E, Taranto NJ, Remondegui CE, et al: Clinical healing of antimony-resistant cutaneous or mucocutaneous leishmaniasis following the combined administration of interferon-gamma and pentavalent antimonial compounds. Trans R Soc Trop Med Hyg 1994;88:95–97.
40. Arana BA, Navin TR, Arana FE, et al: Efficacy of a short course (10 days) of high-dose meglumine antimonate with or without interferon-gamma in treating cutaneous leishmaniasis in Guatemala. Clin Infect Dis 1994;18:381–384.

41. Sharquie KE, Al-Talib KK, Chu AC: Intralesional therapy of cutaneous leishmaniasis with sodium stibogluconate antimony. Br J Dermatol 1988;119:53–57.

42. Bryceson ADM, Murphy A, Moody AH: Treatment of "Old World" cutaneous leishmaniasis with aminosidine ointment: Results of an open study in London. Trans R Soc Trop Med Hyg 1994;88:226–228.

43. Weinrauch L, Cawich F, Craig P, et al: Topical treatment of New World cutaneous leishmaniasis in Belize: A clinical study. J Am Acad Dermatol 1993;29:443–446.

44. Soto J, Fuva P, Herrera R, et al: Topical paromomycin/methylbenzethonium chloride plus parenteral meglumine antimonate as treatment for American cutaneous leishmaniasis: Controlled study. Clin Infect Dis 1998;26(1):56–58.

45. López-Jaramillo R, Ruano C, Rivera J, et al: Treatment of cutaneous leishmaniasis with nitric-oxide donor. Lancet 1998;351:1176–1177.

46. Teklemariam S, Hiwot AG, Frommel D, et al: Aminosidine and its combination with sodium stibogluconate is the treatment of diffuse cutaneous leishmaniasis caused by *Leishmania aethiopica*. Trans R Soc Trop Med Hyg 1994;88:334–339.

47. Salaiza-Suazo N, Volkow P, Tamayo R, et al: Treatment of two patients with diffuse cutaneous leishmaniasis caused by *Leishmania mexicana* modifies the immunohistological profile but not the disease outcome. Trop Med Int Health 1999;4:801–811.

48. Franke ED, Wignall FS, Cruz ME, et al: Efficacy and toxicity of sodium stibogluconate for mucosal leishmaniasis. Ann Intern Med 1990;113(12):934–940.

49. Llanos-Cuentas A, Echevarria J, Cruz M, et al: Efficacy of sodium stibogluconate alone and in combination with allopurinol for treatment of mucocutaneous leishmaniasis. Clin Infect Dis 1997;25:677–684.

50. Sampaio RNR, Marsden PD: [Treatment of the mucosal form of leishmaniasis without response to glucantime, with liposomal amphotericin B]. Rev Soc Bras Med Trop 1997;30:125–128. Portuguese.

51. Jha TK, Olliaro P, Thakur CP, et al: Randomised controlled trial of aminosidine (paromomycin) v sodium stibogluconate for treating visceral leishmaniasis in North Bihar, India. BMJ 1998;316:1200–1205.

52. Thakur CP, Sinha GP, Pandey AK, et al: Do the diminishing efficacy and increasing toxicity of sodium stiboluconate in the treatment of visceral leishmaniasis in Bihar, India, justify its continued use as a first-line drug? An observational study of 80 cases. Ann Trop Med Parasitol 1998;92:561–569.

53. Sundar S, More DK, Singh MK, et al: Failure of pentavalent antimony in visceral leishmaniasis in India: Report from the Center of the Indian Epidemic. Clin Infect Dis 2000;31:1104–1107.

54. Thakur CP, Kumar M, Kumar P, et al: Rationalisation of regimens of treatment of kala-azar with sodium stibogluconate in India: A randomised study. BMJ (Clin Res Ed) 1988;296:1557–1561.

55. Mishra M, Biswas UK, Jha AM, et al: Amphotericin versus sodium stibogluconate in first-line treatment of Indian kala-azar. Lancet 1994;344:1599–1600.

56. Mishra M, Biswas UK, Jha DN, et al: Amphotericin versus pentamidine in antimony-unresponsive kala-azar. Lancet 1992;340:1256–1257.

57. Thakur CP, Sinha GP, Pandey AK, et al: Daily versus alternate-day regimen of amphotericin B in the treatment of kala-azar: A randomized comparison. Bull World Health Organ 1994;72:931–936.

58. Jha TK, Giri YN, Singh TK, et al: Use of amphotericin B in drug-resistant cases of visceral leishmaniasis in north Bihar, India. Am J Trop Med Hyg 1995;52:536–538.

59. Berman JD: U.S. Food and Drug Administration approval of AmBisome (liposomal amphotericin B) for treatment of visceral leishmaniasis [Editorial response]. Clin Infect Dis 1999;28:49–51.

60. Sundar S, Agrawal NK, Sinha PR, et al: Short-course, low-dose amphotericin B lipid complex therapy for visceral leishmaniasis unresponsive to antimony. Ann Intern Med 1997;127:133–137.

61. Thakur CP, Kumar M, Pandey AK: Comparison of regimens of treatment of antimony-resistant kala-azar patients: A randomized study. Am J Trop Med Hyg 1991;45:435–441.

62. Jha SN, Singh NK, Jha TK, et al: Changing response to diamidine compounds in cases of kala-azar unresponsive to antimonial. J Assoc Physicians India 1991;39:314–316.

63. Thakur CP, Olliaro P, Gothoskar S, et al: Treatment of visceral leishmaniasis (kala-azar) with aminosidine (paromomycin)-antimonial combinations: A pilot study in Bihar, India. Trans R Soc Trop Med Hyg 1992;86:615–616.

64. Seaman J, Pryce D, Sondorp HE, et al: Epidemic visceral leishmaniasis in Sudan: A randomized trial of aminosidine plus sodium stibogluconate versus sodium stibogluconate alone. J Infect Dis 1993;168:715–720.

65. Rashid JR, Wasunna KM, Gachihi GS, et al: The efficacy and safety of ketoconazole in visceral leishmaniasis. East Afr Med J 1994;71:392–395.

66. Wali JP, Aggarwal P, Gupta U, et al: Ketoconazole in the treatment of visceral leishmaniasis [letter]. Lancet 1990;336:810–811.

67. Wali JP, Aggarwal P, Gupta U, et al: Ketoconazole in the treatment of antimony- and pentamidine-resistant kala-azar [letter]. J Infect Dis 1992;166:215–216.

68. Sundar S, Kumar P, Singh VP, et al: Ketoconazole in visceral leishmaniasis [letter]. Lancet 1990;336:1582–1583.

69. Sundar S, Singh VP, Agrawal NK, et al: Treatment of kala-azar with oral fluconazole [letter]. Lancet 1996;348:614.

70. Llorente S, Gimeno L, Navarro MJ, et al: Therapy of visceral leishmaniasis in renal transplant recipients intolerant to pentavalent antimonials. Transplantation 2000;70:800–801.

71. Hueso M, Bover J, Seron D, et al: The renal transplant patient with visceral leishmaniasis who could not tolerate meglumine antimoniate: Cure with ketoconazole and allopurinol. Nephrol Dial Transplant 1999;14:2941–2943.

72. Torrus D, Boix V, Massa B, et al: Fluconazole plus allopurinol in treatment of visceral leishmaniasis. J Antimicrob Chemother 1996;37:1042–1043.

73. Laguna F, López-Vélez R, Soriano V, et al: Assessment of allopurinol plus meglumine antimoniate in the treatment of visceral leishmaniasis in patients infected with HIV. J Infect 1994;28:255–259.

74. Singh NK, Jha TK, Singh IJ, et al: Combination therapy in kala-azar. J Assoc Physicians India 1995;43:319–320.

75. Sundar S, Murray HW: Effect of treatment with Interferon-γ alone in visceral leishmaniasis. J Infect Dis 1995;172:1627–1629.

76. Badaro R, Johnson W: The role of interferon-γ in the treatment of visceral and diffuse cutaneous leishmaniasis. J Infect Dis 1993;167(Suppl 1):13–17.

77. Sundar S, Rosenkaimer F, Murray HW: Successful treatment of refractory visceral leishmaniasis in India using antimony plus interferon-γ. J Infect Dis 1994;170:659–662.

78. Sundar S, Singh VP, Sharma S, et al: Response to Interferon-γ plus pentavalent antimony in Indian visceral leishmaniasis. J Infect Dis 1997;176:1117–1119.

79. Sundar S, Rosenkaimer F, Lesser M, et al: Immuno-chemotherapy for a systemic intracellular infection: Accelerated response using interferon-γ in visceral leishmaniasis in India. J Infect Dis 1995;171:992–996.

80. Squires KE, Rosenkaimer F, Sherwood JA, et al: Immunochemotherapy for visceral leishmaniasis: A controlled pilot trial of antimony vs. antimony plus Interferon-γ. Am J Trop Med Hyg 1993;48:666–669.

81. Thakur CP, Kumar K: Efficacy of prolonged therapy with stibogluconate in post kala-azar dermal leishmaniasis. Indian J Med Res 1990;91:144–148.

82. Laguna F, López-Vélez R, Pulido F, et al: Treatment of visceral leishmaniasis in HIV-infected patients: A randomized trial comparing meglumine antimoniate with amphotericin B. Spanish HIV-Leishmania Study Group. AIDS 1999;13:1063–1069.

83. Boletis JN, Pefanis A, Stathakis C, et al: Visceral leishmaniasis in renal transplant recipients: Successful treatment with liposomal amphotericin B (AmBisome). Clin Infect Dis 1999;28:1308–1309.

84. Leiguarda R, Roncoroni A, Taratuto AL, et al: Acute CNS infection by Trypanosoma cruzi (Chagas' disease) in immunosuppressed patients. Neurology 1990;40:850–851.

85. Pizzi TP, De Croizet VA, Smok G, et al: [Chagas' disease in a patient with renal transplantation and immunosuppressive treatment]. Rev Med Chile 1982;110:1207–1211. Spanish.

86. Libow LF, Beltrani VP, Silvers DN, et al: Post-cardiac transplant reactivation of Chagas' disease diagnosed by skin biopsy. Cutis 1991;48:37–40.

87. Bocchi EA, Bellotti G, Uip D, et al: Long-term follow-up after heart transplantation in Chagas' disease. Transplant Proc 1993;25(1 pt2):1329–1330.

88. Bocchi EA, Bellotti G, Mocelin AO, et al: Heart transplantation for chronic Chagas' heart disease. Ann Thorac Surg 1996;61:1727–1733.

89. de Carvalho VB, Sousa EF, Vila JH, et al: Heart transplantation in Chagas' disease. 10 years after the initial experience. Circulation 1996;94:1815–1817.

90. Cohen JE, Tsai EC, Ginsberg HJ, et al: Pseudotumoral chagasic meningoencephalitis as the first manifestation of acquired immunodeficiency syndrome. Surg Neurol 1998;49:324–327.

91. Sartori AM, Shikanai-Yasuda MA, Amato Neto V, et al: Follow-up of 18 patients with human immunodeficiency virus infection and chronic Chagas' disease, with reactivation of Chagas' disease causing cardiac disease in three patients. Clin Infect Dis 1998;26:177–179.

92. Cunha-Neto E, Coelho V, Guilherme L, et al: Autoimmunity in Chagas' disease. Identification of cardiac myosin-B13 Trypanosoma cruzi protein crossreactive T cell clones in heart lesions of a chronic Chagas' cardiomyopathy patient. J Clin Invest 1996;98:1709–1712.

93. Gruppi A, Gea S, Moretti E, et al: Human antibodies against T. cruzi exoantigens recognizing parasite surface antigens and heart tissue components. Int Arch Allergy Appl Immunol 1989;90:119–123.

94. Tarleton RL, Zhang L: Chagas disease etiology: Autoimmunity or parasite persistence? Parasitol Today 1999;15:94–99.

95. Bellotti G, Bocchi EA, de Moraes AV, et al: In vivo detection of Trypanosoma cruzi antigens in hearts of patients with chronic Chagas' heart disease. Am Heart J 1996;131:301–307.

96. Levi GC, Lobo IM, Kallas EG, et al: Etiological drug treatment of human infection by Trypanosoma cruzi. Rev Inst Med Trop São Paulo 1996;38:35–38.

97. Coura JR: [Current prospects of specific treatment of Chagas' disease]. Bol Chil Parasitol 1996;51:69–75. Spanish.

98. Toledo MJ, Guilherme AL, Silva JC: Trypanosoma cruzi: Chemotherapy with benznidazole in mice inoculated with strains from Paraná state and from different endemic areas of Brazil. Rev Inst Med Trop São Paulo 1997;39:283–290.

99. Brener Z, Cançado JR, Galvão LM, et al: An experimental and clinical assay with ketoconazole in the treatment of Chagas disease. Mem Inst Oswaldo Cruz 1993;88:149–153.

100. Moreira AA, De Souza HB, Amato Neto V, et al: [Evaluation of the therapeutic activity of itraconazole in chronic infection, experimental and human, by Trypanosoma cruzi]. Rev Inst Med Trop São Paulo 1992;34:177–180. Portuguese.

101. Apt W, Aguilera X, Arribada A, et al: Treatment of chronic Chagas' disease with itraconazole and allopurinol. Am J Trop Med Hyg 1998;59:133–138.

102. Gallerano RH, Marr JJ, Sosa RR: Therapeutic efficacy of allopurinol in patients with chronic Chagas' disease. Am J Trop Med Hyg 1990;43:159–166.

103. Lauria-Pires L, de Castro CN, Emanuel A, et al: [Ineffectiveness of allopurinol in patients in the acute phase of Chagas disease]. Rev Soc Bras Med Trop 1988;21:79.

104. Grant IH, Gold JW, Wittner M, et al: Transfusion-associated acute Chagas disease acquired in the United States. Ann Intern Med 1989;111:849–851.

105. Cançado JR: Criteria of Chagas disease cure. Mem Inst Oswaldo Cruz 1999;94(Suppl 1):331–335.

106. Teixeira A, Tinoco D, Maneta L, et al: "Os perfis parasitológico, imunológico e eletrocardiográfico de chagásicos crônicos tratados com nitroarenos são indistinguíveis daqueles observados nos chagásicos não tratados". In [6th Annual Meeting on Applied Research in Chagas' Disease. Uberaba, 2–4 November 1989. Program and abstracts]. Rev Soc Bras Med Trop. 1989;22(Suppl 2):1–144. Portuguese.

107. Silveira CA, Castillo E, Castro C: [Evaluation of a specific treatment for Trypanosoma cruzi in children, in the evolution of the indeterminate phase]. Rev Soc Bras Med Trop 2000;33:191–196. Portuguese.

108. Braga MS, Lauria-Pires L, Argañaraz ER, et al: Persistent infections in chronic Chagas' disease patients treated with anti-Trypanosoma cruzi nitroderivatives. Rev Inst Med Trop São Paulo 2000;42:157–161.

109. Andrade AL, Zicker F, Oliveira RM, et al: Randomised trial of efficacy of benznidazole in treatment of early Trypanosoma cruzi infection. Lancet 1996;348:1407–1413.

110. Viotti R, Vigliano C, Armenti H, et al: Treatment of chronic Chagas' disease with benznidazole: Clinical and serologic evolution of patients with long-term follow-up. Am Heart J 1994;127:151–162.

111. Blanche C, Aleksic I, Johanna J, et al: Heart transplantation for Chagas' disease cardiomyopathy. Ann Thorac Surg 1995;60:1406–1408.

112. [Guidelines for the prevention of opportunistic infections in persons with HIV or AIDS in Latin America and the Caribbean. USPHS/IDSA]. Bol Oficina Sanit Panam 1996;121:377–415. Spanish.

113. Ferreira MS, Nishioka SA, Silvestre MTA, et al: Reactivation of Chagas' disease in patients with AIDS: Report of three new cases and review of the literature. Clin Infect Dis 1997;25:1397–1400.

114. Rassi A, Amato Neto V, Siqueira AF, et al: [The influence of corticoids, in chronic Chagas disease, administered in virtue of associated disorders]. Rev Soc Bras Med Trop 1997;30:93–99. Portuguese.

115. Tresoldi AT, Belangero VMS, Silva PEMR, et al: [Congenital Chagas disease: Reactivation by corticosteroid therapy]. Pediatria (São Paulo) 1984;6:207–210. Portuguese.

116. Rassi A, Amato Neto VA, Siqueira AF, et al: [Nifurtimox as a prophylactic drug to prevent reactivation in chronic chagasic patients treated with corticoids for associated diseases]. Rev Soc Bras Med Trop 1998;31:249–255. Portuguese.

117. Rassi A, Amato Neto VA, Siqueira AF, et al: [Protective effect of benznidazole against parasite reactivation in patients chronically infected with Trypanosoma cruzi and treated with corticoids for associated diseases]. Rev Soc Bras Med Trop 1999;32:475–482. Portuguese.

118. World Health Organization: Comunicable disease surveillance and response (CSR) web site *http://www.who.int/emc*.

119. Bryan RT, Waskin HA, Richards FO, et al: African trypanosomiasis in American travelers: A 20 years review. In Steffen R, Lobel HO, Haworth J, Bradley DJ (eds): Travel Medicine. Berlin, Springer-Verlag, 1989.

120. Panosian CB, Cohen L, Bruckner D, et al: Fever, leukopenia, and a cutaneous lesion in a man who had recently traveled in Africa. Rev Infect Dis 1991;13:1131–1138.

121. Kirchhoff LV: Use of a PCR assay for diagnosing African trypanosomiasis of the CNS: A case report. Cent Afr J Med 1998;44:134–136.

122. Dedet JP, Pratlong F: *Leishmania, Trypanosoma* and monoxenous trypanosomatids as emerging opportunistic agents. J Eukaryot Microbiol 2000;47:37–39.

123. Miezan TW, Meda HA, Doua F, et al: Assessment of central nervous system involvement in *gambiense* trypanosomiasis: Value of the cerebrospinal white cell count. Trop Med Int Health 1998;3:571–575.

124. Control and Surveillance of African Trypanosomiasis: Report of a WHO Expert Committee, Geneva, World Health Organization, 1998 (WHO Technical Report Series, no. 881).

125. Pepin J, Milord F: The treatment of human African trypanosomiasis. Adv Parasitol 1994;33:1–47.

126. Neujean G: "Contribution à l'études des liquids rachidiens et céphaliques dans la maladie du sommeil à *Trypanosoma gambiense*". Annales de la Sociéte Belge de Médecine Tropicale 1950;30:1125–1387. French.

127. Neujean G, Evens F: "Diagnostic et traitement de la maladie du sommeil à T. gambiense." Bilan de dix ans d'activité du centre de traitement de Léopoldville, in-80, Tome VII, Fascicule 2. Académie Royale des Sciences Coloniales: Classe des Sciences Naturelles et Médicales. Mémoires, 1958. French.

128. Iten M, Mett H, Evans A, et al: Alterations in ornithine decarboxylase characteristics account for tolerance of *Trypanosoma brucei rhodesiense* to D,L-alpha-difluoromethylornithine. Antimicrob Agents Chemother 1997;41:1922–1925.

129. Milord F, Pepin J, Loko L, et al: Efficacy and toxicity of eflornithine for treatment of *Trypanosoma brucei gambiense* sleeping sickness. Lancet 1992;340:652–655.

130. Doua F, Miezan TW, Sanon Singaro JR, et al: The efficacy of pentamidine in the treatment of early-late *Trypanosoma brucei gambiense* trypanosomiasis. Am J Trop Med Hyg 1996;55:586–588.

131. Pepin J, Milord F, Khonde AN, et al: Risk factors for encephalopathy and mortality during melarsoprol treatment of *Trypanosoma brucei gambiense* sleeping sickness. Trans R Soc Trop Med Hyg 1995;89:92–97.

Malaria and Babesiosis

JAIME R. TORRES, MD, MPH, TM

MALARIA

Malaria is without question the most significant parasitic disease worldwide, accounting for an estimated 300 to 500 million cases of infection and at least 1.5 to 2.7 million deaths annually.[1,2] A steady parallel rise in the magnitude of international travel to and immigration from malaria-endemic areas and in the incidence of drug resistance has been noticed over the last two decades. Therefore an increasing number of travelers are exposed to drug-resistant malaria. Currently 10,000 to 30,000 travelers from industrialized countries are expected to contract malaria each year. Periodically updated information on the local geographic risk of malaria is available from the World Health Organization (WHO).[1,2]

Although four species of the genus *Plasmodium*—*P. falciparum, P. vivax, P. malariae,* and *P. ovale*—can naturally infect humans, most new malaria infections around the world are accounted for by *P. falciparum* and *P. vivax*.[3] Unlike *P. falciparum* malaria, *P. vivax* infection is rarely fatal but may cause debilitating relapsing episodes of a relatively severe illness.

Although successful treatment of patients with malaria depends primarily on effective antimalarial drugs, it also depends on a full complement of supportive strategies as diverse as the maintenance of appropriate blood glucose levels and the use of dialysis. Other crucial issues of the treatment include the proper management of several common complications of severe malaria, such as seizures, pulmonary edema, renal failure, and lactic acidosis.[4]

In general, currently used antimalarials may be classified into any of four wide classes:

1. Quinoline-derived compounds: chloroquine, quinine, quinidine, mefloquine, halofantrine, and primaquine
2. Antifolates: pyrimethamine and proguanil
3. Artemisinin derivatives: artemether, artesunate, and arteether
4. Antimicrobials: sulfonamides, dapsone, clindamycin, tetracyclines, and azithromycin

Drug-resistant *P. falciparum* malaria continues to spread and at present involves almost all areas of transmission worldwide. High levels of resistance to mefloquine and halofantrine have been documented in Southeast Asia, where sensitivity to quinine is also decreasing. On the other hand, strains of *P. vivax* resistant or tolerant to chloroquine and primaquine are well established in Oceania and seem to be spreading to new geographic areas, such as Guyana, Brazil, and parts of Asia. Since infection by *P. falciparum* usually kills people lacking effective acquired immunity or having no access to appropriate chemotherapy, the argument for prescribing chemoprophylaxis to exposed travelers to lessen both morbidity and mortality is most persuasive. Indeed chemoprophylaxis has effected a 10-fold reduction in the risk of malaria for nonimmune travelers visiting hyper-endemic areas of Africa.[5]

Imported malaria-associated deaths are largely preventable. Most cases occur because the traveler fails to use or fails to comply with appropriate chemoprophylactic regimens, because physicians or laboratories misdiagnose the disease, or because the chosen prophylactic regimen was unsuitable.[6-9] The overall case-fatality rate associated with imported *P. falciparum* malaria in recent series has ranged from 0.6% to 3.8%. Yet such rates may be as high as 20% among elderly patients or those who have severe malaria, even when treatment is administered in modern intensive care units.[9]

Chemotherapy and chemoprophylaxis for malaria are complicated by the fact that in the human host, plasmodia go through various distinct stages, and each exhibits unique susceptibilities to antimalarial agents.[3,5,10] For instance, chloroquine is active against asexual blood stages but has no apparent effect on sexual blood stages or asexual liver stages. Similarly, primaquine kills liver stages, has relatively little effect on asexual blood stages, but sterilizes sexual blood forms.

For the purpose of chemotherapy and chemoprophylaxis, human malaria may be divided into two functional groups of clinical relevance: relapsing (*P. vivax* and *P. ovale*) and nonrelapsing (*P. falciparum* and *P. malariae*).[3,5,10] The term *relapse* represents passage from latent to patent infection or disease and refers to the seeding of the bloodstream with proliferative merozoites by secondary tissue schizonts, the so called hypnozoites, arising from quiescent liver forms weeks, months, or years after natural exposure to sporozoites. The prepatent period of malaria, that is, the interval between inoculation of sporozoites and the appearance of trophozoites in the bloodstream of nonimmune patients, is usually 9 to 14 days for *P. falciparum*, *P. vivax*, and *P. ovale*, and for *P. malariae*, it is 15 to 16 days. Among nonimmune persons the usual interval between detectable parasitemia and onset of illness may be as short as a couple of days (up to 10 days for *P. malariae*). In patients with naturally acquired immunity the interval between patent parasitemia and clinical illness is indefinite. The incubation period refers to the interval between inoculation and the onset of clinical illness. Inadequate (regimen or resistance) chemoprophylaxis may prolong this incubation period, especially when long acting drugs such as mefloquine are used. Likewise the use of chemoprophylaxis for *P. vivax* usually prevents the clinical illness through suppression of parasitemia; however, clinical relapses may still occur, especially when a full course of primaquine has not been given after the patient has left the endemic area.[10]

The choice of malaria chemotherapy ultimately will be based on the infecting species, the severity of illness, the patient's age, the degree or lack of background immunity, the likely pattern of susceptibility to antimalarials, and the cost and availability of such drugs. Therefore recommendations vary according to geographic region and should be under constant reappraisal.[4,5,10]

Mechanisms of Drug Action against Plasmodia

The antiparasitic effect of aminoquinolines (chloroquine, quinine, quinidine, amodiaquine, and probably mefloquine) and halofantrine is related to their capacity to inhibit the proteolysis of hemoglobin in the parasite's food vacuole.[10,11] In its soluble form, ferriprotoporphyrin IX, a byproduct of the proteolysis of hemoglobin, may induce lyses of membranes and inhibits a variety of parasitic enzymes. It is potentially toxic to the parasite, as it neutralizes into an insoluble, nontoxic crystalline material (malarial pigment) by the activity of a heme polymerase. Aminoquinolines may inhibit both the heme polymerase[12] and the aspartic and cysteine proteases that degrade hemoglobin and alkalinize the plasmodial food vacuole or secondary lysosome.[13] Artemisinin and its derivatives seem instead to act by binding to the iron in the malarial pigment, yielding free radicals that ultimately will damage parasite proteins in the vicinity of the plasmodial food vacuole.[14,15]

Mechanisms of Drug Resistance in Plasmodia

Laboratory studies suggest a single mechanism of chloroquine resistance: an energy-dependent chloroquine efflux pump, which reduces chloroquine accumulation.[16] Although the genetic basis of chloroquine resistance in *P. falciparum* appears to be a 300-kD protein on chromosome 7,[17] chloroquine resistance is not genetically linked to either of the two multidrug resistance–like genes described in the same species.[18] In vivo the response to chloroquine treatment is graded on the basis of whether standard doses of chloroquine produce a cure (S = susceptible), an initial clearance of the parasitemia followed by recrudescence within 28 days (RI = low-level resistance), an initial decrease of the parasitemia without parasite clearance (RII = intermediate-level resistance), or no impact (either no decrease or an increase) of the parasitemia (RIII = high-level resistance).

Unlike chloroquine resistance, resistance to mefloquine and halofantrine has been associated with amplification of multidrug resistance–like genes but not with a drug efflux process. On the other hand, resistance to antifolates is based primarily on specific point mutations at the active site of the parasite dihydrofolate reductase thymidylate synthase, which would interfere with drug binding to the enzyme.[19-21] There are no known artemisinin-resistant plasmodia.

Neither the nature nor the genetic basis of chloroquine resistance in *P. vivax* has been defined, and it is not clear whether chloroquine-resistant *P. vivax* also has an energy-dependent efflux pump or a different mechanism of chloroquine resistance.

Prevention of Malaria in Travelers

Several issues need to be carefully considered before one decides on the most appropriate alternative to use in preventing travel-associated malaria.[4,5,10] Travelers need to be well aware of the risk of malaria, understand how serious an infection it can be, know how to help prevent it, and realize the importance of seeking prompt medical attention should they develop fever during or after the journey. A travel schedule and any specific potential risk behaviors should be fully discussed in advance with the traveler. Destination may be the most important risk factor to consider, since the chance of acquiring malaria depends on the geographic area visited (sub-Saharan Africa, especially West and East Africa, is considered a particularly risky destination).[5,10] Even within the same geographic area the risk is higher in rural settings and camping accommodations than in urban areas and well-screened or air-conditioned facilities. Other factors associated with an increased risk of malaria are long stays, travel during the local high-transmission season, and visits to areas below 2000 meters above sea level.[4,5,10]

Since naturally acquired malaria requires exposure to infective anophelines, travelers at risk should be encouraged to adopt any measures aimed at reducing exposure to the evening and nighttime feeding female *Anopheles* mosquito. These include use of insecticide-impregnated bed nets (permethrin or deltamethrin treated) unless sleeping quarters are well screened or otherwise completely enclosed and air-conditioned. Treated nets have proven significantly effective in preventing malaria and are safe for children and pregnant women.[22] Nets should be re-treated with permethrin (300 to 500 mg/m^2) or a similar residual insecticide every 6 months to maintain effectiveness.[22]

In addition the use of insect repellent on exposed skin should be strongly encouraged. Insect repellents containing *N,N* diethylmethyltoluamide (DEET) are the most effective. The concentration of DEET in products usually varies from 35% to 95%. Higher concentrations protect for longer periods. Insect repellents with higher percentages of DEET carry a small risk of neurotoxicity (seizures or encephalopathy), particularly if they are used repeatedly on young children. Consequently only preparations with a DEET concentration lower than 35% must be used in children, and the product should always be applied sparingly, only to exposed surfaces, and washed off soon after coming indoors.[22]

Chemoprophylaxis

Given the high global prevalence of malaria and the serious threat it poses to many travelers, malaria prophylaxis is clearly a relevant medical topic. Unfortunately, aspects of malaria prevention are often complicated by the diverse strains of the parasite and the numerous chemoprophylactic agents available. In addition some travelers fail to take nonmedical precautions against malaria.

Several factors need to be assessed when one is selecting an appropriate chemoprophylactic regimen against malaria. The travel itinerary should be reviewed in detail to determine the likelihood that the traveler will be at risk of acquiring malaria. The specific activities (e.g., rural travel, night-time exposure, unscreened accommodations) of the person while he or she is in the endemic area should be considered in estimating the risk of contracting malaria. It is important to establish whether the traveler will be in a drug-resistant *P. falciparum* area and if symptoms of malaria were to occur, whether prompt access to medical care will be possible. It is also important to take into consideration the health of the person (e.g., age, pregnancy, asplenia, use of other medications, immunocompromise, chronic illness, contraindications to the use of a particular antimalarial drug) in determining the risk of severe disease if malaria were to occur and in the selection of an appropriate antimalarial drug for chemoprophylaxis.[5,10,23–28]

Travelers to the following regions should consider the use of chemoprophylactic drugs to reduce the risk of contracting clinical malaria: urban and rural areas of sub-Saharan Africa (except most of South Africa), Oceania (including Papua New Guinea, West Irian, Vanuatu), Nepal (Terai region), India, Bangladesh, Pakistan, and Haiti; evening or overnight exposure in rural, nonresort areas of Southeast Asia, Central and South America, and certain parts of Mexico. Travelers to tourist destinations and most urban areas of Southeast Asia, as well as South and Central America, often require no chemosuppressive drugs.[5,10]

It must be stressed that although antimalarials can markedly decrease the risk that symptomatic malaria will develop, none of these agents can guarantee complete protection against malaria.

Chemoprophylaxis for P. vivax

When only *P. vivax* is a concern, the recommended malarial chemoprophylactic regimen consists of the classic combination of a 4-aminoquinoline, chloroquine phosphate, which interrupts the erythrocytic or blood-feeding phase of the parasite's life cycle (suppressive prophylaxis) but has no effect on the hepatic phase, plus primaquine, an 8-aminoquinoline active against the tissue (liver) stages of malaria. The latter can eliminate *P. vivax* infections that might be developing in the liver (causal prophylaxis).[9,10,23,24]

Chloroquine phosphate salt (Aralen) comes as 250 mg tablets (equivalent to 150 mg chloroquine base). The prophylactic dose for adults is 300 mg base (500 mg salt) weekly, taken with a meal at the same time and on the same day each week. The weekly dose for children is 5 mg/kg. Because of the bitter taste of chloroquine, pediatric dosing is difficult. Liquid suspensions of chloroquine for children are no longer available; therefore a tablet has to be divided to provide the appropriate dose. When administered to children, chloroquine should be crushed and dissolved in a strong-flavored (sweet) drink or mixed with food to disguise the taste. Childproof containers are useful because an accidental dose of chloroquine would be extremely toxic and has provoked severe hypotension and fatal arrhythmias in small children.[10]

The same 300 mg base (500 mg salt) dose of chloroquine per week must be administered for 4 weeks after the traveler returns home. As chloroquine given alone will suppress but not cure an infection with *P. vivax*, illness may still ensue weeks or months after the traveler has returned home.[9,10,23,26]

Side effects of chloroquine include mild nausea, generalized itching, blurred vision, partial alopecia, headache, and psoriasis flare-ups. In addition generalized itching may occur in dark-skinned people. There have been rare reports of nail and mucous membrane discoloration, nerve deafness, photophobia, myopathy, blood dyscrasias, psychosis, and seizures. In dosages higher than 500 mg per week, chloroquine has been associated with retinal degenerative disorders; consequently its use in persons with such disorders is discouraged. In the usual prophylactic dosage the drug is not harmful to the retina. Unusual reactions to chloroquine include agranulocytosis, photosensitivity, and neuropsychiatric alterations.[23,24]

In travelers at risk for the relapsing type of malaria (*P. vivax* or *P. ovale*) a regimen of primaquine 15 mg base (26.3 mg salt) per day for 14 days in adults, or 0.3 mg/kg base (0.5 mg/kg salt) per day for 14 days in children, should be administered to eradicate any surviving latent tissue stage (terminal prophylaxis).[10,23]

Because of the lack of precise information about the relative prevalence of chloroquine-resistant strains of *P. vivax* in those still limited geographic regions where chloroquine-resistance has been reported, chemoprophylaxis recommendations for travel to those areas remain unchanged.[23–28]

In some European countries, hydroxychloroquine sulfate (Plaquenil), a synthetic 4-aminoquinoline derivative commercially available as tablets containing 200 mg of hydroxychloroquine sulfate (equivalent to 155 mg of base), is used as an alternative to Aralen. Peak plasma levels of hydroxychloroquine sulfate are reached within 1 to 3 hours. About 50% of the drug is excreted unmodified in the urine. For chemoprophylaxis of malaria, Plaquenil is given at a dose of 400 mg (310 mg base) every 7 days. If therapy was not initiated 14 days before exposure, an initial loading dose of 800 mg (620 mg base) may be given in two divided doses 6 hours apart. In children a dose of 6.4 mg/kg (not to exceed the adult dose) every 7 days is recommended. If therapy was not initiated 14 days before exposure, an initial loading dose of 12.9 mg/kg may be given in two doses 6 hours apart.[29]

Chemoprophylaxis for *P. falciparum*

Because of the emergence of drug-resistant *P. falciparum* strains, chloroquine has become ineffective in most parts of the world. Indeed, chloroquine is, at present, only indicated for chemoprophylaxis in travelers to endemic areas of *P. falciparum* in the Middle East, Central America, Haiti, and the Dominican Republic. The recommended antimalarial schedule is similar to that described above for *P. vivax*, but terminal prophylaxis with primaquine is unnecessary as hypnozoites do not occur in this species of the parasite.

A practical approach to the selection of a proper chemoprophylactic regimen for travelers at risk of *P. falciparum* malaria is to base it on the knowledge of the drug-resistance patterns of the visited area (Table 34–1).

Chloroquine-Resistant Zones

When a person is traveling to known chloroquine-resistant *P. falciparum* endemic zones, a selection

TABLE 34–1 ■ Malaria Chemoprophylactic Regimens for Persons at Risk According to the Drug-Resistance Pattern Prevalent in the Visited Area

Drug-resistance pattern*	Recommendation	Alternatives
Chloroquine-sensitive	Chloroquine phosphate Adults: 300 mg base weekly Children: 5 mg/kg weekly	Doxycycline
Chloroquine-resistant	Mefloquine Adults: 1 tablet weekly (228 mg base; 250 mg salt) Children <15 kg (33 lb): 5 mg/kg weekly Children 15–19 kg (33–42 lb): 1/4 tablet weekly Children 20–30 kg (44–66 lb): 1/2 tablet weekly Children 31–45 kg (68–99 lb): 3/4 tablet weekly Children >45 kg (99 lb): 1 tablet weekly	First choice: Doxycycline Second choice (less effective): Chloroquine plus proguanil Adults: 200 mg/d Proguanil Children <2 y: 50 mg/d Children 2–6 y: 100 mg/d Children 7–10 y: 150 mg/d Children >10 y: 200 mg/d
Chloroquine- and mefloquine-resistant	Doxycycline: 100 mg/d	

*All drugs are to be taken 1 week before entering malarial areas, continuing during the stay in malarial areas, and for 4 weeks after leaving malarial areas. Exceptions are doxycycline and proguanil, which may be started 1 day before entering malarial areas but must be continued for 4 weeks after departure.

between alternatives such as mefloquine, doxycycline, or to a lesser degree chloroquine plus proguanil will have to be made.

Mefloquine (Lariam), a quinolone methanol derivative, is at present considered the drug of choice for most travelers to these areas. Although mefloquine provides the best current protection against chloroquine-resistant *P. falciparum* malaria, mefloquine-resistant strains already exist in Cambodia and along Thailand's borders with Cambodia and Myanmar (formerly Burma).[30]

Mefloquine is available as 250 mg salt (228 mg base) tablets with a notch in the middle to facilitate pediatric dosing. It has an elimination half-life of 2 to 3 weeks.[31] The dosing schedule is similar to that for chloroquine, including an initial 1- to 2-week "piling up" period before departure, during which a 250 mg tablet once a week is taken, followed by 250 mg once a week during travel and for 4 weeks after returning home.[32,33]

In prophylactic doses, mefloquine usually is well tolerated, and only 1% to 6% of all users may have to discontinue prophylaxis because of adverse effects. Such rates are not significantly different from those seen with other common chemosuppressive regimens. Although approximately 25% to 40% of travelers do experience some side effects from mefloquine, nearly all of them remain mild and self-limited.[34,35] The minor side effects most frequently reported by users are nausea, odd dreams, dizziness, mood changes, insomnia, headache, and diarrhea.[34,35] Neuropsychological adverse events such as anxiety, depression, insomnia, nightmares, paranoid delusions, hallucinations, and even true psychoses, which require drug discontinuation, are reported in less than 1% of users on prophylactic doses. Therapeutic doses (25 mg/kg base) of mefloquine, however, are less well tolerated, and severe neuropsychiatric reactions are reported to occur 10 to 60 times more often than with prophylactic doses. Toxic metabolites of mefloquine do not accumulate, and its long-term use (>1 year) does not seem to be associated with additional adverse effects.[34]

Its effectiveness notwithstanding, mefloquine prophylaxis has some serious shortcomings. The drug is expensive, and there are relative contraindications to its use in pregnant women during the first trimester, in small children (weighing <15 kg), and in occupations that require fine coordination such as aircraft pilots (because the drug may decrease their spatial discrimination ability). In addition quininelike drugs (halofantrine and mefloquine) should not be used simultaneously.[2] Relative contraindications to the use of mefloquine may nevertheless be overcome when the risk of malaria far outweighs the risk of prophylaxis in persons traveling to highly endemic destinations such as Africa.

Since about 70% of neuropsychiatric adverse effects occur within the first three prophylactic doses and most of them disappear on cessation of therapy,[36] a longer trial of mefloquine before departure appears reasonable.[33]

Mefloquine should be used with caution in patients with a history of seizures, cardiac arrhythmias, or psychosis.[32] Therapy with beta blockers or calcium channel blockers is no longer considered a contraindication to the use of mefloquine unless the traveler has an underlying cardiac conduction problem or arrhythmia.[32]

In situations in which the traveler is at high immediate risk of drug-resistant *P. falciparum* malaria, consideration may be given to the use of a loading dose of mefloquine. For this purpose, once daily doses of mefloquine for 3 days are initiated before travel, followed by a once-weekly dose. Such a dose is a well-tolerated and effective way to rapidly achieve therapeutic blood levels of mefloquine (after 4 days, as compared to 7 to 9 weeks with standard weekly dosing).[36–38] Only about 1% to 2% of recipients of this loading dose discontinue mefloquine, and most of them do so during the first week. Loading doses permit an appraisal of drug tolerance before travel and allow a change to a suitable alternative if necessary.

For persons in whom mefloquine cannot be used, doxycycline is the preferred alternative. In travelers to sub-Saharan Africa, chloroquine plus proguanil can also be used. However, even though chloroquine plus proguanil is more effective than chloroquine alone, it is considerably less effective than doxycycline or mefloquine, providing only about 50% to 65% protective efficacy.[34,35,37,38]

Chloroquine- and Mefloquine-Resistant Zones

In chloroquine- and mefloquine-resistant zones, doxycycline (Vibramycin) alone is the chemosuppressive agent of choice. Doxycycline acts against both the pre-erythrocytic phase (occurring in the liver) and the erythrocytic phase of the *Plasmodium* life cycle through ribosomal inhibition. Doxycycline is an effective chemosuppressive agent against mefloquine-sensitive and mefloquine-resistant *P. falciparum* strains. A loading dose before exposure is not required. Thus doxycycline is the prophylactic drug of choice for short-notice travel. The drug is taken in a dosage of 100 mg/d during exposure and should be continued for 4 weeks after the traveler leaves the endemic area. Noncompliance is the major reason for doxycycline failures.[39,40]

Side effects of doxycycline therapy include photosensitivity (the use of hats and sunscreen preparations that block ultraviolet A rays is advised), nausea, esophagitis or esophageal ulceration, and *Candida* vaginitis. Although bothersome, most of these side effects can be minimized with care.

Doxycycline therapy is contraindicated in pregnant and breast-feeding women and in children less than 9 years old.[23]

Doxycycline should be swallowed while standing or sitting in an upright position, and it should be taken with food or a liberal amount of fluid to prevent the tablet from sticking in the esophagus. Both bismuth derivatives and antacids may interfere with the absorption of doxycycline and therefore should not be used simultaneously.[23,39,40] Although the long-term (>3 months) safety of doxycycline has not been established, historically, tetracycline derivatives have been used safely for many years.

Other Prophylactic Options

Primaquine

Primaquine, an 8-aminoquinolone, has long been used to prevent relapses of P. vivax and P. ovale infections (radical cure) and as a gametocidal agent to interrupt the transmission of P. falciparum in endemic areas. Primaquine is active against both the blood and the tissue stages of the parasite and prevents symptomatic or clinical infection. Because primaquine is active against the pre-erythrocytic stages of both P. vivax and P. falciparum, it may be a potential causal prophylactic, eliminating infections that are developing in the liver. Therefore, the need for long postexposure prophylaxis is eliminated, thus enhancing compliance.[41]

Although early studies established the potential of primaquine for prophylaxis, reports of severe adverse effects (methemoglobinemia and severe hemolytic reactions),[42–45] as well as the emergence of chloroquine as a widely used prophylactic agent, reduced its use for prophylactic purposes.

Primaquine appears to be a safe, well-tolerated, and apparently more effective prophylactic agent than either doxycycline or mefloquine. It is important to note, however, that the proportion of P. falciparum infection has been higher than that of other plasmodia among primaquine-failure cases. P. falciparum infection usually develops within 1 month after the traveler returns from the area of endemicity. Adult travelers exposed to malaria may use primaquine in a dosage of 30 mg base (26.3 mg salt) daily starting 1 day before entering a malaria-endemic area, continued while in the area, and for 1 week after departure. The pediatric dose is 0.3 mg/kg base (0.5 mg/kg salt) per day.

The need for a higher dose or a longer duration of treatment might be the reason for the failure of primaquine prophylaxis in some cases.[46,47] Travelers taking prophylactic primaquine should continue it for 48 to 72 hours after leaving the area of endemicity.[46,47]

Primaquine is usually well tolerated. Side effects are mainly gastrointestinal (nausea and abdominal pain) and can be reduced by taking the drug with food. Few of these side effects are severe enough to require withdrawal from treatment. The drug is contraindicated in glucose-6-phosphate dehydrogenase (G6PD)-deficient travelers, who may develop severe oxidant-induced hemolytic anemia with methemoglobinemia, and in pregnant women, but otherwise it is an effective and safe prophylactic drug.[46,47]

Prophylactic schedules based on primaquine appear to be effective in semi-immune children and nonimmune adults. At present, however, there is not enough evidence to recommend its use over other routinely used standard regimens in nonimmune travelers. Because primaquine is a prophylactic causal agent, the need for a 4-week radical cure or terminal chemoprophylaxis following exposure (a common reason for nonadherence with standard regimens) may be avoided. This could be particularly useful for travelers with short exposures (2 to 7 days) in high-risk areas.

Proguanil

Proguanil, or chloroguanide hydrochloride, is manufactured under the brand name of Paludrine. It inhibits the dihydrofolate reductase, thereby disrupting the ability of Plasmodium parasites to synthesize nucleic acids in the pre-erythrocytic phase. Proguanil, at a daily dose of 200 mg taken with food, has served as a less effective alternative to mefloquine in hyperendemic areas of Africa, but it must be taken in conjunction with the weekly chloroquine prophylactic regimen. The traveler should start taking proguanil several days before departure and continue taking the drug (in addition to the weekly chloroquine dose) for 4 weeks after returning home.[23,24]

Proguanil is usually well tolerated, although it may cause gastrointestinal distress and aphthous ulcers. Hematuria has been observed in rare cases. The dosage must be reduced in patients with renal insufficiency. The combined regimen of proguanil and chloroquine is safe for pregnant women and infants. If this regimen is used with folate supplementation, it is a reasonable prophylactic option for pregnant women who travel to Africa.[23,24]

Widespread resistance to proguanil limits its use to Africa. The proguanil-chloroquine regimen is significantly less effective than those including mefloquine or doxycycline.

Atovaquone-Proguanil (Malarone)

Malarone, a fixed synergistic combination of atovaquone (a hydroxynapthoquinone analog of ubiquinone) and proguanil in a single tablet (250 mg atovaquone and 100 mg proguanil), recently has been licensed for malaria prevention and for treatment of all species of malaria, particularly chloroquine-resistant P. falciparum. Atovaquone selectively inhibits the parasite's mitochondrial electron transport. It is recommended for all areas of the world where chloroquine-resistant P. falciparum is a risk.[5,9]

Compared with other standard antimalarial regimens, Malarone has demonstrated excellent safety and tolerance.[9,48–50] Although 8% to 15% of all adults and children taking therapeutic doses experience nausea, vomiting, abdominal pain, or diarrhea and in 5% to 10% transient, asymptomatic elevations in serum transaminases and amylase develop, no definite side effects are evident when Malarone is used for malaria prevention. Nevertheless atovaquone has been shown to be teratogenic in rabbits (FDA category C drug).

Early field trials have demonstrated 100% protective efficacy (95% confidence interval 95% to 100%) of Malarone as a suppressive agent (acting in the blood stage) against P. falciparum malaria in semi-immune adults in Kenya.[48,49] Furthermore preliminary evidence suggests that atovaquone-proguanil may also be a causal prophylactic agent (acting in the liver stage).[48–51] Therefore the need for the traveler to complete 4 weeks of prophylaxis after exposure (a common reason for non-adherence) is thus avoided, and this regimen may be particularly useful for travelers who undergo short or repeated exposures in high-risk areas.

The recommended prophylactic dose of atovaquone-proguanil (Malarone) is a 250 mg/100 mg tablet taken orally once a day starting 1 day before travel and continuing for 1 week after leaving the malarious area. Pregnancy and hypersensitivity to either component are the only contraindications to atovaquone-proguanil.[48–51]

Azithromycin

Azithromycin (Zithromax) is an azalide antimicrobial agent related to erythromycin. In small-scale human challenge studies it has proven to be an effective chemosuppressive agent against *P. vivax*. Its protective efficacy against *P. falciparum* in phase II and III trials (70% to 83%), however, is generally considered to be too low for azithromycin to be relied on as a single agent to prevent *P. falciparum* malaria.[51,52] Like doxycycline, it is not causally prophylactic and needs to be given daily (adult dose: 1 tablet per day) starting on the day before exposure and continued during exposure and for 4 weeks after departure from the malarial region.[51,52]

Azithromycin may ultimately be useful for preventing malaria in selected groups of populations such as young children and pregnant women, for whom other agents are contraindicated or difficult to use. Its potential use in children has been facilitated by the recent availability of an oral suspension. In view of the serious consequences of malaria in pregnancy, however, the use of suboptimal antimalarial agents should not be recommended routinely.

Tafenoquine (WR 238605)

Tafenoquine (Etaquine, WR 238605), an 8-aminoquinoline closely related to primaquine with activity against both asexual (blood and liver) and sexual (gametocyte) stages of the parasite, is currently undergoing phase II and III chemosuppressive trials in semi-immune and non-immune persons. This drug has a long half-life (2 to 4 weeks), allowing for a weekly dosing regimen. Like primaquine, etaquine is contraindicated in G6PD deficiency, but otherwise it seems to be better tolerated than primaquine. Etaquine might also have potential as a transmission-blocking agent.[51,53–56]

Special Situations

Pregnant and Breast-Feeding Women

Malaria poses a serious threat both to the pregnant woman and to her fetus. It increases the risk of maternal death and fetal prematurity, miscarriage, and stillbirth.

Therefore pregnant women are in general advised not to travel to a malaria area unless absolutely necessary.

Chloroquine remains the preferred drug for chemoprophylaxis for pregnant women in malaria areas where it is still effective. In chloroquine-resistant areas, mefloquine may be used instead. Neither chloroquine nor mefloquine has had harmful effects on the fetus during any stage of pregnancy when used in dosages sufficient to prevent malaria.[57,58] On the other hand, doxycycline, atovaquone-proguanil, and primaquine should not be used during pregnancy. Small amounts of antimalarial drugs may be passed on to infants through breast-feeding. Although not harmful to the infant, these small amounts of drug in breast milk are not enough to protect them against malaria; therefore infants need to be given appropriate drugs in dosages according to their weight.[57,58]

Infants and Children

Dosage of antimalarials must be tailored to the child's age or weight. The pharmacist may crush the chloroquine or mefloquine tablets, which have a bitter flavor, and place the powder in gelatin capsules with the calculated pediatric doses. Crushed powder may also be mixed in food, drinks, or desserts. Malarone is now available in a pediatric tablet (250 mg atovaquone and 100 mg proguanil) one-fourth of the strength of the adult tablet. The dosage of pediatric-strength tablets is based on weight: 11 to 20 kg, 1 tablet; 21 to 30 kg, 2 tablets; 31 to 40 kg, 3 tablets. Only doxycycline is not indicated for infants and children less than 8 years old.

Stand-by Treatment of Malaria

The soundness of a self-administered empiric malaria treatment has been a controversial issue for many years, but recent concerns about the potential adverse effects of antimalarials, in particular mefloquine, have again made it a popular concept. Travelers should be made aware that self-treatment is only a temporary measure, however, and medical attention should still be sought as soon as possible.

Under some circumstances, persons may be unable to obtain prompt medical care within 48 hours and may require self-treatment for presumptive malaria. Because of the nonspecific symptoms of malaria, the potentially serious risk of incorrectly treating another disease, and the potential toxicity of malaria therapy, self-treatment should never be undertaken lightly.

The drug selected for self-treatment should not be the same as that used for chemoprophylaxis. Malarone is the drug of choice for self-treatment when it is not being used for prevention. The adult self-treatment regimen with Malarone is 4 tablets once daily for 3 days; the regimen with mefloquine is 5 tablets taken in divided doses over 12 hours.

Mefloquine is seldom recommended for self-treatment because its potential neurologic and psychological side effects are 10 times more common when the drug is used for treatment. Halofantrine is not recommended for self-treatment of malaria because of the risk of cardiotoxicity.[59]

Treatment of Acute Infection

Most patients without acquired immunity and *P. vivax*, *P. ovale*, or *P. malariae* infection and those with partial immunity and uncomplicated *P. falciparum* infection can be treated as outpatients if close follow-up is possible. Contrarily, nonimmune patients with *P. falciparum* infection should be considered a medical emergency and hospitalized until an initial response to treatment has been observed and enough time has elapsed to be certain that cerebral, renal, pulmonary, or other complication is not likely.

In general all cases of *P. vivax* infection and uncomplicated cases of *P. falciparum* may be treated with oral drugs. Chloroquine is the drug of choice for *P. vivax* malaria because its resistance to chloroquine is rare. When the species of *Plasmodium* involved is in doubt or the infection is mixed, *P. falciparum* should be considered. If drug sensitivities are uncertain, any *P. falciparum* infection should be assumed to be chloroquine resistant and resistant to both chloroquine and mefloquine if contracted in Southeast Asia.

Patients with *P. falciparum* disease are considered to suffer from severe malaria and may be at risk of potentially lethal complications if they present with one or more of the following clinical or laboratory features: prostration, impaired consciousness, respiratory distress (acidotic breathing), multiple convulsions (≥ 3 in 24 h), circulatory collapse, radiologic evidence of pulmonary edema, abnormal bleeding, jaundice (total bilirubin >2.5 mg/dl or >43 μmol/L), hemoglobinuria, and severe anemia (hemoglobin <5 g/dl, or hematocrit <15%). Other features indicating a poor prognosis in adult patients with severe malaria include parasitemia greater than 5% (parasite count >250,000/μl), acidosis (plasma bicarbonate <15 μmol/L), azotemia (serum creatinine >3 mg/dl or >265 μmol/L), hypoglycemia (blood glucose <40 mg/dl or 2.2 μmol/L), hyperlactemia (venous lactate >45 mg/dl or >5 μmol/L), and elevated levels of aminotransferases (>3 times normal).[4,31]

It must be stressed that although successful treatment of patients with malaria depends primarily on the proper use of effective antimalarial drugs, ancillary measures as diverse as the infusion of glucose solutions, compensation of acidosis, respiratory support, and dialysis are often required. It is important to monitor the blood glucose level, as hypoglycemia is a common cause of coma and both quinine and quinidine stimulate the release of insulin directly from the beta cells of the pancreas. Steroids are contraindicated in cerebral malaria because they prolong the coma.

An ideal antimalarial drug should be able to reduce parasitemia quickly and maintain effective levels long enough to eliminate all parasites. Consequently the drug must rapidly reach adequate blood concentrations and interfere with the erythrocytic cycle so that no new schizonts are produced. However, even though some drugs, such as quinine, quinidine, and artemisinin, rapidly reach effective blood concentrations, they also have relatively short half-lives. On the other hand, drugs with long half-lives, such as mefloquine, often achieve effective blood levels at a slower rate (chloroquine being an exception). Since nonimmune hosts with *P. falciparum* infection may exhibit high total parasite burdens (up to 10^{12} parasites), even drugs reaching a 4 log or 99.99% killing rate per cycle would take no less than three schizogonic cycles (6 days) to eliminate the last parasite in the blood.[60] If a short half-life drug such as doxycycline is given alone, it should be maintained for at least 6 consecutive days. Contrarily, drugs such as chloroquine, mefloquine, and pyrimethamine-sulfadoxine (Fansidar), which rapidly achieve effective blood concentrations and have long elimination half-lives, may be given at shorter or even single-dose schedules.[4,60]

A common source of confusion in the treatment of malaria is the coexistence of two systems for calculating the dose of an antimalarial drug. Because the therapeutic index of these drugs is low, mistakes in dosing may induce potentially severe complications, such as hypotension and arrhythmias. Therefore to prevent costly nursing or pharmacy errors, it is necessary to establish whether the dose is recommended as a base or as a salt. Traditionally doses of chloroquine, mefloquine, and primaquine are prescribed according to the amount of base, whereas quinine and halofantrine doses are expressed as the amount of salt.[61] Quinidine is better prescribed according to the amount of base because several salt formulations are available.

Recommended doses and schedules of commonly used antimalarials are summarized in Tables 34–2 and 34–3.

Chloroquine-Sensitive Malaria

Chloroquine continues to be the drug of choice for all *P. ovale* and *P. malariae* infections and for sensitive *P. falciparum* and *P. vivax* infections. Uncomplicated infections may be treated orally with a total dose of 25 mg/kg chloroquine base given over 3 days. The usual schedule for adults is 600 mg base chloroquine phosphate initially, 300 mg base 6 hours later, then 300 mg base at 24 and 48 hours. Equivalent pediatric doses are 10 mg/kg base (max. 600 mg base) initially, 5 mg/kg base 6 hours later, then 5 mg/kg base at 24 and 48 hours. The expected cure rates exceed 95%.[62–64]

Patients unable to take oral medications may be treated initially with parenteral chloroquine hydrochloride and then switched to oral chloroquine phosphate when they are able to take oral medications. Even for patients with central nervous system involvement quinine (or other antimalarial agents) offers no advantage over

TABLE 34–2 ■ Recommended Oral Therapeutic Schedules for Commonly Prescribed Antimalarials

Drug	Adult dose	Pediatric dose
Chloroquine	600 mg base at 0 h 600 mg base at 24 h 300 mg base at 48 h	10 mg/kg base at 0 h 10 mg/kg base at 24 h 5 mg/kg base at 48 h
Quinine (sulfate salt)	650 mg salt q8h × 7 d OR 650 mg salt q8h × 3 d (when in combination)*	10 mg/kg salt q8h × 7 d OR 10 mg/kg salt q8h × 3 d
Mefloquine†	5 tablets at 0 h 3 tablets at 8–24 h	15 mg/kg base at 0 h 10 mg/kg base at 8–24 h Some authorities feel 15 mg/kg base is sufficient except in areas of mefloquine resistance or reported prophylaxis failures where 25 mg/kg base should be used
Doxycycline	100 mg q12h × 7 d	2.5 mg/kg qd × 7 d
Artesunate	6 tablets qd × 3 d‡	4 mg/kg qd × 3 d
Halofantrine§	2 tablets q8h × 3 doses; repeat in 1 wk	8 mg/kg q8h × 3 doses; repeat in 1 wk
Sulfadoxine-pyrimethamine‖	3 tablets as a single dose	1 mg/kg (pyrimethamine component) as single dose

See text for toxicities, contraindications, and comments.

*When quinine is used in combination with another slower acting drug, many physicians use only 3 days of quinine to avoid toxicity.
†228 mg mefloquine base = 250 mg mefloquine HCl salt
‡Artesunate should always be used in combination with a slower acting drug. Artesunate, 50-mg tablets, not yet licensed in United States.
§Halofantrine (Halfan), 250 mg base per tablet; licensed in United States but not commercially distributed.
‖One tablet = sulfadoxine 500 mg plus pyrimethamine 25 mg (Fansidar); contraindicated in patients with sulfa allergy; this combination may fail in areas of sulfadoxine resistance.

TABLE 34–3 ■ Recommended Parenteral Schedules for Commonly Prescribed Antimalarials*

Drug	Loading dose	Maintenance dose	Observations
Chloroquine	10 mg/kg base in isotonic fluid by constant rate IV infusion over 8 h, followed immediately by maintenance dose	15 mg/kg base over 24 h	Total dose = 25 mg/kg base High blood concentrations resulting from rapid IV, IM, or SC administration may be hypotensive and negatively inotropic
Quinine	20 mg/kg dihydrochloride salt diluted in 10 ml/kg isotonic fluid by IV infusion over 4 h, followed 8 h later by maintenance dose OR 7 mg/kg salt over 30 min by IV infusion (or pump), followed immediately by maintenance dose	10 mg/kg salt diluted in 10 ml/kg isotonic fluid by IV infusion over 4 h, q8h for maintenance	Maximum maintenance dose 600 mg; loading dose unnecessary if the patient received quinine within the preceding 12 h; all patients, especially pregnant women and children, are at risk of developing hyperinsulinemic hypoglycemia
Quinidine	15 mg/kg base by IV infusion over 4 h, followed 8 h later by maintenance dose OR 6.2 mg/kg base over 1–2 h, followed immediately by maintenance dose	7.5 mg/kg base over 4 h, q8h OR Continuous infusion of base 0.0125 mg/kg/h	Cardiac monitoring indicated during infusion; slow or stop infusion if QRS lengthens >25% of baseline value or QTc >0.500 ms; 100 mg quinidine base = 161 mg quinidine gluconate salt
Clindamycin	Not required	20 mg/kg/d in 2 divided doses × 5 or 7 d	
Artesunate	2.4 mg/kg IV or IM bolus	1.2 mg/kg qd × 5–7 d	Shorter parasite clearance time and less hypoglycemia than quinine has but longer fever resolution time and coma; artemether and arteether derivatives are dissolved in oil for IM use; fatal neurotoxicity in animal studies at high doses
Artemether	3.2 mg/kg IM	1.6 mg/kg IM qd × 5–7 d	

*When improvement is evident and the patient can tolerate oral medications. If parenteral medicines are continued past 48 h, decrease dose by one-third to one-half; in renal failure use normal loading dose but decrease maintenance dose by one-third to one-half.

chloroquine for infections due to chloroquine-susceptible parasites. Chloroquine hydrochloride is available as a solution containing 40 mg/ml of the base. Because of its arrhythmogenic potential,[65,66] intravenous chloroquine must be given as a carefully controlled infusion at constant rates not exceeding 0.83 mg/kg base per hour or in frequent small subcutaneous or intramuscular injections not exceeding 3.5 mg/kg base to achieve a total dose of 25 mg/kg base.

Persons with *P. vivax* or *P. ovale* infection in nonendemic areas usually are treated with primaquine to eradicate hypnozoites in the liver (radical cure), hence preventing eventual relapses. In adults chloroquine must thus be followed by a 2-week course of primaquine phosphate at a dose of 15 mg base per day for 14 days or 45 mg base per week for 8 weeks. The pediatric dose is 0.3 mg/kg base per day for 14 days.[31,50,62,64,67] Primaquine is contraindicated in severe G6PD deficiency, but closely supervised weekly doses of primaquine for 6 to 8 weeks have been used uneventfully in patients with a mild deficiency.[31,49,60–63,67–69]

Chloroquine-Resistant *P. falciparum* and *P. vivax*

Oral intolerance poor general health, and erratic enteric absorption due to splanchnic vasculopathy make the oral therapy less reliable. Therefore severe malaria should always be treated initially with parenteral antimalarials to ensure adequate treatment. This approach excludes drugs such as mefloquine and halofantrine (Halfan).

It is safer to treat all cases of severe *P. falciparum* malaria as chloroquine-resistant unless the sensitivity of the involved strain has been clearly established. Many health providers in endemic regions would prefer to treat partially immune hosts with one shorter course of a rapid acting drug in combination with one slower acting drug to avoid the adverse effects of the rapid acting drug and allow for the steady onset of the parasitic-killing activity of the less toxic slower acting drug.

All antimalarial drugs have a narrow safety range, and excess doses may have serious adverse effects. In addition a larger dose does not offer any superior antimalarial effect. Since most antimalarials have long plasma half-lives, adding a similar drug once the treatment has begun will only add to the adverse effects and not to the therapeutic benefit. Therefore administration of the following combinations concurrently or within a short period, should be avoided: chloroquine plus either quinine or mefloquine; quinine plus mefloquine, primaquine, or halofantrine; and mefloquine plus primaquine.

Combination regimens widely used to treat chloroquine-resistant *P. falciparum* infection include quinine sulfate plus doxycycline (or clindamycin in children less than 10 years old and pregnant women), quinine sulfate plus pyrimethamine-sulfadoxine, quinidine plus doxycycline, or pyrimethamine-sulfadoxine alone (currently recommended only in sub-Saharan Africa).[31,62,68–72] In *P. falciparum* malaria acquired in Southeast Asia, South America, and East Africa where pyrimethamine-sulfadoxine resistance is widespread, chloroquine-resistant *P. falciparum* should be treated with quinine sulfate plus tetracycline or halofantrine (Halfan).[31,70–72]

Quinine remains the drug of choice for severe *P. falciparum* malaria in most of the tropical world.[4,60,73] Quinine causes less hypotension and diarrhea and is less cardiotoxic then quinidine is; therefore electrocardiogram monitoring is not required. Quinine, however, is associated with more hearing impairment than quinidine is. Both drugs cause cinchonism (bitter taste, dysphoria, tinnitus, unsteadiness, and reversible high-tone hearing loss), which seldom requires cessation of therapy.[4,73] Quinine causes hyperinsulinemic hypoglycemia, especially in severely ill children and pregnant women.[62,74,75] Although quinine may induce abortion or premature delivery at high doses, it is safe and does not have teratogenic or oxytocic effects in therapeutic doses.[62,74,75]

Cure rates between 85% and 90% are expected when *P. falciparum* infections are treated with a combination of quinine plus tetracycline for 7 days. Shorter 3-day courses may also be effective but should not be used in nonimmune patients or in infections from areas such as Southeast Asia or the Amazon basin, where *P. falciparum* resistance to quinine is rising.[26,31,72,76,77]

Mefloquine is highly effective (cure rates between 90% and 95%) against chloroquine-resistant *P. falciparum* infections, except those acquired in multidrug-resistant endemic areas of Southeast Asia, for which lower cure rates are to be expected.[62,78,79] Mefloquine may induce vomiting, ataxia, diaphoresis, nightmares, changes of mood or dissociation, and seizures.[27,62] At doses of 25 mg/kg base (or 1250 mg) a severe, usually limited, toxic encephalopathy manifested as anxiety, depression, ataxia, hallucinations, delirium, and seizures may be seen in 0.1% to 1% of patients.[27,80]

Halofantrine should not be used to treat suspected mefloquine-resistant strains, since therapeutic doses (24 mg/kg over 12 hours) cure only 65% of chloroquine-resistant *P. falciparum* malaria in Thailand and Africa.[68,81,82] In addition halofantrine causes a dose-dependent delay in atrioventricular conduction and ventricular repolarization and has caused sudden deaths in patients with prolonged QTc syndromes and in patients taking drugs that can prolong the QT interval.[59]

Pyrimethamine-sulfadoxine (Fansidar: pyrimethamine 25 mg plus sulfadoxine 500 mg) has become the mainstay therapy in sub-Saharan Africa because resistance is still uncommon, side effects are rare, and the cost is reasonable. Unfortunately the combination is currently not useful in most of Southeast Asia and the endemic Amazon regions of South America, where pyrimethamine-sulfadoxine–resistant strains are widespread. Serum folate may further antagonize the drug's effect, so it may be less effective in well-nourished populations. Pyrimethamine-sulfadoxine may be combined with quinine in patients unable to take doxycycline, but the effectiveness of this combination remains unclear.[83] Pyrimethamine-sulfadoxine cures 80% to 90% of sensitive *P. falciparum* infections,[27,34,49,78,84] but it has been abandoned as a once-weekly chemoprophylactic agent because of severe, occasionally fatal, exfoliative dermatitis, erythema multiforme, and Stevens-Johnson syndrome, which is observed in 1 of every 11,000 to 25,000 patients.[54,78] The estimated risk of severe exfoliative dermatitis after a standard three-tablet single dose in adults is 1 in 10 million.[78,85,86]

Chloroquine-resistant *P. vivax* infections consistently respond either to mefloquine or the combination of quinine sulfate plus tetracycline, whereas pyrimethamine-sulfadoxine is less effective.[31,86] Higher doses of primaquine (22.5 to 30 mg base per day for 14 days) are habitually required to eradicate hypnozoites and to prevent relapses of *P. vivax* strains from Southeast Asia.[62,87]

Multidrug-Resistant *P. falciparum*

Uncomplicated, mefloquine-resistant *P. falciparum* infections are best treated with quinine sulfate plus tetracycline (clindamycin for pregnant women).[62,77,78] Quinine-resistant *P. falciparum* infections should be treated with combinations including artemisinin derivatives (artesunate, artemether, or dihydroartemisinin), which are also effective against mefloquine-resistant *P. falciparum* strains.[31,60,78,88–90]

Artemisinin derivatives are potent blood schizotocides that rapidly reduce the parasitemia and the clinical symptoms.[91] A significant inhibiting effect on gametocytogenesis of *P. falciparum* has been demonstrated.[91–94] Cure rates above 95% are usual for *P. falciparum* infections when artemisinin derivatives are combined with tetracycline, clindamycin, or mefloquine to prevent recrudescence.[60,78,90]

Artemisinin derivatives are the fastest acting known antimalarials, and so far no plasmodia have shown resistance.[60] They may be given intramuscularly or by rectal suppository, which facilitates their use in poor and rural endemic areas.[31,60]

In general the most common adverse side effects are nausea, vomiting, itching, and fever; occasionally, bleeding and arrhythmias, including first-degree atrioventricular block, have been noted. Although experimental studies with laboratory animals show that doses above 10 mg/kg may cause fetal resorption,[95] the preclinical studies did not manifest any mutative or teratogenic effects.[94] Despite reports of a devastating experimental brainstem neurotoxicity in rats and monkeys that leads to gait disturbance, dysconjugate eye movements, loss of ocular and pain reflexes, cardiovascular collapse, and death, this feared side effect has not yet been observed in humans.[89,96] Artemisinin derivatives can be used in the second and third trimesters of pregnancy but are not recommended in the first trimester, even in cases with severe and complicated malaria.[91]

Treatment of Severe or Life-Threatening Malaria

Parenteral preparations such as quinine dihydrochloride or quinidine gluconate are considered the drugs of choice for the treatment of life-threatening chloroquine-resistant and mefloquine-resistant *P. falciparum* malaria.[26,31,62,78,97,98] Survival rates as high as 75% to 85% are seen in adults or children with severe and cerebral malaria receiving intravenous quinine or quinidine combined with pyrimethamine-sulfadoxine, mefloquine, or doxycycline.[99,100] Although quinidine gluconate is twice as malariacidal, it is also far more cardiotoxic than quinine dihydrochloride.[99,100] The major toxicities of both drugs are dysrhythmias, hypotension, and hyperinsulinemic hypoglycemia.[31,62] Therapeutic serum concentrations for quinidine range between 4 and 8 mg/L, whereas for quinine they are 8 to 20 mg/L.[31] It must be noted that serum levels of both quinine and quinidine may be elevated in patients with severe malaria and high parasitemia because of a diminution in the volume of distribution and a reduction of their clearance. Therefore to avoid unnecessary toxicity, the dosage of each drug should be decreased by 30% to 50% after 48 hours.[60,62]

Quinine-resistant *P. falciparum* infection is best treated with a combination of parental artemisinin derivatives plus either tetracycline or mefloquine.[78,89,101,102] If artemisinin is not available, parenteral quinidine or quinine combined with tetracycline should be used.[62,99,100] Although artemisinin derivatives clear bloodstream parasites about 20% faster and shorten the period of fever by about 30% more than quinine dihydrochloride does, they confer no survival advantage. Furthermore recovery from coma may be delayed, and the incidence of seizures among children was 11% higher than with quinine dihydrochloride.[60,91,92,94]

Because of its slow antimalarial activity, clindamycin should not be relied on solely, but it may be beneficial as an adjunct to quinine for treating patients with chloroquine-resistant *P. falciparum* infection in whom doxycycline is contraindicated. Indeed cure rates of 50% for chloroquine-resistant *P. falciparum* malaria treated with clindamycin alone at oral doses of 450 mg every 8 hours for 3 days have been reported in Thailand.[85] When clindamycin is combined with quinine, the cure rate increases to 100%, but there is a parallel rise in the frequency of vomiting.[103]

Parenteral chloroquine is as effective as intravenous quinine and is the treatment of choice for severe chloroquine-sensitive *P. falciparum* infections and for those rare cases of life-threatening malaria caused by *P. vivax, P. ovale,* and *P. malariae.*[27,62,64,78,104] Chloroquine must be given by controlled intravenous infusion to avoid severe hypotension.[31,65]

Malaria in Pregnancy

Plasmodium falciparum malaria is particularly dangerous during the first pregnancy of nonimmune women.

Severe malaria may lead to fetal loss and high maternal mortality due to hypoglycemia and acute respiratory distress syndrome. Chloroquine is the only antimalarial agent known to be safe during pregnancy.[105,106] There are no reliable clinical data for most antimalarials to be declared safe for pregnant women.

Even though mefloquine appears to be safe during any trimester of pregnancy,[107] the number of pregnant women studied thus far is limited. Although quinine may be oxytocic at higher doses, it does not induce uterine contractions at the intravenous doses normally used to treat malaria. Indeed therapeutic doses of quinine in pregnant women with chloroquine-resistant *P. falciparum* infection decrease both premature uterine contractions and fever.[74]

Clindamycin, an antibiotic active against resistant strains of *P. falciparum*, is an alternative to tetracycline or doxycycline because it does not produce significant adverse side effects in the pregnant patient or the fetus. The drug is given at a dosage of 20 mg/kg/d divided into two daily doses for a period of 5 or 7 days and can be administered orally or intravenously. Over the last two decades the drug has been used routinely in combination with quinine to treat pregnant patients with multidrug-resistant *P. falciparum* strains in Brazil, and no significant adverse side effects have been observed in either the mothers or the fetuses.[108]

Although concerns remain about chemoprophylaxis, treatment is essential to save symptomatic pregnant women and their pregnancies. There is no indication of increased risk of congenital abnormalities following the use of alternative antimalarials to chloroquine (with the exception of doxycycline) during the first trimester of pregnancy. Artemisinin derivatives have been used in the second and third trimesters of pregnancy, but there are not enough data about their safety. Nevertheless these derivatives should be avoided in the first trimester because of the risk of potential teratogenicity.

Malaria in Children

In areas of intense transmission, severe malaria is more common in children. Coma, convulsions, hypoglycemia, lactic acidosis, and severe anemia frequently are presenting signs of severe malaria in childhood. Malaria in non-immune children is similar to that in the adult population and depends mostly on the infecting species, the level of parasitemia, and in breast-fed children less than 6 months of age, the pre-existence of maternal immunity.[4,75,109]

New Approaches in the Treatment and Prevention of Malaria

Since vaccines historically have been a highly cost-effective means of controlling infectious diseases, the possibility of developing an effective malaria vaccine is very appealing. Accumulating basic and clinical research during the last two decades suggests that it can indeed be accomplished. An ideal malaria vaccine is one that would elicit protective immunity to block infection, and if this is not possible, it should prevent morbidity and interrupt transmission of parasites.

Malaria parasites have complex life cycles that include distinct developmental stages, each with multiple antigens that could serve as potential targets of an immune response. In general, populations residing in endemic areas ordinarily have naturally acquired protective immunity against the disease, which may be passively transferred by immunoglobulins purified from the serum of immune adults. Induction of protective immunity in experimental animals may involve multiple different immune responses, both humoral and cellular.[110,111] Factors such as CD8$^+$ cytotoxic T lymphocytes and T cell–derived cytokines also seem to be involved in the elimination of parasites within hepatocytes, possibly through the induction of mediators such as nitric oxide. Clinical studies have also shown that experimental exposure to attenuated sporozoites can effectively immunize patients against a subsequent malaria infection.

Vaccines against malaria can be designed to work at any of the different stages of the parasite's life cycle. A pre-erythrocytic vaccine would protect against the mosquito-borne sporozoites or inhibit development of the parasite in the liver or both. Nevertheless in previously unexposed persons even one single surviving sporozoite would eventually multiply and result in full-blown illness. An erythrocytic or blood-stage vaccine would instead inhibit parasite multiplication in the red cells, thus preventing, or at least diminishing, severe illness. Sexual-stage vaccines are aimed at interrupting the cycle of transmission by inhibiting the further development of parasites once they, along with antibodies produced in response to the vaccine, are ingested by the mosquito. Transmission-blocking vaccines could be useful as part of a comprehensive strategy to eliminate parasites in low-transmission areas or as a means of protecting drugs directed at pre-erythrocytic or erythrocytic stages against the spread of resistant parasites.

As no single parasitic antigen appears to induce complete protection, an alternative might be the use of a mixture or "cocktail" of antigens derived from several subunits of different parasite stages synthetically put together, that is, a combination vaccine. Safety, efficacy, storage, type of adjuvant, doses, and schedules and routes of administration, among others, remain areas of concern. Furthermore in naturally acquired infection unregulated immune responses may contribute to the pathogenesis of the disease; therefore the potential for enhanced immunopathogenesis must also be taken into account in any vaccine development effort.

Currently more than 30 distinct antigens identified in various stages of the parasite have been proposed at some level as potential malaria vaccine, but only one candidate vaccine, SPf66, based on antigens from both merozoite and sporozoite stages, has undergone extensive field trials.[112,113]

DNA vaccines, based on the stimulation of an immune response through the introduction of foreign genes, which will produce foreign proteins, are a promising new approach as they circumvent the problem of genetic restriction.[114] DNA vaccines are capable of inducing dose-related killer cytotoxic T lymphocyte responses in mice. These vaccines, however, have not been evaluated in humans, and their protective efficacy is unknown. Another innovative approach is to develop vaccines that target molecular receptors used by the malaria parasite for cell invasion and disease progression.

Naturally occurring immunity wanes rapidly in the absence of ongoing parasite exposure. Similar short-lived protective responses have been demonstrated in persons exposed to subunit vaccines. Such a vaccine might be useful for travelers.[115]

Despite these advances, major improvements are still needed. Because of the short-lived immunity induced by currently available vaccines, new technologies or innovative approaches are needed to improve their efficacy. However, it is likely that to be used in endemic areas, vaccines will need to take advantage of boosting immunity provided by parasite exposure to provide long-lived protection.

BABESIOSIS

Babesiosis is a tick-borne infection caused by malaria-like protozoa of the genus *Babesia*. Worldwide more than 70 *Babesia* species are known to infect numerous wild and domestic mammals, birds, and sporadically, humans also. The parasite multiplies in the erythrocytes and may cause fever, hemolysis, and hemoglobinuria. Usually associated with a mild or subclinical illness in the healthy host, babesiosis may be overwhelming in asplenic or immunocompromised patients. Splenectomized patients are more likely to have high-level parasitemia and to be severely ill, but the infection may also be severe in patients with a functional spleen.[116]

Occasionally cases of babesiosis are reported from the United States and Europe (Yugoslavia, France, Russia, Sweden, Ireland, and Scotland). Infection is known to occur in Asia, Africa, and South America as well.[116,117] Only the rodent strain *Babesia microti* and the still uncharacterized strain WA-1 have been positively identified as a cause of human disease in the United States, whereas the cattle strains *Babesia divergens* and *Babesia bovis* have been identified in Europe.[116,117]

Treatment

Most patients infected by *B. microti* develop a mild illness and recover without specific chemotherapy. In patients with serious disease an apparently effective regimen is the combination of either intravenous or intramuscular clindamycin (20 mg/kg/d in children; 300 to 600 mg every 6 hours in adults) and oral quinine (25 mg/kg/d in children; 650 mg every 6 to 8 hours in adults) for 7 to 10 days.[118–120]

Occasional failures have been reported with the clindamycin-quinine combination.[119,120] An assortment of other antimalarial and antiprotozoal drugs have been largely unsuccessful, including chloroquine, primaquine, quinacrine, pyrimethamine, pyrimethamine-sulfadoxine, sulfadiazine, tetracycline, minocycline, pentamidine isethionate, and TMP-SMX.[119]

Atovaquone alone, or in combination with azithromycin, has been shown to be effective in the treatment of experimental babesiosis in hamsters.[121] However, atovaquone monotherapy resulted in recrudescence and resistance. The combination of atovaquone and azithromycin, both for 7 days, appears as effective as that of clindamycin and quinine in clearing parasitemia, but its long-term efficacy remains to be validated.[121] Although the atovaquone-azithromycin regimen may not be as rapidly effective as clindamycin-quinine is, it appears to induce fewer side effects. The usual dose of atovaquone is 750 mg orally taken with a meal twice daily. Doses of 40 mg/kg/d have been used in children. The dose of azithromycin in adults is 500 mg initially, followed by 250 mg daily thereafter.[122]

Exchange transfusions may be used concurrently with chemotherapy in life-threatening infections with high levels of parasitemia and hemolysis in an attempt to reduce the level of parasitemia and remove toxic products and parasites from erythrocytes, or macrophage-produced proinflammatory factors.[123,124] A combination of clindamycin, doxycycline, and azithromycin successfully treated a patient with acquired immunodeficiency syndrome who became allergic to quinine.[125] The combination of pentamidine with TMP-SMX was successful in treating a splenectomized patient in France with *B. divergens* infection.[118]

REFERENCES

1. Kain KC, Keystone JS: Malaria In travelers. Epidemiology, disease, and prevention. Infect Dis Clin North Am 1998;12:267.
2. World Health Organization: International Travel and Health: Vaccination requirements and health advice 1997. Geneva, WHO, 1997.
3. World Health Organization: The World Health Report 1996. Geneva, WHO, 1996.
4. World Health Organization: Trans R Soc Trop Med Hyg 2000; 94:S1/1–S1/90.
5. Svenson JE, MacLean JD, Gyorkos TW, et al: Imported malaria: Clinical presentation and examination of symptomatic travelers. Arch Intern Med 1995;155:861.
6. Centers for Disease Control and Prevention: Summary of notifiable diseases. MMWR Morb Mortal Wkly Rep 1997;46(SS-2).
7. Greenberg A, Lobel HO: Mortality from *Plasmodium falciparum* malaria in travelers from the United States. Ann Intern Med 1990;113:326.
8. Humar A, Sharma S, Zoutman D, et al: Fatal falciparum malaria in Canadian travellers. CMAJ 1997;156:1165.

9. Kain KC: Malaria chemoprophylaxis in the age of drug resistance. I. Currently recommended drug regimens. Clin Infect Dis 2001;33:226.

10. Krogstad DJ: *Plasmodium* species (malaria). In Mandell GL, Bennett JE, Dolin R (eds): Principles and Practice of Infectious Diseases. 5th ed. New York, Churchill Livingstone, 1995, p 2817.

11. Rosenthal PJ, Nelson RG: Isolation and characterization of a cysteine proteinase gene of *Plasmodium falciparum*. Mol Biochem Parasitol 1992;51:143.

12. Slater AF, Cerami A: Inhibition by chloroquine of a novel haem polymerase enzyme activity in malaria trophozoites. Nature 1992;355:167.

13. Krogstad DJ, Schlesinger PH: A perspective on antimalarial action: Effects of weak bases on *Plasmodium falciparum*. Biochem Pharmacol 1986;35:547.

14. Meshnick SR, Yang YZ, Lima V, et al: Iron-dependent free radical generation from the antimalarial agent artemisinin (quinghaosu). Antimicrob Agents Chemother 1993;37:1108.

15. Zhang F, Gosser DK Jr, Meshnick SR: Hemin-catalyzed decomposition of artemisinin (quinghaosu). Biochem Pharmacol 1992;43:1805.

16. Krogstad DJ, Gluzman IY, Kyle DE, et al: Efflux of chloroquine from *Plasmodium falciparum*: Mechanism of chloroquine resistance. Science 1987;238:1283.

17. Su X-Z, Kirkman LA, Fujioka H, et al: Complex polymorphisms in a p330 kDa protein are linked to chloroquine-resistant *Plasmodium falciparum* in Southeast Asia and Africa. Cell 1997;91:591.

18. Wellems TE, Panton LJ, Gluzman IY, et al: Chloroquine resistance not linked to mdr-like genes in a *Plasmodium falciparum* cross. Nature. 1990;345:253.

19. Peterson DS, DiSanti SM, Povoa M, et al: Prevalence of the dihydrofolate reductase Asn-108 mutation as the basis for pyrimethamine-resistant *Plasmodium falciparum* malaria in the Brazilian Amazon. Am J Trop Med Hyg 1991;45:492.

20. Gyang FN, Peterson DS, Wellems TE: *Plasmodium falciparum:* Rapid detection of dihydrofolate reductase mutations that confer resistance to cycloguanil and pyrimethamine. Exp Parasitol 1992;74:470.

21. Peterson DS, Milhous WK, Wellems TE: Molecular basis of differential resistance to cycloguanil and pyrimethamine in *Plasmodium falciparum* malaria. Proc Natl Acad Sci USA 1990;87:3018.

22. Nevill CG, Some ES, Mug'ala VO, et al: Insecticide-treated bed nets reduce mortality and severe morbidity from malaria among children. Trop Med Intl Health 1996;1:139

23. Wyler DJ: Malaria chemoprophylaxis for the traveler. N Engl J Med 1993;329:31

24. Health information for international travel, 1996-97. Atlanta, U.S. Dept of Health and Human Services, Public Health Service, Centers for Disease Control and Prevention, National Center for Infectious Diseases, Division of Quarantine, 1997; HHS publication no. 95-8280.

25. Pang LW, Limsomwong N, Boudrea EF, et al: Prophylactic treatment of vivax and falciparum malaria with low dose doxycycline. J Infect Dis 1988;88:1124.

26. Pasvol G, Newton CR, Winstanley PA, et al: Quinine treatment of severe falciparum malaria in African children: A randomized comparison of three regimens. Am J Trop Med Hyg 1991;45:702.

27. Patchen LC, Campbell CC, Williams SB: Neurologic reactions after a therapeutic dose of mefloquine. N Engl J Med 1989;321:1415.

28. Paxton LA, Slutsker L, Schultz LJ, et al: Imported malaria in Montagnard refugees settling in North Carolina: Implications for prevention and control. Am J Trop Med Hyg 1996;54:54.

29. Koranda FC: Antimalarials. J Am Acad Dermatol 1981;4:650.

30. Mockenhaupt FP: Mefloquine resistance in *Plasmodium falciparum*. Parasitol Today 1995;11:248.

31. White NJ: The treatment of malaria. N Engl J Med 1996;335:800.

32. Wetsteyn JCFM, de Geus A: Comparison of three regimens for malaria prophylaxis in travellers to East, Central, and Southern Africa. BMJ 1993;307:1041.

33. Bradley DJ, Warhurst DC: Malaria prophylaxis: Guidelines for travellers from Britain. BMJ 1995;310:709.

34. Lobel HO, Miani M, Eng T, et al: Long-term malaria prophylaxis with weekly mefloquine. Lancet 1993;341:848.

35. Steffen R, Fuchs E, Schildknecht J, et al: Mefloquine compared with other malaria chemoprophylactic regimens in tourists visiting East Africa. Lancet 1993;341:1299.

36. Davis TME, Dembo LG, Kaye-Eddie SA, et al: Neurological, cardiovascular and metabolic effects of mefloquine in healthy volunteers: A double-blind, placebo-controlled trial. Br J Clin Pharmacol 1996;42:415.

37. Boudreau E, Schuster B, Sanchez J, et al: Tolerability of prophylactic Lariam regimens. Trop Med Parasitol 1993;44:257.

38. Weiss WR, Oloo AJ, Johnson A, et al: Daily primaquine is effective for prophylaxis against falciparum malaria in Kenya: Comparison with mefloquine, doxycycline and chloroquine plus proguanil. J Infect Dis 1996;171:1569.

39. Ohrt C, Richie TL, Widjaja H, et al: Mefloquine compared with doxycycline for the prophylaxis of malaria in Indonesian soldiers: A randomized, double blind, placebo-controlled trial. Ann Intern Med 1997;126:963.

40. Pang LW, Limsomwong N, Boudreau EF, et al: Doxycycline prophylaxis for falciparum malaria. Lancet 1987;1:1161.

41. Schwartz E, Regev-Yochay G: Primaquine as prophylaxis for malaria for nonimmune travelers: A comparison with mefloquine and doxycycline. Clin Infect Dis 1999;29:1502.

42. Clayman CB, Arnold J, Hockwald RS, et al: Toxicity of primaquine in Caucasians. JAMA 1952;149:1563.

43. Georg JN, Sears DA, McCurdy PR, Conrad ME: Primaquine sensitivity in Caucasians: Hemolytic reactions induced by primaquine in G-6-PD deficient subjects. J Lab Clin Med 1967;70:80.

44. Cohen RJ, Sachs JR, Wicker DJ, Conrad ME: Methemoglobinemia provoked by malarial chemoprophylaxis in Vietnam. N Engl J Med 1968;279:1127.

45. Clyde DF: Clinical problems associated with the use of primaquine as a tissue schizonticidal and gametocytocidal drug. Bull World Health Organ 1981;59:391.

46. Lobel HO, Kozarsky PE: Update on prevention of malaria for travelers. JAMA 1997;278:1767.

47. Soto J, Toledo J, Rodríguez M, et al: Primaquine prophylaxis against malaria in nonimmune Colombian soldiers: Efficacy and toxicity. A randomized, double-blind, placebo-controlled trial. Ann Intern Med 1998;129:241.

48. de Alencar FEC, Cerutti C Jr, Durlache RR, et al: Atovaquone and proguanil for the treatment of malaria in Brazil. J Infect Dis 1997;175:1544.

49. Looareesuwan S, Viravan C, Webster HK, et al: Clinical studies of atovaquone alone or in combination with other antimalarial drugs for the treatment of acute uncomplicated malaria in Thailand. Am J Trop Med Hyg 1996;54:62.

50. MacPherson D, Gamble K, Tessier D, et al: Mefloquine tolerance: Randomized double-blind placebo controlled study [abstract]. Fifth Meeting of the International Society for Travel Medicine, Geneva, 1997.

51. Baird JK, Hoffman SL: Prevention of malaria in travelers. Med Clin North Am 1999;83:923.

52. Anderson SL, Berman J, Kuschner R, et al: Prophylaxis of *Plasmodium falciparum* malaria with azithromycin administered to volunteers. Ann Intern Med 1995;123:771.

53. Brueckner RP, Lasseter KC, Lin ET, et al: First-time in-humans safety and pharmacokinetics of WR 238605, a new antimalarial. Am J Trop Med Hyg 1998;58:645.

54. Obaldia N, Rossan RN, Cooper RD, et al: WR 238605, chloroquine, and their combinations as blood schizonticides against a chloroquine-resistant strain of *Plasmodium vivax* in Aotus monkeys. Am J Trop Med Hyg 1997;56:508.

55. Walsh DS, Looareesuwan S, Wilairatana P, et al: Randomized dose-ranging study of the safety and efficacy of WR 238605 (tafenoquine) in the prevention of relapse of *Plasmodium vivax* malaria in Thailand. J Infect Dis 1999;180:1282.

56. Cooper RD, Milhous WK, Rieckmann KH: The efficacy of WR 238605 against the blood stages of a chloroquine-resistant strain of *Plasmodium vivax*. Trans R Soc Trop Med Hyg 1994;88:691.

57. Steketee RW, Wirima JJ, Slutsker L, et al: Malaria treatment and prevention in pregnancy: Indications for use and adverse events associated with use of chloroquine or mefloquine. Am J Trop Med Hyg 1996;55:50.

58. Vanhauwere B, Maradit H, Kerr L: Post-marketing surveillance of prophylactic mefloquine use in pregnancy. Am J Trop Med Hyg 1998;58:17.

59. Nosten F, ter Kuile FO, Luxemburger C, et al: Cardiac effects of antimalarial treatment with halofantrine. Lancet 1993;341:1054.

60. White NJ: Malaria. In Cook GC (ed): Manson's Tropical Diseases, 20th ed. London, WB Saunders, 1996, pp 1087–1164.

61. Warrell DA: Treatment and prevention of malaria. In Gilles HM, Warrell DA (eds): Bruce-Chwatt's Essential Malariology, 3rd ed. London, Edward Arnold, 1993, pp 164–195.

62. Drugs for parasitic infections. Med Lett 1995;37:99.

63. Hoffman SL: Diagnosis, treatment, and prevention of malaria. Med Clin North Am 1992;76:1327.

64. White NJ, Miller KD, Churchill FC, et al: Chloroquine treatment of severe malaria in children. N Engl J Med 1988;319:1493.

65. Looareesuwan S, White NJ, Chanthavanich P, et al: Cardiovascular toxicity and distribution kinetics of intra-venous chloroquine. Br J Clin Pharmacol 1986;22:31.

66. Jaeger A, Sauder P, Kopferschmitt J, et al: Clinical features and management of poisoning due to antimalarial drugs. Med Toxicol Adverse Drug Exper 1987;2:242.

67. Rieckmann KH, Davis DR, Hutton DC: *Plasmodium vivax* resistant to chloroquine. Lancet 1989;2:1183.

68. Kain KC: Chemotherapy and prevention of drug-resistant malaria. Wilderness Env Med 1995;6:307.

69. Stanley J: Malaria. Emerg Med Clin North Am 1997;15:113.

70. Dobertslyn EB, Phintuyothim P, Noeypatimondh S, et al: Single-dose therapy of falciparum malaria with mefloquine or pyrimethamine-sulfadoxine. Bull World Health Organ 1979;57:275.

71. Dourado HV, Abdon NP, Martino SJ: Falciparum malaria: Epidemiology in Latin America, biological and clinical considerations, treatment and prophylaxis. Infect Dis Clin North Am 1994;8:207.

72. Watt G, Loesuttiribool L, Shanks GD, et al: Quinine with tetracycline for the treatment of drug-resistant falciparum malaria in Thailand. Am J Trop Med Hyg 1992;47:108.

73. Miller LH: Malaria. In Warren KS, Mahmoud AAF (eds): Tropical and Geographical Medicine. New York, McGraw-Hill Book Co, 1984, pp 223–239.

74. Looareesuwan S, Phillips RE, White NJ, et al: Quinine in severe falciparum malaria in late pregnancy. Lancet 1985;2:4.

75. White NJ, Warrell DA, Chanthavannich P, et al: Severe hypoglycemia and hyperinsulinemia in falciparum malaria. N Engl J Med 1983;309:61.

76. Looareesuwan S, Charoenpan P, Ho M: Fatal *Plasmodium falciparum* malaria after an inadequate response to quinine treatment. J Infect Dis 1990;161:577.

77. Looareesuwan S, Wilairatana P, Vanijanonta S, et al: Efficacy of quinine-tetracycline for acute uncomplicated falciparum malaria in Thailand. Lancet 1992;339:369.

78. Looareesuwan S, Wiravan C, Vanijanonta S, et al: Randomized trial of artesunate and mefloquine alone and in sequence for acute uncomplicated falciparum malaria. Lancet 1992;339:821.

79. Luxemberger C, terKuile FO, Nosten F, et al: Single day mefloquine-artesunate combination in the treatment of multidrug resistant falciparum malaria. Trans R Soc Trop Med Hyg 1994;88:213.

80. Phillips-Howard PA, terKuile FO: CNS adverse events associated with antimalarial agents—Fact or fiction? Drug Safety 1995;12:370.

81. terKuile FO, Dolan G, Nosten F, et al: Halofantrine versus mefloquine in treatment of multidrug resistant falciparum malaria. Lancet 1993;341:1044.

82. Warrell DA, Molyneaux ME, Beales PF: Severe and complicated malaria. Trans R Soc Trop Med Hyg 1990;84(Suppl):1.

83. Newton CRJC, Winstanley PA, Watkins WM, et al: A single dose of intramuscular sulfadoxine-pyrimethamine as an adjunct to quinine in the treatment of severe malaria: Pharmacokinetics and efficacy. Trans R Soc Trop Med Hyg 1993;87:207.

84. Fryauff DJ, Baird JK, Basri H, et al: Randomised placebo-controlled trial of primaquine for prophylaxis of falciparum and vivax malaria. Lancet 1995; 346:1190.

85. Ortel B, Sivayathorn A, Honigsmann H: An unusual combination of phototoxicity and Stevens-Johnson syndrome due to antimalarial therapy. Dermatologica 1989;178:39.

86. Miller KD, Lobel HO, Satriale RF: Severe cutaneous reactions among American travelers using pyrimethamine-sulfadoxine (Fansidar) for malaria prophylaxis. Am J Trop Med Hyg 1986;35:451.

87. Krotoski WA: Frequency of relapse and primaquine resistance in Southeast Asian vivax malaria. N Engl J Med 1980; 303:587.

88. Hien TT, White NJ: Qinghaosu. Lancet 1993;341:603.

89. White NJ: Artemisinin: Current status. Trans R Soc Trop Med Hyg 1994;88(Suppl):3.

90. Alecrim WD, Espinosa EM, Alecrim MG: *Plasmodium falciparum* infection in the pregnant patient. Infect Dis Clin North Am 2000;14:83–95.

91. World Health Organization: The role of artemisinin and its derivatives in the current treatment of malaria. Report of an Informal Consultation. WHO/MAL 1994;94:1067.

92. Chen PQ, Li GQ, Guo XB, et al: The infectivity of gametocytes of *Plasmodium falciparum* from patients treated with artemisinin. Chin Med J (Engl) 1994;107:709.

93. Mehra N, Bhasin VK: In vitro gametocytocidal activity of artemisinin and its derivatives on *Plasmodium falciparum*. Jpn J Med Sci Biol 1993;46:37.

94. World Health Organization: The use of artemisinin and its derivatives as antimalarial drugs. Report of an Informal Consultation. WHO/MAL/98. 1998;1086.

95. Qinghaosu Antimalarial Coordinating Committee: Antimalarial studies on quinghaosu. Chin Med J (Engl) 1979;92:811.

96. Brewer TG, Grate SJ, Peggins JO, et al: Fatal neurotoxicity of arteether and artemether. Am J Trop Med Hyg 1994;51:251.

97. Miller KD, Greenberg AE, Campbell CC: Treatment of severe malaria in the United States with a continuous infusion of quinidine gluconate and exchange transfusion. N Engl J Med 1989;321:65.

98. Phillips RE, Warrell DA, White NJ, et al: Intravenous quinidine for the treatment of severe falciparum malaria—Clinical and pharmacokinetic studies. N Engl J Med 1985;312:1273.

99. Hensbroek MBV, Onyiorah E, Jaffar S, et al: A trial of artemether or quinine in children with cerebral malaria. N Engl J Med 1996;335:69.

100. Hien TT, Day NPJ, Phu NJ, et al: A controlled trial of artemether or quinine in Vietnamese adults with severe falciparum malaria. N Engl J Med 1996;335:76.

101. Karbwang J, Na-Bangchang K, Thanavibul A, et al: A comparative trial of two different regimens of artemether plus mefloquine in multidrug resistant falciparum malaria. Trans R Soc Trop Med Hyg 1995;89:296.

102. Taylor TE, Wills B, Kazembre P, et al: Rapid coma resolution with artemether in Malawian children with cerebral malaria. Lancet 1993;341:661.

103. Kremsner PG, Winkler S, Brandts C, et al: Clindamycin in combination with chloroquine or quinine is an effective therapy for uncomplicated *Plasmodium falciparum* malaria in children from Gabon. J Infect Dis 1994;169:467.

104. White NJ, Waller D, Crawley J, et al: Comparison of artemether and chloroquine for severe malaria in Gambian children. Lancet 1992;339:317.

105. Levy M, Buskila D, Gladman DD, et al: Pregnancy outcome following first trimester exposure to chloroquine. Am J Perinatol 1991;8:174.

106. Nyirjesy P, Kavasya T, Axelrod P, et al: Malaria during pregnancy: Neonatal morbidity and mortality and the efficacy of chloroquine chemoprophylaxis. Clin Infect Dis 1993;16:127.

107. Steketee RW, Wirima JJ, Slutsker L, et al: Malaria prevention in pregnancy: The effects of treatment and chemoprophylaxis on placental malaria infection, low birth weight and fetal, infant and child survival. CDC-ARTS Publication 0994048. Washington, DC, U.S. Dept of Health and Human Services, 1994.

108. Alecrim WD, Albuquerque BC, Alecrim MGC, et al: Tratamento da malaria *P. falciparum* com clindamicina. II. Esquema posologico de cinco dias. Rev Inst Med Trop Sao Paulo 1982;24(Suppl):40.

109. Phillips RE, Soloman T: Cerebral malaria in children. Lancet 1990;336:1355.

110. Hoffman SL: In Hoffman SL (ed): Malaria Vaccine Development: A Multi-immune Response Approach. Washington, DC, American Society of Microbiologists, 1996.

111. Good MF, Doolan DL: Immune effector mechanisms in malaria. Curr Opin Immunol 1999;11:412.

112. Miller LH, Hoffman SL: Research toward vaccines against malaria. Nature Med 1998;5:520.

113. Facer CA, Tanner M: Clinical trials of malaria vaccines: Progress and prospects. Adv Parasitol 1997;39:1.

114. Weiner DB, Kennedy RC: Genetic vaccines. Sci Am 1999;281:50.

115. Lalvani A, Moris P, Voss G, et al: Potent induction of focused Th1-type cellular and humoral immune responses by RTS,S/SBAS2, a recombinant *Plasmodium falciparum* malaria vaccine. J Infect Dis 1999;180:1656.

116. Dammin GJ: Babesiosis. In Weinstein L, Fields B (eds): Semin Infect Dis, New York, Stratton, 1978, pp 169–199.

117. Gorenflot A, Moubri K, Precigout E, et al: Human babesiosis. Ann Trop Med Parasitol 1998;92:489.

118. Raoult D, Soulayrol L, Toga B, et al: Babesiosis, pentamidine, and cotrimoxazole. Ann Intern Med 1987;107:944.

119. Wittner M, Rowin KS, Tanowitz HB, et al: Successful chemotherapy of transfusion babesiosis. Ann Intern Med 1982;96:601.

120. Centers for Disease Control and Prevention: Clindamycin and quinine treatment for *Babesia microti* infections. MMWR Morb Mortal Wkly Rep 1983;32:65.

121. Wittner M, Lederman J, Tanowitz HB, et al: Atovaquone in the treatment of *Babesia microti* infections in hamsters. Am J Trop Med 1996;55:219.

122. Krause PJ, Telford S, Spielman A, et al: Treatment of babesiosis: Comparison of atovaquone and azithromycin with clindamycin and quinine [Abstract]. In Program and Abstracts of the 46th Annual Meeting of the American Society of Tropical Medicine and Hygiene, Lake Buena Vista, Fla, 1997. Northbrook. III, American Society of Tropical Medicine and Hygiene, 1997, p 247.

123. Machtinger L, Telford SR III, Inducil C, et al: Treatment of babesiosis by red blood cell exchange in an HIV-positive splenectomized patient. J Clin Apheresis 1993;8:78.

124. Jacoby GA, Hunt JV, Kosinski KS, et al: Treatment of transfusion-transmitted babesiosis by exchange transfusion. N Engl J Med 1980;303:1098.

125. Falagas ME, Klempner MS: Babesiosis in patients with AIDS: A chronic infection presenting as fever of unknown origin. Clin Infect Dis 1996;22:809.

INTERNET LOCATIONS FOR OBTAINING ADDITIONAL GENERAL INFORMATION ON MALARIA

- **World Health Organization (WHO) Site on Malaria**

Comprehensive information primarily aimed at doctors and researchers.

http://www.who.int/health-topics/malaria

It also contains details of the geographic distribution of malaria, the recommended drugs for each area,

http://www.who.int/ith/english/map3.htm

and the malaria situation for each country.

http://www.who.int/ith/english/country.htm

- **U.S. Centers for Disease Control and Prevention**

Authorized full adult and pediatric recommendations, including malaria risks and recommendations. See Travelers' Health section. Information also available via telephone (877-FYI-TRIP) or fax (888-232-3299). The CDC book *Health Information for International Travel* (the Yellow Book) can be downloaded from this site.

http://www.cdc.gov/travel/malinfo.htm

- **Malaria Foundation International**

This site provides wide general information about malaria, including a literature database, scientific information, details on global malaria initiatives, and so forth.

http://www.malaria.org

- **The Public Health Laboratory Services—Malaria Reference Laboratory**

In the United Kingdom this laboratory develops national policy on the prevention of imported malaria. This site provides general information for the clinician and the public and offers two telephone help lines. *Guidelines for the Prevention of Malaria in Travelers from the United Kingdom* can be downloaded from this site.

http://www.malaria-reference.co.uk

- **The International Society of Travel Medicine**

This is an organization of professionals dedicated to the advancement of the specialty of travel medicine. Its site has general information on travel health, including information on travel clinics.

http://www.istm.org/

- **Health Canada**

  Reliable recommendations and updates for preventing and treating malaria in travelers.

  http://www.hc-sc.gc.ca/hpb/lcdc/osh/tmp e.html

- **The Virtual Naval Hospital**

  This site enables medical professionals to download the Navy Medical Department Pocket Guide to Malaria Prevention and Control.

  http://www.vnh.org/Malaria/Malaria.html

- **The British Travel Health Association**

  http://www.btha.org

- **The International Society for Infectious Diseases**

  http://www.isid.org

- **The Swiss Tropical Institute**

  http://www.sti.unibas.ch

- **The Asian Collaborative Training Network for Malaria (ACT Malaria)**

  http://www.actmalaria.org

section
11

Zoonoses and Infections Associated with Outdoor Exposure

chapter
35

Rickettsioses, Q Fever, and Ehrlichioses

HAROLD W. HOROWITZ, MD

Infections due to organisms within the Rickettsiaceae family occur globally. Bacteria classified within this family are sometimes divided into the spotted fever group (those that tend to cause rashes), the typhus group, and others that include *Coxiella* and *Ehrlichia spp.* The bacteria (and the eponym[s] for the diseases that they cause) include *Rickettsia rickettsii* (Rocky Mountain spotted fever [RMSF]), *Rickettsia conorii* (boutonneuse fever, Mediterranean spotted fever, Israeli spotted fever, African spotted fever), *Rickettsia australis* (Queensland tick typhus), *Rickettsia sibirica* (North Asian tick typhus), *Rickettsia akari* (rickettsialpox), *Rickettsia prowazekii* (epidemic typhus and Brill-Zinsser disease or louse-borne typhus), *Rickettsia typhi* (endemic or murine typhus), *Orientia tsutsugamushi* (scrub typhus or chigger fever), *Ehrlichia chaffeensis* (human monocytic ehrlichiosis), *Anaplasma phagocytophila* (human granulocytic ehrlichiosis), *Ehrlichia ewingii*, and *Coxiella burnetii* (Q fever) (Table 35–1). With the exception of *C. burnetii*, these organisms have in common a reservoir in mammals and arthropod vectors in nature. Although *C. burnetii* may be found in ticks, it is likely that inhalation of aerosols and not ticks are the source of transmission to humans. Except for *C. burnetii*, they are obligate, intracellular parasites. *C. burnetii* can live outside the host cell for brief periods of time.

These infections tend to occur in relatively discrete geographic locales because of the requirement for specific transmission cycles. An understanding of which of these infections occurs in a particular locale and a detailed travel and exposure history from a febrile patient are important factors in deciding which, if any, of these infections need to be treated rapidly and possibly empirically. Delay in treatment can lead to severe illness and even death from some of these organisms such as *R. rickettsii* and *A. phagocytophila*. Several of the principles of prevention and treatment of these infections are listed in Table 35–2.

PREVENTION

Prevention of infection caused by most of the organisms within the Rickettsiaceae family may occur at several points in the transmission cycle of the specific organism. Public health measures may be required to decrease natural host populations. For instance, improved sanitation can decrease mouse or rat populations, the respective hosts for *R. akari* and *R. prowazekii*. People should use personal protective measures to either avoid or diminish contact with arthropod vectors such as ticks, fleas, and body lice. Use of protective clothing, tucking pants inside of socks, and insecticides can help to diminish the chances of being bitten by arthropod vectors. Depending upon the specific vector, transmission can be interrupted by prompt vector removal (i.e., ticks with tweezers or delousing with lindane powder or dichlorodiphenyltrichloroethane [DDT]).

TABLE 35–1 ■ **Epidemiologic Features of Selected Rickettsioses**

Organism	Disease	Vector	Geographic domains
Spotted fever group			
Rickettsia rickettsii	Rocky mountain spotted fever	Ixodid ticks	Western Hemisphere
Rickettsia conorii	Mediterranean spotted fever Boutonneuse fever	Ixodid ticks	India, Southern Europe, Africa
Rickettsia akari	Rickettsialpox	Mouse mite	Worldwide United States, South Korea, Africa, former Soviet Union
Typhus group			
Rickettsia prowazekii	Epidemic typhus	Human body	Endemic highlands of Americas, Asia, Africa
Rickettsia typhi	Murine typhus	Flea	Worldwide, especially coastal tropical and subtropical areas
Orientia tsutsugamushi	Scrub typhus	Larval mites	Asia, Australia, South Pacific
Coxiella burnetii	Q fever	? Ticks	Worldwide
Ehrlichioses			
Ehrlichia chaffeensis	Human monocytic ehrlichiosis	Lone Star tick	Southeastern United States, Europe
Ehrlichia phagocytophila	Human granulocytic (agent of HGE) ehrlichiosis	Ixodid ticks	United States, Europe
Ehrlichia ewingii		? Lone Star tick	Southern United States

TABLE 35–2 ■ **Principles of Prevention and Treatment of Infections due to Rickettsiaceae Family Bacteria**

PREVENTIVE MEASURES
1. Personal protective measures are important to prevent exposure to vectors.
2. Focal or more broad environmental insecticide use may be required to decrease the vector population.
3. No vaccines are commercially available for these diseases.
4. Pre- or postexposure antibiotic prophylaxis cannot be recommended except in select, extreme circumstances.

TREATMENT
1. Early treatment, empiric in highly endemic areas, may prevent severe sequelae of several of these diseases.
2. Oral therapy is used whenever possible.
3. Doxycycline is the drug of choice for all Rickettsiaceae family infections.
4. In selected situations, such as pregnant women, chloramphenicol may be the drug of choice.
5. For children, short-course doxycycline or chloramphenicol is the recommended antibiotic.
6. Quinolone antibiotics, and in some instances newer macrolides, appear promising for several of these infections.
7. Treatment of 5–10 d is generally used in practice, although single dose doxycycline therapy is effective with some diseases. The exception to this is the prolonged treatment necessary for chronic Q fever.

Pharmacologic intervention with "prophylactic" antibiotic treatment after exposure to specific arthropods is theoretically possible. However, data are lacking on the efficacy of postexposure prophylaxis for most of these infections. If intense exposure to specific vectors is anticipated, preventive antibiotics given prior to exposure may be useful in some diseases, such as scrub typhus.

It is anticipated that vaccination will someday play a major role in the prevention of these infections. It is possible that vaccines that are cross protective between rickettsial species can be developed. This hope is based upon experimental data demonstrating lymphoproliferative responses to antigens shared among several spotted fever group and typhus group species. Vaccines, however, are not currently available.

TREATMENT

Tetracyclines (tetracycline or doxycycline) and in some instances chloramphenicol are the antibiotics of choice for treatment of most of these infections (Table 35–3). Because it is better tolerated, requires fewer doses per day, and is safe for patients with renal impairment, doxycycline is preferred to tetracycline. Furthermore in those infections that can be treated with short-term therapy, doxycycline is preferred in children because it binds calcium considerably less than tetracycline does and therefore has less potential to stain teeth.[1] Because tetracycline staining of teeth is total-dose dependent, short course therapy should reduce the incidence of this complication.[2] Quinolone antibiotics and macrolides may have a role in the treatment of some of these infections, but there are few clinical data to recommend these as first-line agents. Macrolides, and in some scenarios rifampin, may be considered for the treatment of children and pregnant women. Duration of treatment varies for the various organisms within this family. There is little consensus on the optimal duration of therapy for these infections, at least in part because shorter duration of treatment is usually successful but may increase the incidence of relapses. Duration is frequently based upon clinical response. Data for

TABLE 35–3 ■ Antibiotic Choices for Treatment of Rickettsial Family Infections

Organism	Antibiotic and dosing	
	Adults	Children
Rickettsia rickettsii	**Choice:** doxycycline 100 mg bid × 5–7 d or until afebrile 2 d **Alternative:** chloramphenicol* 500 mg qid × 5–7 d or until afebrile 2 d **Pregnancy:** chloramphenicol as above	**Choice:** doxycycline 5 mg/kg/d in two divided doses × 5–7 d **Alternative:** chloramphenicol 50 mg/kg/d in 4 divided doses × 5–7 d†
Rickettsia conorii	**Choice:** doxycycline 100 mg qd × 1–5 d‡ **Alternatives:** chloramphenicol 500 mg qid × 7–10 d OR ciprofloxacin 750 mg bid × 5 d OR ofloxacin 400 mg bid × 5 d **Pregnancy:** chloramphenicol as above	**Choice:** doxycycline 2.5 mg/kg bid × 7 d OR clarithromycin 15 mg/kg/d in 2 divided doses × 7 d OR azithromycin 10 mg/kg/d as single dose × 3 d **Alternative:** chloramphenicol 50 mg/kg/d in 4 divided doses × 5 d
Rickettsia akari	**Choice:** doxycycline 100 mg bid × 2–5 d **Alternative:** chloramphenicol 500 mg qid × 2–5 d **Pregnancy:** chloramphenicol as above	**Choice:** doxycycline 2.5 mg/kg bid × 2–5 d **Alternative:** chloramphenicol 50 mg/kg/d in 4 divided doses × 2–5 d
Rickettsia prowazekii	**Choice:** doxycycline 100 mg bid × at least 5 d and until afebrile 2 d‡ **Alternative:** chloramphenicol 500 mg qid as for doxycycline **Pregnancy:** chloramphenicol as above	**Choice:** doxycycline 2.5 mg/kg bid × 5 d **Alternative:** chloramphenicol 50 mg/kg/d in 4 divided doses × 5–7 d
Rickettsia typhi	**Choice:** doxycycline 100 mg bid × at least 5 d and until afebrile 2 d§ **Alternative:** chloramphenicol 500 mg qid × 5–10 d **Pregnancy:** chloramphenicol as above	**Choice:** doxycycline 2.5 mg/kg qid × 5 d OR chloramphenicol 50 mg/kg/d in 4 divided doses × 5 d
Orientia tsutsugamuchi	**Choice:** doxycycline 100 mg bid × 7 d OR In Northern Thailand where there is doxycycline and chloramphenicol resistance, rifampin 450 mg bid × 7 d **Alternative:** chloramphenicol 500 mg qid × 7 d **Pregnancy:** chloramphenicol or in Northern Thailand as above	**Choice:** chloramphenicol 50 mg/kg/d in 4 divided doses × 5 d OR doxycycline 2.5 mg/kg bid × 5 d In northern Thailand rifampin 10 mg/kg bid (max 600 mg) × 7 d
Coxiella burnetii	**Acute Q fever** **Choice:** doxycycline 100 mg bid × 14–21 d‖ **Alternative:** erythromycin 1 g qid for mild disease × 14 d OR azithromycin 500 mg qid × 3–5 d OR a quinolone × 14 d **Chronic Q fever** **Choice:** doxycycline 100 mg bid plus either ciprofloxacin 750 mg bid or ofloxacin 200 mg tid	**Choice:** erythromycin 10 mg/kg qid × 14–21 d OR azithromycin 10 mg/kg on day 1, then 5 mg/kg qid × 4 d

Continued

TABLE 35–3 ■ Antibiotic Choices for Treatment of Rickettsial Family Infections (*Continued*)

| Organism | Antibiotic and dosing | |
	Adults	Children

	OR
	Any of above drugs plus rifampin 450 mg
	    bid × at least 3 y
	OR
	doxycycline as above plus hydroxychloroquine
	    200 mg tid × at least 2 y[#]
	Pregnancy: TMP-SMX (320 mg TMP plus
	    1600 mg SMX) daily (1 double-strength
	    co-trimazole BID) till term followed by 1 year
	    doxycycline plus hydroxychloroquine	

Ehrlichia chaffeensis	**Choice:** doxycycline 100 mg bid × 10–14 d
	Alternative: chloramphenicol 500 mg qid ×
	    10–14 d
	Pregnancy: consider chloramphenicol
		Choice: doxycycline 2.5 mg/kg bid × 10–14 d
		Alternative: chloramphenicol 50 mg/kg/d in a
		    divided dose × 10–14 d

Ehrlichia phagocytophila	**Choice:** doxycycline 100 mg bid × 10–14 d **Alternative:** possibly rifampin or quinolone **Pregnancy:** possibly rifampin 300 mg bid × 5 d	**Choice:** doxycycline 2.5 mg/kg bid × 5 d **Alternative:** possibly rifampin 10–20 mg/kg (max 600 mg) qd × 5 d
Ehrlichia ewingii	**Choice:** doxycycline 100 mg bid × 10–14 d **Alternative:** ? rifampin **Pregnancy:** ? rifampin	**Choice:** doxycycline 2.5 mg/kg bid × 5 d **Alternative:** ?

[*]Oral chloramphenicol not available in United States.

[†]For children who need intravenous, chloramphenicol 100 mg/kg/d in 4 divided doses.

[‡]Single dose therapy often successful in this disease.

[§]Recurrences with single dose therapy.

[‖]For patients with valvular heart disease consider doxycycline plus hydroxychloroquine regimen as for chronic disease for 21 days.

[¶]In severe pneumonia consider adding rifampin.

[#]Duration based upon serial antibody levels; measure hydroxychloroquine levels to keep 0.8 to 1.2 μg/ml.

recommendations of specific antibiotics are based upon nonstandardized in vitro testing of few isolates, limited in vivo animal studies, and mostly upon anecdotal responses of patients to therapy. Few large-scale, randomized, comparative trials between antimicrobial agents have been published.

RICKETTSIAE

Rickettsia rickettsii (Rocky Mountain Spotted Fever)

Prevention of Infection

INTERRUPTION OF TRANSMISSION CYCLE. *Dermacentor* spp ticks are the vectors for *R. rickettsii* transmission. In the eastern United States and the Far West *Dermacentor variabilis* (the American dog tick) is the major vector, and *Dermacentor andersoni* (the Rocky Mountain wood tick), *Rhipicephalus sanguineus*, and *Amblyomma cajennense* are the main vectors in western states, Mexico, and Central and South America, respectively. Ticks may walk on the body for hours before actually feeding. A good body search after potential exposure to ticks allows one

to remove ticks prior to being bitten. Prompt removal of ticks with a tweezer to remove all tick body parts may help to decrease transmission. Human exposure to ticks may also be decreased by treating household pets such as dogs with insecticides to rid them of *Dermacentor* spp ticks.[3]

ANTIBIOTIC PROPHYLAXIS. Human studies of antibiotic prophylaxis to prevent RMSF have not been made. In a guinea pig model of RMSF a single dose of oxytetracycline prevented disease when it was given within 48 hours of the expected onset of disease. Relapses occurred when treatment was given more than 48 hours before disease onset.[4] Currently, preventive antibiotic therapy prior to exposure or after a tick bite is not recommended.

VACCINATION. No vaccine to prevent *R. rickettsii* infection is currently available.[5] Early attempts to develop a vaccine used either a phenolized suspension of infected ticks[6] or formalin-killed rickettsiae propagated in chick embryos.[7] Neither proved effective in protecting adult human volunteers from *R. rickettsii* infection.[8] More recently, immunodominant surface protein antigens that measure 190- and 135-kDa by SDS-PAGE (Omp A and

Omp B, respectively) have been identified and cloned.[9] Omp A is an adhesin allowing rickettsiae to attach to cells. A protein of the Omp A size has been found in many of the spotted fever group of rickettsiae. An outer membrane protein that seems to be similar to Omp B has been found, cloned, and sequenced in typhus group rickettsiae.[5] The respective proteins from *R. rickettsii* and *R. prowazekii* demonstrate 78% nucleotide and 65% deduced amino acid similarity.[10,11] Immunization with Omp A in a baculovirus vector protects guinea pigs against challenge with *R. rickettsii*.[12] In other studies, vaccinating with a cloned Omp A product has provided some cross-protection between rickettsial strains. Recombinant *R. conorii* rOmp A provided partial protection against infection with *R. rickettsii* in guinea pigs.[13] The duration of immunity induced using these cloned protein products has not been studied. Protection afforded by cloned rOmp B has been less well studied.[5]

Spotted fever group T lymphocyte–stimulating epitopes might provide cross-protection between *R. rickettsii*, *R. typhi*, and *R. prowazekii*. After *R. conorii* infection, lymphoproliferative responses to *R. conorii* antigens as well as antigens from *R. rickettsii* and *R. sibirica* have been demonstrated.[14]

Treatment

Early antibiotic therapy of RMSF is essential to limit the severity of disease.[15] In general, oral therapy should be used unless the patient cannot tolerate oral therapy. A tetracycline antibiotic, in particular doxycycline, is the drug of choice to treat RMSF.[16] The dose of doxycycline is 100 mg twice daily and that for tetracycline is 25 to 50 mg/kg/d. Chloramphenicol also has been used with success at a dose of 50 to 75 mg/kg/d given in four divided doses per day. Chloramphenicol, however, may not be as effective as doxycycline for the treatment of RMSF,[15a] (Table 35–3).

In vitro studies have demonstrated that *R. rickettsii* are susceptible to doxycycline, rifampin, ciprofloxacin, ofloxacin, pefloxacin, josamycin, and clarithromycin.[17] The organism is reported to be resistant to β-lactam antibiotics, TMP-SMX, and gentamicin.[17] Ives et al have demonstrated good in vitro activity of azithromycin, clarithromycin, and roxithromycin against *R. rickettsii*.[18] The active metabolite of clarithromycin, 14-hydroxy-clarithromycin, demonstrates markedly more activity than the parent compound in vitro (minimum inhibitory concentration [MIC] of clarithromycin 8 µg/ml compared to 0.45 µg/ml for 14-hydroxy-clarithromycin).[19]

An animal model using *R. rickettsii* infection of dogs has demonstrated that chloramphenicol, enrofloxacin, and tetracycline are equally active for treatment of RMSF.[20] Another study using the dog model for RMSF has shown that trovafloxacin is equal to doxycycline and more effective than azithromycin for treatment of RMSF.[21] In the latter study, time to defervescence was slower in the azithromycin group and the number of eye lesions was not as low as in controls.[21] Although quinolones and several of the newer macrolide antibiotics (excluding erythromycin) have good in vitro activity against *R. rickettsii*, there are too few data to recommend them as primary agents for RMSF treatment.

In children a short course of doxycycline should not cause significant tooth staining. Doxycycline binds about 10-fold less calcium than tetracycline does.[1] Despite the potential risks of doxycycline, because of the severity of the illness and the fact that at least in the United States oral chloramphenicol is not available, doxycycline is frequently chosen as the drug of choice for RMSF in children. During pregnancy, tetracyclines can retard fetal long bone and tooth growth and rarely cause severe hepatitis or pancreatitis in the pregnant woman; therefore tetracyclines generally are not prescribed for pregnant women. In more severely ill patients, because of its efficacy, doxycycline is probably the preferred agent even during pregnancy.

Duration of therapy for RMSF has not been comprehensively studied. Although a few days of doxycycline may be all that is needed for treatment, many physicians treat for about 5 to 7 days or until 2 to 3 days after a patient is afebrile.[16]

In severely ill patients supportive care is a necessity. Respiratory, cardiac, and renal functions may need to be supported. With antimicrobial therapy, mortality has decreased to less than 5%.[15a,22] Corticosteroids have been used to treat severely ill patients but have not been adequately studied. In a dog model, corticosteroids neither helped nor hindered the response to treatment.[23]

Rickettsia conorii (Boutonneuse Fever, Mediterranean Spotted Fever, Israeli Spotted Fever)

Prevention of Infection

INTERRUPTION OF TRANSMISSION CYCLE. The ixodid tick vector for *R. conorii* is the brown dog tick *Rhipicephalus sanguineus*. Treating dogs with insecticide washes or sprays or treating the animals' living areas with insecticides may help to control the tick population.[3]

ANTIBIOTIC PROPHYLAXIS. Prevention of infection after exposure to ticks that potentially harbor *R. conorii* has not been adequately studied and is not recommended.

VACCINATION. No vaccine is currently available to prevent *R. conorii* infection. A surface protein of 198 kDa that is analogous to the 190-kDa surface protein of *R. rickettsii* has been cloned and expressed in *Escherichia coli*.[24] Guinea pigs immunized with lysates of an *E. coli* strain expressing the recombinant gene product were protected from infection with homologous *R. conorii* strains.[24] Another *R. conorii* 112- to 120-kDa protein that is cytoplasmic and is not related to rOmp A or rOmp B appears to be immunogenic.[25] Lymph node cells from mice immunized with lysates of *E. coli* expressing this recombinant protein proliferate when exposed to *R. conorii* in vitro. Both these proteins may be candidates for a subunit vaccine. Adoptive transfer and cell depletion experiments in a mouse model demonstrate that clearance of *R. conorii* from endothelial cells requires immune CD8[+] T lymphocytes.[26] Therefore any vaccine candidate will likely need to stimulate this T cell subset.

Treatment

Although clinical disease due to *R. conorii* may be self-limited, is rarely fatal, and is generally milder than infection due to *R. rickettsii*,[27] treatment is generally recommended. Two doses of doxycycline 100 mg in one day has been shown to be as effective as a 10-day course of tetracycline for treatment of *R. conorii* infection in a randomized study of 70 patients by Bella-Cueto et al.[28] Doxycycline treatment for 1 to 5 days is the recommended treatment of choice[16,17] (Table 35–3). However, tetracycline (25 mg/kg/d), chloramphenicol (2 g/d for 7 to 10 days), or quinolone antibiotics such as ciprofloxacin (750 mg twice daily) and ofloxacin (200 mg twice daily) have been used with success to treat *R. conorii* infection.[16,29–31] Single dose ofloxacin (400 mg) failed in four patients with Mediterranean spotted fever when 200 mg twice daily was successful.[16] Because response to this dose of ofloxacin was slower than the response to doxycycline or ciprofloxacin, 400 mg twice daily was recommended by the authors.[16]

The activity of erythromycin against *R. conorii* in vitro is limited (MIC values of 4 to 8 μg/ml),[32] and clinical failure has been reported with this agent.[33] In a randomized trial of erythromycin and tetracycline in 81 children, clinical symptoms and fever disappeared more rapidly in the tetracycline arm than in the erythromycin group.[33] Several newer macrolide antibiotics including clarithromycin and azithromycin demonstrate variable activity in vitro activity against *R. conorii*.[18,34] In a study of 75 children with Mediterranean spotted fever clarithromycin at a dose of 15 mg/kg/d orally in two divided doses led to more rapid defervescence than did chloramphenicol 50 mg/kg/d orally in 4 divided doses.[35] Treatment was for 7 days. Clinical outcome was similar in the two groups.[35] In an open-label, randomized study of the treatment of 87 children younger than 8 years with Mediterranean spotted fever, clarithromycin (15 mg/kg/day in 2 divided doses for 7 days) was equivalent to azithromycin (10 mg/kg/day in 1 dose for 3 days).[35a] Azithromycin has the potential advantages in that it is given once daily and could be given for only 3 days. Josamycin, a macrolide not available in the United States, compared favorably to doxycycline in a study comparing 5 days of josamycin to 2 doses of doxycycline.[29] All 59 patients infected with *R. conorii* recovered without problems. Josamycin or other new macrolides may be of use for the treatment of children and pregnant women.

Rifampin has been found to have excellent in vitro activity.[34] However, in comparison to two doses of doxycycline 100 mg, defervescence took longer in patients using rifampin (10 mg/kg every 12 hours).[36] Four of fifteen patients took more than 5 days to become afebrile and were considered clinical treatment failures in a small study by Bella and colleagues.[36] Rifampin should not be considered first-line therapy for this infection.

In pregnant women and children a single dose of doxycycline 200 mg has been recommended.[16] Chloramphenicol is an alternative therapy for children. For pregnant women the role of the newer macrolides has not been established.

Rickettsia akari (Rickettsialpox)

Prevention of Infection

INTERRUPTION OF TRANSMISSION CYCLE. *R. akari* infection is transmitted by bites of the mite *Liponyssoides sanguineus*. The mouse *Mus musculus* is the preferred host for the mite. Rickettsialpox is frequently reported from urban areas because of the mouse habitat. Control of the mouse population from human habitats by antirodent measures can help to reduce transmission. Personal protection measures such as the use of repellents applied to the skin or clothing and spraying of infested terrain with residual insecticides such as hexachlorocyclohexane (HCH), malathion, or propoxur can reduce infection by deterring or reducing the mite population.[3]

ANTIBIOTIC PROPHYLAXIS. No data suggest that antibiotic prophylaxis is successful or warranted, and therefore it is not recommended.

VACCINATION. No vaccine is currently available. Cross-protection between infection with *R. akari* and other spotted-fever group rickettsiae has been postulated because of the high degree of serologic cross-reactivity.[37] Moreover, Coonrod and Shepard demonstrated that lymphocytes from patients infected with *R. rickettsii* proliferate when exposed to *R. akari* antigen.[38] However, guinea pigs infected with *R. akari* were not protected against experimental infection with *R. rickettsii*.[37] There are no well-established human data to suggest such cross-protection. The observation that recrudescence and reinfection with *R. akari* are rare or nonexistent raises the possibility that long-lasting immunity develops in humans. This may allow for the development of a durable vaccine.

Treatment

Rickettsialpox is generally self-limited with resolution occurring within 2 to 3 weeks of infection.[39] Headache and fatigue, however, can last even longer. Death is rare. With a tetracycline antibiotic treatment, symptoms resolve within 48 hours, and recurrence is rare. Treatment of 2 to 5 days appears to be adequate[39,40] (Table 35–3).

Chloramphenicol (50 mg/kg/d in 4 divided doses) has also been employed successfully to treat rickettsialpox.[39] For children and pregnant women a short course of doxycycline (100 mg twice daily) or chloramphenicol would be recommended choices of therapy.

In vitro, clarithromycin and azithromycin have activity against R. akari,[18] and these antibiotics may prove useful for the treatment of children and pregnant women with this infection. Currently, however, no clinical data support the use of these antibiotics for the treatment of R. akari infection.

Rickettsia prowazekii (Epidemic Typhus, Louse-Borne Typhus, Recrudescent Typhus, Brill-Zinsser Disease)

Prevention of Infection

INTERRUPTION OF TRANSMISSION CYCLE. R. prowazekii is transmitted to humans by infected lice and louse feces.[41] Disease can arise in a population when appropriate cultural, political, and socioeconomic conditions develop such that the louse population is high and transmission of lice can be from person to person. Although the frequency of outbreaks has decreased since the Second World War, as recently as 1997 there was a large outbreak of epidemic typhus in Burundi.[41] Other outbreaks occurred in 1997 in Russia and in 1975 in Peru. The disease can be the most epidemic of the rickettsioses but can also occur endemically or sporadically. Nonimmune contacts of louse-infected persons are at risk for contracting the disease, albeit infrequently. Infection with R. prowazekii is an occupational hazard for health care providers. Patients suspected of having lice should be decontaminated. Clothing and bedding can be treated with heat that kills the lice as well as rickettsiae.[41]

Control of the louse population will decrease transmission of R. prowazekii. In a large jail outbreak the immediate control of epidemic typhus was effected by use of insecticides.[42] However, because of the need to repeat insecticide applications every 6 weeks and the large quantity of insecticide needed, this is not always feasible. Bathing and laundering of clothes in hot water can help to eliminate exposure to lice. When meticulous care to avoid lice is not possible, however, use of insecticide dusts such as 1% lindane, 1% malathion, 10% DDT, or newer carbamates on clothing can reduce exposure.[41] Unfortunately louse resistance to several of these insecticides has been reported.[3,43–45] Treating clothing with permethrin or diethyltoluamide is hypothesized, but not proven, to reduce exposure to R. prowazekii.[3] In areas where conditions permit a high population of lice that cannot be controlled, insecticides will be less effective, and resistance may develop. Because lice usually reside mostly in clothing where they lay their eggs, leaving only to feed, delousing of persons is not the main part of eradication. Long-term control of lice depends upon removing the political, cultural, and economic obstacles to cleanliness in the society.

ANTIBIOTIC PROPHYLAXIS. A single dose of doxycycline 100 mg once or twice weekly may provide protection for persons who are intensively exposed for a short time in special conditions.[46] This idea has not been formally tested, and neither the dose nor frequency of antibiotic administration is known. Furthermore, when prophylaxis is discontinued, disease might develop.

VACCINATION. Several inactivated R. prowazekii vaccines were developed in the 1930s and 1940s that were administered subcutaneously and elicited minor local or systemic reactions.[47] For each vaccine, few volunteers were studied, and the vaccine was either partially or completely effective in protecting the volunteers against disease when they were challenged with R. prowazekii.[47] An attenuated vaccine of R. prowazekii, E strain, also provides partial or complete protection against illness. This vaccine is not available currently. No controlled, large-scale studies using these vaccines have been undertaken to demonstrate efficacy.

Subunit vaccines using the cloned gene for the immunodominant 135-kDa surface protein or serotype-specific polypeptide antigen (SPA) are being developed but have not yet been tested in humans.[48] SPA purified by high-performance liquid chromatography (HPLC) from various strains of R. prowazekii provided partial or complete protective immunity from infection with R. prowazekii in a guinea pig model.[5] Other cloned products also can be tested because of the construction of a R. prowazekii gene library.[5]

Treatment

Epidemic typhus is an acute illness that has an associated mortality ranging from less than 10% to nearly 60% depending upon such factors as age, prior infection, and nutritional status. In some instances the causative organism persists in tissues and will recrudesce years after the first episode (Brill-Zinsser disease). Treatment with appropriate antimicrobials generally reduces the duration of illness to 24 to 48 hours and virtually prevents death.[46] For patients able to tolerate oral therapy, doxycycline 100 mg twice daily or chloramphenicol 500 mg four times daily are the recommended agents of choice[16] (Table 35–3). These antibiotics have approximately similar efficacy.[49,50] TMP-SMX worked less well in a clinical trial by Huys et al.[49] For persons too ill to take these medications by mouth, intravenous preparations of these drugs are available. Although a single dose of doxycycline (200 mg) may cure epidemic typhus with few or no relapses,[50–52] it is common to treat epidemic typhus for longer periods.

On the basis of in vitro studies the newer macrolides clarithromycin (MIC 0.125–1 µg/ml) and azithromycin (MIC 0.25 µg/ml) have activity against R. prowazekii. Rifampin (MIC 0.06–0.25 µg/ml) and the quinolones ciprofloxacin (MIC 0.5–1 µg/ml), ofloxacin (MIC 1 µg/ml), and pefloxacin (MIC 1 µg/ml) also have excellent activity against this organism.[17–19] Clinical data are limited for treatment with these antimicrobials, and they cannot at this time be recommended for first-line therapy. A severely ill patient treated with ciprofloxacin 500 mg twice daily died after 1 day of treatment.[53] The duration of treatment was clearly too short to make recommendations about quinolone use based on this single case. Azithromycin failure has been reported in two patients with Brill-Zinsser disease. Therefore this drug cannot be recommended for treatment of this entity until further data are available.[54] These patients were treated for 3 days with 500 mg of azithromycin.

Children are probably best treated with a few doses of doxycycline or chloramphenicol, and pregnant women should be treated with chloramphenicol. The treatment of Brill-Zinsser disease is similar to that of acute infection. However, single dose doxycycline (200 mg) may be adequate in most cases.

Rickettsia typhi (Murine Typhus)

Prevention of Infection

INTERRUPTION OF TRANSMISSION CYCLE. Murine typhus is a zoonosis that is maintained by a cycle in which small animals, primarily rats (*Rattus rattus* and *Rattus norvegicus*), are the hosts upon which fleas (*Xenopsylla cheopis* and others) feed. During subsequent feeds, probably by fleas defecating into the host wounds, the organism is transmitted. *R. typhi* is transmitted transovarially in fleas that are infected for life. Less commonly, it appears that *R. typhi* can be transmitted through inhalation of infected flea or rat feces or in the laboratory. The infection is not spread from person to person. Murine typhus is found worldwide, particularly in coastal areas of temperate and subtropical areas.[55]

Disease can be avoided by avoiding endemic foci where fleas and rats abound. Flea control of pets in endemic areas is another important way to reduce human exposure to fleas. Insecticide sprayed on clothing may also help to decrease transmission. Control of rat and flea populations is critical in interrupting the transmission cycle. During attempts to control the rat population, it is essential to have a flea control program such as an insecticide application. If such a program is not in place, fleas leave their rodent hosts and feed upon humans. Dusts using residual pesticides that kill immature flea stages that live in the homes of animals are the mainstay of most flea control programs. Resistance to organochlorines such as DDT, HCH, and dieldrin among several *Xenopsylla* spp has been reported.[3]

ANTIBIOTIC PROPHYLAXIS. Short-term antibiotic use after exposure to a flea to prevent infection with *R. typhi* is currently not recommended.

VACCINATION. At this time, no vaccine is available to prevent murine typhus. A killed vaccine was developed but was not shown to protect volunteers experimentally infected after vaccination.[55] Both cellular and humoral immunity appear to play a role in protection.[56] Surface proteins of 120 to 135 and 17 kDa and a 68 to 70-kDa polypeptide that may be a heat shock protein are recognized in sera of convalescent infected animals and humans.[55] Whether these are protective is not known. In laboratory animals, immunity may not be sterile because organisms can be grown for prolonged periods after antibiotics are stopped. Whether this occurs in humans is not known.[55]

Treatment

Without treatment, mortality due to murine typhus is reported to be in the range of 1% to 2%.[56] However, fever can last for weeks (average 15 days) in untreated patients.[57,58] Doxycycline (100 mg twice daily) is the first-line agent for treatment of *R. typhi* infection. Oral chloramphenicol (500 mg four times daily) is an alternative but may not be as effective as doxycycline because relapses have been reported.[59] Patients who cannot tolerate oral therapy can be treated with intravenous doxycycline (100 mg twice daily) or chloramphenicol (50 to 75 mg/kg/d in four divided doses). Although single dose doxycycline is effective in most patients,[60] treatment is generally continued for 2 to 3 days after resolution of fever, typically 5 to 10 days. Fever typically resolves within a median of 72 hours after antibiotics are initiated (Table 35–3).

In vitro studies have demonstrated that doxycycline is the most efficacious antibiotic with MIC values of 0.06 to 0.125 μg/ml.[17] Other antibiotics with in vitro activity against *R. typhi* include the quinolones ciprofloxacin (MIC 0.5 to 1 μg/ml), ofloxacin (MIC 1 μg/ml), and pefloxacin (MIC 1 μg/ml), the macrolides erythromycin (MIC 0.125–1 μg/ml), clarithromycin (MIC 0.5–1 μg/ml), and josamycin (MIC 0.5–1 μg/ml), and rifampin (MIC 0.06–0.25 μg/ml).[17] A few clinical cases of murine typhus have been treated successfully with ciprofloxacin.[61,62]

Short courses of doxycycline or chloramphenicol are probably the safest choices for pregnant women and children.

Orientia tsutsugamushi (Formerly Rickettsia tsutsugamushi) (Scrub Typhus)

Prevention of Infection

INTERRUPTION OF TRANSMISSION CYCLE. Scrub typhus is endemic to a broad geographic locale in eastern Asia including eastern China, Taiwan, Vietnam, India, Korea, the Philippines, Sri Lanka, South Pacific islands, New Guinea, and parts of Australia. The reservoir is trombiculid mites, primarily but not exclusively *Leptotrombidium deliense*. Larval forms (chiggers) are the only vectors for this disease and feed only once during their lifetime. Although *Rattus* rats can serve as hosts for infection, in nature *O. tsutsugamushi* is mainly maintained via transovarial transmission in the mite.

O. tsutsugamushi is host specific and does not infect the trombiculid mites in the Americas, Europe, or Africa. Therefore disease is not found in these regions. Because mites reside within a few yards of where they hatch, endemic pockets are highly focal. Scrub typhus is a misnomer as the range of *O. tsutsugamushi* includes rain forests and mountain deserts. Limiting exposure by applying insect repellants such as dibutyl phthalate, diethyltoluamide, and benzyl benzoate to skin and clothing (lower pants and tops of boots and socks) and by not lying or sitting on the ground can be tried but may prove impractical among those who are exposed occupationally.[3] Residual insecticide spraying of infected terrain with malathion, propoxur, or HCH may help control the mite population.[3]

ANTIBIOTIC PROPHYLAXIS. Doxycycline (200 mg weekly) has been tested in exposed troops and in experimental infection with a reasonable degree of success in preventing scrub typhus.[63,64] In a double-blinded and placebo-controlled trial using doxycycline 200 mg weekly among 1125 soldiers exposed to scrub typhus in a hyperendemic area, Olson et al reported a fivefold decrease in the incidence of scrub typhus among treated individuals.[63] In experimentally infected persons studied by Twartz et al an 89% efficacy of weekly doxycycline was found.[64] Mild disease occurred after discontinuation of doxycycline in some patients, and some eschars were found.[64] In a series of placebo-controlled studies, Smadel and colleagues examined the potential of chloramphenicol (in several different dosing regimens from daily through weekly) to prevent scrub typhus.[65,66] Chloramphenicol was markedly less successful than doxycycline.[65,66] After discontinuation of chloramphenicol, relapses occurred long after exposure had ceased. There was no difference in the frequency of scrub typhus or its intensity. However, fewer individuals developed eschars.[65,66] Although data are limited for the use of antibiotics to prevent scrub typhus in persons intensively exposed to *O. tsutsugamushi*, doxycycline chemoprophylaxis can be considered.

VACCINATION. There are currently no effective human vaccines against *O. tsutsugamushi*. This organism has a great amount of genetic heterogeneity with diverse antigenicity even within a defined geographic locale. This antigenic diversity and the fact that infection with one strain does not necessarily provide protection from infection by other strains makes development of a vaccine difficult. A 54- to 56-kDa outer surface protein appears to be the most abundant surface protein.[5] However, other major surface proteins with molecular masses from 25 to 165 kDa have been identified.[4] The 56-kDa protein from *O. tsutsugamushi* (Boryong strain) has been fused with a maltose-binding protein and used to vaccinate mice.[5] Vaccination led to stimulation of T cell– and B cell–dependent immune responses and to protection of mice infected with *O. tsutsugamushi*.[5] Ongoing research is aimed at determining the most immunogenic proteins.

Treatment

Early treatment, often empiric, is essential to reduce the duration of disease and prevent severe disease and mortality. Doxycycline 100 mg twice daily for approximately 7 days is the treatment of choice (Table 35–3). Chloramphenicol in doses of 50 to 75 mg/kg/d is also effective treatment.[16,67,68] With these therapies, defervescence usually occurs within 24 to 36 hours.[67] Tetracyclines, however, appear to reduce symptoms earlier than chloramphenicol does. In a comparative study of chloramphenicol and tetracycline by Sheehy et al 33% of patients given chloramphenicol became afebrile within 24 hours compared to 77% prescribed tetracycline.[67] Doxycycline treatment courses as short as one dose, or two doses separated by 7 days, have been used, and in most cases have been successful.[69] A comparative study of single-dose doxycycline vs. 7 days of tetracycline therapy (500 mg four times a day) demonstrated both to be equally effective without relapse.[69] However, disease recrudescence may be more frequent with shorter courses than with more prolonged treatment.[63] When possible, oral therapy should be used.

Recently in northern Thailand a strain of *O. tsutsugamushi* that is resistant to doxycyline and chloramphenicol was reported.[70] Fever clearance by day 3 of treatment was uniform in a western region of Thailand not harboring this strain, but it cleared in only 5 of 12 patients from the northern region. In a mouse model and cell cultures, strains from this northern Thailand region were less susceptible to chloramphenicol and doxycycline. A treatment trial in this region demonstrated that rifampin in doses of 900 mg daily for 7 days led to more rapid fever clearance and a higher proportion of patients with complete fever resolution by 48 hours than did rifampin 600 mg daily or doxycycline 100 mg twice daily.[71] Furthermore there were two relapses among patients who took doxycycline and none among patients who used rifampin-based therapy. Interestingly a third arm of this randomized study used rifampin plus doxycycline combination therapy. This arm was abandoned because of lack of efficacy.[71] A caveat regarding the use of rifampin monotherapy for 1 week in the developing world is the potential for inducing *Mycobacterium tuberculosis* resistance. If such therapy is contemplated for a given patient, it would be worthwhile to rule out active tuberculosis.

There are few data regarding alternatives to doxycycline, chloramphenicol, and perhaps rifampin for treatment of scrub typhus. Azithromycin has been demonstrated in vitro, using a mouse fibroblast cell culture system, to be more active than doxycycline against doxycycline-susceptible and doxycycline-resistant strains of *O. tsutsugamushi*.[72] In a BalbC mouse model of *O. tsutsugamushi* infection, all animals treated with ciprofloxacin or chloramphenicol survived compared to no survival among gentamicin-treated animals.[73] In one report ciprofloxacin 500 mg twice daily for 3 days was effective in the treatment of scrub typhus in one patient; defervescence occurred within 24 hours.[62] Quinolones may prove to be alternatives to doxycycline and chloramphenicol. More clinical data are needed regarding the efficacy of the quinolones for treatment of scrub typhus before they can be recommended as first-line therapy.

Short course doxycycline is the current treatment of choice for scrub typhus in children and pregnant women. However, if the in vitro data using azithromycin are confirmed in clinical studies and larger studies using rifampin confirm the initial in vivo data with this drug, azithromycin or rifampin or both may offer alternatives to short course doxycycline for the treatment of these specific populations.

Severe illness may occur, particularly among patients infected with drug-resistant organisms or among those with a delay in diagnosis. Supportive care and close attention to fluid management is crucial for the severely ill patients who may be hypotensive with capillary leak syndromes due to vasculitis.

Other Spotted-Fever Rickettsiae

Numerous spotted-fever rickettsiae associated with specific geographic locales are the agents responsible for diseases that frequently carry the name of the region where the disease is present. Examples of these organisms are *Rickettsia australis* (Queensland tick typhus), *Rickettsia sibirica* (Siberian or North Asian tick typhus), *Rickettsia africae* (African tick-bite fever), *Rickettsia honei* (Flinders Island spotted fever), and *Rickettsia japonica* (Japanese or Oriental spotted fever). Other rickettsiae, such as *Rickettsia helvetica*, which is found in Scandinavia, and *Rickettsia felis*, which is found in south and southwestern United States and the Yucatan Peninsula in Mexico, also cause disease in humans. Clinical data on treatment of these diseases is limited. However, in situations in which doxycycline has been used to treat, patients have fared well.

Limited in vitro data demonstrate that *R. sibirica*, *R. australis*, *R. japonica*, *R. honei*, *R. helvetica*, and *R. africae* are susceptible to rifampin, clarithromycin, josamycin, ciprofloxacin, ofloxacin, and pefloxacin.[17]

COXIELLA BURNETII (Q FEVER)

Prevention of Infection

INTERRUPTION OF TRANSMISSION CYCLE. *C. burnetii* is found worldwide, and humans are infected by inhalation of aerosolized particles containing the organism. There are numerous reservoirs for *C. burnetii* including mammals, birds, and ticks. Cattle, goat, and sheep are the major sources of human infection. Exposures to the placentas of infected mammals, contaminated wool, and aerosols from newborn animals have been implicated in transmission to humans. Raw milk is also a potential route of infection because pregnant mammals can shed *C. burnetii* in milk. Although tick bite transmission is hypothesized, tick bites have not been reported to directly transmit *C. burnetii*. Rarely *C. burnetii* has been reported to have spread between humans after contact with infected parturient women, by blood transfusion, or via inhalation of infectious particles at autopsy.[74]

Decreasing exposure to *C. burnetii*-infected animals is considered a major way to avoid infection. Culture of *C. burnetii* should be done with careful laboratory security (biosafety level 3 conditions), and research animals should be free of infection, that is, seronegative, before transfer to laboratories. Drinking only pasteurized milk and ectoparasite control of sheep, cattle, and goats are measures that may also help decrease transmission of *C. burnetii*. Infected female sheep, goats, and cattle should be isolated, and it is important to disinfect their placentas. Spread of *C. burnetii* to health care workers or within hospitals due to aerosolization of particles is rare, and patients with suspected infection need not be isolated.

VACCINATION. *C. burnetii* is unique among rickettsiae because it demonstrates host-dependent phase variation. In fresh isolates and animals, phase I is found. Phase II develops after repeated passage in embryonated chicken eggs. The two phases differ in several ways including the organism's ability to agglutinate, resistance to phagocytosis, staining properties, and antigens. An immune response to phase I antigens has been associated with protective immunity. A commercially available vaccine made from a phase I formalin-inactivated whole cell strain (Henzerling strain) of *C. burnetii* prepared by the Ormsbee method[75] has been shown to provide nearly complete protection from acute Q fever. These studies have been performed in the high-risk group of abattoir workers in Australia.[75,76] The duration of protection is at least 5 years.[76] This vaccine preparation is not available in the United States.

A problem with the formalin-inactivated vaccine preparation is that sterile abscesses, granulomas, and severe local reactions may develop in patients who have existing antibodies to *C. burnetii*. Therefore vaccinees require preliminary immunologic testing for prior *C. burnetii* exposure. A chloroform-methanol extraction of phase I whole cells (chloroform-methanol residue vaccine [CMR]) was developed to try to alleviate this problem. In a hairless guinea pig model the CMR vaccine led to fewer local reactions than the whole cell vaccine did[77] and was efficacious when guinea pigs were exposed to *C. burnetii* aerosol.[78] The dose required to protect 50% of mice was one-third that of the whole cell vaccine but four times the dose of the whole cell vaccine in guinea pigs.[78] In goats and sheep with prior antibodies to *C. burnetii* no severe reactions were noted with the CMR vaccine.[79]

This suggests that the vaccine is safe in animals previously exposed to *C. burnetii*. Humans tested with the CMR vaccine developed some local erythema and induration at higher doses (120 and 240 µg).[80] The vaccine appears immunogenic in humans. IgG responses were seen in up to 40% of individuals given the 240-µg dose. Peripheral blood T cell proliferative responses to *C. burnetii* recall antigens were of low magnitude and transient in 40% of recipients at the 240-µg dose.[80] Although this vaccine is still being tested, the results so far have been disappointing. Even with this more highly purified vaccine, prior skin testing may be required because the doses that confer immunity produce local reactions.

An outer membrane protein of 67 kDa from phase I *C. burnetii* QiYi strain has been purified and led to anti–67 K antibody production and in vitro lymphocyte stimulation responses in guinea pigs and mice.[81] Furthermore intraperitoneal immunization with the 67 K protein led to 100% protection from challenge in mice and guinea pigs.[81] This protein may be a candidate for a subunit vaccine against Q fever.

Although epidemiologic data are limited regarding the extent of the population at high risk for exposure to *C. burnetii*, persons such as abattoir workers and veterinarians who work with infected animals are clearly high-risk groups that should be considered for vaccination when a safe vaccine becomes available.

ANTIBIOTIC PROPHYLAXIS. Studies evaluating the use of antibiotic prophylaxis after exposure to *C. burnetii* are lacking. Currently there are no recommendations to give such therapy.

Treatment

Q fever may present as an acute infection,[81a] typically pneumonia but rarely hepatitis or meningoencephalitis, or as a chronic infection.[82,82a] Chronic Q fever most typically is manifested by endocarditis. Endovascular infections of aneurysms or vascular prostheses, infection of bone, and rarely chronic lung and liver infection also have been reported as forms of chronic Q fever.[74]

ACUTE DISEASE. Diagnosis of acute Q fever is difficult. Therefore it is often treated empirically based upon potential exposure. Although patients with acute Q fever often have self-limited disease that can be treated symptomatically, because of the fear of chronic disease, therapy is generally preferred. In acutely infected cells, all antibiotics tested to date are bacteriostatic, except perhaps for quinolones.[83,84] For patients with acute disease, even bacteriostatic therapy is generally sufficient to allow recovery.

Tetracyclines, particularly doxycycline (100 mg twice daily), have been recommended as the treatment of choice for acute Q fever[82] (Table 35–3). Chloramphenicol has also been used to treat acute Q fever.[85] A few persons have been treated with pefloxacin, ofloxacin, or levofloxacin

with cure of infection.[86,87] During treatment of acute Q fever pneumonia tetracycline and the quinolones have been reported to decrease the duration of disease by 2 days.[86,88] In one study this effect was limited to patients presenting within the first 3 days of cough.[88] In vitro studies indicate that *C. burnetii* is resistant to erythromycin. However, clinical responses to macrolides have been reported for milder disease.[89–91] Marrie has noted that severe pneumonia does not respond to erythromycin even at high doses.[82] Addition of rifampin 300 mg twice daily to erythromycin led to cure of patients failing erythromycin therapy.[82] Azithromycin as a single dose of 1.5 g or 500 mg daily for 3 days for the treatment of community-acquired pneumonia led to cure of the six patients with serologically documented *C. burnetii*.[91] Five of these patients received the single dose therapy.

Recently Fenollar and colleagues reported that patients with acute Q fever treated with doxycycline (100 mg twice daily) plus hydroxychloroquine (200 mg three times daily) had fewer episodes of endocarditis than patients treated with doxycycline alone.[92] The authors suggested that this regimen be considered for the treatment of acute Q fever, particularly for patients with cardiac valve abnormalities, who have a markedly increased incidence of endocarditis after acute Q fever than those without such lesions have.[92]

For children, short course treatment with doxycycline, rifampin, or azithromycin is a possible alternative to longer courses of doxycycline for treatment of acute Q fever.

Q FEVER IN PREGNANCY. Acute Q fever during pregnancy can lead to catastrophic outcomes if untreated or treated inadequately.[92a] Abortions, neonatal death, premature births, low birth weights, or in 29% of cases no abnormalities have been reported.[92b,92c] Both chronic infections and relapses have also been reported after acute disease during pregnancy.[92b] The outcome is affected by the trimester of infection, with first trimester infections leading to poorer outcomes than later trimester infections. Treatments with long-term doxycycline and quinolone antibiotics are contraindicated in pregnancy. Raoult et al recently reported that treatment of pregnant women developing acute Q fever during pregnancy with TMP-SMX (320 mg of trimethoprim in combination with 1600 mg of sulfamethoxazole) until term protected against abortion but not colonization of the placenta.[92a] This regimen also did not protect against the development of chronic infection in the women.[92a] Treatment with doxycycline plus hydroxychloroquine for a year after pregnancy led to elimination of infection and susequent pregnancies were normal.[92a]

The strategy of using TMP-SMX for the duration of pregnancy followed by doxycycline plus hydroxychloroquine may be the preferred regimen for treating pregnant women with acute Q fever until further data are forthcoming.

CHRONIC DISEASE. In vitro studies using a persistently infected fibroblast L929 cell line have demonstrated that the quinolones (ciprofloxacin, difloxacin, and oxolinic acid) and rifampin are the most effective antibiotics.[93] Doxycycline, chloramphenicol, and trimethoprim appear to be less effective.[93] Tetracycline, gentamicin, erythromycin, sulfamethoxazole, and penicillin G were ineffective in this model.[93] Models of chronic Q fever that use cyclohexamide to block cell division (thereby causing persistent cell line infection) or that use persistently infected cell lines have shown that quinolones are less effective in this setting than in models of acute infection.[83,94] During chronic in vitro culture conditions, no antibiotic is bactericidal for *C. burnetii*. Attempts to demonstrate synergism between antibiotics in chronically infected cells have shown that ciprofloxacin plus doxycycline was not synergistic but that ciprofloxacin plus rifampin acted synergistically.[82]

Endocarditis is the most common and serious form of chronic Q fever. It is estimated to occur in approximately 5% to 7.5% of patients with Q fever.[92,95] Most persons with Q fever endocarditis have underlying valvular disease; patients frequently have prosthetic valves in place.[96–98] Although the interval between acute disease and the development of endocarditis has not been well defined, Q fever is often overlooked in the differential diagnosis of culture-negative endocarditis, leading to estimated delays in diagnosis of more than 12 months. Diagnostic clues to Q fever endocarditis are not specific and include hypergammaglobulinemia, liver involvement, and thrombocytopenia.[99] Steroids have also been implicated in delaying the diagnosis of Q fever endocarditis because of symptom and fever suppression.[100] Steroids have also been suspected of exacerbating quiescent disease.[101]

Serologic studies are most commonly used to make the diagnosis of Q fever endocarditis. A complement fixation antibody of 1:200 or higher or an indirect immunofluorescence antibody titer of 1:400 or higher to phase I antigen is considered diagnostic for Q fever endocarditis. In acute Q fever, antibody titers to phase I antigens do not reach this level. An IgG antibody titer of 1:800 or higher to phase I antigen by microimmunofluorescence was found by Fournier et al to be diagnostic of Q fever endocarditis.[102] Peacock and colleagues have reported that high phase-specific IgA antibody titers by indirect immunofluorescence were diagnostic for Q fever endocarditis.[103]

Serologic studies are also used to monitor disease progression. Mortality is significant with rates varying from 5% to over 60%.[97,104,105] Optimal treatment regimens are not known, and relapse of infection has been reported after prolonged treatment regimens and heart valve replacement.[106] This poor cure rate is probably at least in part due to the lack of bactericidal effects of antibiotics against *C. burnetii*.

Tetracycline or doxycycline has been used with some success to treat Q fever endocarditis.[88] Although doxycycline can produce some clinical improvement while it is being taken, disease can recur even after years of therapy.[95,104,107] In fact, treatment may need to be indefinite when valve replacement is not performed. Mortality is still in the range of 50% with tetracycline or doxycycline monotherapy. TMP-SMX has been reported to be successful in the treatment of several cases of Q fever endocarditis.[97,99,108] Ciprofloxacin monotherapy (500 mg orally twice daily) led to defervescence, decreased splenomegaly, and a decreased sedimentation rate in one patient reported by Yebra et al.[109] At the time of that report the patient had been on 18 months of continuous therapy. Others have reported successful treatment of Q fever endocarditis with quinolone monotherapy in a few patients.[110,111]

Because of poor responses to monotherapy, combination drug therapies have been used with variable success. Rifampin plus TMP-SMX did not lead to cure after 5 months of combination therapy in one patient reported by Subramanya and colleagues.[112] Combination therapy using a quinolone (pefloxacin or ofloxacin [200 mg three times daily] plus doxycycline (100 mg twice daily) enhanced patient survival in a group of 32 patients reported by Levy et al.[113] In that study, 6 of 9 patients treated with doxycycline alone were considered treatment failures compared to 1 of 16 patients who received doxycycline plus a quinolone. Raoult et al reported five patients receiving doxycycline plus ofloxacin who were cured after more than 4 years of therapy.[105] However, one patient died and seven had relapses among the 14 patients treated with this combination. Tetracycline plus rifampin (450 mg twice daily) has shown some efficacy in the treatment of Q fever endocarditis.[98,114] Doxycycline combined with rifampin for 6 months followed by doxycycline alone appeared to be more efficacious than doxycycline alone in one small study by Raoult and colleagues.[115] For patients who undergo valve replacement, rifampin may be problematic for long-term treatment because of its interaction with coumadin.

Doxycycline plus chloroquine is an intriguing combination therapy based upon the alkalinizing effects of chloroquine in lysosomes. Raoult and colleagues demonstrated that bactericidal activity of doxycycline could be restored when cells were incubated with chloroquine in vitro.[98] A clinical trial subsequently was performed employing this principle.[105] Twenty-one patients took doxycycline 100 mg twice daily plus hydroxychloroquine 200 mg three times a day (maintaining levels of 0.8 to 1.2 μg/ml by drug level monitoring). Of the 18 patients with data collection complete at the time of the report, cure was achieved in 17 patients. There was one death due to surgical complications. Of note is the fact that no patient treated for longer than 18 months had a relapse. In this study the mortality was only 5% in the two comparator arms, doxycycline plus ofloxacin vs. doxycycline plus hydroxychloroquine. Four of the treatment failures in the doxycycline plus ofloxacin cohort were switched to doxycycline plus hydroxychloroquine. Three of these patients were cured. In both treatment groups hyperphotosensitivity was reported in nearly all patients. Patients taking hydroxychloroquine should have intermittent retinal exam inations because of potential retinal accumulation of drug. Only one patient had to stop drug for this reason in Raoult and colleagues' experience.

The recent studies reporting decreased mortality with the use of quinolones in combination with other antibiotics or doxycycline plus hydroxychloroquine must be interpreted in light of the fact that the investigators reporting these data are well versed in the clinical presentation and diagnostic evaluation of Q fever endocarditis. It is likely that the time to diagnosis of infection was shorter in these studies than in earlier reports. Therefore responses may have been better than in prior reports.

A major question that remains unanswered is the duration of treatment for Q fever endocarditis. Antibody titers are followed during treatment. Raoult and Marrie believe that levels of phase I IgA and IgG of 1:200 or lower indicate cure.[74] In 1991 Levy et al recommended that treatment continue at least 3 years because none of the 32 patients they followed who had Q fever endocarditis were cured after 2 years of therapy.[113] It is of note that Raoult and Marrie have not observed decreases of antibody levels to 1:200 or lower within 3 years.[74] This recommendation was modified in 1999 when the doxycycline plus chloroquine results were published. At that time Raoult and colleagues recommended that regimens using doxycycline and ofloxacin should be prescribed for at least 4 years.[105] However, doxycycline plus chloroquine should be given for 18 months to no longer than 4 years[105] (Table 35–3).

Surgical treatment is required for patients with cardiac decompensation or recurrent emboli. After surgery it is probably best to continue therapy for at least several years because prosthetic valve infection occurs when therapy is discontinued even years after the prosthetic valve placement.[116]

EHRLICHIAE

Members of the genus *Ehrlichia* share a common ancestor with members of the genus *Rickettsia*. These two genera, however, can be differentiated genetically by differing antigenic components and by the cells that they infect. *Ehrlichia* spp form clusters in host cell vacuoles termed *morulae*. The major ehrlichial pathogens in the United States and Europe are zoonoses that are transmitted by tick bites. These organisms have only recently been reported to cause human disease: *Ehrlichia sennetsu* (1953 in Japan),[117] *Ehrlichia chaffeensis* (1986 in the United States),[118] the *Anaplasma phagocytophila* Agent (1994 in the United States),[119] and *Ehrlichia ewingii* (1999 in the United States).[120]

Although the specific taxonomy is still being characterized, organisms within the genus *Ehrlichia* can be divided into three genetic-antigenic groups.[121] The first group comprises *E. chaffeensis*, *E. ewingii*, *Ehrlichia canis*, *Ehrlichia muris*, and *Cowdria ruminatium*. *E. chaffeensis* is the major human pathogen within this group. However, a few cases of *E. ewingii* have been reported in the United States.[120] *E. muris* infects Japanese voles and ticks, and *C. ruminantium* infects ruminants. The second major cluster includes *A. phagocytophila*, which is nearly identical to *Ehrlichia equi*; *Ehrlichia platys*; and *Anaplasma marginale*. The human granulocytic ehrlichiosis agent is the only human pathogen within this group and is nearly identical to the bacteria *E. phagocytophila* and *E. equi*. The last ehrlichial group includes *E. sennetsu*, *Ehrlichia risticii*, and *Neorickettsia helminthoeca*. *E. sennetsu* is the only human pathogen within this group. This latter group differs genetically from the other two enough that it may soon be reclassified as another genus.[121]

Ehrlichia chaffeensis (Human Monocytic Ehrlichiosis)

Prevention of Infection

INTERRUPTION OF TRANSMISSION CYCLE. *E. chaffeensis* appears to be transmitted by the Lone Star tick, *Amblyomma americanum*, in the south central and southeastern United States.[122] In other areas of the United States such as the Midwest and Northwest and in Europe and Africa *D. variabilis* ticks are infected and may be the vector.[121] At least in the southern area of the United States where *E. chaffeensis* is found, white-tailed deer may be the major reservoir for *E. chaffeensis*. Infection can be found naturally and induced experimentally in these deer. Prevention of infection depends upon wearing appropriate clothing to avoid tick exposure, using insect repellents, and early removal of ticks via careful body searches.

ANTIBIOTIC PROPHYLAXIS. There are no studies to date to indicate that use of antibiotics after a tick bite will prevent *E. chaffeensis*.

VACCINATION. To date no vaccines have been developed for protection against *E. chaffeensis* infection. Major outer membrane proteins such as p30 have been identified. However, the ability of these antigens to stimulate a protective host immune response is not known. Experimentally, dogs can be reinfected with the closely related organism *E. canis* when rechallenged after cure from a prior infection.[123] Although dogs may self-cure *E. canis* infection even without antibiotic treatment, chronic, subclinical *E. canis* infection has been reported in dogs.[124] If the immune response in humans to infection with *E. chaffeensis* parallels that of dogs to *E. canis*, then it is likely that a vaccine will be difficult to develop against *E. chaffeensis*.

Treatment

In cell culture assays using DH82 cells, doxycycline and rifampin are rapidly bactericidal for *E. chaffeensis*; minimum bactericidal concentrations of these antibiotics are 0.5 μg/ml and 0.125 μg/ml, respectively.[125] Chloramphenicol, ciprofloxacin, erythromycin, cotrimazole, penicillin, and gentamicin are ineffective in vitro.[125] There are no published randomized, comparative trials for the treatment of human monocytic ehrlichiosis (HME). However, data on treatment have been collected in observational cohort studies. The choice of antibiotics has been based at least in part upon treatment of canine ehrlichiosis. In dogs experimentally infected with *E. canis*, tetracycline and doxycycline generally lead to rapid clinical improvement during acute infection.[123,126,127] Alternatively, chloramphenicol, penicillin, sulfadimethoxine, and sulfacetamide have been ineffective in the treatment of *E. canis* in dogs.[128] *E. canis* can be identified after treatment of acute infection in dogs even after clinical improvement and also can be isolated after doxycycline treatment in some chronically infected dogs.[121]

In a review of the clinical, epidemiologic, and laboratory findings of 40 patients identified as infected with *E. canis* (now designated *E. chaffeensis*) doxycycline, tetracycline, and chloramphenicol were all effective treatment choices.[129] The median range to defervescence was 2 days for tetracycline or doxycycline, chloramphenicol, and the aminoglycosides. Defervescence occurred by day 4, 6, 8, and 10 for cephalosporins, penicillins, erythromycin, and TMP-SMX, respectively. Hospitalization appeared to be prevented by the early use of antibiotics.[129] Fishbein and associates expanded upon the initial study cited above.[129] In 1994 they reported the results of treatment of 237 patients with *E. chaffeensis* infection.[130] In this review, patients who were prescribed tetracycline or chloramphenicol within 8 days of illness were less likely to require hospitalization and less likely to die.[130] Furthermore patients who were severely ill had more rapid recovery after hospitalization if they were given one of these antibiotics as opposed to other antibiotics.

In a study by Schutze et al doxycycline (4 mg/kg/d in two divided doses) was used to treat 12 children less than 15 years of age (range 7 months to 13½ years) with rapid recovery in eight.[131] Four patients who presented with shock had complicated courses. The children were treated for 10 to 14 days without short-term adverse reactions.[131] Although shorter courses of doxycycline might be effective for treatment of HME and might have less potential for tooth staining, until further data are available, 10 days of treatment is probably warranted in children.

Besides an acute febrile illness that can lead to death, particularly in the elderly if untreated, *E. chaffeensis*

can cause a more indolent infection and be identified as a fever of unknown origin. Roland et al reported that 6 of 41 patients who were not promptly diagnosed had prolonged fevers of 17 to 51 days prior to diagnosis.[132] In two cases, ciprofloxacin therapy failed. However, doxycycline in a dose of 100 mg twice daily led to clinical improvement rapidly, within 3 to 5 days in four patients and 7 days in another patient. Time to defervescence was not reported in the other patient.

On the basis of the limited clinical data available, doxycycline 100 mg twice daily is the agent of choice for HME (Table 35–3). Treatment is generally prescribed for approximately 14 days.

Anaplasma phagocytophila (the Human Granulocytic Ehrlichiosis Agent)

Prevention of Infection

INTERRUPTION OF TRANSMISSION CYCLE. HGE has been reported in those regions where Lyme borreliosis occurs. In the United States the disease is mainly found in the upper Midwest and the Northeast with some cases also reported from the Northwest. It has also been reported in many areas of Europe. *A. phagocytophila* is transmitted by the bites of *Ixodes* spp ticks.[133] These ticks also are the vectors for the transmission of *Borrelia burgdorferi* and *Babesia microti*. It appears that *A. phagocytophila* is transmitted after bites by either adult or nymphal ticks. Therefore the transmission season tends to extend beyond that for Lyme disease.

Mouse models of HGE agent transmission have revealed somewhat differing results regarding the time for larvae to transmit the HGE agent.[134,135] Hodzik et al reported larval transmission of infection to mice occurred between 40 and 48 hours after attachment.[134] Des Vignes and colleagues reported a shorter time before transmission, 24 hours.[135] This difference is significant with regard to the potential role that tick removal may play in preventing infection due to these bacteria. Measures to prevent tick bites such as the use of insect repellents and the use of long-sleeved shirts and long pants with the end of the pants tucked into socks may reduce tick exposure. Furthermore careful searches of the entire body for attached ticks and prompt removal may prevent transmission of *A. phagocytophila* by limiting the time of feeding.

ANTIBIOTIC PROPHYLAXIS. No data suggest that treatment either before or after exposure is protective against infection. Therefore antibiotic prophylaxis after a tick bite is not recommended. However, with the recent report of successful prevention of Lyme disease with one dose (200 mg) of doxycycline,[136] it can be expected that prophylaxis for tick bites will become more widespread. It will be interesting to determine whether this is protective for HGE also.

VACCINATION. To date no vaccine is available for the HGE agent. A 44-kDa immunodominant outer surface protein has been identified by several groups.[137,138] Limited data in a mouse model suggest that passive immunization with monoclonal antibodies to this antigen provide protection to challenge with the HGE agent.[139] In the short term, prior infection can lead to immunity. Barlough et al demonstrated that prior infection of a horse with the HGE agent led to protection from reinfection with the closely related species *E. equi* 8 weeks after the initial infection.[140] However, prior infection does not provide complete immunity. In horses and sheep infected with *E. equi*, there is partial but not complete protection when animals are rechallenged.[141,142] Antibody responses decline to low levels in approximately 50% of humans during the first year after infection.[143,144] Furthermore reinfection with the HGE agent has been demonstrated in a human approximately 1 year after the first infection at a time when antibody responses had waned.[143] Therefore because natural infection does not necessarily provide durable immunity, a protective vaccine may be difficult to develop.

Treatment

In vitro studies of the susceptibility of *A. phagocytophila* to antibiotics are limited. To date only nine isolates have been tested with some or all of the antibiotics reported below.[145,146] Because the organism only recently has been cultivated[147] and the cell culture assay is time consuming, antibiotic susceptibility testing on this organism rarely has been performed. In vitro, *E. phagocytophila* is uniformly susceptible to doxycycline, rifampin, and quinolone antibiotics including ciprofloxacin, trovafloxacin, ofloxacin, and levofloxacin.[145,146] In vitro, *E. phagocytophila* is resistant to chloramphenicol, amoxicillin, ceftriaxone, erythromycin, azithromycin, clarithromycin, amikacin, gentamicin, clindamycin, TMP-SMX, and imipenem-cilastatin.[145,146]

In vivo responses in animals have demonstrated that dwarf goats infected with *E. phagocytophila* respond to treatment with oxytetracycline and sulfadimidine but not to ampicillin.[148] Horses infected with *E. equi* have rapid clinical and laboratory improvement when treated with tetracycline.[149]

No controlled studies of the treatment of HGE infection have been reported. In studies of cohorts of patients who were followed with serial clinical and laboratory evaluations, doxycycline 100 mg twice daily was rapidly effective[144,151] (Table 35–3). Clinical improvement including defervescence frequently occurs within 48 hours, even in extremely ill patients.[145] Rifampin has been used in two pregnant women with apparent success.[152] In several patients ampicillin treatment did not lead to defervescence after 1 to 2 weeks of therapy.[151] However, fever resolved within 24 to 48 hours after switching to doxycycline.[151] Treatment failures with erythromycin[144] and cephalosporins[145] have been reported.

Studies reporting limited numbers of patients must be interpreted with caution because HGE may be self-limited in most patients. In seroprevalence studies from Wisconsin, nearly 15% of people tested had antibodies demonstrating prior infection. However, none of these seropositive people gave a clinical history compatible with HGE infection.[153] Because this disease can be quite serious, leading to intensive care unit admission and even death,[144,151,154] particularly in the elderly, treatment should be offered to patients suspected clinically of having HGE.

Duration of treatment is generally 10 to 14 days. However, much shorter duration of treatment may lead to cure. Treatment for as little as 1 day may be sufficient to cure *A. phagocytophila* infection.[146] Because coinfection with the HGE agent and *B. burgdorferi* has been demonstrated in humans,[155] longer treatment duration for HGE is often prescribed.

Rifampin may be an alternative to doxycycline in children and pregnant women. Alternatively a short course of doxycycline in children or pregnant women may be advisable. An infected neonate was treated successfully with a 5-day course of doxycycline.[156] On the basis of in vitro data, quinolones may be alternative antibiotics for patients with intolerance to tetracyclines for the treatment of HGE. However, no cases of successful quinolone treatment of humans with HGE have been reported.

Ehrlichia ewingii

Prevention of Infection

INTERRUPTION OF TRANSMISSION CYCLE. *E. ewingii* appears to be transmitted by the Lone Star tick, *A. americanum*. Personal protective methods to avoid tick exposure and early removal of feeding ticks should decrease the chance of infection.

ANTIBIOTIC PROPHYLAXIS. No data support the use of antibiotics to prevent infection when persons are either bitten by ticks or are exposed to Lone Star ticks. Use of such prophylaxis is not recommended.

VACCINATION. No vaccine is currently available.

Treatment

Dogs with *E. ewingii* infection respond to treatment with doxycycline.[157] To date only four human *E. ewingii* infections have been reported.[120] These patients all responded to doxycycline. The two patients who had data reported on duration of therapy received approximately 14 days of doxycycline. Data on clinical response to other antibiotics have not been reported. Doxycycline 100 mg twice daily would be the recommended treatment at this time (Table 35–3).

REFERENCES

1. Forti G, Benincori C: Doxycycline and the teeth. Lancet 1969;1:782.
2. Grossman ER, Walchek A, Freedman H: Tetracyclines and permanent teeth: The relation between dose and tooth color. Pediatrics 1971;47:567–570.
3. Robert LL: Control of arthropods of medical importance. In Strickland GT (ed): Hunter's Tropical Medicine and Emerging Infectious Diseases, 8th ed. Philadelphia, WB Saunders, 2000, pp 1019–1034.
4. Kenyon RH, Williams RG, Oster CN, et al: Prophylactic treatment of Rocky Mountain spotted fever. J Clin Microbiol 1978;8:102–104.
5. Schuenke KW, Walker DH: Vaccine development for rickettsial infections: Rocky Mountain spotted fever, epidemic typhus, and scrub typhus. In Plotkin SA, Orenstein WA (eds): Vaccines, 3rd ed. Philadelphia, WB Saunders, 1999, pp 527–543.
6. Spencer RR, Parker RR: Rocky Mountain spotted fever. Vaccination of monkeys and man. Public Health Rep 1925;40:2159–2167.
7. Cox HR: Rocky Mountain spotted fever. Protective value for guinea pigs of vaccine prepared from rickettsiae cultivated in embryonic chick tissues. Public Health Rep 1939;54:1070–1077.
8. DuPont HL, Hornick RB, Dawkins AT, et al: Rocky Mountain spotted fever: A comparative study of the active immunity induced by inactivated and viable pathogenic Rickettsia rickettsii. J Infect Dis 1973;128:340–344.
9. Vishwanath S: Antigenic relationships among the rickettsiae of the spotted fever and typhus groups. FEMS Microbiol Lett 1991;65:341–344.
10. Carl M, Dobson ME, Ching WM, et al: Characterization of the gene encoding the protective paracrystalline-surface layer protein of Rickettsia prowazekii: Presence of a truncated identical homolog in Rickettsia typhi. Proc Natl Acad Sci USA 1990;87:8237–8241.
11. Gilmore RD Jr, Cieplak W Jr, Policastro PF, et al: The 120 kilodalton outer membrane protein (rOmpB) of Rickettsia rickettsii is encoded by an unusually long open reading frame: Evidence for protein processing from a large precursor. Mol Microbiol 1991;5:2361–2370.
12. Sumner JW, Sims KG, Jones DC, et al: Protection of guinea pigs from experimental Rocky Mountain spotted fever by immunization with baculovirus-expressed Rickettsia rickettsii rOmpA protein. Vaccine 1995;13:29–35.
13. Vishwanath S, McDonald GA, Watkins NG: A recombinant Rickettsia conorii vaccine protects guinea pigs from experimental boutonneuse fever and Rocky Mountain spotted fever. Infect Immun 1990;58:646–653.
14. Jerrells TR, Jarboe DL, Eisemann CS: Cross-reactive lymphocyte responses and protective immunity against other spotted fever group rickettsiae in mice immunized with Rickettsia conorii. Infect Immun 1986;51:832–837.
15. Fishbein DB, Frontini MG, Giles R, et al: Fatal cases of Rocky Mountain spotted fever in the United States, 1981–1988. Ann NY Acad Sci 1990;590:246–247.
15a. Holman RC, Paddock CD, Curns AT, et al: Analysis of risk factors for fatal Rocky Mountain spotted fever: Evidence for superiority of tetracycline therapy. J Infect Dis 2001;184:1437–1444.
16. Raoult D, Drancourt M: Minireview: Antimicrobial therapy of rickettsial diseases. Antimicrob Agents Chemother 1991;35:2457–2462.
17. Rolain JM, Maurin M, Vestris G, et al: In vitro susceptibilities of 27 rickettsiae to 13 antimicrobials. Antimicrob Agents Chemother 1998;42:1537–1541.

18. Ives TJ, Manzewitsch P, Regnery RL, et al: In vitro susceptibilities of Bartonella henselae, B. quintana, B. elizabethae, Rickettsia rickettsii, R. conorii, R. akari, and R. prowazekii to macrolide antibiotics as determined by immunofluorescent antibody analysis of infected Vero cell monolayers. Antimicrob Agents Chemother 1997;41:578–582.
19. Ives TJ, Marston EL, Regnery RL, et al: In vitro susceptibilities of Rickettsia and Bartonella spp. to 14-hydroxy-clarithromycin as determined by immunofluorescent antibody analysis of infected Vero cell monolayers. J Antimicrob Chemother 2000;45:305–310.
20. Breitschwerdt EB, Davidson MG, Aucoin DP, et al: Efficacy of chloramphenicol, enrofloxacin, and tetracycline for treatment of experimental Rocky Mountain spotted fever in dogs. Antimicrob Agents Chemother 1991;35:2375–2381.
21. Breitschwerdt EB, Papich MG, Hegarty BC, et al: Efficacy of doxycycline, azithromycin, or trovafloxacin for treatment of experimental Rocky Mountain spotted fever in dogs. Antimicrob Agents Chemother 1999;43:813–821.
22. Kirk JL, Fine DP, Sexton DJ, et al: Rocky Mountain spotted fever: A clinical review based on 48 confirmed cases, 1943–1986. Medicine 1990;69:35–45.
23. Breitschwerdt EB, Davidson MG, Gegarty BC, et al: Prednisolone at anti-inflammatory or immunosuppressive dosages in conjunction with doxycycline does not potentiate the severity of Rickettsia rickettsii infection in dogs. Antimicrob Agents Chemother 1997;41:141–147.
24. Vishwanath S, McDonald GA, Watkins NG: A recombinant Rickettsia conorii vaccine protects guinea pigs from experimental boutonneuse fever and Rocky Mountain spotted fever. Infect Immun 1990;58:646–653.
25. Schuenke KW, Walker DH: Cloning, sequencing and expression of the gene coding for an antigenic 120-kilodalton protein of Rickettsia conorii. Infect Immun 1994;62:904–909.
26. Feng J-m, Popov VL, Yuoh G, et al: Role of T lymphocyte subsets in immunity to spotted fever group rickettsiae. J Immunol 1997;158:5314–5320.
27. Font-Creus B, Bella-Cueto F, Espejo-Arenas E, et al: Mediterranean spotted fever: A cooperative study of 227 cases. Rev Infect Dis 1985;7:635–642.
28. Bella-Cueto F, Font-Creus F, Segura-Porta F, et al: Comparative, randomized trial of one-day doxycycline versus 10-day tetracycline therapy for Mediterranean spotted fever. J Infect Dis 1987;155:1056–1058.
29. Bella F, Font B, Uriz S, et al: Randomized trial of doxycycline versus josamycin for Mediterranean spotted fever. Antimicrob Agents Chemother 1990;34:937–938.
30. Raoult D, Gallais H, De Micco P, et al: Ciprofloxacin therapy for Mediterranean spotted fever. Antimicrob Agents Chemother 1986;30:606–607.
31. Bernard E, Carles M, Politano S, et al: Rickettsiosis caused by Rickettsia conorii: treatment with ofloxacin. Rev Infect Dis 1989;11(Suppl 5):S989–S991.
32. Raoult D, Roussellier P, Tamalet J: In vitro evaluation of josamycin, spiramycin, and erythromycin against Rickettsia rickettsii and R. conorii. Antimicrob Agents Chemother 1988;32:255–256.
33. Munoz-Espin T, Lopez-Pares P, Espejo-Arenas E, et al: Erythromycin versus tetracyline for treatment of Mediterranean spotted fever. Arch Dis Child 1986;61:1027–1029.
34. Raoult D, Roussellier P, Vestris G, et al: In vitro antibiotic susceptibility of Rickettsia rickettsii and Rickettsia conorii: Plaque assay and microplaque colorimetric assay. J Infect Dis 1987;155:1059–1062.
35. Cascio A, Colomba C, Di Rosa D, et al: Efficacy and safety of clarithromycin as treatment for Mediterranean spotted fever in children: A randomized controlled trial. Clin Infect Dis 2001;33:409–411.

35a. Cascio A, Colomba C, Antinori S, et al: Clarithromycin vs. Azithromycin in the treatment of Mediterranean spotted fever in children. Clin Infect Dis 2002;34:154–158.

36. Bella F, Espejo E, Uriz S, et al: Randomized trial of 5-day rifampin versus 1-day doxycycline therapy for Mediterranean spotted fever. J Infect Dis 1991;164:433–434.

37. Heubner RJ, Stamps P, Armstrong C: Rickettsialpox. A newly recognized rickettsial disease. I. Isolation of the etiological agent. Public Health Rep 1946;61:1605–1614.

38. Coonrod JD, Shepard CC: Lymphocyte transformation in rickettsioses. J Immunol 1971;106:209–216.

39. Brettman LR, Lewin S, Holzman RS, et al: Rickettsialpox: Report of an outbreak and a contemporary review. Medicine 1981;60:363–372.

40. Rose HM: The treatment of rickettsialpox with antibiotics. Ann NY Acad Sci 1952;55:1019–1026.

41. Raoult D, Roux V: The body louse as a vector of reemerging human disease. Clin Infect Dis 1999;29:888–911.

42. Bis G, Coninx R: Epidemic typhus in a prison in Burundi. Trans R Soc Trop Med Hyg 1997;91:133–134.

43. Clark PH, Cole MM: Resistance of body lice to carbaryl. J Econ Entomol 1967;60:398–400.

44. Miller RN, Wisseman CL, Sweeney GW, et al: First report of resistance of human body lice to malathion. Trans R Soc Trop Med Hyg 1972;66:372–375.

45. Sholdt LL, Seibert DJ, Holloway ML, et al: Resistance of human body lice to malathion in Ethiopia. Trans R Soc Trop Med Hyg 1976;70:532–533.

46. Olson JG: Epidemic louse-borne typhus. In Strickland GT (ed): Hunter's Tropical Medicine and Emerging Infectious Diseases, 8th ed. Philadelphia, WB Saunders, 2000, pp 430–433.

47. Woodward TE: Rickettsial vaccines with emphasis on epidemic typhus: Initial report of an old vaccine trial. S Afr Med J 1986;11(Suppl);73–76.

48. Dasch A: Isolation of species-specific protein antigens of *Rickettsia typhi* and *Rickettsia prowazekii* for immunodiagnosis and immunoprophylaxis. J Clin Microbiol 1981;14:333–341.

49. Huys J, Freyens P, Kayihigi J, et al: Treatment of epidemic typhus: A comparative study of chloramphenicol, trimethoprim-sulfamethoxazole, and doxycycline. Trans R Soc Trop Med Hyg 1973;67:718–721.

50. Krause DW, Perine PL, McDade JE, et al: Treatment of louse-borne typhus fever with chloramphenicol, tetracycline or doxycycline. E Afr Med J 1975;52:421–427.

51. Perine PL, Awoke S, Krause DW, McDade JE: Single-dose doxycycline treatment of louse-borne relapsing fever and epidemic typhus. Lancet 1974;ii:742–744.

52. Raoult D, Ndihokubwayo JB, Tissot-Dupont H, et al: Outbreak of epidemic typhus associated with trench fever in Burundi. Lancet 1998;352:353–358.

53. Zanetti G, Francioli P, Tagan D, et al: Imported epidemic typhus. Lancet 1998;352:1709.

54. Turcinov D, Kuzman I, Herendic B: Failure of azithromycin in treatment of Brill-Zinsser disease. Antimicrob Agent Chemother 2000;44:1737–1738.

55. Higgins JA, Azad AF: Murine flea-borne typhus. In Strickland GT (ed): Hunter's Tropical Medicine and Emerging Infectious Diseases, 8th ed. Philadelphia, WB Saunders, 2000, pp 434–435.

56. Murphy JR, Wisseman CL, Fiset P: Mechanisms of immunity in typhus infection: Analysis of immunity to *Rickettsia mooseri* infection of guinea pigs. Infect Immun 1980;27:730–738.

57. Stuart BM, Pullen RL: Endemic (murine) typhus fever: Clinical observations of 180 cases. Ann Intern Med 1945;23:520–536.

58. Bernabeu-Wittel M, Pachon J, Alarcon A, et al: Murine typhus as a common cause of fever of intermediate duration. Arch Intern Med 1999;159:872–876.

59. Shaked Y, Samra Y, Maier MK, et al: Relapse of rickettsial Mediterranean spotted fever and murine typhus after treatment with chloramphenicol. J Infect Dis 1989;18:35–37.

60. Silpapojakul K, Chayakul P, Krisanapan S, et al: Murine typhus in Thailand: Clinical features, diagnosis, and treatment. QMJ 1993;86:43–47.

61. Strand O, Stromberg A: Ciprofloxacin treatment of murine typhus. Scand J Infect Dis 1990;22:503–504.

62. Eaton M, Cohen MT, Shlim DR, et al: Ciprofloxacin treatment of typhus. JAMA 1989;262:772–773.

63. Olson JG, Bourgeois AL, Fang RCY, et al: Prevention of scrub typhus: Prophylactic administration of doxycycline in a randomized double blind trial. Am J Trop Med Hyg 1980;29:989–997.

64. Twartz JC, Selvaraju SG, Saunders JP, et al: Doxycycline prophylaxis for human scrub typhus. J Infect Dis 1982;146:811–818.

65. Smadel JE, Traub R, Ley HL Jr, et al: Chloramphenicol (chloromycetin) in the chemoprophylaxis of scrub typhus (tsutsugamushi disease). II. Results with volunteers exposed in hyperendemic areas of scrub typhus. Am J Hyg 1949;50:75–91.

66. Smadel JE, Traub R, Frick LP, et al: Chloramphenicol (chloromycetin) in the chemoprophylaxis of scrub typhus (tsutsugamushi disease). III. Suppression of overt disease by prophylactic regimens of four-week duration. Am J Hyg 1950;51:216–228.

67. Sheehy TW, Hazlett D, Turk RE: Scrub typhus: A comparison of chloramphenicol and tetracycline in its treatment. Arch Intern Med 1973;132:77–80.

68. Smadel JE, Woodward TE, Ley HL Jr, et al: Chloramphenicol (chloromycetin) in the treatment of tsutsugamushi disease (scrub typhus). J Clin Invest 1949;28:1196–1215.

69. Brown GW, Saunders JP, Singh S, et al: Single dose doxycycline therapy for scrub typhus. Trans Roy Soc Trop Med Hyg 1978;72:412–416.

70. Watt G, Chouriyagune C, Ruangweerayud R, et al: Scrub typhus infections poorly responsive to antibiotics in northern Thailand. Lancet 1996;348:86–89.

71. Watt G, Kantipong P, Jongsakul K, et al: Doxycycline and rifampcin for mild scrub-typhus infections in northern Thailand: A randomized trial. Lancet 2000;356:1057–1061.

72. Strickman D, Sheer T, Salata K, et al: *In vitro* effectiveness of azithromycin against doxycycline-resistant and susceptible strains of *Rickettsia tsutsugamushi*, etiologic agent of scrub typhus. Antimicrob Agents Chemother 1995;39:2406–2410.

73. McClain JB, Joshi B, Rice R: Chloramphenicol, gentamicin, and ciprofloxacin against murine scrub typhus. Antimicrob Agents Chemother 1988;32:285–286.

74. Raoult D, Marrie T: Q fever. Clin Infect Dis 1995;20:489–496.

75. Marmion BP, Kyrkou M, Worswick D, et al: Vaccine prophylaxis of abattoir-associated Q fever. Lancet 1984;ii:1411–1414.

76. Ackland JR, Worswick DA, Marmion BP: Vaccine prophylaxis of Q fever. A follow-up study of the efficacy of Q-Vax (CSL) 1985–1990. Med J Aust 1994;160:704–708.

77. Elliott JJ, Ruble DL, Zacha GM, et al: Comparison of Q fever cellular and chloroform-methanol residue vaccines as skin test antigens in the sensitized guinea pig. Acta Virol 1998;42:147–155.

78. Waag DM, England MJ, Pitt ML: Comparative efficacy of a *Coxiella burnetii* chloroform-methanol residue (CMR) vaccine and a licensed cellular vaccine (Q-Vax) in rodents challenged by aerosol. Vaccine 1997;15:1779–1783.

79. Williams JC, Peacock MG, Waag DM, et al: Vaccines against coxiellosis and Q fever. Development of a chloroform:methanol residue subunit of phase I *Coxiella burnetii* for the immunization of animals. Ann NY Acad Sci 1992;653:88–111.

80. Fries LF, Waag DM, Williams JC: Safety and immunogenicity in human volunteers of a chloroform-methanol residue vaccine for Q fever. Infect Immun 1993;61:1251–1258.

81. Zhang YX, Zhi N, Yu SR, et al: Protective immunity induced by 67 K outer membrane protein of phase I *Coxiella burnetii* in mice and guinea pigs. Acta Virol 1994;38:327–332.

82. Marrie TJ: *Coxiella burnetii* (Q fever). In Mandell GL, Bennett JE, Dolin R (eds): Mandell, Douglas, and Bennett's Principles and Practice of Infectious Diseases, 5th ed. Philadelphia, Churchill Livingstone, 2000, vol 2, pp 2043–2050.

82a. Bernit E, Pouget J, Jambon F, et al: Neurologic involvement in acute Q fever: A report of 29 cases and review of the literature. Arch Intern Med 2002;162:693–700.

83. Yeaman MR, Roman MJ, Naca OG: Antibiotic susceptibilities of two *Coxiella burnetii* isolates implicated in distinct clinical syndromes. Antimicrob Agents Chemother 1989;33:1052–1057.

84. Raoult D, Bres P, Drancourt M, et al: In vitro susceptibilities of *Coxiella burnetii*, *Rickettsia rickettsii*, and *Rickettsia conorii* to the fluoroquinolone sparfloxacin. Antimicrob Agents Chemother 1991;34:88–91.

85. Pierce TH, Yucht SC, Gorin AB, et al: Q fever pneumonitis: Diagnosis by transbronchoscopic lung biopsy. West J Med 1979;130:453–455.

86. Bertrand A, Janbon F, Jonquet O, et al: Infections par les rickettsiales et fluoroquinolones. Pathol Biol (Paris) 1988;36:493–495.

87. Raffi F: Q fever endocarditis. Lancet 1989;ii:1336–1337.

88. Powell OW, Kennedy KP, McIver M, et al: Tetracycline in the treatment of "Q" fever. Aust Ann Med 1962;11:184–188.

89. D'Angelo LG, Hetherington R: Q fever treated with erythromycin. BMJ 1979;2:305–306.

90. Ellis ME, Dunbar EM: *In vivo* response of acute Q fever to erythromycin. Thorax 1982;37:867–868.

91. Schonwald S, Kusman I, Oreskovic K, et al: Azithromycin: Single 1.5 g dose in the treatment of patients with atypical pneumonia syndrome—a randomized study. Infection 1999;27:198–202.

92. Fenollar F, Fournier P-E, Carrieri MP, et al: Risks factors and prevention of Q fever endocarditis. Clin Infect Dis 2001;33:312–316.

92a. Raoult D, Fenollar F, Stein A: Q fever during pregnancy: Diagnosis, treatment, and follow-up. Arch Intern Med 2002;162:701–704.

92b. Ludlam H, Wreghitt TG, Thornton S, et al: Q fever in pregnancy. J Infect 1997;34:75–78.

92c. Marrie TJ: Q fever in pregnancy: Report of two cases. Infect Dis Clin Pract 1993;2:207–209.

93. Yeaman MR, Mtischer LA, Baca OG: *In vitro* susceptibility of *Coxiella burnetii* to antibiotics, including several quinolones. Antimicrob Agents Chemother 1987;31:1079–1084.

94. Jabarit-Aldighieri N, Torres H, Raoult D: Susceptibility of *Rickettsia conorii*, *R. rickettsii*, and *Coxiella burnetii* to PD 127,391, PD 131,628, pefloxacin, ofloxacin, and ciprofloxacin. Antimicrob Agents Chemother 1992;36:2529–2532.

95. Stein A, Raoult D: Q fever endocarditis. Eur Heart J 1995;16(Suppl B):19–23.

96. Brouqui P, DuPont HT, Drancourt M, et al: Chronic Q fever—ninety-two cases from France, including 27 cases without endocarditis. Arch Intern Med 1993;153:642–648.

97. Varma MPS, Adgey AAJ, Connolly JH: Chronic Q fever endocarditis. Br Heart J 1980;43:695–699.

98. Raoult D, Etienne J, Massip P, et al: Q fever endocarditis in the south of France. J Infect Dis 1987;155:570–573.

99. Tobin MJ, Cahill N, Gearty G, et al: Q fever endocarditis. Am J Med 1982;72:396–400.

100. Shafer RW, Braverman ER: Q fever endocarditis: Delay in diagnosis due to an apparent clinical response to corticosteroids. Am J Med 1989;86:729.

101. Lev BI, Shachar A, Segev S, et al: Quiescent Q fever endocarditis exacerbated by cardiac surgery and corticosteroid therapy. Arch Intern Med 1988;148:1531–1532.

102. Fournier PE, Casalta JP, Habib G, et al: Verification of the diagnostic criteria proposed by the Duke Endocarditis Service to permit improved diagnosis of Q fever endocarditis. Am J Med 1996;100:629–633.

103. Peacock MG, Philip RN, Williams JC, et al: Serological evaluation of Q fever in humans: Enhanced phase I titers of immunoglobulins G and A are diagnostic for Q fever endocarditis. Infect Immun 1983;41:1089–1098.

104. Wilson HG, Neilson GH, Galea EG, et al: Q fever endocarditis in Queensland. Circulation 1976;53:680–684.

105. Raoult D, Houpikian P, DuPont HT, et al: Treatment of Q fever endocarditis: Comparison of 2 regimens containing doxycycline and ofloxacin or hydroxychloroquine. Arch Intern Med 1999;159:167–173.

106. Pedoe HDT: Apparent recurrence of Q fever endocarditis following homograft replacement of aortic valve. Br Heart J 1970;32:568–570.

107. Turck WPG, Howitt G, Turnberg LA, et al: Chronic Q fever. QJM 1976;45:193–217.

108. Freeman R, Hodson ME: Q fever endocarditis treated with trimethoprim and sulfamethoxazole. BMJ 1972;12:419–420.

109. Yebra M, Ortigosa J, Albarran F, et al: Ciprofloxacin in a case of Q fever endocarditis. N Engl J Med 1990;323:614.

110. Haldane EV, Marrie TJ, Faulkner RS, et al: Endocarditis due to Q fever in Nova Scotia: Experience with five patients in 1981–1982. J Infect Dis 1983;148:978–985.

111. Ellis ME, Smith CC, Moffat MA: Chronic or fatal Q-fever infection: A review of 16 patients seen in North-East Scotland (1967–1980). QJM 1983;52:54–66.

112. Subramanya NI, Wright JS, Khan MAR: Failure of rifampcin and co-trimoxazole in Q fever endocarditis. BMJ 1982;285:343–344.

113. Levy PY, Drancourt M, Etienne J, et al: Comparison of different antibiotic regimens for therapy of 32 cases of Q fever endocarditis. Antimicrob Agents Chemother 1991;35:533–537.

114. Kimbrough RC III, Ormsbee RA, Peacock M, et al: Q fever endocarditis in the United States. Ann Intern Med 1979;91:400–402.

115. Raoult D, Levy PY, Harle JR, et al: Chronic Q fever: Diagnosis and follow-up. Ann NY Acad Sci 1990;590:51–60.

116. Fernandez-Guerrero ML, Muelas JM, Aguado JM, et al: Q fever endocarditis on porcine bioprosthetic valves—clinicopathologic features and microbiologic findings in three patients treated with doxycycline, co-trimoxazole, and valve replacement. Ann Intern Med 1988;108:209–213.

117. Misao T, Kobayashi Y: Studies on infectious mononucleosis (glandular fever). I. Isolation of etiologic agent from blood, bone marrow, and lymph node of a patient with infectious mononucleosis by using mice. Kyushu J Med Sci 1955;6:145–152.

118. Maeda K, Markowitz N, Hawley RC, et al: Human infection with *Ehrlichia canis*, a leukocytic rickettsia. N Engl J Med 1987;316:853–856.

119. Bakken JS, Dumler JS, Chen S-M, et al: Human granulocytic ehrlichiosis in the upper Midwest United States: A new species emerging? JAMA 1994;272:212–218.

120. Buller RS, Arens M, Hmiel SP, et al: *Ehrlichia ewingii*, a newly recognized agent of human ehrlichiosis. N Engl J Med 1999;341:148–155.

121. Walker DH, Dumler JS: *Ehrlichia chaffeensis* (human monocytotropic ehrlichiosis), *Ehrlichia phagocytophila* (human granulocytotropic ehrlichiosis), and other ehrlichiae. In Mandell GL, Bennett JE, Dolin R (eds): Mandell, Douglas, and Bennett's Principles and Practice of Infectious Diseases, 5th ed. Philadelphia, Churchill Livingstone, 2000, vol 2 pp 2057–2064.

122. Anderson BE, Sims KG, Olson JG, et al: *Amblyomma americanum*: A potential vector of human ehrlichiosis. Am J Trop Med Hyg 1993;49:239–244.

123. Breitschwerdt EB, Hegarty BC, Hancock SI: Doxycycline hyclate treatment of experimental canine ehrlichiosis followed by challenge inoculation with two *Ehrlichia canis* strains. Antimicrob Agents Chemother 1998;42:362–368.

124. Harrus S, Waner T, Aizenberg I, et al: Therapeutic effect of doxycycline in experimental subclinical canine monocytic ehrlichiosis. J Clin Microbiol 1998;36:2140–2142.

125. Brouqui P, Raoult D: *In vitro* antibiotic susceptibility of the newly recognized agent of ehrlichiosis in humans, *Ehrlichia chaffeensis*. Antimicrob Agents Chemother 1992;36:2799–2803.

126. Buhles WC Jr, Huxsoll DL, Ristic M: Tropical canine pancytopenia: Clinical, hematologic, and serological response of dogs to *Ehrlichia canis* infection, tetracycline therapy, and challenge inoculation. J Infect Dis 1974;130:357–367.

127. Amyx HL, Huxsoll DL, Zeiler DC, et al: Therapeutic and prophylactic value of tetracycline in dogs infected with the agent of tropical canine pancytopenia. J Am Vet Med Assoc 1971;159:1428–1432.

128. Buckner RG, Ewing SA: Experimental treatment of canine ehrlichiosis and haemobartonellosis. J Am Vet Med Assoc 1967;150:1524–1530.

129. Eng TR, Harkess JR, Fishbein DB, et al: Epidemiologic, clinical, and laboratory findings of human ehrlichiosis in the United States, 1988. JAMA 1990;264:2251–2258.

130. Fishbein DB, Dawson JE, Robinson LE: Human ehrlichiosis in the United States, 1985 to 1990. Ann Intern Med 1994;120:736–743.

131. Schutze GE, Jacobs RF: Human monocytic ehrlichiosis in children. Pediatrics 1997;100(1):E10.

132. Roland WE, McDonald G, Caldwell CW, et al: Ehrlichiosis—a cause of prolonged fever. Clin Infect Dis 1995;20:821–825.

133. Telford SR, Dawson JE, Katavolos P, et al: Perpetuation of the agent of human granulocytic ehrlichiosis in a deer tick–rodent cycle. Proc Natl Acad Sci USA 1996;93:6209–6214.

134. Hodzic E, Fish D, Maretzki CM, et al: Acquisition and transmission of the agent of human granulocytic ehrlichiosis by *Ixodes scapularis* ticks. J Clin Microbiol 1998;36:3574–3578.

135. des Vignes F, Piesman J, Heffernan R, et al: Effect of tick removal on transmission of *Borrelia burgdorferi* and *Ehrlichia phagocytophila* by *Ixodes scapularis* nymphs. J Infect Dis 2001;183:773–778.

136. Nadelman RB, Nowakowski J, Fish D, et al: Prophylaxis with single-dose doxycycline for the prevention of Lyme disease after an *Ixodes scapularis* tick bite. N Engl J Med 2001;345:79–84.

137. Zhi N, Rikihisa Y, Kim HY, et al: Comparison of major antigenic proteins of six strains of the human granulocytic ehrlichiosis agent by Western immunoblot analysis. J Clin Microbiol 1997;35:2606–2011.

138. Asanovich KM, Bakken JS, Madigan JE, et al: Antigenic diversity of granulocytic *Ehrlichia* isolates from humans in Wisconsin and New York and a horse in California. J Infect Dis 1997;176:1029–1034.

139. Kim H-Y, Rikihisa Y: Characterization of monoclonal antibodies to the 44-kilodalton major outer membrane protein of the human granulocytic ehrlichiosis agent. J Clin Microbiol 1998;36:3278–3284.

140. Barlough JE, Madigan JE, DeRock E, et al: Protection against *Ehrlichia equi* infection is conferred by prior infection with the human granulocytotropic *Ehrlichia* (HGE agent). J Clin Microbiol 1995;33:3333–3334.

141. Gribble DH: Equine ehrlichiosis. J Am Vet Med Assoc 1969;155:462–469.

142. Stamp JT, Watt JA: Tick-borne fever as a cause of abortion in sheep-part I. Vet Rec 1950;62:465–468.

143. Bakken JS, Krueth J, Wilson-Nordskog C, et al: Clinical and laboratory characteristics of human granulocytic ehrlichiosis. JAMA 1996;275:199–205.

144. Horowitz HW, Aguero-Rosenfeld M, Dumler JS, et al: Reinfection with the agent of human granulocytic ehrlichiosis. Ann Intern Med 1998;129:461–463.

145. Klein MB, Nelson CM, Goodman JL: Antibiotic susceptibility of the newly cultivated agent of human granulocytic ehrlichiosis: Promising activity of quinolones and rifamycins. Antimicrob Agents Chemother 1997;41:76–79.

146. Horowitz HW, Hsieh T-C, Aguero-Rosenfeld ME, et al: Antimicrobial susceptibility of *Ehrlichia phagocytophila*. Antimicrob Agents Chemother 2001;45:786–788.

147. Goodman JL, Nelson C, Vitale B, et al: Direct cultivation of the causative agent of human granulocytic ehrlichiosis. N Engl J Med 1996;334:209–215.

148. Anika SM, Nouws JFM, Van Gogh H, et al: Chemotherapy and pharmacokinetics of some antimicrobial agents in healthy dwarf goats and those infected with *Ehrlichia phagocytophila* (tick-borne fever). Res Vet Sci 1986;41:386–390.

149. Madigan JE, Gribble D: Equine ehrlichiosis in northern California: 49 cases (1968–1981). J Am Vet Med Assoc 1987;190:445–448.

150. Hossain D, Aguero-Rosenfeld ME, Horowitz HW, et al: Clinical and laboratory evolution of a culture-confirmed case of human granulocytic ehrlichiosis. Conn Med 1999;63:265–270.

151. Aguero-Rosenfeld ME, Horowitz HW, Wormser GP, et al: Human granulocytic ehrlichiosis: A case series from a medical center in New York State. Ann Intern Med 1996;125:904–908.

152. Buitrago MI, Ijdo JW, Rinaudo P, et al: Human granulocytic ehrlichiosis during pregnancy treated successfully with rifampin. Clin Infect Dis 1998;27:213–215.

153. Bakken JS, Goellner P, Van Etten M, et al: Seroprevalence of human granulocytic ehrlichiosis among permanent residents of Northwestern Wisconsin. Clin Infect Dis 1998;27:1491–1496.

154. Hardalo CJ, Quagliarello V, Dumler JS: Human granulocytic ehrlichiosis in Connecticut: Report of a fatal case. Clin Infect Dis 1995;21:910–914.

155. Nadelman RB, Horowitz HW, Hsieh T-C, et al: Simultaneous human granulocytic ehrlichiosis and Lyme borreliosis. N Engl J Med 1997;337:27–30.

156. Horowitz HW, Kilchevsky E, Haber S, et al: Perinatal transmission of the agent of human granulocytic ehrlichiosis. N Engl J Med 1998;339:375–378.

157. Stockham SL, Schmidt DA, Curtis KS, et al: Evaluation of granulocytic ehrlichiosis in dogs of Missouri, including serologic status to *Ehrlichia canis*, *Ehrlichia equi*, and *Borrelia burgdorferi*. Am J Vet Res 1992;53:63–68.

Tularemia, Leptospirosis, Borreliosis, and Brucellosis

E. DALE EVERETT, MD

TULAREMIA

Tularemia is a bacterial illness caused by a fastidious, aerobic gram-negative rod. Two biovars, *Francisella tularensis* bv. *tularensis* or bv. *palaearctica*, are responsible for most human tularemia. Tularemia occurs in several geographic areas including North America, most European countries, the former Soviet Union, China, Japan, and others. It has been reported from all 49 continental states, but Arkansas, Missouri, and Oklahoma generally account for most of the cases. *Francisella* can infect more than 100 vertebrate and nonvertebrate hosts. Lagomorphs, rodents, and ticks are important in the transmission of tularemia in North America, and mosquitoes are principal vectors in Europe. Humans are an incidental host of tularemia and acquire the illness from ticks, biting flies, and mosquitoes, from handling infected animals, notably rabbits, squirrels, or muskrats, ingestion of contaminated water or meat that has not been thoroughly cooked, and occasionally from the bite of another animal, often a cat. Microbiology laboratory workers are at risk for inhalation of the organism when handling cultures that unexpectedly contain *Francisella*. After an incubation period of 2 to 10 days, several clinical syndromes, ulceroglandular, glandular, typhoidal, pneumonic, oropharyngeal, and oculoglandular, have been associated with *Francisella* infections. Diagnosis is usually confirmed by serum agglutination or enzyme-linked immunosorbent assay (ELISA) testing, occasionally by culture, and recently by polymerase chain reaction (PCR). Often cases need to be treated on the basis of the clinical presentation, since confirmation by serologic tests may take 2 to 4 weeks. It is uncommon for cultures to be positive, and PCR is not widely available.

No prospective controlled or randomized trials of therapy for tularemia have been performed. Neither has the optimal duration of therapy been established. Streptomycin has long been considered the drug of choice for treatment of tularemia. The lack of availability of streptomycin in the early 1990s led Enderlin et al to review the literature related to the treatment of tularemia with streptomycin as well as alternative agents.[1] Although there have been hundreds of cases of tularemia treated in the United States and other countries, only a small number of cases were found by these authors. Specifically they found 224 cases treated with streptomycin, 50 with tetracyclines, 43 with chloramphenicol, and 36 with gentamicin. Fewer than 10 cases each were found that were treated with tobramycin, fluoroquinolones, ceftriaxone, or imipenem-cilastatin. Since their review, additional cases treated with fluoroquinolones have been reported.[2–5] Two cases of tularemia have been reported to respond to erythromycin.[6, 7]

It has been held that relapses occur more frequently with bacteriostatic antimicrobials such as tetracyclines and chloramphenicol. Although the number of reported cases treated with these agents is small, results from Enderlin's review support this contention.[1] However, some patients appear to have received short courses of less than 7 to 10 days of treatment. The fewest relapses have been seen after streptomycin therapy.

A caveat in selecting treatment for tularemia is that it appears to be one of those microorganisms for which in vitro susceptibilities may not predict in vivo results. Despite favorable in vitro sensitivities, ceftriaxone therapy has been shown to be ineffective.[8] Other β-lactams were also ineffective therapy except for a single case that responded to imipenem–cilastatin.[9]

On the basis of the published literature and personal experience, I recommend the following options for treatment of tularemia.

In severe disease, whether in children or adults, an aminoglycoside, preferably streptomycin or gentamicin, should be used. Only six cases have been reported that were treated with tobramycin, and the cure rate was only 50% with two deaths.[1] In adults 30 mg/kg/d of streptomycin divided into two doses given intramuscularly for 7 to 10 days is recommended. In children 30 mg/kg/d intramuscularly given in two divided doses is recommended. Dosage should not exceed 2 g daily. Gentamicin 3 to 5 mg/kg/d given in three divided doses intravenously or intramuscularly for 7 to 10 days can be used in adults. For children 6 mg/kg/d in three divided doses is recommended.[10] Aminoglycoside dosages may need to be modified according to renal function. No data are available on the treatment of tularemia with a single daily dose of aminoglycosides.

Several choices of therapy for mild-to-moderate illness are available. One can use aminoglycoside therapy, but oral treatment is more convenient to administer. Tetracycline 500 mg four times daily or doxycycline 100 mg twice daily can be used. My anecdotal experience suggests that completion of at least 14 days of treatment with these agents may reduce the incidence of relapse. Chloramphenicol 2 to 3 g/d in four divided doses has been used in adults. However, an oral preparation of chloramphenicol is no longer available in the United States. Furthermore chloramphenicol's rare but serious consequence of bone marrow aplasia makes it a less desirable agent.

Fluoroquinolones have been reported to be effective treatment for tularemia, but experience is relatively limited.[2–5] A report from Spain disclosed a 50% relapse rate in 14 cases treated with ciprofloxacin.[5] Fluoroquinolones generally have not been recommended for use in children. Nevertheless a report indicates an excellent response in 10 children treated with 15 to 20 mg/kg/d of ciprofloxacin in two divided doses for 10 to 14 days.[3] In my opinion levofloxacin 500 mg daily or ciprofloxacin 750 mg twice daily orally for 10 to 14 days is a reasonable choice for mild-to-moderate disease. Giving fluoroquinolones to children remains controversial, but they could be used under circumstances in which other therapies are not feasible. With timely therapy, mortality ranges between 2% and 4%. Most patients respond promptly to therapy, becoming afebrile within 72 hours.

Complications are uncommon but can include spontaneous drainage of suppurative lymph nodes, pericarditis, meningitis, acute respiratory distress syndrome, and rhabdomyolysis. Some patients with large, painful, fluctuant nodes benefit from aspiration for pain relief.

Two situations deserve special attention: tularemia during pregnancy and tularemia meningitis. There is no published experience with tularemia in pregnancy. In mild disease a trial of erythromycin 500 mg four times daily can be undertaken. Otherwise I believe that an aminoglycoside regimen should be used. About 12 cases of tularemia meningitis have been reported with approximately 50% of these occurring after antimicrobial therapy was available. On the basis of limited data an aminoglycoside regimen plus chloramphenicol or doxycycline for 14 days would be appropriate therapy.[11]

Prevention of tularemia is largely avoidance of vectors, of handling infected animals, and of ingestion of contaminated food or water. No effective vaccine is available in the United States.

LEPTOSPIROSIS

Leptospirosis is an illness with protean manifestations. It is caused by a spirochete, *Leptospira interrogans*, of which there are over 200 serovars. In nature, *Leptospira* spp infect both wild and domestic animals, especially rodents, cattle, swine, dogs, horses, sheep, and goats. After infection, animals excrete the organism in their urine for a long time, thus contaminating the environment, especially water. Man becomes infected after cuts, abraded skin, mucous membrane, or conjunctiva is exposed to animal urine, contaminated water and soil, or infected animal tissue. On rare occasions infection may be acquired by ingestion of food contaminated by animal urine or by aerosols.

Between 2 and 26 days after exposure, there is an abrupt onset of fever, chills, myalgias and headache. About one-fourth of patients exhibit a cough, and approximately one-half experience nausea, vomiting, and diarrhea. About 50% of untreated patients will manifest the classic biphasic illness. Physical examination is nonspecific, although the finding of conjunctival suffusion raises the diagnostic possibility of leptospirosis.

Routine laboratory findings are not diagnostic, with white blood cell counts ranging between 3000 and 26,000/mm³. A febrile illness accompanied by some combination of abnormal urinalysis, impaired renal function, abnormal liver studies, and elevated creatine kinase levels should raise the possibility of leptospirosis. After about 1 week of illness, from 50% to 85% of patients have pleocytosis.

Diagnosis is usually established by acute and convalescent serologic studies performed by several techniques, which include microscopic agglutination test, macroscopic agglutination test, indirect hemagglutination, or ELISA. Other ways to establish the diagnosis but less available than serology include culture of blood or urine or both in special media and by PCR. Like a number of other infectious diseases, therapy often needs to be instituted on the basis of the clinical setting and before confirmation of the diagnosis.

In most cases, leptospirosis is a self-limited disease; however, severe complications such as renal failure, hepatic failure, transverse myelitis, myocarditis, and a hemorrhagic diasthesis, especially pulmonary hemorrhage, can occur. Mortality ranges between 2.2% and 9.7%.

Controversy over whether antimicrobial agents alter the course of leptospirosis persisted for several years. Another contention was that antimicrobial therapy was beneficial only when administered within 3 or 4 days of the onset of the illness. In vitro and experimental animal evidence suggest that penicillin, chloramphenicol, tetracyclines, erythromycin, and ciprofloxacin might be effective treatment. Although suffering from small numbers, two controlled trials strongly suggest that antimicrobial therapy is indicated for shortening the course of leptospirosis. McClain et al showed that administering doxycycline 100 mg twice daily within a mean time of 45 hours of illness shortened the illness by 2 days as compared to placebo.[12] A few years later, Watt et al showed that penicillin 6 MU per day for 7 days started at any point during severe illness resulted in faster defervescense, more rapid decline in serum creatinine, shortened hospital stay, and reduction of leptospiruria as compared to placebo.[13] On the basis of the above, I would recommend doxycycline 100 mg twice daily for 7 days for mild-to-moderate disease or penicillin 6 MU daily for adults with leptospirosis. No data were found that addressed treatment of leptospirosis in pregnancy, but the penicillin regimen would seem appropriate. For children, adjustment of the dosage of penicillin or a 1-week course of doxycycline would be reasonable. The Jarisch-Herxheimer reaction may complicate the treatment of leptospirosis. The management of this complication will be addressed in the borreliosis discussion of this chapter.

In addition to antimicrobial therapy, ancillary measures such as hemodialysis and ventilator support may be necessary. A case report of a patient with leptospirosis and severe lung injury suggested benefit from inhaled nitric oxide and hemofiltration.[14]

Prevention of leptospirosis, like many other zoonoses, is avoidance of contaminated environments. Two studies using 200 mg of doxycycline weekly showed benefit in reducing symptomatic infection in a nonimmune population and a reduction of clinical illness in a partially immune population.[15,16] An unsubstantiated recommendation of 200 mg of doxycycline as postexposure prophylaxis, for example, veterinarian students exposed to dog urine or to a known contaminated water source, has been suggested. No effective vaccine for human use is available.

BORRELIOSIS

Spirochetes of the genus *Borrelia* are the cause of borreliosis or relapsing fever. As suggested by the latter terminology, the illness is characterized by fever, often high grade, for a few days punctuated by a period of no fever for several days followed by recrudescence of fever. There are two varieties of relapsing fever, tick-borne (TBRF) and louse-borne (LBRF). TBRF occurs in North America, especially the western part of the United States. TBRF also occurs in other countries. LBRF occurs in developing countries and is transmitted from person to person by the body louse, *Pediculus humanus*.

Although fever and relapses are the cardinal features of the disease, headache, neck stiffness, muscle aches, arthalgias, cough, and nausea may also accompany the syndrome. Neurologic symptoms such as dizziness, unsteady gait, delirium, apathy, stupor, coma, facial palsy, myelitis, and radiculopathy can also occur. Neurologic symptoms are more common in TBRF than in LBRF. Nosebleeds, petechiae, and ecchymoses are common in LBRF but not TBRF. Other findings in LBRF and TBRF may include hepatosplenomegaly and myocarditis. The number of relapses average about three, but as many as 13 have been reported. Fever lasts for 1 to 6 days with afebrile interludes of 4 to 10 days.

Routine laboratory studies are nonspecific. White blood cell counts are usually normal but range from leukopenia to moderate elevation. Thrombocytopenia can be a prominent feature. Liver enzymes may be elevated, and clotting parameters may be prolonged. Patients with signs of meningitis or meningoencephalitis may have pleocytosis.

If the diagnosis of relapsing fever is suspected, thick and thin smears stained with Wright or Giemsa stains should be examined microscopically to detect the thread-like spirochete. Stains with acridine orange or flourescein-labeled antibody followed by examination under ultraviolet light can also be used. Spirochetes can be cultivated by injecting blood intraperitoneally into animals or by inoculating blood or plasma into Barbour-Stoener-Kelly media. Serologic studies are fraught with nonspecificity and are performed by few laboratories. PCR will likely be useful in the future. In the past in the United States, where relapsing fever is uncommon and sporadic, the diagnosis was commonly made by an astute technician while examining a peripheral blood smear microscopically. With today's automated blood count procedures this is unlikely to happen since microscopic examinations are not done unless requested or there are abnormalities in the automated results that precipitate a microscopic review.

LBRF is a more severe disease than TBRF with mortality ranging from 30% to 70% for LBRF and 4% to 10% for TBRF. Relapsing fever during pregnancy increases maternal and fetal mortality. Congenital infection does occur. Several antimicrobials have been used to treat relapsing fever including penicillin, tetracyclines, chloramphenicol, erythromycin, aminoglycosides, and ceftriaxone (one case).[17,18] As a rule of thumb, TBRF seems to be more refractory to treatment than LBRF; that is, more doses of drug are needed to prevent relapse. Treatment with any drug regimen, although more common with tetracyclines, produces a high incidence of Jarisch-Herxheimer reaction (JHR). Such a reaction is seen perhaps 33% to 50% of the time in TBRF and from 5% to 100% of the time with LBRF. JHR is not a trivial matter, with case fatality rates of 4% to 6%.

Most of the published literature reflects treatment with tetracyclines or penicillin.[18,19] In the United States no systematic study of the treatment of TBRF has been done. Many regimens have been successful in the treatment of LBRF, but no consensus as to the best treatment has been reached. Penicillin regimens seem to result in fewer JHRs but more relapses. Single dose therapy can be successful in most LBRF cases. On the basis of the review by Rahlenbeck and Gebre-Yohannes, the following treatment regimens can be recommended.[18,19]

1. Single dose, oral:

    a. Tetracycline 250 or 500 mg
    b. doxycycline 100 mg
    c. Erythromycin 500 mg
    d. Chloramphenicol 500 mg (Because of potential side effects and lack of universal availability, chloramphenical is not recommended unless it is the only choice.)

2. Single dose parenteral: tetracycline 250 mg or presumably doxycycline 100 mg (no data) or procaine penicillin G 600,000 U intramuscularly. (Various doses of procaine penicillin have been used, but for convenience and efficacy 600,000 U seems reasonable.)

A ploy to try to reduce the JHR is to give a low dose of procaine penicillin, for example, 100,000 to 400,000 U, followed by tetracycline for one or more doses. The erythromycin regimen is recommended for pregnant women.

TBRF seems to be more refractory to treatment than LBRF. In particular, single dose regimens are said to be less efficacious than in LBRF. The numbers of patients and drugs used that are recorded in the literature are considerably fewer than those for LBRF. A general theme is that TBRF should be treated with 5- to 10-day courses of antimicrobials.[20] Although standardized doses of drugs were not used, several regimens appear to be effective in TBRL in pregnancy. These included procaine penicillin intramuscularly, oral erythromycin, and low-dose penicillin (400,000 U) followed by erythromycin.[21] Neonatal relapsing fever is uncommon, but perinatal mortality is high. It is unclear what the effects of treatment are on perinatal mortality. Although appearing to vary somewhat, maternal mortality does not seem to be substantially higher than in nonpregnant controls infected with *Borrelia*.[21] On the basis of less than optimal data, the following recommendations are made for the antimicrobial treatment of TBRL:

1. Oral for 5 to 10 days

    a. Tetracycline 500 mg four times daily
    b. doxycycline 100 mg twice daily
    c. Erythromycin 500 mg four times daily

2. Intramuscular: procaine penicillin G 600,000 U twice daily for 7 to 10 days

The appropriate formulation of the foregoing agents can be given intravenously if circumstances preclude oral or intramuscular administration. In pregnancy, penicillin or erythromycin or a combination regimen seems reasonable to administer. One case of TBRL that relapsed after 14 days of intravenous penicillin 14 mu per day apparently was cured with ceftriaxone 1 g intramuscularly twice daily for 10 days.[22]

JHR is common following drug treatment of relapsing fever and much less common after drug treatment of leptospirosis. The reaction is characterized by the onset of restlessness, apprehension, and intense chills 1 to 2 hours after receiving a therapeutic agent and lasting for 10 to 30 minutes. Temperature, respiratory and pulse rates, and blood pressure rise. This is followed by profuse sweating, a fall in blood pressure, and a slow decline in temperature over a few hours. Because of the possible severity of the reaction, including mortality, it is recommended that patients be kept under close observation with resuscitation support available following the initial dose of antimicrobial for relapsing fever. Steroids and antipyretics do not prevent the reaction. Two agents—meptazinol, an opioid antagonist with some agonist properties, and sheep-derived polyclonal Fab antibody fragments against tumor necrosis factor alpha—when given prophylactically reduce the severity of JHR.[23,24] Neither are currently commercially available for use.

Prevention of TBRL is to avoid the tick vector or to use insect repellent. Prevention of LBRL depends upon improvement of impoverished areas and personal hygiene.

BRUCELLOSIS

Brucellois is an illness characterized by fever and often nonspecific complaints. Human disease is caused by one of four species of aerobic gram-negative rods, *Brucella abortus*, *Brucella suis*, *Brucella canis*, and *Brucella melitensis*. Worldwide, *B. melitensis* is the most common cause of disease. Major reservoirs of *Brucella* spp include cattle, swine, sheep, and goats. Nondomesticated ungulates such as deer, bison, and elk may also harbor the organism. The principal reservoir for *B. canis* is dogs. Humans become infected from handling infected animals or tissues or by ingestion of unpasteurized dairy products. Consequently, farm workers, veterinarians, abbatoir workers, and those who consume raw milk or cheeses made from raw milk are at highest risk for acquiring the illness. Following acquisition of the organism, illness may occur within a few days, but more often it occurs after 30 to 60 days of incubation. Fever (continuous, intermittent, or irregular) is a cardinal feature of the disease. Accompanying symptoms may include headache, chills, sweating, arthralgias, depression, and weight loss. Localization to an organ system may result in presentation of a febrile illness with focal signs, for example, osteoarticular, epididymoorchitis, meningitis, endocarditis, or liver abscess. Each of these conditions has its own causes that are more common than brucellosis; therefore the differential diagnosis may be broad. In the United States, brucellosis is uncommon, with approximately 100 cases reported annually (not all states require reporting).

Diagnosis may be established by cultures of blood, other body fluids, or tissue, for example, bone marrow. *Brucella* tends to grow slowly, and not all cases are culture positive. Serologic testing by a number of different methods, although not as specific as culture, may support the diagnosis sufficiently to warrant a course of therapy. PCR shows promise as a diagnostic test, but insufficient clinical experience and lack of availability of the test hamper its use at the present time.

The treatment of brucellosis needs to be individualized. The following regimens are adequate for adult cases of uncomplicated brucellosis with or without sacroilitis:

1. Doxycycline 200 mg PO daily for 42 to 45 days plus streptomycin 1 g IM daily for 21 days.[25-27] Relapse rates are 5% or less with this regimen.
2. Doxycycline 100 mg PO twice daily for 42 to 45 days plus streptomycin 1 g IM daily for 14 or 15 days.[28-30] Relapse rates are similar to those for regimen 1.
3. Doxycycline 100 mg twice daily plus rifampin 600 or 900 mg or 15mg/kg for 42 to 45 days.[26,29-31] Relapse rates varied from 16% to as low as 3.2%. Failure to respond to therapy appears to be slightly higher with this regimen than with streptomycin-containing regimens.
4. Ofloxacin 400 mg plus rifampin 600 mg once daily for 42 days produced cure rates similar to those of doxycycline 200 mg and rifampin 600 mg once daily.

Thirty-one patients were in the fluoroquinolone group, and 30 in the doxycycline plus rifampin group. In each group there was one therapeutic failure and one relapse.[31] Despite favorable in vitro susceptibilities, monotherapy with fluoroquinolones has been disappointing.[32]

TMP-SMX when used as a single agent has been fraught with high relapse rates unless used for a prolonged time. Montejo et al, using a moderately high dose of TMP-SMX, 160 mg TMP/800 mg SMX, every 8 hours for 10 days, followed by the same dose every 12 hours for 4 weeks, followed by 80 mg TMP/400 mg SMX encompassing a 6-month course, cured 52 of 64 patients. There were two relapses and four therapeutic failures, and six dropped out for other reasons.[27]

Ceftriaxone displays good in vitro activity against *B. melitensis*. Results of therapy have been variable, but therapeutic failure and relapses are relatively common, especially if a dose of 2 g daily is used.[33] If one is placed

in the position that ceftriaxone needs to be used, a dosage of 2 g every 12 hours is recommended and presumably for 4 to 6 weeks (my suggestion). It cannot be recommended as a first-line drug.

Therapy of brucellosis in children younger than 8 years requires special attention, since prolonged use of tetracyclines should be avoided in this age group. In a study of 1100 children, 598 were treated with non-tetracycline-containing regimens. The number of cases under 8 years of age is unclear. TMP-SMX alone, TMP-SMX plus streptomycin, TMP-SMX plus gentamicin, TMP-SMX plus rifampin, rifampin alone, rifampin plus streptomycin, and rifampin plus gentamicin were used in varying numbers of patients. The authors concluded that TMP-SMX, 10 mg/kg TMP and 50 mg/kg SMX, orally per day in two divided doses for 3 weeks along with 5 mg/kg of gentamicin in two divided doses for the first 5 days of treatment was a preferred regimen.[34] Khuri-Bulos et al treated 113 children, 66 of whom were less than 9 years of age, with TMP-SMX, 10 to 12 mg/kg TMP and 50 to 60 mg/kg SMX, plus rifampin 15 to 20 mg/kg/d, both orally in two divided doses. Results were quite good with only a 3.5% relapse rate.[35] In my opinion, either of these regimens appears adequate for children 8 years of age and younger, and one of the non-quinolone regimens used in adults can be given to children over 8 years of age.

Certain *Brucella* infections may be viewed as occurring under unusual circumstances, (e.g., pregnancy or in an HIV-infected patient) or as complicated (e.g., endocarditis, foreign body infection, neurobrucellosis, or some cases of spondylitis). Additionally, persons can be exposed to *Brucella* live attenuated vaccines, RB 51, Rev-1, or S19 used to immunize animals, particularly by accidental injection. Data on appropriate therapy of brucellosis in pregnancy is not available. Suggested regimens have included rifampin 900 mg once daily for 6 weeks or rifampin plus TMP-SMX for 4 weeks.[36] If this latter regimen is used, perhaps one TMP-SMX double-strength tablet (160/800 mg) three times daily plus rifampin 900 mg once daily would be reasonable. Depending upon the acuity of the illness, allergies, drug intolerances, and so forth, and as in other situations in which risk vs. benefit needs to be weighed, a tetracycline plus streptomycin regimen might be used after thorough discussion with the patient.

Moreno et al reported 12 HIV-infected patients and an additional five cases found in a literature review who were infected with *Brucella*. Most of the patients, on the basis of CD4 counts when available, did not have far advanced HIV disease. The response rate to commonly used adult *Brucella* treatment regimens was excellent. Patients apparently were not placed on long-term suppressive therapy.[37]

Both native valve and prosthetic valve endocarditis have been caused by *Brucella*. The general recommendation for native valve endocarditis has been antimicrobial therapy and valve replacement. Cohen et al reported one case and found 12 others that were cured with antimicrobial agents without surgery.[38] Absence of congestive heart failure, mild extravalvular cardiac involvement, and a short disease history may be markers for successful nonsurgical treatment. Treatment consisting of a tetracycline, an aminoglycoside, sulfonamides, or rifampin for 10 days to 9 months was successful. They also reviewed 49 cases of surgically treated disease, 14 of which were prosthetic valve endocarditis. Treatment consisted of variable preoperative antimicrobials and replacement of the prosthetic valve followed by further antimicrobial treatment for 2 weeks to 13 months after surgery.[38] Combinations of tetracyclines, streptomycin, and TMP-SMX or rifampin were given postoperatively for a mean time of about 3 months. Two cases of pacemaker infection with *Brucella* have been reported. One was successfully treated by removal of the apparatus, a temporary pacemaker, and a 45-day course of doxycycline and rifampin plus 21 days of streptomycin. One week after completion of antimicrobials a permanent pacemaker was reinserted successfully.[39] The other case failed a 6-week course of doxycycline and streptomycin and an 8-week course of doxycycline and rifampin. The pacemaker was removed, but the patient died in the postoperative period of complications of a perforated ulcer and gastrointestinal hemorrhage.[40]

Other foreign body infections include three cases of total knee arthroplasty infections and one prosthetic hip infection. The knee infections responded to 6 weeks to 19 months of antimicrobial treatment without prosthesis removal.[41–43] The hip prosthesis was removed followed by long-term antimicrobials.[44]

Neurobrucellosis, usually manifested as meningitis but occasionally as meningovascular disease, polyradiculitis, myelopathy, or optic neuropathy, is an uncommon complication of brucellosis.[45,46] A three- or four-drug regimen consisting of agents that cross the blood-cerebrospinal fluid barrier is generally recommended plus or minus streptomycin for 14 to 21 days. TMP-SMX, tetracyclines, and rifampin are recommended. It is recommended that treatment be continued until clinical recovery occurs and cerebrospinal fluid parameters, especially glucose and cell counts, return to normal. Some would also recommend concomitant steroid administration. Duration of antimicrobial therapy is often 2 to 4 months and sometimes longer.[46]

Although some cases of *Brucella* spondylitis may respond to regimens used in uncomplicated brucellosis, some observations suggest that a doxycycline-streptomycin regimen is superior[29,30] and that the therapy, at least the nonaminoglycoside part of therapy, may need to be continued for 3 months or longer.[47] Like other causes of infectious spondylitis, surgery for decompression of the spinal cord, stabilization of the spine, or drainage of paravertebral abscesses may be needed.

Because all treatment regimens for brucellosis have some incidence of relapse, follow-up of patients is highly desirable. Most relapses occur within the first 3 months and almost all within 6 months after therapy. Approximately 80% of patients have acute clinical relapses with fever and other symptoms, but a small percentage may be afebrile and have nonspecific symptoms. At the end of therapy base line serologies should be obtained. In those patients who have clinical relapse and those with persistent malaise, blood cultures should be performed and serologies repeated.[48] Preliminary findings indicate that PCR may be useful for detecting relapses when it becomes more widely available.[49]

Finally, humans, especially veterinarians, may be exposed to live attenuated vaccines, S19, Rev-1, or RB 51. Most commonly exposures are accidental inoculation or conjunctival splashes. Although there are no good studies of efficacy, it is recommended that a full course of treatment be given in those with such exposures.[50] For S19 or Rev-1 a 6-week course of doxycycline 100 mg twice daily and rifampin 600 to 900 mg once daily seems reasonable. Recommendations are to give doxycycline 100 mg twice daily for 21 days for RB 51 exposure (RB 51 is resistant to rifampin in vitro) with additional drugs added should symptoms of infection occur.[51]

Prevention of brucellosis is mainly through control of infections in animals and pasteurization of dairy products.

REFERENCES

1. Enderlin G, Morales L, Jacobs RF, Cross JT: Streptomycin and alternative agents for the treatment of tularemia: Review of the literature. Clin Infect Dis 1994;19:42–47.
2. Limaye AP, Hooper CJ: Treatment of tularemia with fluoroquinolones: Two cases and review. Clin Infect Dis 1999;29:922–924.
3. Johansson A, Berglund L, Gothefors L, et al: Ciprofloxacin for treatment of tularemia in children. Pediatr Infect Dis J 2000;10:449–453.
4. Arav-Boger R: Cat-bite tularemia in a seventeen-year-old girl treated with ciprofloxacin. Pediatr Infect Dis J 2000;19:583–584.
5. Chocarro A, Gonzalez A, Gracia I: Treatment of tularemia with ciprofloxacin. Clin Infect Dis 2000;31:623.
6. Westerman EL, McDonald J: Tularemia pneumonia mimicking Legionnaires' disease: isolation of organisms on CYE agar and successful treatment with erythromycin. South Med J 1980;75:1169–1170.
7. Harrell RE Jr, Simmons HF: Pleuropulmonary tularemia: Successful treatment with erythromycin. South Med J 1990;83:1363–1364.
8. Cross JT, Jacobs RF: Tularemia: Treatment failures with outpatient use of ceftriaxone. Clin Infect Dis 1993;17:976–980.
9. Lee HC, Horowitz E, Linder W: Treatment of tularemia with imipenem/cilastatin sodium. South Med J 1991;84:1277–1278.
10. Cross JT Jr, Schulze GE, Jacobs RF: Treatment of tularemia with gentamicin in pediatric patients. Pediatr Infect Dis J 1995;14:151–152.
11. Rodgers BL, Duffield RP, Taylor T, et al: Tularemic meningitis. Pediatr Infect Dis J 1998;17:439–441.

12. McClain BL, Ballow WR, Harrison SM, Steinway DL: Doxycycline therapy for leptospirosis. Ann Intern Med 1984;100:696–698.
13. Watt G, Tuazon ML, Santiago E, et al: Placebo-controlled trial of intravenous penicillin for severe and late leptospirosis. Lancet 1988;1:433–435.
14. Borer A, Metz I, Riesenberg K, et al: Massive pulmonary haemorrhage caused by leptospirosis successfully treated with nitric oxide inhalation and haemofiltration. J Infect 1999;38:42–45.
15. Takafuji ET, Kirkpatrick JW, Miller RN, et al: An efficacy trial of doxycycline chemoprophylaxis against leptospirosis. N Engl J Med 1984;310:497–500.
16. Sehgal SC, Suguwan AP, Murhekar MV, et al: Randomized controlled trial of doxycycline prophylaxis against leptospirosis in an endemic area. Int J Antimicrob Agents 2000;13:249–255.
17. Cadavid D, Barbour AG: Neuroborreliosis during relapsing fever: Review of the clinical manifestations, pathology, and treatment of infections in humans and experimental animals. Clin Infect Dis 1998;21:151–164.
18. Rahlenbeck SI, Gebre-Yohannes A: Louse-borne relapsing fever and its treatment. Trop Med Int Health 1995;47:49–52.
19. Seboxa T, Rahlenbeck SI: Treatment of louse-borne relapsing fever with low dose penicillin or tetracycline: A clinical trial. Scand J Infect Dis 1995;27:29–31.
20. Horton JM, Blaser MJ: The spectrum of relapsing fever in the Rocky Mountains. Arch Intern Med 1985;145:871–875.
21. Jongen VHWM, Roosmalen JV, Tiems J, et al: Tick-borne relapsing fever and pregnancy outcome in rural Tanzania. Acta Obstet Gynecol Scand 1997;76:834–838.
22. Nassif X, Dupont B, Fleury J: Coftriaxonein relapsing fever (letter). Lancet 1988;2:394.
23. Tekhu B, Habte-Michael A, Warrell DA, et al: Meptazinol diminishes the Jarisch-Herxheimer reaction of relapsing fever. Lancet 1983;1:835–839.
24. Fekade D, Knox K, Hussein K, et al: Prevention of Jarisch-Herxheimer reactions by treatment with antibodies against tumor necrosis factor α. N Engl J Med 1996;335:311–315.
25. Lulu AR, Araj GF, Khateeb MI, et al: Human brucellosis in Kuwait: A prospective study of 400 cases. QJM 1988;66(249):39–54.
26. Acocella G, Bertrand A, Beytout J, et al: Comparison of three different regimens in the treatment of acute brucellosis: A multicenter multinational study. J Antimicrob Chemother 1989;23:433–439.
27. Montejo JM, Alberola I, Glez-Zarate P, et al: Open, randomized therapeutic trial of six antimicrobial regimens in the treatment of human brucellosis. Clin Infect Dis 1993;16:671–676.
28. Cisneros JM, Viciana P, Calmenero J, et al: Multicenter prospective study of treatment of Brucella melitensis brucellosis with doxycycline for 6 weeks plus streptomycin for 2 weeks. Antimicrob Agents Chemother 1990;34:881–883.
29. Ariza J, Gudiol F, Pallares R, et al: Treatment of human brucellosis with doxycycline plus rifampin or doxycycline plus streptomycin. Ann Intern Med 1992;117:25–30.
30. Solera J, Rodriguez-Zapata M, Geijo P, et al: Doxycycline-rifampin versus doxycycline-streptomycin in treatment of human brucellosis due to Brucella melitensis. Antimicrob Agents Chemother 1995;39:2061–2067.
31. Akova M, Ömrüm U, Akalin HE, et al: Quinolones in treatment of human brucellosis: Comparative trial of ofloxacin-rifampin versus doxycycline-rifampin. Antimicrob Agents Chemother 1993;37:1831–1843.
32. Lang R, Rubinstein E: Quinolones for treatment of brucellosis. J Antimicrob Chemother 1992;29:357–360.
33. Lang R, Dagan R, Potasman I, et al: Failure of ceftriaxone in the treatment of acute brucellosis. Clin Infect Dis 1992;14:506–509.
34. Lubani MM, Dudin KI, Sharda DC, et al: A multicenter therapeutic study of 1100 children with brucellosis. Pediatr Infect Dis J 1989;8:75–78.
35. Khuri-Bulos NA, Daoud AF, Azab SM: Treatment of childhood brucellosis: Results of a prospective trial on 113 children. Pediatr Infect Dis J 1993;12:377–381.
36. Solera J, Martinez-Alfaro E, Espinosa A: Recognition and optimum treatment of brucellosis. Drugs 1997;53:245–256.
37. Moreno S, Ariza J, Espinosa FJ, et al: Brucellosis in patients infected with the human immunodeficiency virus. Eur J Clin Microbiol Infect Dis 1998;17:319–326.
38. Cohen J, Golik A, Alon I, et al: Conservative treatment for Brucella endocarditis. Clin Cardiol 1997;20:291–294.
39. de la Fuente A, Sanchez JR, Uriz J, et al: Infection of a pacemaker by Brucella melitensis. Tex Heart Inst J 1997;24: 129–130.
40. Francia E, Domingo P, Sambeat MA, et al: Pacemaker infection by Brucella melitensis: A rare cause of relapsing brucellosis. Arch Intern Med 2000;160:3327–3328.
41. Agarwal S, Kadhi SKM, Rooney RJ: Brucellosis complicating total knee arthroplasty. Clin Orthop 1991;269:179–181.
42. Orti A, Roig P, Alcala R, et al: Brucellar prosthetic arthritis in a total knee replacement. Eur J Clin Microbial Infect Dis 1997;16:843–845.
43. Malizos KN, Makris CA, Soucacos PN: Total knee arthroplasties infected by Brucella melitensis: A case report. Am J Orthop 1997;26:283–285.
44. Jones RE, Berryhill WH, Smith J, et al: Secondary infection of a total hip replacement with Brucella abortus. Orthopedics 1983;6:184–186.
45. Bashir R, Al-Kawi MZ, Harder EJ, Jinkins J: Nervous system brucellosis: Diagnosis and treatment. Neurology 1985;35:1576–1581.
46. McLean DR, Russell N, Khan MY: Neurobrucellosis: Clinical and therapeutic features. Clin Infect Dis 1992;15:582–590.
47. Lifeso RM, Hardor E, McCorkell SJ: Spinal brucellosis. J Bone Joint Surg Br 1985;67:345–351.
48. Ariza J, Corredoira J, Pallares R, et al: Characteristics of risk factors for relapse of brucellosis in humans. Clin Infect Dis 1995;20:1241–1249.
49. Morate P, Queipo-Ortúño MI, Reguera JM, et al: Post treatment follow-up of brucellosis by PCR assay. J Clin Microbiol 1999;37:4163–4166.
50. Young EJ: An overview of human brucellosis. Clin Infect Dis 1995;21:283–289.
51. Human exposure to Brucella abortus strain RB51—Kansas, 1997. MMWR Morb Mortal Wkly Rep 1998;47:172–175.

Bartonellosis

JENNIFER S. DALY, MD

HISTORY

The genus *Bartonella* contains its original member, *Bartonella bacilliformis*, the etiologic agent of Oroya fever and verruga peruana, the organisms previously classified as *Rochalimaea* spp and *Grahamella* spp, and the newer species including those that have been shown to cause cat scratch disease (CSD), endocarditis, and bacillary angiomatosis.[1] These organisms are related not only in the laboratory but also in the clinical characteristics of the diseases produced in humans and in animals, which are similar in members of the genus. There are now 15 described species in the genus *Bartonella* (See Table 37–1). Although the genus *Bartonella* has been classified in the family Bartonellaceae within the order Rickettsiales, some of the closest relatives to the expanded genus *Bartonella* are the *Brucella* spp.[2]

CLINICAL DISEASE

Classic Bartonellosis

Bartonella spp produce a variety of clinical manifestations from endocarditis to vascular proliferative lesions, lymphadenopathy, and reticuloendothelial system lesions. The oldest recognized species, *B. bacilliformis*, causes two distinct syndromes (an acute febrile illness and a chronic skin eruption) that are characteristic of the genus. The chronic form of bartonellosis is verruga peruana or warts of the Andes. Fever, bacteremia, and hemolysis characterize the acute form, called Oroya fever. In many patients *B. bacilliformis* produces a biphasic illness, in that over months the patients experience both the acute and chronic manifestations. Chronic bartonellosis is characterized by vascular proliferation (verruga peruana) histologically similar to bacillary angiomatosis, an illness caused by *Bartonella quintana* and *Bartonella henselae*. The organism grows in the vascular epithelium of the skin. Skin lesions consist of nodules exhibiting active proliferation of newly formed capillaries, dilated venules, and precapillary vessels with endothelial hyperplasia.[3] The lesions may be found in bones, mucous membranes, lungs, liver, spleen, brain, and lymph nodes and may undergo spontaneous regression. In the preantibiotic era mortality was high, with 40% of patients dying of bacterial superinfection, particularly bacteremic salmonellosis. Treatment with chloramphenicol appears to be beneficial,[4] but a recent analysis of an epidemic suggests that there are many more mild or asymptomatic cases than previously described. Only 4.8% of the patients in this outbreak developed skin lesions (the chronic form of the disease) weeks to months after presenting with the acute febrile phase. In other studies up to 15% of patients may exhibit prolonged, asymptomatic

TABLE 37-1 ■ *Bartonella* Species Causing Human Disease

Organism	Major human diseases	Reservoir	Vectors	Possible treatment
B. bacilliformis	Verruga peruana Oroya fever (Carrión's disease)	Humans	Sandfly	Chloramphenicol/Rifampin ?
B. quintana	Trench fever Bacillary angiomatosis/ visceral peliosis Fever / bacteremia Endocarditis Lymphadenopathy	Humans	Body louse	Doxycycline/Chloramphenicol Macrolides Doxycycline ?Ampicillin and gentamicin Ceftriaxone and gentamicin ?Plus doxycycline Unknown
B. henselae	Fever / bacteremia Bacillary angiomatosis/ visceral peliosis Cat-scratch disease Endocarditis	Cats	Fleas	Doxycycline or macrolides Doxycycline or macrolides None vs azithromycin or various other agents ?Ampicillin and gentamicin Ceftriaxone and gentamicin ?Plus doxycycline
B. elizabethae	Endocarditis	Rats		Unknown
B. clarridgeiae	Cat-scratch disease	Cats		None/unknown
B. vinsonii subsp. *berkhoffi*	Endocarditis	Dogs/coyotes		Unknown
B. vinsonii subsp *arupensis*	Fever	Unknown		Unknown
B. grahamii	Neuroretinitis	Unknown		Unknown

bacteremia, similar to that seen with the more recently described species. Physicians need to consider the diagnosis in travelers who may develop skin lesions weeks to months after return from an endemic area. *B. bacilliformis* is transmitted by phlebotomine sandflies of the genus *Lutzomyia verrucarum* and geographically is limited to the western slopes of the Andes Mountains at elevations between 500 and 3375 m in Colombia, Ecuador, Peru, Chile, Bolivia, and probably Guatemala.

Trench Fever

B. quintana is the organism that produces trench fever, initially recognized during World War I. Although it resulted in significant loss of manpower, as soldiers were frequently ill for 5 to 6 weeks, death was uncommon. Occasionally soldiers developed a relapsing or prolonged fever. After World War II, small epidemics and sporadic cases were noted in Europe, but epidemics were not recognized in the United States until 1994 when eight cases were reported in homeless men in Seattle[5] and then in France. A modern description of this illness involved eight patients with *B. quintana* bacteremia who had febrile illnesses compatible with trench fever and two patients with endocarditis. Many of these patients were homeless, used alcoholic beverages, and had lice or scabies. The organism has been found in several different geographic areas including Europe, North America, Ethiopia, and China. In addi-

tion to its role as etiologic agent in cases of trench fever and cases of fever of unknown origin, *B. quintana* has been isolated from skin lesions of patients with bacillary angiomatosis, detected in the livers of patients with peliosis hepatis, and cultured from the blood of patients with endocarditis.[6,7]

Bacillary Angiomatosis

Bacillary angiomatosis is a vasculoproliferative disease primarily affecting immunocompromised patients. It was first diagnosed in 1983 in an HIV-infected man with subcutaneous nodules, fever, and weight loss.[8,9] Clinical manifestations of the illness are similar to those seen in patients with *B. bacilliformis* infection and those with cat scratch disease.[10] Patients most commonly present with multiple, angiomatous, tender papules or subcutaneous nodules. Patients with peliosis often complain of fever, abdominal pain, and weight loss and exhibit hepatomegaly or splenomegaly or both. Bone lesions, which are lytic, most frequently involve the long bones. Lesions may occur in the mouth, stomach, large or small intestine, and the respiratory tract. Central nervous system and retinal lesions have been documented. Cases have been described of neuroretinitis, or Leber's stellate neuroretinitis, a form of optic neuropathy manifest as optic nerve swelling with a macular star of exudate, similar to that seen in CSD, and in some normal hosts. These patients had serologic evidence of *Bartonella* infection, and the retinitis resolved with or without therapy and often with little visual damage.[11,12] Patients with bacillary angiomatosis may have prolonged bacteremia that can be documented by processing the blood cultures to detect *Bartonella* spp. Systemic signs and symptoms include fever, chills, malaise, headache, anorexia, and weight loss and may be present weeks to months before the diagnosis is made. Occasional patients relapse with fever, bacteremia, or skin lesions when treatment is stopped. Both *B. quintana* and *B. henselae* have been found in patients with bacillary angiomatosis.[13] There is one report of neuroretinitis in a patient with serologic evidence and molecular sequence evidence of infection with *B. vinsonii* subsp *arupensis*.[14,15]

Cat-Scratch Disease

Bartonella spp, most commonly *B. henselae* and sometimes *B. clarridgeiae*, cause most CSD. *B. henselae* was first isolated in 1986 from the blood of two patients with fever and symptomatic human immunodeficiency virus (HIV)-1 infection.[16] It was then found in patients with bacillary angiomatosis, typical CSD, and endocarditis.[10] The similarity between bacillary angiomatosis and CSD was first noted in HIV-infected patients, and serologic studies provided confirmation of this association.[17] *B. henselae* has been cultured from the lymph nodes of patients with CSD, and with polymerase chain reaction (PCR) techniques it was detected in patients with CSD. In addition, *Bartonella*-specific sequences have been detected in the material used for the CSD skin test. *B. henselae* and *B. clarridgeiae* have been isolated from the blood of cats, and antibody to *B. henselae* has been found in cats owned by patients with CSD.[18] The extent of disease due to *B. clarridgeiae* has not been determined, but hopefully with the use of a specific antibody test using antigen from the polar flagella (not present in *B. henselae*) more information will become available.[19] Other *Bartonella* species, including *B. quintana*, may produce syndromes similar to CSD,[20] but further research is needed.

The most common presenting symptom of a patient with CSD is lymphadenopathy in the region draining the primary inoculation. Sites usually involved (in order of frequency) are the upper extremity, head and neck, and groin. The papule at the inoculation site is often unrecognized by physicians not used to dealing with the disease or may disappear by the time the lymphadenopathy is recognized.[21] The lymphadenopathy develops within 2 to 3 weeks but sometimes is not noticed for up to 8 weeks. Approximately 30% to 50% of the patients have fever, and as many as 9% have temperatures as high as 38.4°C to 40.5°C (102°F to 105°F).[4,5,6,22] In more than three quarters of the patients the disease is mild, although these patients may have generalized achiness, malaise, and anorexia.[22] The lymphadenopathy usually disappears within 2 to 4 months. About 10% of the nodes suppurate and may require drainage or drain spontaneously. A few patients exhibit more unusual presentations, including

Parinaud's ocular glandular fever, central nervous system manifestations including neuroretinitis, fever of unknown origin, granulomatous hepatitis, pulmonary symptoms, or persistent fatigue.[23–26] Some patients present with meningoencephalitis, with seizures (including status epilepticus) as the first feature of CSD. Patients who are immunocompromised may develop widespread disease, including the skin lesions of bacillary angiomatosis, peliosis or microabscesses of the liver and spleen, lytic bone lesions, lymphadenopathy, or persistent bacteremia.

Endocarditis

Several *Bartonella* spp have been shown to cause endocarditis. Cases are difficult to diagnose, as the organisms grow slowly and standard blood cultures are frequently negative. *B. henselae*, *B. quintana*, *Bartonella elizabethae*, and several *B. vinsonii* subspecies have been proven to cause endocarditis.[27–29] Patients often have abnormal heart valves and are difficult to cure without surgery. The organism is difficult to culture, and diagnosis relies on high clinical suspicion, serology, culture, and PCR techniques. An example of the difficulty in diagnosis of cases of endocarditis is the history of the discovery of *B. elizabethae*, a species that could not be identified when first isolated in 1986 from a patient with endocarditis treated at Saint Elizabeth's Hospital in Boston.[28] The organism was initially subcultured from Bactec blood culture bottles with the subculture plates incubated for 10 days in 5% CO_2. In 1992 after the microbiologic and molecular characteristics of *B. henselae* had been reported, it was found to be a unique organism related to the *Bartonella* species by phenotypic characteristics, cellular fatty acid content, DNA relatedness data, and 16S rRNA sequence analysis. Other isolates of this species have been found in rats in the United States and in Peru, and serologic responses to this organism have been detected in patients using intravenous drugs and a patient with fatal myocarditis. Recently subspecies of *B. vinsonii* have been shown to cause endocarditis first in a dog and then in humans.[27,30]

TABLE 37–2 ■ Nomenclature of *Bartonella* Species Originally Designated as Different Species

Current name	Previous designations
HUMAN PATHOGENS	
B. bacilliformis	
B. quintana	*Rochalimaea quintana*
	Rickettsia quintana
B. henselae	*Rochalimaea henselae*
B. elizabethae	*Rochalimaea elizabethae*
ANIMAL ASSOCIATED	
B. vinsonii	Vole agent
	Rochalimaea vinsonii
B. talpae	*Grahamella talpae*
B. peromysci	*Grahamella peromysci*

ANIMAL SPECIES

Like *B. vinsonii*, the organisms originally classified as *Grahamella* species (*Bartonella talpae, Bartonella peromysci, Bartonella grahamii, Bartonella taylorii,* and *Bartonella doshiae*) have been found only in animals and in the past were named for the animal host.[31–33] These organisms are erythrocyte-associated bacteria that were first observed in 1905 by G. S. Graham-Smith in moles. They have been found most commonly in rodents, were first cultured in 1932, and were poorly characterized until 1994 when Birtles and co-workers reported isolation of several species from the blood of two-thirds of small mammals trapped in Shropshire, United Kingdom.[34]

EPIDEMIOLOGY

A number of epidemiologic associations with insect vectors and animals are known. *B. bacilliformis* infection is associated with transmission by the bite of the sand fly; *B. quintana* has been cultured from wild body lice, and *B. henselae* can be transmitted from cat to cat by fleas,[35] *B. vinsonii* subsp *berkhoffii* has been found in domestic dogs and wild coyotes,[36] and *B. elizabethae* has been cultured from rats.[37] There may be more than one vector for each species. Five of the ten patients bacteremic with *B. quintana* in the report by Spach and co-workers had scabies, and one had lice.[5] Prevalence of the *Bartonella* bacteremia in animals is most common in summer and early autumn when flea infestations are heaviest, and there seems to be a parallel seasonal increase in the incidence of CSD in humans. Several *Bartonella* spp have been found in ticks.[38] *B. bacilliformis* is found in a limited geographic region, whereas *B. quintana* and *B. henselae* are found worldwide. It is not known if asymptomatic, chronically infected humans serve as a reservoir for some of these organisms.

DIAGNOSIS

Microbiology

The members of this genus are thin, aerobic, slightly curved rods that stain weakly gram-negative but can be stained with the Warthin-Starry, Giemsa, and Gimenez stains. *B. bacilliformis* grows best at 25°C, and the other species grow at 35°C to 37°C. Isolation of these nutritionally fastidious organisms from the blood of patients can be accomplished with commercially available blood culture systems and subcultured with prolonged incubation of subculture plates (chocolate agar, anaerobic blood agar, and freshly prepared brain heart infusion agar with 5% rabbit blood) in an atmosphere of 5% CO_2 with high humidity. After initial isolation the organisms will grow in haemophilus test medium and specially prepared blood-free media. After several passages, incubation time decreases, and colonies become larger and less adherent. A MicroScan Rapid Anaerobe Identification Panel can be used along with phenotypic characteristics to suggest to the technologist that *Bartonella* spp have been isolated, but determination of cellular fatty acids or molecular techniques are needed to confirm the identification. Techniques available in research laboratories include reactivity with specific antiserum, cellular fatty acid analysis, 16S rRNA gene sequencing, restriction fragment length polymorphism after PCR amplification of the citrate synthase gene, the riboflavin synthetase gene, the 16S-23S rRNA gene ITS, and pulsed-field gel electrophoresis.[39,40] The organisms parasitize the erythrocytes of their hosts (*B. bacilliformis* and animal species), and smears are used for direct detection of *B. bacilliformis* in endemic areas. *B. bacilliformis* and *B. clarridgeiae* are the only members of the genus that have polar flagella. Several species may be distinguished from each other with commercial tests to detect specific preformed enzymes. Isolation of the organism from tissue is more difficult than from blood.[41] Cocultivation with an endothelial cell monolayer has been used to aid recovery. Direct plating of tissue has yielded *B. henselae*, but in some cases only after up to 60 days incubation.[42]

Serology

Serologic tests are available to aid in the diagnosis of infection with these organisms and have been used in patients with bacillary angiomatosis, fever or bacteremia, and CSD.[43–46] Indirect fluorescent antibody tests are available from the Centers for Disease Control and Prevention (CDC). A commercial enzyme immunoassay for the detection of antibodies to *B. henselae* is available from the Specialty Laboratories, Santa Monica, California. An immunoblot technique that can detect both IgM and IgG to *B. henselae* has been developed, and new antibody tests for differentiation of the species remain to be validated clinically. Serum from patients with CSD shows antibodies against both *B. quintana* and *B. henselae*, probably the result of cross-reactivity. Patients with *B. bacilliformis* infection may have reactions to serology for brucellosis (40%). Further epidemiologic study including studies of the rate of antibody response to these organisms is needed. The initial serology may be negative, but patients may exhibit a rise in titer over time.[47]

Histology

The diagnosis can be suggested by histologic findings in tissue from skin lesions, lymph nodes, spleen, or liver. In chronic bartonellosis due to *B. bacilliformis*, lesions consist of nodules that exhibit active proliferation of newly formed capillaries, dilated venules, and precapillary vessels with endothelial hyperplasia.[3] These nodules may be found in bones, mucous membranes, lungs, liver, spleen, brain, and lymph nodes. In patients with bacillary angiomatosis, nodules show proliferating endothelial and histiocytic cells in a framework of weakly formed capillaries. The lesions contain bacteria that stain with the Warthin-Starry stain and may be few in numbers or widely disseminated.[48] Some patients may have only skin mucosal lesions, and others have histologically similar lesions in bone, lung, liver, spleen, lymph nodes, and the central nervous system. Bacillary angiomatosis–associated lesions in the liver and spleen, bacillary peliosis hepatis, or bacillary peliosis splenitis show cystic, blood-filled spaces, foci of necrosis, or granulation-like tissue. In contrast, immunocompetent patients with CSD are often diagnosed clinically or by serologic tests. If a biopsy is done, the histology of the lesions reflects the host response to the organism. Initially there is a neutrophilic response and bacteria can be seen around vessels and in microabscesses. Later in the disease, as the node enlarges, lymphoid hyperplasia occurs with stellate necrotizing granulomata. Some lymph nodes have caseous necrosis. In the later stages, few organisms are found in the tissue with the silver stain. The pathologic findings are nonspecific, and without the finding of the organism on Warthin-Starry staining or probing of the tissue with a *Bartonella*-specific primer, the diagnosis can only be suggested.

TREATMENT

Antibiotics are known to decrease mortality in Oroya fever. Chloramphenicol, penicillins, and aminoglycosides have been used, but it is not known if the improved outcome has been due to therapy of the *Bartonella* infection or because of efficacy against secondary pathogens such as *Salmonella* spp. Antibiotics (a macrolide or a tetracycline) appear to be beneficial in patients with bacillary angiomatosis, peliosis hepatis, and bacteremia and fever but not in most patients with CSD. One study suggests the volume of affected lymph nodes during therapy with azithromycin is lower than in controls with no treatment. Other agents have appeared to be successful, although penicillins and first-generation cephalosporins appear to be the least active.[49–51] Various agents have been tried in patients with CSD, including TMP-SMX, rifampin, ciprofloxacin, and gentamicin. Only aminoglycosides have bactericidal activity.[50] There are no studies to help determine optimal treatment for *Bartonella* endocarditis. Before the discovery of this organism as a cause of endocarditis, it is thought that *Bartonella* cases were included in the group of patients treated for culture-negative endocarditis and responded to therapy with ampicillin and gentamicin. Isolated cases have been treated with combinations of ceftriaxone, doxycycline, and gentamicin for at least 4 weeks, and 6 to 9 months of therapy with macrolide agents has been used after valve replacement.

The optimal duration of therapy is not known, but prolonged treatment from weeks to months, even lifelong, may be needed in HIV-infected patients. Fever and bacteremia in immunocompetent persons initially appeared to be cured after relatively brief courses (7 to 10 days) of antibiotics. Lucey et al, however, reported two immunocompetent patients (one with aseptic meningitis) with clinical relapses after treatment that were cured after re-treatment.[52] This spectrum of clinical disease is similar to that seen in patients with trench fever and infection with *B. bacilliformis*. The influence of antibiotic treatment on the course and duration of chronic disease is not well understood. In vitro testing reveals that the organisms are susceptible to several classes of antimicrobials and does not reflect clearly clinical experience. It is thought that the intracellular growth of bacteria and perhaps inhibitory rather than bactericidal activity of the agents may explain clinical relapses and failure.

SUMMARY

As laboratories become aware of the growth characteristics of *Bartonella* species and physicians better understand the illnesses caused by these pathogens, it is likely that more cases will be recognized. With the increase in detection, more in vitro information about antimicrobial susceptibility and in vivo data about clinical risk factors for infection will emerge to help clinicians correctly diagnose and treat patients with infection with these organisms.

REFERENCES

1. Daly J: *Bartonella* species. In Gorbach S, Bartlett J, Blacklow N (eds): Infectious Diseases, 2nd ed. Philadelphia, W. B. Saunders, 1998.
2. Brenner DJ, O'Connor SP, Winkler HH, Steigerwalt AG: Proposals to unify the genera *Bartonella* and *Rochalimaea*, with descriptions of *Bartonella quintana* comb. nov., *Bartonella vinsonii* comb. nov., *Bartonella henselae* comb. nov., and *Bartonella elizabethae* comb. nov., and to remove the family Bartonellaceae from the order Rickettsiales. Int J Syst Bacteriol 1993;43:777–786.
3. Arias-Stella J, Lieberman PH, Erlandson RA, Arias-Stella J Jr: Histology, immunohistochemistry, and ultrastructure of the verruga in Carrion's disease. Am J Surg Pathol 1986;10:595–610.
4. Gray GC, Johnson AA, Thornton SA, et al: An epidemic of Oroya fever in the Peruvian Andes. Am J Trop Med Hyg 1990;42:215–221.
5. Spach DH, Kanter AS, Dougherty MJ, et al: *Bartonella (Rochalimaea) quintana* bacteremia in inner-city patients with chronic alcoholism. N Engl J Med 1995;332:424–428.
6. Drancourt M, Mainardi JL, Brouqui P, et al: *Bartonella (Rochalimaea) quintana* endocarditis in three homeless men. N Engl J Med 1995;332:419–423.
7. Spach DH, Callis KP, Paauw DS, et al: Endocarditis caused by *Rochalimaea quintana* in a patient infected with human immunodeficiency virus. J Clin Microbiol 1993;31:692–694.
8. Slater LN, Welch DF, Min KW: *Rochalimaea henselae* causes bacillary angiomatosis and peliosis hepatis. Arch Intern Med 1992;152:602–606.

9. Slater LN, Welch DF, Hensel D, Coody DW: A newly recognized fastidious gram-negative pathogen as a cause of fever and bacteremia. N Engl J Med 1990;323:1587–1593.

10. Adal KA, Cockerell CJ, Petri WA Jr: Cat scratch disease, bacillary angiomatosis, and other infections due to *Rochalimaea*. N Engl J Med 1994;330:1509–1515.

11. Earhart KC, Power MH: *Bartonella* Neuroretinitis. N Engl J Med 2000;343:1459.

12. Chrousos G: Neuroretinitis in cat scratch disease. J Clin Neuroophthalmol 1990;10:92–94.

13. Koehler JE, Sanchez MA, Garrido CS, et al: Molecular epidemiology of *Bartonella* infections in patients with bacillary angiomatosis-peliosis. N Engl J Med 1997;337:1876–1883.

14. Welch DF, Carroll KC, Hofmeister EK, et al: Isolation of a new subspecies, *Bartonella vinsonii* subsp. *arupensis*, from a cattle rancher: Identity with isolates found in conjunction with *Borrelia burgdorferi* and *Babesia microti* among naturally infected mice. J Clin Microbiol 1999;37:2598–2601.

15. Houpikian P, Fournier PE, Raoult D: Phylogenetic position of *Bartonella vinsonii* subsp. *arupensis* based on 16S rDNA and gltA gene sequences. Int J Syst Evol Microbiol 2001;51:179–182.

16. Slater L, Welch D, Hensel D, et al: A newly recognized fastidious gram-negative pathogen as a cause of fever and bacteremia. N Engl J Med 1990;323:1587.

17. Regnery R, Tappero J: Unraveling mysteries associated with cat-scratch disease, bacillary angiomatosis, and related syndromes. Emerg Infect Dis 1995;1:16–21.

18. Breitschwerdt EB, Kordick DL: *Bartonella* infection in animals: Carriership, reservoir potential, pathogenicity, and zoonotic potential for human infection. Clin Microbiol Rev 2000;13:428–438.

19. Sander A, Zagrosek A, Bredt W, et al: Characterization of *Bartonella clarridgeiae* flagellin (FlaA) and detection of antiflagellin antibodies in patients with lymphadenopathy. J Clin Microbiol 2000;38:2943–2948.

20. Case records of the Massachusetts General Hospital. Weekly clinicopathological exercises. Case 1–1998. An 11-year-old boy with a seizure. N Engl J Med 1998;338:112–119.

21. Margileth AM: Dermatologic manifestations and update of cat scratch disease. Pediatr Dermatol 1988;5:1–9.

22. Carithers HA: Cat-scratch disease. An overview based on a study of 1200 patients. Am J Dis Child 1985;139:1124–1133.

23. Dangman BC, Albanese BA, Kacica MA, et al: Cat scratch disease in two children presenting with fever of unknown origin: Imaging features and association with a new causative agent, *Rochalimaea henselae*. Pediatrics 1995;95:767–771.

24. Kahr A, Kerbl R, Gschwandtner K, et al: Visceral manifestation of cat scratch disease in children. A consequence of altered immunological state? Infection 2000;28:116–118.

25. Marra CM: Neurologic complications of *Bartonella henselae* infection. Curr Opin Neurol 1995;8:164–169.

26. Wong MT, Dolan MJ, Lattuada CP Jr, et al: Neuroretinitis, aseptic meningitis, and lymphadenitis associated with *Bartonella (Rochalimaea) henselae* infection in immunocompetent patients and patients infected with human immunodeficiency virus type 1. Clin Infect Dis 1995;21:352–360.

27. Roux V, Eykyn SJ, Wyllie S, Raoult D: *Bartonella vinsonii* subsp. *berkhoffii* as an agent of afebrile blood culture–negative endocarditis in a human. J Clin Microbiol 2000;38:1698–1700.

28. Daly JS, Worthington MG, Brenner DJ, et al: *Rochalimaea elizabethae* sp. nov. isolated from a patient with endocarditis. J Clin Microbiol 1993;31:872–881.

29. Raoult D, Fournier PE, Drancourt M, et al: Diagnosis of 22 new cases of *Bartonella* endocarditis. Ann Intern Med 1996;125:646–652.

30. Breitschwerdt EB, Kordick DL, Malarkey DE, et al: Endocarditis in a dog due to infection with a novel *Bartonella* subspecies. J Clin Microbiol 1995;33:154–160.

31. Birtles RJ, Canales J, Ventosilla P, et al: Survey of *Bartonella* species infecting intradomicillary animals in the Huayllacall Valley, Ancash, Peru, a region endemic for human bartonellosis. Am J Trop Med Hyg 1999;60:799–805.

32. Bermond D, Heller R, Barrat F, et al: *Bartonella birtlesii* sp. nov., isolated from small mammals (*Apodemus* spp.). Int J Sys Evol Microbiol 2000;6:1973–1979.

33. Birtles RJ, Hazel SM, Bennett M, et al: Longitudinal monitoring of the dynamics of infections due to *Bartonella* species in UK woodland rodents. Epidemiol Infect 2001;126:323–329.

34. Birtles R, Harrison T: *Grahamella* in small woodland mammals in the U.K.: Isolation, prevalence and host specificity. Ann Trop Med Parasitol 1994;88:317.

35. Higgins JA, Radulovic S, Jaworski DC, Azad AF: Acquisition of the cat scratch disease agent *Bartonella henselae* by cat fleas (Siphonaptera:Pulicidae). J Med Entomol 1996;33:490–495.

36. Chang CC, Kasten RW, Chomel BB, et al: Coyotes (*Canis latrans*) as the reservoir for a human pathogenic *Bartonella* sp.: molecular epidemiology of *Bartonella vinsonii* subsp. *berkhoffii* infection in coyotes from central coastal California. J Clin Microbiol 2000;38:4193–4200.

37. Ellis BA, Regnery RL, Beati L, et al: Rats of the genus *Rattus* are reservoir hosts for pathogenic *Bartonella* species: An Old World origin for a New World disease? J Infect Dis 1999;180:220–224.

38. Chang CC, Chomel BB, Kasten RW, et al: Molecular evidence of *Bartonella* spp. in questing adult *Ixodes pacificus* ticks in California. J Clin Microbiol 2001;39:1221–1226.

39. Renesto P, Gouvernet J, Drancourt M, et al: Use of rpoB gene analysis for detection and identification of *Bartonella* species. J Clin Microbiol 2001;39:430–437.

40. Joblet C, Roux V, Drancourt M, et al: Identification of *Bartonella (Rochalimaea)* species among fastidious gram-negative bacteria on the basis of the partial sequence of the citrate-synthase gene. J Clin Microbiol 1995;33:1879–1883.

41. Brenner SA, Rooney JA, Manzewitsch P, Regnery RL: Isolation of *Bartonella (Rochalimaea) henselae*: Effects of methods of blood collection and handling. J Clin Microbiol 1997;35:544–547.

42. Wong MT, Thornton DC, Kennedy RC, Dolan MJ: A chemically defined liquid medium that supports primary isolation of *Rochalimaea (Bartonella) henselae* from blood and tissue specimens. J Clin Microbiol 1995;33:742–744.

43. Maurin M, Eb F, Etienne J, Raoult D: Serological cross-reactions between *Bartonella* and *Chlamydia* species: Implications for diagnosis. J Clin Microbiol 1997;35:2283–2287.

44. Nadal D, Zbinden R: Serology to *Bartonella (Rochalimaea) henselae* may replace traditional diagnostic criteria for cat-scratch disease. Eur J Pediatr 1995;154:906–908.

45. Guibal F, de La Salmoniere P, Rybojad M, et al: High seroprevalence to *Bartonella quintana* in homeless patients with cutaneous parasitic infestations in downtown Paris. J Am Acad Dermatol 2001;44:219–223.

46. Del Prete R, Fumarola D, Fumarola L, et al: Prevalence of antibodies to *Bartonella henselae* in patients with suspected cat scratch disease (CSD) in Italy. Eur J Epidemiol 1999;15:583–587.

47. Karem KL: Immune aspects of *Bartonella*. Crit Rev Microbiol 2000;26:133–145.

48. Perkocha L, Geaghan S, Benedict Yen T, et al: Clinical and pathological features of bacillary peliosis hepatis in association with human immunodeficiency virus infection. N Engl J Med 1990;323:1581.

49. Maurin M, Gasquet S, Ducco C, Raoult D: MICs of 28 antibiotic compounds for 14 *Bartonella* (formerly *Rochalimaea*) isolates. Antimicrob Agents Chemother 1995;39:2387–2391.

50. Rolain JM, Maurin M, Raoult D: Bactericidal effect of antibiotics on *Bartonella* and *Brucella* spp.: Clinical implications. J Antimicrob Chemother 2000;46:811–814.

51. Sobraques M, Maurin M, Birtles RJ, Raoult D: In vitro susceptibilities of four *Bartonella* bacilliformis strains to 30 antibiotic compounds. Antimicrob Agents Chemother 1999;43:2090–2092.

52. Lucey D, Dolan MJ, Moss CW, et al: Relapsing illness due to *Rochalimaea henselae* in immunocompetent hosts: Implication for therapy and new epidemiological associations. Clin Infect Dis 1992;14:683–688.

Toxoplasma gondii and Toxoplasmosis

ELAINE PETROF, MD

RIMA MCLEOD, MD

Toxoplasma gondii is an obligate, intracellular, protozoan parasite, first described in 1908.[1] It is a member of the subphylum Apicomplexa and thus is related to other pathogenic apicomplexan parasites, such as *Plasmodium* (malaria), *Cryptosporidium*, and *Babesia*. *T. gondii* is the parasite; toxoplasmosis is the disease. Infection does not always result in recognized illness.[2–4]

LIFE CYCLE, MODES OF TRANSMISSION, AND EPIDEMIOLOGY

Life Cycle

T. gondii infects animals worldwide. Cats are the definitive hosts. Three forms of *T. gondii* are infectious to humans: tachyzoites, bradyzoites, and oocysts containing sporozoites (Fig. 38–1). The oocyst is highly infectious and is encountered in materials contaminated with cat excrement. *T. gondii* infects almost all animal species. Bradyzoite and tachyzoite forms infect all animal-tested cells except fat head minnow cells (Pfefferkorn, personal communication, 1980).[3,5–7]

When a cat is infected for the first time with cysts containing bradyzoites or oocyst containing sporozoites, the parasite undergoes its complete sexual cycle within the cat intestine. The numbers of female macrogametes are much more abundant than the male microgametes; macrogametes and microgametes make schizonts; up to 10 million oocysts can be excreted in a single day.[8–11] Oocyst production peaks between 5 and 8 days after the cat is infected, and these oocysts are shed over 7 to 20 days.[9] Depending on the temperature of the soil, sporulation of oocysts occurs in 1 to 21 days, and sporulated oocysts can remain infectious for up to 18 months in warm, moist soil. Humans may contract infection by ingestion of any material contaminated with cat feces containing oocysts. This can be an unrecognized exposure, for example, with contaminated fruits and vegetables that have not been thoroughly washed in water.

The tachyzoite is haploid, asexual, rapidly dividing, invasive, and destroys cells and tissues. Infection with tachyzoites develops shortly after ingestion of either bradyzoites or oocysts during acute infection. Tachyzoites are the form of the parasite that produces clinical manifestations of toxoplasmosis. Acute infection may be asymptomatic. Once acute infection resolves, *T. gondii* persists in all infected hosts as bradyzoites in tissue cysts.[2,6,7]

The bradyzoite is the latent, more slowly growing form of *T. gondii*. Bradyzoites are found in tissue cysts, which may be present in any organ but most frequently involve the central nervous system and muscle. Since cysts are relatively resistant to gastric acid and acidic pH, transmission results from eating meat that contains cysts

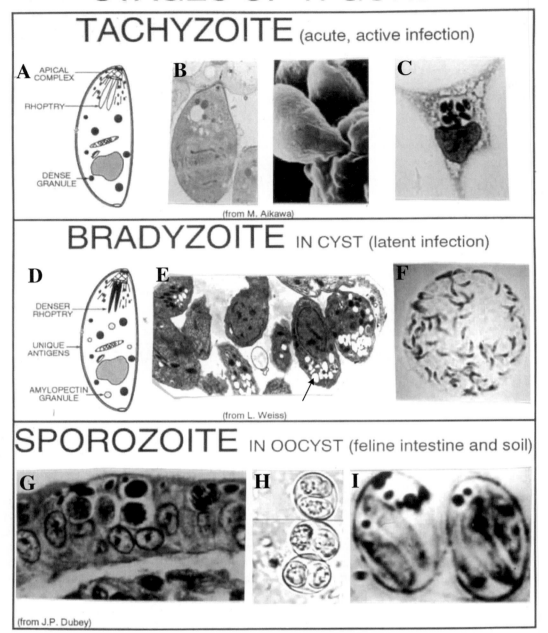

FIGURE 38–1. Stages of *Toxoplasma gondii*. **A**, Schematic diagram of tachyzoite. **B**, Transmission and scanning electron micrographs of tachyzoite invading a host cell. **C**, Light micrograph of tachyzoites replicating within a parasitophorous vacuole in the host cell cytoplasm. **D**, Schematic diagram of bradyzoite. **E**, Transmission electron micrograph of cyst containing bradyzoites (*arrow* indicates amylopectin granules). **F**, Light micrograph of cyst containing bradyzoites. **G**, Development of oocysts in cat intestine. **H**, oocysts in lumen of cat intestine. **I**, Sporulating oocysts that contain sporozoites. (*A* from McLeod R, Mack D, Brown C: New advances in cellular and molecular biology of *Toxoplasma gondii*. Exp Parasitol 1991; 72: 109–121. *B* from Aikawa M, Komata Y, Asai T, Midorikawa O: Transmission and scanning electronmicroscopy of host cell entry by *Toxoplasma gondii*. Am J Pathol 1977; 87: 285–296. *E* from Weiss LW, LaPlace D, Takvorian P, et al: A cell culture system for study of development of *Toxoplasma gondii* bradyzoites. J Eur Microbiol 1995; 42: 150–157. *F* from Remington JS: In discussion, Lainson R: Observations on the nature and transmission of *Toxoplasma gondii* in light of its wide host and geographical range. Toxoplasmosis. Surv Ophthalmol 1961; 6:721–758, *G* from Gardner CH, Fayer R, Dubey JP: An Atlas of Protozoan Parasites in Animal Tissues. Agriculture Handbook No 651. Washington, DC, U.S. Department of Agriculture, 1988; *H* and *I* from Dubey JP, Miller NL, Frenkel JK: The *Toxoplasma gondii* oocysts from cat feces. J Exp Med 1970; 132:636–662, composite from Boyer K, McLeod R: Toxoplasmosis. Long S, Pickering L, Proeber C [eds]: Principles and Practice of Pediatric Infectious Diseases. New York, Churchill Livingstone, 1997.)

and that has not been cooked to "well-done." Bradyzoites persist for the life of an infected animal or person.

When cysts rupture in an immunocompetent person, the immune system eradicates the rapidly proliferating parasites. In the immunocompromised host, however, it is usually reactivation of this latent form, associated with cyst rupture, that leads to acute infection with tachyzoites and the development of toxoplasmosis.

Epidemiology

Estimates of infection with *T. gondii* worldwide are based on seroprevalence data, and it is estimated that between one-third and one-half of the world's population is infected with this parasite (Fig. 38–2). There can be considerable variability in incidence even within the same geographic area. In the United States the Rocky Mountain States appear to have a lower incidence of infection.[12] Toxoplasmosis has been identified as the second most frequent single cause of food-borne-associated death in the United States[13] and as one of the most costly food-borne pathogens, with associated morbidities being responsible for $3.3 billion to $7.8 billion per year in health care and other costs.[13,14] Toxoplasmosis is not a reportable illness in the United States, and thus there is no accurate information about the numbers of cases of *T. gondii* infection. Family clusters of acute infection occur.[15] Epidemics have been reported in association with ingestion of contaminated food,[16–19] with a dusty riding rink in a stable with kittens in a nearby barn,[20] with water in Panama,[21] and without a clearly identifiable source when a water supply was suspected in Victoria, BC, Canada,[22] and in Brazil in a large epidemic of 176 cases.[23] Three clonal types of *T. gondii* have differing virulence in murine models, two of which are found in humans.[24,25] Type I and hybrid crosses of clonal types of parasites have been reported to be associated with more virulent disease in mice.[26] In Erecim, Brazil, there is a high incidence of retinal disease due to *T. gondii*.[27] Eighteen percent of the population have retinal disease that appears to be toxoplasmic chorioretinitis, and 99% of these persons have serum antibodies to *T. gondii*.[27] It appears that one of the three clonal types[24,25] of greater virulence for mice and certain recombinant parasites may be associated with more virulent ocular disease.[28] Interestingly, predominantly clonal type I parasites were identified recently in chickens in Sao Paulo, Brazil.[29] Human infections with clonal type I parasites have been identified in infants with congenital toxoplasmosis whose mothers had no evidence of increased pathogenicity or retinal disease (McLeod, unpublished observations). It is likely that clonal type, dose, route of infection, and immunogenetics all will be found to influence the outcome of *T. gondii* infection in humans.[24,25,30–38]

In congenital infections, monozygotic twins are often both infected with similar manifestations, whereas dizygotic twins are often discordant for occurrence and

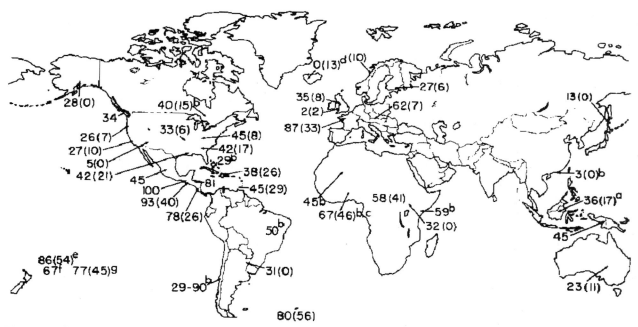

FIGURE 38–2. Prevalence of antibodies against *T. gondii* in persons in selected locales. Unless otherwise specified, figures outside parentheses represent the percentage of seropositive adults of approximately 30 to 40 years of age; figures inside parentheses are percentage of seropositive children younger than 10 years. **a**, IHA antibodies, others were IFA or dye test; **b**, adults with either age range not clearly specified or wider age range than approximately 30 to 40 years; **c**, juveniles; **d**, 14 persons 30 to 39 years of age having no *Toxoplasma* antibody, 29% of 14 persons 40 to 49 years of age with *Toxoplasma* antibody; **e**, Society Island; **f**, American Somoa; **g**, Tahiti. (From Remington JS, McLeod R: Toxoplasmosis. In Braude IA, Davis CE, Fierer J [eds]: Infectious Diseases and Medical Microbiology 2nd ed. Philadelphia, WB Saunders, 1986, pp 1521–1535).

manifestations of infection.[2,3,39] In both congenital infections and in patients with AIDS and toxoplasmic encephalitis, HLA DQ3 appears to be associated with increased susceptibility.[30,34] Chronically infected women who are immunologically normal rarely transmit the infection if it is acquired before conception,[3] and vaccines in animals can reduce congenital infections.[40]

Transmission

Routes of transmission to humans include the following:

- *Ingestion* of meat containing tissue cysts (i.e., to render bradyzoites in cysts noninfectious, meat must be cooked to well done, 56°C) or of vegetables or food products contaminated with oocysts is a common route of transmission.[41–43]
- *Congenital*, transplacental transmission during pregnancy from an acutely infected immunocompetent or an acutely or chronically infected immunocompromised mother to fetus.[3,5]

Other modes of transmission are

- *Organ transplantation*, usually from a seropositive donor organ to a seronegative recipient.[44–49] Reactivation from encysted organisms with immunosuppression also is a significant source of disease.[46,50–55]
- *Blood transfusion* of contaminated blood products.[56,57]
- *Laboratory accidents*, which usually involve accidental self-inoculation with the parasite (e.g., needle sticks).[58,59]
- *Autopsy accidents*, transmission from cadavers to the pathologist performing the autopsy has been reported.[60]

Routes of transmission are illustrated in Figure 38–3.

INFECTION IN THE IMMUNOCOMPETENT HOST

Incidence and Clinical Manifestations

On the basis of serologic data from the 1994 National Health and Nutrition Examination Survey (NHANES), it has been estimated that at least 1.5 million people in the United States experience an acute infection caused by *T. gondii* each year.[41] Thirty to fifty percent of the world population is infected with *T. gondii*. Only ten to twenty percent of acutely infected persons have had symptoms recognized as toxoplasmosis.[61–63] Lymphadenopathy, most often cervical and without associated symptoms, is the most common manifestation.[63–66] It is noteworthy that in an epidemic in Atlanta, Georgia, of 35 infected persons, 32 felt ill enough to seek medical attention, but the physicians evaluating these patients correctly diagnosed this infection in only 3 cases.[20] Rarely, pectoral nodes may be mistaken for breast malignancy, and mesenteric nodes with fever can mimic acute appendicitis.[66] *T. gondii* infection may also present as a mononucleosis-like syndrome, with fever, malaise, lymphadenopathy, and lymphocytosis

with atypical lymphocytes seen on peripheral blood smear.[66] Rash, hepatomegaly, and splenomegaly, although less common, have been reported. *T. gondii* is a cause of heterophil-negative mononucleosis-like syndromes, second only to cytomegalovirus. Guillain-Barré syndrome has occurred with toxoplasmosis.[67] Adenopathy with or without fever and fatigue can persist for more than a year.[66] In immunologically competent persons *T. gondii* infection rarely causes significant end-organ damage such as encephalitis, brain abscess or meningitis,[68] chorioretinitis,[69–71] myocarditis, acute or chronic pericarditis,[72] hepatitis,[20] and polymyositis[73,74] or death.[75,76] Although murine studies provide some precedent, recent reports of acute acquired and chronic toxoplasmosis causing behavioral abnormalities in humans require further corroboration.

Diagnosis

Diagnosis is made by demonstration of a pattern of antibody response characteristic of acute acquired infection.[4,5,77–89] This includes seroconversion, fourfold rise in serum antibody titer, IgM, IgA, or IgE specific to *T. gondii*,[5,77,81,90,91] and a characteristic pattern in the differential agglutination test.[4,86,92] The IgG antibody avidity test may be especially useful in establishing the time of acquisition of *T. gondii* relative to gestation,[93–99] as presence of high avidity antibody demonstrates that infection occurred more than 12 to 16 weeks earlier.[100] A lymph node biopsy has characteristic histopathology with epithelioid histiocytes and monocytoid cells encroaching on and blurring the margins of germinal centers.[101] Isolation of *T. gondii* or demonstration of parasites by polymerase chain reaction (PCR) from amniotic fluid or body fluids such as cerebrospinal fluid (CSF), bronchoalveolar lavage, or blood is also indicative of acute infection.[102–106] There are newer methods to distinguish stage of parasite and strain of parasite,[107,108] but these have not yet been used clinically.

Treatment

Acute *Toxoplasma* infection in the immunocompetent host does not require treatment when it is a self-limited illness.[84] Following are indications for therapeutic intervention:

1. Ocular disease.
2. Other vital end-organ damage such as myocarditis, pericarditis, hepatitis, encephalitis, meningitis, polymyositis.[20,68,72,74,79]
3. Persistence of severe constitutional symptoms.
4. Acquisition of infection from blood transfusion[57] or laboratory accident, which present the risks of exposure to an unusual parenteral route of transmission with a high parasite burden and to a rapid parenteral exposure to the tachyzoite form of the parasite, may result in more severe illness.

If the decision is made to treat, administration of pyrimethamine, sulfadiazine, and leucovorin for 4 to 6

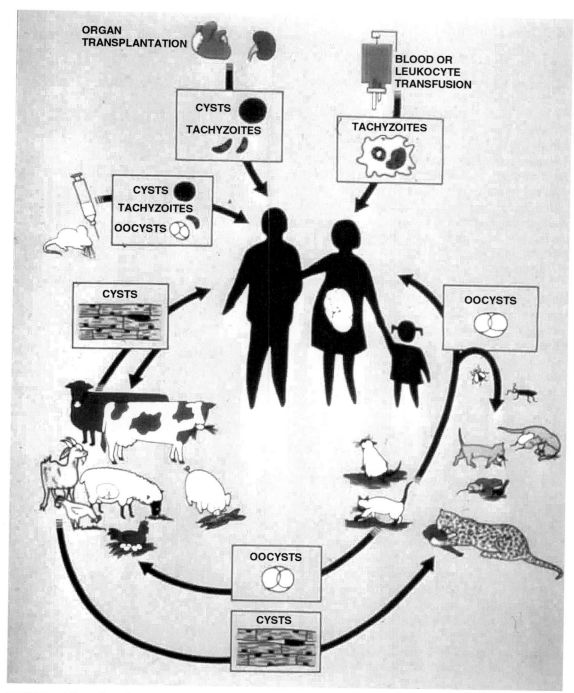

FIGURE 38–3. Life cycle and modes of transmission of *Toxoplasma gondii*. Infection in man and other animals occurs primarily after ingestion of either the cyst or the oocyst. Released organisms invade the intestinal epithelium, spread to tissue (either hematogenously or via lymphatics), and from cysts. When humans or other animals (including the cat) eat infected tissues (from any animal) or mature oocysts (excreted only by members of the cat family), the life cycle is completed. Laboratory accidents, organ transplantation, and blood and white blood cell transfusion also have been implicated in transmission of the organism. (From Remington JS, McLeod R: Toxoplasmosis. In Braude IA, Davis CE, Fierer J [eds]: Infectious Diseases and Medical Microbiology, 2nd ed. Philadelphia, WB Saunders, 1986, pp 1521–1535.)

weeks is usually associated with resolution of signs and symptoms. Establishing whether an acutely infected woman is pregnant or has family members or other close household contacts who are pregnant (as common risk factors often exist, causing infections to occur in family clusters)[15] is important because it influences the approach to treatment of the patient and her contacts. As pyrimethamine may be teratogenic in the first trimester, first-trimester pregnancy should be excluded before treatment with pyrimethamine is initiated.

OCULAR TOXOPLASMOSIS

Incidence and Clinical Manifestations

It has been estimated that *T. gondii* is the most frequent single cause of posterior uveitis, accounting for 30% to 50% of cases in the United States; it is one of the leading causes of posterior granulomatous uveitis in many countries.[109–113] Both congenital infection and acute acquired infection can cause retinal lesions, but whereas chorioretinitis is a uniform sequela of untreated congenital infection,[114–117] retinal disease is not common with acute acquired infection.[112,118–121] Certain clonal types, that is, the more virulent type I parasites, and certain recombinations of clonal types of parasites may be associated with more severe ocular disease.[26] The exact mechanisms whereby ocular disease is initiated and recurs remain to be determined, although both hematogenous and retrograde neuronal spread have been proposed as feasible routes for the parasite to take to reach the eye.[109,112,113] The presence of *T. gondii* cysts in an otherwise normal retina and the observation of new lesions that are satellites of older lesions suggest that cyst rupture is part of the pathogenesis of ocular disease.

Ocular toxoplasmosis most often is due to reactivation of congenital lesions[122] but also occurs in acute (primary acquired) infection with *T. gondii*.[62,123,124] Ocular lesions due to infections acquired postnatally seem to be more prevalent in certain geographic locales. It was estimated that 17.9% of adults in Erecim, Brazil, for example, had postnatally acquired ocular toxoplasmosis.[27,71] Serum antibodies to *T. gondii* were found in 99% of persons with ocular lesions and in 77% of those who did not have ocular lesions. In contrast, two separate studies in the United States found that 0.6% of residents in areas of Maryland and Alabama had evidence of ocular toxoplasmosis.[125,126] The estimated incidence in the United Kingdom was 0.1% to 1% in one report.[127] Chorioretinitis was the sentinel illness leading to identification of an outbreak of *T. gondii* in British Columbia, Canada.[70] It is estimated that there are between 300 and 2100 new cases of acquired ocular toxoplasmosis annually in the United States.[41] It is likely that the prevalence of ocular toxoplasmosis in these countries is underestimated because the diagnosis is missed, and the disease is not a reportable one.

The diagnosis of ocular toxoplasmosis usually is made clinically (Fig. 38–4) on the basis of characteristic findings of funduscopic examination in a person who has serum antibodies to *T. gondii*.[112,128] The typical feature of active, initial disease is an oval-shaped, cream-colored lesion that may progress to involve all layers of the retina, as well as the retinal pigment epithelium and choroid (Fig. 38–4A). The margins of the active lesions are blurred, and the vitreous fluid may become hazy because of inflammatory cells and cellular debris when infection is acute or active. Patients complain of "floaters" and a decrease in visual acuity, especially if the lesion involves the macula. Pain is

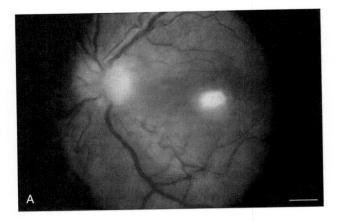

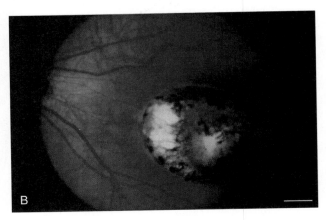

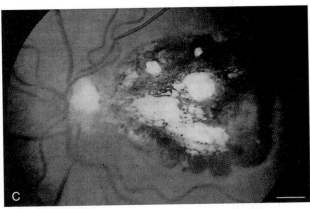

FIGURE 38–4. Active toxoplasmic chorioretinitis in a patient with acute acquired infection (**A**). Quiescent toxoplasmic retinochoroidal scar in a congenitally infected patient (**B**). Toxoplasmic chorioretinitis in a patient with HIV infection (**C**). (*A* kindly provided by Dr. Jack S. Remington; courtesy of Dr. M. Polis, National Institutes of Health, and Dr. R.B. Nussenblatt, National Eye Institute.) Scale bars ≅ 1.5 μm. (With permission from Roberts F and McLeod R. Pathogenesis of Toxoplasmic Retinochoroiditis. Parasitology Today 15:51-7, 1999.)

uncommon. Isolated involvement of uveal tissue and anterior segment structures of the eye does not occur in immunocompetent patients.[124] In immunocompromised hosts the lesions progress more rapidly and often appear adjacent to retinal blood vessels rather than close to retinal scars, suggesting hematogenous spread.[50,112,124,129]

Congenital infection with untreated *T. gondii*[130] is almost always associated with eye involvement, and often there is recrudescence.[114–116] Congenital lesions are often bilateral with multiple scarred areas and clustered lesions, whereas postnatally acquired ocular toxoplasmosis often is unilateral with single lesions. The active lesion of ocular toxoplasmosis appears similar in congenital and postnatally acquired ocular toxoplasmosis, although in congenital infection there are often new lesions contiguous to older scars.

Without treatment congenital ocular toxoplasmosis is a recurrent, recrudescent disease and a frequent manifestation of infection in children who have symptoms at birth.[131,132] In the treatment trials of the Toxoplasmosis Collaborative Study Group, 76% of children referred to this study in the newborn period with congenital toxoplasmosis had ocular involvement at birth, determined by fundoscopic examination.[131] In infants with subclinical infection detected by obstetric or neonatal serologic screening programs, 20% already had retinal lesions at birth.[133,134] In two separate studies of children who were untreated or treated for only 1 month, more than 90% of those with subclinical infection at birth had retinal lesions by 9 years of age[116] or adolescence.[114,115]

In children followed by the Toxoplasmosis Collaborative Study Group who had recrudescent eye disease and who were promptly treated with pyrimethamine and sulfadiazine, symptoms resolved and their visual acuity returned to prerecrudescent illness levels.[131] In a small study of chorioretinitis due to acute, postnatally acquired *T. gondii* infection, 14 (89%) of 16 patients had complete or partial improvement of visual acuity, with pyrimethamine-sulfadiazine, pyrimethamine-clindamycin, or atovaquone treatment.[78] Two patients did not regain their preillness visual acuity because of substantial macular involvement.

In the otherwise healthy patient with ocular toxoplasmosis, as the active lesion heals, it becomes white and atrophic with a surrounding border of retinal epithelial cells that create the characteristic hyperpigmented "ring" (Fig. 38–4*b*). In our experience with children treated with pyrimethamine and sulfadiazine, lesions usually become quiescent within approximately 10 days.[131] Scarring of the retina and underlying choroid are common; scotomas occur, and visual field defects may be detected on visual field testing. Satellite lesions close to previously healed, scarred areas may develop.[112,131] New lesions in retina that has appeared normal previously also occur.[112,131]

Diagnosis

Serologic studies are helpful in establishing whether infection with *T. gondii* is acute or chronic in immunocompetent patients. When test results guide therapeutic decisions, confirmatory testing in a reference laboratory is needed.[77,81,100,135,136] Serologic tests usually are positive for the presence of *T. gondii* infection in immunocompromised patients, but occasionally they can be negative even with severe ocular disease.[137] Vitreous fluid analysis may prove helpful. PCR techniques have been used successfully to diagnose ocular toxoplasmosis.[80,138] One study has shown local IgG production in patients with toxoplasmic chorioretinitis.[139,140] Another recent study suggested that *T. gondii* DNA is identified by PCR,[102] more frequently in primary-acquired than in congenital ocular toxoplasmosis.[111] Historically a test used when diagnosis was difficult was a quotient demonstrating local antibody production in the eye.[139] The *T. gondii* antibody levels in aqueous humor were compared to serum *T. gondii* antibody levels. A quotient greater than 1 was suggestive of active ocular disease.[128,139] This test has now been largely replaced by PCR.[78,80,81] A recent study of Brazilian children with ocular toxoplasmosis described lower peripheral blood lymphocyte blastogenic responses to *Toxoplasma* antigens in the subset of children felt to have congenital, rather than acute acquired infection.[141]

Treatment

Although there is some debate in the literature about whether peripheral retinal disease due to *T. gondii* requires treatment, we treat all active *T. gondii* retinal lesions for the following reasons:

1. Macular vision is needed.
2. Peripheral vision is needed, and visual field defects cause morbidity.
3. New lesions, often satellites of older ones, and even lesions that begin in the peripheral retina, may become progressive, recurrent, satellite lesions contiguous to or within the macula over time.
4. In children our experience has been that active lesions resolve within approximately 10 days after initiation of treatment with pyrimethamine-sulfadiazine, with restoration of preillness visual acuity in almost all instances.[131] Without treatment, active lesions may persist considerably longer than 10 to 14 days.

There is general agreement that ocular toxoplasmosis should always be treated under the following circumstances:[131,142,143]

1. Lesion in the papillomacular area or optic disc
2. Large retinal lesion with pronounced vitritis
3. Peripheral lesions that cause dragging of the macula and thus compromise visual acuity
4. Compromised immunity (see Immunocompromised Patients)

We treat any active retinal lesions due to *T. gondii* whether they are central or peripheral in the retina.

One group reported that ocular toxoplasmosis is a self-limiting illness (median time to resolution is 8 weeks) regardless of whether antimicrobial agents were used,[144] and these authors concluded that there is little or no benefit in treatment.[145]

Although occasional development of new lesions that are first detected as healed scars is part of our experience,[83,131] it has not been our experience that ocular toxoplasmosis is always a self-limiting illness that rapidly heals without consequence in the absence of antimicrobial therapy. We have cared for a number of children and young adults who present with active retinal disease several weeks to months after they first noted their new symptoms, which progressively worsened. Adverse sequelae of untreated ocular toxoplasmosis are often substantial.[114,115,130,131] In contrast, active lesions almost always become quiescent, sharply demarcated, and pigmented within 10 to 14 days after treatment with pyrimethamine, sulfadiazine, and leucovorin is initiated.

The medications that have been used to treat ocular disease are the same as those used to treat other forms of toxoplasmosis: most commonly, pyrimethamine (with leucovorin) and sulfadiazine (or triple sulfonamides [sulfapyrazine, sulfamethazine, and sulfamerazine]) and less commonly, when there is allergy or toxicity to sulfonamides, clindamycin.[112,131] Some case reports of azithromycin and atovaquone use have been published.[145,146] The optimal doses of any of these drugs or even the optimal duration of treatment for ocular toxoplasmosis has never been determined in randomized, controlled trials, but treatment for 1 week beyond active appearance of lesions (usually 3 to 4 weeks of therapy) has been recommended.[144] In our experience with children there is usually response to treatment with pyrimethamine and sulfadiazine within approximately 10 days, and we then continue treatment for at least 1 week after the lesions become quiescent in appearance (i.e., resolution of vitreous inflammation and lesions with sharply demarcated borders).[131] Leucovorin is continued for another week after discontinuation of treatment because of the long serum half-life of pyrimethamine (60 to 90 hours).[147]

It should be emphasized that available medications treat only tachyzoite-stage parasites and do not eradicate the latent encysted form of *T. gondii*. Since the bradyzoite form within cysts is responsible for disease reactivation in the eye, recurrences of ocular disease cannot be prevented with the medicines currently available. Azithromycin, a drug shown to have modest in vitro activity against bradyzoites,[148] does not appear to provide any benefit in preventing recurrent ocular toxoplasmosis.[145]

Corticosteroids are given in combination with pyrimethamine, sulfadiazine, and leucovorin to help alleviate intraocular inflammation if the lesions are in or near the macula or optic nerve and thus threaten vision. Their use has been standard practice for a variety of ophthalmologic conditions involving intraocular inflammation or when vision is threatened. There are no controlled studies documenting the utility of steroids in the treatment of ocular toxoplasmosis, and there are no controlled trials comparing treatment with and without steroids.[149] Starting dosages range from 20 to 150 mg/d prednisone in adults and 1 mg/kg/d (0.5 mg/kg twice daily) in infants.[131,150] There is considerable evidence that the use of steroids in adults without anti-*Toxoplasma* medications adversely affects the outcome in ocular toxoplasmosis.[119] Corticosteroids should never be used for treatment of ocular toxoplasmosis without concomitant administration of antimicrobial treatment effective against *T. gondii* infection.[120,151,152] It may be unnecessary to use steroids in the immunocompromised patient if there is little associated ocular inflammation.

CONGENITAL TOXOPLASMOSIS

Incidence and Clinical Manifestations

Since the incidence of *T. gondii* infection varies markedly not only from country to country but also within different communities within the same city and since neither the disease nor the infection is reported, there is little accurate data concerning the true incidence of *T. gondii* as a cause of congenital infection in the newborn in most countries. A study from France (1982–1983) calculated the risk of *T. gondii* infection in newborns to be 6.4 per 1000 live births. Unlike France, the United States has no universal screening program to test pregnant women for the acquisition of *T. gondii* infection. Data from the Third NHANES of military recruits suggests, however, that there may be approximately 3500 children born each year in the United States with toxoplasmosis[12]; other estimates range from 400 to 6000 affected infants born annually.[3,14,133] Congenital *T. gondii* infection in HIV-infected persons may resemble other congenital *T. gondii* infection or be especially fulminant.[153,154]

Congenital toxoplasmosis is transmitted by an immunocompetent or immunocompromised mother who is infected for the first time while she is pregnant.[2,3,89,134,155] Infection occasionally may be transmitted to the fetus from a chronically infected and severely immunocompromised pregnant woman. Infection rarely may be transmitted to the fetus when the infection is acquired in the months just before conception.[156–158] Congenital transmission of *T. gondii* from an acutely infected mother to her fetus occurs least frequently but has the most severe consequences for the fetus in the first trimester of pregnancy; transmission occurs more frequently but has less severe manifestations in the third trimester. The fetus is infected transplacentally.[62,159–162] During acute infection, when there is maternal parasitemia, the organism is able to reach the placenta, where it multiplies and subsequently infects the fetus via the fetal circulation. There can be a delay between placental infection and transmission to the fetus, termed the "prenatal incubation period," which means that the fetus may be at risk of acquiring the disease following a hiatus after the time the mother acquired the infection. The delay between acquisition of the fetal infection and acquisition of the maternal infection can be as long as 16 weeks.[3]

Although less commonly transmitted in the first trimester, the sequelae of *T. gondii* infection to the fetus are more severe if transmission occurs during the early weeks of gestation.[134] Brain necrosis and hydrocephalus are most commonly seen in the neonate who has acquired infection during the first trimester. Transmission to the fetus is relatively infrequent during weeks 1 to 10.[3] Thereafter the incidence of transmission of congenital infection rises in relation to gestational age. The period of highest risk for transmission associated with severe clinical illness is gestational weeks 10 to 24.[3] In contrast, the incidence of transmission is highest during the third trimester of pregnancy (weeks 26 to 40). Infection during the latter part of the third trimester usually results in either a subclinical infection or in a mild form of the disease in the newborn, although without treatment, sequelae almost always occur later.

The issue of frequency of transmission of *T. gondii* from a chronically infected mother with AIDS was addressed in a small study of 28 women with HIV, chronic *T. gondii* infection, and a CD4 count less than 200.[54] No transmission was observed, and the authors concluded that transmission in this scenario is not a common phenomenon. A number of such infected infants are described in the literature[137,153] and have been noted in our personal experience, however.

Congenital toxoplasmosis presents with the classic triad of hydrocephalus, chorioretinitis, and intracranial calcifications in only a minority of cases.[3,4,114–116,134,150,163–168] When the disease is clinically apparent at birth, central nervous system signs are often present.[3,169,170] Other signs of systemic disease (e.g., intrauterine growth retardation, being small for gestational age, petechiae, blueberry muffin rash, jaundice, fever, pneumonia, hepatitis, hepatosplenomegaly, anemia, thrombocytopenia, neutropenia, atypical lymphocytes, eosinophilia, and pleocytosis) may also be found.[150,169]

As most infants are infected later in gestation, most often congenital toxoplasmosis is subclinical and most children appear superficially normal at birth. However, nearly all such children will subsequently develop signs of *T. gondii* infection weeks to years later in life. Neurologic disease may develop from 3 to 12 months after birth or later, and ocular abnormalities may occur months to years later.[114–116,171] Deafness, seizure disorders, psychomotor retardation, developmental delay, and hydrocephalus have all been reported.[116,169,171] Ocular manifestations include chorioretinitis, strabismus, and loss of sight.[112,122,131,132,169,171] If congenitally infected infants are untreated, between 82% and 95% of them develop chorioretinal lesions by the time they reach adolescence.[114–116,130] Diminution of cognitive function also was reported for untreated children,[130,172] but this does not appear to occur in children treated in the first year of life.[173–175] Retinal disease has recurred in a small number of children over 1 year of age who were treated in the first year of life.[131] To date, data are insufficient to predict later ocular outcome for treated children with subclinical infection with *T. gondii*.[3,83] Normal cognitive and motor function appear to be sustained for many children with congenital toxoplasmosis who were treated in the first year of life.[117,173]

Diagnosis

Diagnosis is made on the basis of consistent physical findings in the infant and on serologic test results in the mother. Confirmation is by one or more of the following:[3,81,102,176–179] *T. gondii*–specific IgM or IgA antibodies in the serum or CSF of the infant: parasitemia, parasites in the CSF, amniotic fluid, or placenta demonstrated by subinoculation of the placenta or peripheral white blood cells (or blood clot) or CSF cell pellet into mice or tissue culture; PCR of amniotic fluid, peripheral white blood cells, CSF or urine; isolation of parasites from the placenta; or compatible illness in a child of a mother with serologic evidence of acute acquired *T. gondii* infection. PCR for the *T. gondii* B1 gene using amniotic fluid is most sensitive in midgestation and less sensitive earlier and later in gestation. Overall sensitivity is about 85%.[180] Tests used are shown in Table 38–1.[2–4,87] Recognition of different *Toxoplasma* antigens by IgM and IgG antibodies in sera of mothers and their congenitally infected infants[86] and lymphocyte blastogenic response to *Toxoplasma* antigens[130,181–184] have sometimes been useful in establishing the diagnosis. Lymphocyte blastogenesis in response to *Toxoplasma* antigens is not present uniformly.

Treatment of the Mother to Prevent and Treat Infection in the Fetus

Couvreur, Desmonts, Daffos, Holfeld, Thulliez, Romand, Merlissi, and others in Paris have performed a series of important, elegant, and careful studies.[3,134,170,178,180,185–189] In this work they initially[170] demonstrated that there were 50% fewer *T. gondii* infected infants born to a cohort of mothers with gestational, acute, acquired *T. gondii* infection treated with spiramycin than in a cohort in the previous decade when mothers were not treated (*P*<.05).[170] In a related study in Austria[190–192] it was demonstrated that treatment of the acutely infected pregnant woman with pyrimethamine and sulfadiazine reduced the incidence of congenital infection from 15% to 5% (*P*<.05). In similar supporting evidence that treatment in utero reduces parasite burden,[193,194] it was demonstrated that the *T. gondii* isolation rates from placentas of acutely infected women who were treated with spiramycin (80% isolation rate) or pyrimethamine and sulfadiazine (50% isolation rate) were lower than the rate from placentas of acutely infected women who were not treated (95% isolation rate).[185,193,194] Spiramycin is less effective in animal models and should not be used to treat encephalitis in immunocompromised humans[195] but is concentrated in the placenta and reduces placental infection in animal models and in humans. Schoondermark–Van de Ven et al demonstrated high concentrations of spiramycin in the placenta and a reduction in transmission in a study of acutely infected pregnant primates.[196,197] These studies of placentas from acutely infected women[193,194] and acutely infected pregnant primates[196,197] who were treated provide a logical

TABLE 38–1A ■ Guidelines for Interpretation of Serologic Tests for Toxoplasmosis

Test	Positive titer	Titer in congenital infection (infant); acute infection (older child, adult)	Titer in chronic infection	Duration of elevation of titer
IgG				
Sabin-Feldman dye test	Undiluted	NC, S OCA, 1:4 to ≥1:1,000 (usual)	1:4 to 1:2,000	Years
Direct agglutination test	≥1:20	NC, S OCA, rises slowly from negative to low to high titer (1:512)	Stable (≥1:1,000) or slowly decreasing titer	≥1 year
Indirect fluorescent for IgG antibody	≥1:10	NC, S OCA, ≥1:1,000	1:8 to 1:2,000	Years
Indirect hemagglutination test	≥1:16	NC, S OCA, ≥1:1,000	1:16 to 1:256	Years
Complement fixation	≥1:4	NC, S OCA, varies among laboratories	Negative to 1:8	Years
IgM				
Indirect fluorescent for IgM	≥1:10, adults	OCA, ≥1:80 (use only for OCA, not NC)	Negative to 1:20	Weeks to months, occasionally years, can be ≥1 year
Double-sandwich IgM ELISA	≥0.2, newborns, fetuses ≥1.7, older children, adults	NC, ≥0.2 OCA, ≥1.7	Negative to 1:7 (OCA)	
Immunosorbent test for IgM	≥3, infants; 8, adults	NC, ≥3 OCA, >8	Negative to 1	Unknown, can be ≥1 year
IgA				
IgA, ELISA	≥1.0, infants; ≥1.4, adults	NC, ≥1.0 OCA, >1.4	Negative to <1.0 Negative to ≤1.3	Weeks to months, occasionally longer
IgE				
IgE, ELISA	≥1.9 infants and adults	NC and OCA, ≥1.9	Negative	Weeks to months, occasionally longer
Immunosorbent test for IgE	≥4 infants and adults	NC and OCA, ≥4	Negative	Weeks to months, occasionally longer
AC/HS	See Table 38–1B	See Table 38–1B	See Table 38–1B	Usually <9 months
PCR (amniotic fluid; CSF)	Positive	Positive	Negative	Only when *Toxoplasma* DNA present during active infection

AC/HS, differential agglutinin test; *CSF*, cerebrospinal fluid. *ELISA*, enzyme-linked immunosorbent assay; *NC*, titer in newborn with congenital infection; *OCA*, titer in older child or adult with acute, acquired infection; *PCR*, polymerase chain reaction; *S*, usually the same as the mother.

Values are those of one reference laboratory: each laboratory must provide its own standards and interpretation of results in each clinical setting.

From Boyer K, McLeod R: Toxoplasmosis. In Principles and Practice of Pediatric Infectious Diseases. Prober C, Pickering L (eds). New York, Churchill Livingstone, 2002.

TABLE 38–1B ■ Interpretation of ACHS Test

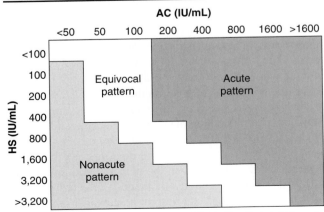

Adapted from Dannenmann BR, Vaughan WC, Thulliez P, et al: Differential agglutination test for diagnosis of recently acquired infection with *Toxoplasma gondii*. J Clin Microbiol 28:1928–1933, 1990.

explanation for reduced transplacental transmission noted in studies of treated women.[170,190–192,198,199]

Many cohort studies of the effect of treatment during gestation on the prevention of congenital toxoplasmosis used historical controls for comparison to their treatment groups. The validity of these studies has been questioned,[200] and data that demonstrate that spiramycin decreases transmission of *T. gondii* infection to the fetus has been disputed.[200] Wallon et al describes 144 cases of proven *T. gondii* infection during pregnancy in which there was no correlation between the incidence of transmission and any other variable except gestational age; that is, a variety of treatment regimens did not appear to affect transmission rates.[200] The Cochrane database, which screened 2591 published studies on treatment of toxoplasmosis during pregnancy, found no randomized controlled trials (RCTs) to

TABLE 38–2 ■ **Paris Approach to Prenatal Prevention, Diagnosis, and Treatment**

Diagnosis mother:	Systematic serologic screening, before conception and intrapartum
Treatment of mother:	If acute serology, spiramycin reduces transmission
	Untreated 94 (60%) of 154 vs. treated 91 (23%) of 388
Treatment of fetus:	Pyrimethamine, sulfadiazine, or termination
	N = 54 livebirths; 34 terminations
Diagnosis fetus:	Ultrasounds; amniocentesis, PCR at ≥18 weeks' gestation
	Sensitivity 37 (97%) of 38; specificity 301 of 301
Outcome:	All 54 normal development; initial report was 19% subtle findings:
	7 (13%) intracranial calcifications, 3 (6%) chorioretinal scars;
	follow-up of 18 children (median age 4.5 y; range, 1–11 y)*: 39%
	retinal scars, most scars were peripheral

Adapted from Roberts F, McLeod R, Boyer K: Toxoplasmosis. In Katz S, Gershon A, Hotez P (eds): Krugman's Infectious Diseases of Children, 10th ed. St. Louis, CV Mosby, 1998, pp 538–570.
*Brezin A, Thulliez P, McLeod R: Mets M. In Press, 2002.

demonstrate that antenatal treatment prevents transmission during pregnancy.[201]

Such analyses[200,201] identify limitations in currently available data but do not obviate the usefulness of studies in which data provide information relevant to clinical decision making. Data that provide part of a conceptual and empiric basis for initiating prevention and treatment of congenital toxoplasmosis during gestation as soon as is feasible after infection, when meningoencephalitis[3,131,133,170,202] and retinal damage[132] commonly occur, include the following:

1. Antimicrobial agents are effective against *T. gondii* tachyzoites in tissue culture.[4,147,203–210]
2. Antimicrobial agents are effective in animal models of acute toxoplasmosis.[104,148,208,211–224]
3. Antimicrobial agents are effective in other clinical settings*
4. Data described above indicate efficacy following treatment in utero and in the first year of life.[†]
5. Data also provide both a rationale for and empiric evidence of efficacy of available antimicrobial agents in preventing or treating manifestations of fetal toxoplasmosis.
6. It is not currently possible to eradicate latent infection once *T. gondii* is transmitted to an infected fetus, and thus the person infected in utero is vulnerable to life-long illness that threatens sight, cognition, and motor function.

Because careful studies have demonstrated a decreased incidence of fetal infection and diminution in manifestations of fetal infections with currently available treatments,[3] although the available data are not from RCTs with placebo groups, institutional review boards (IRBs) may not sanction future placebo-controlled RCTs.

Currently available data leave no question that the available methods for diagnosis are 85% sensitive (more sensitive in midgestation than in early or late gestation) and 100% specific and that the available medicines reduce infection in the placenta and parasite destruction of the fetal brain and associated meningitis.[62,178,188] Perhaps when medicines become available that eliminate tachyzoites and bradyzoites more efficiently and with less toxicity, their results could be compared in cohorts followed with randomization to (1) the current standard French approach (Table 38–2) discussed in Remington et al (2000), to (2) the current U.S. standard of care in which no systematic serologic screening is provided during pregnancy,[116,228] or to (3) the serologic screening of newborn infants that currently takes place in Massachusetts, adding screening of all mothers at term.[133] Informed consent for a placebo-controlled RCT appears to us to remain problematic, however, as this would involve explaining to a mother why she should allow herself and her child to be placed in a group in which diagnostic measures with known sensitivity and specificity and treatment with known efficacy would not be available. Lack of treatment for diagnosed and treatable fetal toxoplasmic meningoencephalitis, chorioretinitis, or systemic infection appears to breach the standard for a placebo-controlled RCT: that there would be no irreversible harm, no serious but reversible harm, and no serious discomfort so that the best interests of the patient are protected.

Treatment of the Fetus and Neonate

Several studies provide evidence that treatment during pregnancy is of benefit in decreasing the number of severe sequelae from *T. gondii* infection in the newborn[3,83,178,188,233] (Tables 38–2 and 38–3). Although treatment failures occur, the sooner treatment is received by the infected mother, the milder the child's symptoms are at birth[234] (Table 38–3). Delays in maternal treatment during gestation were reported to result in more brain and eye disease in the infant.[3,233] Pyrimethamine together with sulfadiazine appears to be the most effective treatment for *T. gondii* infection in the fetus and newborn. Because of the potential teratogenic effects of

*References 47, 50, 55, 78, 79, 83, 84, 137, 150, 225–230.
†References 3, 83, 87, 117, 150, 170, 173, 178, 188, 194, 196, 197, 231, 232.

TABLE 38–3 ■ Significant Correlations of Brain Hyperechogenic Areas in Fetal and Newborn Ultrasounds with Other Clinical Aspects of Congenital Toxoplasmosis

	Cerebral hyperechogenicity*	No cerebral hyperechogenicity	Total OR [significance of difference]
Interval between diagnosis of maternal and fetal infection	8.5 Weeks	6.5 Weeks	[P=.03]
Interval between maternal infection and beginning pyrimethamine and sulfadiaxine	9.5 Weeks	8.5 Weeks	[P=.06]
Ocular lesions	9/37 (24%)†	7/96 (7%)	16/133 (12%) [P<.008]
New eye lesions	7/37 (18%)	5/67 (7%)	12/104 (12%) [P<.058]

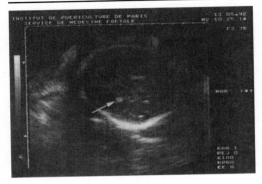

*The ultrasound displays hyperechogenecity (arrow).

†Number with finding or number in group (%). Maximum duration of follow-up was until 2 years old. *Note:* delays in diagnosis and treatment were associated with cerebral hyperechogenicity on brain ultrasound, and such hyperechogenicity was associated with more ocular lesions and development of new eye lesions. From Mirlesse, et al: Long-term follow-up of fetuses and newborn with congenital toxoplasmosis diagnosed and treated prenatally, in preparation; and Remington JS, McLeod R, Thulliez P, and Desmonts G: Toxoplasmosis, In Infectious Diseases of the Fetus and Newborn Infant. Remington J and Klein J (eds); Philadelphia, WB Saunders, 2002, pp 205–346.

pyrimethamine, which have been reported in animal studies, spiramycin or sulfonamides alone have been used until at least 12 (and usually 17) weeks' gestation before diagnostic procedures are attempted and therapy is changed to pyrimethamine-sulfadiazine.[3] The use of pyrimethamine appears to be safe after 17 weeks' gestation.[3,178,188,235] Treatment recommendations are summarized in Table 38–4. Treatment of an infected infant during the first year of life resolves signs of active disease in the first weeks of treatment. Outcomes (i.e., cognitive and motor function, hearing) today appear to be better for many *T. gondii*–infected children who were treated for one year relative to outcomes for similarly affected children in earlier decades who were untreated or treated for only a month.[83,150,173,231] Prompt correction of hydrocephalus by ventriculoperitoneal shunt is also an important adjunct to medical treatment of congenital toxoplasmosis with hydrocephalus (Fig. 38–5). Intracerebral calcifications may diminish in size or resolve in treated infants[236] (Fig. 38–6).

Methods for preparation of medicines and their formulation are shown in Figure 38–7 and Table 38–5. Telephone numbers and websites that will aid in obtaining advice concerning medicines or information concerning prevention and treatment of congenital toxoplasmosis are in Table 38–6. Comparison of the more favorable outcomes for children who were treated during the first year of life (and in some instances in utero)[83] vs. those who were untreated or treated for 1 month[130,169] are in Tables 38–7 and 38–8.

INFECTION IN PATIENTS WITH HIV/AIDS

Incidence and Clinical Manifestations

In 95% of HIV patients with toxoplasmosis, latent *T. gondii* infection causes their disease.[237] Central nervous system (CNS) toxoplasmosis (Fig. 38–8) remains a major AIDS presenting illness even in the age of highly active anti-retroviral therapy (HAART) and TMP-SMX prophylaxis.[52,136,137,238–242] The incidence of toxoplasmosis varies according to the prevalence of exposure to *T. gondii* (i.e., as reflected in *Toxoplasma* IgG serum antibodies in any given population). In Africa, Haiti, France, Switzerland, and Central and South America, where *T. gondii* infection is more common, there are more cases of toxoplasmic encephalitis in patients with AIDS than in patients with AIDS the United States, where the incidence of chronic infections is less. The numbers of cases of toxoplasmosis in patients with AIDS in the United States has been steadily decreasing over the past several years, most likely because of the increased use of TMP-SMX prophylaxis against *Pneumocystis carinii* and of HAART.[137]

Even in the age of HAART and TMP-SMX prophylaxis, however, *T. gondii* causes 20% of intracerebral infections in AIDS patients and is the most common cause of focal neurologic lesions in AIDS patients. The lifetime risk that CNS toxoplasmosis will develop in AIDS patients is 6% to 12%, with a mortality of 50% and infection undiagnosed until autopsy.[240–242]

TABLE 38–4 ■ Treatment of Toxoplasmosis

Manifestation of infection	Medication	Dosage	Duration of therapy
Pregnant women with acute toxoplasmosis First 17 wk of gestation or until term if fetus not infected	Spiramycin*	1 g q8h without food	Until fetal infection is documented or excluded at 17–20 wk; continued until term if no fetal infection
Fetal infection confirmed after 17th wk of gestation or if maternal infection acquired in last few weeks of gestation (after amniocentesis and PCR to determine whether there is *Toxoplasma* infection in the fetus)	Pyrimethamine Sulfadiazine Leucovorin (folinic acid)	Loading dose: 100 mg/d in two divided doses for 2 d, then 50 mg/d 100 mg/kg/d in two or four divided doses (maximum 4 g/d) 5–20 mg/d‡	Until term (leucovorin is continued 1 wk after pyrimethamine is discontinued)
Congenital *Toxoplasma* infection in infants	Pyrimethamine§ Sulfadiazine§ Leucovorin§	Loading dose: 2 mg/kg/d for 2 d, then beginning third day, 1 mg/kg/d for 2 or 6 mo,‖ then this dose every Monday, Wednesday, and Friday 100 mg/kg/d in two divided doses 5–10 mg three times weekly‡	1 y¶ (leucovorin is continued 1 wk after pyrimethamine is discontinued)
CSF protein value ≥1 g/dl or active chorioretinitis that threatens vision	Corticosteroids (prednisone)	1 mg/kg/d in two divided doses#	Until resolution of elevated CSF protein level to < 1 g/dl or active chorioretinitis
Active chorioretinitis in older children	Pyrimethamine Sulfadiazine Leucovorin Corticosteroids	Loading dose: 2 mg/kg/d (maximum 50 mg) for 2 d, then beginning third day maintenance, 1 mg/kg/d (maximum 25 mg) 50 mg/kg every 12 h (maximum 4 g/d) 5–20 mg three times weekly‡ 1 mg/kg/d of prednisone in two divided doses#	Usually 1–2 wk beyond resolution of signs and symptoms (leucovorin is continued 1 wk after pyrimethamine is discontinued) Until resolution#

Immunologically normal children
  Lymphadenopathy
  Significant organ damage that is life threatening
	No therapy
	Pyrimethamine, sulfadiazine, leucovorin
		Same as above for active chorioretinitis in older children; no corticosteroids	Usually 4–6 wk or 2 wk beyond resolution of signs and symptoms

Immunocompromised children Non-AIDS	Pyrimethamine, sulfadiazine, leucovorin	Same as above for active chorioretinitis in older children; no corticosteroids	Usually 4–6 wk beyond complete resolution of signs and symptoms
AIDS	Pyrimethamine, sulfadiazine, leucovorin Clindamycin in place of sulfadiazine	Same as above for active chorioretinitis in older children; no corticosteroids Reported trials for adults, but not infants and children	Until CD4 count >200 for 6 mo beyond the complete resolution of signs and symptoms

*Available only on request from the U.S. Food and Drug Administration; telephone 301-443-5680.

†The only studies are those of Hohlfeld, et al. However, because Hohlfeld and colleagues found pyrimethamine-sulfadiazine therapy to be superior to spiramycin for treatment of the fetus, continuous therapy with pyrimethamine, sulfadiazine, and leucovorin should be considered in the third trimester.

‡Adjusted for megaloblastic anemia, granulocytopenia, or thrombocytopenia; blood counts, including platelets, should be monitored as described in text.

Continued

TABLE 38–4 ■ Treatment of Toxoplasmosis (*Continued*)

§Optimal dosage, feasibility, and toxicity are currently being evaluated or planned in ongoing Chicago-based National Collaborative Treatment Trial; telephone 773-834-4152.

∥These two regimens are currently being compared in a randomized National Collaborative Treatment Trial. Data are not yet available to determine which, if either, is superior. Both regimens appear to be feasible and relatively safe.

¶In infants with AIDS. The duration of therapy is unknown. Please see discussion in section on congenital toxoplasmosis and AIDS.

#Corticosteroids should be continued until signs of inflammation (high CSF protein value ≥1 g/dL) or active chorioretinitis that threatens vision have subsided; dosage can then be tapered and discontinued; use only with pyrimethamine, sulfadiazine, and leucovorin.

From Roberts F, Boyer KM, McLeod R: Toxoplasmosis. In Krugman S, Gershon AA, Katz SL, et al (eds): Infectious Diseases of Children, 10th ed. St. Louis, Mosby-Year Book, 1997.

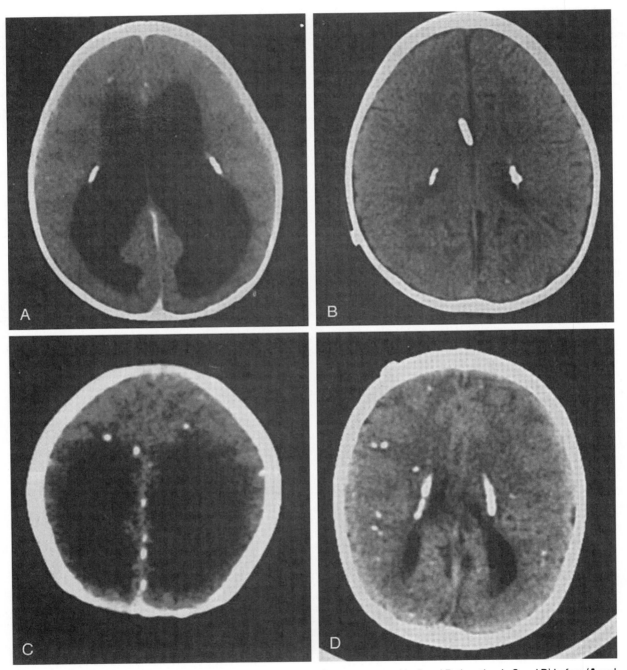

FIGURE 38–5. Brain computed tomography (CT) scans of two infants (one represented in **A** and **B**, the other in **C** and **D**) before (**A** and **C**) and after (**B** and **D**) placement of ventriculoperitoneal shunts. Both of these infants initially developed normally. The child in **CD** has had subsequent cognitive delay. These CT scans and the subsequent normal (**AB**) and near-normal (**CD**) later development of these children indicate that it is not possible to predict ultimate cognitive outcome from the initial appearance of the CT scan. From Boyer KM, McLeod RL: *Toxoplasma gondii* [toxoplasmosis]. In Long SS, Prober CG, Pickering LK (eds): Principles and Practice of Pediatric Infectious Diseases. New York, Churchill Livingstone, 1997, pp 1421–1448.

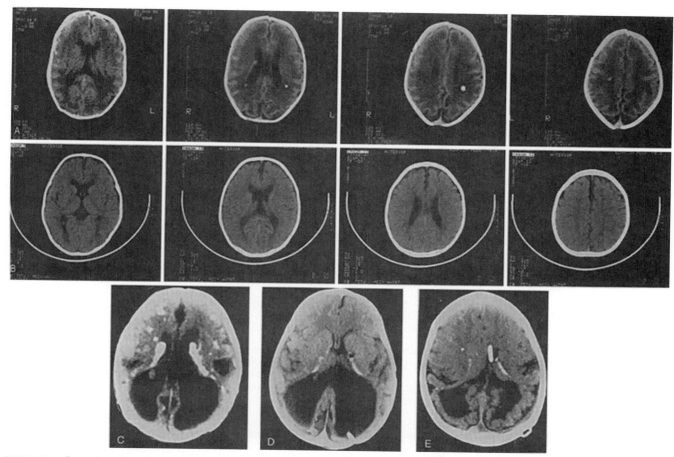

FIGURE 38–6. Examples of cranial computed tomography (CT) scans that demonstrate resolution of calcifications in treated children. **A** and **B**, CT scans in a treated infant obtained at birth, August 1992 (**A**), and August 1993 (**B**). **C** to **E**, Diminution or resolution of large areas of calcification are seen in these representative cranial CT scans from another treated infant. Cranial CT scans in this treated infant obtained (**C**) at birth, February 1987, (**D**) at follow-up, May 1988, and (**E**) July 1991. (From Patel, et al: Resolution of intracranial calcifications in infants with treated congenital toxoplasmosis. Radiology 1996, 199:433–440.)

TABLE 38–5 ■ Oral Suspension Formulations for Pyrimethamine and Sulfadiazine in the United States

Pyrimethamine, 2 mg/ml suspension*
1. Crush four 25-mg pyrimethamine tablets in a mortar to a fine powder.
2. Add 10 ml of syrup vehicle.[†]
3. Transfer mixture to an amber bottle.
4. Rinse mortar with 10 ml of sterile water and transfer.
5. Add enough of the serum vehicle to make 50 ml final volume.
6. Shake well until this is a fine suspension.
7. Label and give a 7-d expiration.
8. Store refrigerated.

Sulfadiazine, 100 mg/ml suspension[‡]
1. Crush ten 500-mg sulfadiazine tablets in a mortar to a fine powder.
2. Add enough sterile water to make a smooth paste.
3. Slowly triturate the syrup vehicle[†] close to the final volume of 50 ml.
4. Transfer the suspension to a larger amber bottle.
5. Add sufficient syrup vehicle to make 50 ml final volume.
6. Shake well.
7. Label and give a 7-d expiration.
8. Store refrigerated.

---

*Pyrimethamine: 25-mg tablets (Daraprim, GlaxoSmithkline, Inc.) NDC #0173-0201-55.

[†]Syrup vehicle: suggest 2% sugar suspension for pyrimethamine. If the infant is not lactose intolerant, 2% sugar suspension can be 2 g lactose per 100 ml distilled water. Suggest simple syrup or alternatively cherry syrup for sulfadiazine suspension.

[‡]Sulfadiazine: 500-mg tablets (Eon Labs Manufacturing, Inc.) NDC #00185-0757-01.

WEIGH BABY <u>EACH</u> WEEK.
INCREASE MEDICATIONS ACCORDINGLY.

Dispensing caps

Medication syringe marked with number of milliliters
to be given in each dose during that week

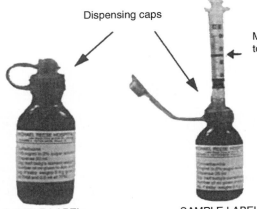

	SAMPLE LABEL:	SAMPLE LABEL:	SAMPLE LABEL:
MEDICATION:	Sulfadiazine	Pyrimethamine	Folinic acid (calcium leucovorin)
CONCENTRATION:	100 mg/ml*	2 mg/ml*	5 mg tablets
DISPENSE:	50 ml	25 ml	30 tablets
DOSAGE:	Sig: half baby's current weight equals number of milliliters given in AM and PM. for example: if baby weighs 5 kg give 2.5 ml at 7AM and 2.5 ml at 7PM	Sig: half baby's current weight in kilograms equals number of milliliters given once each day. for example: if baby weighs 5 kg, give 2.5 ml daily	Sig: 10 mg (2 tablets) on Monday, Wednesday and Friday. Crush and give with formula, milk, or apple juice in one dosage

*Suspended in sugar solution. Suspension at usual concentration must be made up each week. Store refrigerated.

FIGURE 38–7. Preparation of pyrimethamine, sulfadiazine, and leucovorin in treatment of congenital toxoplasmosis. (Adapted from McAuley J, Roizen N, Patel D, et al: Early and longitudinal evaluation of treated infants and children and untreated historical patients with congenital toxoplasmosis: The Chicago Collaborative Treatment Trial. Clin Infect Dis 1994, 18:38–72. University of Chicago.)

TABLE 38–6 ■ Some Pertinent Resources and Phone Numbers/Internet Sites

Reference laboratory for serology, isolation, and PCR (U.S.)	650-853-4828
Reference laboratory for serology, isolation, and PCR (France)	33-1-40-44-39-41
FDA for IND number to obtain spiramycin for treatment of a pregnant woman (U.S.)	301-827-2335
FDA Public Health Advisory	301-594-3060
Spiramycin (Rhone Poulenc) for treatment of a pregnant woman (U.S.)	610-454-8469
Congenital Toxoplasmosis Study Group (U.S.)	773-834-4152
Education Pamphlet/The March of Dimes (U.S.)	312-435-4007 or 1-800-323-9100
Educational pamphlet: "Congenital Toxoplasmosis: The Hidden Threat"	301-496-5717
Educational pamphlet: "Toxoplasmosis," NIH publication No. 83-308	www.niaid.nih.gov
Information concerning AIDS and congenital toxoplasmosis (U.S.)	305-243-6522
Information for European families: The Toxoplasmosis Trust (U.K.)	44-171-713-0663
Educational information on the Internet	http://www.lit.edu/≈toxo/pamphlet

In countries, for example, in Africa, where infection with *T. gondii* and HIV are common and TMP-SMX and HAART are less readily available, toxoplasmosic encephalitis (TE) remains common in patients with AIDS.

About 30% to 50% of patients with AIDS who also have *T. gondii* latent infection, as demonstrated by positive serologies, and who do not receive HAART or TMP-SMX will subsequently develop TE.[237] Interestingly,

persons with the HLA DQ3 haplotype have a higher incidence of TE than do those with HLA DQ1 haplotypes, suggesting immunogenetic factors play a role in susceptibility.[34] This is similar to the increased prevalence of HLA DQ3 in infants with congenital toxoplasmosis and hydrocephalus with causality demonstrated with murine class II Knockout, HLA DQ1 or DQ3 transgenic mice.[30]

Usually patients with HIV develop toxoplasmosis when their CD4 count is less than 100, although this is

TABLE 38–7 ■ Comparison of Ophthalmologic, Developmental, and Audiologic Outcomes with Postnatal Treatment

Author(s), year of publication [reference]	Treatment	No. studied	Mean age in years when data tabulated (range)	Percent with finding or impairment					
				Ophthalmologic			Neurologic		
				Lesions[a]	Vision[b]	New[c]	Cognitive	Motor or seizures	Audiologic
Eichenwald, 1959	0 or 1 mo P, S	104	4 (minimum)	NA	0, 42, 67[d]	NA	50, 81, 89[d]	0, 58, 76[d]	0, 10, 17[d]
Wilson et al, 1980	0 or 1 mo P, S	23	8.5 (1–17)	93	47	22	55 (20 severe)	20	22, 30[e]
Koppe et al, 1986	0 or 1 mo P, S	12	20 (NA)	80	NA	NA	0	0	NA
Labadie and Hazemann, 1984	0	17	1 (NA)	28	NA	NA	NA	NA	NA
Couvreur et al, 1984	1 y P, S, Sp	172	NA (2–11)	NA	NA	8	NA	NA	NA
Hohlfeld, 1989	Prenatal, 1 y P, S, Sp	43	NA (0.5–4)	12	NA	NA	0	0	NA
Villena, 1998	F, Sp	47	NA [born 1980–89]	–	–	15/45 (33)[f]	–	–	–
	1 y F	19	NA [born 1990–96]	–	–	2/18 (11)	–	–	–
	2 y F	12	NA [born 1990–97]	–	–	1/11 (9)	–	–	–
Peyron, 1996	F'	121	12 (5–22)	–	–	37/121 (31)	–	–	–
Chicago study (historical patients)	0	7	5.6 (2–10)	100	86	29	25	25	14
Chicago study (treated patients)	Most for 1 y P, S	37[g]	3.4 (0.3–10)	81	81	8	0, 24[h]	0, 24	0

F = Fansidar (pyrimethamine 1.25 mg/kg each 14 d); F' = Fansidar (in utero and postnatally pyrimethamine 6 mg/5 kg each 10 d; small numbers also treated in utero); NA = not available; P = pyrimethamine; S = sulfonamides; Sp = spiramycin.

[a]Lesions = any chorioretinal lesions.

[b]Vision = vision impaired.

[c]New = new lesions.

[d]Subclinical, generalized, neurologic.

[e]Subclinical, generalized, neurologic.

[f]Number with finding/number in group (%).

[g]These data are for the first 37 children studied before May 1991.

[h]First number is percentage for children who had subclinical or systemic signs without severe neurologic disease; second number is percentage for children who had severe neurologic disease at birth.

Adapted from McAuley J, Boyer KM, Patel D, et al: Early and longitudinal evaluations of treated infants and children and untreated historical patients with congenital toxoplasmosis: The Chicago Collaborative Treatment Trial. Clin Infect Dis 1994;18:38–72.

not always the case. In addition there have been at least three cases reported of patients with cerebral toxoplasmosis that developed within 3 months of the patients' being started on HAART therapy. One of these patients had a CD4 count over 200.[243] This phenomenon of opportunistic pathogen infection "flares" associated with the initiation of HAART usually has been noted with viruses such as CMV or hepatitis virus. Close monitoring and great vigilance in the use of *Toxoplasma* prophylaxis is

thus required in *Toxoplasma*-seropositive HIV patients beginning HAART, even if there is no evidence of severe immunosuppression.

In countries where prevalence is high, seronegative patients with HIV are also at risk of acquiring *T. gondii* and development of acute toxoplasmosis. In France in a study of seronegative patients the authors report a *T. gondii* seroconversion rate of 5.5% over a median follow-up of 28 months. All seronegative patients should be

TABLE 38–8 ■ **Early Outcomes for Children ≥5 Years Old in the United States (Chicago) National Collaborative Treatment Trial**

A	% IN LITERATURE 5 Y, 10 Y[c]	HISTORICAL PATIENTS[d]	Mild[a] TREATMENT A[b] FEASIBILITY	TREATMENT A[b] RANDOMIZED	TREATMENT C[b] FEASIBILITY	TREATMENT C[b] RANDOMIZED
Vision <20/20	25, 50	11/14 (79)[e]	0/4	0/3	0/0	0/0
New retinal lesions	25, 85	5/9 (56)	0/4	1/3	0/0	0/0
Motor abnormality	10, 10	0/14 (0)	0/4	0/3	0/0	0/0
IQ < 70	0–50, 0–50	0/13 (0)	0/4	0/3	0/0	0/0
ΔIQ ≥ 15	50, 50	0/5 (0)	0/4	1/3	0/0	0/0
Hearing loss	30, 30	0/14 (0)	0/4	0/3	0/0	0/0

B	% IN LITERATURE 5 Y, 10 Y[f]	HISTORICAL PATIENTS	Severe[a] TREATMENT A FEASIBILITY	TREATMENT A RANDOMIZED	TREATMENT C[b] FEASIBILITY	TREATMENT C[b] RANDOMIZED
Vision <20/20	70, 70	10/10 (100)	7/9 (78)	8/9 (89)	1/2	6/9 (67)
New retinal lesions	50, 90	4/9 (44)	3/9 (33)	1/8 (13)	2/2	0/9 (0)
Motor abnormality	60, 60	1/10 (10)	3/9 (33)	2/9 (22)	0/2	1/9 (11)
IQ < 70	90, >90	1/10 (10)	4/9 (44)	4/9 (44)	0/2	2/9 (22)
ΔIQ ≥ 15	95, 95	0/8 (0)	0/9 (0)	2/9 (22)	0/2	1/9 (11)
Hearing loss	30, 30	0/10 (0)	0/9 (0)	0/9 (0)	0/2	0/9 (0)

Note: Percentages not shown when ≤4 patients per group.

[a]Clinical disease considered "Mild" if infant is apparently normal and develops normally on follow-up (e.g., but has isolated nonmacular retinal scars or < 3 intracranial calcifications on CT). Clinical disease considered "Severe" if neurologic signs or symptoms present, symptomatic chorioretinitis that threatened vision, ≥3 intracranial calcifications on CT.

[b]Treated children received 2 months (Treatment A) or 6 months (Treatment C) of daily pyrimethamine and sulfadiazine, followed by pyrimethamine on Monday, Wednesday, and Friday and continued daily sulfadiazine for the remainder of the year of therapy. Feasibility patients were treated in the early phase of the study before randomized study.

[c]Data from Wilson et al.[116]

[d]Historical patients were untreated patients diagnosed after 1 year of age.

[e]Number with abnormality/number in group (% affected). No differences between treatment regimens achieved statistical significance ($P > .05$ using Fisher Exact test).

[f]Data from Eichenwald HG: A study of congenital toxoplasmosis, with particular emphasis on clinical manifestations, sequelae, and therapy. In Human Toxoplasmosis. Copenhagen, Munksgaard, 1960, pp. 41–49.

From MCLeod R et al.[83]

counseled on appropriate preventive measures to minimize their risk of acquiring *T. gondii*.

T. gondii most frequently causes CNS disease in patients with AIDS.[137] *T. gondii* produces a multifocal necrotizing encephalitis that rarely involves the meninges (Fig. 38–8). CSF studies often reveal only elevated protein and leukocytes with normal glucose if any abnormalities are present.[244] TE initially may present as a diffuse encephalitis, but focal neurologic signs usually develop over time as the disease progresses. Although any area of the brain may be involved, *T. gondii* commonly affects the basal ganglia.[245] Toxoplasmic chorioretinitis can develop[246] with or without TE and sometimes heralds the onset of TE, but it is not common.[247] Only 1% of 781 patients with AIDS and ocular complications of HIV were found to have active *T. gondii* retinal infection; over half of those with ocular involvement also had concurrent TE.[248] Spinal cord *Toxoplasma* infection and myelitis have also been described but are rare.[249,250]

The second most commonly reported serious manifestation of toxoplasmosis in patients with AIDS is pneumonitis.[251–253] The clinical manifestations are similar to those of PCP, including fever, dyspnea, and nonproductive cough that may rapidly progress to acute respiratory failure.[251,254] Diffuse bilateral interstitial infiltrates are the most common finding on chest radiograph. Bronchoalveolar lavage (BAL) has been described only occasionally in the United States. A study of BAL specimens in 169 AIDS patients in France reported an incidence of *T. gondii* of 5%.[252] Whether this discrepancy reflects underdiagnosis in the United States, or simply the lower incidence of latent infection in the United States, or other factors is not known.

Some cases of *T. gondii* infection presenting as a fever of unknown origin in patients with AIDS who were receiving TMP-SMX prophylaxis have been reported.[255] Diagnosis was made by PCR, and symptoms resolved with treatment with pyrimethamine and clindamycin.

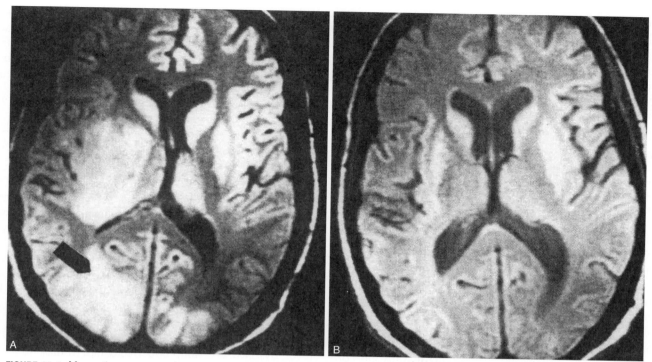

FIGURE 38–8. Magnetic resonance imaging of the brain of a patient with AIDS and toxoplasmic encephalitis before (*A*) and after (*B*) antimicrobial therapy. Note that large areas of necrosis and inflammation in *A* (*arrow*) have resolved in *B*. From McLeod R, Wisner J, Boyer K: Toxoplasmosis. In Krugman S, Katz S, Wilfert C, Gershon A, (eds.): Infectious Diseases of Children, 9ᵗʰ ed. St. Louis, Mosby, 1992, p 526.

Other clinical manifestations (e.g., orchitis, pancreatitis, hepatic and gastrointestinal involvement) have been described in detailed reviews of the various clinical presentations of *T. gondii* infection in the patient with HIV infection.[137,256–258]

Diagnosis

Given the technical difficulties and morbidity often associated with brain biopsy, initial treatment of TE is usually based on presumptive clinical diagnosis in the presence of serum antibodies against *T. gondii* and characteristic findings on brain computed tomography (CT) or magnetic resonance imaging (MRI). Although the incidence of TE has decreased in developed countries since the introduction of TMP-SMX and HAART, there are still rare reports of toxoplasmic brain abscesses developing in AIDS patients even while they are receiving prophylactic medication.[259] Therefore we still recommend a trial of anti–*T. gondii* treatment. This approach has been critically examined and widely used for over 10 years as an acceptable management strategy.[260]

BAL has been successful for diagnosing *Toxoplasma* pneumonitis, although the sensitivity of this test is not known. In a few isolated reports, PCR testing of BAL specimens has also shown promise.

In a group of 22 patients the sensitivity of PCR in detecting *T. gondii* in peripheral blood was 86.6% and in CSF was 60% in patients not taking TMP-SMX but was 25% in peripheral blood and 16.7% in CSF in patients receiving prophylactic therapy.[261] Another group calculated a positive predictive value of 100% and a negative predictive value of 40% on the basis of their experience using PCR to diagnose TE from CSF.[262] However, no comment was made on whether these patients were receiving TMP-SMX prophylaxis.

In patients with a presumptive diagnosis of TE given empiric therapy a clear clinical response should be apparent within 7 to 14 days.[263] If there is no improvement within this time, a brain biopsy should be obtained to confirm the diagnosis. This is particularly important as CNS lymphoma can mimic TE, and coinfection with other pathogens has also been reported. In addition the probability that a focal brain lesion is due to *Toxoplasma* infection is less if the patient is taking TMP-SMX prophylaxis.[264] A study of TE cases in France showed the rate of TE in patients on TMP-SMX prophylaxis was 45% as compared to 75% in patients not taking PCP prophylaxis.[265] Another study examining the etiologic trends of focal brain lesions in patients with AIDS and *T. gondii* IgG serum antibodies found that the probability that TE was the correct diagnosis was 0.87 if the patients were not taking prophylaxis. However, this probability dropped to 0.59 if patients were taking prophylactic medicines.[266] Lymphoma was most commonly misdiagnosed as TE. In cases in which AIDS patients taking prophylaxis present with focal brain lesions, CSF should be sent for Epstein-Barr virus (EBV) PCR to rule out lymphoma.[264] Similarly, if there is a single lesion on MRI with mass effect and no clinical response after 1 week of anti-*Toxoplasma* treatment, a brain biopsy to rule out lymphoma is recommended.[237,263,266] Any patient with worsening neurologic signs and symptoms or the development of new neurologic signs while receiving treatment for TE should also have a brain biopsy.[237,263]

Treatment

The treatment of choice for TE is pyrimethamine (loading dose of 100 to 200 mg, then 50 to 75 mg daily in adults) and sulfadiazine (adult dose of 1 to 1.5 g every 6 hours, not to exceed 6 g daily); leucovorin (10 mg daily starting dose in adults) is given to minimize the marrow toxicity associated with pyrimethamine. No other antimicrobial agent regimen has been shown to be as efficacious as this combination in treating toxoplasmosis.[84,258,267] Unfortunately these antimicrobial agents are associated with a high rate of adverse reactions,[268,269] and up to one-third of patients are unable to tolerate these medications. Other possible choices are pyrimethamine with clindamycin,[226,270] atovaquone,[270–272] dapsone,[224,273,274] or macrolides such as clarithromycin[275] or azithromycin.[276–279] Relapse rates tend to be higher with these alternative regimens. Pyrimethamine (50 mg daily) and clindamycin (600 mg every 6 hours) were found to have efficacy comparable to that of pyrimethamine-sulfadiazine in treating TE but were associated with a higher relapse rate.[270] The few randomized clinical trials that have compared these alternatives with pyrimethamine and sulfadiazine are summarized in Table 38–9.[226,272,280–283] Medications that have been used in nonrandomized clinical trials or that have been described in case reports are briefly discussed under Medications used for treatment of *T. gondii* infection.

Anti-*Toxoplasma* Prophylaxis and Maintenance Therapy

Because of the high incidence of disease reactivation, all AIDS patients with CD4 counts less than 200 and positive *T. gondii* serology should receive prophylaxis.[84] Fortunately agents used for prophylaxis against *Pneumocystis carinii* (e.g., TMP-SMX, dapsone, atovaquone) also have activity against *T. gondii*. Although not specifically designed to address the issue of toxoplasmosis, several studies examining the efficacy of PCP prophylaxis regimens have reported (as a secondary outcome measure) success with these same regimens in preventing *T. gondii* infection (Table 38–10).[230,273,274,284–291]

Various prophylactic regimens have been reported to be successful.* Recently it has been shown that for patients taking HAART, *T. gondii* prophylactic therapy may be discontinued once CD4 counts are consistently maintained

above 200 as measured on at least two separate occasions, 3 months apart, that is, for 4 to 6 months, with no adverse sequelae.[284,308] Recently, patients with immune reconstitution who have already been treated for toxoplasmosis (thus considered more susceptible to relapse) discontinued their lifelong maintenance therapy successfully.

INFECTION IN TRANSPLANT PATIENTS

Incidence and Clinical Manifestations

T. gondii infection in patients with tissue or organ transplantation and its associated immunosuppression often presents with nonspecific signs, and the diagnosis may easily be missed. It usually develops within the first 6 months after transplantation, with the incidence being highest in the first 2 to 3 months of the post-transplantation period.[309–313] Fever is the single most common finding. Pneumonitis, encephalitis, and myocarditis are the most frequently described clinical syndromes.

Toxoplasma pneumonitis typically presents with fever, dyspnea, and nonproductive cough. It may be clinically indistinguishable from other opportunistic infections that commonly present in this same time period in immunosuppressed transplant patients such as those with *Pneumocystis carinii* pneumonia (PCP). LDH levels are often elevated, as they are with PCP, and chest radiographs generally show diffuse bilateral interstitial infiltrates, although other abnormalities (e.g., pleural effusions) have been reported.[314]

Unlike in HIV patients, in post-transplant patients, CNS toxoplasmosis often presents with general, rather than focal, neurologic signs.[315–317] Headaches, fever, altered mental status, and lethargy are the most commonly described findings, and the CSF may be unremarkable or there may be pleocytosis (with polymorphonuclear leukocytes as well as lymphocytes). Retinal disease due to *Toxoplasma* has also been documented in patients who have received organ transplants.[318–320] Patients usually present with visual disturbances, which lead to diagnosis on ophthalmologic examination; if disease is restricted to the eye, patients generally respond well to therapy.[321,322]

Cardiac toxoplasmosis may present as pericarditis or myocarditis progressing to heart failure refractory to vasopressor support. Fever, a low cardiac output, and an elevated pulmonary artery wedge pressure may be the only clues. In heart transplant recipients, cardiac toxoplasmosis may mimic organ rejection. Diagnosis may be made in these instances by endomyocardial biopsy.

Special Problems of Toxoplasmosis During Bone Marrow Transplantation

The incidence of positive *T. gondii* serologic tests in recipients of bone marrow transplants varies by region. A French study found an incidence of *T. gondii* IgG

---

*References 227, 228, 230, 259, 270, 271, 280–282, 285–290, 292–307.

TABLE 38–9 ■ Randomized Controlled Trials (RCT) Addressing Treatment and Maintenance Therapy of Toxoplasmosis in Patients with HIV Infection

Reference	Objective or question asked	Design, setting, outcome measures	Patient population	Intervention	Results	Conclusions
Katlama, 1996	How effective is C compared to S for acute treatment or maintenance therapy of TE?[a]	ITT, U	N = 299	6 wk: P + L PLUS	Complete clinical response in 103 (68%) of P-C and 112 (76%) of PS	No difference in survival
		F/u NS	Includes a,b,d	C (n = 152) OR	Cross-over to other treatment arm secondary to lack of response more common with C	Trend in favor of better response to S but not of statistical significance between the two groups
		B, F, CC (n = 31)	Excludes 1–3	S (n = 147)	Maintenance phase risk of relapse 2.16 higher in C	P-S better prevents TE relapse
		D, A, R		M = 50% (n = 175)	Adverse events rate: severe reactions S (30%), C (11%)	
Torre, 1998	Which therapy, TMP-SMX or P-S is best for treatment of first episode TE?[b]	Not ITT, U	N = 77	30 d* P + L$_1$ + S$_1$ (n = 37) OR	No mortalities Complete clinical response in 23 (65.7%) of P-S and 23 (62%) at 30 d of TMP-SMX	No difference detected between the two treatment groups
		F/u = 3 mo	Includes a,b,d	TMP-SMX	1 relapse in TMP-SMX group	Not analyzed by intention to treat
		I	Excludes 1–6	M = 50% × 3	Adverse reactions P-S (37.8%) (skin rash most common) and TMP-SMX (12.5%)	Pilot study but lacking adequate power (numbers in each group small)
		D, A, R				
Podzamczer, 1995	Is twice weekly P sufficient for maintenance therapy to prevent relapse of TE?[c]	ITT	N = 105	S$_2$ + L$_2$ PLUS	11 (10.4%) diagnosed relapse, 3 in daily group and 8 in twice weekly	Twice weekly P maintenance therapy not as effective as daily for prevention of relapse of TE
		F/u = 11 mo	Includes a,c,d	P$_1$ (n = 60) OR/C	Estimated adjusted relapse 30% (twice weekly) and 6% (daily regimen) (adjusted risk ratio = 5.6)	
		Sp, 8 UH	Excludes 4	P$_2$ (n = 45)	Adverse reactions: (rash, GI intolerance) in 6	
		D, A, R				
Podzamczer, 2000	Is × 3/wk maintenance therapy with P as efficacious as daily to prevent TE relapse?[d]	ITT	N = 124	S$_3$ + L$_2$ PLUS	No relapses if CD4>100	Higher than expected rates of relapse, even in daily treated group (?compliance)
		F/u = 11 mo	Includes a,c,d	P$_3$ (n = 66) OR	16 diagnosed with relapse, 7 (17%) daily; 9 (19%) in × 3/wk	
		Sp, UH, 12	Excludes 4	P$_1$ (n = 58)	Not receiving HAART associated with relapse (r.r. = 4.08)	No significant difference between relapse rates in two regimens
		D, A, R, PCP			Adverse reactions in 14 (rash, GI most common)	

Continued

TABLE 38–9 ■ RCT Trials Addressing Treatment and Maintenance Therapy of Toxoplasmosis in Patients with HIV Infection (*Continued*)

Reference	Objective or question asked	Design, setting, outcome measures	Patient population	Intervention	Results	Conclusions
Dannemann, 1992	Treatment of TE with C-P vs. P-S,[e]	IIT, U USMC UH	26 P-C 33 P-S	6-wk treatment P, F, S OR P, F, C (C IV × 3 wk)	Survival greater P-S; D not related directly to TE P-C more likely to achieve complete clinical and radiologic response A; skin rash P-C 6, 11-P-S	Similar efficacy resolution of abnormal mental status, fever, headache
Chirgwin, 2002	Activity, safety tolerance; atovaquone (suspension) and pyrimethamine; atovaquone and sulfadiazine,[f]	IIT, R, U, N		P or S PLUS Atovaquone	77% response; 28% intolerance (nausea, vomiting) taste bad 1/2 relapse 21/28 P(75%) 9/11 S(82%)	Equivalent to P-S

Design

B, blinded; ITT, intention to treat; U, unblinded.

Setting

B, Belgium; CC, clinical center; F, France; I, Italy; Sp, Spain; UH, University teaching hospital; USMC, United States MultiCenter.

Outcome measures

A, adverse reactions to medications; D, death; F/u, follow-up (median); F/uNS, follow-up not specified, median survival 12 months; R, relapse of disease.

Inclusion criteria

a, CD4 <200; b, acute episode of TE; c, previous episode of TE; d, HIV.

Exclusion criteria

1, previous episode of TE; 2, severe hematologic abnormalities; 3, intolerance to study drugs; 4, any patients taking atovaquone, clarithromycin, azithromycin, TMP-SMX; 5, pregnant; 6, under 18 years old; 7, another diagnosis; 8, did not meet early criteria.

Treatment interventions

C, clindamycin 600 mg q6h.

L, leucovorin 50 mg/wk; L_1, leucovorin 10 mg qd; L_2, leucovorin 15 mg qd.

M, maintenance treatment (percent of treatment dose).

P, pyrimethamine 50 mg qd; P_1, pyrimethamine 25 mg qd; P_2, pyrimethamine 25 mg × 2/wk; P_3, pyrimethamine 50 mg × 3/wk.

S, sulfadiazine 1 g q6h; S_1, sulfadiazine 60 mg/kg/d; S_2, sulfadiazine 500 mg q6h; S_3, sulfadiazine 1 g bid.

T, TMP 10 mg/kg/d; SMX, 50 mg/kg q12h.

*Most in both arms also received steroids for cerebral edema; none received HAART during treatment period.

a, Katlama.

b, Torre.

c, Podzamczer.

d, Podzamczer.

e, Dannemann.

f, Chirgwin.

antibodies of 67% in their pretransplant population.[44] In contrast, two U.S. studies found a lower incidence of *T. gondii* IgG antibodies (23% in a study from New York[315] and 15% in the Seattle series[323] of transplant recipients). The incidence of post-transplant disseminated toxoplasmosis is significantly lower, ranging from 0.1% to 6%.[44,315,323] Disseminated toxoplasmosis is not a common complication of bone marrow transplant.[319,324–326] When it does occur, however, the case fatality rate is high (over 90% in one series).[315] Most cases of toxoplasmosis

are due to reactivation of latent infection already present in the bone marrow transplant recipient.

Using a logistic regression model, Small et al were able to identify an association between the development of toxoplasmosis and having an unrelated donor (odds ratio [OR] = 5.48, 95% confidence interval [CI] 1.61–55), having a recipient with positive IgG serology and a donor with negative serology (OR = 7.80, 95% CI 1.45–41.83), or having both a recipient and donor with positive IgG titres (OR = 9.41, 95% CI 1.61–55).[315] The

TABLE 38–10 ■ Randomized Controlled Trials Addressing Efficacy of Primary Prophylaxis for Prevention of Toxoplasmic Encephalitis (TE) in Patients with HIV Infection

Reference	Objective/ question asked	Design, f/u, setting	Patients N CD4 Ig+	Treatment intervention	Outcome measures	Results	Conclusions
Mussini, 2000	When can prophylaxis for PCP/TE be safely discontinued?	ITT F/u = 6 mo MC, I, F	N = 708 CD4 > 200* IgG + = 46.6% (discontinued), 52% (continued) Excluded 1, 4	Discontinuation of primary prophylaxis‡	PCP, TE, M	TE: none	It is safe to discontinue prophylaxis for TE in patients started on HAART once CD4 > 200 for more than 3 mo
Leport, 1996	Can P be used as primary prophylaxis for TE?	ITT tte, F/u = 3 y Sp, US, F	N = 554 CD4 < 200 (a) Excluded	P_1 X 3/wk + L (N = 274) OR X + L + AP (N = 280)	TE AR	Terminated early TE: Incidence lower in P (4%) than X (12%); no difference in the 2 groups after 1 y	P at this dose not recommended for TE prophylaxis
Podzamczer, 1995	Is primary prophylaxis with D-P comparable to TMP-SMX for TE?	ITT F/u = 14 mo Sp	N = 230, CD4 < 200, IgG + = 65%, Excluded 1, 2, 4	D_1 + P_1 X 2/wk OR TMP-SMX bid, X 3/wk	PCP, TE, M AR	TE: 1 TMP-SMX, 2 D-P, Similar (9.3% and 9.6%) discontinuation of treatment because of AR	Both regimens appear effective; no conclusions re D-P vs. TMP-SMX for prophylaxis as event rates TE too low in both groups
Opravil, 1995	Can once-a-week P-D be used for prophylaxis of TE?	ITT F/u = 483 d Sw, I, F	N = 533 CD4 ~ 116 (P-D), ~ 105 (A), IgG + = 46% (P-D) and 49% (A) Excluded	P_2 + D X 2/wk OR AP	PCP, TE, AR	AR: 30% D-P (nausea, rash, and headache most common)	No difference in TE between two groups; D-P regimen poorly tolerated
Jacobson, 1994	Can P be used as primary prophylaxis for TE?	ITT F/u = 15 mo	N = 396, CD4 < 200†, IgG + = all, Excluded 3, 4	P X 3 wk OR X §	TE, M	Clinical Course: P vs. X Mortality: P >> X; study terminated early	No protective advantage of P for TE prophylaxis seen, but TE event rate low Increased mortality with P, possibly due to marrow-suppressing effect of P (increased mortality in anemic patients taking zedovudine; L administration no protective effect)
Antinori, 1995	Primary prophylaxis PCP + *T. gondii* and P vs. TMP-SMX vs. D-P	ITT tte, F/u = 7.7 mo	N = 197, CD4 < 200 (b), IgG + = 18/64 (PYR), 29/66 (TMP-SMX),	TMP-SMX qod (N = 63) OR D_1 qwk + P X 2/wk ‖(N = 63)	PCP, M, TE^2, AR	Excess PCP and M in D-P; trial discontinued prematurely; results therefore interpreted by "on-treatment" analysis; incidence of TE per 100	"On-treatment" analysis to evaluate TE, but large number of patients changed therapies

Continued

TABLE 38-10 ■ Randomized Controlled Trials Addressing Efficacy of Primary Prophylaxis for Prevention of Toxoplasmic Encephalitis (TE) in Patients with HIV Infection (Continued)

Reference:	Objective/question asked	Design, f/u, setting	Patients N CD4 Ig+	Treatment intervention	Outcome measures	Results	Conclusions
			26/59 (D-P), Excluded 1, 4, 5, 6	OR P (N = 68)		patient-years was 15.8 in P group, 6.2 in TMP-SMX group, and 2.5 in D-P group. AR?	
Brossard, 1994	How important is L to prevent hematologic toxicity from P and what is optimal dose?	F/u = 6 mo F	N = 30, Karnofsky score >80, IgG+ = all Excluded 2, 7	P_1 X 3/wk + L_1 OR L_2 OR X	H, O	Hemoglobin placebo >> L appeared after 3 mo of treatment WBC, platelets similar at 6 mo Opportunistic infections?	P hematologic toxicity if without L Lower dose (5 mg) L worked as well as higher dose (25 mg) in preventing marrow toxicity from P
Torres, 1993	Can D be used for primary prophylaxis of TE?	ITT F/u = 43 wk	N = 278, CD4 <250, IgG = (cl), Excluded 2, 4, 5	D_1 X 2/wk (N = 126) OR P (N = 152)	PCP, D, TE[2], AR	6 patients in P group developed TE, none in D group Toxoplasmosis-free survival at 1 y AR (rash, hepatitis, hemolytic anemia) in 14 d	Kaplan-Meier estimate shows trend favoring D but not statistically significant
Girard, 1993	Primary prophylaxis D-P vs. AP	ITT F/u = 539 d F	N = 347 CD4? IgG+ = 262 Excluded 1, 4	D qd + P_1 qwk (N = 173) (L?) OR AP (N = 176)	PCP TE D AR	TE in 32/176 in AP and 19/173 in D-P With serum IgG antibody to *T. gondii*, Relative risk = 2.37 higher for TE if AP AR more common D-P(42) than AP(3)	Patients with positive serum IgG antibody to *T. gondii*, Relative risk = 2.37 higher to develop TE if A
Durant, 1995	Primary prophylaxis R	F	N = 52, CD4?, Toxo IgG?	R (N = 17) OR A + R (N = 17) OR AP (N = 18)	PCP TE MAI AR	Patients developing TE: 5/18 AP 1/17 AP + R 0/17 R AR 14.7% (nausea, abdominal pain, elevated liver function test results, skin allergy)	Small study but shows promise
Payen 1997	Primary prophylaxis w/D vs. P-S	ITT (b)	CD4 <200/mm³	D_1 OR F	PCP TE AR		No conclusion for TE prophylaxis (=for PCP)

Design

F/u, duration of follow-up (mean f/u given for Torres 1993; the rest are reported as median f/u); ITT, intention to treat; tte, trial terminated early.

Setting

B, Belgium; F, France; I, Italy; MC, multicenter; Sp, Spain; Sw, Switzerland; US, United States.

Serologic data—comments

(a) No information on toxoserologies provided.

(b) IgG Toxoplasma serologies not done on everyone.

(c) IgG Toxoplasma serologies not determined, but all patients with TE had positive serologies.

Patient characteristics—comments

* Majority of patients with undetectable viral load at time of enrollment.

† Average CD4<100 or history of AIDS-defining illness.

Medications

AP, Aerosolized pentamidine; D, dapsone; L, leucovorin; P, pyrimethamine; R, Roxithromycin; S, sulfadiazine.

Outcome measures

AR, adverse reactions to medications; H, hematologic toxicity; M, mortality; MAI, *Mycobacterium avium-intracellulare*; O, any opportunistic infection; PCP, episode of *Pneumocystis carinii* pneumonia; TE, episode of toxoplasmic encephalitis; [2] a secondary endpoint.

Exclusion criteria

1, previous episode of PCP; 2, major laboratory abnormalities (including severe hematologic abnormalities); 3, history of central nervous system disease; 4, previous episode of TE; 5, history of asthma or COPD; 6, pregnant; 7, malnourished or chronic diarrhea.

Treatment interventions

‡Discontinuation of primary prophylaxis with TMP-SMX (77.3%, 80.1% continued), aerosolized pentamidine (19.3%, 16.8% continued), or dapsone-pyrimethamine (3.4%, 3.1% continued with treatment).

§the same PCP prophylaxis was continued, i.e., for pyrimethamine / placebo: T-S (53.8% / 57.6%), A (29.2% / 30.3%), D (17% / 12.1%)

AP, aerosolized pentamidine given for PCP prophylaxis.

D, dapsone 50 mg; D_1, dapsone 100 mg; D_2, dapsone 200 mg.

F, Fansidar+of week.

L, leucovorin; L_1, leucovorin 25 mg X3/wk; L_2, leucovorin 5 mg X3/wk.

P, pyrimethamine 25 mg; P_1, pyrimethamine 50 mg; P_2, pyrimethamine 75 mg.

R, roxithromycin 300 mg tid qwk.

TMP, 160 mg; SMX, 800 mg.

X, placebo.

∥Folinic acid given only if signs of hematologic toxicity developed.

situation of recipient negative and donor positive was not discussed, as none of the patients in their study were in this category. In another recent review, toxoplasmosis occurred almost exclusively in *Toxoplasma*-seropositive allogeneic marrow recipients.[327] Additional risk factors for developing toxoplasmosis include severe graft-vs.-host disease (GVHD) and corticosteroid treatment.[328]

Because of the difficulties associated with diagnosis (see below), most cases of toxoplasmosis in bone marrow transplant recipients are diagnosed only at autopsy, and the disease is 100% fatal without treatment. Given the high mortality associated with this disease, physicians caring for recipients of bone marrow transplants need to maintain a high index of suspicion concerning toxoplasmosis. Efforts should be directed toward aggressive early diagnosis and treatment to improve outcomes.

Diagnosis of toxoplasmosis in bone marrow transplant recipients may be difficult.[44,46] Pretransplant serologic testing is useful. Serologic tests are unreliable after transplant because of intense immunosuppression. There have been several documented cases of patients who were known to have IgG antibodies to *T. gondii* before transplant who were seronegative on repeat testing after transplant (Table 38–11).[44,45,309,316,321,329] Invasive procedures that may be needed for diagnosis (e.g., brain biopsy, BAL, open lung biopsy) are not always easy to achieve because of thrombocytopenia in bone marrow transplant recipients. As a result no single test is reliably diagnostic of *T. gondii* infection, and investigators have had the most success using a combined battery of tests, including serologies, mouse inoculation, cell culture, immunohistochemistry, and PCR. One study of bone marrow transplant patients showed that PCR combined with immunohistochemistry improved diagnostic sensitivity to 90%, better than either method alone.[330] PCR has shown promise as a diagnostic tool, both for early detection[331] and in difficult cases in which the diagnosis is initially missed.[325,332] Toxoplasmic empyema was described recently in a patient with a bone marrow transplant.[333]

Special Problems of Toxoplasmosis in Recipients of Solid Organ Transplants

Heart

Toxoplasmosis is a well-recognized infectious complication in heart transplant recipients.[47,309,329,334–337] Unlike toxoplasmosis in bone marrow transplant recipients, the majority (two-thirds) of toxoplasmosis occurring in heart transplant recipients is due to infection acquired by a seronegative recipient from a seropositive donor,[47] rather than reactivation of latent infection already present in the recipient (Table 38–11). One study showed that toxoplasmosis developed in 3 (17%) of 18 seronegative recipients who received a heart from a seropositive donor (Table 38–11). Reactivation of latent infection in the heart transplant recipient also has been described, particularly in

patients receiving intensive courses of immunosuppressive therapy to prevent organ rejection.[151] In seropositive recipients who receive a heart from a seropositive donor, *T. gondii* serum IgG and IgM titres may rise without clinical illness.[329] These persons need to be monitored closely, even though usually toxoplasmosis does not develop (Table 38–11).

Cardiac toxoplasmic infection can be confused with acute organ rejection. Endomyocardial biopsy may show diffuse lymphocytic infiltrates mimicking acute rejection.[321] Usually the presence of *Toxoplasma* associated with the inflammation will be seen with immunoperoxidase staining, which helps to distinguish between these two entities.[84,258,321,338]

A case of polymyositis in a heart transplant recipient presenting with proximal muscle weakness has been reported.[73] Diagnosis was confirmed by electromyography (EMG) studies and by skeletal muscle biopsy. Endomyocardial biopsy showed inflammation with multiple *Toxoplasma* cysts. No information on donor or recipient serologies was available. This patient was already receiving TMP-SMX as prophylaxis at the time of diagnosis; medications were changed to pyrimethamine plus sulfadiazine, and the patient subsequently improved.

Overall the outcomes and survival rates of heart transplant recipients with toxoplasmosis are excellent when the diagnosis is made and treatment is initiated promptly, in contrast to outcomes for toxoplasmosis in recipients of bone marrow transplants. This may be related to less intensive immunosuppressive therapy and heightened awareness of the disease in this group, as it is more common than among bone marrow transplant patients. In addition, many experts now begin therapy when seroconversion is detected, even when there is no evidence of clinical disease, and so treatment is begun early. Prophylaxis against *Toxoplasma* is now recommended in seronegative recipients of hearts from seropositive donors.[310] Serologic tests are more reliable in this group than in bone marrow transplant recipients, for the reasons discussed previously.

Kidney

Toxoplasmosis in renal transplant recipients has been reported but is rare.[339–341] In two studies (n = 69, n = 73) there was no overt clinical disease, although seroconversion did occur[45,316] (Table 38–11). Data from a recent review of case reports of renal transplant patients with toxoplasmosis showed that a seronegative recipient receiving a kidney from a seropositive donor is at highest risk that overt clinical disease will develop.[340,341] Ten of eleven treated patients (either with pyrimethamine-sulfadiazine or pyrimethamine-clindamycin) survived. There are at least two separate case reports of transplantation of a donor kidney from a seropositive person; toxoplasmosis developed in both recipients.[339] As is the case with heart transplants, serologic tests were found to be

TABLE 38–11 ■ Toxoplasmosis in Recipients of Transplants

Type of transplant	Country	No. of patients	Serology (% of total); no. (%) with clinical disease				No. with increase in serum antibody to Toxoplasma				Type of immunosuppressive therapy	Outcome
			R-D-	R-D+	R+D-	R+D+	R-D-	R-D+	R+D-	R+D+		
Heart*	USA	50	27(54%); 0	4(8%); 3(75%)	12(24%); 0	7(14%); 0	0	4	10/19(53%)	None	a,b,e or c,b,e	66% (2/3), M
Heart† heart-lung	England	217H 33HL	154; 0	21(8%); 6(28%)	44; 0	31; 0	0	7A	0	2A	a,e,b or c,e or c,a or c,a	33% (2/6), M
Heart‡	Switzerland	121	34(28%); 1(6%)	18(15%); 3(17%)	59(49%); 2(3%)	10(8%); 0	0	11(8A)	4(2A)	1A i.e., 11/16 (69%) MSe	b or d (to day 14) then c,b,e	Reactivation R+, SC
Bone marrow§	France	80	16(20%); 1(6%)	10(13%); 0	29(36%); (24%)	25(31%); 1(4%)	Serologies after transplant unreliable; R+, 30/54+ and 16/54				c,e (plus b or d for acute GVHD)	M n/a
Kidney‖	France	73	24(33%); 0		49(67%); 0		2/24(8%)SC		13/49(13%)MSe		a,e or a,b,e or	M none
Kidney¶	France	69	15(22%); 0		54(78%); 0		O SC		3/54(6%)MSe		a,b,f or a,d,e	M none

a, azathiaprine; A, asymptomatic; b, ATG; c, cyclosporin; d, OKT3; D, donor; e, steroids; f, ibuprofen; H, heart; HL, heart-lung; l, donor T. gondii serologic test results not provided or incomplete; M, mortality; MSe, amount of T. gondii-specific antibody increased without disease; PCR, early diagnosis made by PCR; R, recipient; SC, seroconversion; T, toxoplasmosis with mortality.

‖Derouin 1987
¶Renoult 1992
*Luft 1983
†Wreghitt 1989
§Derouin 1986
‡Gallino 1996

helpful in diagnosis, and the prognosis for both recipients was better than that for patients who have received a bone marrow transplant, likely because of less profound immunosuppression and early recognition and treatment of disease. There is one report of bone marrow aspiration being successfully used to diagnose acute toxoplasmosis in a kidney transplant recipient.[342]

Liver

Toxoplasmosis in recipients of liver transplants is not common.[343,344] *Toxoplasma* pneumonitis and encephalitis have both been reported.[314,345] Interestingly, two cases of primary acquired ocular toxoplasmosis were described in liver transplant recipients.[318,345] As with recipients of heart and renal transplants, most case reports describe a donor who is seropositive and a recipient who is seronegative. Disease is usually seen in the context of intense immunosuppression effected with antirejection agents such as OKT3. In all cases in which this information was available, liver biopsies showed no evidence of *T. gondii* infection. Diagnosis was made by serology, by ophthalmologic examination, or at autopsy.

Pancreas

There is one case report of *Toxoplasmic* pneumonitis that developed in a recipient of a pancreas transplant after she completed a course of immunosuppressive therapy for transplant rejection.[346] The initial presentation was fever; diagnosis was made by BAL. She responded favorably to treatment with pyrimethamine and clindamycin. No information about the serologic status of the donor or recipient was provided.

Special Treatment Considerations

As toxoplasmosis is a relatively uncommon infection in patients with transplants, RCTs on the treatment or prevention of this disease in transplant recipients have not yet been performed. Toxoplasmosis in transplant recipients has been treated successfully with pyrimethamine-sulfadiazine.[340,341]

Since pyrimethamine is known to cause bone marrow suppression, there is a theoretical risk that this drug may be more problematic in bone marrow transplant patients. Close monitoring of complete blood counts is strongly recommended, and amounts of folinic acid adequate to minimize bone marrow toxicity are of paramount importance.

In the patient who has received a kidney transplant, careful monitoring of renal function is important when sulfadiazine is used, as this medication may cause crystalluria and renal stones.[347-349] Maintaining adequate fluid intake with nonacidic liquids should be stressed, as hydration decreases the risk of these side effects, which may have serious consequences in the renal transplant patient. Alkalinization of urine by ingestion of NaHCO$_3$ has also been used.

For maintenance therapy and *T. gondii* prophylaxis, TMP-SMX has been used successfully. Fansidar has been used for *T. gondii* prophylaxis in bone marrow transplant recipients in Europe.[350]

OTHER IMMUNOCOMPROMISED PATIENTS

The clinical manifestations of *T. gondii* infection in patients with cancer most frequently involve the CNS (including the eye), the heart, and the lung. Cases of widely disseminated *T. gondii* infection have been reported.[351,352]

The incidence of toxoplasmosis in cancer patients is not known, but it is not common.[351,352] Toxoplasmosis most often is the result of reactivation of latent disease in cancer patients and most often has been associated with lymphoproliferative disorders and hematologic malignancies. In a review of 128 cases of toxoplasmosis in patients with malignancies, 46% had Hodgkin's lymphoma.[351,352] Most of these patients presented with fever and signs of neurologic involvement, including 11% with chorioretinitis. Development of toxoplasmosis is thought to be due to a combination of the defects in cell-mediated immunity caused by Hodgkin's disease itself and the immunosuppressive treatment used to treat Hodgkin's lymphoma. Since both Hodgkin's disease and toxoplasmosis can present with similar signs (fever, lymphadenopathy), serologic tests or a lymph node biopsy or both are needed to distinguish between the two entities.

Toxoplasmosis has also been reported in non-Hodgkin's lymphoma, acute and chronic leukemias, myeloma, and hairy cell leukemia, among others.[351,352] Patients with leukemia and toxoplasmosis usually present with fever. Transfusion-related transmission of acute toxoplasmosis (e.g., from white blood cells of persons with chronic myelogenous leukemia), although uncommon, has been demonstrated on at least two separate occasions.[57] Myocarditis due to *T. gondii* has been reported more frequently in patients with acute lymphocytic leukemia than in patients with other hematologic malignancies.[351] Ocular toxoplasmosis, when it occurs in cancer patients, is usually due to reactivation of latent infection.[351,352] It has been reported most frequently in cases of Hodgkin's and non-Hodgkin's lymphoma and should be suspected in any immunocompromised patient who complains of decreased visual acuity.

Toxoplasmosis can also occur in patients with solid tumors, especially those receiving chemotherapy or other immunosuppressive treatment. A review at Sloan-Kettering showed that most patients (85%) were receiving alkylating agents, antimetabolites, radiation therapy, or steroids when they were diagnosed with toxoplasmosis.[353,354]

Toxoplasmosis in cancer patients is almost always fatal if left untreated. A review of 74 cases of toxoplasmosis in cancer patients showed a mortality of 98% (45/46) in patients who were not treated. In those instances in which the diagnosis was made early enough to institute treatment, 68% (19/28) improved.[351,352] As with transplant and other immunocompromised patients, early diagnosis and timely treatment improve the outcome.

Patients with connective tissue disease (e.g., rheumatoid arthritis, systemic lupus erythematosus [SLE]) also develop toxoplasmosis.[351,352] These patients are often taking long-term immunosuppressive therapy with steroids. Both serum rheumatoid factor and antinuclear antibodies (e.g., ANA test for lupus), which are often high in this group of patients, can produce false-positive IgM indirect fluorescent antibody (IFA) serologic tests for toxoplasmosis.[355] IgM capture assays may obviate the confounding results for rheumatoid factor.[356] Neither capture ELISAs nor the dye test obviate the possible confounding results due to cross-reactive ANAs.

CD40 deficient patients may also be at risk for toxoplasmosis.[357]

Special Treatment Considerations

Since concomitant administration of pyrimethamine and cytostatic agents used in chemotherapy (e.g., cytarabine, daunorubicin) has caused fatal bone marrow aplasia, these agents should not be used together. Similarly, pyrimethamine should not be used together with methotrexate. Since toxoplasmosis left untreated carries a high mortality in immunocompromised patients, treatment of *T. gondii* infection should take precedence over the use of other medications, and alternative chemotherapeutic or immunosuppressive regimens should be sought during the treatment period. Two sulfonamides should not be used simultaneously because of the increased risk of bone marrow toxicity.

Corticosteroids are often used to treat connective tissue disorders, but steroids used alone have been shown to exacerbate both ocular and disseminated *T. gondii* infections.[358,359] For this reason, if there is evidence of *T. gondii* infection and steroids are to be used for treatment of connective tissue disorders, they should always be used together with a full regimen of anti-*Toxoplasma* therapy.[351,352]

MEDICATIONS USED FOR TREATMENT OF *T. GONDII* INFECTION

When used together, pyrimethamine and sulfadiazine remain the treatment of choice for *T. gondii* infections. No other therapeutic regimen has been found to be as effective in treating acute toxoplasmosis. These drugs inhibit sequential steps in the biosynthesis of tetrahydrofolic acid and thus disrupt the biosynthesis of protozoal nucleic acids. Pyrimethamine and sulfadiazine, as well as several other alternatives and some experimental options, are discussed below. Desensitization to sulfadiazine has also been

used,[360] although some agents (e.g. didanosine, atovaquone, azithromycin) may possess some activity against cysts and bradyzoites in vitro,[208,361] to date there is no treatment available that is capable of eradicating the bradyzoite or latent cyst form of *T. gondii* from animals.

Pyrimethamine

Pyrimethamine acts by inhibiting the enzyme dihydrofolate reductase (DHFR), a critical step in folate synthesis.[362] Recently it has been shown that apicomplexans cannot increase production of DHFR in the presence of inhibitors of DHFR, whereas mammals can.[363,364]

Dosages for infants are discussed under treatment of Congenital Toxoplasmois and in Table 38–4. In adults, the serum half-life of pyrimethamine is about 100 hours, and in infants, the half-life is approximately 60 hours.[147] In adults the average serum levels found 4 hours after a dose of 25 to 50 mg are on the order of 1000 to 2000 ng/mL.[147,365] In patients with AIDS, however, pyrimethamine displays variable absorption and pharmacokinetics.[365–369] For adults a loading dose of 50 mg twice daily for 2 days is given, followed by 50 to 75 mg a day until 1 week beyond the time when signs of acute infection have resolved. A loading dose is important, as the time to reach therapeutic steady state levels is lengthened to 14 days if the loading dose is omitted.[370] If there is evidence of CNS involvement, the higher dose of pyrimethamine should be used for optimal CNS penetration. In infants, levels achieved in the CSF are usually 10% to 20% of those measured in serum. Caution should be used in treating young children, in whom seizures have been described with serum levels above 5000 ng/mL.[147] In the case of patients on immunosuppressive therapy, maintenance therapy for *T. gondii* should be given after treatment of the acute episode until immunosuppressive agents can be discontinued.

Because of the frequent occurrence of bone marrow toxicity, biweekly blood counts should be performed on all patients taking pyrimethamine. Folinic acid (leucovorin) should always be given when pyrimethamine is administered to minimize bone marrow toxicity caused by pyrimethamine. Leucovorin should also be administered for 1 additional week after discontinuation of pyrimethamine therapy because of the long half-life of pyrimethamine. Starting doses for leucovorin are 10 mg daily in adults and 10 mg Monday, Wednesday, and Friday in infants. It is important to emphasize that folic acid should *not* be used, as *T. gondii* can use folic acid, and this may decrease the efficacy of pyrimethamine.[203] In contrast, leucovorin does not interfere appreciably with the action of pyrimethamine on *T. gondii* at the usual doses administered.[147]

Since pyrimethamine is metabolized in the liver by the cytochrome P450 enzymes, any medications that affect the cytochrome P450 system will have an effect on serum pyrimethamine levels. Phenobarbital, which activates cytochrome P450 enzymes, is one example of an agent that will induce the cytochrome P450 system and thus will accelerate the degradation of pyrimethamine and decrease pyrimethamine serum levels.[147]

Side effects from pyrimethamine include gastrointestinal discomfort, headaches, vomiting, seizures, and bone marrow suppression. The most common toxicity is neutropenia; anemia and thrombocytopenia have also been described.[362] Folinic acid (leucovorin) is given to minimize bone marrow toxicity (see above).

Pyrimethamine is teratogenic in animal models, causing congenital malformations in rats at doses higher than those used for humans (e.g., cranial and brain developmental abnormalities, hydrocephalus, hydrops, growth retardation). In these studies, pyrimethamine was given early in gestation. Because of its potential for teratogenicity, pyrimethamine is not recommended for treatment of toxoplasmosis during the first trimester in acutely infected pregnant women.

Sulfadiazine

Sulfadiazine is a sulfonamide that inhibits the enzyme dihydropteroate synthase, which is an earlier step in the folate biosynthetic pathway than DHFR is (Fig. 38–9).[371] Sulfadiazine used in combination with pyrimethamine is synergistic, with the combination being eight times more active than either medication alone.[211,212,214] Sulfadiazine should be used together with pyrimethamine and should not be used as a single agent to treat *T. gondii* infection. In infants and older children the usual dose is 100 mg/kg/d orally divided into two or four equal doses. In adults a typical dose would be 1 to 1.5 g every 6 hours, not to exceed a total daily dose of 4 to 6 g daily.

Sulfadiazine also may be given in two divided doses per day as the half-life is approximately 15 hours.

Rash, hypersensitivity reactions, and renal stones are the most common side effects. As with all sulfonamides, sulfadiazine may induce photosensitivity reactions. It has been associated with severe cutaneous reactions such as erythema multiforme, Stevens-Johnson syndrome, and toxic epidermal necrolysis. Bone marrow suppression has also been reported.[362] Pre-existing megaloblastic anemia is a relative contraindication to receiving sulfadiazine. Other pre-existing conditions that require caution include glucose-6-phosphate dehydrogenase (G-6-PD) deficiency (sulfonamides may precipitate hemolysis), and porphyria (sulfonamides may precipitate an acute attack of porphyria). Exacerbations of kernicterus in the newborn have been described with sulfonamide treatment, but as these reports involved infants with many complicated medical problems,[372] a cause-and-effect relationship has not been proven. We and others have used sulfadiazine safely to treat pregnant women and to treat infants with total serum bilirubin levels up to 15 mg/dl (McLeod, unpublished data, 2002). Above this level we replace sulfadiazine with clindamycin. Since sulfonamides may cause crystalluria and kidney stone formation, patients should be advised to increase their fluid intake (e.g., in adults, 8 glasses of water or nonacidic beverages daily) to maintain adequate hydration. Patients should be cautioned to avoid consuming acidic beverages such as orange juice, as these increase the risk of renal stone formation. Sodium bicarbonate may be used to alkalinize urine to prevent crystalluria[373] and renal stones in this setting.

There has been one sulfonamide resistant clinical isolate reported recently.

C. Folate synthesis

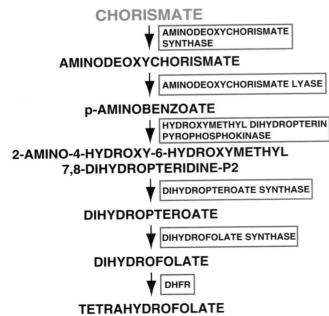

FIGURE 38–9. Synthesis of folate from chorismate. Sulfadiazine inhibits dihydropteroate synthase and pyrimethamine inhibits dihydrofolate reductase. From McLeod R, et al: The shikimate pathway and its branches in apicomplexan parasites. (CIDCS) Chicago, University of Chicago Press, 2002.

Other Sulfonamides

Other sulfonamides that have been shown to have efficacy comparable to that of sulfadiazine include the combination of sulfapyrazine, sulfamethazine, and sulfamerazine.[362] Sulfadoxine (the agent in Fansidar) is less effective, and because of the long half-life of sulfadoxine, if toxicity occurs, it is present for a longer time. An one study of AIDS patients with TE treated with pyrimethamine-clindamycin who were switched to the pyrimethamine-sulfadoxine combination, 7% (4/56) experienced a relapse. Other sulfonamides such as sulfapyridine, sulfadimidine, sulfathiazole, sulfisoxazole, and sulfamethoxazole[210] are not as effective and should not be used for treatment.

Fansidar

A fixed combination of 25 mg pyrimethamine and 500 mg sulfadoxine, Fansidar acts on the same enzyme pathway that pyrimethamine-sulfadiazine does (see above) to deplete parasite stores of folic acid, an essential cofactor in the biosynthesis of nucleic acids. It was once commonly used for malaria prophylaxis, but the incidence of Stevens-Johnson and other severe cutaneous reactions associated with Fansidar and its longer half-life have caused it to fall out of favor for this use. Although in vitro data suggest that it is less active against *T. gondii* than pyrimethamine-sulfadiazine is, there have been studies reporting success with this medication in bone marrow transplant recipients and pregnant women,[350] and its use in infants has been reported.[200,374] Sulfadoxine has a substantially longer half-life than sulfadiazine has, and the fixed dose provides a suboptimal dose of pyrimethamine.[204] Adverse effects are essentially the same as those described for pyrimethamine-sulfadiazine (see above), but sulfadoxine persists longer.[375] Fansidar has the potential for serious toxicity, as the sulfadoxine persists for a substantially longer time than sulfadiazine does. Thus because of the lesser efficacy in vitro and the fixed combination that provides a suboptimal dose of pyrimethamine and the sulfonamide sulfadoxine, which has a longer half-life and increases the risk for more sustained toxicity, we do not recommend Fansidar for the treatment of toxoplasmosis.

Dapsone

Dapsone is a sulfone chemically related to the sulfonamides. It has been used as an antimicrobial agent for several decades, most notably for the treatment of leprosy. The first trial of dapsone against *Plasmodium falciparum*, another apicomplexan parasite related to *T. gondii*, was in 1943.[362]

Like sulfadiazine, dapsone acts by inhibiting dihydropteroate synthase.[362] In combination with pyrimethamine, it has been successfully used in some instances to treat cerebral toxoplasmosis in AIDS patients.[224] More recently, dapsone has been used as an alternative for PCP prophylaxis in HIV patients unable to tolerate TMP-SMX. It has a half-life of 10 to 50 hours, with a mean half-life of 28 hours. Urinary excretion is variable. Peak serum concentrations are reached 1 to 3 hours after a dose is given. The average serum level obtained following a dose of 100 mg/d is 2 μg "free" dapsone per gram of blood; 50% is protein bound.[362,376]

Hemolysis is the most well-known side effect of dapsone; methemoglobinemia is also not uncommon. Hemolysis occurs, to varying degrees, in almost every person treated with high doses of dapsone (200 to 300 mg/d). In the absence of G-6-PD deficiency, a dose of 100 mg usually does not cause an appreciable hemolysis. The risk increases in persons with G-6-PD deficiency, even at low levels of 50 mg/d. In a person with G-6-PD deficiency, however, doses of 50 mg or less are usually well tolerated.[377] Complete blood count (CBC) should be monitored during treatment with dapsone.

Side effects are mostly dose related and include anorexia, nausea, and vomiting. The "dapsone syndrome," although rare, can be fatal if unrecognized. It tends to occur in the first 6 weeks of treatment and is characterized by fever, eosinophilia, lymphadenopathy, leucovorinpenia, jaundice or hepatitis, and exanthematous skin eruptions that may progress to Stevens-Johnson syndrome.[362,377]

Clindamycin

Clindamycin is a lincosaminide. Pfefferkorn et al found that clindamycin was effective against *T. gondii* in vitro.[209,378] It has been used as an alternative to sulfadiazine, in conjunction with pyrimethamine, in patients who have significant allergic reactions to sulfonamide drugs.[226,379,380] The combination of pyrimethamine and clindamycin has been used successfully to treat patients with AIDS and TE who have allergies to sulfonamide drugs. This combination appears comparable in efficacy to pyrimethamine-sulfadiazine in treating acute infection but has displayed higher relapse rates (Table 38–9).

In bacteria, clindamycin binds to the 50S subunit of the bacterial ribosome and disrupts protein synthesis. Its mechanism of action in *T. gondii* appears to be through inhibition of protein synthesis in the plastid organelle of the parasite.[381,382] In bacteria, several antimicrobials act at the same site (50S subunit) even though they are not structurally related, and thus concurrent administration of these antibiotics (clindamycin, chloramphenicol, and the macrolide erythromycin) may act antagonistically to inhibit binding of the others.[362] It is currently not known whether a similar phenomenon occurs in *T. gondii*. Therefore none of these drugs should be used together. In tissue culture, lethality requires several days, that is, clindamycin appears to have a cumulative effect over time but with a slower initial effect. This has also been noted for other antimicrobial agents that affect plastid-associated enzymes.[383–385] Active retinal lesions in children treated with pyrimethamine and clindamycin seem to resolve more slowly than they do in children treated with pyrimethamine and sulfadiazine, but this has not been proven in RCTs or other controlled studies.

Clindamycin is well absorbed with oral administration. Its half-life is 2.5 hours, with 90% or more being bound to plasma protein. Penetration of clindamycin is excellent in most tissues including pigmented retina. It readily crosses the placenta.[362] Although significant levels are not attained in CSF, brain tissue concentrations attained are high enough to treat brain abscesses. Most of the compound is inactivated by hepatic metabolism and then excreted in urine and bile. Caution should be used in patients with severe hepatic failure, as drug accumulation can be greater in this group.[362] Dose adjustment is not required in patients with renal failure.

The most common side effect of clindamycin is diarrhea, and the most serious side effect is pseudomembranous colitis, which can be life threatening. Pseudomembranous colitis is due to intestinal overgrowth with the pathogen *Clostridium difficile* and is characterized by fevers, abdominal pain, and profuse diarrhea, often with blood or mucus. As this complication can be lethal, clindamycin should be immediately discontinued if pseudomembranous colitis develops. Treatment of severe *C. difficile* colitis with oral metronidazole should be initiated. Skin rashes occur in 10% of patients receiving clindamycin.[362]

Macrolides

In bacteria, macrolides act by inhibiting bacterial protein synthesis by binding to the 50S ribosomal subunit.[362] The mechanism of action of macrolides in *T. gondii* is not known, and investigators have proposed a plastid mechanism of action.[386,387] It has been shown that macrolides must penetrate phagocytic cells to be effective against *T. gondii*.[386,388] The macrolides azithromycin and roxithromycin have been shown to reach concentrations in macrophages that are over 200 times higher than levels measured in serum.[386,387] A stimulating effect of macrolides on macrophages and other phagocytic cells, which may enhance the immune function and render these cells more effective at killing the parasite, has been proposed by some investigators.[386,387]

Spiramycin is a macrolide antibiotic with a bacterial spectrum of action similar to that of erythromycin.[389] As it is concentrated in the placenta, spiramycin has been used to decrease transmission of toxoplasmosis from mother to fetus (60% transmission in those untreated vs. 23% transmission in those treated).[170] Its use for this indication has been challenged (see discussion under treatment in pregnancy). There is no other indication for its use in the treatment of toxoplasmosis. It does not penetrate the CSF or brain tissue and cannot be used to treat TE. TE has occurred in patients receiving spiramycin.[195] An optimal dose has never been established, but the current recommendation for the acutely infected pregnant woman is 1 g three times a day. This is based in part on studies[193] that demonstrated a much higher placental concentration (6.2 μg/ml) with 3 g total daily dose as opposed to 2 g daily (2.75 μg/ml). Common complaints are abdominal discomfort, nausea, vomiting, diarrhea, and paraesthesias. As with erythromycin, allergies (skin rash, hives), QT prolongation, and arrhythmias have been described.[390,391]

In combination with pyrimethamine, both azithromycin and clarithromycin have been used with some degree of success in treating AIDS patients with TE in small, clinical pilot studies.[137,275,276] Experimental models have shown that azithromycin possesses activity against the bradyzoite form of *T. gondii*, which has led to considerable interest in this medication for clinical use.[148,386] Significant differences in susceptibility have been reported in different strains of tachyzoites,[387] and mutations conferring resistance to macrolides have been described.[378] Currently two clinical trials are in progress (one with azithromycin alone, the other with azithromycin plus pyrimethamine) to evaluate the clinical efficacy of this medication in treating TE in patients with AIDS (AIDS database 2000).

Atovaquone

Atovaquone is a hydroxynaphthoquinone that acts by selectively inhibiting the third cytochrome complex (cytochrome bc [1] complex) of the mitochondrial respiratory chain of *T. gondii*.[392] It has been reported to have in vitro activity against both the tachyzoite and bradyzoite forms of the parasite.[148,393] Concentrations 100-fold higher were reported to kill bradyzoites in vitro.[148,361,394]

The tablet form of this drug has been used successfully to treat AIDS patients with cerebral toxoplasmosis, but high relapse rates have been reported.[393] In a study of 65 patients treated for TE, atovaquone used as maintenance therapy in patients unable to tolerate other regiments resulted in a relapse rate of 26%.[393] Atovaquone was used as single agent therapy in 75% of these cases. Atovaquone should not be used as single agent therapy to treat *T. gondii* but rather should be used in combination with another drug such as pyrimethamine. Salvage regimens consisting of atovaquone and pyrimethamine have been effective.[393]

Atovaquone comes in a tablet[393] or suspension form.[283] The tablet form was poorly aqueous soluble,[395] and its absorption increased at least three-fold when given with a high-fat meal.[396] The suspension formulation has an approximately two-fold greater bioavailability whether administered with or without food, and for this reason its use has replaced that of the tablets.[397,398] Atovaquone has a long serum half-life (57 to 77 hours).[393,399] Serum levels higher than 18.5 μg/ml correlated with therapeutic response in the treatment of toxoplasmosis.[393] Atovaquone effect in murine models is augmented by use of pyrimethamine or sulfadizine.[400] A recent study[283] of atovaquone suspension (1500 mg orally twice daily) administered with either pyrimethamine (200 mg loading dose followed by 75 mg daily) or sulfadiazine (1500 mg four times daily) resulted in an approximately 77% response rate; 28% discontinued treatment as a result of adverse events, including nausea, vomiting, and intolerance of the taste of atovaquone, with 1 of 20 patients experiencing relapse during maintenance. These outcomes are similar to outcomes with other treatment regimens including pyrimethamine and sulfadizine and pyrimethamine and clindamycin.

Most of the compound is hepatically metabolized, and less than 0.6% is renally excreted. Although CSF/plasma ratios of drug levels of less than 1% indicate that atovaquone does not cross the blood-brain barrier, its successful use in treating cerebral toxoplasmosis suggests that it is able to penetrate brain tissue in infected patients.[393]

Side effects most commonly experienced with atovaquone are headache, rash, nausea, vomiting, diarrhea, and elevated liver enzymes.[399] Rifampin should not be given with atovaquone, as rifampin decreases atovaquone plasma concentrations to subtherapeutic levels.

OTHER MEDICATIONS

Other compounds have shown promise in experimental models. These are briefly discussed.

Ketolides

The new generation of macrolide antibiotics, the ketolides, have been studied in murine models of *T. gondii* infection. When used at a concentration of 50 mg/kg, ketolides protected 30% of mice lethally infected and provided 100% protection at 10 days when used in combination with clindamycin, atovaquone, or sulfadiazine.[222] In another study, doses needed to effectively treat infection in mice were lower than those required for the macrolides azithromycin and roxithromycin, suggesting that ketolides may be more potent against *T. gondii* than other macrolides.[221] As yet no data are available on the use of ketolide antibiotics in treating *T. gondii* infection in humans.

Fluoroquinolones

Of the fluoroquinolones, in vitro data show that gatifloxacin is active against *T. gondii* with a 50% inhibitory concentration (IC_{50}) of 5.1 mg/L, moxifloxacin with an IC_{50} of 5.1 mg/L, and trovafloxacin with an IC_{50} of 0.4 mg/L.[401] Only trovafloxacin, however, has been shown to possess activity against *T. gondii* both in vitro and in

vivo.[402,403] The U.S. Food and Drug Administration (FDA) removed trovafloxacin from the market because of several reports of fatal liver toxicity attributed to this medication. Thus far no information is available on the efficacy of the newer quinolones against *T. gondii* in humans.

Epiroprim

Epiroprim, like pyrimethamine, inhibits DHFR and interferes with this step of folate synthesis. It has been used successfully in animal models to treat *T. gondii* infections, either alone or in combination with dapsone.[404-406] There is no data available on its use for this indication in humans.

Rifamycin Derivatives

Rifapentine and rifabutin are both derivatives of rifamycin. In vitro and in vivo mouse studies have shown these medications are able to inhibit intracellular replication of *T. gondii*.[219,220] In murine studies, relapses were reported in mice treated with rifabutin.[219] Some synergy was observed when atovaquone and rifabutin were given in combination.[407] There is no data on the use of rifapentine or rifabutin to treat toxoplasmosis in humans.

Synercid

Synercid, or quinupristin-dalfopristin, has recently been shown to possess in vitro activity against *T. gondii*.[408] A 200 mg/kg dose for 10 days achieved 100% survival in mice infected with *T. gondii*.[403] No data is available on its in vivo efficacy in humans.

Protease Inhibitors

A recent report showed that certain protease inhibitors have in vitro activity against *T. gondii*.[409] The mechanism of action for this effect is unknown. Ritonavir was found to have an IC_{50} of 5.4 mg/L, and nelfinavir, an IC_{50} of 4 mg/L; indinavir was found to be only partially inhibitory, even at high concentrations.[409]

MISCELLANEOUS

A number of inhibitors of metabolic pathways and enzymes present in apicomplexan parasites but not in mammals demonstrate in vitro activity against *T. gondii*; some have been shown to protect mice from *T. gondii* infections.[410,411] These include inhibitors of the shikimate pathway such as glyphosate, which inhibits 5-enolpyruvylshikimate-3-phosphate (EPSP) synthase and is an active ingredient in many herbicide preparations, inhibitors of fatty acid synthesis such as Triclosan (an active ingredient in many antibacterial handsoaps),[385] and the herbicide Clodinafop.[384] An inhibitor of isoprenoid synthesis has been shown to be efficacious in vitro and in mice.[412] These compounds show promise as lead compounds in the development of antimicrobial agents against *T. gondii*, but no data are yet available on their use in humans. Organelles present in apicomplexans but not animals[382,413] also offer another potential for developing novel antimicrobial agents.

Cytokines

Interferon-gamma has been shown to be effective in the treatment of *T. gondii* infections. Interferon-gamma has been shown to have a synergistic effect with the macrolide roxithromycin in treating *T. gondii* infection in animal models.[414] Interleukin-12 has also shown some promise.[415] The use of these and other cytokines in the treatment of *T. gondii* infections is under study.[416]

CONCLUSIONS AND THE FUTURE

Antimicrobial treatment and prophylaxis has improved the outcome for congenitally infected and immunocompromised persons. Better, nontoxic medicines that eliminate tachyzoites and bradyzoites are urgently needed. The sequence of the *Toxoplasma* genome should result in new targets for development of novel antimicrobial agents. Understanding which metabolic pathways and enzymes are unique to apicomplexans and parasite life cycel stages as well as mechanisms involved in subcellular organelle targeting and function provide a conceptual basis for preparation of inhibitory compounds. Serologic screening programs should permit earlier diagnosis and treatment of congenitally infected persons.

ACKNOWLEDGMENTS We thank Esther Castro, Ernest Mui, and Julie Mastbrook for their assistance in the preparation of this manuscript. This work was supported by R01 16945, R01 27530, and R01 43228.

REFERENCES

1. Nicole C, Manceaux L: Sur une infection a corps de Leishman (ou organisme Voisins) du gondii. C.R. Acad Sci 1908; 147:763–766.
2. Remington JS, Mcleod R, Desmonts G: Toxoplasmosis. In Remington J, Klein J (eds): Infectious Diseases of the Fetus and Newborn Infant. Philadelphia, WB Saunders, 1995, pp 140–268.
3. Remington JS, McLeod R, Thulliez P, Desmonts G: Toxoplasmosis. In Remington JS (ed): Infectious Diseases of the Fetus and Newborn Infant. Philadelphia, WB Saunders, 2001, pp 205–346.
4. Roberts CW, McLeod R: *Toxoplasma gondii.* In Bartlett J, Gorbach S, Blacklow N (eds): Infectious Diseases in Medicine and Surgery. Philadelphia, WB Saunders, 2002.
5. Boyer K, McLeod R: Toxoplasmosis. Long S, Proeber C, Pickering L (eds): In Principles and Practice of Pediatric Infectious Diseases. New York, Churchill Livingstone, 2002.
6. Dubey JP, Lindsay DS, Speer CA: Structures of *Toxoplasma gondii* tachyzoites, bradyzoites, and sporozoites and biology and development of tissue cysts. Clin Microbiol Rev 1998;11:267–299.
7. Ferguson DJ, Hutchison WM: The host-parasite relationship of *Toxoplasma gondii* in the brains of chronically infected mice. Virchows Arch 1987;411:39–43.
8. Frenkel JK, Dubey JP, Miller NL: *Toxoplasma gondii* in cats: Fecal stages identified as coccidian oocysts. Science 1970; 167:893–896.
9. Dubey JP, Miller NL, Frenkel JK: Characterization of the new fecal form of *Toxoplasma gondii.* J Parasitol 1970; 56:447–456.
10. Frenkel JK, Dubey JP, Miller NL: *Toxoplasma gondii*: Fecal forms separated from eggs of the nematode *Toxocara cati.* Science 1969;164:432–433.
11. Hutchinson WM, Dunachie JF, Work K: The fecal transmission of *Toxoplasma gondii* (brief report). Acta Pathol Microbiol Scand 1968;74:462–464.
12. Smith KL, Wilson M, McAuley J: Prevalence of *Toxoplasma gondii* antibodies in US military recruits in 1989: Comparison with data published in 1965. Clin Infect Dis 1996;23: 1182–1183.
13. DeWaal CS, Birkett D, Enga Z: Unexpected consequences: Miscarriage and birth defects from tainted food. Center for Science in the Public Interest, 2000, pp. 1–18.
14. Roberts T, Frenkel JK: Estimating income losses and other preventable costs caused by congenital toxoplasmosis in people in the United States. J Am Vet Med Assoc 1990;196: 249–256.
15. Luft BJ, Remington JS: Acute *Toxoplasma* infection among family members of patients with acute lymphadenopathic toxoplasmosis. Arch Intern Med 1984;144:53–56.
16. Kean BH, Kimball AC, Christenson WN: An epidemic of acute toxoplasmosis. JAMA 1969;208:1002–1004.
17. Choi WY, et al: Foodborne outbreaks of human toxoplasmosis. J Infect Dis 1997;175:1280–1282.
18. Desmonts G, et al: Epidemiological study on toxoplasmosis: The influence of cooking slaughter-animal meat on the incidence of human infection. Rev Fr Etud Clin Biol 1965; 10:952–958.
19. Edelhofer R, Aspock H: Modes and sources of infections with *Toxoplasma gondii* in view of the screening of pregnant women in Austria. Mitt Osterr Ges Tropenmed Parasitol 1996; 18:59–70.
20. Teutsch SM, et al: Epidemic toxoplasmosis associated with infected cats. N Engl J Med 1979;300:695–699.
21. Benenson MW, et al: Oocyst-transmitted toxoplasmosis associated with ingestion of contaminated water. N Engl J Med 1982;307:666–669.
22. Bowie WR, et al: Outbreak of toxoplasmosis associated with municipal drinking water. The Toxoplasma Investigation Team. Lancet 1997;350:173–177.
23. Taverne J: Toxoplasmosis in Brazil. Trends Parasitol 2002;18: 203–204.
24. Howe DK, Sibley LD: *Toxoplasma gondii* comprises three clonal lineages: Correlation of parasite genotype with human disease. J Infect Dis 1995;172:1561–1566.
25. Darde ML, Bouteille B, Pestre-Alexandre M: Isoenzyme analysis of 35 *Toxoplasma gondii* isolates and the biological and epidemiological implications. J Parasitol 1992;78:786–794.
26. Grigg M, et al: Success and virulence in toxoplasma as the result of sexual recombination between two distinct ancestries. Science 2001;294:161–165.
27. Glasner PD, et al: An unusually high prevalence of ocular toxoplasmosis in southern Brazil. Am J Ophthalmol 1992;114: 136–144.

28. Grigg M, et al: Unusual abundance of atypical strains associated with human ocular toxoplasmosis. J Infect Dis 2001;184:633–639.

29. Dubey JP, et al: Biological and genetic characterisation of *Toxoplasma gondii* isolates from chickens (Gallus domesticus) from Sao Paulo, Brazil: Unexpected findings. Int J Parasitol 2002;32:99–105.

30. Mack D, et al: HLA-class II genes modify outcome of *Toxoplasma gondii* infection. Int J Parasitol 1999;29:1351–1358.

31. Brown CR, McLeod R: Class I MHC genes and CD8+ T cells determine cyst number in *Toxoplasma gondii* infection. J Immunol 1990;145:3438–3441.

32. Brown C, et al: Definitive identification of a gene that confers resistance against Toxoplasma cyst burden and encephalitis. Immunology 1995;85:419–428.

33. Johnson JJ, et al: Genetic analysis of influences on survival following *Toxoplasma gondii* infection. Int J Parasitol 2001;31:109–113.

34. Suzuki Y, et al: Evidence for genetic regulation of susceptibility to toxoplasmic encephalitis in AIDS patients. J Infect Dis 1996;173:265–268.

35. Johnson JJ, et al: In vitro correlates of Ld restricted resistance to toxoplasmic encephalitis and their critical dependence on parasite strain. J Immunol 2002;169:966–973.

36. McLeod R, et al: Genetic regulation of early survival and cyst number after peroral *Toxoplasma gondii* infection of AXB/BXA recombinant inbred and B10 congenic mice. J Immunol 1989;143:3031–3034.

37. McLeod R, et al: Immunogenetics in pathogenesis of and protection against toxoplasmosis. In Gross U, (ed): Current Topics in Microbiology and Immunology. New York, Springer-Verlag, 1996, pp. 95–112.

38. Brown C, et al: Effects of human class I transgenes on *Toxoplasma gondii* cyst formation. J Immunol 1994;152:4537–4541.

39. Couvreur J, Desmonts G, Girre JY: Congenital toxoplasmosis in twins: A series of 14 pairs of twins: absence of infection in one twin in two pairs. J Pediatr 1976;89:235–240.

40. McLeod R, et al: Subcutaneous and intestinal vaccination with tachyzoites of *Toxoplasma gondii* and acquisition of immunity to peroral and congenital Toxoplasma challenge. J Immunol 1988;140:1632–1637.

41. Mead PS, et al: Food-related illness and death in the United States: Reply to Dr. Hedberg. Emerg Infect Dis 1999;5:607–625.

42. Dubey JP, et al: Effect of high temperature on infectivity of *Toxoplasma gondii* tissue cysts in pork. J Parasitol 1990;76:201–204.

43. Swartzberg JE, Remington JS: Transmission of toxoplasma. Am J Dis Child 1975;129:777–779.

44. Derouin F, et al: Toxoplasma infection after human allogeneic bone marrow transplantation: Clinical and serological study of 80 patients. Bone Marrow Transplant 1986;1:67–73.

45. Derouin F, et al: Toxoplasma antibody titers in renal transplant recipients. Transplantation 1987;44:515–518.

46. Derouin F, et al: Toxoplasmosis in bone marrow-transplant recipients: Report of seven cases and review. Clin Infect Dis 1992;15:267–270.

47. Ryning FW, et al: Probable transmission of *Toxoplasma gondii* by organ transplantation. Ann Intern Med 1979;90:47–49.

48. Gottesdiener KM: Transplanted infections: Donor-to-host transmission with the allograft. Ann Intern Med 1989;110:1001–1016.

49. Jurges E, et al: Transmission of toxoplasmosis by bone marrow transplant associated with Campath-1G. Bone Marrow Transplant 1992;9:65–66.

50. Masur H, et al: Salvage trial of trimetrexate-leucovorin for the treatment of cerebral toxoplasmosis in patients with AIDS. J Infect Dis 1993;167:1422–1426.

51. Mathews WC, Fullerton SC: Use of a clinical laboratory database to estimate toxoplasma seroprevalence amoung human immunodeficiency virus-infected patients: Overcoming bias in secondary analysis of clinical records. Arch Pathol Lab Med 1994;118:807–810.

52. Marra CM, et al: Diagnostic accuracy of HIV-associated central nervous system toxoplasmosis. Int J STD AIDS 1998;9:761–764.

53. Millogo A, et al: Toxoplasma serology in HIV infected patients and suspected cerebral toxoplasmosis at the Central Hospital of Bobo-Dioulasso (Burkina Faso). Bull Soc Pathol Exot 2000;93:17–19.

54. Minkoff H, et al: Vertical transmission of toxoplasma by human immunodeficiency virus-infected women. Am J Obstet Gynecol 1997;176:555–559.

55. Deleze M, Mintz G, Del Carmen Mejia M: *Toxoplasma gondii* encephalitis in systemic lupus erythematosus. A neglected cause of treatable nervous system infection. J Rheumatol 1985;12:994–996.

56. Raisanen S: Toxoplasmosis transmitted by blood transfusion. Transfusion 1978;18:329–332.

57. Siegel SE, et al: Transmission of toxoplasmosis by leukocyte transfusion. Blood 1971;37:388–394.

58. Remington JS, Gentry LO: Acquired toxoplasmosis: Infection versus diseases. Ann NY Acad Sci 1970;174:1006–1017.

59. Strom J: Toxoplasmosis due to laboratory infection in two adults. Acta Med Scand 1951;139:244–252.

60. Neu HC: Toxoplasmosis transmitted at autopsy. JAMA 1967;202:844–845.

61. Remington JS: Toxoplasmosis in the adult. Bull NY Acad Med 1974;50:211–227.

62. Remington JS, McLeod R, Desmonts G: Toxoplasmosis. In Remington J, Klein J (eds.): Infectious Diseases of the Fetus and Newborn Infant. Philadelphia, WB Saunders, 1995, pp. 140–267.

63. Labadie MD, Hazeman JJ: Aport des bilans de sante de l'enfant pour le depistage et l'etude epidemiologique de la toxoplasmose congenitale. J Pediatr 1984;70:714–723.

64. Brooks RG, McCabe R, Remington JS: Role of serology in the diagnosis of toxoplasmic lymphadenopathy. Rev Infect Dis 1987;9:1055–1062.

65. Fleck DG: Annotation: Diagnosis of Toxoplasmosis. J Clin Pathol 1989;42:191–193.

66. McCabe R, et al: Clinical spectrum in 107 cases of toxoplasmic lymphadenopathy. Rev Infect Dis 1987;9:754–774.

67. Bossi P, et al: *Toxoplasma gondii* associated Guillain-Barré syndrome in an immuno-competent patient. J Clin Microbiol 1998;36:3724–3725.

68. Townsend JJ, et al: Acquired toxoplasmosis. A neglected cause of treatable nervous system disease. Arch Neurol 1975;32:335–343.

69. Couvreur J, Thulliez P: Toxoplasmose acquise a localisation oculaire ou neurologique. Presse Med 1996;25:438–442.

70. Burnett AJ, et al: Multiple cases of acquired toxoplasmosis retinitis presenting in an outbreak. Ophthalmology 1998;105:1032–1037.

71. Silveira C, et al: Acquired toxoplasmic infection as the cause of toxoplasmic retinochoroiditis in families. Am J Ophthalmol 1988;106:362–364.

72. Theologides A, Kennedy BJ: Toxoplasmic myocarditis and pericarditis. Am J Med 1969;47:169–174.

73. Cuturic M, et al: Toxoplasmic polymyositis revisited: Case report and review of literature. Neuromuscul Dis 1997;7:390–396.

74. Greenlee JE, et al: Adult toxoplasmosis presenting as polymyositis and cerebellar ataxia. Ann Intern Med 1975;82:367–371.

75. Darde ML, Foudrinier F, Beguinot I: Disseminated toxoplasmosis acquired in French Guyana in an immunocompetent patient with isoenzyme typing of the Toxoplasma isolate. J Clin Microbiol 1998;36:324.

76. Debord T, Eono P, Rey JL: Les risques infectieux chez les militaires en operation. Medecine et Maladies Infectieuses 1996;26:402–407.

77. Montoya JG, Remington JS: Studies on the serodiagnosis of toxoplasmic lymphadenitis. Clin Infect Dis 1995;20: 781–789.

78. Montoya JG, Remington JS: Toxoplasmic chorioretinitis in the setting of acute acquired toxoplasmosis. Clin Infect Dis 1996; 23:277–282.

79. Montoya JG, et al: Toxoplasmic myocarditis and polymyositis in patients with acute acquired toxoplasmosis diagnosed during life. Clin Infect Dis 1997;24:676–683.

80. Montoya, JG, et al: Use of the polymerase chain reaction for diagnosis of ocular toxoplasmosis. Ophthalmology 1999;106: 1554–1563.

81. Montoya JG: Laboratory diagnosis of Toxoplasma gondii infection and toxoplasmosis. J Infect Dis 2002;185(Suppl 1): S73–S82.

82. Naot Y, Desmonts G, Remington JS: IgM enzyme-linked immunosorbent assay test for the diagnosis of congential Toxoplasma infection. J Pediatr 1981;98:32–336.

83. McLeod R, et al: The child with congenital toxoplasmosis. In Remington JS, Swartz MN (eds): Current Clinical Topics in Infectious Diseases. Boston, Blackwell Science, 2000, pp. 189–208.

84. Beaman MH, et al: Toxoplasma gondii. In Mandell GL, Bennett JE, Dolin R (eds): Principles and Practice of Infectious Diseases. New York, Churchill Livingstone, 1995, pp. 2455–2475.

85. Remington JS, Desmonts G: Toxoplasmosis. In Remington KT (ed): Infectious Diseases of the Fetus and Newborn Infant. Philadelphia, WB Saunders, 1976, p 1121.

86. Remington JS, Araujo FG, Desmonts G: Recognition of different Toxoplasma antigens by IgM and IgG antibodies in mothers and their congenitally infected newborns. J Infect Dis 1985;152:1020–1024.

87. Remington JS, McLeod R: Toxoplasmosis. In Bartlett JG, Gorbach S, Blacklow N (eds): Infectious Diseases in Medicine and Surgery. Philadelphia, WB Saunders, 2002.

88. Naessens A, et al: Diagnosis of congenital toxoplasmosis in the neonatal period: A multicenter evaluation. J Pediatr 1999; 135:714–719.

89. Jenum PA, et al: Incidence of Toxoplasma gondii infection in 35,940 pregnant women in Norway and pregnancy outcome for infected women. J Clin Microbiol 1998;36: 2900–2906.

90. Boyer K, McAuley J: Congenital toxoplasmosis. Semin Pediatr Dis 1994;5:42–51.

91. Wong SY, et al: Role of specific immunoglobulin E in diagnosis of acute Toxoplasma infection and toxoplasmosis. J Clin Microbiol 1993;31:2952–2959.

92. Dannemann B, et al: Differential agglutination test for diagnosis of recently acquired infection with Toxoplasma gondii. J Clin Microbiol 1990;28:1928–1933.

93. Rossi CL: A simple, rapid enzyme-linked immunosorbent assay for evaluating immunoglobulin G antibody avidity in toxoplasmosis. Diagn Microbiol Infect Dis 1998;30: 25–30.

94. Lappalainen M, et al: Toxoplasmosis acquired during pregnancy: Improved serodiagnosis based on avidity of IgG. J Infect Dis 1993;167:691–697.

95. Pelloux H, et al: Determination of anti-Toxoplasma gondii immunoglobulin G avidity: Adaptation to the Vidas system (bioMerieux). Diagn Microbiol Infect Dis 1998;32:69–73.

96. Jenum PA, Stray-Pedersen B, Gundersen AG: Improved diagnosis of primary Toxoplasma gondii infection in early pregnancy by determination of antitoxoplasma immunoglobulin G avidity. J Clin Microbiol 1997;35:1972–1977.

97. Ashburn D, et al: Do IgA, IgE, and IgG avidity tests have any value in the diagnosis of toxoplasma infection in pregnancy? J Clin Pathol 1998;51:312–315.

98. Cozon GJ, et al: Estimation of the avidity of immunoglobulin G for routine diagnosis of chronic Toxoplasma gondii infection in pregnant women. Eur J Clin Microbiol Infect Dis 1998;17:32–36.

99. Hedman K: Avidity of IgG in serodiagnosis of infectious diseases. Rev Med Microbiol 1993;4:123–129.

100. Liesenfeld O, et al: Effect of testing for IgG avidity in the diagnosis of Toxoplasma gondii infection in pregnant women: Experience in a US reference laboratory. J Infect Dis 2001;183: 1248–1253.

101. Dorfman RF, Remington JS: Value of lymph node biopsy in the diagnosis of acute acquired toxoplasmosis. N Engl J Med 1973;289:878–881.

102. Grover CM, et al: Rapid prenatal diagnosis of congenital Toxoplasma infection by using polymerase chain reaction and amniotic fluid. J Clin Microbiol 1990;28:2297–2301.

103. Bretagne S, et al: Detection of Toxoplasma gondii by competitive DNA amplification of bronchoalveolar lavage samples. J Infect Dis 1993;168:1585–1588.

104. Kirisits MJ, Mui EJ, McLeod R: Measurement of the efficacy of vaccines and antimicrobial therapy against infection with Toxoplasma gondii. Int J Parasitol 2000;30:149–155.

105. Gratzl R, et al: Follow-up of infants with congenital toxoplasmosis detected by polymerase chain reaction analysis of amniotic fluid. Eur J Clin Microbiol Infect Dis 1998;17:853–858.

106. Burg JL, et al: Direct and sensitive detection of a pathogenic protozoan, Toxoplasma gondii, by polymerase chain reaction. J Clin Microbiol 1989;27:1787–1792.

107. Lyons RE, et al: Construction and validation of a polycompetitor construct (SWITCH) for use in competitive RT-PCR to assess tachyzoite-bradyzoite interconversion in Toxoplasma gondii. Parasitology 2001;123(Pt 5):433–439.

108. Lyons RE, McLeod R, Roberts CW: Toxoplasma gondii tachyzoite-bradyzoite interconversion. Trends Parasitol 2002;18:198–201.

109. Holland GN: Reconsidering the pathogenesis of ocular toxoplasmosis. Am J Ophthalmol 1999;128:502–505.

110. Hay J, Dutton GN: Toxoplasma and the eye. BMJ 1995;310: 1021–1022.

111. Ongkosuwito JV, et al: Serologic evaluation of patients with primary and recurrent ocular toxoplasmosis for evidence of recent infection. Am J Ophthalmol 1999;128:407–412.

112. Roberts F, McLeod R: Pathogenesis of toxoplasmic retinochoroiditis. Parasitol Today 1999;15:51–57.

113. Holland GN, et al: Intraocular inflammatory reactions without focal necrotizing retinochoroiditis in patients with acquired systemic toxoplasmosis. Am J Ophthalmol 1999; 128:413–420.

114. Koppe JG, Kloosterman GJ, DeRoéver-Bonnet H: Toxoplasmosis and pregnancy, with a long-term follow-up of the children. Eur J Obstet Gynecol Reprod Biol 1974;413: 101–110.

115. Koppe JG, Loewer-Sieger DH, DeRoéver-Bonnet H: Results of 20-year follow-up of congenital toxoplasmosis. Lancet 1986;1:254–256.

116. Wilson CB, et al: Development of adverse sequelae in children born with subclinical congenital Toxoplasma infection. Pediatrics 1980;66:767–774.

117. Swisher CN, Boyer KM, McLeod R: Congenital toxoplasmosis. The Toxoplasmosis Study Group. Semin Pediatr Neurol 1994;1:4–25.

118. Hogan MJ: Ocular toxoplasmosis. New York, Columbia University Press, p. 1951, 86.

119. O'Connor GR, Frenkel JK: Editorial: Dangers of steroid treatment in toxoplasmosis. Periocular injections and systemic therapy. Arch Ophthalmol 1976;94:213.

120. O'Connor G: Factors related to the initiation and recurrence of uveitis. XL Edward Jackson memorial lecture. Am J Ophthalmol 1983;96:577–599.

121. McMenamin PG: The ultrastructural pathology of congenital toxoplasmic retinochoroiditis. Part 1: The localization and morphology of Toxoplasma cysts in the retina. Exp Eye Res 1986;43:529–543.

122. Brezin AP, et al: Ocular toxoplasmosis in the fetus. Immunohistochemistry analysis and DNA amplication. Retina 1994;14:19–26.

123. D'Amico DJ: Diseases of the retina. N Engl J Med 1994; 331:95–106.

124. Holland GN, et al: Ocular toxoplasmosis in patients with the acquired immunodeficiency syndrome. Am J Ophthalmol 1988;106:653–667.

125. Smith RE, Ganley JP: Ophthalmic survey of a community 1: Abnormalities of the ocular fundus. Am J Ophthalmol 1972; 74:1126–1130.

126. Maetz HM, et al: Estimated prevalence of ocular toxoplasmosis and toxocariasis in Alabama. J Infect Dis 1987;156: 414.

127. Perkins ES: Ocular toxoplasmosis. Br J Ophthalmol 1973; 57:1–17.

128. Nussenblatt R, Belfort R Jr: Ocular toxoplasmosis: An old disease revisited. JAMA 1994;271:304–307.

129. Holland GN, et al: Ocular toxoplasmosis in immunosuppressed nonhuman primates. Invest Opthalmol Vis Sci 1988; 29:835–842.

130. Wilson CB, et al: Lymphocyte transformation in the diagnosis of congenital Toxoplasma infection. N Engl J Med 1980; 302:785–788.

131. Mets M, et al: Eye manifestations of congenital toxoplasmosis. Am J Opthalmol 1996;122:309–324.

132. Roberts F, et al: Histopathological features of ocular toxoplasmosis in the fetus and infant. Arch Ophthalmol 2001; 119:51–58.

133. Guerina NG, et al: Neonatal serologic screening and early treatment for congential *Toxoplasma gondii* infection. The New England Regional Toxoplasma Working Group. N Engl J Med 1994;330:1858–1863.

134. Couvreur J: Prospective study of acquired toxoplasmosis in pregnant women with a special reference to the outcome of the fetus. In D. Hentsch, (ed): Toxoplasmosis. Bern, Huber Publishers, 1971, pp. 119–136.

135. Liesenfeld O, et al: Confirmatory serologic testing for acute toxoplasmosis and rate of induced abortions among women reported to have positive Toxoplasma immunoglobulin M antibody titers. Am J Obstet Gynecol 2001;184:140–145.

136. Liesenfeld O, et al: False-positive results in immunoglobulin M (IgM) Toxoplasma antibody tests and importance of confirmatory testing: The Platelia Toxo IgM test. J Clin Microbiol 1997;35:174–178.

137. Liesenfeld O, Wong SY, Remington JS: Toxoplasmosis in the setting of AIDS. In Bartlett JG, Merigan TC, Bolognesi D (eds): Textbook of AIDS Medicine. Baltimore, Williams & Wilkins, 1999.

138. Brezin AP, et al: Analysis of aqueous humor in ocular toxoplasmosis. N Engl J Med 1991;324:699.

139. Desmonts G, Baron A, Offret G: La production locale d'anticorps au cours de la toxoplasmose oculaire. Arch Ophthalmol 1960;20:137–145.

140. Desmonts G: Definitive serological diagnosis of ocular toxoplasmosis. Arch Ophthalmol 1966;76:839–851.

141. Yamamoto JH, et al: Discrimination between patients with acquired toxoplasmosis and congenital toxoplasmosis on the basis of the immune response to parasite antigens. J Infect Dis 2000;181:2018–2022.

142. Rothova A, et al: Therapy for ocular toxoplasmosis. Am J Ophthalmol 1993;115:517–523.

143. St Georgiev V: Opportunistic/nosocomial infections. Treatment and developmental therapeutics. Toxoplasmosis. Med Res Rev 1993;13:529–568.

144. Rothova A: Ocular involvement in toxoplasmosis. Br J Ophthalmol 1993;77:371–377.

145. Rothova A, et al: Azithromycin for ocular toxoplasmosis. Br J Ophthalmol 1998;82:1306–1308.

146. Lopez JS, et al: Orally administered 566C80 for treatment of ocular toxoplasmosis in a patient with the acquired immunodeficiency syndrome. Am J Ophthalmol 1992;113: 331–333.

147. McLeod R, et al: Levels of pyrimethamine in sera and cerebrospinal and ventricular fluids from infants treated for congenital toxoplasmosis. Antimicrob Agents Chemother 1992;36:1040–1048.

148. Araujo FG, Huskinson J, Remington JS: Remarkable in vitro and in vivo activities of the hydroxynaphthoquinone 566C80 against tachyzoites and tissue cysts of *Toxoplasma gondii*. Antimicrob Agents Chemother 1991;35:293–299.

149. Bosch-Driessen EH, Rothova A: Sense and nonsense of corticosteroid administration in the treatment of ocular toxoplasmosis. Br J Ophthalmol 1998;82:858–860.

150. McAuley J, et al: Early and longitudinal evaluations of treated infants and children and untreated historical patients with congenital toxoplasmosis: The Chicago Collaborative Treatment Trial. Clin Infect Dis 1994;18:38–72.

151. Frenkel JK, Nelson BM, Arias-Stella J: Immunosuppression and toxoplasmic encephalitis: Clinical and experimental aspects. Hum Pathol 1975;6:97–111.

152. Nicholson DH, Wolchok EB: Ocular toxoplasmosis in an adult receiving long-term corticosteroid therapy. Arch Ophthalmol 1976;94:248–254.

153. Mitchell CD, et al: Congenital toxoplasmosis occurring in infants perinatally infected with human immunodeficiency virus 1. Pediatr Infect Dis J 1990;9:512–518.

154. Mitchell W: Neurological and developmental effects of HIV and AIDS in children and adolescents. Ment Retard Dev Disabil Res Rev 2001;7:211–216.

155. Beazley DM, Egerman RS: Toxoplasmosis. Semin Perinatol 1998;22:332–338.

156. Desmonts G, Couvreur J, Thulliez P: Congenital toxoplasmosis. 5 cases of mother-to-child transmission of pre-pregnancy infection. Presse Med 1990;19:1445–1449.

157. Vogel NP, et al: Congenital toxoplasmosis transmitted from an immunologically competent mother infected before conception. Clin Infect Dis 1996;23:1055–1060.

158. Garcia AG: Congenital toxoplasmosis in two successive sibs. Arch Dis Child 1968;43:705–710.

159. Beckett RS, Flynn, FJ Jr: Toxoplasmosis report of two new cases, with a classification and with a demonstration of the organisms in the human placenta. N Engl J Med 1953;249: 345–350.

160. Boyer KM, McLeod R: *Toxoplasma gondii* (toxoplasmosis). Etiologic Agents of Infectious Disease 2000;3: 1421–1448.

161. Feldmann HA, Miller LT: Congenital human toxoplasmosis. Ann NY Acad Sci 1956;64:180–184.

162. Boyer K, et al: Toxoplasmosis. In Cherry J, Feigin, RD (eds): Pediatric Infectious Diseases. Philadelphia, WB Saunders, 2002.

163. Sabin AB: Toxoplasmic encephalitis in children. JAMA 1941;116:801–807.

164. Wolf A, Cowen D, Paige BH: Human toxoplasmosis. Occurrence in infants as an encephalomyelitis. Science 1939; 89:226–227.

165. Wolf A, Cowen D, Paige BH: Toxoplasmic encephalomyelitis. Trans Am Neural Assoc 1939;65:76–79.

166. Miller MJ, Seaman E, Remington JS: The clinical spectrum of congenital toxoplasmosis: Problems in recognition. J Pediatr 1967;70:714–723.

167. Pratt-Thomas HR, Cannon WM: Systemic infantile toxoplasmosis. Am J Pathol 1946;22:779–795.

168. Sever JL: Perinatal infections affecting the developing fetus and newborn. In HG Eichenwald (ed): The Prevention of Mental Retardation Through Control of Infectious Diseases. Public Health Service Publication No. 1692, U.S. Government Printing Office, 1968, 37–68.

169. Eichenwald HG: A study of congenital toxoplasmosis, with particular emphasis on clinical manifestations, sequelae and therapy. In Human Toxoplasmosis. Copenhagen, Munksgaard, 1960, pp. 41–49.

170. Desmonts G, Couvreur J: Congenital toxoplasmosis. N Engl J Med 1974;291:365–366.

171. Wilson CB, Remington JS: What can be done to prevent congenital toxoplasmosis? Am J Obstet Gynecol 1980;138: 357–363.

172. Saxon SA, et al: Intellectual deficits in children born with subclinical congenital toxoplasmosis: A preliminary report. J Pediatr 1973;82:792–797.

173. Roizen N, et al: Neurologic and developmental outcome in treated congenital toxoplasmosis. Pediatrics 1995;95: 11–20.

174. Roizen N, et al: Impact of visual impairment of measures of cognitive function for children with congenital toxoplasmosis: Compensatory intervention strategies. American Society of Pediatric Meeting – Abstract, 2002. X: p. Y.

175. Roizen N, et al: Impact of visual impairment of measures of cognitive function for children with congenital toxoplasmosis: Compensatory intervention strategies. In preparation.

176. Desmonts G, Naot Y, Remington JS: Immunoglobulin M-immunosorbent agglutination assay for diagnosis of infectious diseases: diagnosis of acute congenital and acquired toxoplasma infections. J Clin Microbiol 1981;14:486–491.

177. Decoster A, Darcy F, Caron A: IgA antibodies against P30 as markers of congenital and acute toxoplasmosis. Lancet 1988; 2:1104–1107.

178. Hohlfeld P, et al: Prenatal diagnosis of congenital toxoplasmosis with a polymerase-chain-reaction test on amniotic fluid. N Engl J Med 1994;331:695–699.

179. Wallon M, et al: Diagnosis of congenital toxoplasmosis at birth: What is the value of testing for IgM and IgA? Eur J Pediatr 1999;158:645–649.

180. Romand S, et al: Prenatal diagnosis using polymerase chain reaction on amniotic fluid for congenital toxoplasmosis. Obstet Gynecol 2001;97:296–300.

181. Purner MB, et al: CD4-mediated and CD8-mediated cytotoxic and proliferative immune responses to *Toxoplasma gondii* in seropositive humans. Infect Immun 1996;64: 4330–4338.

182. Subauste CS, et al: Preferential activation and expansion of human peripheral blood gamma delta T cells in response to *Toxoplasma gondii* in vitro and their cytokine production and cytotoxic activity against *T. gondii*-infected cells. J Clin Invest 1995;96:610–619.

183. Subauste CS, et al: Alpha beta T cell response to *Toxoplasma gondii* in previously unexposed individuals. J Immunol 1998; 160:3403–3411.

184. McLeod R, Mack D, Boyer K: Phenotypes and functions of lymphocytes in congenital toxoplasmosis. J Lab Clin Med 1990;116:623–635.

185. Couvreur J, Desmonts G, Thulliez P: Prophylaxis of congenital toxoplasmosis. Effects of spiramycin on placental infection. J Antimicrob Chemother 1998;22(Suppl B):B193–B200.

186. Couvreur J, Desmonts G, Aron-Rosa D: Le pronostic oculaire de la toxoplasmosis congenital. Ann Pediatr 1994;31: 855–858.

187. Couvreur J, et al: Fetal toxoplasmosis. In utero treatment with pyrimethamine sulfamides. Arch Fr Pediatr 1991;48: 397–403.

188. Hohlfeld P, Daffos F, Thulliez P: Fetal toxoplasmosis: Outcome of pregnancy and infant follow-up after in utero treatment. J. Pediatr 1989;115(5 Pt 1):765–769.

189. Couvreur J, et al: In utero treatment of toxoplasmic fetopathy with the combination pyrimethamine-sulfadiazine. Fetal Diagn Ther 1993;8:45–50.

190. Kraubig H: Preventive method of treatment of congenital toxoplasmosis. In Kirchhoff H, Kraubig H (eds): Toxoplasmose: Praktische Fragen und Ergebnisse. Stuttgart, Georg Thieme, 1966, pp. 104–122.

191. Kraubig H: Erste praktische erfahrungen mit der prophylaze der konnatalen toxoplasmose. Med Klin 1963;58:1361–1364.

192. Aspock H: Prevention of congenital toxoplasmosis by serological surveillance during pregnancy: Current strategies and future perspectives. In Lang W, Marget W, Gabler-Sandberger E (eds): Parasitic Infections, Immunology, Mycotic Infections, General Topics. Munich, MMVM, 1986.

193. Forestier F, et al: Fetomaternal therapeutic follow-up of spiramycin during pregnancy. Arch Fr Pediatr 1987;44: 539–544.

194. Foulon W, et al: Treatment of toxoplasmosis during pregnancy: A multicenter study of impact on fetal transmission and children's sequelae at age 1 year. Am J Obstet Gynecol 1999;180(2 Pt 1):410–415.

195. Leport C, et al: Failure of spiramycin to prevent neurotoxoplasmosis in immunosuppressed patients. JAMA 1986;255: 2290.

196. Schoondermark-Van de Ven E, Galama J, Camps W, et al: Pharmacokinetis of spiramycin in the rhesus monkey: Transplacental passage and distribution in tissue in the fetus. Antimicrob Agents Chemother 1994;38:1922–1929.

197. Schoondermark-Van de Ven EN, Melchess W, Camps W, et al: Effectiveness of spiramycin for treatment of congenital *Toxoplasma gondii* infection in rhesus monkeys. Antimicrob Agents Chemother 1994;38:1930–1936.

198. Thalhammer O: Prevention of congenital toxoplasmosis (French). Neuropediatrie 1973;4:233–237.

199. Thalhammer O: Congenital toxoplasmosis in Vienna. In Colloque sure la Toxoplasmosede la Femme Enceinte et la Prevention de la Toxoplasmose Congenitale. Lyon, Medical, 1969, pp. 109–129.

200. Wallon M, et al: Congenital toxoplasmosis: Systematic review of evidence of efficacy of treatment in pregnancy. BMJ 1999;318:1511–1514.

201. Peyron F, et al: Treatments for toxoplasmosis in pregnancy. 2000, Cochrane Database of Systematic Reviews (computer file).

202. Alford CA, et al: Subclinical central nervous system disease of neonates: A prospective study of infants born with increased levels of IgM. J Pediatr 1969;75:1167–1178.

203. Allegra CJ, et al: Potent in vitro and in vivo antitoxoplasma activity of the lipid-soluble antifolate trimetrexate. J Clin Invest 1987;79:478–482.

204. Mack D, McLeod R: New micromethod to study the effect of antimicrobial agents on *Toxoplasma gondii*: Comparison of sulfadoxine and sulfadiazine individually and in combination with pyrimethamine and study of clindamycin, metronidazole, and cyclosporin A. Antimicrob Agents Chemother 1984;26:26–30.

205. Estes R, et al: Paclitaxel arrests growth of intracellular *Toxoplasma gondii*. Antimicrob Agents Chemother 1998;42: 2036–2040.

206. Hohlfels E, et al: In vitro effects of artemisinin ether, cycloguanil hydrochloride (alone and in combination with sulfadiazine), quinine sulfate, mefloquine, primaquine phosphate, trifluoperazine hydrochloride, and verapamil on *Toxoplasma gondii*. Antimicrob Agents Chemother 1994;38: 1392–1396.

207. Chang HR, Pechere JC: In-vitro effects of four macrolides (roxithromycin, spiramycin, azithromycin [CP-62, 993], and A-56268) on *Toxoplasma gondii*. Antimicrob Agents Chemother 1988;32:524–529.

208. Derouin F, Santillana-Hayat M: Anti-Toxoplasma activity antiretroviral drugs, interactions with pyrimethamine and sulfadiazine in vitro. Presented at International Congress of Antimicrobial Agents and Chemotherapy, 2000, Toronto.

209. Pfefferkorn ER, Nothnagel RF, Borotz SE: Parasiticidal effect of clindamycin on *Toxoplasma gondii* grown in cultured cells and selection of a drug-resistant mutant. Antimicrob Agents Chemother 1992;36:1091–1096.

210. Grossman PL, Remington J: The effect of trimethoprim and sulfamethoxasol on *Toxoplasma gondii* in vitro and in vivo. Am J Trop Med Hyg 1979;28:445–455.

211. Eyles DE, Coleman M: Synergistic effect of sulfadiazine and Daraprim against experimental toxoplasmosis in the mouse. Antibiot Chemother, 1953;3:483–90.

212. Eyles DE, Coleman M: An evaluation of the curative effects of pyrimethamine and sulfadiazine, alone and in combination, on experimental mouse toxoplasmosis. Antibiot Chemother 1955;3:483–490.

213. Eyles DE, Coleman M: The relative activity of the common sulfonamides against experimental toxoplasmosis in the mouse. Am J Trop Med Hyg 1959;2:54–63.

214. Garin JP, et al: Effect of pyrimethamine sulfadoxine (Fansidar) on an avirulent cystogenic strain of *Toxoplasma gondii* (Prugniaud strain) in white mice. Bull Soc Pathol Exot Filiales 1985;78(5 pt 2):821–824.

215. Garin JP, Paillard B: Experimental toxoplasmosis in mice. Comparative activity of clindamycin, midecamycin, josamycin, spiramycin, pyrimethamine-sulfadoxine, and trimethoprim-sulfamethoxazole. Ann Pediatr 1984;31: 841–845.

216. Harper JS, III, London WT, Sever JL: Five drug regimens for treatment of acute toxoplasmosis in squirrel monkeys. Am J Trop Med Hyg 1985;34:50–57.

217. Mathur LK, et al: In vivo-in vitro correlations for trisulfapyrimidine suspensions. J Pharm Sci 1983;72:1071–1072.

218. Araujo FG, Guptill DR, Remington JS: Azithromycin, a macrolide antibiotic with potent activity against *Toxoplasma gondii*. Antimicrob Agents Chemother 1988;32:755–757.

219. Araujo FG, Slifer T, Remington JS: Rifabutin is active in murine models of toxoplasmosis. Antimicrob Agents Chemother 1994;38:570–575.

220. Araujo FG, Khan AA, Remington JS: Rifapentine is active in vitro and in vivo against *Toxoplasma gondii*. Antimicrob Agents Chemother 1996;40:1335–1337.

221. Araujo FG, Hunter CA, Remington JS: Treatment with interleukin 12 in combination with atovaquone or clindamycin significantly increases survival of mice with acute toxoplasmosis. Antimicrob Agents Chemother 1997;41: 188–190.

222. Araujo FG, et al: Use of ketolides in combination with other drugs to treat experimental toxoplasmosis. Antimicrob Chemother 1998;42:665–667.

223. Frenkel JK, Weber RW, Lunde MN: Acute toxoplasmosis. Effective treatment with pyrimethamine, sulfadiazine, leucovorin calcium and yeast. JAMA 1960;173:1471–1476.

224. Derouin F, et al: Anti-Toxoplasma effects of dapsone alone and combined with pyrimethamine. Antimicrob Agents Chemother 1991;35:252–255.

225. Brun-Pascaud M, et al: Experimental evaluation of combined prophylaxis against murine pneumocystosis and toxoplasmosis. J Infect Dis 1994;107:653–658.

226. Dannemann B, et al: Treatment of toxoplasmic encephalitis in patients with AIDS. A randomized trial comparing pyrimethamine plus clindamycin to pyrimethamine plus sulfadiazine. The California Collaborative Treatment Group. Ann Intern Med 1992;116:33–43.

227. McCabe R, Chirurgi V: Issues in toxoplasmosis. Infect Dis Clin North Am 1993;7:587–604.

228. McCabe R, Oster S: Current recommendations and future prospects in the treatment of toxoplasmosis. Drugs 1989;38: 973–987.

229. McCabe R, Remington JS: Toxoplasmosis: The time has come. N Engl J Med 1988;318:313–315.

230. Leport C, et al: Pyrimethamine for primary prophylaxis of toxoplasmic encephalitis in patients with human immunodeficiency virus infection: A double-blind, randomized trial. ANRS 005-ACTG 154 Group Members. Agence Nationale de Recherche sur le SIDA. AIDS Clinical Trial Group. J Infect Dis 1996;173:91–97.

231. McGee T, et al: Absence of sensorineural hearing abnormalities in treated infants with congenital toxoplasmosis. Otolaryngol Head Neck Surg 1992;106:75–80.

232. Chakraborty P, et al: Toxoplasmosis in women of child bearing age and infant follow up after in-utero treatment. Indian J Pediatr 1997;64:879–882.

233. Mirlessi V, Daffos F: Long-term follow-up of fetuses and newborns with congenital toxoplasmosis diagnosed and treated prenatally. In preparation.

234. Brezin AP, et al: Ophthalmic outcome after pre and postnatal treatment of congenital toxoplasmosis. In preparation.

235. Daffos F, et al: Prenatal management of 746 pregnancies at risk for congenital toxoplasmosis. N Engl J Med 1988;318: 271–275.

236. Patel DV, et al: Resolution of intracranial calcifications in infants with treated congenital toxoplasmosis. Radiology 1996;199:433–440.

237. Luft BJ, Remington JS: Toxoplasmic encephalitis in AIDS. Clin Infect Dis 1992;15:211–222.

238. Raffi F, et al: A prospective study of criteria for the diagnosis of toxoplasmic encephalitis in 186 AIDS patients. The BIOTOXO Study Group. AIDS 1997;11: 177–184.

239. Lanska DJ: Epidemiology of human immunodeficiency virus infection and associated neurologic illness. Semin Neurol 1999;19:105–111.

240. Ives NJ, Gazzard BG, Easterbrook PJ: The changing pattern of AIDS-defining illnesses with the introduction of highly active antiretroviral therapy (HAART) in a London clinic. J Infect 2001;42:134–139.

241. Kirkman LA, Weiss LM, Kim K: Cyclic nucleotide signaling in *Toxoplasma gondii* bradyzoite differentiation. Infect Immun 2001;69:148–153.

242. Weiss L, Kim K: The development and biology of bradyzoites of *Toxoplasma gondii*. Front Biosci 2000;5: D391–405.

243. Rodriguez-Rosado R, et al: Opportunistic infections shortly after beginning highly active antiretroviral therapy. Antivir Ther 1998;3:229–231.

244. Cohen BA: Neurologic manifestations of toxoplasmosis in AIDS. Semin Neurol 1999;19:201–211.

245. Levy RM, Rosenbloom S, Perrett LV: Neuroradiologic findings in AIDS: A review of 200 cases. AJR Am J Roentgenol 1986;147:977–983.

246. Polis MA: Differential diagnosis of retinal lesions in persons with HIV infection. Opportun Infect Interact 1994;3:1–3.

247. Rodgers CA, Harris JR: Ocular toxoplasmosis in HIV infection. Int Journal STD AIDS 1996;7:307–309.

248. Jabs DA: Ocular manifestations of HIV infection. Trans Am Ophthalmol Soc 1995;93:623–683.

249. Resnick DK, et al: Isolated toxoplasmosis of the thoracic spinal cord in a patient with acquired immunodeficiency syndrome. Case report. J Neurosurg 1995;82:493–496.

250. Lortholary O, et al: Myelitis due to *Toxoplasma gondii* in a patient with AIDS. Clin Infect Dis 1994;19:1167–1168.

251. Rabaud C, et al: Pulmonary Toxoplasmosis in patients infected with human immunodefiency virus: A French national survey. Clin Infect Dis 1996;23:1249–1254.

252. Derouin F, et al: Prevalence of pulmonary toxoplasmosis in HIV-infected patients. AIDS 1990;4:1036.

253. Pomeroy C, Filice GA: Pulmonary toxoplasmosis: A review. Clin Infect Dis 1992;14:863–870.

254. Campagna AC: Pulmonary toxoplasmosis. Semin Respir Infect 1997;12:98–105.

255. Zylberberg H, et al: Prolonged isolated fever due to attenuated extracerebral toxoplasmosis in patients infected with human immunodeficiency virus who are receiving trimethoprim-sulfamethoxazole as prophylaxis. Clin Infect Dis 1995;21:680–681.

256. Kofman E, et al: Gastric toxoplasmosis: Case report and review of the literature. Am J Gastroenterol 1996;91:2436–2438.

257. Bonacini M, Kanel G, Alamy M: Duodenal and hepatic toxoplasmosis in a patient with HIV infection: Review of the literature. Am J Gastroenterol 1996;91:1838–1840.

258. McCabe R, Remington JS: Toxoplasmosis. In Dolin RG, Mandell BJ (eds): Principles and Practice of Infectious Diseases. New York, Churchill Livingstone, 1995.

259. Katlama C: The impact of the prevention of cerebral toxoplasmosis. J Neuroradiol 1995;22:193–195.

260. Cohn JA, et al: Evaluation of the policy of empiric treatment of suspected Toxoplasma encephalitis in patients with the acquired immunodeficiency syndrome. Am J Med 1989;86:521–527.

261. Foudrinier F, et al: Detection of *Toxoplasma gondii* in immunodeficient subjects by gene amplification: influence of therapeutics. Scand J Infect Dis 1996;28:383–386.

262. Gianotti N, et al: Diagnosis of toxoplasmic encephalitis in HIV-infected patients. AIDS 1997;11:1529–1530.

263. Luft BJ, et al: Toxoplasmic encephalitis in patients with acquired immunodeficiency syndrome. Members of the ACTG 077p/ANRS 009 Study Team. N Engl J Med 1993;329:995–1000.

264. Ammassari A, et al: Changing disease patterns in focal brain lesion-causing disorders in AIDS. J Acquir Immune Defic Syndr Hum Retrovirol 1998;18:365–371.

265. Davies J, et al: HIV-associated brain pathology: A comparative international study. Neuropathol Appl Neurobiol 1998;24:118–124.

266. Antinori A, et al: Diagnosis of AIDS-related focal brain lesions: a decision-making analysis based on clinical and neurological characteristics combined with polymerase chain reaction assays in CSF. Neurology 1997;48:687–694.

267. Fung HB, Kirschenbaum HL: Treatment regimens for patients with toxoplasmic encephalitis. Clin Ther 1996;18:1037–1056.

268. Caumes E, et al: Adverse cutaneous reactions to pyrimethamine/sulfadiazine and pyrimethamine/clindamycin in patients with AIDS and toxoplasmic encephalitis. Clin Infect Dis 1995;21:656–658.

269. Ioannidis JP, et al: A Meta-analysis of the relative efficacy and toxicity of *pneumocystis carinii* prophylactic regimens. Arch Intern Med 1996;156:177–188.

270. Katlama C, et al: Pyrimethamine-clindamycin vs. Pyrimethamine-sulfadiazine as acute and long-term therapy for toxoplasmic encephalitis in patients with AIDS. Clin Infect Dis 1996;22:268–275.

271. Torres RA, et al: Atovaquone for salvage treatment and suppression of toxoplasmic encephalitis in patients with AIDS. Clin Infect Dis 1997;24:422–429.

272. Katlama C, et al: Atovaquone as long-term suppressive therapy for toxoplasmic encephalitis in patients with AIDS and multiple drug intolerance. Atovaquone Expanded Access Group. AIDS 1996;10:1107–1112.

273. Antinori A, et al: Aerosolized pentamidine, cotrimoxazole and dapsone-pyrimethamine for primary prophylaxis of *Pneumocystis carinii* pneumonia and toxoplasmic encephalitis. AIDS 1995;9:1343–1350.

274. Opravil M, et al: Once-weekly administration of dapsone/pyrimethamine vs. aerosolized pentamidine as combined prophylaxis for *Pneumocystis carinii* pneumonia and toxoplasmic encephalitis in human immunodeficiency virus-infected patients. Clin Infect Dis 1995;20:531–541.

275. Fernandez-Martin J, et al: Pyrimethamine-clarithromycin combination for therapy of acute Toxoplasma encephalitis in patients with AIDS. Antimicrob Agents Chemother 1991;35:2049–2052.

276. Saba J, et al: Pyrimethamine plus azithromycin for treatment of acute toxplasmic encephalitis in patients with AIDS. Eur J Clin Microbiol Infect Dis 1993;12:853–856.

277. Nasta P, Chiodera S: Azithromycin for relapsing cerebral toxoplasmosis in AIDS. AIDS 1997;11:1188.

278. Wynn R, Leen CL, Brettle RP: Azithromycin for cerebral toxoplasmosis in AIDS. Lancet 1993;341:243–244.

279. Wiselka MJ, Read R, Finch RG: Response to oral and intravenous azithromycin in a patient with Toxoplasma encephalitis and AIDS. J Infect 1996;33:227–229.

280. Torre D, et al: A retrospective study of treatment of cerebral toxoplasmosis in AIDS patients with trimethoprim-sulphamethoxazole. J Infect 1998;37:15–18.

281. Podzamczer D, et al: Twice-weekly maintenance therapy with sulfadiazine-pyrimethamine to prevent recurrent toxoplasmic encephalitis in patients with AIDS. Spanish Toxoplasmosis Study Group. Ann Intern Med 1995;123:175–180.

282. Podzamczer D, et al: Thrice-weekly sulfadiazine-pyrimethamine for maintenance therapy of toxoplasmic encephalitis in HIV-infected patients. Spanish Toxoplasmosis Study Group. Eur J Clin Microbiol Infect Dis 2000;19:89–95.

283. Chirgwin K, et al: Randomized phase II trial of atovaquone with pyrimethamine or sulfadiazine for treatment of toxoplasmic encephalitis in patients with acquired immunodeficiency syndrome: ACTG 237/ANRS 039 Study. AIDS Clinical Trials Group 237/Agence Nationale de Recherche sur le SIDA, Essai 039. Clin Infect Dis 2002;34:1243–1250.

284. Mussini C, et al: Discontinuation of primary prophylaxis for *Pneumocystis carinii* pneumonia and toxoplasmic encephalitis in human immunodeficiency virus type I-infected patients: the changes in opportunistic prophylaxis study. J Infect Dis 2000;181:1635–1642.

285. Podzamczer D, et al: Intermittent trimethoprim-sulfamethoxazole compared with dapsone-pyrimethamine for the simultaneous primary prophylaxis of pneumocystis pneumonia and toxoplasmosis in patients infected with HIV. Ann Intern Med 1995;122:755–761.

286. Jacobson MA, et al: Primary prophylaxis with pyrimethamine for toxoplasmic encephalitis in patients with advanced human immunodefiency virus disease: Results of a randomized trial. Terry Beirn Community Programs for Clinical Research on AIDS. J Infect Dis 1994;169:384–394.

287. Brossard G, et al: Prophylaxie primaire de la toxoplasmose cerebrale efficacite de l'acide folinique dans la prevention de la toxicite hematologique de la pyrimethamine. Presse Med 1994;23:613–615.

288. Torres RA, et al: Randomized trial of dapsone and aerosolized pentamidine for the prophylaxis of *Pneumocystis carinii* pneumonia and toxoplasmic encephalitis. Am J Med 1993;95:573–583.

289. Girard PM, et al: Dapsone-pyrimethamine compared with aerosolized pentamidine as primary prophylaxis against *Pneumocystis carinii* pneumonia and toxoplasmosis in HIV infection. The PRIO Study Group. N Engl J Med 1993;328: 1514–1520.

290. Durant J, et al: Prevention of *Pneumocystis carinii* pneumonia and of cerebral toxoplasmosis by roxithromycin in HIV-infected patients. Infection 1995;23(Suppl 1):S33–S38.

291. Payen MC, et al: A controlled trial of dapsone versus pyrimethamine-sulfadoxine for primary prophylaxis of *Pneumocystis carinii* pneumonia and toxoplasmosis in patients with AIDS. Biomed Pharmacother 1997;51: 439–445.

292. Bucher HC, et al: Meta-analysis of prophylactic treatments against *pneumocystis carinii* pneumonia and toxoplasma encephalitis in HIV-infected patients. J Acquir Immune Defic Syndr Hum Retrovirol 1997;15:104–114.

293. Chene G, et al: Intention-to-treat vs. on-treatment analysis of clinical trial data: Experience from a study of pyrimethamine in the primary prophylaxis of toxoplasmosis in HIV-infected patients. ANRS 005/ACTG 154 trial group. Control Clin Trials 1998;19:233–248.

294. Richards FO Jr, Kovacs JA, Luft BJ: Preventing toxoplasmic encephalitis in persons infected with human immunodeficiency virus. Clin Infect Dis 1995;21(Suppl 1): S49–S56.

295. Sande MA, et al: Evaluation of new anti-infective drugs for the treatment of toxoplasma encephalitis. Infectious Diseases Society of America and the Food and Drug Administration. Clin Infect Dis 1992;15(Suppl 1):S200–S205.

296. Ruf B, et al: Efficacy of pyrimethamine/sulfadoxine in the prevention of toxoplasmic encephalitis relapses and *Pneumocystis carinii* pneumonia in HIV-infected patients. Eur J Clin Microbiol Infect Dis, 1993;12:325–329.

297. Teira R, et al: Pyrimethamine and sulfadoxine as a preventive treatment for *Pneumocystis carinii* and Toxoplasma encephalitis. Enferm Infecc Microbiol Clin 1999;17: 347–349.

298. Bossi P, et al: Epidemiologic characteristics of cerebral toxoplasmosis in 399 HIV-infected patients followed between 1983 and 1994. Rev Med Interne 1998;19:313–317.

299. Guex AC, Radziwill AJ, Bucher HC: Discontinuation of secondary prophylaxis for toxoplasmic encephalitis in human immunodeficiency virus infection after immune restoration with highly active antiretroviral therapy. Clin Infect Dis 2000;30:602–603.

300. Smadja D, et al: Efficacite et bonne tolerance du cotrimoxazole comme traitement de la toxoplasmose cerebrale au cours de SIDA. Presse Med 1998;27:1315–1320.

301. Jones JL, et al: Toxoplasmic encephalitis in HIV-infected persons: Risk factors and trends: The Adult/Adolescent Spectrum of Disease Group. AIDS 1996;10.

302. Mariuz P, Bosler EM, Luft BJ: Toxoplasmosis in individuals with AIDS. Infect Dis Clin North Am 1994;8:365–381.

303. Rabaud C, et al: Extracerebral toxoplasmosis in patients infected with HIV. A French National Survey. Medicine 1994;73:306–314.

304. Weigel HM, et al: Cotrimoxazole is effective as primary prophylaxis for toxoplasmic encephalitis in HIV-infected patients: A case control study. Scand J Infect Dis 1997;29:499–502.

305. Torre D, et al: Randomized trial of trimethoprim-sulfamethoxazole versus pyrimethamine-sulfadiazine for therapy of toxoplasmic encephalitis in patients with AIDS. Italian Collaborative Study Group. Antimicrob Agents Chemother 1998;42:1346–1349.

306. Ribera E, et al: Comparison of high and low doses of trimethoprim-sulfamethoxazole for primary prevention of toxoplasmic encephalitis in human immunodeficiency virus-infected patients. Clin Infect Dis 1999;29:1461–1466.

307. Zeller V, et al: Discontinuation of secondary prophylaxis against disseminated *Mycobacterium avium* complex infection and toxoplasmic encephalitis. Clin Infect Dis 2002;34: 662–667.

308. Miro J, Lopez JC, Podzamczer D: Discontinuation of toxoplasmic encephalitis prophylaxis is safe in HIV-1 and *T. gondii* co-infected patients after immunologic recovery with HAART. In 7th Conference on Retroviruses and Opportunistic Infections. San Francisco, Foundation for Retrovirology and Human Health, 2000.

309. Wreghitt TG, et al: Toxoplasmosis in heart and heart and lung transplant recipients. J Clin Pathol 1989;42:194–199.

310. Soave R: Prophylaxis strategies for solid-organ transplantation. Clin Infect Dis 2001;33(Suppl 1):S26–S31.

311. Orr KE, et al: Outcome of *Toxoplasma gondii* mismatches in heart transplant recipients over a period of 8 years. J Infect 1994;29:249–253.

312. Michaels MG, et al: Toxoplasmosis in pediatric recipients of heart transplants. Clin Infect Dis 1992;14:847–851.

313. Holliman RE, et al: Toxoplasmosis and heart transplantation. J Heart Lung Transplant 1991;10:608–610.

314. Mayes JT, et al: Transmission of *Toxoplasma gondii* infection by liver transplantation. Clin Infect Dis 1995;21: 511–515.

315. Small TN, et al: Disseminated toxoplasmosis following T cell-depleted related and unrelated bone marrow transplantation. Bone Marrow Transplant 2000;25:969–973.

316. Renoult E, et al: Evolution and significance of *Toxoplasma gondii* antibody titers in kidney transplant recipients. Transplant Proc 1992;24:2754–2755.

317. Seong DC, et al: Leptomeningeal toxoplasmosis after allogeneic marrow transplantation. Case report and review of the literature. Am J Clin Oncol 1993;16:105–108.

318. Singer MA, Hagler WS, Grossniklaus HE: *Toxoplasma gondii* retinochoroiditis after liver transplantation. Retina 1993;13:40–45.

319. Yadlapati S, et al: Ocular toxoplasmosis after autologous peripheral-blood stem-cell transplantation. Clin Infect Dis 1997;25:1255–1256.

320. Brinkman K, et al: Toxoplasma retinitis/encephalitis 9 months after allogeneic bone marrow transplantation. Bone Marrow Transplant 1998;21:635–636.

321. Gallino A, et al: Toxoplasmosis in heart transplant recipients. Eur J Clin Microbiol Infect Dis 1996;15:389–393.

322. Peacock JE, Jr, et al: Reactivation toxoplasmic retinochoroiditis in patients undergoing bone marrow transplantation: Is there a role for chemoprophylaxis? Bone Marrow Transplant 1995;15:983–987.

323. Slavin MA, et al: *Toxoplasma gondii* infection in marrow transplant recipients: A 20-year experience. Bone Marrow Transplant 1994;13:549–557.

324. Martino R, et al: Toxoplasmosis after hematopoietic stem cell transplantation. Clin Infect Dis 2000;31:1188–1195.

325. Bretagne S, et al: Late toxoplasmosis evidenced by PCR in a marrow transplant recipient. Bone Marrow Transplant 1995; 15:809–811.

326. Maschke M, et al: Opportunistic CNS infection after bone marrow transplantation. Bone Marrow Transplant 1999;23: 1167–1176.

327. Chandrasekar PH, Momin F: Disseminated toxoplasmosis in marrow recipients: A report of three cases and a review of the literature. Bone Marrow Transplant Team. Bone Marrow Transplant 1997;19:685–689.

328. Zver S, et al: Case report: Cerebral toxoplasmosis—a late complication of allogeneic haematopoietic stem cell transplantation. Bone Marrow Transplant 1999;24:1363–1365.

329. Luft BJ, et al: Primary and reactivated toxoplasma infection in patients with cardiac transplants. Clinical spectrum and problems in diagnosis in a defined population. Ann Intern Med 1983;99:27–31.

330. Held TK, et al: Diagnosis of toxoplasmosis in bone marrow transplant recipients: Comparison of PCR-based results and immunohistochemistry. Bone Marrow Transplant 2000;25: 1257–1262.

331. Khoury H, et al: Successful treatment of cerebral toxoplasmosis in a marrow transplant recipient: Contribution of a PCR test in diagnosis and early detection. Bone Marrow Transplant 1999;23:409–411.

332. Sing A, et al: Pulmonary toxoplasmosis in bone marrow transplant recipients: Report of two cases and review. Clin Infect Dis 1999;29:429–433.

333. Dawis, MA, et al: Unsuspected *Toxoplasma gondii* empyema in a bone marrow transplant recipient. Clin Infect Dis 2002;34:37–39.

334. Candolfi E, Derouin F, Kien T: Detection of circulating antigens in immunocompromised patients during reactivation of chronic toxoplasmosis. Eur J Clin Microbiol 1987;6:44–48.

335. Couvreur J, et al: Transplantation cardiaque ou cardiopulmonaire et toxoplasmose. Presse Med 1992;21: 1569–1574.

336. McGregor CGA, et al: Disseminated toxoplasmosis in cardiac transplantation. J Clin Pathol 1984;37:74–77.

337. Spes CH, et al: Sulfadiazine therapy for toxoplasmosis in heart transplant recipients decreases cyclopsporine concentration. Clin Invest 1992;70:752–754.

338. Conley FK, Jenkins KA, Remington JS: *Toxoplasma gondii* infection of the central nervous system. Use of the peroxidase-antiperoxidase method to demonstrate toxoplasma in formalin fixed, paraffin embedded tissue sections. Hum Pathol 1981;12:690–698.

339. Renoult E, et al: Transmission of toxoplasmosis by renal transplant: A report of four cases. Transplant Proc 1996;28: 181–183.

340. Renoult E, et al: Toxoplasmosis in kidney transplant recipients: A life-threatening but treatable disease. Transplant Proc 1997;29:821–822.

341. Renoult E, et al: Toxoplasmosis in kidney transplant recipients: Report of six cases and review. Clin Infect Dis 1997;24: 625–634.

342. Feron D, et al: Bone marrow aspiration as a diagnostic tool for acute toxoplasmosis in a kidney transplant recipient. Transplantation 1990;50:1054–1055.

343. Kusne S, et al: Infections after liver transplantation. An analysis of 101 consecutive cases. Medicine 1988;67:132–143.

344. Chiquet C, et al: Acquired ocular toxoplasmosis (panuveitis) after liver transplantation. J Fr Ophtalmol 2000;23: 375–379.

345. Singh N, Gayowski T, Marino IR: *Toxoplasma gondii* pneumonitis in a liver transplant recipient: Implications for diagnosis. Liver Transpl Surg 1996;2:299–300.

346. Munir A, Zaman M, Eltorky M: *Toxoplasma gondii* pneumonia in a pancreas transplant patient. South Med J 2000;93: 614–617.

347. Carbone LG, Bendixen B, Appel GB: Sulfadiazine-associated obstructive nephropathy occurring in a patient with the acquired immunodeficiency syndrome. Am J Kidney Dis 1988;12:72–75.

348. Simon DI, Brosius FC, Rothstein DM: Sulfadiazine crystalluria revisited. The treatment of toxoplasma encephalitis in patients with acquired immunodeficiency syndrome. Arch Intern Med 1990;150:2379–2384.

349. Molina JM, et al: Sulfadiazine-induced crystalluria in AIDS patients with toxoplasma encephalitis. AIDS 1991;5: 587–589.

350. Foot AB, et al: Prophylaxis of toxoplasmosis infection with pyrimethamine/sulfadoxine (Fansidar) in bone marrow transplant recipients. Bone Marrow Transplant 1994;14:241–245.

351. Israelski DM, Remington JS: Toxoplasmosis in patients with cancer. Clin Infect Dis 1993;17(Suppl 2):S423–S435.

352. Israelski DM, Remington JS: Toxoplasmosis in the non-AIDS immunocompromised host. Curr Clin Topics Infect Dis 1993;13:322–356.

353. Carey RM, et al: Toxoplasmosis. Clinical experiences in a cancer hospital. Am J Med 1973;54:30–38.

354. Hakes TB, Armstrong D: Toxoplasmosis. Problems in diagnosis and treatment. Cancer 1983;52:1535–1540.

355. Hyde B, Barnett EV, Remington JS: Method for differentiation of nonspecific from specfic toxoplasma IgM fluorescent antibodies in patients with rheumatoid factor. Proc Soc Exp Biol Med 1975;148:1184–1188.

356. Stepick-Biek P, et al: IgA antibodies for diagnosis of acute congenital and acquired toxoplasmosis. J Infect Dis 1990;162:270–273.

357. Subauste CS, Wessendarp M: Human dendritic cells discriminate between viable and killed *Toxoplasma gondii* tachyzoites: Dendritic cell activation after infection with viable parasites results in CD28 and CD40 ligand signaling that controls IL-12-dependent and -independent T cell production of IFN-gamma. J Immunol 2000;165: 1498–1505.

358. Frenkel JK: Effects of cortisone, total body irradiation, and nitrogen mustard on chronic latent toxoplasmosis. Am J Pathol 1957;33:618–619.

359. Gallant JE, Chaisson RE, Moore RD: The effect of adjunctive corticosteroids for the treatment of *Pneumocystis carinii* pneumonia on mortality and subsequent complications. Chest 1998;114:1258–1263.

360. Tenant-Flowers, M, et al: Sulphadiazine desensitization in patients with AIDS and cerebral toxoplasmosis. AIDS 1991;5:311–315.

361. Huskinson-Mark J, Araujo FG, Remington JS: Evaluation of the effect of drugs on the cyst form of *Toxoplasma gondii*. J Infect Dis 1991;164:170–171.

362. Hardman JG, Limbird LL, Gilman AG: Pharmacological Basis of Therapeutics. 10th ed. New York, McGraw Hill, 2001, pp. 2147.

363. Goldberg DE: Parasitology: When the host is smarter than the parasite. Science 2002;296:482–483.

364. Zhang K, Rathod PK: Divergent regulation of dihydrofolate reductase between malaria parasite and human host. Science 2002;296:545–547.

365. Weiss LM, et al: Pyrimethamine concentrations in serum and cerebrospinal fluid during treatment of acute Toxoplasma encephalitis in patients with AIDS. J Infect Dis 1988;157: 580–583.

366. Jacobson JM, et al: Pyrimethamine pharmacokinetics in human immunodeficiency virus-positive patients seropositive for *Toxoplasma gondii*. Antimicrob Agents Chemother 1996;40:1360–1365.

367. Winstanley P, et al: Marked variation in pyrimethamine disposition in AIDS patients treated for cerebral toxoplasmosis. J Antimicrob Chemother 1995;36:435–439.

368. Gatti G, et al: Penetration of clindamycin and its metabolite N-demethyclindamycin into cerebrospinal fluid following

intravenous infusion of clindamycin phosphate in patients with AIDS. Antimicrob Agents Chemother 1998;42:3014–3017.

369. Klinker H, Langmann P, Richter E: Plasma pyrimethamine concentrations during long-term treatment for cerebral toxoplasmosis in patients with AIDS. Antimicrob Agents Chemother 1996;40:1623–1627.

370. Kaufman HE, Caldwell LA: Pharmacological studies of pyrimethamine (Daraprim) in man. Arch Ophthalmol 1959;61:885–890.

371. Roberts CW, et al: The Shikimate pathway and its branches in apicomplexan parasites. J Infect Dis 2002;185(Suppl 1):S25–S36.

372. Fichter EG, Curtis JA: Sulfonamide administration in newborn and premature infants. Pediatrics 1956;18:50–58.

373. Colebunders R, et al: Obstructive nephropathy due to sulfa crystals in two HIV seropositive patients treated with sulfadiazine. JBR-BTR 1999;82:153–154.

374. Villena I, et al: Pyrimethamine-sulfadoxine treatment of congenital toxoplasmosis: Follow-up of 78 cases between 1980 and 1997. Reims Toxoplasmosis Group. Scand J Infect Dis 1998;30:295–300.

375. Dorangeon PH, et al: The risks of pyrimethamine-sulfadoxine combination in the prenatal treatment of toxoplasmosis. J Gynecol Obstet Biol Reprod 1992;21:549–556.

376. Gatti G, et al: Penetration of dapsone into cerebrospinal fluid of patients with AIDS. J Antimicrob Chemother 1997;40:113–115.

377. DeGowin RL: A review of therapeutic and hemolytic effects of dapsone. Arch Intern Med 1967;120:242–248.

378. Pfefferkorn ER, Borotz SE: Comparison of mutants of *Toxoplasma gondii* selected for resistance to azithromycin, spiramycin, or clindamycin. Antimicrob Agents Chemother 1994;38:31–37.

379. Fichera ME, Bhopale MK, Roos DS: In vitro assays elucidate peculiar kinetics of clindamycin action against *Toxoplasma gondii*. Antimicrob Agents Chemother 1995;39:1530–1537.

380. Derouin F, et al: Determination of the inhibitory effect on toxoplasma growth in the serum of AIDS patients during acute therapy for toxoplasmic encephalitis. J Acquir Immune Defic Syndr Hum Retrovirol 1998;19:50–54.

381. Beckers CJ, et al: Inhibition of cytoplasmic and organellar protein synthesis in *Toxoplasma gondii*. Implications for the target of macrolide antibiotics. J Clin Invest 1995;95:367–376.

382. Kohler S, et al: A plastid of probably green algal origin in Apicomplexan parasites. Science 1997;275:1485–1489.

383. Fichera ME, Roos DS: A plastid organelle as a drug target in apicomplexan parasites. Nature 1997;390:407–409.

384. Zuther E, et al: Growth of *Toxoplasma gondii* is inhibited by aryloxphenoxypropionate herbicides targeting acetyl-CoA carboxylase. Proc Natl Acad Sci USA 1999;96:13387–13392.

385. McLeod R, et al: Triclosan inhibits the growth of *Plasmodium falciparum* and *Toxoplasma gondii* by inhibition of Apicomplexan Fab I. Int J Parasitol 2001;31:109–113.

386. Chang HR: The potential role of azithromycin in the treatment of prophylaxis of toxoplasmosis. Int J STD AIDS 1996:7(Suppl 1):S18–S22.

387. Araujo FG, Shepard RM, and Remington JS: In vivo activity of the macrolide antibiotics azithromycin, roxithromycin and spiramycin against *Toxoplasma gondii*. Eur J Clin Microbiol Infect Dis 1991;10:519–524.

388. Romand, S, et al: In-vitro and in-vivo activities of roxithromycin in combination with pyrimethamine or sulphadiazine against *Toxoplasma gondii*. J Antimicrob Chemother 1995;35:821–832.

389. Vergani P, et al: Congenital toxoplasmosis: Efficacy of maternal treatment with spiramycin alone. Am J Reprod Immunol 1998;39:335–340.

390. Stramba-Badiale M, et al: QT interval prolongation and cardiac arrest during antibiotic therapy with spiramycin in a newborn infant. Am Heart J 1993;126(3 Pt 1):740–742.

391. Stramba-Badiale M, et al: QT interval prolongation and risk of life-threatening arrhythmias during toxoplasmosis prophylaxis with spiramycin in neonates. Am Heart J 1997;133:108–111.

392. McFadden DC, et al: Characterization of cytochrome b from *Toxoplasma gondii* and Q(o) domain mutations as a mechanism of atovaquone-resistance. Molecul Biochem Parasitol 2000;108:1–12.

393. Spencer CM, Goa KL: Atovaquone: A review of its pharmacological properties and therapeutic efficacy in opportunistic infections. Drugs 1995;50:176–196.

394. Araujo FG, et al: In vitro and in vivo activities of the hydroxynaphthoquinone 566C80 against the cyst form of *Toxoplasma gondii*. Antimicrob Agents Chemother 1992;36:326–330.

395. Kovacs J: Efficacy of atovaquone in treatment of toxoplasmosis in patients with AIDS. The NIAID-Clinical Center Intramural AIDS Program. Lancet 1992;340:637–638.

396. Rolan PE, et al: Examination of some factors responsible for a food-induced increase in absorption of atovaquone. Br J Clin Pharmacol 1994;37:13–20.

397. Dixon R, et al: Single-dose and steady-state pharmacokinetics of a novel microfluidized suspension of atovaquone in human immunodeficiency virus-seropositive patients. Antimicrob Agents Chemother 1996;40:556–560.

398. Rolan PE, et al: Disposition of atovaquone in humans. Antimicrob Agents Chemother 1997;41:1319–1321.

399. Hughes WT, et al: Safety and pharmacokinetics of 566C80, a hydroxynaphthoquinone with anti-*Pneumocystis carinii* activity: A phase I study in human immunodeficiency virus (HIV)-infected men. J Infect Dis 1991;163:843–848.

400. Araujo FG, Lin T, Remington JS: The activity of atovaquone (566C80) in murine toxoplasmosis is markedly augmented when used in combination with pyrimethamine or sulfadiazine. J Infect Dis 1993;167:494–497.

401. Gozalbes R, Brun-Pascaud M, Garcia-Domenech R: Anti-Toxoplasma activities of 24 quinolones and fluoroquinolones in vitro. Prediction of activity by molecular topolgy and virtual computational techniques. Presented at International Congress of Antimicrobial Agents and Chemotherapy. Toronto, Canada, 2000.

402. Khan AA, et al: Activity of trovafloxacin in combination with other drugs for treatment of acute murine toxoplasmosis. Antimicrob Agents Chemother 1997;41:893–897.

403. Khan AA, et al: Anti-*Toxoplasma gondii* activities and structure-activity relationships of novel fluoroquinolones related to trovafloxacin. Antimicrob Agents Chemother 1999;43:1783–1787.

404. Brun-Pascaud M, et al: Combination of PS-15, epiroprim, or pyrimethamine with dapsone in prophylaxis of *Toxoplasma gondii* and *Pneumocystis carinii* dual infection in a rat model. Antimicrob Agents Chemother 1996;40:2067–2070.

405. Martinez A, Allegra CJ, Kovacs JA: Efficacy of epiroprim (roll-9858), a new dihydrofolate reductase inhibitor, in the treatment of acute toxoplasma infection in mice. Am J Trop Med Hyg 1996;54:249–252.

406. Chang HR, et al: Activity of Epiroprim (RO 11-8958), a dihydrofolate reductase inhibitor, alone and in combination with dapsone against *Toxoplasma gondii*. Antimicrob Agents Chemother 1994;38:1803–1807.

407. Romand S, et al: In vitro and in vivo effects of rifabutin alone or combined with atovaquone against *Toxoplasma gondii*. Antimicrob Agents Chemother 1996;40:2015–2020.

408. Khan AA, et al: Quinupristin-dalfopristin is active against *Toxoplasma gondii*. Antimicrob Agents Chemother 1999;43:2043–2045.

409. Derouin F, et al: Cotrimoxazole for prenatal treatment of congenital toxoplasmosis. Parasitol Today 2000;16:254–256.

410. Roberts F, et al: Evidence for the shikimate pathway in apicomplexan parasites. Nature 1998;393:801–805.

411. Stokkermans TJ, et al: Inhibition of *Toxoplasma gondii* replication by dinitroaniline herbicides. Exp Parasitol 1996;84:355–370.

412. Jomaa H, et al: Inhibitors of the nonmevalonate pathway of isoprenoid biosynthesis as antimalarial drugs. Science 1999;285:1573–1576.

413. Sato S, Tews I, Wilson RJ: Impact of a plastid-bearing endocytobiont on apicomplexan genomes. Int J Parasitol 2000;30:427–439.

414. Hofflin JM, Remington JS: In vivo synergism of roxithromycin (RU 965) and interferon against *Toxoplasma gondii*. Antimicrob Agents Chemother 1987;31:346–348.

415. Araujo FG, et al: The ketolide antibiotics HMR 3647 and HMR 3004 are active against *Toxoplasma gondii* in vitro and in murine models of infection. Antimicrob Agents Chemother 1997;41:2137–2140.

416. Hunter CA, Subauste CS, Remington JS: The role of cytokines in toxoplasmosis. Biotherapy 1994;7:237–247.

Lyme Disease

GARY P. WORMSER, MD

DURLAND FISH, PHD

Lyme disease (also known as Lyme borreliosis), caused by the spirochete *Borrelia burgdorferi*,[1–3] is the most common tick-borne infection in North America and is also widespread throughout northern regions of Europe and Asia.[4,5] The infection is transmitted by the usually asymptomatic bite of certain ticks of the genus *Ixodes*. *Ixodes* ticks have a three-stage life-cycle: larval, nymphal, and adult stages. Ticks acquire infection from the white-footed mouse and other small mammals or birds.[6–11] Migrating birds may have a role in the spread of ticks and *B. burgdorferi* to new locations.[12] Despite reports of Lyme disease–like illness in Australia, Africa, and South America, *B. burgdorferi* has not been isolated from patients there, and these locations should not be considered endemic for this infection.[13]

Lyme disease occurs with similar frequency in males and females in the United States and affects people of all ages.[14] A bimodal age distribution has been described in the United States with highest rates in children ages 5 to 9 years old and in adults 45 to 54 years old.[14] Lyme disease is concentrated in limited geographic areas in the United States, with cases occurring in certain areas of the Northeast, Mid-Atlantic, Midwest, and Far West regions. Just ten states account for over 90% of cases, and in the state with the largest number of cases (New York), more than 80% of cases are reported from just 5 of 62 counties.[14] Human *B. burgdorferi* infection has not been documented in the Southeast and South Central United States, although there are many reported cases of a Lyme disease–like illness in that region that appears to be associated with the bite of a different tick species (*Amblyomma americanum*).[15–17]

The particular geographic location in which an *Ixodes* bite occurs not only determines the risk of acquiring *B. burgdorferi* infection but also other pathogens besides *B. burgdorferi* that infect members of this tick species. In the United States, potential coinfecting microorganisms include the agent of human granulocytic ehrlichiosis (HGE) and *Babesia microti*, whereas in Europe possible coinfecting agents include the HGE agent, *Babesia divergens*, and the tick-borne encephalitis virus. Coinfections may influence disease manifestation and severity.[18,19] In Europe Lyme disease may be caused by other genospecies of *Borrelia* in addition to *B. burgdorferi* such as *B. garinii* and *B. afzelii*.[20] Reference to *B. burgdorferi* sensu stricto (s.s.) (strict sense), as well as to the related genospecies, is made by the designation *B. burgdorferi* sensu lato (s.l.) (broad sense). Increasing evidence suggests that the particular genospecies of *Borrelia* causing infection will affect clinical presentation.[21,22] Two dermatologic manifestations of Lyme disease, borrelial lymphocytoma and acrodermatitis chronica atrophicans, are rarely if ever seen in the United States because the genospecies that cause these clinical manifestations are exclusively found in Eurasia.[23]

VECTORS

Lyme disease spirochetes are transmitted exclusively by hard ticks of the genus *Ixodes*.[24] Hard ticks differ from the distantly related soft ticks, which transmit relapsing fever spirochetes, in that feeding occurs only once during each developmental stage of hard ticks and that host seeking is widespread in the environment rather than confined to host burrows or nests, as with soft ticks.[25] Although many species within the genus *Ixodes* ticks transmit *B. burgdorferi* s.l. in enzootic natural maintenance cycles, only those species belonging to the *Ixodes persulcatus* group of *Ixodes* ticks transmit *B. burgdorferi* s.l. to humans.[26,27] Tick species in this group include *I. persulcatus* in Eurasia, *Ixodes ricinus* in Europe, *Ixodes pacificus* in the western United States and *Ixodes scapularis* in the middle and eastern United States.[24] These ticks are characterized by having high humidity requirements for off-host survival[28] and a broad host range for all feeding stages (larva, nymph, and adult), which often includes humans.[29] The broad host range of these species makes them efficient vectors of zoonotic pathogens, as they form a transmission bridge from wildlife reservoir hosts to humans.

The black-legged or deer tick, *I. scapularis*, is responsible for more than 95% of Lyme disease cases in the United States.[30] Larval ticks become infected with *B. burgdorferi* when they feed on infected wildlife. The white-footed mouse, *Peromyscus leucopus*, is thought to be the primary source of infection for *I. scapularis* because of its ubiquity in forested environments and because it can maintain *B. burgdorferi* infection for life.[6,7] However, other mammals, such as chipmunks, and some bird species, such as robins, may also serve as sources of infection.[8–11] *I. scapularis* larvae host-seek and feed in late summer.[31] This stage does not pose a risk of *B. burgdorferi* infection for humans. After 2 to 3 days of feeding, engorged larvae drop to the ground, molt into the nymphal stage, and overwinter unfed until the following spring.[29] Larvae may be distinguished from nymphs both by their smaller size and the presence of only 6 legs, which is characteristic of insects (Hexopoda). Nymph and adult ticks (and mites) always have 8 legs, in contrast to true insects. Nymphs begin feeding in late spring, and depending upon the vertebrate host species composition in a given area, infection prevalence in host-seeking nymphs can reach as high as 30%.[32,33] The peak season for *B. burgdorferi* transmission to both wildlife and humans occurs during June and July when *I. scapularis* seeks a blood meal as a nymph.[34] Transmission to wildlife completes the enzootic cycle by infecting reservoir hosts just prior to peak larval feeding in August.

Adult *I. scapularis* has two opportunities for acquiring *B. burgdorferi* infection, first as a larva and second as a nymph. Consequently infection prevalence in adults commonly exceeds 50%.[32,33] Transmission by adults is an ecological dead end, however, since the preferred host for adults, white-tailed deer, are incapable of maintaining *B. burgdorferi* infection.[35] Adult ticks are also poor vectors of human infection for reasons described in a later discussion. The apple-seed size of adult *I. scapularis* ticks makes them more visible on clothing and pets, however, and provides a cause for concern of exposure to nymphs, which are the size of poppy seeds and much less noticeable. Although adults host-seek primarily in the fall and spring months when nymphs are absent, they are usually excellent indicators of eminent risk from summer nymphs.

PREVENTION

Risk Assessment

Knowledge of the seasonal and geographic distribution of Lyme disease risk is essential for effective prevention. Methods for Lyme disease prevention have their own costs in terms of financial burden, inconvenience, and vigilance, and targeting prevention efforts to high-risk populations or individuals is important for reducing disease incidence.[36] The seasonality of Lyme disease risk is dictated by the onset and duration of host-seeking activity by nymphal *I. scapularis*.[29,34] These parameters are predictable, since onset is photocontrolled by a critical day length, which in the northeastern United States occurs in late May, and duration, while dependent upon local climate, rarely lasts until September.[29] Thus the seasonal period of risk is roughly equivalent each year.

The geographic distribution of Lyme disease risk is less precisely defined, and evidence for an expanding range of *I. scapularis* in the upper Midwest and Northeast suggests that risk is not geographically stable.[37,38] The prevalence of infection with *B. burgdorferi* in *I. scapularis* nymphs is geographically variable, with only rare infections found in the southern states, in contrast to persistently high infection prevalence in the Northeast and upper Midwest.[39] The incidence of human Lyme disease closely follows this pattern with more than 90% of cases reported from the Northeast and upper Midwest.[14] The National Lyme Disease Risk Map produced for the CDC[40] (Fig. 39–1) provides information on Lyme disease risk at the national level. This map places all counties within the contiguous United States within one of four risk categories ranging from high to low or none. Even within high-risk counties, risk at the local level is dependent upon habitat suitability for the establishment and maintenance of vector ticks and human activities that result in exposure.[32,41] In the Northeast the risk is primarily from peridomestic exposure due to the expansion of suburban developments into forested areas and an overabundance of deer, which contribute to high densities of *I. scapularis* ticks.[10,42,43] However, exposure to infected ticks from recreational activities appears to be the

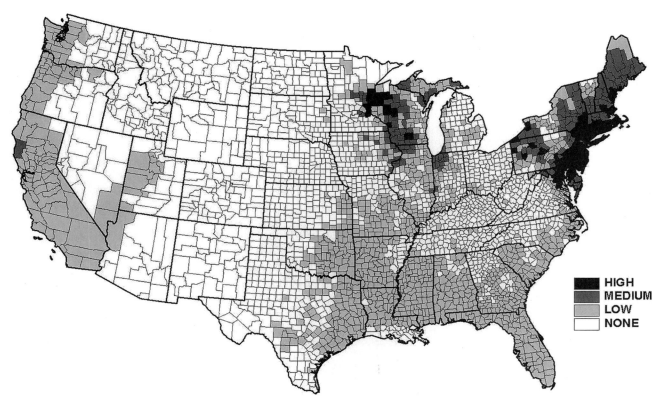

FIGURE 39–1. National Lyme Disease Risk Map differentiated into counties with high, moderate, low, or minimal to no risk.

predominant mode of acquiring Lyme disease in the upper Midwest.[44] Information on the local distribution of *I. scapularis* and delineation of areas of high human risk for exposure can frequently be obtained from local or state departments of public health.

Vector Control

Prevention of a vector-borne disease traditionally is facilitated by reduction or elimination of the vector species. Three approaches have been found to be effective for controlling ticks in the environment: area application of insecticides, wildlife host management, and environmental alteration. Several replicated studies have demonstrated the efficacy of applying insecticides to tick-infested areas to reduce Lyme disease risk.[45–49] Representatives of all three currently used categories of insecticides have been tested with acceptable results: organophosphates, carbamates, and pyrethroids. In a replicated experiment involving 101 residential properties in Westchester County, NY, chlorpyrifos, carbaryl, and cyfluthrin reduced nymphal *I. scapularis* densities on individual properties by 78.1%, 97.4%, and 92.2% respectively, compared to untreated control properties, with a single application during early June.[48] Granular formulations are more effective and more easily applied than are liquid formulations of these insecticides.[45] Although adult ticks pose little risk of Lyme disease, a second application of insecticide during September will reduce the densities of both fall and spring adults. Chlorpyrifos recently was banned in the United States, but studies have shown that almost any insecticide registered for lawn insect control will also control ticks.[50] A single application is effective when targeted against nymphal ticks in early spring because new nymphs will not appear until they are produced by larvae later in the summer, and these nymphs will not feed until the following summer.[48] Nymphs already attached to animals will complete feeding and molt into adults. Once eradicated from an area, there is no mechanism for recruitment of new nymphs until the next year. Therefore persistent insecticides are not necessary; those with short periods of activity are equally as effective.

Management of wildlife hosts that maintain the tick population and *B. burgdorferi* infection in ticks would seem a daunting task, but carefully selected options may be considered. The dependence of adult stage *I. scapularis* upon deer as a definitive reproductive host provides the option of eliminating deer as a host for tick population maintenance.[51–53] Removing deer by killing or capture is impractical for Lyme disease risk reduction, but excluding deer from high risk residential or recreational areas can be accomplished by fencing. Replicated studies in New York and Connecticut have shown that deer exclusion by fencing individual residential properties reduces the abundance of nymphal *I. scapularis* by 47% to 83%.[31,54] Exclusion must be total, since a single deer can support more than 100 female ticks, each of which can produce 3000 larvae. Fencing may be limited to the winter months (October to April) to coincide with the activity period of adult *I. scapularis*.[29]

Other options include products that prevent immature *I. scapularis* from feeding upon mammalian hosts that serve as sources of infection for nymphs. Such products include cotton treated with pyrethin insecticide, which is collected by mice for nesting material, and bait-boxes that attract and directly treat small mammals with insecticide.[55] Wholesale control or elimination of such hosts is not practical, and these products are designed only to reduce infection prevalence in nymphal ticks and not to reduce or eliminate the tick population. However, such products so far have had limited success in independent studies.[56–58]

Altering residential or recreational environments to create habitats less attractive to wildlife and less suitable for tick survival is another option. Studies on clearing leaf litter and providing an inhospitable barrier for mammals and ticks by surrounding the property with a narrow strip of wood chips has been found to reduce nymphal abundance by more than 70% in residential properties.[36,59] Lowering humidity levels near the ground by litter removal and thinning canopy trees and shrubs will reduce the survival of overwintering ticks.[28,51] A combination of deer reduction, insecticide use, and vegetation management has been demonstrated to be effective in reducing populations of the Lone Star tick *A. americanum* in recreational areas in the Southeast.[60] A similar integrated approach may also be effective for *I. scapularis* reduction over large areas in the Northeast. Research is currently in progress to evaluate the efficacy of such integrated community-based vector control programs in reducing the incidence of Lyme disease in the Northeast.

Personal Protection

In the absence of effective control of infected ticks in the environment, preventing contact between ticks and human skin to reduce opportunities for attachment and feeding are essential if tick-infested areas cannot be avoided. Personal protection methods include wearing clothing tightly fitted at the ankles and wearing socks over the cuffs of trousers to prevent tick entry.[32] Ticks do not fly or jump but instead seek hosts by ascending blades of grass or brush and awaiting a passing animal. Host-seeking height varies by stage with larvae and nymphs, usually ascending less than 0.5 m (20 inches) and adults from 0.5 to 1 m (20 to 40 inches).[29] Nymphal ticks are more likely to ascend under clothing and attach on the legs or trunk of the body, whereas adult ticks are more likely to ascend outside clothing and attach near the head.[61] The low host-seeking height and the tick's small size make access restriction below the knees extremely important for preventing nymphs from contacting skin. Light colored clothing further facilitates prevention of

tick attachment by making crawling ticks more visible, thus providing greater opportunity for removal from the body.

Insect repellents are effective in preventing ticks from contacting and crawling upon clothing or skin.[62–65] Repellents containing DEET (*N,N*-diethyl-*m*-toluamide) can be used directly on exposed skin or on clothing. DEET should be applied to exposed skin only and not to skin underneath clothing. Face and hands need not be treated, since these are unlikely places for ticks to attach without notice. The duration of effectiveness depends upon physical activity and concentration of the product. One to several hours of protection can be expected with concentrations of 30% active ingredient. Lower concentrations are recommended for children.[66]

Clothing, but not skin, can also be treated with 1% permethrin, which effectively repels ticks for many hours or even days.[63] Permethrin-treated shoes and socks in combination with DEET application to exposed skin provides the best protection in warm weather when wearing long trousers tucked into socks but is not practical or comfortable. Neither protective clothing nor a combination of protective clothing and repellents is 100% effective in preventing tick bites.

Outdoor clothing and domestic animals, particularly cats, are frequent sources of nymphal *I. scapularis* inside the home.[67] Clothing should be placed in a clothes dryer for 30 minutes to kill ticks that may have been inadvertently collected during forays into tick-infested areas. Pets should be brushed to remove unattached ticks before entry into the house. A variety of veterinary products are available for protecting pets from ticks.[68] Because of high humidity requirements for prolonged survival of *I. scapularis*, infestations within houses have not been reported and are not likely possible. Likewise, engorged ticks dropping from pets after feeding are not likely to survive until molting inside houses, and female ticks will not survive long enough to lay eggs.

Daily inspections and prompt removal of attached ticks is the best defense against tick bites, even when all other preventive measures are followed. Complete body searches are recommended, as ticks may become attached in inaccessible areas.[61] Removal is best facilitated by using a fine-tipped forceps to pull the tick away from the attachment site at an angle perpendicular to the skin.[69] It is important to grab the tick as close to the skin as possible to avoid damaging the tick body, as damage to the tick might facilitate the introduction of tick-borne pathogens. Complete removal of the mouth parts (hypostome) may not be possible because of associated barbs (denticles). Surgical removal of mouth parts is not recommended, and retention of these parts does not cause complications if antiseptic is promptly applied. Removed ticks may be sent to the local health department, cooperative extension service, or academic entomology department if identification is in doubt.

Testing of removed ticks for the presence of pathogens is not practical. Few commercial laboratories provide this service, and those that do are not tested for proficiency. Blood accumulated in the gut of feeding ticks even after 24 hours of feeding can complicate the sensitivity of both immunofluorescent and molecular-based pathogen detection methods.[33,70]

Chemoprophylaxis

Four prospective, randomized, placebo-controlled studies of antibiotic prophylaxis for prevention of Lyme disease in patients who had recent *I. scapularis* tick bites have been conducted (Table 39–1).[71–74] Efficacy of antibiotics in preventing erythema migrans at the tick bite site (the most reliable indicator of transmission of *B. burgdorferi* by a specific tick bite) varied from 87% to 100%. Antibiotics were not significantly more effective than placebo, however, in three of the studies despite an efficacy rate of 100% in each of the studies.[71–73] This is attributable to the relatively small number of subjects enrolled and the low risk of transmission of *B. burgdorferi* from tick bites that are recognized and removed (1.1% to 3.2%). Transmission of *B. burgdorferi* is a slow process that can be interrupted successfully by removing the tick during the feeding process.[75–77] In animal experiments, transmission rarely occurs until the tick has been feeding for 36 hours. In addition, two studies have demonstrated that the frequency of transmission to humans is significantly greater after tick bites in which the ticks were estimated to have fed for 72 hours or longer compared to shorter feeding periods. The risk of Lyme disease in humans after *I. scapularis* tick bites in which the estimated duration of feeding was 72 hours or longer was 20% among patients bitten on Long Island, NY,[79] and 25% among patients bitten in Westchester County, NY,[74] both areas endemic for Lyme disease. In a study of *I. scapularis* ticks removed from humans, approximately 63% were removed before 24 hours, 9% between 24 and 48 hours, 15% between 48 and 72 hours, and 13% were removed after 72 hours of feeding based on the degree of blood engorgement of the tick, an experimentally validated estimate of the duration of feeding.[80] The infrequency of feeding durations of 72 hours or longer is probably the explanation for the low risk of

Lyme disease among placebo recipients in the chemoprophylaxis trials. Paradoxically, transmission of *B. burgdorferi* by adult *I. scapularis* is much less frequent than by nymphal stage ticks despite a higher infection rate with *B. burgdorferi*, presumably because adult ticks are larger and therefore more readily observed and removed more quickly. In one study, the estimated median duration of attachment of 115 nymphal ticks removed from humans was 30 hours compared to 10 hours for 76 adult ticks ($P < .001$).[74] In addition the number of bites due to nymphal stage ticks exceeds that due to adult stage ticks for several reasons, including the greater number of nymphal stage ticks in the environment (>10-fold higher than adult stage ticks)[29] and seasonal differences in the abundance of nymphal vs. adult stage ticks pertinent to human exposure.[34]

In most of the studies on chemoprophylaxis of tick bites,[71–73] as well as in a cost-effectiveness analysis,[81] a 10- to 14-day course of antibiotics was prescribed after the tick bite, which is the same duration of antibiotic therapy found to be effective for treatment of early Lyme disease.[82,83] In a departure from this approach, however, Nadelman and colleagues randomized 482 patients to receive either a single 200-mg dose of doxycycline or an identical appearing placebo.[74] The rationale for use of single dose therapy was the established success of this approach in prevention of syphilis[84] or leptospirosis[85] in exposed persons. In the Nadelman study[74] 3.2% of placebo recipients, including 5.6% of 142 patients bitten by nymphal stage ticks and 0 of 97 patients bitten by adult stage ticks, developed erythema migrans at the tick bite site. Only one doxycycline-treated patient developed erythema migrans at the tick bite site (this patient was bitten by a nymphal stage tick) for a treatment efficacy rate of 87% (95% CI 25% to 98%) (P value < .04).

Before publication of the single dose doxycycline study, our practice had been not to offer antibiotic prophylaxis and instead to monitor patients with tick bites for signs and symptoms of tick-borne illness for up to 30 days after the bite, and specifically for the occurrence of erythema migrans at the tick bite site, or fever (which might suggest HGE or babesiosis). The success of single dose doxycycline therapy warrants a re-evaluation of this

---

TABLE 39–1 ■ Randomized, Placebo-Controlled Trials of Chemoprophylaxis for *Borrelia burgdorferi* Infection from *Ixodes scapularis* Tick Bites

Author (year)	Number of subjects	Antibiotic and duration	Incidence of erythema migrans*		Efficacy rate of antibiotic
			Antibiotic (%)	Placebo (%)	
Costello et al[73] (1989)	56	Penicillin × 10 d	0	3.0	100
Shapiro et al[71] (1992)	365	Amoxicillin × 10 d	0	1.2	100
Agre and Schwartz[72] (1993)	179	Penicillin or tetracycline × 10 d	0	1.1	100
Nadelman et al[74] (2001)	482	Doxycycline × 1 dose	0.4	3.2	87

*Either stated or presumed to occur at tick bite site.

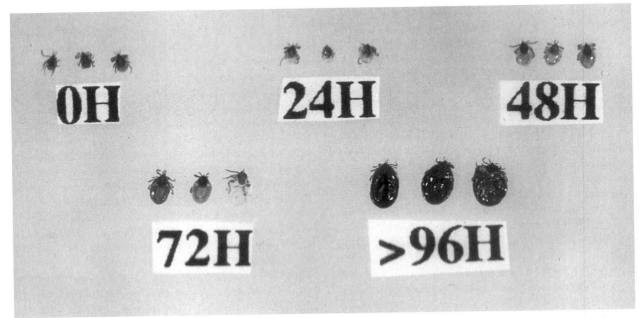

FIGURE 39–2. Nymphal *Ixodes scapularis* ticks demonstrating changes in blood engorgement after various durations of attachment to an animal host (see Color Plate 3). (Photograph is a generous gift from Dr. Richard Falco.)

approach, and our current practice is to offer a single 200-mg dose of doxycycline (with food for better gastrointestinal tolerance[85]) to adult patients who have removed an engorged nymphal stage *I. scapularis* tick and who have no contraindications to receipt of tetracycline antibiotics. Because pregnant or lactating women and children <8 years of age are not eligible to receive tetracyclines, they should not be offered single-dose doxycycline. On the basis of a crude extrapolation from the single dose doxycycline study, a 72-hour course of amoxicillin may be offered to persons who are unable to tolerate tetracyclines, although this regimen has never been systematically studied. Chemoprophylaxis of *I. pacificus* tick bites may not be justified because the infection rate with *B. burgdorferi* is low (≤6%) throughout the distribution of these ticks with the exception of one California county.[86–89] Single dosage doxycycline chemoprophylaxis would probably be effective for *I. ricinus* or *I. persulcatus* tick bites (the vectors of Lyme borreliosis in Eurasia), since all genospecies of *B. burgdorferi* are highly susceptible to doxycycline in vitro,[90] but no data are available to substantiate this hypothesis. Chemoprophylaxis for larval stage *Ixodes* ticks is not necessary, since this stage is usually uninfected with *B. burgdorferi* because of the rarity of transovarian transmission of the spirochete.[91]

Chemoprophylaxis for tick bites has a number of limitations. There is no evidence that such treatment would prevent transmission of other potential tick-borne pathogens. In addition single dose therapy is not 100% effective, and insufficient numbers of patients with tick bites have been treated with doxycycline to establish with certainty the precise efficacy rate of prophylaxis. Further even single dose antibiotic treatment can cause an array

TABLE 39–2 ■ **Chronology of Selected Events Culminating in U.S. Food and Drug Administration (FDA) Approval of a Lyme Disease Vaccine**

1977	First description of Lyme disease
1982	*Borrelia burgdorferi* identified as agent of Lyme disease
1986	Immunoprophylaxis successful in laboratory animal
1990	Whole cell dog vaccine developed
1990	OspA vaccine studies in laboratory animals reported
1994	OspA vaccine entered human trials
1998	OspA vaccine received FDA approval

of potential adverse effects including, but not limited to, allergic reactions, nausea, and vomiting.[74] In addition many practitioners and patients may not be able to reliably differentiate an engorged from an unengorged nymphal stage tick (Fig. 39–2 and Color Plate 3). Also, scabs and insects may be confused with ticks, and vector-tick species may not be distinguished from nonvector species, leading to unwarranted use of antibiotic prophylaxis.[79,92]

Immunoprophylaxis

A fundamental limitation of chemoprophylaxis is that approximately 75% of patients with Lyme disease do not recognize the tick bite in the first place.[93] In this situation immunoprophylaxis is a much more logical option. Johnson and colleagues first showed that active immunization with an inactivated whole cell *B. burgdorferi* preparation could protect laboratory animals against challenge by isolates of *B. burgdorferi* (Table 39–2).[94,95] These findings paved the way for introduction of an inactivated whole cell *B. burgdorferi* vaccine for use in dogs.[96–98] Development of an inactivated whole cell vaccine for use in humans has not been pursued because of theoretical concerns that such a vaccine preparation might cause unintended immunologic sequelae for the host.[99–103] Immune responses to spirochetal antigens that cross-react with host proteins might lead to chronic inflammatory conditions and tissue damage. Antibodies to *B. burgdorferi* are known to cross-react in vitro with nerve cell axons, synovial cells, hepatocytes, and cardiac and skeletal muscle protein.[93–96] The *B. burgdorferi* antigens thought to be principally responsible for the molecular mimicry are the 41-kD flagellin protein and heat shock proteins.

Subunit vaccines were considered to have the greatest promise for prevention of Lyme disease in humans. Proteins expressed via recombinant DNA technology in *Escherichia coli*, particularly certain outer surface proteins (Osp) of *B. burgdorferi*, such as OspA, OspB, and OspC, are highly protective when used as immunogens in experimental animals.[99–110] The most extensively studied of the recombinant single protein vaccines has been OspA. Active and passive immunization studies with OspA immunogens in various strains of mice have shown high levels of protection.[109,111–119]

Functional Immunity

In experimental animals, humoral immunity is sufficient for protection against *B. burgdorferi*,[112–114,120–127] and in some model systems, passive immunization may also ameliorate or eliminate pre-existent infection.[124,128–130] The mechanism(s) by which antibodies provide protection has not been established. Direct activity of antibodies against *B. burgdorferi* can be measured by assays that assess spirochetal immobilization, agglutination, growth inhibition, or killing.[123,131,132] Antibodies may also facilitate phagocytosis by macrophage-monocytes through binding to Fc receptors.[102,133,134] Hypothetically, antibodies may block attachment of *B. burgdorferi* to structures of the extracellular matrix or to endothelial cells and thereby prevent penetration into tissue.[112,135–141] Growth-inhibiting antibody titers directly correlated with protection in several experimental studies of laboratory animals vaccinated with an OspA vaccine preparation.[142,143] Efficient spirochete killing by OspA antibody is dependent on the presence of complement.[144–147] Antibodies to OspA that are protective in mice bind specifically to epitopes located within the carboxyl end of the protein.[148–153] These epitopes appear to be distinct from the immunodominant epitope on OspA recognized by T helper cells in synovial fluid of patients with antibiotic-refractory Lyme arthritis (see below).[152]

Complement proteins may immobilize *B. burgdorferi* independent of antibodies via the alternative complement pathway. This role of complement may be a factor in the determination of which wildlife species are reservoir competent for this microorganism.[154,155] The importance of cell-mediated immunity in preventing Lyme disease in humans and animals has not been determined conclusively,[103,108] and in certain animal models cellular immune responses may in fact be detrimental to the host.[156]

Vaccine Studies

In December 1998 an aluminum hydroxide adjuvanted lipidated recombinant OspA vaccine known as LYMErix was granted U.S. Food and Drug Administration (FDA) approval.[157] The pivotal efficacy study that led to approval of this vaccine recruited a total of 10,936 subjects ages 15 to 70 years who received 3 doses of the vaccine administered intramuscularly into the deltoid muscle at time 0, 1 month, and 12 months.[158] Eleven percent of the vaccine recipients had a history of Lyme disease, and 2.3% were seropositive for IgG antibodies to *B. burgdorferi* on enrollment. The subjects were then followed for 20 months over two Lyme disease transmission seasons from the time of the first injection. Primary end points were the incidences of definite and asymptomatic Lyme disease. Patients with definite Lyme disease had to have objective clinical manifestations such as erythema migrans or neurologic, cardiovascular, or musculoskeletal manifestations, plus laboratory results indicative of *B. burgdorferi* infection. Laboratory support of the diagnosis could include a positive culture for *B. burgdorferi*, detection of borrelial DNA by polymerase chain reaction (PCR) from a skin biopsy sample, or seroconversion by IgM or IgG immunoblot (using criteria specified in the study). Subjects were defined as having asymptomatic infection if there was no recognizable clinical manifestation but if IgG seroconversion by immunoblot occurred between months 2 and 12 of the first year or between months 12 and 20 of the second year.

The OspA vaccine preparation was significantly more effective than placebo for prevention of definite Lyme disease in both year 1 (49% efficacy) ($P = .009$) and year 2 (76% efficacy) ($P < .001$).[158] Efficacy in preventing asymptomatic infection was 83% after 2 doses of vaccine ($P = .004$) and 100% ($P = .001$) after 3 doses. Improvement in vaccine efficacy from year 1 to 2 could be explained by the enhanced antibody response after 3 doses compared with 2 doses of the OspA vaccine preparation. Repeat antibody titers at month 13, 1 month after the third vaccine dose, revealed a marked anamnestic response to OspA with 99% of the recipients tested producing detectable antibody to OspA. Statistical studies by the vaccine manufacturer have suggested that a titer of at least 1400 ELISA U/ml of IgG antibody to the OspA antigen before the start of tick season is associated with protection from disease for that tick season,[159] but this type of testing is not commercially available. Approximately 90% of the subjects in the efficacy trial who had serologic testing reported had a titer of at least 1400 ELISA U/ml 1 month after receipt of the third vaccine dose.

Although data are limited, the clinical features of patients who have developed Lyme disease despite OspA vaccination appear to be identical to those in unvaccinated patients.[160,161]

Side effects of the LYMErix vaccine preparation in the efficacy trial were primarily limited to discomfort at the injection site and self-limited systemic reactions. Significantly more subjects in the vaccine group reported soreness at the injection site (24.1%) than did those who received placebo (adjuvant in buffered saline) (7.6%) (*P* value < .001).[158] It should be noted that the incidence of local reactions at the injection site may have been underestimated in the efficacy study because these symptoms were spontaneously reported rather than solicited. In other studies of the same vaccine preparation in adults in which symptoms were actively solicited from each subject, the frequency of local reactions was higher (up to 85%).[159,162,163]

Vaccine recipients in the efficacy trial were significantly more likely to report systemic complaints (19.4%) such as fever, chills, and myalgias than were the placebo group (15.1%) (*P* value < .001).[158] For the subgroup of 938 volunteers for whom systemic symptoms during the 72-hour period following vaccination were solicited by diary cards, 63% of the vaccine recipients vs. 53% of placebo recipients recorded symptoms possibly or probably related to the injection (*P* = .004). Systemic complaints occurred within 48 hours after vaccination and lasted a median of 3 days. They were typically mild or moderate in severity, and the severity usually did not increase with subsequent injections. Of note, reports of arthritis or neurologic events were no more frequent in vaccine recipients than in the placebo group.[157,158] This is an important finding, because in natural infection, OspA antibodies are principally found in patients with Lyme arthritis.[164] In addition, since in genetically predisposed patients a T cell response to OspA may cross-react with a human antigen (leukocyte function–associated antigen 1 [LFA-1]), autoimmune phenomena may play an etiologic role in the small subgroup of patients with Lyme arthritis who do not improve with antibiotic therapy.[165–168] Therefore concerns have been raised that a vigorous immunologic response to OspA from vaccination might cause joint inflammation. The safety profile for subjects seropositive for antibodies to *B. burgdorferi* on enrollment and for those with a history of Lyme disease was no different from those for other vaccinees.[158] The lack of serious adverse effects observed in the efficacy trial was similar to that obtained in a smaller phase II prospective study in which varying dosages of the same vaccine preparation were given on a 0, 1 month, 2 month schedule to 30 healthy volunteers who previously, following antimicrobial therapy, had recovered from a well-documented episode of Lyme disease.[162]

On the basis of the available evidence from the vaccine trial, immunization with this recombinant OspA preparation is safe and will reduce the frequency of but will not eliminate Lyme disease in adults. However, additional information on the safety of vaccines is collected through a passive surveillance system known as the Vaccine Adverse Events Reporting System (VAERS). Reports to VAERS associated with LYMErix, from the date of its licensure in December 1998 through July 2000, were reviewed by the Centers for Disease Control and Prevention and the FDA (CDC unpublished data). During this time 1.4 million doses were distributed and 905 adverse events were reported. The review detected no unexpected pattern of adverse events compared to clinical trials except that there were rare hypersensitivity reactions including urticaria and occasional reports of dyspnea.[169,170] The number of reports of arthritis was well below what would have been expected on the basis of the rates of arthritis reported in the efficacy trial.[170]

The FDA-approved dosage schedule is for the vaccine to be given at 0, 1, and 12 months, a schedule identical to that used in the efficacy study. The three dose vaccine regimen given over 1 year is disadvantageous for patients because of the long delay in development of the maximum protective response. Shorter course regimens (0, 1 month, 6 months[159] or 0, 1 month, 2 months[171]), although apparently as well tolerated and capable of eliciting a protective immunologic response more rapidly, have not received FDA approval. To achieve maximal protection using the 0, 1 month, 12 month schedule, the second and third doses of the Lyme disease vaccine should each be administered approximately 1 month before the start of the local Lyme disease season.[157,172] The vaccine is administered intramuscularly into the deltoid area. The effect of concurrent administration of other vaccines is unknown. The vaccine is not approved for children under 15 years of age, but safety and immunogenicity studies in pediatric populations (children 5 to 15 years old were studied in one trial[173] and children 2 to 5 years old in another[174]) have shown results similar to those seen in adults except that the vaccine is more immunogenic in children, suggesting that a two-dose schedule might be protective. Recommendations for use of the Lyme disease vaccine derived from the Advisory Committee on Immunization Practices (ACIP) are shown in Table 39–3.[172]

Several studies have examined the cost-effectiveness of the Lyme disease vaccine. Meltzer et al reported a net cost of vaccination of $4467 per case of Lyme disease averted when the annual cost of vaccination was assumed to be $100 and the probability of contracting Lyme disease was 0.01.[175] Shadick and colleagues evaluated the cost-effectiveness of vaccination in terms of cost per quality-adjusted life-year gained; this analysis reflects the relative impact on the patient's time with symptoms.[176] In population groups with a seasonal incidence of Lyme disease of 1% the additional cost of vaccination per quality-adjusted life-year gained compared with no vaccination was $62,300. If a yearly booster shot were necessary to maintain protection, the cost per quality-

TABLE 39–3 ■ Indications for Use of Lyme Disease Vaccine

1. Vaccinated persons should continue to practice personal protection measures against ticks and should seek early diagnosis and treatment of suspected tick-borne infections.
2. Lyme disease vaccination should be considered for persons 15 to 70 years of age who engage in activities that require frequent or prolonged exposure to tick-infested habitat in areas of high or moderate risk of Lyme disease in the United States (see Fig. 39–1), including travelers to such areas with similar exposures.
3. Lyme disease vaccination may be considered for persons 15 to 70 years of age in areas of high or moderate risk for Lyme disease in the United States who are exposed to tick-infested habitat but whose exposure is neither frequent nor prolonged.
4. Lyme disease vaccination is not recommended
    a. For persons who have minimal or no exposure to tick-infested habitat
    b. For persons who have exposure only in areas of low or no risk of Lyme disease
    c. For persons <15 years old or >70 years old
    d. For pregnant women
    e. For patients with treatment-resistant Lyme arthritis
5. No information is available on the safety or efficacy of Lyme disease vaccination in
    a. Persons with immunodeficiency
    b. Persons with musculoskeletal diseases, for example, rheumatoid arthritis, or illnesses associated with diffuse musculoskeletal pain
    c. Persons with chronic neurologic disease related to Lyme disease or with other manifestations of active Lyme disease such as heart block

Modified from Centers for Disease Control and Prevention: Recommendations for the use of Lyme disease vaccine: Recommendations of the Advisory Committee on Immunization Practices (ACIP). MMWR Morb Mortal Wkly Rep 1999;48:1–25.

adjusted life-year gained increased to $72,700. To place this figure in perspective, these investigators compared their findings with other cost utilities such as mammography screening (vs. no population-based screening) in women 45 to 69 years old, which was $18,000, or preoperative autologous donation of 2 units of blood (vs. no autologous donations) for patients undergoing primary, elective coronary artery bypass graft surgery, which was $590,000. Both Shadick et al[176] and Meltzer et al[175] concluded that vaccination against Lyme disease was economically attractive only for persons who have a yearly risk of *B. burgdorferi* infection of 1% or higher. Such high incidence rates may occur focally but not in most geographic areas as large as counties or states (e.g., from 1992 to 1998 the highest mean annual incidence among all counties in the United States was 1009.9/100,000 persons, and the highest mean annual incidence rate among states was 67.9/100,000 in Connecticut[14]).

Mechanism of Action of OspA Vaccine

In unattached and unfed ticks, *B. burgdorferi* present in the midgut expresses abundant quantities of OspA. During the feeding process, however, a major phenotypic change occurs, resulting in down-regulation of expression of OspA and up-regulation of expression of another outer surface protein (OspC).[177–179] Presumably for this reason, tick-borne infection initially elicits antibody to OspC in the host but not to OspA. Down-regulation of OspA continues in vivo, so that antibody production to this antigen is delayed or never occurs at all.[103,106,164,180–182]

Assuming that this sequence of events is correct, why would an OspA vaccine be clinically effective if the infecting spirochete is not expressing OspA antigen? The answer appears to be that the vaccine's protective effect actually occurs in the tick during the grace period from

onset of feeding to spirochete transmission. Microscopic examination has demonstrated that *B. burgdorferi* is eliminated or substantially reduced in number in ticks that have taken a blood meal from an OspA-immunized animal host.[116,117,150,183–187] Furthermore in one study the spirochete could no longer be detected in the tick even by culture of midgut contents.[153]

Therefore, the effectiveness of OspA vaccination appears to be principally based on an ex vivo mechanism of action, so that the tick can no longer transmit the spirochete to the host. A particular benefit of this mode of action is that it seems to be highly potent, with immunity extending to diverse strains of *B. burgdorferi*.[150] In addition this mechanism of action may explain why immunization appears to prevent both clinical illness and asymptomatic infection.[111,116,117] There are, however, some potential scenarios that might result in vaccine failure. For example, if the spirochete had already migrated to the salivary gland of the tick before attachment to the host, it might escape inactivation by OspA antibody present in the blood meal.[99,188,189] The frequency with which such an event occurs is unknown but is probably low. In addition, because IgG antibodies have been shown to pass through the midgut epithelium of ticks, it is possible that OspA-expressing spirochetes would be targeted for destruction even after migration to the salivary glands.[190] Of greater concern is that Lyme disease probably would not be prevented in the absence of a significant titer of OspA antibody in the host at the time of the tick bite. If immunity fails to be maintained continuously, even a vigorous anamnestic response following exposure to the microorganism may not be rapid enough to prevent infection. In addition, on the basis of the previously described phenotypic shift from OspA to OspC in the spirochetes residing in the tick during the blood meal, it is unlikely that an OspA immune response would be sustained by repeated tick bites alone. Only approximately one-half of vaccinees will maintain protective levels of OspA antibody by 12 months following the third dose of vaccine.[157] Periodic booster doses of vaccine will be necessary, although data on safety are limited.[171] The frequency with which these doses would be required has not been established but might be as often as every 12 to 24 months. Administration of booster doses has not received FDA approval.

Limitations of Lyme Disease Vaccine

There are a number of additional limitations to the use of a single protein recombinant OspA vaccine preparation. Among these is the inherent heterogeneity of this protein among borrelial isolates.[149,191–199] Most, but not all,[172] evidence indicates that a monovalent *B. burgdorferi*–derived OspA vaccine is unable to provide protection against the wide diversity of borrelial strains present in Eurasia, especially for the genospecies *B. garinii* and *B. afzelii*.[113,119,142] Experimentally, however, a polyvalent OspA vaccine preparation has shown promise for protection of laboratory animals against all three genospecies.[200] Because the Lyme disease vaccine is not 100% effective and because it will not prevent infection due to other *Ixodes*-borne pathogens,[18,19,201,202] it is important that practitioners advise their vaccinated patients to maintain personal protection measures for prevention of tick bites and to remove any attached ticks as expeditiously as possible. A reduction in precautions or vigilance for tick bites because of a false sense of security from being vaccinated might paradoxically increase the risk of acquiring *Ixodes*-transmitted infections.

In addition, receipt of an OspA vaccine has important implications for serologic testing for Lyme disease. Current guidelines call for two-stage testing in which a positive or equivocal first-stage test (enzyme-linked immunosorbent assay [ELISA] or an immunofluorescent assay) is followed by immunoblot as the second stage test.[203] For someone to be regarded as seropositive, both the first and second stage tests must be positive. ELISAs usually consist of whole cell sonicates of *B. burgdorferi* and hence include OspA antigen. Immunoblot preparations also contain OspA antigen. Consequently OspA vaccination almost uniformly causes false-positive results on first-stage tests and may produce diverse effects on immunoblotting (as a function of the specific immunoblot preparation employed), making immunoblot test results difficult to interpret in some patients, potentially resulting in false-negative or false-positive readings.[204–206] Great impetus has been placed on developing serologic assays that do not incorporate OspA, and a few such assays are now becoming available commercially. A general approach for the prevention of Lyme disease is shown in Table 39–4. In February 2002 the manufacturer discontinued production of LYMErix due to poor sales.

TABLE 39–4 ■ **Prevention of Lyme Disease**

PREVENTION OF TICK BITES
Risk Assessment
  Avoid tick-infested areas
  Avoid high-risk time periods
Vector Control
  Insecticides
  Wildlife management
  Environmental alteration
Personal Protection
  Protective clothing
  Insect repellents
  Inspections for ticks
  Protect pets

CHEMOPROPHYLAXIS
Doxycycline 200 mg × 1 dose within 72 hours of removing an engorged nymphal *Ixodes scapularis* tick*

IMMUNOPROPHYLAXIS
Recombinant Osp A vaccination, 3 dose series†

*A 72-hour course of amoxicillin may be considered for doxycycline-intolerant patients such as children <8 y of age or pregnant or lactating women.

†Booster doses are likely to be needed, but the frequency and safety are as yet unknown. In February 2002 the manufacturer discontinued production of the vaccine.

TREATMENT

Although most manifestations of Lyme disease resolve spontaneously without treatment, antibiotics are recommended to hasten the resolution of symptoms and to prevent disease progression. With rare exceptions, relatively short courses of antibiotics (10 to 28 days) are successful for treatment of patients with Lyme disease.[82] Although techniques for in vitro susceptibility testing have not been standardized, available studies suggest that *B. burgdorferi* is highly susceptible to a variety of antimicrobial agents including tetracyclines, penicillin, amoxicillin, second- and third-generation cephalosporins, and macrolides.[90,207,208] These microorganisms are resistant to quinolones such as ciprofloxacin, rifampin, and first-generation cephalosporins.[209]

Erythema Migrans

The most common objective clinical manifestations of Lyme disease include cutaneous lesions such as erythema migrans (Fig. 39–3 and Color Plate 3) (at University Medical Centers in the United States, approximately 90% of cases that satisfy the CDC surveillance definition of Lyme disease have erythema migrans[210]), early and late neurologic conditions, carditis, and arthritis (Table 39–5).[13,211] With regard to therapy the best studied clinical manifestation of Lyme disease is erythema migrans. At least eight randomized prospective trials have addressed the treatment of early Lyme disease associated with erythema migrans in the United States alone, and many additional studies have been conducted in Europe.[83,212–218] Several

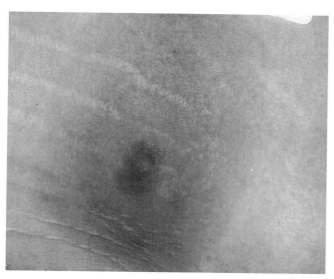

FIGURE 39–3. Example of most common clinical manifestation of Lyme disease, erythema migrans (see Color Plate 3).

TABLE 39–5 ■ Principal Clinical Manifestations of Lyme Disease

CUTANEOUS
Erythema migrans
Acrodermatitis chronica atrophicans
Lymphocytoma

NEUROLOGIC (EARLY)
Cranial neuropathy
Radiculopathy
Meningitis

NEUROLOGIC (LATE)
Peripheral neuropathy
Encephalopathy
Encephalomyelitis

CARDIAC
Myocarditis (typically with atrioventricular block)

RHEUMATOLOGIC
Arthritis
Tendonitis

conclusions can be drawn from these studies. Doxycycline, amoxicillin, and cefuroxime axetil, when given for time periods ranging from 10 to 21 days, are highly effective in the treatment of this manifestation (Tables 39–6 and 39–7).[82] Most patients respond promptly and completely. Compared to oral antibiotic therapy, a parenteral drug such as ceftriaxone offers no additional benefit to such patients.[83,218] Despite excellent activity against *B. burgdorferi* in vitro,[219] certain macrolides may be less effective clinically.[82,220] Erythromycin and azithromycin in studies from the United States[212,217] and roxithromycin in a study performed in Europe[221] have been found to be less effective than other therapeutic agents. Azithromycin has appeared to be as efficacious as comparators in several European trials[222–226]; whether this is a function of the different genospecies of *Borrelia* causing disease there or due to methodologic limitations in study design such as small sample size has not been determined.

Clarithromycin has not been studied in a controlled trial.[227] Approximately 10% of treated patients have or develop subjective complaints despite therapy that otherwise appears curative.[83,228] Such complaints are often referred to as post–Lyme disease syndrome and sometimes as chronic Lyme disease. Less than 5% of infected persons fail to respond to antibiotic therapy, however, as evidenced by objective manifestations of persistent infection (e.g., development of Lyme arthritis), and repeat treatment with antimicrobials is rarely required.[82] In general, patients who are more systemically ill (have more numerous and severe symptoms) or who have multiple erythema migrans lesions at the time of diagnosis are more liable to have persistent or intermittent subjective complaints.[228] Coinfection with other tick-borne infections or inadequately recognized central nervous system infection may be the explanation for antibiotic failures in some cases.[13,18,19]

TABLE 39–6 ■ Recommended Antimicrobial Regimens for Treatment of Patients with Lyme Disease

Recommendation, drug	Dosage for adults	Dosage for children
Preferred oral		
Amoxicillin	500 mg PO tid	50 mg/kg/d PO divided into 3 doses (maximum 500 mg per dose)
Doxycycline	100 mg PO bid*	Age <8 y: not recommended
		Age ≥8 y: 1–2 mg/kg/bid PO (maximum 100 mg per dose)
Alternative oral: cefuroxime axetil	500 mg PO bid	30 mg/kg/d PO divided into 2 doses (maximum 500 mg per dose)
Preferred parenteral: ceftriaxone	2 g IV once daily	75–100 mg/kg/d IV in a single dose (maximum 2 g)
Alternative parenteral		
Cefotaxime	2 g IV tid	150–200 mg/kg/d IV divided into 3 or 4 doses (maximum 6 g/d)
Penicillin G	18–24 MU/d IV divided into 6 doses given q4h†	200,000–400,000 U/kg/d IV divided into 6 doses given q4h† (maximum 18–24 MU/d)

*Tetracyclines are relatively contraindicated for pregnant or lactating women.
†The penicillin dosage should be reduced for patients with impaired renal function.
From Wormser GP, Nadelman RB, Dattwyler RJ, et al: Practice guidelines for the treatment of Lyme disease. Clin Infect Dis 2000;31(Suppl 1):S1–S14.

TABLE 39–7 ■ Recommended Therapy for Patients with Lyme Disease

Indication	Treatment	Duration (days)
Cutaneous lesions		
Erythema migrans	Oral regimen[†‡]	10–21
Lymphocytoma	Oral regimen[†‡]	14–21
Acrodermatitis chronica atrophicans[*]	Oral regimen[†]	28
Acute neurologic disease		
Meningitis or radiculopathy	Parenteral regimen[†§]	14–28
Cranial nerve palsy	Oral regimen[†]	14–21
Cardiac disease		
First- or second-degree heart block	Oral regimen[†]	14–21
Third-degree heart block	Parenteral regimen[†‖]	14–21
Late disease		
Arthritis without neurologic disease	Oral regimen[†]	28
Recurrent arthritis after oral regimen	Oral regimen[†] or	28
	parenteral regimen[†]	14–28
Persistent arthritis after 2 courses of oral antibiotics or 1 course of a parenteral antibiotic	Symptomatic therapy	
Central nervous system or peripheral nervous system disease	Parenteral regimen	14–28
Post–Lyme disease syndrome	Symptomatic therapy	

[*]Oral therapy is not recommended if patients have concomitant neurologic disease. These patients should be treated with parenteral therapy.

[†]See Table 39–5.

[‡]For adult patients who are intolerant of amoxicillin, doxycycline, and cefuroxime axetil, alternatives are azithromycin 500 mg/d PO × 7–10 d; erythromycin 500 mg PO qid × 14–21 d; or clarithromycin 500 mg PO bid × 14–21 d (except during pregnancy). The recommended dosages of these agents for children are as follows: azithromycin 10 mg/kg/d PO (maximum 500 mg/d); erythromycin 12.5 mg/kg PO qid (maximum 500 mg per dose); clarithromycin 7.5 mg/kg PO bid (maximum 500 mg per dose). Patients treated with macrolides should be closely followed.

[§]For nonpregnant adult patients intolerant of both penicillin and cephalosporins, doxycycline 200–400 mg/d PO (or IV if oral medications cannot be taken) divided into 2 doses may be adequate.

[‖]A temporary pacemaker may be required.

Modified from Wormser GP, Nadelman RB, Dattwyler RJ, et al: Practice guidelines for the treatment of Lyme disease. Clin Infect Dis 2000; 31(Suppl 1):S1–S14.

Within 24 hours of initiating appropriate antibiotic therapy for patients with erythema migrans, approximately 15% of patients experience arthralgias, an increase in temperature, or malaise.[82] Such Jarisch-Herxheimer-like reactions are not seen in patients treated for later manifestations of Lyme disease.

All antimicrobials effective for treatment of patients with erythema migrans are associated with a low frequency of serious adverse effects.[82] Drug-induced rashes occur with both amoxicillin and cefuroxime axetil. Doxycycline may cause photosensitivity, which may be problematic since erythema migrans occurs during the summer months. However, an advantage of doxycycline over β-lactam drugs is that this drug is also effective against the HGE agent, which is transmitted by the same tick species that transmits *B. burgdorferi*.[229] Patients who have Lyme disease and HGE simultaneously are well described.[19,230] Persons treated with doxycycline are advised to avoid exposure to the sun while receiving therapy. In addition, doxycycline is relatively contraindicated for children under 8 years of age and for women who are pregnant or breast-feeding. Cefuroxime axetil is much more expensive than doxycycline or amoxicillin, making it a less attractive agent for first-line therapy.[82] In contrast to the second-generation cephalosporin cefuroxime and to certain third-generation cephalosporins (e.g., ceftriaxone

or cefotaxime), first-generation cephalosporins such as cephalexin are ineffective clinically.[209]

None of the prospective treatment trails enrolled pregnant patients. Nevertheless there are no data to suggest, and little rationale to believe, that pregnant patients should be treated differently from other patients with Lyme disease, except that tetracycline therapy should be avoided.[82,231–233]

Early Neuroborreliosis

Relatively few studies exist on therapy of early neurologic Lyme disease, and most of them are reported from Europe, where this manifestation of Lyme disease may be more common.[13,82] Patients with Lyme meningitis or acute radiculopathy respond to parenteral antimicrobial therapy. Doxycycline administered orally has also been used successfully in Europe, but experience with this agent for treatment of patients with meningitis due to Lyme disease in the United States is limited.[82]

Given the generally accepted standard of treating patients with neurologic Lyme disease with antimicrobials, it may be surprising to learn that there has never been documentation that such patients actually need to be treated.[234] No placebo-controlled studies have ever been (nor will be) done. When antibiotic-treated patients are compared to historical series of untreated patients or patients treated with only corticosteroids, the data are conflicting as to whether there is an advantage favoring antibiotics.[235–240] Most studies have suggested that the rate of resolution of motor weakness is unaffected by antibiotics (the mean time for complete resolution is approximately 2 months).[234–237] The natural history of untreated patients is slow resolution of clinical and cerebrospinal fluid (CSF) abnormalities over the course of 2 to 6 or more months.[235,237,241] Clinical findings typically fluctuate in intensity over this period. Pain is a particularly prominent symptom among European cases of early neuroborreliosis, and according to some investigators this symptom responds better to corticosteroids than to high-dose parenteral penicillin.[237,238,240] In one United States study, 12 patients treated with parenteral penicillin were compared retrospectively to 15 patients previously treated only with corticosteroids.[235] Resolution of headache and stiff neck began by the second day of antibiotic therapy and was significantly faster in the penicillin-treated cases. In other studies, clinical improvement has been noted in most patients by the third to fifth day of antimicrobial therapy.[242]

Probably to a large extent because of the benign outcome of early neuroborreliosis, there is no evidence of superiority for any particular antibiotic regimen, including oral or IV doxycycline, high-dose parenteral penicillin, cefotaxime, or ceftriaxone, or of an advantage of early vs. delayed antibiotic therapy.[234,235,237,242–250] This statement should be tempered by the knowledge that no large-scale, double-blind, multicenter prospective studies have been done.[234]

"Standard" management is to use parenteral antibiotic therapy for adult patients with early neuroborreliosis, with once daily IV administration of ceftriaxone being the most convenient regimen (because of the drug's long serum half-life) (Tables 39–6 and 39–7).[82] Ceftriaxone is also highly effective for children with neuroborreliosis.[244,249,250]

An exception to the use of parenteral therapy is the patient with uncomplicated seventh nerve palsy for whom oral antibiotic therapy may be sufficient (Tables 39–6 and 39–7).[82] According to an expert panel, patients with seventh nerve palsy for whom there is a strong clinical suspicion of central nervous system involvement (i.e., those with severe headache or meningismus) should undergo a lumbar puncture.[82] If the CSF examination is found to be abnormal, then these patients should be treated with parenteral antibiotic therapy. Because the frequency and rate of recovery of seventh nerve palsy in patients who are treated with antibiotics appear to be the same as in untreated patients, the principal goal of therapy is to prevent later development of clinical manifestations.[236] Parenteral antibiotic therapy (i.e., ceftriaxone) is often used for other Lyme disease patients whose neurologic manifestations appear to involve only the peripheral nervous system. Given the absence of data or a clear rationale to justify parenteral therapy, comparative studies with oral regimens appear warranted.[234]

Lyme Carditis

There are no controlled studies on the treatment of cardiac manifestations of Lyme disease, but an expert panel has recommended that patients with first- or second-degree heart block resulting from Lyme disease be treated with oral antibiotic therapy (Tables 39–6 and 39–7).[82] Because of the potential for life-threatening complications, patients with third-degree heart block should be closely monitored, preferably in a hospital setting.[251] These patients usually are treated at least initially with parenteral antibiotic therapy, and insertion of a temporary pacemaker also may be necessary.[82]

Lyme Arthritis

Both oral and intravenous antibiotic therapy are effective for patients with Lyme arthritis (Tables 39–6 and 39–7).[82,252,256] In a cost-effectiveness analysis, oral therapy was found to be more cost effective than intravenous therapy for patients with Lyme arthritis, since intravenous therapy is more likely to result in serious complications and is substantially more expensive.[257] The authors of that analysis concluded that oral antibiotics are preferred in the initial treatment of Lyme arthritis in the absence of concurrent neurologic involvement. Approximately 90% of patients with Lyme arthritis can be expected to respond to antibiotic therapy or to improve spontaneously.[258] In one treatment trial, however, in none of the 16 patients with Lyme arthritis who were treated with ceftriaxone did the arthritis resolve within 3 months after completion of therapy.[259] That study's enrollment requirement of continuous joint swelling for at least 3 months despite treatment with other recommended parenteral or oral antibiotic regimens differs from requirements in previous studies. These 16 patients were also found to have distinctive immunogenetic and immune markers, including a high frequency of human leukocyte antigen–DR4 specificity and of antibody reactivity with OspA of the spirochete.[166] Data based on PCR testing of serial joint fluid samples suggest that arthritis may persist in up to 10% of patients despite eradication of the spirochete.[260] The observation that there are epitopes of OspA that cross-react with human LFA-1 suggests that autoimmunity may explain the persistent joint inflammation in these cases.[165]

For patients who have persistent or recurrent joint swelling after a 28-day course of oral antibiotic therapy, an expert panel recommended repeat treatment with another 28-day course of oral antibiotics or with a 14- to 28-day course of ceftriaxone (Tables 39–6 and 39–7).[82] In general, re-treatment should be postponed until approximately 3 months after the initial course of therapy because of the anticipated slow resolution of inflammation.

Arthroscopic synovectomy has been used successfully in the treatment of patients whose arthritis persists despite antibiotic therapy. Of 20 patients who underwent this procedure for refractory chronic Lyme arthritis of the knee, the joint inflammation resolved in 16 (80%) during the first month following surgery or soon thereafter.[261] The remaining 4 patients (20%) had persistent or recurrent synovitis.

Late Neuroborreliosis

The natural history of untreated late peripheral neuropathy and encephalopathy is less well understood, but these manifestations appear to progress slowly.[260] How often spontaneous resolution may occur is unclear, but most of these patients and those with encephalomyelitis improve coincident with antibiotic therapy, although often without complete resolution of signs and symptoms.[262,263] Two comparative studies have suggested that the third-generation cephalosporins ceftriaxone or cefotaxime are more efficacious than parenteral penicillin in late Lyme disease.[254,264] These studies included some patients with only rheumatologic complications of Lyme disease. Because of this and other methodologic concerns, it cannot be considered proven that cephalosporins are superior to high-dose IV penicillin for patients with late neuroborreliosis.[234] Although cefotaxime has to be administered three to four times daily (compared with once daily administration of ceftriaxone), it does not cause the biliary complications that have been associated with ceftriaxone therapy.[265]

There is little need, however, to restudy whether penicillin is more or less effective than third-generation cephalosporins are, as the convenience of once daily dosing makes ceftriaxone the preferred agent (Tables 39–6 and 39–7).[82] Following antibiotic therapy, patients with late neuroborreliosis improve slowly over the course of several months.[254,262,263,266] Adjunctive use of steroids is reported to hasten recovery but has never been systematically evaluated.[237]

In a trial conducted from 1987 to 1989, 27 adult patients with Lyme encephalopathy, polyneuropathy, or both were treated with intravenous ceftriaxone for 2 weeks.[262] In addition to clinical signs and symptoms, outcome measures included CSF analyses and neuropsychological tests of memory. Response to therapy was usually gradual and did not begin until several months after treatment. When response was measured 6 months after treatment, 17 patients (63%) had uncomplicated improvement, 6 (22%) had improvement but then relapsed, and 4 (15%) had no change in their condition.

In a subsequent study, 18 adult patients with Lyme encephalopathy were treated with a longer course of intravenous ceftriaxone for 30 days.[263] As determined 6 months after treatment, 14 (93%) of the 15 patients examined had diminished symptoms, and verbal memory scores for the 15 patients were significantly improved

(*P* value < .01). CSF protein values were reduced significantly for the 10 patients who had follow-up analyses (*P* value < 0.05). One patient was retreated at 8 months. At 12 to 24 months all patients had returned to normal or had improved. The authors concluded that Lyme encephalopathy may be associated with active infection of the nervous system and that infection in most patients can be treated successfully with a 30-day course of intravenous ceftriaxone. Whether a 30-day course is superior to 14 days of treatment is unclear.[82] Although the data are much more limited, the conditions of children with neurocognitive abnormalities attributed to Lyme disease also appear to improve after 2 to 4 weeks of intravenous ceftriaxone.[267]

Post–Lyme Disease Syndrome

Regardless of the manifestation of Lyme disease being treated, a small proportion of patients following therapy may experience either constantly or intermittently a variety of subjective complaints such as myalgia, arthralgia, or fatigue. Although some of these patients have been classified as having post–Lyme disease syndrome or chronic Lyme disease, a strict case definition for these entities is lacking.[13,82] The frequency and type of complaints reported are indistinguishable from those that occur in otherwise healthy matched controls without Lyme borreliosis.[268] Two treatment trials of patients with 6 months or longer of post–Lyme disease symptoms were reported recently.[269] In one trial, seropositive patients were randomized to receive 1 month of intravenous ceftriaxone followed by 2 months of oral doxycycline vs. identical appearing placebo therapies.[269] Both of these antimicrobials are active against *B. burgdorferi* and able to cross the blood-brain barrier. The second trial was identical to the first except that the patients were seronegative.[269] The primary end point of these studies was symptom improvement based on patient responses to a health-related quality of life questionnaire given 90 days after they completed the course of antibiotic treatment or placebo. Both studies were terminated early by a data and safety monitoring board because of lack of efficacy of the antibiotic therapy. Overall in these studies, approximately one-third improved, approximately one-third remained unchanged, and approximately one-third worsened, regardless of whether antibiotic or placebo was administered. During these trials, CSF and blood samples were tested systematically from 129 patients for evidence of active *B. burgdorferi* infection by use of culture and PCR techniques. No evidence of persistent *B. burgdorferi* infection could be found in any of the patients. The investigators concluded that the cause of the patients' subjective complaints was not active *B. burgdorferi* infection and that it would be highly unlikely that different antibiotic regimens involving either alternative antimicrobial agents or longer durations of therapy would be beneficial. To our knowledge, *B. burgdorferi* has not been recovered from any patient in the United States following a recommended course of antibiotic treatment,[270,271] and only rarely has this phenomenon been reported in Europe.[272] Symptomatic therapy is the recommended approach for management of patients with post–Lyme disease syndrome (Table 39–7).[82]

Duration of Treatment

In 1983 Steere et al reported on an open-label study of 49 patients with erythema migrans who were randomized to receive 10 vs. 20 days of tetracycline therapy.[212] No significant difference in outcome for these patients was observed. Nevertheless, over time recommendations for the duration of treatment of patients with erythema migrans have increased to as long as 30 days.[273] For example, the *Medical Letter* has published treatment recommendations on 3 separate occasions in 1992, 1997, and most recently in 2000.[274–276] Over this 9-year period the recommended minimum duration of treatment of erythema migrans increased from 10 to 21 days, despite the absence of additional prospective controlled trials evaluating duration of therapy. Indeed the findings in the only other comparative study to address specifically duration of treatment in patients with erythema migrans provided evidence against the notion that longer courses of therapy improve outcome. In this retrospective study reported in 1995, Nowakowski et al compared the outcome over 1 year of follow-up in 38 patients who were treated with doxycycline (300 mg/d) for 20 days with 21 patients who received the same antimicrobial (200 mg/d for 6 patients and 300 mg/d for 15 patients) for 14 days.[277] No significant difference in treatment efficacy was observed.

It is likely that recommendations for prescribing longer treatment courses were motivated by the presumption that more prolonged therapy would eliminate or reduce the frequency and severity of post–Lyme disease subjective complaints.[278] Other factors that may have been influential include the speculation that *B. burgdorferi* may be in some way inherently resistant to antibiotic therapy or that the spirochete might lodge in sanctuaries protected from antimicrobial effects. Attempts to find evidence in support of the latter hypothesis have motivated a number of investigations aimed at discovering the putative sanctuary or demonstrating other ways in which *B. burgdorferi* might elude the bactericidal effects of antimicrobial treatment.[279] To date, convincing evidence in support of this theory is lacking. In addition there is no evidence that *B. burgdorferi* has acquired (or can acquire) resistance to the antimicrobials conventionally used for treatment.[82]

Furthermore there is no precedent for use of prolonged courses of antibiotics for other spirochetal infections.[220] Other borrelial infections such as louse-borne relapsing fever may be treated with courses of antibiotics as short as one dose of tetracycline or erythromycin, and tick-borne relapsing fever is routinely treated with a 5- to 10-day course of these antimicrobials.[280]

In light of the results of the recently published study of patients with post–Lyme disease subjective complaints

in which no evidence of active *B. burgdorferi* infection could be demonstrated,[269] a critical reappraisal of the need for, and desirability of, 21- to 30-day courses of antibiotics for patients with early Lyme disease is warranted. A prospective, double-blind, controlled study of 180 adult patients with erythema migrans from New York State has provided important new information pertinent to this issue. This study compared 10 days of doxycycline (100 mg orally twice daily) with either 10 days of oral doxycycline plus one initial dose of intravenous ceftriaxone (2 g), or 20 days of doxycycline (100 mg orally twice daily).[83] This treatment trial differed in significant ways from other therapeutic trials for Lyme disease in that follow-up was extended to 30 months (from the usual 6 to 12 months), and volunteers underwent serial detailed neurologic examinations and neurocognitive testing. Results of this study based on both an intent-to-treat analysis and an analysis of on-study patients showed no significant difference in efficacy rates among the three treatment groups at any time point.[83] There was only a single treatment failure during the study, which occurred in a patient who was diagnosed with presumed Lyme meningitis 8 days after completing the 10-day course of doxycycline. A significantly greater frequency of diarrhea was reported by the patients who received ceftriaxone ($P < .001$), which indicates that there are potential risks from administration of even a single dose of an antibiotic. Similarly, adverse events from administration of a single dose of oral doxycycline for prevention of Lyme disease after an *I. scapularis* tick bite have been described.[74]

Evidence from Europe indicates that even shorter courses of antibiotic therapy are effective for patients with erythema migrans. Weber et al randomized 73 German patients with erythema migrans in an open label study to receive either 5 days of ceftriaxone (1 g/d) or 12 days of an oral penicillin preparation.[281] The 5-day course of ceftriaxone was found to be equally as effective as the penicillin therapy.

Preliminary results of a study that compared duration of antimicrobial therapy for patients with late Lyme disease also found that the shorter duration treatment regimen had similar efficacy to a longer course of therapy.[255] In this open-label, randomized, multicenter study, 143 evaluable patients with manifestations of late Lyme disease, primarily Lyme arthritis, were treated with 2 g/d of intravenous ceftriaxone for either 2 or 4 weeks. In 76% of those treated for 2 weeks and 70% of those treated for 4 weeks, symptoms resolved after treatment. The most common persistent symptoms were arthralgia, pain, weakness, malaise, and fatigue.

Animal Studies

Studies in animals are consistent with the premise that short courses of antimicrobial therapy are efficacious for *B. burgdorferi* infection. In experimental studies of rodents a 5- to 10-day course of ceftriaxone successfully eradicated *B. burgdorferi* infection; confirmation of the eradication was based on the inability to recover the spirochete by culture of tissues at time of sacrifice.[282–285] A 5-day course of ceftriaxone was also uniformly effective in mice immunosuppressed by corticosteroids.[284] Short courses of ceftriaxone were also highly effective in eradicating *B. burgdorferi* infection in even more highly immunocompromised animals. Kazragis et al demonstrated that a 9-day course of ceftriaxone reliably eradicated *B. burgdorferi* infection in mice with severe combined immunodeficiency (scid mice).[285]

The pharmacokinetics of ceftriaxone in mice and humans appear to have substantial differences. The serum half-life of ceftriaxone in humans is approximately 7 hours,[284] which is much longer than that reported in mice.[287,288] On the basis of this information, Pavia et al abbreviated the treatment regimen for *B. burgdorferi*-infected C3H mice to 5 doses of ceftriaxone administrated over just 24 hours.[284] Administration of ceftriaxone on an every-6-hour schedule should have maintained inhibitory blood levels continuously during the treatment period despite the short half-life in mice. Based on negative cultures of bladder and ear tissue samples obtained at the time of sacrifice (5 to 7 days after completion of the ceftriaxone treatment), all of the mice were cured. The 24-hour treatment regimen was estimated to maintain a level of ceftriaxone in mouse serum in excess of the minimum bactericidal concentration of the particular infecting strain of *B. burgdorferi* for a period of time less than would be expected from a single 125-mg dose of ceftriaxone given to humans.

CONCLUSION

Lyme disease is the most common tick-borne disease in North America and parts of Europe and Northern Asia. Strategies for prevention of Lyme disease include avoiding *Ixodes* tick bites, prompt removal of attached *Ixodes* ticks, chemoprophylaxis with a single 200-mg dose of doxycycline for patients who remove engorged nymphal *I. scapularis* ticks and who have no contraindications to receiving this drug, and up until recently immunoprophylaxis with the Lyme disease vaccine for selected persons with frequent or prolonged exposure to tick-infested habitat in areas of high or moderate risk of Lyme disease in the United States (Table 39–4).

Almost all patients with objective manifestations of Lyme disease respond to conventional 10- to 28-day courses of antibiotics (Tables 39–6 and 39–7).[82,83] Oral regimens are preferred for patients with cutaneous and rheumatologic manifestations. Patients with neurologic manifestations other than uncomplicated cranial nerve palsy and patients with advanced heart block usually are treated with parenteral antibiotics for 14 to 28 days. Symptomatic therapy is recommended for post–Lyme disease subjective symptoms and patients with Lyme arthritis in whom 2 courses of antibiotic therapy have failed.

ACKNOWLEDGMENTS We thank Eleanor Bramesco, Lisa Giarratano, Joan Laden, John Nowakowski, and Robert Nadelman for their assistance.

REFERENCES

1. Burgdorfer W, Barbour AG, Hayes SF, et al: Lyme disease—a tick borne spirochetosis? Science 1982;216:1317–1319.
2. Benach JL, Bosler EM, Hanrahan JP, et al: Spirochetes isolated from the blood of two patients with Lyme disease. N Engl J Med 1983;308:740–742.
3. Steere AC, Grodzicki RL, Kornblatt AN, et al: The spirochetal etiology of Lyme disease. N Engl J Med 1983;308:733–740.
4. Centers for Disease Control and Prevention: Lyme disease—United States, 1999. MMWR Morb Mortal Wkly Rep 2001;50:181–185.
5. O'Connell S, Granstrom M, Gray JS, Stanek G: Epidemiology of European Lyme borreliosis. Zentralbl Bakteriol 1998;287:229–240.
6. Donahue JG, Piesman J, Spielman A: Reservoir competence of white-footed mice for Lyme disease spirochetes. Am J Trop Med Hyg 1987;36:92–96.
7. Levine JF, Wilson ML, Spielman A: Mice as reservoirs of the Lyme disease spirochete. Am J Trop Med Hyg 1985;34:355–360.
8. Mannelli A, Kitron U, Jones CJ, Slajchert TL: Role of the eastern chipmunk as a host for immature *Ixodes dammini* (Acari: Ixodidae) in northwestern Illinois. J Med Entomol 1993;30:87–93.
9. Slajchert T, Kitron UD, Jones CJ, Mannelli A: Role of the eastern chipmunk (*Tamias striatus*) in the epizootiology of Lyme borreliosis in northwestern Illinois, USA. J Wildl Dis 1997;33:40–46.
10. Falco RC, Fish D: Prevalence of *Ixodes dammini* near the homes of Lyme disease patients in Westchester County, New York. Am J Epidemiol 1988;127:826–830.
11. Richter DS, Komar A, Matuschka N: Competence of American robins as reservoir hosts for Lyme disease spirochetes. Emerg Infect Dis 2000;6:133–138.
12. Smith RP, Rand PW, Lacombe EH, et al: Role of bird migration in the long-distance dispersal of *Ixodes dammini*, the vector of Lyme disease. J Infect Dis 1996;174:221–224.
13. Nadelman RB, Wormser GP: Lyme borreliosis. Lancet 1998;352:557–565.
14. Orloski KA, Hayes EB, Campbell GL, Dennis DT: Surveillance for Lyme disease—United States, 1992–1998. MMWR Morb Mortal Wkly Rep 2000;49(SS-3):1–12.
15. James AM, Liveris D, Wormser GP, et al: *Borrelia lonestari* infection after a bite by an *Amblyomma americanum* tick. J Infect Dis 2001;183:1810–1814.
16. Felz MW, Chandler FW Jr, Oliver JH Jr, et al: Solitary erythema migrans in Georgia and South Carolina. Arch Dermatol 1999;135:1317–1326.
17. Masters E, Granter S, Duray P, Cordes P: Physician-diagnosed erythema migrans and erythema migrans–like rashes following Lone Star tick bites. Arch Dermatol 1998;134:955–960.
18. Krause PJ, Telford SR III, Spielman A, et al: Concurrent Lyme disease and babesiosis: Evidence for increased severity and duration of illness. JAMA 1996;275:1657–1660.
19. Nadelman RB, Horowitz HW, Hsieh T-C, et al: Simultaneous human ehrlichiosis and Lyme borreliosis. N Engl J Med 1997;337:27–30.

20. Barbour AG: Borrelia: A diverse and ubiquitous genus of tick-borne pathogens. In Scheld WM, Craig WA, Hughes JM (eds): Emerging Infections, ed 5. Washington, DC, American Society of Microbiology, 2001, pp 154–174.

21. Van Dam AP, Kuiper H, Vos K, et al: Different genospecies of *Borrelia burgdorferi* are associated with distinct clinical manifestations of Lyme borreliosis. Clin Infect Dis 1993; 17:708–717.

22. Strle F, Nadelman RB, Cimperman J, et al: Comparison of culture-confirmed erythema migrans caused by *Borrelia burgdorferi* sensu stricto in New York State and by *Borrelia afzelii* in Slovenia. Ann Intern Med 1999;130:32–36.

23. Wang G, Van Dam AP, Schwartz I, Dankert J: Molecular typing of *Borrelia burgdorferi* sensu lato: Taxonomic, epidemiologic, and clinical implications. Clin Microbiol Rev 1999;12:633–653.

24. Barbour AG, Fish D: The biological and social phenomenon of Lyme disease. Science 1993;260:1610–1616.

25. Sonenshine DE: *Biology of Ticks*. New York, Oxford University Press, 1991, vol 1.

26. Telford SR III, Spielman A: Enzootic transmission of the agent of Lyme disease in rabbits. Am J Trop Med Hyg 1989;41:482–490.

27. Maupin GO, Gage KL, Piesman J: Discovery of an enzootic cycle of *Borrelia burgdorferi* in *Neotoma mexicana* and *Ixodes spinipalpis* from northern Colorado, an area where Lyme disease is nonendemic. J Infect Dis 1994;170:636–643.

28. Stafford KC III: Survival of immature *Ixodes scapularis* (Acari: Ixodidae) at different relative humidities. J Med Entomol 1994;31:310–314.

29. Fish D: Population ecology of *Ixodes dammini*. In Ginsberg H, (ed): *Ecology and Environmental Management of Lyme Disease*. New Brunswick, NJ, Rutgers University Press, 1993; pp 25–42.

30. Dennis DT, Nekomoto TS, Victor JC, et al: Reported distribution of *Ixodes scapularis* and *Ixodes pacificus* (Acari: Ixodidae) in the United States. J Med Entomol 1998;35:629–638.

31. Daniels TJ, Fish D, Schwartz I: Reduced abundance of *Ixodes scapularis* (Acari: Ixodidae) and Lyme disease risk by deer exclusion. J Med Entomol 1993;30:1043–1049.

32. Fish D: Environmental risk and prevention of Lyme disease. Am J Med 1995;98:2S–7S.

33. Schwartz I, Fish D, Daniels TJ: Prevalence of the rickettsial agent of human granulocytic ehrlichiosis in ticks from a hyperendemic focus of Lyme disease. N Engl J Med 1997;337:49–50.

34. Falco RC, McKenna DF, Daniels TJ, et al: Temporal relation between *Ixodes scapularis* abundance and risk for Lyme disease associated with erythema migrans. Am J Epidemiol 1999; 149:771–776.

35. Telford SR III, Mather TN, Moore SI, et al: Incompetence of deer as reservoirs of the Lyme disease spirochete. Am J Trop Med Hyg 1988;39:105–109.

36. Hayes EB, Maupin GO, Mount GA, Piesman J: Assessing the prevention effectiveness of local Lyme disease control. J Public Health Manag Pract 1999;5:84–92.

37. Bouseman JK, Kitron U, Kirkpatrick CE, et al: Status of *Ixodes dammini* (Acari: Ixodidae) in Illinois. J Med Entomol 1990;27:556–560.

38. White DJ, Chang HG, Benach JL, et al: The geographic spread and temporal increase of the Lyme disease epidemic. JAMA 1991;266:1230–1236.

39. Piesman J, Clark KL, Dolan MC, et al: Geographic survey of vector ticks (*Ixodes scapularis* and *Ixodes pacificus*) for infection with the Lyme disease spirochete, *Borrelia burgdorferi*. J Vector Ecol 1999;24:91–98.

40. Fish D, Howard C: Methods used for creating a national Lyme disease risk map. MMWR Morb Mortal Wkly Rep 1999; 48(RR07):21–24.

41. Mount G, Haile DG, Daniels E: Simulation of backlegged tick (Acari: Ixodidae) population dynamics and transmission of *Borrelia burgdorferi*. J Med Entomol 1997;34:461–484.

42. Maupin GO, Fish D, Zultowsky J, et al: Landscape ecology of Lyme disease in a residential area of Westchester County, New York. Am J Epidemiol 1991;133:1105–1113.

43. Dister SW, Fish D, Bros SM, et al: Landscape characterization of peridomestic risk for Lyme disease using satellite imagery. Am J Trop Med Hyg 1997;57:687–692.

44. Kitron U, Kazmierczak JJ: Spatial analysis of the distribution of Lyme disease in Wisconsin. Am J Epidemiol 1997; 145:558–566.

45. Schulze TL, Taylor GC, Jordan RA, et al: Effectiveness of selected granular acaricide formulations in suppressing populations of *Ixodes dammini* (Acari: Ixodidae): short-term control of nymphs and larvae. J Med Entomol 1991;28:624–629.

46. Schulze TL, Jordan RA, Vasvary LM, et al: Suppression of *Ixodes scapularis* (Acari: Ixodidae) nymphs in a large residential community. J Med Entomol 1994;31:206–211.

47. Schulze TL, Jordan RA, Hung RW, et al: Efficacy of granular deltamethrin against *Ixodes scapularis* and *Amblyomma americanum* (Acari: Ixodidae) nymphs. J Med Entomol 2001; 38:344–346.

48. Curran KL, Fish D, Piesman J: Reduction of nymphal *Ixodes dammini* (Acari: Ixodidae) in a residential suburban landscape by area application of insecticides. J Med Entomol 1993; 30:107–113.

49. Stafford KC III: Effectiveness of carbaryl applications for the control of *Ixodes dammini* (Acari: Ixodidae) nymphs in an endemic residential area. J Med Entomol 1991;28:32–36.

50. Maupin GO, Piesman J: Acaricide susceptibility of immature *Ixodes scapularis* (Acari: Ixodidae) as determined by the disposable pipet method. J Med Entomol 1994;31:319–321.

51. Wilson ML: Reduced abundance of adult *Ixodes dammini* (Acari: Ixodidae) following destruction of vegetation. J Econ Entomol 1986;79:693–696.

52. Wilson ML, Levine JF, Spielman A: Effect of deer reduction on abundance of the deer tick (*Ixodes dammini*). Yale J Biol Med 1984;57:697–705.

53. Deblinger RD, Wilson ML, Rimmer DW, Spielman A: Reduced abundance of immature *Ixodes dammini* (Acari: Ixodidae) following incremental removal of deer. J Med Entomol 1993;30:144–150.

54. Stafford KC III: Reduced abundance of *Ixodes scapularis* (Acari: Ixodidae) with exclusion of deer by electric fencing. J Med Entomol 1993;30:986–996.

55. Mather TN, Ribeiro JM, Spielman A: Lyme disease and babesiosis: Acaricide focused on potentially infected ticks. Am J Trop Med Hyg 1987;36:609–614.

56. Daniels TJ, Fish D, Falco RC: Evaluation of host-targeted acaricide for reducing risk of Lyme disease in southern New York State. J Med Entomol 1991;28:537–543.

57. Stafford KC III: Third-year evaluation of host-targeted permethrin for the control of *Ixodes dammini* (Acari: Ixodidae) in southeastern Connecticut. J Med Entomol 1992;29:717–720.

58. Stafford KC III: Effectiveness of host-targeted permethrin in the control of *Ixodes dammini* (Acari: Ixodidae). J Med Entomol 1991;28:611–617.

59. Schulze TL, Jordan RA, Hung RW: Suppression of subadult *Ixodes scapularis* (Acari: Ixodidae) following removal of leaf litter. J Med Entomol 1995;32:730–733.

60. Barnard DR, Mount GA, Koch HG, Garris GI: Management of the Lone Star tick in recreation areas. United States Department of Agriculture Handbook 682,1988, p 33.

61. Falco RC, Fish D: Ticks parasitizing humans in a Lyme disease endemic area of southern New York State. Am J Epidemiol 1988;128:1146–1152.

62. Lane RS, Anderson JR: Efficacy of permethrin as a repellent and toxicant for personal protection against the Pacific Coast tick and the Pajaroello tick (Acari: Ixodidae and Argasidae). J Med Entomol 1984;21:692–702.

63. Schreck CE, Fish D, McGovern T: Activity of repellents applied to skin for protection against *Amblyomma americanum* and *Ixodes scapularis* ticks (Acari: Ixodidae). J Am Mosq Control Assoc 1995;11:136–140.

64. Fradin MS: Mosquitoes and mosquito repellents: A clinician's guide. Ann Intern Med 1998;28:931–940.

65. US Environmental Protection Agency, Office of Pesticide Programs: Using insect repellents safely. Publication EPA-735/F-93-052R. Washington, DC, US Environmental Protection Agency, 1996.

66. Brown M, Herbert AA: Insect repellents: An overview. J Am Acad Dermatol 1997;36:243–249.

67. Curran KL, Fish D: Increased risk of Lyme disease for cat owners. N Engl J Med 1989;320:183.

68. Taylor MA: Recent developments in ectoparasiticides. Vet J 2001;161:253–268.

69. Needham GR: Evaluation of five popular methods for tick removal. Pediatrics 1985;75:997–1002.

70. Piesman J, Mather TN, Donahue JG, et al: Comparative prevalence of *Babesia microti* and *Borrelia burgdorferi* in four populations of *Ixodes dammini* in eastern Massachusetts. Acta Tropica 1986;43:263–270.

71. Shapiro ED, Gerber MA, Holabird NB, et al: A controlled trial of antimicrobial prophylaxis for Lyme disease after deer-tick bites. N Engl J Med 1992;327:1769–1773.

72. Agre F, Schwartz R: The value of early treatment of deer tick bites for the prevention of Lyme disease. Am J Dis Child 1993;147:945–947.

73. Costello CM, Steere AC, Pinkerton RE, Feder HM Jr: A prospective study of tick bites in an endemic area for Lyme disease. J Infect Dis 1989;159:136–139.

74. Nadelman RB, Nowakowski J, Fish D, et al: Prophylaxis with single-dose doxycycline for the prevention of Lyme disease after an *Ixodes scapularis* tick bite. N Engl J Med 2001;345:79–86.

75. Piesman J, Mather TN, Sinsky RJ, Spielman A: Duration of tick attachment and *Borrelia burgdorferi* transmission. J Clin Microbiol 1987;25:557–558.

76. Piesman J, Maupin GO, Campos EG, Happ CM: Duration of adult female *Ixodes dammini* attachment and transmission of *Borrelia burgdorferi* with description of a needle aspiration isolation method. J Infect Dis 1991;163:895–897.

77. Ribeiro JM, Mather TN, Piesman J, Spielman A: Dissemination and salivary delivery of Lyme disease spirochetes in vector ticks (Acari: Ixodidae). J Med Entomol 1987:24:201–205.

78. des Vignes F, Piesman J, Heffernan R, et al: Effect of tick removal on transmission of *Borrelia burgdorferi* and *Ehrlichia phagocytophila* by *Ixodes scapularis* nymphs. J Infect Dis 2001;183:773–778.

79. Sood SK, Salzman MB, Johnson BJB, et al: Duration of tick attachment as a predictor of the risk of Lyme disease in an area in which Lyme disease is endemic. J Infect Dis 1997:175:996–999.

80. Falco RC, Fish D, Piesman J: Duration of tick bites in a Lyme disease–endemic area. Am J Epidemiol 1996;143:187–192.

81. Magid D, Schwartz B, Craft J, Schwartz JS: Prevention of Lyme disease after tick bites. A cost-effectiveness analysis. N Engl J Med 1992;327:534–541.

82. Wormser GP, Nadelman RB, Dattwyler RJ, et al: Practice guidelines for the treatment of Lyme disease. Clin Infect Dis 2000;31(Suppl 1):S1–S14.

83. Nadelman RB, Ramanathan R, Nowakowski J, et al: Duration of antibiotic therapy for early Lyme disease: A double-blind, prospective, randomized study. 39th Annual Meeting of the Infectious Diseases Society of America, San Francisco, California, October 25–28, 2001.

84. Schroeter AL, Turner RH, Lucas JB, Brown WJ: Therapy for incubating syphilis: Effectiveness of gonorrhea treatment. JAMA 1971;218:711–713.

85. Takafuji ET, Kirkpatrick JW, Miller RN, et al: An efficacy trial of doxycycline chemoprophylaxis against leptospirosis. N Engl J Med 1984;310:497–500.

86. Clover JR, Lane RS. Evidence implicating nymphal *Ixodes pacificus* (Acari: Ixodidae) in the epidemiology of Lyme disease in California. Am J Trop Med Hyg 1995;53:237–240.

87. Lane RS, Piesman J, Burgdorfer W: Lyme borreliosis: Relation of its causative agent to its vectors and hosts in North America and Europe. Annu Rev Entomol 1991;36:587–609.

88. Li X, Peavey CA, Lane RS: Density and spatial distribution of *Ixodes pacificus* (Acari: Ixodidae) in two recreational areas in north coastal California. Am J Trop Med Hyg 2000;62:415–422.

89. Burkot TR, Clover JR, Happ CM, et al: Isolation of *Borrelia burgdorferi* from *Neotoma fuscipes, Peromyscus maniculatus, Peromyscus boylii* and *Ixodes pacificus* in Oregon. Am J Trop Med Hyg 1999;60:453–457.

90. Baradaran-Dilmaghani R, Stanek G: In vitro susceptibility of thirty *Borrelia* strains from various sources against eight antimicrobial chemotherapeutics. Infection 1996;24:60–63.

91. Piesman J, Donahue JG, Mather TN, Spielman A: Transovarially acquired Lyme disease spirochetes (*Borrelia burgdorferi*) in field-collected larval *Ixodes dammini* (Acari: Ixodidae). J Med Entomol 1986;23:219.

92. Falco RC, Fish D, D'Amico V: Accuracy of tick identification in a Lyme disease endemic area. JAMA 1998;280:602–603.

93. Nadelman RB, Nowakowski J, Forseter G, et al: The clinical spectrum of early Lyme borreliosis in patients with culture-confirmed erythema migrans. Am J Med 1996;100:502–508.

94. Johnson RC, Kodner C, Russell M: Active immunization of hamsters against experimental infection with *Borrelia burgdorferi*. Infect Immun 1986;54:897–898.

95. Johnson RC, Kodner CL, Russell ME: Vaccination of hamsters against experimental infection with *Borrelia burgdorferi*. Zentralbl Bakteriol 1986;263:45–48.

96. *Borrelia burgdorferi* bacterin. Lyme Vax. Package insert. Fort Dodge, Iowa, Fort Dodge Laboratories, 1994.

97. Levy SA, Lissman BA, Ficke CM: Performance of a *Borrelia burgdorferi* bacterin in borreliosis-endemic areas. J Am Vet Med Assoc 1993;202:1834–1838.

98. Chu H-J, Chavez LG Jr, Blumer BM, et al: Immunogenicity and efficacy study of commercial *Borrelia burgdorferi* bacterin. J Am Vet Med Assoc 1992;201:403–411.

99. Wormser GP: Vaccination as a modality to prevent Lyme disease. A status report. Infect Dis Clin North Am 1999;13:135–148.

100. Edelman R: The Sixth International Conference on Lyme Borreliosis: Progress on the development of Lyme disease vaccines. Vaccine 1995;13:133–135.

101. Keller D, Koster FT, Marks H, et al: Safety and immunogenicity of recombinant outer surface protein A Lyme vaccine. JAMA 1994;271:1764–1768.

102. Szczepanski A, Benach JL: Lyme borreliosis: Host responses to *Borrelia burgdorferi*. Microbiol Rev 1991;55:21–34.

103. Wormser GP: Prospects for a vaccine to prevent Lyme disease in humans. Clin Infect Dis 1995;21:1267–1274.

104. Sigal LH, Tatum AH: Lyme disease patients' serum contains IgM antibodies to *Borrelia burgdorferi* that cross-react with neuronal antigens. Neurology 1988;38:1439–1442.

105. Aberer E, Brunner C, Suchanek G, et al: Molecular mimicry and Lyme borreliosis: A shared antigenic determinant between *Borrelia burgdorferi* and human tissue. Ann Neurol 1989;26:732–737.

106. Sigal LH: Immunology of Lyme disease. N EngJ J Med 1990;87:567–571.

107. Fikrig E, Berland R, Chen M, et al: Serologic response to the *Borrelia burgdorferi* flagellin demonstrates an epitope common to a neuroblastoma cell line. Proc Natl Acad Sci USA 1993;90:183–187.

108. Preac-Mursic V, Wilske B, Patsouris E, et al: Active immunization with pC protein of *Borrelia burgdorferi* protects gerbils against *B. burgdorferi* infection. Infection 1992; 20:342–349.

109. Fikrig E, Barthold SW, Marcantonio N, et al: Roles of OspA, OspB and flagellin in protective immunity to Lyme borreliosis in laboratory mice. Infect Immun 1992;60:657–661.

110. Gilmore RD Jr, Kappel KJ, Dolan MC, et al: Outer surface protein C (Osp C), but not p39, is a protective immunogen against a tick-transmitted *Borrelia burgdorferi* challenge: Evidence for a conformational protective epitope in Osp C. Infect Immun 1996;64:2234–2239.

111. Fikrig E, Barthold SW, Kantor FS, Flavell RA: Long-term protection of mice from Lyme disease by vaccination with OspA. Infect Immun 1992;60:773–777.

112. Simon MM, Schaible UE, Kramer MD, et al: Recombinant outer surface protein A from *Borrelia burgdorferi* induces antibodies protective against spirochetal infection in mice. J Infect Dis 1991;164:123–132.

113. Schaible UE, Wallich R, Kramer MD, et al: Immune sera to individual *Borrelia burgdorferi* isolates or recombinant OspA thereof protect SCID mice against infection with homologous strains but only partially, or not at all against those of different OspA/OspB genotype. Vaccine 1993;11:1049–1054.

114. Schaible UE, Kramer MD, Eichmann K, et al: Monoclonal antibodies specific for the outer surface protein A (OspA) of *Borrelia burgdorferi* prevent Lyme borreliosis in severe combined immunodeficiency (scid) mice. Proc Natl Acad Sci Si USA 1990;87:3768–3772.

115. Fikrig E, Barthold SW, Kantor FS, Flavell RA: Protection of mice against the Lyme disease agent by immunizing with recombinant OspA. Science 1990;250:553–556.

116. Gern L, Rais O, Capiau C, et al: Immunization of mice by recombinant OspA preparations and protection against *Borrelia burgdorferi* infection induced by *Ixodes ricinus* tick bites. Immunol Lett 1994;39:249–258.

117. Telford SR III, Kantor FS, Lobet Y, et al: Efficacy of human Lyme disease vaccine formulations in a mouse model. J Infect Dis 1995;171:1368–1370.

118. Probert WS, Crawford M, Cadiz RB, LeFebvre RB: Immunization with outer surface protein (Osp) A, but not Osp C, provides cross-protection of mice challenged with North American isolates of *Borrelia burgdorferi*. J Infect Dis 1997;175:400–405.

119. Golde WT, Burkot TR, Piesman J, et al: The Lyme disease vaccine candidate outer surface protein A (OspA) in a formulation compatible with human use protects mice against natural tick transmission of *B. burgdorferi*. Vaccine 1995; 13:435–441.

120. Johnson RC, Kodner C, Russell M: Passive immunization of hamsters against experimental infection with the Lyme disease spirochete. Infect Immun 1986;53:713–714.

121. Johnson RC, Kodner C, Russell M, Duray PH: Experimental infection of the hamster with *Borrelia burgdorferi*. Ann NY Acad Sci 1988;539:258–263.

122. Fikrig E, Bockenstedt LK, Barthold SW, et al: Sera from patients with chronic Lyme disease protect mice from Lyme borreliosis. J Infect Dis 1994;169:568–574.

123. Callister SM, Schell RF, Case KL, et al: Characterization of the borreliacidal antibody response to *Borrelia burgdorferi* in humans: A serodiagnostic test. J Infect Dis 1993;167:158–164.

124. Hansen MS, Cassatt DR, Guo BP, et al: Active and passive immunity against *Borrelia burgdorferi* decorin binding protein A (DbpA) protects against infection. Infect Immun 1998;66:2143–2153.

125. Barthold SW, Bockenstedt LK: Passive immunizing activity of sera from mice infected with *Borrelia burgdorferi*. Infect Immun 1993;61:4696–4702.

126. Fikrig E, Barthold SW, Chen M, et al: Protective antibodies in murine Lyme disease arise independently of CD40 ligand. J Immunol 1996;157:1–3.

127. Barthold SW: Specificity of infection-induced immunity among *Borrelia burgdorferi* sensu lato species. Infect Immun 1999;67:36–42.

128. Zhong W, Stehle T, Museteanu C, et al: Therapeutic passive vaccination against chronic Lyme disease in mice. Proc Natl Acad Sci USA 1997;94:12533–12538.

129. Zhong W, Gern L, Stehle T, et al: Resolution of experimental and tick-borne *Borrelia burgdorferi* infection in mice by passive, but not active immunization using recombinant Osp C. Eur J Immunol 1999;29:946–957.

130. Barthold SW, de Souza M, Feng S: Serum-mediated resolution of Lyme arthritis in mice. Lab Invest 1996;74:57–67.

131. Šadžiene A, Thompson PA, Barbour AG: In vitro inhibition of *Borrelia burgdorferi* growth by antibodies. J Infect Dis 1993;167:165–172.

132. Luke CJ, Marshall MA, Zahradnik JM, et al: Growth-inhibiting antibody responses of humans vaccinated with recombinant outer surface protein A or infected with *Borrelia burgdorferi* or both. J Infect Dis 2000;181:1062–1068.

133. Montgomery RR, Nathanson MH, Malawista SE: Fc- and non-Fc-mediated phagocytosis of *Borrelia burgdorferi* by macrophages. J Infect Dis 1994;170:890–893.

134. Benach JL, Fleit HB, Habicht GS, et al: Interactions of phagocytes with the Lyme disease spirochete: Role of the Fc receptor. J Infect Dis 1984;150:497–507.

135. Ma Y, Sturrock A, Weis JJ. Intracellular localization of *Borrelia burgdorferi* within human endothelial cells. Infect Immun 1991;59:671–678.

136. Comstock LE, Thomas DD: Characterization of *Borrelia burgdorferi* invasion of cultured endothelial cells. Microb Pathog 1991;10:137–148.

137. Szczepanski A, Furie MB, Benach JL, et al: Interaction between *Borrelia burgdorferi* and endothelium in vitro. J Clin Invest 1990;85:1637–1647.

138. Comstock LE, Thomas DD: Penetration of endothelial cell monolayers by *Borrelia burgdorferi*. Infect Immun 1989;57:1626–1628.

139. Thomas DD, Comstock LE: Interaction of Lyme disease spirochetes with cultured eucaryotic cells. Infect Immun 1989;57:1324–1326.

140. Guo BP, Norris SJ, Rosenberg LC, Hook M: Adherence of *Borrelia burgdorferi* to the proteoglycan decorin. Infect Immun 1995;63:3467–3472.

141. Brown EL, Wooten RM, Johnson BJB, et al: Resistance to Lyme disease in decorin-deficient mice. J Clin Invest 2001;107:845–852.

142. Padilla ML, Callister SM, Schell RF, et al: Characterization of the protective borreliacidal antibody response in humans and hamsters after vaccination with a *Borrelia burgdorferi* outer surface protein A vaccine. J Infect Dis 1996;174:739–746.

143. Chang Y-F, Appel MJG, Jacobson RH, et al: Recombinant OspA protects dogs against infection and disease caused by *Borrelia burgdorferi*. Infect Immun 1995;63:3543–3549.

144. Montgomery RR, Malawista SE: *Borrelia burgdorferi* and the macrophage: Routine annihilation but occasional haven? Parasitol Today 1994;10:154–157.

145. Pavia CS, Kissel V, Bittker S, et al: Antiborrelial activity of serum from rats injected with the Lyme disease spirochete. J Infect Dis 1991;163:656–659.

146. Kochi SK, Johnson RC: Role of immunoglobulin G in killing of *Borrelia burgdorferi* by the classical complement pathway. Infect Immun 1988;56:314–321.

147. Nowling JM, Philipp MT: Killing of *Borrelia burgdorferi* by antibody elicited by OspA vaccine is inefficient in the absence of complement. Infect Immun 1999;67:463–465.

148. Bockenstedt LK, Fikrig E, Barthold SW, et al: Inability of truncated recombinant Osp A proteins to elicit protective immunity to *Borrelia burgdorferi* in mice. J Immunol 1993;151:900–906.

149. Fikrig E, Barthold SW, Persing DH, et al: *Borrelia burgdorferi* strain 25015: Characterization of outer surface protein A and vaccination against infection. J Immunol 1992; 148:2256–2260.

150. Fikrig E, Telford SR III, Wallich R, et al: Vaccination against Lyme disease caused by diverse *Borrelia burgdorferi*. J Exp Med 1995;181:215–222.

151. Sears JE, Fikrig E, Nakagawa TY, et al: Molecular mapping of Osp-A mediated immunity against *Borrelia burgdorferi*, the agent of Lyme disease. J Immunol 1991;147:1995–2000.

152. Ding W, Huang X, Yang X, et al: Structural identification of a key protective B-cell epitope in Lyme disease antigen Osp A. J Mol Biol 2000;302:1153–1164.

153. Golde WT, Piesman J, Dolan MC, et al: Reactivity with a specific epitope of outer surface protein A predicts protection from infection with the Lyme disease spirochete, *Borrelia burgdorferi*. Infect Immun 1997;65:882–889.

154. Kurtenbach K, Sewell H-S, Ogden NH, et al: Serum complement sensitivity as a key factor in Lyme disease ecology. Infect Immun 1998;66:1248–1251.

155. Kuo MM, Lane RS, Gicias PC: A comparative study of mammalian and reptilian alternative pathway of complement-mediated killing of the Lyme disease spirochete (*Borrelia burgdorferi*). J Parasitol 2000;86:1223–1228.

156. McKisic MD, Redmond WL, Barthold SW: Cutting edge: T-cell-mediated pathology in murine Lyme borreliosis. J Immunol 2000;165:6096–6099.

157. Onrust SV, Goa KL: Adjuvanted Lyme disease vaccine. A review of its use in the management of Lyme disease. Drugs 2000;59:281–299.

158. Steere AC, Sikand VK, Meurice F, et al: Vaccination against Lyme disease with recombinant *Borrelia burgdorferi* outer-surface lipoprotein A with adjuvant. N Engl J Med 1998;339:209–215.

159. Van Hoecke C, Lebacq E, Beran J, Parenti D: Alternative vaccination schedules (0,1 and 6 months versus 0, 1 and 12 months) for a recombinant Osp A Lyme disease vaccine. Clin Infect Dis 1999;28:1260–1264.

160. Wormser GP, Nowakowski J, Nadelman RB, et al: Efficacy of an OspA vaccine preparation for prevention of Lyme disease in New York State. Infection 1998;26:208–212.

161. Smith RP, Schoen RT, Rahn DW, et al: Clinical characteristics and treatment outcome of early Lyme disease in patients with microbiologically confirmed erythema migrans. Ann Intern Med 2002;136:421–428.

162. Schoen RT, Meurice F, Brunet CM, et al: Safety and immunogenicity of an outer surface protein A vaccine in subjects with previous Lyme disease. J Infect Dis 1995;172:1324–1329.

163. Van Hoecke C, Comberback M, De Grave D, et al: Evaluation of the safety, reactogenicity and immunogenicity of three recombinant outer surface protein (Osp A) Lyme vaccines in healthy adults. Vaccine 1996;14:1620–1626.

164. Craft JE, Fischer DK, Shimamoto GT, Steere AC: Antigens of *Borrelia burgdorferi* recognized during Lyme disease. Appearance of a new immunoglobulin M response and expansion of the immunoglobulin G response late in the illness. J Clin Invest 1986;78:934–939.

165. Gross DM, Forsthuber T, Tary-Lehmann M, et al: Identification of LFA-1 as a candidate autoantigen in treatment resistant Lyme arthritis. Science 1998;281:703–706.

166. Kalish RA, Leong JM, Steere AC: Association of treatment-resistant chronic Lyme arthritis with HLA-DR4 and antibody reactivity to OspA and OspB of *Borrelia burgdorferi*. Infect Immun 1993;61:2774–2779.

167. Lengl-JanBen B, Strauss AF, Steere AC, Kamradt T: The T helper cell response in Lyme arthritis: Differential recognition of *Borrelia burgdorferi* outer surface protein A in patients with treatment-resistant or treatment-responsive Lyme arthritis. J Exp Med 1994;180:2069–2078.

168. Steere AC, Gross D, Meyer AL, Huber BT: Autoimmune mechanisms in antibiotic treatment–resistant Lyme arthritis. J Autoimmun 2001;16:263–268.

169. Parenti D: Outer surface protein A and arthritis in hamsters. Infect Immun 2000;68:7212.

170. Hayes EB, Schriefer ME: Lyme disease vaccine. In Gray JS, Kahl O, Lane R, Stanek G (eds): Lyme Borreliosis: Biology of the Infectious Agents and Epidemiology of the Disease. Wallingford, OXON, UK, CAB International, 2002, pp. 281–293.

171. Schoen RT, Sikand VK, Caldwell MC, et al: Safety and immunogenicity profile of a recombinant outer-surface protein A Lyme disease vaccine: Clinical trial of a 3-dose schedule at 0, 1, and 2 months. Clin Ther 2000;22:315–325.

172. Centers for Disease Control and Prevention: Recommendations for the use of Lyme disease vaccine: Recommendations of the Advisory Committee on Immunization Practices (ACIP). MMWR Morb Mortal Wkly Rep 1999;48:1–25.

173. Feder HM, Beran J, Van Hoecke C, et al: Safety and immunogenicity in children and adolescents of a recombinant *Borrelia burgdorferi* outer-surface protein A vaccine against Lyme disease. J Pediatr 1999;135:575–579.

174. Beran J, DeClercq N, Dieussaert I, Van Hoecke C: Reactogenicity and immunogenicity of a Lyme disease vaccine in children 2–5 years old. Clin Infect Dis 2000;31:1504–1507.

175. Meltzer MI, Dennis DT, Orloski KA: The cost-effectiveness of vaccinating against Lyme disease. Emerg Infect Dis 1999;5:321–328.

176. Shadick MA, Liang MH, Phillips CB, et al: The cost-effectiveness of vaccination against Lyme disease. Arch Intern Med 2001;161:554–561.

177. deSilva AM, Fikrig E: Arthropod and host-specific gene expression by *Borrelia burgdorferi*. J Clin Invest 1997;99:377–379.

178. Schwan TG, Piesman J: Temporal changes in outer surface proteins A and C of the Lyme disease-associated spirochete, *Borrelia burgdorferi*, during the chain of infection in ticks and mice. J Clin Microbiol 2000;38:382–388.

179. Schwan TG, Piesman J, Golde WT, et al: Induction of an outer surface protein on *Borrelia burgdorferi* during tick feeding. Proc Natl Acad Sci USA 1995;92:2909–2913.

180. Golde WT, Kappel KJ, Dequesne G, et al: Tick transmission of *Borrelia burgdorferi* to inbred strains of mice induces an antibody response to p39 but not to outer surface protein A. Infect Immun 1994;62:2625–2627.

181. Barthold SE, de Souza MS, Janotka JL, et al: Chronic Lyme borreliosis in the laboratory mouse. Am J Pathol 1993; 143:959–971.

182. Yang X, Goldberg MS, Papova TG, et al: Interdependence of environmental factors influencing reciprocal patterns of gene expression in virulent *Borrelia burgdorferi*. Mol Microbiol 2000;37:1470–1479.

183. Telford SR III, Fikrig E, Barthold SW, et al: Protection against antigenically variable *Borrelia burgdorferi* conferred by recombinant vaccines. J Exp Med 1993;178:755–758.

184. Shih C-M, Spielman A, Telford SR III: Mode of action of protective immunity to Lyme disease spirochetes. Am J Trop Med Hyg 1995;52:72–74.

185. Fikrig E, Telford SR III, Barthold SW, et al: Elimination of *Borrelia burgdorferi* from vector ticks feeding on Osp-A immunized mice. Proc Natl Acad Sci USA 1992; 89:5418–5421.

186. de Silva AM, Telford SR, Brunet LR, et al: *Borrelia burgdorferi* OspA is an arthropod-specific transmission blocking Lyme disease vaccine. J Exp Med 1996;183:271–275.

187. de Silva AM, Zeidner NS, Zhang Y, et al: Influence of outer surface protein A antibody on *Borrelia burgdorferi* within feeding ticks. Infect Immun 1999;67:30–35.

188. Shih C-M, Liu L-P: Differential efficacy of passive immunization against infection by Lyme disease spirochetes transmitted by partially fed vector ticks. J Med Microbiol 1998;47:773–779.

189. Zung JL, Lewengrub S, Rudzinska MA, et al: Fine structural evidence for the penetration of the Lyme disease spirochete *Borrelia burgdorferi* through the gut and salivary tissues of *Ixodes dammini*. Can J Zool 1989;67:1737.

190. Wang H, Nuttall PA: Excretion of host immunoglobulin in tick saliva and detection of IgG-binding proteins in tick haemolymph and salivary glands. Parasitology 1994;109:525–530.

191. Wilske B, Barbour AG, Bergström S, et al: Antigenic variation and strain heterogeneity in *Borrelia* spp. Res Microbiol 1992;143:583–596.

192. Dykhuizen DE, Polin DS, Dunn JJ, et al: *Borrelia burgdorferi* is clonal: Implications for taxonomy and vaccine development. Proc Natl Acad Sci USA 1993;90:10163–10167.

193. Milch LJ, Barbour AG: Analysis of North American and European isolates of *Borrelia burgdorferi* with antiserum to a recombinant antigen. J Infect Dis 1989;160:351–353.

194. Wilske B, Preac-Mursic V, Göbel UB, et al: An OspA serotyping system for *Borrelia burgdorferi* based on reactivity with monoclonal antibodies and OspA sequence analysis. J Clin Microbiol 1993;31:340–350.

195. Lovrich SD, Callister SM, Lim LCL, et al: Seroprotective groups of Lyme borreliosis spirochetes from North America and Europe. J Infect Dis 1994;170:115–121.

196. Wallich R, Helmes C, Schaible UE, et al: Evaluation of genetic divergence among *Borrelia burgdorferi* isolates by use of OspA, *fla*, HSP60 and HSP70 gene probes. Infect Immun 1992;60:4856–4866.

197. Wilske B, Preac-Mursic V, Schierz G, et al: Antigenic variability of *Borrelia burgdorferi*. Ann NY Acad Sci 1988;539:126–143.

198. Marconi RT, Garon CF: Phylogenetic analysis of the genus *Borrelia burgdorferi*. J Bacteriol 1992;174:241–244.

199. Mathiesen DA, Oliver JH Jr, Kolbert CP, et al: Genetic heterogeneity of *Borrelia burgdorferi* in the United States. J Infect Dis 1997;175:98–107.

200. Gern L, Hu CM, Voet P, et al: Immunization with a polyvalent OspA vaccine protects mice against *Ixodes ricinus* tick bites infected by *Borrelia burgdorferi* ss, *Borrelia garinii* and *Borrelia afzelii*. Vaccine 1997;15:1551–1557.

201. Spielman A, Wilson ML, Levine JF, Piesman J: Ecology of *Ixodes dammini*–borne human babesiosis and Lyme disease. Annu Rev Entomol 1985;30:439–460.

202. Piesman J, Hicks TC, Sinsky RJ, Obin G: Simultaneous transmission of *Borrelia burgdorferi* and *Babesia microti* by individual nymphal *Ixodes dammini* ticks. J Clin Microbiol 1987;25:2012–2013.

203. Centers for Disease Control and Prevention: Recommendations for test performance and interpretation from the Second National Conference on Serologic Diagnosis of Lyme Disease. MMWR Morb Mortal Wkly Rep 1995;44:590–591.

204. Aguero-Rosenfeld ME, Roberge J, Carbonaro CA, et al: Effects of OspA vaccination on Lyme disease serologic testing. J Clin Microbiol 1999;37:3718–3721.

205. Fawcett PT, Rose CD, Budd SM, Gibney KM: Effect of immunization with recombinant OspA on serologic tests for Lyme borreliosis. Clin Diag Lab Immunol 2001;8:79–84.

206. Molloy PJ, Berardi VP, Persing DH, Sigal LH: Detection of multiple reactive protein species by immunoblotting after recombinant outer surface protein A Lyme disease vaccination. Clin Infect Dis 2000;31:42–47.

207. Johnson RC, Kodner C, Russell M: In vitro and in vivo susceptibility of the Lyme disease spirochete, *Borrelia burgdorferi*, to four antimicrobial agents. Antimicrob Agents Chemother 1987;31:164–167.

208. Nowakowski J, Wormser GP: Treatment of early Lyme disease: Infection associated with erythema migrans. In Coyle PK (ed): Lyme Disease. St. Louis, Mosby Yearbook, 1993, pp 149–162.

209. Nowakowski J, McKenna D, Nadelman RB, et al: Failure of treatment with cephalexin for Lyme disease. Arch Fam Med 2000;9:563–567.

210. Gerber MA, Shapiro ED, Burke GS, et al: Lyme disease in children in southeastern Connecticut. N Engl J Med 1996;335:1270–1274.

211. Steere AC: Lyme disease. N Engl J Med 2001;345:115–125.

212. Steere AC, Hutchinson GJ, Rahn DW, et al: Treatment of early manifestations of Lyme disease. Ann Intern Med 1983;99:22–26.

213. Dattwyler RJ, Volkman DJ, Conaty SM, et al: Amoxicillin plus probenecid versus doxycycline for treatment of erythema migrans borreliosis. Lancet 1990;336:1404–1406.

214. Massarotti EM, Luger SW, Rahn DW, et al: Treatment of early Lyme disease. Am J Med 1992;92:396–403.

215. Nadelman RB, Luger SW, Frank E, et al: Comparison of cefuroxime axetil and doxycycline in the treatment of early Lyme disease. Ann Intern Med 1992;117:273–280.

216. Luger SW, Paparone P, Wormser GP, et al: Comparison of cefuroxime axetil and doxycycline in treatment of patients with early Lyme disease associated with erythema migrans. Antimicrob Agents Chemother 1995;39:661–667.

217. Luft BJ, Dattwyler RJ, Johnson RC, et al: Azithromycin compared with amoxicillin in the treatment of erythema migrans: A double-blind, randomized, controlled trial. Ann Intern Med 1996;124:785–791.

218. Dattwyler RJ, Luft BJ, Kunkel M, et al: Ceftriaxone compared with doxycycline for the treatment of acute disseminated Lyme disease. N Engl J Med 1997;337:289–294.

219. Dever LL, Jorgensen JH, Barbour AG: Comparative in vitro activities of clarithromycin, azithromycin, and erythromycin against *Borrelia burgdorferi*. Antimicrob Agents Chemother 1993;37:1704–1706.

220. Wormser GP: Lyme disease: Insights into the use of antimicrobials for prevention and treatment in the context of experience with other spirochetal infections. Mt. Sinai J Med 1995;62:188–195.

221. Hansen K, Hovmark A, Lebech A-M, et al: Roxithromycin in Lyme borreliosis: Discrepant results of an in vitro and in vivo animal susceptibility study and a clinical trial in patients with erythema migrans. Acta Derm Venereol 1992;72:297–300.

222. Barsic B, Maretic T, Majerus L, Strugar J: Comparison of azithromycin and doxycycline in the treatment of erythema migrans. Infection 2000;28:153–156.

223. Strle F, Maraspin V, Lotric-Furlan S, et al: Azithromycin and doxycycline for treatment of *Borrelia* culture-positive erythema migrans. Infection 1996;24:64–68.

224. Weber K, Wilske B, Preac-Mursic V, Thurmayr R: Azithromycin versus penicillin V for treatment of early Lyme borreliosis. Infection 1993;21:367–372.

225. Strle F, Ruzic E, Cimperman J: Erythema migrans: Comparison of treatment with azithromycin, doxycycline and phenoxymethyl penicillin. J Antimicrob Chemother 1992;30:543–550.

226. Strle F, Preac-Mursic V, Cimperman J, et al: Azithromycin versus doxycycline for treatment of erythema migrans: Clinical and microbiologic findings. Infection 1993;21:83–88.

227. Dattwyler RJ, Grunwaldt E, Luft BJ: Clarithromycin in treatment of early Lyme disease: A pilot study. Antimicrob Agents Chemother 1996;40:468–469.

228. Nowakowski J, Nadelman RB, Sell R, et al: Outcome of culture-confirmed cases of Lyme disease: Report of 94 patients with 96 episodes of erythema migrans followed prospectively for up to 9 years. (Manuscript submitted).

229. Telford SR III, Dawson JE, Katavalos P, et al: Perpetuation of the agent of human granulocytic ehrlichiosis in a deer tick–rodent cycle. Proc Natl Acad Sci USA 1996; 93:6209–6214.

230. Duffy J, Pittlekow MR, Kolbert P, et al: Coinfection with *Borrelia burgdorferi* and the agent of human granulocytic ehrlichiosis. Lancet 1997;349:399.

231. Maraspin V, Cimperman J, Lotric-Furlan S, et al: Treatment of erythema migrans in pregnancy. Clin Infect Dis 1996;22:788–793.

232. Williams CL, Strobino B, Weinstein A, et al: Maternal Lyme disease and congenital malformation: A cord blood serosurvey in endemic and control areas. Paediatr Perinat Epidemiol 1995;9:320–330.

233. Strobino BA, Williams CL, Abid S, et al: Lyme disease and pregnancy outcome: A prospective study of 2000 prenatal patients. Am J Obstet Gynecol 1993;169:367–374.

234. Wormser GP: Treatment and prevention of Lyme disease, with emphasis on antimicrobial therapy for neuroborreliosis and vaccination. Semin Neurol 1997;17:45–52.

235. Steere AC, Pachner AR, Malawista SE: Neurologic abnormalities of Lyme disease: Successful treatment with high-dose intravenous penicillin. Ann Intern Med 1983;99:767–772.

236. Clark JR, Carlson RD, Sasaki CT, et al: Facial paralysis in Lyme disease. Laryngoscope 1985;95:1341–1345.

237. Kruger H, Kohlhepp W, Konig S: Follow-up of antibiotically treated and untreated neuroborreliosis. Acta Neurol Scand 1990;82:59–67.

238. Pfister HW, Einhaupl KM, Franz P, Garner C: Corticosteroids for radicular pain in Bannwarth's syndrome. A double-blind, randomized, placebo-controlled trial. Ann NY Acad Sci 1988;539:485–487.

239. Kristoferitsch W: Neuropathien bei Lyme-borreliose. Berlin, Springer-Verlag, 1989.

240. Pfister HW, Einhaupl KM, Garner C, Herberl R: Corticosteroids versus penicillin in the treatment of meningoradiculitis of Bannwarth (Bannwarth's syndrome). J Neurol (Suppl) 1985;231:293.

241. Reik L, Steere AC, Bartenhagen NH, et al: Neurologic abnormalities of Lyme disease. Medicine 1979;58:281–294.

242. Pfister H-W, Preac-Mursic V, Wilske B, et al: Randomized comparison of ceftriaxone and cefotaxime in Lyme neuroborreliosis. J Infect Dis 1991;163:311–318.

243. Pfister HW, Preac-Mursic V, Wilske B, Einhaupl KM: Cefotaxime vs penicillin G for acute neurologic manifestations in Lyme borreliosis: A prospective randomized study. Arch Neurol 1989;46:1190–1194.

244. Dotevall L, Alestig K, Hanner P, et al: The use of doxycycline in nervous system *Borrelia burgdorferi* infection. Scand J Infect Dis Suppl 1988;53:74–79.

245. Dotevall L, Hagberg L: Successful oral doxycycline treatment of Lyme disease–associated facial palsy and meningitis. Clin Infect Dis 1999;28:569–574.

246. Karlsson M, Hammers-Berggren S, Lindquist L, et al: Comparison of intravenous penicillin G and oral doxycycline for treatment of Lyme neuroborreliosis. Neurology 1994;44:1203–1207.

247. Kohlhepp W, Oschmann P, Mertens H-G: Treatment of Lyme borreliosis: Randomized comparison of doxycycline and penicillin G. J Neurol 1989;236:464–469.

248. Rohacova H, Hancil J, Hulinska D, et al: Ceftriaxone in the treatment of Lyme neuroborreliosis. Infection 1996; 24:90–92.

249. Bingham PM, Galetta SL, Athreya B, Sladky J: Neurological manifestations in children with Lyme disease. Pediatrics 1995;96:1053–1056.

250. Krbkova L, Stanek G: Therapy of Lyme borreliosis in children. Infection 1996;24:170–177.

251. Steere AC, Batsford WP, Weinberg M, et al: Lyme carditis: Lyme carditis: Cardiac abnormalities of Lyme disease. Ann Intern Med 1980;93:8–16.

252. Steere AC, Green J, Schoen RT, et al: Successful parenteral penicillin therapy of established Lyme arthritis. N Engl J Med 1985;312:869–874.

253. Dattwyler RJ, Halperin JJ, Pass H, Luft BJ: Ceftriaxone as effective therapy for refractory Lyme disease. J Infect Dis 1987;155:1322–1325.

254. Dattwyler RJ, Halperin JJ, Volkman DJ, Luft BJ: Treatment of late Lyme borreliosis: Randomized comparison of ceftriaxone and penicillin. Lancet 1988;1:1191–1194.

255. Dattwyler RJ, Luft BJ, Maladorno D, et al: Treatment of late Lyme disease—a comparison of 2 weeks vs 4 weeks of ceftriaxone [abstract 662]. In Proceedings of the Seventh International Congress on Lyme Borreliosis (San Francisco), June 16–21, 1996.

256. Eichenfield AH, Goldsmith DP, Benach JL, et al: Childhood Lyme arthritis: Experience in an endemic area. J Pediatr 1986;109:753–758.

257. Eckman MH, Steere AC, Kalish RA, Pauker SG: Cost effectiveness of oral as compared with intravenous antibiotic treatment for patients with early Lyme disease or Lyme arthritis. N Engl J Med 1997;337:357–363.

258. Steere AC, Schoen R, Taylor E: The clinical evolution of Lyme arthritis. Ann Intern Med 1987;107:725–731.

259. Steere AC, Levin RE, Molloy PJ, et al: Treatment of Lyme arthritis. Arthritis Rheum 1994;37:878–888.

260. Nocton JJ, Dressler F, Rutledge BJ, et al: Detection of *Borrelia burgdorferi* by polymerase chain reaction in synovial fluid from patients with Lyme arthritis. N Engl J Med 1994;330:229–234.

261. Schoen RT, Aversa JM, Rahn DW, Steere AC: Treatment of refractory chronic Lyme arthritis with arthroscopic synovectomy. Arthritis Rheum 1991;34:1056–1060.

262. Logigian EL, Kaplan RF, Steere AC: Chronic neurologic manifestations of Lyme disease. N Engl J Med 1990;323:1438–1444.

263. Logigian EL, Kaplan RF, Steere AC: Successful treatment of Lyme encephalopathy with intravenous ceftriaxone. J Infect Dis 1999;180:377–383.

264. Hassler D, Zoller L, Haude A, et al: Cefotaxime versus penicillin in the late stage of Lyme disease: Prospective, randomized therapeutic approach. Infection 1990;18:16–20.

265. Ettestad PJ, Campbell GL, Welbel SF, et al: Biliary complications in the treatment of unsubstantiated Lyme disease. J Infect Dis 1995;171:356–361.

266. Logigian EL, Steere AC: Clinical and electrophysiologic findings in chronic neuropathy of Lyme disease. Neurology 1992;42:303–311.

267. Bloom BJ, Wyckoff PM, Meissner HC, Steere AC: Neurocognitive abnormalities in children after classic manifestations of Lyme disease. Pediatr Infect Dis J 1998;17:189–196.

268. Seltzer EG, Gerber MA, Cartter ML, et al: Long-term outcomes of persons with Lyme disease. JAMA 2000;283:609–616.

269. Klempner MS, Hu LT, Evans J, et al: Two controlled trials of antibiotic treatment in patients with persistent symptoms and a history of Lyme disease. N Engl J Med 2001;345:85–92.

270. Nadelman RB, Nowakowski J, Forseter G, et al: Failure to isolate *Borrelia burgdorferi* after antimicrobial therapy in culture-documented Lyme borreliosis associated with erythema migrans: report of a prospective study. Am J Med 1993;94:583–588.

271. Berger BW, Johnson RC, Kodner C, Coleman L: Failure of *Borrelia burgdorferi* to survive in the skin of patients with antibiotic-treated Lyme disease. J Am Acad Dermatol 1992;27:34–37.

272. Preac-Mursic V, Weber K, Pfister HW, et al: Survival of *Borrelia burgdorferi* in antibiotically treated patients with Lyme disease. Infection 1989;17:355–359.

273. Steere AC. *Borrelia burgdorferi* (Lyme disease, Lyme borreliosis). In Mandell, GL, Bennett JE, Dolan R (eds): Mandell, Douglas, and Bennett's Principles and Practice of Infectious Diseases, 5th ed. Philadelphia, Churchill Livingston, 2000, pp 2504–2518.

274. Treatment of Lyme disease. Med Lett Drugs Ther 1992;34:95–97.

275. Treatment of Lyme disease. Med Lett Drugs Ther 1997;39:47–48.

276. Treatment of Lyme disease. Med Lett Drugs Ther 2000;42:37–39.

277. Nowakowski J, Nadelman R, Forseter G, et al: Doxycycline versus tetracycline therapy for Lyme disease associated with erythema migrans. J Am Acad Dermatol 1995; 32:223–227.

278. Wormser GP, Nowakowski J, Nadelman RB: Duration of treatment for Lyme borreliosis: Time for a critical reappraisal. Wien Klin Wochenschr 2002;114:613–615.

279. Klempner MS, Noring R, Rogers RA: Invasion of human skin fibroblasts by the Lyme disease spirochete, *Borrelia burgdorferi*. J Infect Dis 1993;167:1074–1081.

280. Butler T, Jones PK, Wallace CK: *Borrelia recurrentis* infection: Single-dose antibiotic regimens and management of Jarisch-Herxheimer reaction. J Infect Dis 1978;137:573–577.

281. Weber K, Preac-Mursic V, Wilske B, et al: A randomized trial of ceftriaxone versus oral penicillin for the treatment of early European Lyme borreliosis. Infection 1990;18:91–96.

282. Moody KD, Adams RL, Barthold SW: Effectiveness of antimicrobial treatment against *Borrelia burgdorferi* infection in mice. Antimicrob Agents Chemother 1994;38:1567–1572.

283. Mursic VP, Wilske B, Schierz G, et al: In vitro and in vivo susceptibility of *Borrelia burgdorferi*. Eur J Clin Microbiol 1987;6:424–426.

284. Pavia C, Inchiosa MA Jr, Wormser GP: Efficacy of short-course ceftriaxone therapy for *Borrelia burgdorferi* infection in C3H mice. Antimicrob Agents Chemother 2002;46:132–134.

285. Kazragis RJ, Dever LL, Jorgensen JH, Barbour AG: In vivo activities of ceftriaxone and vancomycin against *Borrelia* spp. in the mouse brain and other sites. Antimicrob Agents Chemother 1996;40:2632–2636.

286. Patel IH, Kaplan SA: Pharmacokinetic profile of ceftriaxone in man. Am J Med 1984;77(4C):17–25.

287. Van Ogtrop ML, Mattie H, Guiot HFL, et al: Comparative study of the effects of four cephalosporins against *Escherichia coli* in vitro and in vivo. Antimicrob Agents Chemother 1990;34:1932–1937.

288. Gombert ME, Berkowitz LB, Aulicino TM, DuBouchet L: Therapy of pulmonary nocardiosis in immunocompromised mice. Antimicrob Agents Chemother 1990;34:1766–1768.

Bioterrorism

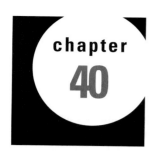

Plague, Anthrax, and Smallpox

MARK G. KORTEPETER, MD, MPH
THEODORE J. CIESLAK, MD

HISTORY OF BIOLOGIC WEAPONS AND BIOTERRORISM

In the fall of 2001, the use of envelopes containing *Bacillus Anthracis* spores as a vehicle for spreading disease intentionally has increased concern about the use of biologic pathogens as weapons for terrorism and warfare.

Despite the recent interest in biologic weapons and bioterrorism in the lay press, popular media, and literature the concept of using biologic pathogens to kill or incapacitate one's adversaries has arisen periodically throughout history.[1] Before the advent of modern microbiologic techniques, armies used various crude methods to spread biologic weapons and contagion among the adversary's forces. Methods could be as unsophisticated as smearing excrement on sharpened stakes ("pungi sticks"), as was used by the Viet Cong during the Vietnam War, or contaminating an adversary's well with feces or carcasses.[1,2]

Biologic warfare is defined as the use of organisms or toxins derived from living organisms to produce death or disability in humans, animals, or plants.[3] Therefore biologic weapons not only can kill or incapacitate humans but also have the potential to be used as weapons of economic warfare against animal and crop industries. The 2001 outbreak of foot and mouth disease in Great Britain provides a good example of the devastating impact of animal diseases on an economy. This chapter will deal only with the treatment and prevention of human disease. When one discusses bioterrorism, then, typically one refers to persons or groups that use biologic weapons for a specific religious, political, or ideological motivation. This distinguishes the use of pathogens in acts of terrorism from their use in the perpetration of a crime for motives other than terrorism per se.[4]

One of the earliest attempted uses of a biologic weapon occurred in 1346 in the Crimean port city of Kaffa (now Feodosia, Ukraine). Tatar invaders laid siege to the city but had an outbreak of bubonic plague occur in their ranks. They came upon the idea of catapulting their dead over the city's walls.[5] The Genoese defenders within the walls subsequently suffered an outbreak of plague and fled to Italy. They brought with them to the continent of Europe the notorious "black death," which wiped out approximately one-third of the population. Another commonly cited example of biologic weapon use occurred during the French and Indian War in North America. The British, under the command of Sir Jeffrey Amherst, gave blankets and handkerchiefs contaminated with smallpox to Indian allies of the French under the guise of "gifts." Subsequent outbreaks of smallpox among the Indians may have been related to the gifts. Although both stories are popularly cited, they exemplify the difficulty in verifying that an endemic disease was spread intentionally.[2] Our knowledge of plague

The opinions and assertions contained herein are the private views of the authors and are not to be construed as official or as necessarily reflecting the views of the Department of Defense, the United States Army, or the U.S. Army Medical Research Institute of Infectious Diseases.

TABLE 40–1 ■ Estimated Illness due to Release of 50 kg of an Agent Along a 2-km Front, Upwind of a City of 500,000 People in a Developing Country

Agent	Downwind carriage (km)	Deaths	Incapacitated, including deaths
Venezuelan equine encephalitis	1	400	35,000
Tick-borne encephalitis	1	9,500	35,000
Influenza	1	100	35,000
Epidemic typhus	5	19,000	85,000
Rocky Mountain spotted fever	5	11,500	85,000
Brucellosis	10	500	100,000
Plague	10	55,000	100,000
Q fever	>20	150	125,000
Tularemia	>20	30,000	125,000
Anthrax	>>20	95,000	125,000

From WHO Group of Consultants: Health Aspects of Chemical and Biological Weapons. Geneva, World Health Organization, 1970.

information from the vast Internet database. In addition numerous "how to" manuals detail the steps necessary, for example, to extract the biologic toxin ricin from castor beans. Finally, concerns have been raised that persons previously employed by state-funded biological warfare programs may be recruited by countries that sponsor terrorism or directly by terrorist organizations.[4] With the crumbling economy of the former Soviet Union, many scientists have found themselves unemployed or at best underpaid and may be susceptible to such recruitment.[15]

BARRIERS TO USE OF BIOWEAPONS

Although there are many reasons terrorists might choose a bioweapon, one must recognize that there are certain constraints, which in many cases present formidable barriers to their production and employment, at least as far as large-scale releases and mass casualty production are concerned. Because biologic weapons are living organisms or proteins, they are generally sensitive to environmental conditions such as wind, sunlight, heat, and rain. An effective release over a large population requires specific conditions such as a slow, steady wind and atmospheric inversion conditions. An inversion tends to keep particles close to the ground and increases the chance of contact with the target population. Although biologic pathogens can be obtained and produced relatively easily if one has the appropriate training and equipment, one difficult hurdle the terrorist must overcome concerns the need to produce an agent of the requisite particle size necessary to optimally infect the human respiratory tract. The biologic weapons programs of the United States and the Soviet Union spent millions of dollars and years of research developing such capabilities. Most terrorists would likely not have the ability to produce better than a crude biologic weapon. In fact some would argue that the money being spent on bioterrorism defense is ill advised, partly because of such hurdles.[23,24] The requirement for specific weather conditions may have an impact on

whether a biologic weapon might be used tactically on the battlefield; however, in the case of a terrorist attempting an indoor release, the hindrance of weather and other environmental conditions is of less importance.

POTENTIAL BIOWEAPONS—THE THREAT LIST

Hundreds of pathogens can produce disease in humans, but only a handful cause concern as potential weapons. Many of these pathogens are zoonotic, affecting both humans and animals. A number of properties of biologic pathogens or toxins must be considered when evaluating them as potential weapons. The most efficient way to infect or intoxicate large numbers of humans is through an airborne release resulting in inhalational exposure. Therefore the stability of a pathogen in aerosol form is a key consideration. Another requisite property is that it retain its virulence while being mass produced. Although many pathogens may cause devastating disease, an agent that causes a high illness-to-infection ratio is desirable for an efficient weapon. This explains why a virus such as Venezuelan equine encephalitis virus, an incapacitating pathogen that causes clinical illness in nearly 100% of infected individuals, is on the weapons threat list, whereas another agent such as Japanese encephalitis virus is not. The latter causes a large number of subclinical infections for every symptomatic infection it produces, making it potentially less attractive to the weaponeer. Whether a lethal or incapacitating pathogen is preferable to the perpetrator would depend on his or her motives. In the context of warfare an incapacitating pathogen could have a more detrimental effect than a lethal one because of the logistical requirement for personnel to care for the victims. Thirty-nine pathogens are listed in a NATO handbook dealing with potential biologic warfare agents and toxins.[25] A group of Russian scientists also compiled a list of what they termed "especially dangerous pathogens."[26] They used a scoring system that rated potential pathogens according to several criteria: infective dose by aerosol, environmental stability, contagiousness, disease severity, rapid diagnostics capabilities, prophylaxis, and treatment methods. The top four pathogens listed by the Russians, from highest to lowest were smallpox, plague, anthrax, and botulism.

Unfortunately one cannot predict which specific properties a terrorist might be interested in and therefore which agent might be chosen to infect or intoxicate a person or a population. Moreover terrorists might employ "weapons of opportunity," that is, weapons that are readily available to a member of a group. Therefore rather than focusing on terrorist motivations, public health authorities have concentrated their efforts on evaluating which pathogens could potentially cause mass casualties that would overwhelm medical capabilities and cause widespread fear and civil unrest. The similarities in the threat lists that were developed by working groups of U.S. experts in this field are interesting. Two separate working groups from the Center for Civilian Biodefense at Johns Hopkins University[27,28] and the Centers for Disease Control and Prevention (CDC)[29,30] came up with lists similar to the one developed by the group of Russian scientists.[26] The CDC panel considered numerous factors in putting together their agent threat list, including the impact on public health; pathogen stability; ease of production; requirements for dissemination; stockpiling needs for treatment, antidotes, surveillance, and diagnosis; and the public's perception and potential for civil disorder related to panic.

The CDC working group placed putative threat agents into three categories. Category A agents are those with the greatest potential for eliciting fear and disruption and having public health impact, necessitating the most intense preparedness requirements. The agents in category A are the same as those on the Johns Hopkins list: smallpox, anthrax, plague, tularemia, botulinum toxin, and certain viral hemorrhagic fevers. Category B includes agents, such as C. burnetii and Brucella spp, with potential for aerosol dissemination but with fewer requirements for additional preparedness measures. Category C agents are those that constitute potential emerging public health threats, such as nipah virus and Hantavirus. The balance of this chapter will focus on the diseases at the top of Category A as they relate to bioterrorism: anthrax, smallpox, and plague. Readers are referred to the complementary or other texts for more in-depth coverage of other aspects of those diseases.

The three diseases share several important properties: All have high fatality rates. All can potentially be produced in large quantities and stabilized for aerosol dissemination. All three are known historical scourges that have devastated the human population at some time in history. The names anthrax, smallpox, and plague all conjure up images of horrific illness in the affected population that would likely influence the public's reaction and potential panic should an outbreak occur with any one of them. All are rarely, if ever, seen in the United States; therefore most clinicians have little if any experience diagnosing and managing patients

with these diseases. Availability of vaccines for all is currently limited or nonexistent. All have been developed for weaponization by a major world power.[11,13,15,16]

ANTHRAX

The name anthrax derives from the Greek word for coal and is so named because of the black eschar typically seen in cutaneous disease. Over the centuries, animals (herbivores, including sheep, goats, cattle) have been primarily affected by the disease, caused by infection with *Bacillus anthracis*, a nonmotile, gram-positive, sporulating bacillus. Humans generally become infected as a result of occupational exposures when they work with animals in the wool, bone meal, or tannery industries—hence the synonyms woolsorter's or ragpicker's disease.

In the early 20th century approximately 130 cases of human anthrax were reported annually in the United States, most of which were of the cutaneous form.[31] In the fall of 2001, an outbreak occurred of 11 cases of inhalation anthrax related to *B. Anthracis*-contaminated letters. Before that, the last case of inhalational anthrax in the United States was reported in 1978.[32] Control measures, including inspection and vaccination of livestock and vaccination of veterinarians and textile workers, and the decline of the wool mill industry have led to a decline in human and animal cases of anthrax. Even so, anthrax periodically causes devastating disease in humans as well as animals. An outbreak of anthrax in Zimbabwe from October 1979 through March 1980 caused over 6000 reported human cases[33–35] and has been alleged to have been intentionally fostered.[36] In addition, exposures occasionally are related to viable spores dormant in the soil in various parts of the United States. In 2000 a cow suffering from anthrax was slaughtered in Minnesota, and the meat subsequently was consumed by the owner's family. The family was provided ciprofloxacin prophylaxis, and there were no confirmed human cases as a result of the exposures.[37] The first confirmed human case of cutaneous anthrax in the United States since 1992 occurred in 2000 as a result of animal contact during a large livestock epizootic in North Dakota.[38] Additional cases occurred concomitant with the inhalation outbreak in 2001.

Three forms of anthrax may occur in humans. Although each presents different clinical manifestations, the pathogenesis of the three forms is similar, regardless of the route of infection. Spores gain entry into the body through abraded skin, ingestion, or inhalation. Spores are then engulfed by local macrophages, where they then germinate. After germination the vegetative bacteria may replicate in the local area (cutaneous disease) or may be transported to the regional lymph nodes in the gastrointestinal tract or lungs. Bacteria further replicate in the lymph nodes and concomitantly release three proteins: edema factor, lethal factor, and protective antigen (PA). PA serves as the binding component for the two factors. Once bound to PA, the factors become edema toxin and lethal toxin. The toxins affect the host as their names imply: edema toxin acts as an adenylate cyclase causing local edema; lethal toxin causes tissue necrosis. The bacteria also possess a polyglutamic acid capsule that is antiphagocytic.

Cutaneous anthrax, which occurs in at least 95% of naturally occurring reported cases, rarely is fatal with appropriate treatment but has a 20% case fatality rate without treatment. Gastrointestinal disease occurs after ingestion of undercooked meat and has a higher case fatality rate, partly because of the delay in recognition of the disease. A new form of the disease, caused by inhalation of spores, was recognized during the industrial revolution. Inhalational anthrax is the form of the disease of greatest concern to bioterrorism response planners.

Anthrax has a number of properties that keep it at the top of biologic weapon threat lists. Inhalational anthrax is nearly universally fatal if not treated before the onset of symptoms. The organism can maintain virulence in a highly stable spore form for decades. Therefore it can be produced in large quantities and stored for long periods of time. The ideal particle size for infecting deep areas of the lungs is approximately 1 to 5 μm; anthrax spores can be milled to this particle size. Various legitimate supply houses around the world sell anthrax, and it can be obtained from soil in regions where anthrax is enzootic. One property that potentially hinders the use of anthrax as a biologic weapon is its high infective dose. Most of the pathogens considered viable biologic threats require small numbers of organisms to infect humans. The dose lethal for half of an exposed population (LD_{50}) for inhalational anthrax is estimated to be 8000 to 10,000 spores and is perhaps as high as 55,000 inhaled spores.[39] Although this may appear to be good news, that amount could potentially be inhaled with one deep breath in a concentrated spore cloud (personal communication, Dr. Louise Pitt, USAMRIID, 2000). Also, the 2001 inhalational anthrax outbreak has caused scientists to re-evaluate the lethal dose, especially in more vulnerable populations such as the elderly.

In 1980, reports of a 1979 outbreak of anthrax in the former Soviet town of Sverdlovsk (now Ekaterinberg, Russia) surfaced in the Western press. Although initially purported by the Russians to be a natural outbreak of gastrointestinal anthrax, epidemiologic and pathologic evidence pointed toward an inhalation source. Various reports have since concluded it was the result of an accidental release of spores from a biologic weapons research facility in Sverdlovsk.[15,40–43] This is the largest documented outbreak of inhalational anthrax, with at least 66 human fatalities as well as numerous animal deaths. Documentation of persons affected up to 4 km downwind and animals up to 50 km downwind validated concerns that humans could be infected great distances downwind if anthrax were ever released in an aerosol.

The incubation period for inhalation anthrax historically has been placed at 1 to 6 days. In the Sverdlovsk outbreak, however, some persons reportedly became ill up to 43 days after the time the exposure is thought to have occurred.[40] The reason for the long incubation period is not known, although in inhalation challenge trials with nonhuman primates, viable spores have been recovered in the mediastinum up to 100 days after exposure.[44] It is plausible that antibiotic treatment may have prevented symptoms until it was withdrawn, after which time viable anthrax spores sequestered in lymph nodes may have germinated to cause active disease. In inhalational anthrax, clinical manifestations generally begin with nonspecific symptoms such as fever, cough, malaise, and chest discomfort. Patients become progressively worse over 24 to 48 hours. Mediastinal lymph nodes become edematous and hemorrhagic and eventually rupture, allowing blood, lymphatic fluid, and organisms to enter the mediastinum. Some patients may exhibit a brief period of improvement before a sudden downhill course marked by the onset of cyanosis, dyspnea, stridor, and ultimately respiratory failure. Early in the clinical illness, physical findings are generally nonspecific. The pathognomonic radiographic sign is a widened mediastinum, although this may only be seen in approximately 60% of patients and may not be recognized in time to affect clinical management of the patient. Pneumonia is not typically a feature of anthrax, although hemorrhagic pleural effusions may develop. Without adequate treatment during the incubation phase or early in the clinical phase of the disease, bacteremia and toxemia will occur. Metastatic foci develop throughout the body, including distal sites such as the gastrointestinal tract and meninges. In the Sverdlovsk epidemic, 50% of 42 victims studied on autopsy exhibited involvement of the meninges with hemorrhagic meningitis.[42] In the inhalational anthrax outbreak in 2001, in a summary of 10 cases, the presenting symptoms included most commonly fevers and chills, fatigue, malaise, cough, nausea or vomiting, dyspnea, and chest discomfort or pleuritic pain. Twenty percent or fewer noted a sore throat or rhinorrhea, which may make those symptoms an important disguishing feature from common upper respiratory illnesses. All 10 persons had abnormal chest x-rays. These included features such as pleural effusion (80%), and mediastinal widening or infiltrates (70%).[42a] Chest CT was utilized with success to confirm chest x-ray findings.

Only encapsulated vegetative bacilli are found in the body during acute infection. These bacilli and their toxins appear in the bloodstream late on day 2 or early on day 3 after exposure in nonhuman primates. Leukocyte counts become elevated along with the appearance of toxin in the bloodstream.

In the acute disease, identifying bacilli by Gram stain or culture can be useful in establishing a diagnosis. Potential clinical samples include peripheral blood, cerebrospinal fluid, or pleural fluid (Fig. 40–1 and Color Plate 4). Sputum Gram stains are not useful because the organisms generally are not found in pulmonary secretions. Serology generally is only useful in establishing a diagnosis retrospectively. Use of newer techniques, such as fluorescent antibody or

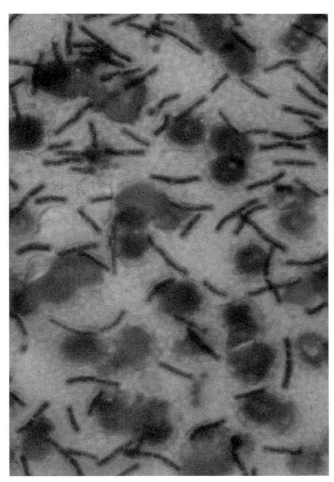

FIGURE 40–1. Peripheral blood smear from a rhesus macaque that succumbed to inhalation anthrax. (Gram stain × 1000.) (Courtesy of CoL Arthur Friedlander, MD, USAMRIID.) (See Color Plate 4.)

polymerase chain reaction (PCR), will likely play an increasing role in establishing a rapid diagnosis. If care providers are presented with patients suspected of having been recently exposed to aerosolized anthrax spores, the spores may be recovered in oropharyngeal secretions or the hairy portions of the face within the first 24 hours or longer after exposure and in stool within 24 to 72 hours after exposure.[45] Since gram-positive bacilli are often considered culture contaminants, clinicians need to alert the laboratory if they suspect anthrax.

Treatment and Prevention

Naturally occurring anthrax strains are generally susceptible to penicillin[46,47]; therefore the drug of choice for endemic anthrax, which is usually cutaneous, historically has been aqueous penicillin G, 2 MU every 2 hours or 4 MU every 4 to 6 hours.[48] Because of concerns that penicillin resistance can be induced relatively easily in the laboratory, the drug of choice for anthrax in the context of bioterrorism (in the absence of sensitivity data) is intravenous ciprofloxacin at 400 mg every 12 hours.[39]

Ciprofloxacin has also been recommended by the military as the drug of choice in the biologic warfare setting.[45,49] Tetracyclines and erythromycin are alternatives in patients allergic to penicillin, assuming the strains are found to be susceptible. Based on information from the 2001 outbreak, newer recommendations call for treatment with intravenous ciprofloxacin (at the dose noted above) or doxycycline 100 mg every 12 hours *plus* 1 or 2 additional antimicrobials such as rifampin, vancomycin, penicillin, ampicillin, chloramphenicol, imipenem, clindamycin, or clarithromycin.[49a] Recent reviews cover the treatment and prophylaxis of special populations including children and pregnant women.[39,50,51] Patients suspected of having anthrax should begin empiric treatment as soon as possible; as the disease progresses, the possibility of a beneficial outcome diminishes, despite treatment. Treatment should continue for 60 days, and patients may be changed to oral therapy as their clinical condition improves. Other modalities that may be required include fluid resuscitation, vasopressors for shock, and management of hypoxemia.

There are reports of the possibility for transmission of cutaneous anthrax by direct contact with a patient's open wound and by biting flies.[52] Subsequent laboratory studies have confirmed this possibility.[53] There is no evidence, however, that inhalational anthrax can be spread person to person; therefore standard precautions are recommended in dealing with inhalational anthrax in the patient-care setting.[54]

Persons with suspected exposure to anthrax should be given postexposure prophylaxis. Ciprofloxacin is the drug of choice in the bioterrorism setting[22,39] and recently was approved by the U.S. Food and Drug Administration (FDA) for this purpose—the first medication formally approved for postexposure prophylaxis against a weapon of mass destruction.[55] Potential alternative prophylactic medications include doxycycline, penicillin, or amoxicillin.[39] In licensing ciprofloxacin the FDA recommended it be given for 60 days after an exposure.[55] Shortly after the inhalational anthrax outbreak in 2001 was recognized, the FDA also licensed penicillin and doxycycline for postexposure prophylaxis. The FDA does not address any difference in duration of prophylaxis in vaccinated individuals; however, a study by Friedlander et al indicated that rhesus monkeys receiving prophylaxis who also received vaccination at the time of aerosol challenge fared better after medications were later discontinued than those given either prophylaxis or vaccination alone.[56]

There is a licensed vaccine in the United States (Anthrax Vaccine Adsorbed) against anthrax. The vaccine derives from the sterile fluid supernatant of an attenuated anthrax strain culture. The licensed initial vaccine series consists of six 0.5-ml subcutaneous injections at 0, 2, and 4 weeks and 6, 12, and 18 months, followed by annual boosters as long as someone remains at risk.[57] In the past the vaccine has been used primarily by personnel at occupational risk of anthrax exposure such as veterinarians, laboratory personnel at USAMRIID, and workers in wool-mill and tannery industries. Current U.S. military policy now calls for vaccination of personnel in high-threat areas and the eventual vaccination of all service members against anthrax because of biologic warfare concerns.

Efficacy of Anthrax Vaccine Adsorbed against cutaneous anthrax was demonstrated in a human clinical trial with New England wool-mill workers.[58] Several animal studies subsequently demonstrated efficacy of the vaccine against anthrax spores in an aerosol challenge of up to 760 LD_{50}. In these studies, protection was provided up to 2 years after vaccination, even after only one or two doses of vaccine.[59,60]

It is common for vaccine recipients to experience local side effects such as tenderness, erythema, induration, and pruritus. Systemic side effects are far less common.[61,62] Next-generation vaccines have been evaluated for protection against anthrax in animals. Three different approaches have been studied: (1) recombinant vaccines, wherein the gene for PA is cloned into minimally pathogenic organisms, such as *B. subtilis*; (2) vaccines composed of mutants of the Sterne *B. anthracis* strain, which require compounds not found in humans for replication; and (3) preparations of purified PA combined with different adjuvants.[63–65] In addition a pilot study with the current licensed vaccine found that subjects receiving the vaccine intramuscularly rather than subcutaneously had fewer local side effects but had no significant difference in mean antibody titers. Moreover the same study demonstrated that antibody titers did not decrease when the 2-week dose was omitted from the regimen (unpublished data, Philip R. Pittman, USAMRIID, 2002). A larger study in accordance with FDA requirements is under way to confirm these findings.

SMALLPOX

No other disease has had as significant an impact on the human species as has smallpox.[66] One of mankind's greatest public health triumphs occurred when the World Health Assembly declared the world free of smallpox in 1980. Sadly the cessation of smallpox vaccination programs after this declaration created the possibility that smallpox could be used as a weapon.

Smallpox (variola) virus is a member of the Orthopoxvirus genus and is related to other orthopoxviruses causing cowpox, vaccinia, and monkeypox. The organism appears bricklike on an electron micrograph and is a large (0.25 μm) DNA virus.

Concerns about smallpox were heightened in recent years after Soviet defector Ken Alibek revealed that the Soviet Union had the capability to produce the variola virus by the metric ton.[15] Apparently the Soviets saw the end of vaccination as an opportunity for future exploitation and even had smallpox ready for loading into intercontinental ballistic missiles directed at the United States. Concerns have also been raised that other nations may have stored old quantities of smallpox virus rather than destroying or surrendering them after the conclusion of the eradication effort.[67]

Civilians and military personnel ceased receiving smallpox vaccinations in the United States in 1972 and in the mid-1980s, respectively. Consequently a minority of the population now is estimated to have, at best, residual protection as a result of the decline of immunity with time.[28] Therefore we must be concerned that a terrorist armed with variola and the knowledge to employ it effectively in aerosol could infect thousands of susceptible victims. Smallpox's communicability gives it the potential to spread logarithmically beyond the initial victims.[68]

Smallpox can be acquired by several different routes. Most patients are probably infected by droplet exposure during face-to-face contact with smallpox victims. A 1970 outbreak in a hospital in Meschede, Germany, demonstrated the potential for spread by aerosol (small droplet nuclei).[69] This mode of spread is thought to be the exception rather than the rule. Other means of infection include direct contact of mucous membranes with a patient's lesions or secretions and rarely virus-contaminated fomites from patient secretions or, less likely, desquamated scabs. Risk of transmission increases if the patient aerosolizes virus by sneezing or coughing or in the presence of hemorrhagic disease. Examples exist of up to 10 to 20 secondary cases emanating from a single case.[70] The challenge of containing an outbreak is compounded if the initial cases go unrecognized. A 1972 outbreak in the former Yugoslavia provides a good illustration. One single imported case in an undiagnosed mildly symptomatic person led to 11 second-generation cases and a total of 175 cases before the outbreak was contained.[71] That occurred in a well-vaccinated population. Therefore one must consider that a similar occurrence today in a susceptible population could be much more severe.

In a smallpox infection, virus gains access through the respiratory mucosa, then moves to regional lymph nodes. After local replication for 3 to 4 days a primary, asymptomatic viremia occurs with clearance of the virus by the reticuloendothelial system. Replication continues, followed by a secondary or major viremia several days later. At this point, virus seeds the skin and patients become symptomatic with a prodrome of fever, headache, muscle aches, and vomiting. The characteristic rash manifests within 2 to 3 days of the secondary viremia and signals the onset of the communicable period. The incubation period (time from infection to prodrome) averages 12 to 14 days but ranges from 7 to 17 days. The rash develops initially on the face and distal extremities before progressing to the trunk. As it remains more prominent on the distal extremities and face, it is often termed a centrifugal rash (Fig. 40–2 and Color Plate 4). Early on the rash was

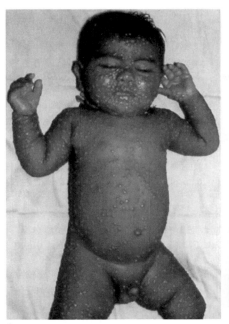
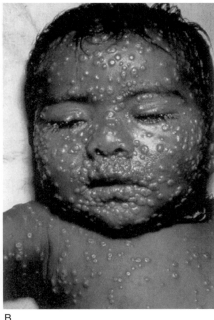
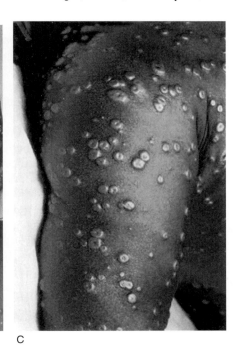

A   B   C

FIGURE 40–2. A, Full view of child with smallpox, day 7 of the rash, demonstrating more lesions on the face and extremities than on the trunk. **B,** Face of child with smallpox, day 7 of the rash, demonstrating confluence of pustules. **C,** Upper extremity of child with smallpox, day 7 of the rash, demonstrating umbilicated pustules. (From Fenner F, Henderson DA, Arita A, et al: Smallpox and its eradication. Geneva, World Health Organization, 1988.) (See Color Plate 4.)

frequently mistaken for varicella; however there are some distinguishing features. Varicella generally causes a centripetal rash, with lesions more prominent on the trunk than on the face or distal extremities, and the rash for varicella develops in a series of crops, thus yielding macules, papules, and pustules at a given point in time. The lesions in the smallpox rash develop in synchrony through the stages of macule, vesicle, umbilicated pustule, and scab. In contrast to varicella, which is no longer communicable by the time all lesions have scabbed, smallpox patients are deemed potentially infectious until all the lesions have fallen off, as the scabs are potentially infectious.

Smallpox is known to have widespread clinical variation, from asymptomatic disease to the highly fatal, hemorrhagic or flat-type smallpox. The disease of concern after a biologic weapon attack is *Variola major*, which historically caused case fatality rates of 20% to 40% in the unvaccinated. The illness can cause a variety of complications, including encephalitis, adult respiratory-distress syndrome (ARDS), blindness, facial scarring, and bony abnormalities, especially in children.

A clinical diagnosis of smallpox is made upon recognition of the characteristic rash. Eosinophilic inclusions (Guarnieri bodies) can be seen on light microscopy of biopsy specimens; however, even experienced technicians may have difficulty recognizing these microscopic features. Electron microscopy of lesion scrapings will demonstrate virus but will not distinguish variola from other orthopoxviruses. Viral culture or PCR is thus required for definitive diagnosis. Nonetheless, any patient with compatible clinical features and a finding of orthopoxvirus on electron microscopy should prompt concern; local and state public-health authorities and the CDC should be notified immediately in such an eventuality. One case of smallpox would constitute an international emergency.

Treatment and Prevention

Unfortunately, supportive care is the only mainstay of treatment of most smallpox victims. Recent work done by USAMRIID scientists at the CDC has looked at other potential therapies. In small studies, rhesus monkeys exposed to monkeypox and mice exposed to cowpox were protected from disease when the antiviral medication cidofovir was administered at the time of infection (personal communication, John Huggins, USAMRIID, 2001). Such findings hold potential promise for similar treatment of human smallpox. Cidofovir is administered intravenously; therefore large-scale administration in the event of a bioterrorist attack could prove logistically difficult.

Because smallpox has the potential to spread by aerosol, infection-control measures in hospitals should include negative-pressure isolation, vaccination of healthcare providers, contact precautions, and high-efficiency particulate air (HEPA)–filter masks.[54] In a large outbreak in the absence of sufficient negative-pressure isolation rooms, consideration would be given to cohort isolation.

Other measures might include having patients cared for by vaccinated family members at home or possibly in dedicated smallpox hospitals, as was done in various locations when smallpox was endemic.

In the absence of a proven, licensed treatment the best method of control is prevention. The licensed vaccine against smallpox is derived from the vaccinia virus, an orthopoxvirus closely related to variola. The vaccine has proven its effectiveness in the global eradication effort. The Advisory Committee on Immunization Practices has published guidelines regarding the use of smallpox vaccination in laboratory researchers and animal-care workers working with nonvariola orthopoxviruses.[72] Vaccinia vaccine was used after a person had been exposed to the disease during the smallpox eradication effort and was shown to prevent or ameliorate disease.[73] After a bonafide exposure, personnel should be vaccinated or boosted as soon as possible.[70] A key aspect of outbreak control in addition to vaccination will include epidemiologic evaluation to identify exposed persons and to appropriately isolate cases to prevent further spread.

Vaccine production was discontinued shortly after the disease was eradicated, and vaccine production facilities subsequently were dismantled. Therefore our national vaccine stockpile of 15.4 million doses in 100-dose vials is aging[74] and currently represents around 6 to 7 million doses[67,75] if one takes into account variations in administration and wastage, which might occur as vaccine is distributed. Given that over 6 million doses were used in New York City to quell a 1947 outbreak of smallpox, which led to 12 cases with two deaths, the limited supply is a topic of concern. Prior production methods of growing virus in calf lymph are crude when compared to today's vaccine production methods and are likely unacceptable for new vaccine production. Therefore to provide more vaccine for the national pharmaceutical stockpile, contracts were awarded in 2000 to produce 40 million doses of a cell-culture-derived vaccinia vaccine. The first lots are due to be produced by 2004. FDA licensure of this new product may prove difficult to obtain given the inability to conduct a human efficacy trial. To shore up contingencies for an event in the interim period clinical trials have been conducted to evaluate whether the existing vaccine could be diluted 10- or 100-fold and still be effective clinically.[74] At the time of this writing it appears that a five fold dilution would allow an acceptable percentage of vaccinated persons with a good vaccine "take." The licensed vaccine contains live virus and thus can cause predictable side effects in certain populations. Patients with dermatologic conditions such as eczema are prone to the development of life-threatening eczema vaccinatum, and immunocompromised persons may develop fatal vaccinia necrosum after receiving the vaccine or after contact with a recently immunized person, thus complicating any vaccination effort.[76] The cell-culture-derived vaccine in development is also live; therefore resumption of routine vaccination probably would

present significant challenges, especially given that the population of immunocompromised people in this country has increased since the time when smallpox vaccine was given routinely.[74] As of this writing the CDC is drafting plans to vaccinate a cadre of medical first responders across the country as a precautionary measure to get a head start on containing a smallpox outbreak.

PLAGUE

Plague's potential for devastating the human populations has been well demonstrated in three pandemics, the most recent of which began in 1898 and continues to this day. The second pandemic, which is perhaps the most notorious, decimated a third of the European population during the Middle Ages. A suspected outbreak of pneumonic plague in India in 1994 demonstrated the ongoing potential for this agent to cause unprecedented fear and economic disruption.[77,78] Care providers abandoned hospitals, medication supplies were depleted, and people fled afflicted areas. In neighboring nations, responses varied, from enhancing surveillance to closing borders or embargoing goods or flights arriving from India. India's economy consequently suffered from loss of tourism and trade.

The causative organism for plague is the nonmotile, gram-negative coccobacillus *Y. pestis*. The organism demonstrates bipolar staining, yielding a "safety pin" appearance under light microscopy. Given that *Y. pestis* does not sporulate, it is far less robust in the environment than *B. anthracis* is; however, the inhaled lethal dose is far lower than that of *B. anthracis*.

Each year several cases of human plague are reported in the western United States. Most of these cases are bubonic in their presentation. Humans generally are dead-end hosts of bubonic disease and are not required for maintaining the plague cycle in nature. Most cases occur when subjects spend time in areas where rodents live or pets bring infected fleas into their household. The few cases of pneumonic plague reported recently in the United States have been associated with close contact with infected cats.[79]

During World War II the Japanese conducted biologic warfare field trials on Chinese cities with plague-infected fleas. Other countries have also examined the potential use of plague as a weapon. For example, the Soviet Union stockpiled plague and targeted the disease for use against the United States and other Western powers.[15] During its offensive research program the United States also evaluated plague as a potential weapon. Research on the organism was discontinued when technical obstacles to maintaining virulence could not be overcome (Personal communication, Mr. William Patrick, 2001).[15]

Plague and smallpox are the only two pathogens on the CDC's category A threat list that are communicable from person-to-person. A terrorist employing one of these pathogens could take advantage of their ability to propagate through a population. Conversely, a contagious agent might be less useful on the battlefield because of the possibility that troops could become infected either by contact with an ill adversary or through contact with infected local rodent populations.

Bubonic plague is the most common endemic form of three possible clinical presentations. In this form of the disease, plague bacilli enter the lymphatics and multiply in regional lymph nodes after inoculation by an infected flea. The result is the development of a bubo, which is an extremely tender, inflamed lymph node. Patients will often attempt to minimize pain by limiting movement of the affected extremity. Without prompt treatment, organisms can spread beyond the lymph node and cause a secondary high-grade bacteremia and septicemia, although septicemic plague also occurs in the absence of a bubo. Pneumonic plague is the least common form and can occur either secondarily when the lungs are hematogenously seeded from bubonic or septicemic plague or primarily if patients inhale infected droplets from animals or other persons who have pneumonic plague. The primary concern of bioterrorism-response planners is plague being spread in an aerosol and causing primary pneumonic plague.

Unlike the case of *B. anthracis*, plague organisms can be identified in respiratory secretions, accounting for their ability to be transmitted from person-to-person. Pneumonia is often seen on chest radiograph. Diagnosis can be made by stains (Gram, Wright-Giemsa, Wayson) of sputum, blood, or a bubo fluid aspirate. A specific direct fluorescent antibody stain for *Y. pestis* is available. Clinical signs generally precede antibody response, so enzyme-linked immunosorbent (ELISA) and passive hemagglutination (PHA) assays are generally only useful in retrospect.[80]

Treatment and Prevention

Streptomycin, despite its limited availability, is the drug of choice for plague in a bioterrorism setting, at a dose of 1 g IM two times a day for 10 days. Requests for the drug can be made directly to Pfizer Pharmaceuticals. Gentamicin has also been recommended as a preferred choice by a public health consensus panel at a dose of 5 mg/kg IM or IV once a day or 2 mg/kg load, then 1.7 mg/kg IM or IV three times a day. Alternative treatments include doxycycline 100 mg IV twice a day, ciprofloxacin, 400 mg IV twice a day, or chloramphenicol 25 mg/kg IV four times a day.[81] The drug of choice for plague meningitis is chloramphenicol because of its superior penetration into the cerebrospinal fluid. Animal studies have demonstrated that β-lactam antibiotics may accelerate death, so generally they are not recommended.[82] Therapy for plague must be initiated promptly, possibly before culture confirmation, as plague mortality increases dramatically if treatment is delayed beyond 24 hours from symptom onset.

Infection control procedures employed in approaching patients with pneumonic plague are not significantly different from those used in the management of other diseases transmitted by droplets, such as meningococcal meningitis. Patients with pneumonic plague transmit the disease through fairly large droplets that tend to fall out of the air readily. Therefore care providers need to wear a mask when within 3 feet (1 m) of a patient. Some facilities may require a mask to be worn by persons entering the patient's room. These precautions need to be maintained until patients have had at least 48 hours of treatment or until they have a favorable response.[54,81,83]

For prophylaxis in patients exposed to aerosolized plague or treatment of patients in a mass casualty setting when bioterrorism is suspected, 100 mg of doxycycline or 500 mg of ciprofloxacin orally can be given twice a day.[81] In addition, others at risk of developing pneumonic plague, such as household or face-to-face contacts of pneumonic plague victims, should be offered prophylaxis.[83] Medications that have been suggested for this purpose include tetracycline (15 to 30 mg/kg) or chloramphenicol (30 mg/kg) orally four times a day or doxycycline (100 mg) orally two times a day for a week after the end of exposure. Personnel traversing borders may be detained up to 6 days if there is a suspicion of exposure to plague or an ongoing plague epidemic.[81,83]

The vaccine that previously was licensed for plague was a whole cell preparation developed in the 1940s. Production of the vaccine was discontinued in 1998. There is anecdotal evidence that it was effective during World War II and the Vietnam War in protecting U.S. service members against bubonic plague.[84-86] Animal studies, however, failed to demonstrate protection against aerosolized organisms.[87,88] Therefore, even if the vaccine were available, it would have little utility after a bioterrorist release of aerosolized organisms. Next-generation vaccine candidates containing F1 or V antigens of *Y. pestis* or both have been evaluated in animals. Some of these candidates appear promising for preventing infection by the respiratory route.[89]

RECOGNITION AND EPIDEMIOLOGIC CLUES

Successful management of a bona fide biologic event is likely to revolve around the issue of recognition. Unlike victims of conventional explosives or chemical agents, biologic agent casualties, owing to the inherent incubation periods of the agents involved, are likely to present to scattered clinics, emergency rooms, and medical providers removed in time and space from the point of exposure. Care providers may not consider an intentionally spread agent when they first encounter an outbreak but may be inclined to consider other possible causes, such as an endemic disease, a new or re-emerging disease, or a laboratory accident.[90] After all, physicians are taught that common diseases occur commonly and should be considered first. With this in mind and given the nonspecific nature of the symptoms associated with many potential bioterrorism agents, it is clear that recognition and accurate diagnosis will rely heavily on the provider's maintenance of a healthy "index of suspicion."[45,91] It is useful, then, for health care providers to be able to distinguish features of an unnatural event from a natural event. Certain clues are useful in making this distinction; some of these are listed in Table 40–2.[45,92] The absence of any particular feature does not necessarily mean that an untoward event has not occurred. Nor does their presence specifically indicate bioterrorism. Certainly, however, the finding of multiple clues should be cause for heightened suspicion. This list is not exhaustive; the reader is referred to other sources for additional discussion of the epidemiology of bioterrorism.[90,93]

The first recognition of an event may not come from a physician or through public health surveillance systems. Instead the recognizing authority may be a facility that receives requests from multiple physicians for services, such as a laboratory receiving excessive requests for a certain test or a pharmacy receiving an unusually large number of requests for a specific medication (such as doxycycline or ciprofloxacin).[90] Alternatively veterinarians might be the first to notice unusual illness or death in the animal population. The 1999 West Nile encephalitis outbreak in New York City provides a good example of the need to monitor animal disease activity. In that outbreak it was recognized that death among crows in the city and exotic birds in the Bronx Zoo was temporally related to cases of human illness. Because many of the diseases that are considered high-threat biologic weapons are zoonotic, animals can serve as sentinels for human illness. In a typical zoonotic disease outbreak, humans often become ill after the disease is circulating in an animal epizootic. Humans then become secondarily affected through direct animal contact or by means of an insect vector. In a bioweapon release, illness may be simultaneous in humans and animals, or human illness may precede animal illness.

After a bioweapon release, one would expect to see the typical features of a point-source outbreak,[90] that is, a fairly acute angled rise, brief plateau, and quick drop in the numbers of ill patients. In fact this epidemic curve may be more compressed than usual, as patients may be exposed within a short time frame or may receive a higher inoculum than would occur naturally. It may be instructive to look at the epidemiologic features of a 1984 criminal case that represents the only confirmed act of bioterrorism on U.S. soil before 2001.[94] In 1981, followers of an Indian guru, the Bhagwan Shree Rajneesh, set up a commune in the town of Antelope, Oregon in The Dalles County. New construction in the commune was limited by legal challenges, and the commune members felt the county commissioner elections in November 1984 could have a potential impact on the commune. A large outbreak of *Salmonella typhimurium* occurred in the The Dalles County seat in September and October 1984, with 751 documented cases. Evidence eventually led to the conclusion that the outbreak was intentionally spread. Commune members ultimately admitted to contaminating salad bars

---

TABLE 40–2 ■ Potential Clues of a Bioterrorist Attack

- A large point-source epidemic, especially in a discrete population
- Many cases of unexplained illnesses or deaths
- More severe disease than is expected for a specific pathogen
- Failure to respond to standard therapy for a specific pathogen
- Unusual route of exposure for a pathogen, such as the inhalation route for a disease that normally is contracted from other types of exposures
- An unusual disease for a given geographic area or transmission season
- A disease transmitted by a vector that is not present in the local area
- Multiple simultaneous or serial epidemics in the same population
- A single case of disease by an uncommon agent (e.g., smallpox, some viral hemorrhagic fevers)
- A disease that is unusual for a given age group
- Unusual strains or variants of organisms or antimicrobial resistance patterns different from those circulating
- Similar genetic type among agents isolated at different times or locations
- Higher attack rates in those exposed in certain areas, such as inside a building if agent is released indoors
- Lower attack rates in those inside a building with a protected air supply if agent is released outdoors
- Simultaneous disease in humans and animals or human disease preceding animal disease
- Intelligence of a potential attack, claims by an aggressor of a release, and discovery of munitions or tampering

Adapted from Kortepeter MG, Christopher GW, Cieslak TF, et al: USAMRIID's Medical Management of Biological Casualties Handbook, 4th ed. 2001. Found at www.usamriid.mil.

and coffee creamers in local restaurants in a trial run to see if they could influence the election results by keeping voters from going to the polls because of illness. Several epidemiologic features of the outbreak in The Dalles warrant comment. The outbreak curve actually demonstrated two classic point-source outbreaks, probably resulting from multiple contaminations over several weeks. Further investigation determined that the outbreak was not associated with water consumption. Other factors such as errors in food rotation, inadequate refrigeration, and infected employees, although possibly contributing factors, were ruled out as primary causes of the outbreak. Most cases were associated with the patients' having eaten at 10 restaurants, and the implicated restaurants were more likely to have salad bars. The epidemiologic red flag in the investigation was that different restaurants were implicated nearly simultaneously even though they lacked common food supply sources. A vial of commercial stock culture was also later identified in a laboratory in the commune. The culture was purchased before the outbreak and matched the outbreak strain.

The work-up of an unnatural outbreak would not differ significantly from that undertaken after a natural event and should be handled through normal public-health channels.[90] Of note, however, when bioterrorism is suspected, law-enforcement personnel should be alerted immediately. With the numerous threats and hoaxes perpetrated throughout the United States over the past few years, public-health and law-enforcement communities have had to come together on this issue and recognize the importance of ongoing dialogue.[95]

Existing disease surveillance systems in this country have a number of limitations, including reliance on case definitions of illness, lack of physician reporting, and lack of automation. Consequently data capture is incomplete and illness reporting may be delayed. In a large-scale bioterrorism event these delays may lead to subsequent delays in the administration of therapeutic and prophylactic modalities, resulting in increased morbidity and mortality. For these reasons, military and public health authorities are evaluating syndrome-based pilot surveillance systems for real-time detection of outbreaks, both natural and man made. Some of these systems have been tested at large, high-profile events, such as the 1999 World Trade Organization meeting in Seattle or the campaign 2000 national political conventions.[96]

RESPONSE

To respond optimally to a potential terrorist act, relevant governmental and institutional entities must be properly trained, equipped, and integrated. In addition, individual medical personnel, public health officials, and other responders must have a working knowledge of personal protection, infection control, decontamination, specimen handling, and other response elements. In this discussion we describe both individual and institutional (local, state, and federal) response to a potential biologic incident.

Individual Response

Once a bioterrorist event is recognized, in many instances (particularly those that are unannounced by the perpetrator) the health care provider becomes the first responder. In certain other situations, such as the announced threat or presumed hoax, public health officials and traditional first responders may need to approach the scene of a potential biologic release. Such responders must first take steps to protect themselves. Because most biologic pathogens are not dermally active, respiratory protection alone often suffices. Although first responders may have the luxury of donning protective suits with HEPA and charcoal filters and although such suits might be warranted if the nature of the threat is unknown (for example, if a chemical incident cannot be ruled out), a simple surgical mask provides adequate protection against most biologic agents. This would apply when approaching a package or device alleged to contain a biologic agent and when treating patients with potential biologic agent–induced diseases. Some have advocated the use of level D protection for health care responders dealing with patients acutely contaminated with infectious biologic agents. Level D consists of normal work clothes with latex gloves, eye protection, and an N-95 respiratory mask.[97] As most of the agents potentially useful to the terrorist are not contagious, no respiratory protection is needed when caring for victims of anthrax, tularemia, brucellosis, Q-fever, botulism, other toxin-mediated conditions, and many other potential threat diseases. Notable exceptions previously mentioned include pneumonic plague, which requires droplet precautions (including a simple surgical mask)[54,98] and smallpox, which would require contact and airborne precautions (including, ideally, a HEPA-filtered mask).[54] In addition certain viral hemorrhagic fevers, such as those caused by Ebola and Marburg viruses, would require the use of contact precautions, which may need to be upgraded to airborne precautions if patients have extensive hemorrhaging, cough, diarrhea, or emesis.[99,100]

In the past, victims of various bioterrorist threats have been subjected to distressing and embarrassing attempts at "decontamination." In some instances these attempts have included forced public disrobing and scrubbing with bleach solutions.[21] Because of the incubation periods of biologic agents, which separate symptoms from exposure by several days in most cases, symptomatic biologic casualties almost never require such decontamination. In all likelihood victims have already bathed and changed clothing several times between exposure and onset of illness. In addition many agents are unable to survive for long periods of time ex vivo and lack volatility (a characteristic that separates them from potential agents of chemical terrorism), thus limiting the risk of exposure to agent reaerosolization. In the few cases in which removing the agent might be warranted (the situation wherein a substance spills from an envelope onto the recipient's skin), simple soap and water cleansing is almost always adequate. Questions often arise regarding the risk to persons from potential environmental contamination. Biologic aerosols in the 1- to 5-μm range have little fallout in the environment, and those that do tend to adhere to larger particles as a result of electrostatic forces. Studies performed at Dugway Proving Ground in Utah noted a low risk of reaerosolization of anthrax spores by wind, vehicles, or other means of energy generation.[101]

The announced threat or hoax differs from the situation involving symptomatic patients in that there is a definitive crime scene and the need to preserve evidence and maintain a chain of custody when handling that evidence. Although human and environmental health protection would certainly take precedence over law-enforcement concerns, threat and hoax scenarios nonetheless require the early involvement of law-enforcement personnel and a respect for the need to maintain an uncompromised crime scene. Moreover, although one might be tempted to "decontaminate" the affected area, care must be taken not to destroy vital evidence.

In the case of a telephoned threat, where no device is apparent, local law-enforcement and public health authorities should be alerted. An envelope containing nothing other than a written threat poses little risk, and the situation should be handled in the same manner as a telephoned threat. As the envelope constitutes evidence in a crime, however, further manipulation should be left to law-enforcement professionals. In these cases no further action is necessary pending results of the legal and public health investigation. If a threat is subsequently deemed credible, public health authorities should contact potentially exposed persons, obtain appropriate information, and consider instituting prophylaxis or therapy.

When a package is found to contain powder, liquid, or other physical material, response should be individualized. In most cases the room should be vacated, additional untrained persons should be prohibited from handling the material or approaching the scene, and law-enforcement and public health officials should again be contacted. Persons coming in physical contact with package contents should remove clothing as promptly as is feasible and seal the clothes in a plastic bag for retention as evidence. Such persons should then wash with soap and water[22] and, in most cases, may be sent home, provided adequate instructions are given and contact information obtained. Specific antibiotic therapy would rarely be necessary before the preliminary identification of package contents by a competent laboratory. Floors, walls, and furniture need not and should not be treated with any decontamination solution before laboratory analysis is completed. Nonporous contaminated personal items such as eyeglasses and jewelry may be washed with soap and water or wiped clean with 0.5% hypochlorite

(household bleach diluted 10-fold) if a foreign substance has contacted the items.

In the event that a device or other evidence of a credible aerosol threat is discovered, the room (and potentially the building) should be vacated. Law-enforcement and public health personnel should be notified immediately and further handling of the device left to personnel with highly specialized training, such as the U.S. Federal Bureau of Investigation's (FBI) Hazardous Materials Response Unit. Contact information should be obtained from potential victims and detailed instructions provided. Clothing removal, soap and water showering, and decontamination of personal effects should be accomplished as above. Decisions regarding institution of empiric therapy should be left to local and state public health authorities, pending determination of the nature of the threat and identification of the involved biologic agents.

In providing a rational and measured response to each situation, public health and law-enforcement personnel can assist in minimizing the disruption and cost associated with biologic threats and hoaxes. Large-scale decontamination, costly HAZMAT unit involvement, broad institution of therapeutic interventions, and widespread panic hopefully can be avoided by a measured and logical response to these increasingly frequent threats.

Institutional (Local, State, and Federal) Response

The institutional response to a WMD event and in fact the response to any disaster, natural or man made, begins at the local level, where preparation efforts are perhaps most critical.[102] Control of such local response rests with a designated local-incident commander, often the fire or police chief. This incident commander can often summon groups of volunteer first responder and medical personnel, organized into metropolitan medical strike teams (MMSTs) under the auspices of the Department of Health and Human Services' (DHHS) Office of Emergency Preparedness.[103] MMSTs, under contract with the mayor, are located in many larger municipalities and can provide assistance with medical control, the extraction of victims, decontamination, triage, and medical treatment.

Specimens originating from a potential bioterrorist event must, again, undergo proper evidence-handling procedures, and sampling should be coordinated with the local-incident commander. The Association of Public Health Laboratories and the CDC have developed a network of public and private laboratories prepared to respond to potential bioterrorist attacks.[104] Under this system, local hospital laboratories, known as level A laboratories, would be capable of ruling out the presence of certain biologic threat agents in clinical specimens. Level B laboratories in certain municipalities and regions would then be capable of isolating potential threat agents and performing susceptibility testing.

When response requirements exceed local capabilities, the local-incident commander may request assistance from the state through the state coordinating officer (SCO). This SCO can then advise the governor to make available various state-level assets. These assets might include the law-enforcement capabilities of the state police and National Guard. Many state guards now include military Weapons of Mass Destruction—Civil Support (WMD-CS) teams, which can offer expert advice and provide liaison to more robust military assets at the federal level. Moreover, most state guards can provide public works assistance and mobile field hospitalization capability. Forensics laboratories are typically available through the state police or other state-level agencies. Level C laboratories are capable of providing sophisticated confirmatory diagnosis and typing of biologic agents; they in many cases are available through the state health departments.

When response requirements exceed the capabilities available at the state level, the state coordinating officer may contact the federal coordinating officer (FCO). The FCO may activate a federal response under the auspices of the Federal Response Plan (FRP),[105] which implements Public Law 93-288, the Robert T. Stafford Disaster Relief and Emergency Assistance Act, providing the authority for federal disaster response. Under the provisions of the FRP, response at the federal level is divided into a crisis management phase, under the direction of the FBI, and a consequence management phase, under the auspices of the Federal Emergency Management Agency (FEMA).

Under the FRP, federal-consequence management is organized into 12 emergency-support functions (ESFs), with each ESF being the responsibility of a specific federal agency. In addition, 29 different federal agencies can be tasked to provide assistance to these lead agencies. Federal disaster medical support is provided for under ESF 8 and is primarily the responsibility of the DHHS, which administers such support through its Office of Emergency Preparedness. This office oversees the National Disaster Medical System (NDMS),[106] which includes numerous disaster medical-assistance teams (DMATs), consisting of trained medical volunteers that can arrive at a disaster site within 8 to 16 hours. The NDMS is also capable of providing surge hospital bed capacity at numerous Department of Veterans Affairs, military, and civilian hospitals throughout the nation.

Myriad other federal agencies would potentially contribute to disaster response and to bioterrorism response in particular. The CDC and USAMRIID provide level D reference laboratories capable of sophisticated biologic threat agent analysis. These laboratories, capable of banking strains, probing for genetic manipulations, and operating at biosafety level 4, would provide backup to level C laboratories at the state health departments.[107] Epidemiologic consultation is also available from the CDC, as are crucial drugs and vaccines necessary to combat a large bioterrorist attack. These pharmaceuticals are stockpiled at several locations throughout the country and are available via CDC's National Pharmaceutical Stockpile program for rapid deployment to an affected area.

In the event of a bioterrorist attack the military could provide several forms of assistance as part of the federal response. In addition to laboratory support, threat evaluation and medical consultation are available through USAMRIID. Moreover the military can provide advice and support to civilian authorities through the Chemical/Biological Rapid Response Team (CBRRT) and the Chemical/Biological Incident Response Force (CBIRF), a Marine Corps unit capable of reconnaissance, decontamination, and field treatment. Both the CBRRT and the CBIRF can be en route to a disaster site within a few hours of notification. Military support, when requested, would be subordinate to federal civilian authorities and would be tailored by the Joint Task Force for Civil Support, a military command designed to provide command and control for all military assets involved in disaster-response missions and contingencies within the United States.

Response to a bioterrorist attack likely would constitute a complex undertaking requiring extensive cooperation among medical practitioners, civilian authorities, and officials at various levels of government as occurred in the fall of 2001. Health care providers will require a thorough understanding of the principles of infectious disease diagnosis and treatment and of personal protection and infection control procedures. Moreover they will also need a working knowledge of the components of our local, state, and federal response systems to function optimally in the event of an attack in their local area.

SUMMARY

As microbiology and techniques for genetic manipulation become ever more sophisticated, the challenge of defending against bioterrorism becomes increasingly complex. To successfully perpetrate a biologic attack on a large population, a terrorist would require a fair amount of knowledge and sophistication. It took years and millions of dollars for the United States and the Soviet Union to develop organism production and dispersal mechanisms. We have seen in examples such as the Aum Shinrikyo that even with millions of dollars at one's disposal, it is difficult to carry out a bioterrorist attack effectively. Nonetheless it would appear that there is little room for complacency, especially after the events in the fall of 2001. During the TOPOFF ("top officials") exercise in May 2000, which used a pneumonic plague scenario in Denver to test response capabilities, many difficulties were noted in the response effort.[108] Specific problem areas identified included flow of information, decision making, prioritizing and distributing antibiotics, overwhelming numbers of casualties, and civil unrest. Certainly we have a way to go in working out planning contingencies, but if one looks at how the United States would have fared only 5 years ago, we have come a long way. It has been argued that training is the key defense against bioterrorism[109] in order to alert health care providers to maintain an index of suspicion for bioterrorism so that they can recognize an event early. It is hoped that health-care providers will never need the ability to recognize and manage an actual bioterrorism event again. Regardless, the training and preparations will likely have benefit beyond bioterrorism preparation for recognition and response to other new and re-emerging endemic disease threats and disasters.

REFERENCES

1. Christopher GW, Cieslak TJ, Pavlin JA, et al: Biological warfare, a historical perspective. JAMA 1997;278:412–417.
2. Robertson AG, Robertson LJ: From asps to allegations: Biological warfare in history. Mil Med 1995;160:369–373.
3. Mobley JA: Biological warfare in the twentieth century: Lessons from the past, challenges for the future. Mil Med 1995;160:547–553.
4. Carus WS: Bioterrorism and biocrimes: The illicit use of biological agents in the 20th century. Working paper. Washington, DC, Center for Counterproliferation Research, National Defense University. August, 1998, revised July, 1999.
5. Derbes VJ: DeMussis and the Great Plague of 1348, a forgotten episode of bacteriological warfare. JAMA 1966;196:179–182.
6. Harris SH: Factories of death. New York, Routledge, 1994.
7. Harris S: Japanese biological warfare research on humans: A case study of microbiology and ethics. Ann NY Acad Sci 1992;666:21–52.
8. Yamaguchi M: Doctor testifies at war crimes trial. Washington Post, Jan 24, 2001.
9. Manchee RJ, Stewart WDP: The decontamination of Gruinard Island. Chem in Brit 1988;July:690–691.
10. Covert NM: Cutting edge, a history of Fort Detrick, Maryland. Fort Detrick, Md, Public Affairs Office (MCHD-PA), 1997.
11. Department of the Army: U.S. Army Activity in the U.S. Biological Warfare Programs, vol II. Publication DTIC B193427L, Washington, DC, 1977.
12. Convention on the prohibition of the development, production, and stockpiling of bacteriological (biological) and toxin weapons and on their destruction, signed 10 April 1972. In Dando M: Biological Warfare in the 21st Century, Biotechnology and the Proliferation of Biological Weapons. New York, Macmillan Publishing Co, 1994, pp 234–239.
13. Zilinskas RA: Iraq's biological weapons, the past as future? JAMA 1997;278:418–424.
14. Myers SL, Schmitt E: Iraq rebuilt weapons factories, officials say. New York Times. Jan 22, 2001.
15. Alibek K, Handelman S: Biohazard. New York, Random House, 1999.
16. Davis CJ: Nuclear blindness: An overview of the biological weapons programs of the former Soviet Union and Iraq. Emerg Infect Dis 1999;5:509–512.
17. Olson KB: Aum Shinrikyo: Once and future threat?. Emerg Infect Dis 1999;5:513–516.
18. Australia Group of export controls on materials used in the manufacture of chemical and biological weapons, control list of dual-use chemicals: Commercial and military application. November 7, 1995.
19. Chemical-Biological Expert Panel. United Nations, 1969.
20. WHO Group of Consultants: Health Aspects of Chemical and Biological Weapons. Geneva, World Health Organization, 1970.
21. Cole LA: Bioterrorism threats: Learning from inappropriate responses. J Public Health Management Practice 2000;6:8–18.
22. Centers for Disease Control and Prevention: Bioterrorism alleging use of anthrax and interim guidelines for management—United States, 1998. MMWR Morbid Mortal Wkly Rep 1999;48:69–74.
23. Cohen HW, Gould RM, Sidel VW: Bioterrorism initiatives: Public health in reverse? Am J Public Health 1999;89:1629–1631.
24. Cohen HW, Sidel VW, Gould RM: Prescriptions on bioterrorism have it backwards (letter). BMJ 2000;320:1211.
25. Departments of the Army, Navy, and Air Force: NATO Handbook on the Medical Aspects of NBC Defensive Operations: AmedP-6(B). Washington, DC, Departments of the Army, Navy, and Air Force, 1996.
26. Vorobjev AA, Cherkassey BL, Stepanov AV, et al: Key problems of controlling especially dangerous infections. In Proceedings of the International Symposium of Severe Infectious Diseases: Epidemiology, Express—Diagnostics and Prevention. Kirov, Russia, State Scientific Institution, Volgo-Vyatsky Center of Applied Biotechnology, June 1997.
27. Kortepeter MG, Parker GW: Potential biological weapons threats. Emerg Infect Dis 1999;5:523–527.
28. Henderson DA: The looming threat of bioterrorism. Science 1999;283:1279–1282.
29. National Center for Infectious Diseases, Centers for Disease Control and Prevention: Critical biological agents for public health preparedness, summary of selection process and recommendations. July 16, 1999.
30. Khan AS, Ashford, DA, Craven RB, et al: Biological and chemical terrorism: Strategic plan for preparedness and response. Recommendations of the CDC Strategic Planning Workgroup. MMWR Morb Mortal 2000;49(RR04):1–14.
31. Pile JC, Malone JD, Eitzen EM, et al: Anthrax as a potential biological warfare agent. Arch Intern Med 1998;158:429–434.
32. Brachman PS: Inhalation anthrax. Ann NY Acad Sci 1980;353:83–93.
33. Turner M: Anthrax in humans in Zimbabwe. Cent Afr J Med 1980;26:160–161.
34. Davies JCA: A major epidemic of anthrax in Zimbabwe. Cent Afr J Med 1983;29:8–12.
35. Levy LM, Baker N, Meyer MP, et al: Anthrax meningitis in Zimbabwe. Cent Afr J Med 1981;27:101–104.
36. Nass M: Anthrax epizootic in Zimbabwe, 1978–1980: Due to deliberate spread? PSR Q 1992;2:198–209.
37. Centers for Disease Control and Prevention: Human ingestion of *Bacillus anthracis*–contaminated meat—Minnesota, August 2000. MMWR Morb Mortal Wkly Rep 2000; 49:813–816.
38. Dull PM, Gomez T, White L, et al: Human anthrax associated with an epizootic—North Dakota, 2000: What's the risk? Programs and abstracts of the 50th Annual Epidemic Intelligence Service Conference. Atlanta, Centers for Disease Control and Prevention, 2001, pp 30–31.
39. Inglesby TV, Henderson DA, Bartlett JG, et al: Anthrax as a biological weapon, medical and public health management. JAMA 1999;281:1735–1745.
40. Meselson M, Gillemin J, Hugh-Jones M, et al: The Sverdlovsk anthrax outbreak of 1979. Science 1994;209:1202–1208.
41. Jackson PJ, Hugh-Jones ME, Adair DM, et al: PCR analysis of tissue samples from the 1979 Sverdlovsk anthrax victims: The presence of multiple *Bacillus anthracis* strains in different victims. Proc Natl Acad Sci USA 1998; 95:1224–1229.
42. Abramova FA, Grinberg LM, Yampolskaya, et al: Pathology of inhalational anthrax in 42 cases from the Sverdlovsk outbreak of 1979. Proc Natl Acad Sci USA 1993; 90:2291–2294.

42a. Jernigan J, Stephens D, Ashford D, et al: Bioterrorism-related inhalation anthrax: the first 10 cases reported in the United States. Emerg Infect Dis 2001;7:933–944.

43. Guillemin J: Anthrax: The investigation of a deadly outbreak. Berkeley, University of California Press, 1999.

44. Henderson DW, Peacock S, Belton FC: Observations on the prophylaxis of experimental pulmonary anthrax in the monkey. J Hygiene 1956;54:28–36.

45. Kortepeter MG, Christopher GW, Cieslak TJ, et al: USAMRIID's Medical Management of Biological Casualties Handbook, 4th ed. 2001. Available at www.usamriid.mil.

46. Odendaal MW, Pieterson PM, DeVos V, et al: The antibiotic sensitivity patterns of Bacillus anthracis isolated from the Kruger National Park. Onderstepoort J Vet Res 1991;58:17–19.

47. Lightfoot NF, Scott RJD, Turnbull PCB: Antimicrobial susceptibility of Bacillus anthracis. Salisbury Med Bul 1990;68:95–98.

48. Lew DP: Bacillus anthracis (anthrax). In Mandell GL, Bennett JE, Dolin R (Eds): Principles and practice of infectious diseases, 5th ed. Philadelphia, Churchill Livingstone, 2000.

49. Headquarters, Departments of the Army, the Navy, and the Air Force, and Commandant, Marine Corps: Army FM 8-284, Navy NAVMED P-5042, Air Force AFMAN(I) 44-156, Marine Corps MCRP 4-11.1C: Treatment of biological warfare agent casualties. Washington, DC, 17 July 2000.

49a. Inglesby TV, O'Toole T, Henderson DA, et al: Anthrax as a biological weapon, 2002—updated recommendations for management. JAMA 2002;287:2236–2252.

50. Dixon TC, Meselson M, Guillemin, et al: Anthrax. N. Engl J Med 1999;341:815–826.

51. Henretig FM, Cieslak TJ, Madsen JM, et al: The emergency department response to incidents of biological and chemical terrorism. In Textbook of Pediatric Emergency Medicine, 4th ed. Philadelphia, Lippincott Williams & Wilkins, 2000.

52. McKendrick DRA: Anthrax and its transmission to humans. Cent Afr J Med 1980;26:126–129.

53. Turell MJ, Knudson GB: Mechanical transmission of Bacillus anthracis by stable flies (Stomoxys calcitrans) and mosquitoes (Aedes aegypti and Aedes taeniorhynchus). Infect Immun 1987;55:1859–1861.

54. English JF, Cundiff MY, Malone JD, et al: Bioterrorism readiness plan: A template for healthcare facilities. April 13, 1999. Available at http://www.apic.org/bioterror/, accessed 26 March 2001.

55. Food and Drug Administration, U.S. Department of Health and Human Services: Approval of Cipro for use after exposure to inhalational anthrax. FDA Talk Paper, August 31, 2000. Available at http://www.fda.bov/bbs/topics/ANSWERS/ANS01030.html, accessed 30 March 2001.

56. Friedlander AM, Welkos SL, Pitt MLM, et al: Postexposure prophylaxis against experimental inhalation anthrax. J Infect Dis 1993;167:1239–1242.

57. Package insert: Anthrax Vaccine Adsorbed, Rev. March, 1999. U.S. License No. 1260. Bioport Corporation, Lansing Mich.

58. Brachman PS, Gold H, Plotkin SA, et al: Field evaluation of a human anthrax vaccine. Am J Public Health 1962;52:632–645.

59. Ivins BE, Fellows PF, Pitt MLM: Efficacy of standard human anthrax vaccine against Bacillus anthracis aerosol spore challenge in rhesus monkeys. Salisbury Med Bull 1996;87:125–126.

60. Ivins BE, Pitt MLM, Fellows PF, et al: Comparative efficacy of experimental anthrax vaccine candidates against inhalation anthrax in rhesus monkeys. Vaccine 1998;16:1141–1148.

61. Friedlander AM, Pittman PR, Parker GW: Anthrax vaccine: Evidence for safety and efficacy against inhalational anthrax. JAMA 1999;282:2104–2106.

62. Centers for Disease Control and Prevention: Surveillance for adverse events associated with anthrax vaccination—U.S. Department of Defense, 1998–2000. MMWR Morb Mortal Wkly Rep 2000;49:341–345.

63. Ivins BE, Welkos SL: Cloning and expression of the Bacillus anthracis protective antigen gene in Bacillus subtilis. Infect Immun 1986;54:537–542.

64. Ivins BE, Welkos SL, Knudson GB, et al: Immunization against anthrax with aromatic compound-dependent (Aro-) mutants of Bacillus anthracis and with recombinant strains of Bacillus subtilis that produce anthrax protective antigen. Infect Immun 1990;58:303–308.

65. Ivins B, Fellows P, Pitt L, et al: Experimental anthrax vaccines: Efficacy of adjuvants combined with protective antigen against an aerosol Bacillus anthracis spore challenge in guinea pigs. Vaccine 1995;13:1779–1784.

66. Barquet N, Domingo P: Smallpox: The triumph over the most terrible of the ministers of death. Ann Intern Med 1997;127:635–642.

67. Henderson DA: Smallpox: Clinical and epidemiologic features. Emerg Infect Dis 1999;5:537–539.

68. O'Toole T: Smallpox: An attack scenario. Emerg Infect Dis 1999;5:540–546.

69. Helfand HM, Posch J: The recent outbreak of smallpox in Meschede, West Germany. Am J Epidemiol 1971;93:234–237.

70. Henderson DA, Inglesby TV, Bartlett JG, et al: Smallpox as a biological weapon: Medical and public health management. JAMA 1999;281:2127–2137.

71. Fenner F, Henderson DA, Arita A, et al: Smallpox and Its Eradication. Geneva, World Health Organization, 1988.

72. Centers for Disease Control and Prevention: Vaccinia (smallpox) vaccine: Recommendations of the immunization practices advisory committee (ACIP). MMWR Morb Mortal Wkly Rep 1991;40(RR-14):1–10.

73. Dixon CW: Smallpox in Tripolitania, 1946: An epidemiological and clinical study of 500 cases, including trials of penicillin treatment. J Hygiene 1948;46:351–377.

74. LeDuc JW, Becher J: [letter] Emerg Infect Dis 1999;5:593.

75. Russell PK: Vaccines in civilian defense against bioterrorism. Emerg Infect Dis 1999;5:531–533.

76. Lane M, Ruben FL, Neff JM, et al: Complications of smallpox vaccination, 1968: Results of ten statewide surveys. J Infect Dis 1970;122:303–309.

77. Campbell GL, Hughes JM: Plague in India: A new warning from an old nemesis. Ann Intern Med 1995;122:151–153.

78. Deodhar NS, Yemul VL, Banerjee K: Plague that never was: A review of the alleged plague outbreaks in India in 1994. J Public Health Policy 1998;19:184–199.

79. Centers for Disease Control and Prevention: Fatal human plague—Arizona and Colorado, 1996. MMWR Morb Mortal Wkly Rep 1997;46:617–620.

80. McGovern TW, Friedlander AM: Plague. In Sidell FR, Takafuji ET, Franz DR (Eds): Textbook of Military Medicine: Medical Aspects of Chemical and Biological Warfare. Washington, DC, Borden Institute, 1997, pp 479–502.

81. Inglesby TV, Dennis DT, Henderson DA: Plague as a biological weapon—medical and public health management. JAMA 2000;283:2281–2290.

82. Byrne WR, Welkos SL, Pitt ML, et al: Antibiotic treatment of experimental pneumonic plague in mice. Antimicrob Agents Chemother 1998;42:675–681.

83. Chin J (Ed): Control of Communicable Diseases Manual, 17th ed. Washington, DC, American Public Health Association, 2000.

84. Meyer KF, Cavanaugh DC, Barelloni PJ, et al: Plague immunization. I. Past and present trends. J Infect Dis 1974;29(Suppl):S13–S18.

85. Butler T: Plague and other *Yersinia* infections. New York, Plenum Medical Book Co, 1983.

86. Meyer KF: Effectiveness of live or killed plague vaccines in man. Bull World Health Organ 1970;421:653–656.

87. Ehrenkranz NF, Meyer KF: Studies on immunization against plague. VIII: Study of three immunizing preparations in protecting primates against pneumonic plague. J Infect Dis 1955;96:138–144.

88. Pitt MLM, Estep JE, Welkos SL, et al: Efficacy of killed whole-cell vaccine against a lethal aerosol challenge of plague in rodents. Annual meeting, American Society for Microbiology 1994. Las Vegas, NV. Abstract E-45.

89. Heath DG, Anderson GW, Mauro JM, et al: Protection against experimental bubonic and pneumonic plague by a recombinant capsular F1-V antigen fusion protein vaccine. Vaccine 1998;16:1131–1137.

90. Pavlin JA: Epidemiology of bioterrorism. Emerg Infect Dis 1999;5:528–530.

91. Cieslak TJ: Medical consequences of biological warfare: The ten commandments of management. Mil Med 2001;166(12 Suppl):11–12.

92. U.S. Army Medical Research Institute of Infectious Diseases (USAMRIID), Centers for Disease Control and Prevention (CDC), and Food and Drug Administration (FDA): Biological warfare and terrorism: The military and public health response. Satellite Television Broadcast Student Handbook. September 21–23, 1999.

93. Wiener SL, Barrett J: Biological warfare defense. In Trauma Management for Civilian and Military Physicians. Philadelphia, WB Saunders, 1986, pp 508–509.

94. Torok TJ, Birkness KA, Foster LR, et al: A large community outbreak of salmonellosis caused by intentional contamination of restaurant salad bars. JAMA 1997;278(5):389–395.

95. National Disaster Preparedness Office, Department of Defense: Criminal and epidemiological investigation report, Soldier Biological Chemical Command Biological Warfare Improved Response Program. Meeting held on January 19–21, 2000.

96. McClam E: Web-based terrorist surveillance eyed. April 23, 2001. Available at www.washingtonpost.com/wp-srv/aponline/20010423/aponline175500_000.htm accessed April 25, 2001.

97. Macintyre AG, Christopher GW, Eitzen E, et al: Weapons of mass destruction events with contaminated casualties: Effective planning for health care facilities. JAMA 2000;283:242–249.

98. Garner JS: Guideline for isolation precautions in hospitals. Infect Control Hosp Epidemiol 1996;17:54–80.

99. Centers for Disease Control and Prevention: Management of patients with suspected viral hemorrhagic fever. MMWR Morb Mortal Wkly Rep 1988;37(S-3):1–16.

100. Centers for Disease Control and Prevention: Update: Management of patients with suspected viral hemorrhagic fever—United States. MMWR Morb Mortal Wkly Rep 1995;44:475–479.

101. Chinn KS: Reaerosolization Hazard Assessment for Biological Agent–Contaminated Hardstand Areas, Life Sciences Division. Dugway Proving Ground, Utah. U.S. Department of the Army, 1996, 1–40. Pub DPG/JCP-96/012.

102. Garrett LC, Magruder C, Molgard CA: Taking the terror out of bioterrorism: Planning for a bioterrorist event from a local perspective. J Public Health Management Pract 2000;6:1–7.

103. Department of Health and Human Services: Department of Health and Human Services Health and Medical Services Support Plan for the Federal Response to Acts of Chemical/Biological Terrorism. June 21, 1996.

104. Gilchrist MJR: A national laboratory network for bioterrorism: Evolution of a prototype network of laboratories for performing routine surveillance. Mil Med 2000;165(Suppl 2):28–31.

105. Federal Emergency Management Agency: The federal response plan for public law 93-288, as amended. April 1992.

106. Moritsugu KP, Reutershan TP: The National Disaster Medical System: A concept in large-scale emergency medical care. Ann Emerg Med 1986;15:1496–1498.

107. Centers for Disease Control and Prevention: Biological and chemical terrorism: Strategic plan for preparedness and response. MMWR Morb Mortal Wkly Rep 2000;49 (RR-04):1–14.

108. Inglesby TV, Grossman R, O'Toole T: A plague on your city: Observations from TOPOFF. Clin Infect Dis 2001; 32:436–445.

109. Eitzen EM: Education is the key to defense against bioterrorism. Ann Emerg Med 1999;34:221–223.

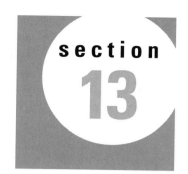

section

13

Fungal Infections

Candidiasis

YOAV GOLAN, MD
LEON LAI, MD
SUSAN HADLEY, MD

The treatment of *Candida* infections remains a challenge despite the increasing availability of antifungal agents. Insufficient culture sensitivity is associated with treatment delays and missed diagnoses. Increasing drug resistance across *Candida* spp and the emergence of the more drug-resistant, non-*albicans* species results in treatment failures. A growing number of critically ill and immunosuppressed patients are predisposed to infections by opportunistic pathogens such as *Candida* spp by virtue of the advent of aggressive cancer therapies, greater numbers of organ and bone marrow transplantation, and improved life support. These patients are also exposed to broad-spectrum antibiotics and central vascular catheters, which further increase their odds of *Candida* infections. As a result, *Candida* spp are currently the fourth most common blood isolate in hospitals, and their prevalence is steadily increasing.[1]

Invasive *Candida* infections are associated with 40% to 70% mortality, even when correctly diagnosed and treated.[2–4] To minimize treatment delays and missed diagnoses, methods other than the traditional culture-proven strategy are being developed. The empiric addition of an antifungal agent to the treatment of neutropenic fever has decreased mortality due to *Candida* infections in this patient population. Similar strategies are being evaluated for intensive care unit patients. The availability of new antifungal agents during the last decade has significantly increased treatment options. Until recently, amphotericin B was the only effective medication for the treatment of invasive *Candida* infections. The addition of fluconazole revolutionized systemic antifungal treatment by virtue of its high safety profile. Several newer triazole and echinocandin compounds show an enhanced spectrum of activity against *Candida* spp and are being extensively evaluated for the treatment of *Candida* infections. A better understanding of treatment approaches and options is necessary to favorably alter the unacceptably high mortality associated with invasive *Candida* infections.

This chapter is divided into two parts: treatment of invasive *Candida* infections and treatment of mucocutaneous and urinary *Candida* infections. Special considerations for patients with HIV, bone marrow and solid organ transplantation, or neutropenia and for patients in the intensive care unit are outlined.

INVASIVE *CANDIDA* INFECTIONS

Results of large-scale randomized trials are available for *Candida* bloodstream infections in immunocompetent hosts. For other forms of invasive *Candida* infections and for bloodstream infections in immunosuppressed hosts, data are mainly from small trials and case series. Treatment recommendations made in this chapter are based on the best available data and particularly rely on practice guidelines published by the Infectious Diseases Society of America (IDSA) in April 2000.[5]

Amphotericin B and fluconazole are the only two medications that have been extensively studied for the therapy of invasive *Candida* infections. Although amphotericin B is active against most azole-resistant *Candida* spp, its administration is frequently associated with severe toxicity.[6,7] Some *Candida glabrata*, *Candida lusitaniae*, and *Candida krusei* isolates exhibit resistance to amphotericin B.[8–10] Fluconazole has an excellent safety profile; however, it is not active against *C. krusei* and approximately 15% of *C. glabrata* isolates.[11] It is active, though, against amphotericin B–resistant *C. lusitaniae*. High fluconazole blood levels are rapidly achieved by administration of twice the daily dose as a loading dose. Daily doses of 12 mg/kg are required to gain efficacy against *C. glabrata* isolates that express dose-dependent susceptibility.[12,13] Three lipid formulations of amphotericin B are available in the United States: amphotericin B colloidal dispersion (ABCD, Amphotec), amphotericin B lipid complex (ABLC, Abelcet), and liposomal amphotericin B (AmBisome). ABCD is associated with acute infusion-related reactions and is not approved for *Candida* infection.[14] All three compounds are less nephrotoxic than the deoxycholate formulation; however, their high cost relegates them to secondary use in candidiasis.[15,16]

ABLC (5 mg/kg/d) or AmBisome (3 to 5 mg/kg/d) is indicated for patients who cannot tolerate amphotericin B, patients who are at high risk for developing kidney dysfunction if given amphotericin B (because of pre-existing kidney dysfunction or concomitant administration of a nephrotoxic drug such as an aminoglycoside, cyclosporin, or cisplatin), or patients who do not improve despite treatment with amphotericin B.[5] The efficacy of the higher doses for each lipid formulation compares favorably with standard amphotericin doses (0.7 mg/kg/d).[15,17] The combination of 5-flucytosine with either amphotericin B or fluconazole may have a synergistic effect. It is not, however, commonly used, and data from clinical trials to support such combinations are limited. Studies of itraconazole, voriconazole, and caspofungin as therapy for invasive candidiasis are in progress but are, at the time of this writing, incomplete, and the clinical experience with these medications is limited. Thus these medications will not be included in the discussion of treatment options.

Candida Bloodstream Infection (Candidemia)

The incidence of candidemia has risen dramatically over recent years in association with the rise in the number of compromised hosts and critically ill patients. Aggressive interventions such as broad-spectrum antibiotics, cytotoxic chemotherapy, hemodialysis, and central venous catheterization are used to manage these patients, putting them at increased risk of invasive candidiasis. *Candida* spp have become the fourth most common bloodstream isolates in hospitals.[1] The isolation of *Candida* from blood is associated with sepsis and a mortality of 30% to 70%.[2–4] Hematogenous seeding of *Candida* may further complicate the course of infection, resulting in organ dysfunction.

The first step in the management of candidemia, if possible, is the removal of all central venous lines.[18,19] Infected lines are frequently the source of candidemia, particularly in immunocompetent patients, and can serve as an ongoing source of *Candida* infection in persistent or relapsing candidemia. Current data suggest that catheter removal alone is insufficient, even in the noncompromised patient, to prevent metastatic hematogenous dissemination to visceral organs.[18,19] Thus the need to treat all patients with candidemia is now widely accepted.[20,21]

Randomized clinical trials and a recent meta-analysis suggest that fluconazole is comparable to amphotericin B for the treatment of candidemia in immunocompetent patients.[7] In a randomized trial by Rex et al treatment of candidemia in immunocompetent patients with amphotericin B at 0.5 to 0.6 mg/kg/d and fluconazole at 400 mg/d was successful in 79% and 70% of cases, respectively, and had a mortality of 40% and 33%, respectively.[22] These differences were not statistically different. In another randomized trial by Anaissie et al amphotericin B was compared to fluconazole for the treatment of proven and presumed invasive *Candida* infections in 164 patients, of whom 60 were neutropenic.[23] Response rates for amphotericin B and fluconazole were 64% and 66%, respectively.

The choice of initial therapy, that is, before the infecting *Candida* species is identified, is discussed separately from the choice of species-based therapy, that is, when the species is known. The three crucial factors when choosing therapy are the patient's immune status (neutropenic or not), the patient's clinical condition (hemodynamically stable or unstable), and the infecting *Candida* species. Although *Candida albicans* is the most common blood isolate, the recent emergence of non-*albicans* species, especially *C. glabrata*, which frequently expresses dose-dependent susceptibility to fluconazole, is relevant to the choice of treatment.[24,25] Prior or current therapies with fluconazole and high hospital rates of non-*albicans* species are associated with higher rates of infection with non-*albicans* species.[26]

For initial treatment of unstable or neutropenic patients, amphotericin B at 0.7 mg/kg/d or higher is recommended by most experts because of its broader spectrum.[20] Flucytosine at 100 mg/kg/d can be given in combination with amphotericin B. Simultaneous administration of these two drugs can result in bone marrow suppression and diarrhea. Serum levels should be monitored with a goal of 50 to 100 μg/ml.[27] The role of combination therapy with fluconazole and flucytosine or fluconazole and amphotericin B has yet to be established.

Several in vitro and in vivo studies demonstrated that pre-exposure of *C. albicans* to fluconazole reduces fungal susceptibility to amphotericin B. The length of fluconazole pre-exposure and whether amphotericin B is subsequently used alone or in combination with fluconazole determine the duration of induced resistance to amphotericin B.[28] Contrary to prior reports, however, a recent randomized trial found that fluconazole may not be antagonistic to amphotericin B when given in combination and may rather have an additive effect.[29]

For initial treatment of stable non-neutropenic patients, fluconazole at 6 mg/kg/d (for a 70-kg patient: 800 mg on day 1 followed by 400 mg/d thereafter) is advocated by most experts.[5,20] For species-based treatment, *C. albicans*, *Candida parapsilosis*, and *Candida tropicalis* may be treated with either fluconazole at 6 mg/kg/d or amphotericin B at 0.6 mg/kg/d.[5] *C. krusei* is treated with amphotericin B at 1 mg/kg/d. *C. lusitaniae* is treated with fluconazole at 6 mg/kg/d.[5] The treatment of candidemia should be continued for 2 weeks after the last positive culture and resolution of signs and symptoms of infection. Longer treatment should be considered if an infected line could not be removed. Amphotericin B can be switched to fluconazole (IV or PO) for completion of therapy. The choice and duration of treatment for patients with visceral involvement is discussed later in this chapter.

Candida Endocarditis

Although endocarditis caused by *Candida* species is uncommon, its incidence has markedly increased during the last decade along with other forms of invasive *Candida* infections.[30] In a report of 22 hospital-acquired endocarditis cases during a 6-year period, 9% were caused by *Candida* spp.[31] In another series of 97 autopsy cases with hospital-acquired endocarditis, 12% were caused by *Candida* spp, of which 39% were diagnosed before death.[32] Patient groups at highest risk for *Candida* endocarditis are those with cardiovascular prosthetic devices (valves, indwelling central catheters, pacemakers, or left ventricular assist devices), the immunosuppressed or critically ill, intravenous drug abusers, and premature infants.[33–38]

Recent case reports describe prosthetic valve endocarditis (PVE) as the main entity of *Candida* endocarditis. In two recent reports, 1% of patients who underwent valve replacement developed fungal PVE; *Candida* spp were the offending pathogens in more than 75% of these cases.[39,40] *C. albicans* and *C. parapsilosis* are the most common isolates from patients with *Candida* endocarditis. Other less common causes are *C. tropicalis*, *C. glabrata*, and *C. lusitaniae*.[41,42]

Treatment of *Candida* endocarditis is based on descriptive data and extrapolation from treatment of *Candida* bloodstream infections and bacterial endocarditis, rather than on results of clinical trials. Most treatment experience is with PVE; information is scarce on the treatment of native valve endocarditis. Without treatment, *Candida* endocarditis is uniformly fatal.[43] Surgery is the mainstay in the management of *Candida* endocarditis. Before the introduction of surgery in the management of this disease the mortality was 90% despite medical therapy. With combined surgical and medical therapy, mortality has decreased to 35% to 45%.[41,43,44] Early surgery (preferably within 48 to 72 hours) is advocated because of the threat of major emboli, ring abscess formation, and myocardial invasion.[45–47] Surgery includes radical resection of all infected tissue and cardiac reconstruction using biologic tissue when possible.[48] Intraoperative amphotericin B irrigation after excision and before prosthetic valve insertion is advocated by some authors.[43]

Aggressive amphotericin B treatment is an adjunct to surgery in the treatment of *Candida* PVE. The optimal dose and length of treatment are not well defined. A dose of 0.7–1 mg/kg, however, is commonly used, and treatment is usually continued for at least 6 to 10 weeks.[41] Experience with fluconazole for the initial treatment of *Candida* endocarditis is limited. Other anti-*Candida* medications are rarely described for this purpose. In the rabbit model of *C. albicans* endocarditis, amphotericin B at 1 mg/kg was more effective then fluconazole at 50 mg/kg in reducing fungal vegetation densities when given daily for 9 or 12 days, regardless of time of initiation of therapy (34 to 60 hours after infection). In a daily dose of 100 mg/kg for 21 days, fluconazole was twice as effective as 12 days of amphotericin B in reducing intravegetation *Candida* densities.[49] Using a similar rabbit model, Louie reported that amphotericin B therapy decreased valvular *Candida* load significantly more than fluconazole after 5, 14, and 21 days.[50] In the *C. tropicalis* rabbit endocarditis model, amphotericin B was more rapidly fungicidal than fluconazole, but the overall effect was equal for amphotericin and fluconazole.[51] Amphotericin was still detected in all vegetations 48 hours after last dose, whereas fluconazole was detected in only one.[52]

Flucytosine may be added to amphotericin B or fluconazole for synergism; however, there have been no controlled trials in *Candida* endocarditis to evaluate whether combination therapy has a better outcome. In the *C. albicans* rabbit model, flucytosine plus fluconazole demonstrated better killing in cardiac vegetations than fluconazole or flucytosine as monotherapy. Similarly the combination of amphotericin B and fluconazole was more active than fluconazole alone in reducing the fungal density in cardiac vegetations ($P<.03$).[50] Another in vivo assessment of the combination of amphotericin B and fluconazole using the rabbit *C. albicans* endocarditis model found no increased or decreased effect as compared with amphotericin B alone.[53] The combination of cyclosporine and fluconazole was demonstrated to be synergistic and superior to amphotericin B in achieving intravegetation drug levels in the rat model.[54] The role of this combination in the treatment of *Candida* endocarditis is not established. However, long-term cure of *Candida* PVE is difficult to substantiate. Late relapses are well described despite combined medical and surgical intervention. Risk factors for relapse remain poorly defined. In the reported cases, *C. parapsilosis* or *C. albicans* was isolated, and the time to relapse was as long as 11 years after the initial episode.[41] Multiple relapses in one patient were described as well.[41] Relapses are treated with valve replacement and amphotericin B followed by long-term suppression therapy with fluconazole. Long-term suppressive therapy with fluconazole (from several months to life-long) has been used to prevent first relapse after an initial PVE.[41]

Suppressive therapy is required in nonsurgical candidates in whom it may be impossible to eliminate infection. Several reports have documented favorable results using fluconazole for *C. parapsilosis* PVE after an initial clinical response had been achieved with amphotericin B.[46,55–57] Most authors advocate life-long treatment.

The effectiveness of prophylactic treatment for the prevention of *Candida* endocarditis in predisposed persons is not yet determined. In the rabbit *C. albicans* endocarditis model a single dose of amphotericin B (1 mg/kg) administered before *Candida* challenge was more effective than a one- or two-dose regimen of fluconazole at both 50 mg/kg and 100 mg/kg (given before challenge and 24 hours after challenge).[49] In a non-*albicans* rabbit endocarditis model, neither amphotericin B at 1 mg/kg nor fluconazole at 100 mg/kg was effective at preventing endocarditis when it was administered in a single dose regimen 1 hour before *Candida* challenge. Their effectiveness increased substantially when a second dose was given 24 hours after challenge.[58]

In summary, *Candida* endocarditis is most often associated with PVE. Radical surgical débridement and valve replacement with amphotericin B at 1 mg/kg/d followed by long-term suppressive therapy with an azole is the recommended treatment at this time.

Peripheral and Central Venous Thrombophlebitis Caused by *Candida*

Peripheral suppurative thrombophlebitis caused by *Candida* is a rare condition that occurs among critically ill patients with vascular lines and exposure to broad-spectrum antibiotics. This condition is difficult to diagnose and may thus be overlooked. It should be suspected in patients with persistent or relapsing candidemia despite treatment with systemic antifungals. In a recently described series of eight patients from Los Angeles with suppurative thrombophlebitis, multiple sites frequently were involved, and septic shock was common. Treatment experience is limited and suggests that surgery, that is, phlebectomy, is required, along with systemic anti-*Candida* therapy. Persistent candidemia may suggest incomplete phlebectomy requiring reoperation. A mild

form of *Candida*-related peripheral thrombophlebitis in seven children was reported recently. Purulent material was aspirated from the infected vein in five of the children, and in only one child was a more extensive incision and drainage performed. All survived.[59]

Catheter-related thrombosis and thrombophlebitis of the central veins, with or without candidemia, is known to be a frequent complication of central venous lines. Treatment includes line removal, anticoagulation, and intravenous administration of amphotericin B, possibly in combination with 5-flucytosine, or administration of fluconazole.[60,61] Comparative data is unavailable, and treatment is based solely on descriptive data. Occasionally conservative treatment fails. Failure is indicated by persistent candidemia, progression of thrombosis, and extension of infection into adjacent perivenous tissues with possible abscess formation.[62] Further complications may include septic embolism and superior vena cava obstruction. These conditions are associated with high mortality and poor response to medical therapy.[63] Once recognized, caval thrombectomy and ligation or resection of the involved vein should be considered.[30]

Candida Skeletal Infections

Infection of bones and joints by *Candida* is an uncommon event. It usually occurs in patients with candidemia, patients with a history of joint replacement or intra-articular injections, and, most commonly, in intravenous drug users. *Candida* spp were the second most common isolate in a series of 20 HIV-infected intravenous drug users who were diagnosed with skeletal infections.[64] Costochondral involvement is common. Osteomyelitis was observed in 75% of a series of 26 intravenous drug users with candidemia and costochondral involvement.[65] When skeletal infection is the result of hematogenous spread of candidemia, it commonly involves the lower thoracic and lumbar spine.[66] Although such complications usually occur at the time or soon after the occurrence of candidemia, they may present a year or more later.[67] *Candida* species described as the etiologic agent in skeletal infections include *C. albicans, C. parapsilosis, C. tropicalis, C. glabrata, C. krusei, C. guilliermondii,* and *C. zeylanoides.*

The choice of treatment for *Candida*-related osteomyelitis and septic arthritis is based on data from case reports and on extrapolation both from treatments of other forms of invasive candidiasis and of osteomyelitis and septic arthritis caused by other pathogens. Untreated joint infection usually destroys the joint. The difficulty of eradicating *Candida* from bones and joints and the high morbidity associated with treatment failure mandate an aggressive surgical approach. In *Candida* osteomyelitis all infected tissues should be débrided.[5] Initial treatment with intravenous amphotericin B at 0.5 to 1 mg/kg/d for 6 to 10 weeks has been used successfully.[68,69] Successful treatment with intravenous fluconazole at 6 mg/kg/d has also been described;[70–72] however, the experience with this compound as initial therapy is limited. Based on existing data, a rational approach to the therapy of osteomyelitis would include initial administration of amphotericin B for 2 to 3 weeks followed by fluconazole for a total duration of therapy of 6 to 12 weeks.[5] For the treatment of native joint infection, adequate repeated drainage is critical.[73] The administration of high-dose intravenous amphotericin B or fluconazole produces substantial synovial fluid drug-levels, and thus intra-articular drug administration seems unnecessary.[5] Treatment length is similar to that for osteomyelitis.[5] The management of prosthetic joint infections requires the removal of all hardware[5,74–76] with subsequent administration of antifungals similar to the treatment of native joint infection. Reimplantation of a new prosthesis should be delayed until infection is eradicated and adequate time is allowed to ensure that infection does not recur after discontinuation of therapy.[5]

Candida Peritonitis

Candida peritonitis usually is a complication of peritoneal dialysis or abdominal surgery or trauma. *Candida* spp are rare causes of spontaneous peritonitis in patients with liver cirrhosis.[77,78] For peritonitis secondary to dialysis, intraperitoneal amphotericin B at a concentration of 2 to 4 mg/kg/ml in dialysate fluid has been used successfully.[79] Its administration, though, can be painful and is not tolerated by many patients. Systemic fluconazole was used successfully for this indication.[80–82] Removal of the peritoneal dialysis catheter is frequently necessary for the treatment of *Candida* peritonitis and prevention of relapse.[80,83,84] The role of *Candida* isolated from the abdominal cavity of patients with abdominal trauma or operation is controversial. *Candida* spp usually are associated with a polymicrobial infection. When the organism is isolated from a patient with a clinical presentation suggestive of intra-abdominal infection or in an immunosuppressed patient, treatment with either amphotericin B or fluconazole is recommended.[79,85,86] When *Candida* is isolated after adequate repair of an acutely perforated viscus in otherwise healthy nonseptic patients, treatment generally is not recommended.[5] Similarly, treatment is also not usually recommended for *Candida* isolated from an abdominal drain placed at the time of gastrointestinal surgery.[20]

Hepatosplenic Candidiasis

Hepatosplenic candidiasis usually is detected soon after recovery from neutropenia.[87] Amphotericin B,[88,89] lipid formulations of amphotericin B,[90,91] and fluconazole[92] successfully treat this condition. Nevertheless failure rates are high. Initial therapy with amphotericin B is recommended by some experts,[20] but as prolonged therapy is required for this hard-to-eradicate condition, oral nontoxic treatment is an attractive alternative.[5] Rex et al in the recently published IDSA practice guidelines for the treatment of candidiasis recommend fluconazole at 6 mg/kg/d for stable patients. Amphotericin B at 0.6 to 0.7 mg/kg/d is recommended for unstable patients or patients with refractory disease.[5] Relapses are common when treatment is discontinued prematurely, particularly in patients who remain immunosuppressed. Therefore treatment should be continued until such time as symptoms resolve and there is radiographic evidence of calcification of the lesions.[5] For those patients requiring ongoing chemotherapy, treatment of hepatosplenic candidiasis should continue.[5,89] Although medical management is the mainstay of therapy, splenectomy may be required for the eradication of large or refractory abscesses.

Candida Central Nervous System Infections

Candida is a rare cause of meningitis. It most often complicates neonatal candidemia.[93,94] *Candida* was also reported to be a common cause of brain abscesses in bone marrow transplant patients (33% of 58 abscesses)[95,96] and in solid-organ transplant recipients with brain lesions.[95,96] *Candida* brain abscesses are associated with a mortality of 85% or higher regardless of treatment regimen.[95,96] The aggressive course of central nervous system (CNS) candidiasis mandates aggressive therapy. Limited treatment data from case reports support the use of intravenous amphotericin B at 0.7 to 1 mg/kg/d in combination with flucytosine at 25 mg/kg/d for initial therapy.[5] Intravenous fluconazole may also be effective. Because this infection tends to relapse, treatment should be continued for at least 4 weeks after all disease manifestations have resolved.[5] When *Candida* meningitis is complicating a neurosurgical procedure, therapy should include the removal of all prosthetic material plus the administration of antifungals as discussed previously.[5]

Candida Ocular Infections

Ocular candidiasis may present as focal necrotizing retinitis, chorioretinitis, or endophthalmitis. Loss of vision in the affected eye has been described in 25% to 45% of patients with *Candida* endophthalmitis.[97–99] Endophthalmitis may develop as the result of exogenous or endogenous transmission. Endogenous endophthalmitis is a consequence of candidemia. Rates of up to 26% have been reported in candidemic patients,[100] suggesting that endophthalmitis is a common complication of candidemia. As the incidence of candidemia increases, so does that of *Candida* endophthalmitis. A dilated retinal examination at baseline, preferably by an ophthalmologist, is thus recommended for all patients with candidemia. Examination should be repeated in 2 weeks, as patients can manifest endophthalmitis as long as 2 weeks after diagnosis of candidemia.[100] For patients with endophthalmitis of unknown origin a diagnostic vitreal aspirate is recommended.[5]

Among the sources for exogenous endophthalmitis are surgical or nonsurgical trauma and extension of a fungal keratitis with or without perforation of the cornea. The presentation of exogenous *Candida* endophthalmitis, as opposed to bacterial endophthalmitis, may be delayed for several weeks after trauma occurs. Outbreaks of exogenous endophthalmitis as a result of exposure to contaminated ocular irrigating solutions have also been described.[101,102]

Treatments for ocular infections include intravenous, oral, and intravitreal administration of an antifungal medication and vitrectomy. For endogenous endophthalmitis, intravenous amphotericin B with or without flucytosine is the standard treatment. In a rabbit model for the treatment of *Candida* endophthalmitis, intravenous amphotericin B demonstrated superior efficacy.[103] Successful treatment with intravenous and oral fluconazole has been described, however, particularly in cases in which the vitreous is not involved.[104] The maximal doses of amphotericin B and fluconazole appropriate for other forms of invasive candidiasis are recommended and should maximize penetration into the eye.[5] Treatment courses of 6 to 12 weeks usually are required to completely resolve visible disease or achieve convincing stabilization of the eye.[5]

Vitreitis or involvement of the anterior chamber poses a high risk for vision loss despite medical therapy. Early concomitant vitrectomy is often required.[105] A recent report of *C. albicans* endophthalmitis in heroin addicts suggests that vitrectomy performed within a week of infection that was preceded and followed by intravenous amphotericin B or fluconazole has better outcomes than late vitrectomy or no vitrectomy.[106] Some ophthalmologists inject intravitreal amphotericin B, but the role of intravitreal antifungals in endogenous endophthalmitis is unclear.[5] The effectiveness of vitrectomy for exogenous *Candida* endophthalmitis has not been studied systematically. Extrapolations from the Endophthalmitis Vitrectomy Study[107] to evaluate the role of immediate vitrectomy and intravenous antibiotics in the management of postcataract extraction bacterial endophthalmitis may be inappropriate. In this large study, all patients received an intravitreal injection of antibiotics and were randomly assigned to treatment with vitrectomy or vitreous tap and to treatment with or without intravenous antibiotics. No differences in final visual acuity or media clarity with or without the intravenous antibiotics were observed. For patients with initial light perception–only vision, immediate vitrectomy produced a threefold increase in the frequency of achieving 20/40 or better acuity and a 50% decrease in the frequency of severe visual loss. Patients with postoperative *Candida* endophthalmitis, however, often present with chronic, rather than acute, infection.[108] In these cases, culturing the specific organism can be difficult, and usually a vitrectomy is required to obtain an adequate specimen.[105] In addition, sterilization is more likely with surgical removal by vitrectomy than with

intraocular antibiotics alone.[105] Available data suggest that early vitrectomy may be of benefit to most patients with *Candida* endophthalmitis.

Prophylaxis to Prevent Invasive *Candida* Infections

Risk groups for whom prophylaxis of invasive candidiasis has been studied include neutropenic bone marrow transplant recipients, neutropenic patients with hematologic malignancies, liver-transplant recipients, and critically ill intensive care unit patients. The risk of developing an invasive *Candida* infection is not equal between and within risk groups and should be assessed on an individual patient basis using established risk factors.[109,110] Intravenous amphotericin B and intravenous and oral fluconazole are effective agents. Intravenous itraconazole, voriconazole, and other new azole and echinocandin compounds are under investigation and may provide additional treatment options.

Several controlled trials demonstrated a reduction in fungal-associated mortality in allogeneic bone marrow transplant recipients receiving oral fluconazole at 400 mg/d.[111,112] In the recently published IDSA practice guidelines for the treatment of candidiasis, Rex et all recommend fluconazole 400 mg/d during the period of neutropenia as prophylaxis for high-risk neutropenic patients.[5] This includes patients receiving chemotherapy for acute myelogenous leukemia, recipients of allogeneic bone marrow transplantation, and high-risk recipients of autologous bone marrow transplantation. It is important to note that neutropenic patients are also at risk of infections due to fungi other than *Candida* and may not respond to treatment with fluconazole. Breakthrough fungemia in patients receiving antifungal prophylaxis is also well described.[113,114]

Among patients undergoing solid-organ transplantation the risk of invasive fungal infections is highest among liver and pancreas recipients. Liver recipients at highest risk are those who have two or more of the following risk factors: retransplantation, serum creatinine clearance above 2 mg/dl, choledochojejunostomy, intraoperative use of 40 units or more of blood products, and *Candida* colonization detected within the first 3 days after transplantation.[115–117] Several randomized trials suggest that prophylactic treatment with fluconazole at 400 mg/d, amphotericin B 10 to 20 mg/d, or liposomal amphotericin B (AmBisome) at 1 mg/kg/d may reduce the incidence of invasive candidiasis among liver transplant recipients.[118–121] Treatment should be given during the early postoperative period.[5]

Approximately half of all hospital-acquired invasive *Candida* infections occur in immunocompetent patients, mostly critically ill patients in the intensive care unit. This patient population is heterogeneous in terms of risk of developing invasive candidiasis. Trials evaluating the effectiveness of fluconazole prophylaxis of *Candida* infections in this patient population are inconclusive. Incorporation of described risk factors into a predictive tool will enable the identification of subsets of patients who will benefit from prophylactic antifungal therapy.

MUCOCUTANEOUS AND URINARY INFECTIONS

Oropharyngeal Candidiasis

The risk factors and *Candida* spp typically involved in oropharyngeal candidiasis are presented in Table 41–1. The six major presentations of oropharyngeal candidiasis and their treatments are described in Table 41–2. Some important general points must be kept in mind. Acute pseudomembranous candidiasis, the most common presentation of oropharyngeal candidiasis, can often be asymptomatic, but treatment is mandatory, as failure to treat can increase discomfort from progressive colonization and predispose the patient to more invasive disease, such as esophageal candidiasis.[122] Perlèche, or angular cheilitis, commonly affects elderly patients with deepening wrinkles at the corners of the mouth, as this creates a chronically moist microenvironment.[123] These lesions can be associated with bacterial superinfection. Assessment of nutritional status should be taken at the same time as empiric therapy is begun to rule out associated riboflavin, pyridoxine, or niacin deficiency.

Candida remains of uncertain significance in the other presentations. For example, acute atrophic candidiasis and median rhomboid glossitis can be indistinguishable from B_{12}, folate, niacin, riboflavin, and protein deficiency. Chronic hyperplastic candidiasis is considered premalignant, and *Candida* spp are not always found in these lesions, raising questions about whether the yeast is merely a colonizer. Therefore biopsies of these lesions usually are required while empiric therapy is initiated. There is little value in performing swab cultures of these lesions because of the high rates of nonpathogenic candidal carrier states in the population.[124] To quantify candidal carriage, have patients rinse for 60 seconds with phosphate buffered saline, and a colony count can be obtained when the expectorant is centrifuged and cultured. More than 200 cfu/ml is more indicative of infection than of simple carriage.[125]

TABLE 41–1 ■ Risk Factors and Typical Species Associated with Mucocutaneous Candidiasis Syndromes

Syndrome	Risk factors	Usual organisms (most to least frequent)
Oropharyngeal candidiasis[126,201–214]	HIV, infancy, age, diabetes mellitus (particularly poorly controlled disease), leukemia, terminal illness, immune suppression (systemic corticosteroids and inhaled corticosteroids), antibiotic use, decreased salivary flow (Sjögren's syndrome, hypothyroidism, hypoadrenalism, anticholinergics, head and neck radiation), dentures (for atrophic candidiasis), and dietary insufficiency of iron or folate (for angular cheilitis).	*Candida albicans*, non-*albicans* (26% in HIV, 46% in cancer, associated with prior episodes, azole therapy, decrease in CD4 count): *Candida glabrata*, *Candida kruseii*, *Candida dubliniensis* (associated with HIV and IV drug use)
Refractory "thrush"[12,136]	As above, but increased risk with severe HIV disease (T cell counts less than 50/ml)	*C. albicans*, *C. glabrata*, *C. kruseii*
Esophageal candidiasis[123,171,208,215–221]	HIV, chemotherapy, hematologic malignancy, concomitant oropharyngeal candidiasis, immunosuppression, antibiotic use	*C. albicans* (53%–80%), *Candida tropicalis*, *Candida pseudotropicalis*, *C. glabrata*, *Candida parapsilosis*, and *C. kruseii*
Vulvovaginal[158,165,211,222–230]	Diabetes mellitus, HIV disease or other immunosuppression, pregnancy, antibiotic use, high-dose estrogen oral contraceptives (but not the current, lower dose hormonal oral contraceptives), obesity, and drug addiction	*C. albicans*, *C. glabrata*, other non-*albicans* strains (increased risk in recurrent disease)
Urinary tract infection[170,183,231–236]	Antibacterial therapy, duration of indwelling urinary catheters, anatomic urinary tract abnormalities, urinary tract manipulation or urologic procedures, female sex, diabetes (particularly poorly controlled diabetes), extremes of age, radiation therapy, and immunosuppression or immunosuppressive therapy, location in intensive care units, neonatal intensive care units, and hematology-oncology wards	*C. albicans*; risk of non-*albicans* species goes up with diabetes, urinary tract abnormalities, malignancies, and, most strongly, with concomitant nonfungal infections treated with antibiotics: *C. glabrata*, *C. kruseii*, *C. tropicalis*, *C. psuedotropicalis*.

HIV, human immunodeficiency virus.

TABLE 41–2 ■ Diagnosis and Therapy of Oropharyngeal and Esophageal Candidiasis

Syndrome	Diagnosis/notes	Therapy
Angular cheilitis, "perlèche"	White, raw, and weeping fissures at one or both corners of the mouth; occasionally in isolation, but usually associated with on-going thrush or denture stomatitis Can be associated with vitamin B deficiency or bacterial superinfection Associated with increased age, moisture in folds at corners of mouth Diagnostic appearance	**14-d course of one of the following**: Nystatin ointment 100,000 U/g tid–qid Clotrimazole 1% cream or ointment tid–qid Nystatin–diphenhydramine ointment tid–qid Nystatin–triamcinolone acetonide ointment tid–qid If disease persists, rule out bacterial superinfection and move to fluconazole 200 mg qd × 14 d
Denture stomatitis or chronic atrophic candidiasis	Lesions are usually localized but may be generalized in tissues that are covered by dentures, particularly the upper dentures; severity varies from asymptomatic mild inflammation to painful lesions with an extreme inflammatory reaction and the formation of highly vascularized papillary nodules	Dental referral Aggressive denture cleaning: brush or ultrasonic cleaning tank qd and overnight soaking (0.12% chlorhexidine solution, commercial denture cleanser with alkaline peroxide or benzoic acid, 10% bleach solution if no metal is present) Clotrimazole troche 5 times daily × 14 d OR Nystatin swish and swallow 5 ml qid × 14 d OR Nystatin 1–2 troches 4 to 5 times daily × 14 d OR Fluconazole 100 mg qd × 10 d
Acute atrophic candidiasis	Burning sensation in the mouth or on the tongue; examination reveals bright red tissues and loss of filiform papillae on the tongue, giving it a glossy appearance Need to rule out malignancy and vitamin deficiency	Clotrimazole troche 5 times daily × 14 d OR Nystatin swish and swallow 5 ml qid × 14 d OR Nystatin 1–2 troches 4–5 times daily × 14 d Biopsy and check B_{12}, folate, niacin, riboflavin, and protein status If disease persists, move to fluconazole 200 mg qd × 14 d
Chronic hyperplastic candidiasis	Discrete, raised lesions on the buccal mucosa or the lateral surfaces of the tongue Need to rule out malignancy and vitamin deficiency	Clotrimazole troche 5 times daily × 14 d OR Nystatin swish and swallow 5 ml qid × 14 d Nystatin 1–2 troches 4–5 times daily × 14 d OR Biopsy and check B_{12}, folate, niacin, riboflavin, and protein status If disease persists, fluconazole 200 mg qd × 14 d
Median rhomboid glossitis	Chronic, elevated, symmetrical area of hypoplasia or atrophy of the filiform papillae of the tongue anterior to the circumvalate papillae Need to rule out malignancy and vitamin deficiency	Clotrimazole troche 5 times daily × 14 d OR Nystatin swish and swallow 5 ml qid × 14 d OR Nystatin 1–2 troches 4–5 times daily × 14 d Biopsy and check B_{12}, folate, niacin, riboflavin, and protein status Persistent disease: fluconazole 200 mg qd × 14 d
Acute Pseudomembranous candidiasis, "thrush"	Discrete, white, raised patches in the oral mucosa that reveal an erythematous or bleeding base when wiped with gauze or scraped with a tongue blade Diagnostic appearance	**Uncomplicated and CD4 > 50**: Clotrimazole troche 5 times daily × 14–28 d OR Nystatin swish and swallow 5 ml qid × 14–28 d OR Nystatin 1–2 troches 4–5 times daily × 14–28 d OR Amphotericin B swish and swallow 1 ml qid given between meals 14–28 d **Complicated or CD4 < 50**: Fluconazole (tablets or suspension) 200 mg PO qd × 14 d OR Itraconazole oral solution (without food) 200 mg PO bid × 14 d

TABLE 41–2 ■ Diagnosis and Therapy of Oropharyngeal and Esophageal Candidiasis (*Continued*)

Syndrome	Diagnosis/notes	Therapy
Refractory thrush	Failure to respond to 14 d of systemic therapy with fluconazole, itraconazole, or amphotericin B Screen for hypothyroidism, hypoadrenalism, anticholinergic medications, low salivary flow conditions such as Sjögren's syndrome or local radiation therapy and the need for salivary replacement Consider culture and sensitivity testing	Improve host factors (maximally manage HIV, diabetes, nutrition, etc.) Fluconazole tablet or suspension 400–800 mg PO qd × 14–28 d Itraconazole solution 200 mg PO bid–tid × 14–28 d Amphotericin B swish & swallow 1 ml PO qid × 14–28 d Amphotericin B 0.3–0.6 mg/kg IV qd × 14 d Gentian violet paint topically bid × 14–28 d
Thrush prophylaxis	Only for severe and recurrent disease	Fluconazole 200 mg PO qd
Esophageal candidiasis	Odynophagia, dysphagia, chest pain in adults; nausea, vomiting, drooling, upper gastrointestinal bleeding in preverbal children May have concomitant oral thrush	Endoscopic diagnosis in immunocompetent patients In HIV patients, empiric therapy: Fluconazole suspension 200 mg PO qd × 14–28 d OR Itraconazole 200 mg PO bid × 14–28 d Failure should prompt endoscopic diagnosis Caspofungin 70 mg IV once, then 50 mg IV daily × 14–28 d
Refractory esophageal candidiasis	Failure of 14–28 d of azole therapy	Switch to fluconazole or itraconazole (as above) if it has not been tried OR Amphotericin B 0.3–0.5 mg/kg IV qd × 14–28 d OR Fluconazole 400–800 mg PO qd × 14–28 d Voriconazole 200 mg PO bid × 14 d

References 122, 123, 126 to 130, 134 to 136, 146 to 150a, 152, 237 to 240.

Empiric treatment with oral agents such as clotrimazole troches or nystatin swish and swallow solution should accompany diagnostic and nutritional evaluation in cases of acute atrophic candidiasis, chronic hyperplastic candidiasis, and median rhomboid glossitis. Angular cheilitis may be treated with the topical application of antifungal creams. Proper denture fit and hygiene are important adjunctive interventions for patients with denture stomatitis. Topical treatment may be effective and is facilitated when patients refrain from wearing dentures while taking the medication. Alternatively, once a day fluconazole at 50 to 100 mg for 10 days has been used with success.[126]

Treatment of acute pseudomembranous candidiasis is more complicated because of the increase in the prevalence of azole-resistant species and the greater degree of immunosuppression in these patients. The first step, if possible, is to treat the underlying immunosuppression or salivary dysfunction. Pharmacologic treatment should begin concurrently. Topical therapy with clotrimazole or nystatin swish and swallow is reasonable initial treatment for patients with uncomplicated disease, no prior history of thrush or only rare and intermittent recurrences, and HIV patients with a CD4 count greater than 50/mm³. Follow-up should occur at 2 weeks, and therapy can be extended for another 2 weeks if infection persists.[122] Patients who have complicated disease (concurrent gastrointestinal illness or recurrent disease, and HIV patients with CD4 counts less than 50/mm³) or in whom topical oral therapy fails should be treated with systemic antifungals. In these cases fluconazole has proven efficacy over clotrimazole troches and nystatin swish and swallow.[127–130] Patients with esophageal symptoms should be treated empirically for esophageal candidiasis as outlined in the next discussion. If the episode is part of frequent recurrences, consideration should be given to isolating the yeast and testing it for antifungal susceptibility.

Unless there is prior knowledge of species or resistance profile, fluconazole is a reasonable first-line systemic agent for the treatment of oropharyngeal candidiasis because of its ease of administration, improved safety and interaction profile, and excellent absorption.[131–133] Now that a more bioavailable oral solution has been produced, itraconazole at 200 mg twice a day is an effective alternative.[134,135] Oral amphotericin B suspension is also now available, and one trial demonstrated clinical efficacy similar to that of fluconazole oral suspension.[135]

Refractory oropharyngeal candidiasis is defined as failure of oropharyngeal candidiasis to respond to a 14-day course of systemic therapy: itraconazole 200 mg twice a day, fluconazole 200 mg a day, amphotericin B oral solution 500 mg four times a day, or IV amphotericin B 1 mg/kg/d.[136] Treatment for refractory disease remains problematic. Itraconazole used for fluconazole-refractory disease had a 55% to 65% response rate, but at 2 months the relapse rate was 36% to 100%.[137,138] Similar response and relapse rates have occurred with oral amphotericin B solution.[139] Administration of intravenous amphotericin B may be required when both of these options have been exhausted. However, its adverse reactions, nephrotoxicity, and requirement for intravenous access lessen the desirability of this option. Improving host factors by maximizing antiretroviral therapy and aggressively treating malnutrition is critical to treatment success. Even then, clinical failures with intravenous amphotericin B can occur. In these situations, there have been some reports of success with doses of fluconazole up to 800 mg/d.[13] Also, one can attempt treatment with topical gentian violet 1% to 2% solution (painted on the oropharynx with a swab twice a day), but the staining effect is too unattractive for most patients. There is a single case report of successful treatment of fluconazole-, itraconazole-, and parenteral amphotericin B–refractory oropharyngeal candidiasis with a bovine lactoferrin– and lysozyme-containing mouthwash (which show in vitro activity against *Candida* spp) and itraconazole therapy.[140] There is also a small trial that showed some mild success for refractory disease (16.7% cure rate) with Melaleuca oral solution, a derivative from an Australian tea leaf that shows in vitro activity against *Candida* spp.[141]

Minimizing azole resistance is important to avoid problems with refractory oropharyngeal candidiasis. Targeted prophylaxis of oropharyngeal candidiasis with fluconazole at 200 mg/d restricted to patients with severe, recurrent disease is a reasonable strategy.[142] Once weekly fluconazole has been proposed but is associated with a risk of relapse.[143] A large prospective clinical trial comparing long-term suppressive therapy with episodic treatment is in the final phase of analysis at the time of this writing; it is hoped it will define the optimal strategy for prevention of relapse and address development of azole resistance by treatment strategy.

Esophageal Candidiasis

Please see Tables 41–1 and 41–2 for risk factors, *Candida* species, presentation, diagnosis, and treatment recommendations for esophageal candidiasis. The definitive diagnosis of esophageal candidiasis is made by endoscopy. Macroscopic findings include yellow-to-tan (and rarely black-green) plaques on the esophageal mucosa. In severe cases these plaques can coalesce circumferentially to coat the mucosal surface and can even impinge upon the esophageal lumen. Pathology is diagnostic. Concomitant ulcers are not uncommon, but in HIV patients, only about 10% of these are due to *Candida* alone; usually another agent is present (cytomegalovirus, herpes simplex, or idiopathic ulcers).[144] Complications of *Candida* esophagitis are rare but include esophageal hemorrhage, lumenal obstruction secondary to fibrosis and stricture formation, fistulization into the bronchial tree, and esophageal perforation into the mediastinum.[145]

Most comparative treatment studies on esophageal candidiasis are based on cohorts of patients with HIV. Presumptive treatment with fluconazole of patients with HIV disease and esophageal symptoms without endoscopic confirmation is cost effective and safe.[146] Fluconazole at 200 mg/d is the first-line therapy of choice, as it is more efficacious than flucytosine, ketoconazole, or itraconazole capsules.[147,148] Studies have shown, however, that itraconazole oral solution (200 mg twice a day) or itraconazole solution plus flucytosine are equivalent to fluconazole in efficacy.[149,150] Now that fluconazole solution is available and seems to be effective, it is an attractive option for patients having difficulty swallowing pills.[151] A recent study demonstrated that voriconazole, a new azole antifungal, is as effective as Fluconazole in treating candida esophagitis.[150a] Treatment courses should last 14 to 28 days depending upon response. Failure of response to fluconazole or itraconazole solution should prompt an endoscopic diagnosis if not already undertaken.

In esophageal candidiasis, as in oropharyngeal candidiasis, refractory disease or mycologic resistance may occur. A switch to higher dose fluconazole or to itraconazole solution may be effective, but treatment with low-dose parenteral amphotericin B (0.3 to 0.5 mg/kg/d) may be required.[152] Newer agents such as the broad-spectrum triazoles or echinocandins are exciting alternatives. Voriconazole and caspofungin are as effective as fluconazole.[153,154]

Vulvovaginal Candidiasis

Vulvovaginal candidiasis (VVC) is the most common form of mucocutaneous candidiasis in women.[155,156] Table 41–1 lists risk factors and species that are typically involved and Table 41–3 lists presentations and diagnostic features. Recurrent vulvovaginal candidiasis (RVVC) is defined as four or more symptomatic episodes per year. This occurs in less than 5% of healthy women in their reproductive years. Underlying risks are the same as for simple VVC.[155,157] Recurrent disease, however, can occur in the absence of any risk factors.[158] The most likely cause is the re-emergence of disease from residual yeast remaining after initial therapy.[159,160] Although *C. albicans* remains the most common species isolated, resistant non-*albicans* spp may emerge.[155,157,161] Morbid physical sequelae from recurrent disease have not been well documented; however, significant psychological consequences of depression, decreased satisfaction with life, decreased self-esteem, and increased stress have been described.[162]

Multiple preparations are available for the treatment of VVC (Table 41–4). The major classes available include the topical azoles, the topical polyene antifungal nystatin, and the systemic azoles. For recurrent disease, boric acid and gentian violet can be used. The choice of therapy depends upon the characteristics and preferences of the patient being treated. Cure rates are similar for acute and uncomplicated disease except for nystatin, which is only slightly less effective for acute disease.[163] For severe disease, systemic fluconazole has been proven to be marginally superior.[164]

TABLE 41–3 ■ Presentation and Diagnosis of Vulvovaginal Candidiasis[155,158]

	Presentation	Laboratory tests	Differential
Vulvovaginal candidiasis	Vulvar itching/burning, soreness, discharge, superficial dyspareunia, erythema, edema, fissuring, curdy discharge, satellite lesions	Negative whiff test (amine test), normal pH (4–4.5), no increase in inflammatory cells, yeast forms under microscopy (best on Gram stain but can use KOH or wet prep), positive fungal culture	Bacterial vaginosis, *Trichomonas* vaginitis, atrophic vaginitis
Recurrent vulvovaginal candidiasis	As above with ≥4 episodes within 12 mo	Fungal culture and sensitivity, consider biopsy	Seborrheic dermatitis, eczema, lichen sclerosus et atrophicus, hypersensitivity vulvitis, psoriasis

Topical therapy provides more immediate relief of local symptoms. Oral therapy is more inconvenient and less messy, but there is an increased risk of drug interaction and adverse effects. In all of these cases it is important to note whether these treatments are compatible with latex contraceptives (condoms and diaphragms) and their safety in pregnancy. For the most part the topical azoles have been assumed to be safe in the second and third trimester of pregnancy. Some are systemically absorbed, however, and should be avoided in the first trimester. The systemic azoles should be avoided in pregnancy if possible. The drug that has the longest history and that is known to be quite compatible with latex contraceptives is nystatin.

Other principles of management include attending to possible exacerbating factors, such as avoiding perfumed products that may act as local irritants and tight-fitting clothing that may increase the moisture of the local environment. Blood sugar should be aggressively managed in patients with diabetes. It is important to note that the systemic azoles elevate serum levels of the sulfonylureas and can potentiate hypoglycemic reactions, sometimes with deleterious results.[165] HIV infection should be aggressively managed in infected patients. They are sometimes treated with prophylactic fluconazole because of recurrent oropharyngeal or vulvovaginal disease; it has been shown to reduce the incidence of recurrence, although the advantages need to be weighed against the risk of increasing colonization with resistant species.[166]

The management of clinically defined RVVC is based upon induction of remission followed by 6 months of maintenance therapy to break the cycle of re-emergence. Please see Figure 41–1 for a recommended treatment algorithm and Table 41–4 for the dosing regimens. The regimens recommended are mostly derived from anecdotal data or specialists' opinions, as there have been few adequately powered clinical trials. It is also important to

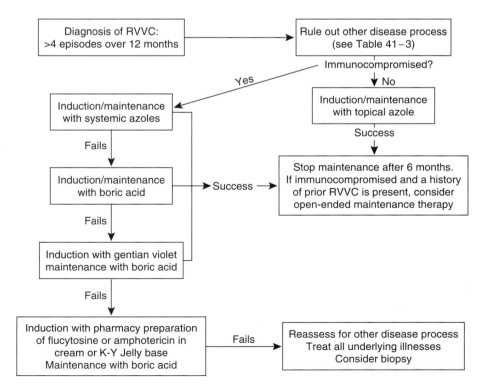

FIGURE 41–1. Algorithm for treatment of RVVC. 1, More than 4 episodes of VVC over 12 months → RVVC. 2, Rule out other diseases (see differential diagnosis, Table 41–3). 3, If immunocompetent, try induction/maintenance with topical azole. If this fails or patient is immunocompromised, go to step 4. 4, Induction/maintenance with systemic azoles. 5, If systemic azoles fail, attempt use of boric acid for induction/maintenance. 6, If boric acid fails, attempt use of gentian violet for induction followed by boric acid for maintenance. 7, If gentian violet fails, try a pharmacy preparation of flucytosine or amphotericin mixed in cream or K-Y Jelly applied topically bid/tid for 14 days, followed by boric acid for maintenance.

TABLE 41–4 ■ Therapeutic Options for Vulvovaginal Candidiasis (VVC)

Dosage in acute VVC	Dosage in recurrent disease: induction	Dosage in recurrent disease: maintenance	Pregnancy, lactation	Safe with latex contraceptives
TOPICAL AZOLES				
Butoconazole				
2% cream 5 g × 3 d	2% cream 5 g × 14 d		avoid in first trimester	No
Clotrimazole				
Pessary 500 mg × 1 d	Cream 1% 5 g × 14 d	Pessary 500 mg/wk × 6 mo	Safe	?
Pessary 200 mg × 3 d		Pessary 200 mg × 2/w × 6 mo		
Pessary 100 mg × 7 d				
Vaginal cream 10% 5 g × 1				
Cream 1% 5 g × 7–14 d				
Econazole				
Pessary 150 mg × 1 d	Pessary 150 mg × 14 d		Class C, uncertain	No
Pessary 150 mg × 3 d				
Fenticonazole				
Pessary 600 mg × 1 d	Cream 2% 5 g × 14 d		Safe	No
Pessary 200 mg × 3 d				
Cream 2% 5 g × 7 d				
Isoconazole				
Two 300-mg vaginal tablets × 1			Class C, not recommended	?
Miconazole				
Pessary 100 mg × 14 nights	Pessary 100 mg × 14 nights		Class C, avoid in first trimester	No
Cream 2% 5 g × 7 d				
Vaginal suppository 100 mg × 7 d				
Vaginal suppository 200 mg × 3 d				
Vaginal suppository 1200 mg × 1 d				
Terconazole				
Cream 0.5% 5 g × 7 d	Cream 0.5% 5 g × 14 d	Cream 0.8% 5 g once q wk	avoid in first trimester	?
Cream 0.8% 5 g × 3 d				
Vaginal suppository 80 mg × 3 d				
Tioconazole				
Cream 2% 5 g × 3 d			Class C, uncertain	No
Cream 6.5% 5 g × 3 d				
POLYENES				
Nystatin				
Vaginal cream 100,000 U 4 g × 14 nights			Safe	Yes
Pessary 100,000 U 1–2 pessaries at night × 14 nights				
SYSTEMIC AZOLES				
Fluconazole				
150 mg tablet × 1	200 mg tablet × 14 d	100 mg tablet qwk × 6 mo	Not safe	Yes
		200 mg tablet qwk × 6 mo		
		150 mg tablet qmo × 6 mo		
Itraconazole				
200 mg bid × 1 d	200 mg bid × 14 d	400 mg/mo × 6 mo	Not safe	Yes
200 mg qd × 3 d		200 mg/mo × 6 mo		
		100 mg/d × 6 mo		

TABLE 41–4 ■ Therapeutic Options for Vulvovaginal Candidiasis (VVC)
(Continued)

Dosage in acute VVC	Dosage in recurrent disease: induction	Dosage in recurrent disease: maintenance	Pregnancy, lactation	Safe with latex contraceptives
Ketoconazole 200 mg bid × 5 d	200 mg qd × 14 d 400 mg qd × 14 d	100 mg/d × 6 mo 200 mg/d × 5 d after menses × 6 mo 100 mg/d × 6 mo	Not safe	Yes
MISCELLANEOUS Boric acid	Vaginal suppository 600 mg bid × 14 d Vaginal suppository 600 mg qd × 14 d	Vaginal suppository 600 mg qd during the 5 d of menstruation × 6 mo	Not safe	?
Gentian violet	Tampon 5 mg × 3–4 h bid × 12–14 d (may leave in overnight if refractory) Avoid intercourse during therapy		Not safe	No

References 155, 158, 159, 164, 167, 241, 242.

treat underlying conditions, such as HIV infection or diabetes.[159] One should also give consideration to empiric antifungal coverage whenever the patient requires a course of antibiotics.[167]

Given the long course of maintenance therapy, there have been concerns about potentiating the rise of resistant isolates, but this has not been demonstrated clinically.[168] An alternative to the long maintenance phase, however, is simply to treat recurrences symptomatically as they occur. This was examined in a small trial of 44 women with clotrimazole, and although there were more breakthroughs with empiric therapy than with maintenance therapy, patient satisfaction and cost-saving were improved with empiric therapy.[169]

Candida Urinary Tract Infections

Urinary tract infections with *Candida* spp are for the most part nosocomial infections that target specific populations and usually are associated with urinary catheters. Indeed *Candida* spp are responsible for 2% to 15% of all nosocomial urinary tract infections.[170–172] Risk factors are presented in Table 41–1. Potential complications of *Candida* urinary tract infections are multiple. Ascending infection can lead to the development of fungus balls, also known as fungal bezoars, that may cause ureteral or cystic obstruction. *Candida* pyelonephritis is usually the result of candidemia and dissemination, but patients with abnormal urinary tracts or those who undergo urologic procedures while colonized are also at higher risk for this complication.[173,174] Candidemia that is a complication of urinary tract infection occurs in less than 10% of cases and usually is associated with urinary obstruction or anatomic abnormalities.[172,175] Emphysematous cystitis, prostatitis, and prostatic abscesses, although uncommon,

do occur, usually in patients with diabetes.[173,176,177] Several cases of candidal epididymo-orchitis have been reported, often in association with penile prostheses.[178]

Most patients with urinary candidiasis are asymptomatic; thus, the significance of a single positive urine culture is unclear. Clues that a positive culture is more than just contamination or colonization of a urinary catheter include a colony count of more than 10,000 cfu/ml and a second positive confirmatory culture or the presence of pyuria on urinalysis. If fever, sepsis, dysuria, hematuria, suprapubic tenderness, or leukocytosis is present, infection should be presumed and treated.[173] In patients with symptomatic urinary candidiasis, blood cultures should be obtained to rule out systemic candidemia, and radiographic imaging should be obtained to rule out complicated upper urinary tract disease, pyelonephritis, or locally invasive disease (emphysematous cystitis, prostatitis, or epididymo-orchitis).[173,178] Patients with pyelonephritis can present with signs and symptoms indistinguishable from bacterial pyelonephritis, such as fever, leukocytosis, and costovertebral angle tenderness.[173] The best imaging modality for upper urinary tract disease is either computed tomography with parenteral contrast or renal ultrasonography, although an intravenous pyelogram may be required in difficult cases.[179,180]

In the past, therapy for urinary tract disease has been controversial.[181] These infections may be organized into five clinical syndromes and managed accordingly. The clinical syndromes are asymptomatic infection in an immunocompetent host, symptomatic infection in an immunocompetent host, infection in a compromised host (defined as patients who have undergone renal transplantation, low-birth-weight infants, neutropenic patients, patients with urinary tract abnormalities or who are about to undergo urologic manipulation, and critically ill patients), ascending infection, and renal candidiasis

TABLE 41–5 ■ Therapy of *Candida* Urinary Tract Infections

Syndrome	First-line therapy	Second-line therapy
Asymptomatic candiduria, immunocompetent host	Remove or change urinary catheter Address host risk factors Usually resolves spontaneously with these changes, low risk of complications	Fluconazole 200 mg qd × 7–14 d (only if necessary)
Asymptomatic candiduria, compromised host	Fluconazole 400 mg × 1 followed by 200 mg/d × 7–14 d (treatment with fluconazole reduces risk of dissemination and improves survival)	Amphotericin B bladder irrigation (50 mg/l) at 42 ml/h × 3–5 d Amphotericin B 0.3 mg/kg IV × 1
Symptomatic *Candida*, cystitis	Fluconazole 400 mg × 1 followed by 200 mg/d × 7–14 d (better sustained cure rate, treats upper tract disease), double dose for resistant species, do not renally adjust (because of decreased urine levels in renal disease)	Amphotericin B bladder irrigation (50 mg/l) at 42 ml/h × 3–5 d (more rapid clearance of candiduria but does not treat upper tract disease) Amphotericin B 0.3 mg/kg IV × 1 Flucytosine 25 mg/kg/d × 7–14 d with amphotericin (not enough experience with lipid preparations to warrant recommendations at this time)
Ascending pyelonephritis	Surgical drainage & removal of fungal balls, nephrostomy tubes if necessary (can serve as a mode of antibiotic delivery) PLUS Fluconazole 6 mg/kg/d (maximum 400 mg) × 2–6 wk OR Amphotericin B 0.6 to 1 mg/kg/d × 2–6 wk	
Renal candidiasis	Fluconazole 6 mg/kg/d (maximum 400 mg) × 2–6 wk OR Amphotericin B 0.6–1 mg/kg/d × 2–6 wk Imaging to rule out perinephric abscess, blood cultures to rule out candidemia	

References 172, 173, 179, 182 to 184, 186, 188, 233, 243 to 249.

TABLE 41–6 ■ Topical Antifungal Therapies

Antifungal	Directions	Preparations
Clotrimazole (Lotrimin, Mycelex)	Apply topically bid × 14 d	Cream 1% (15, 30, 45, 90 g), solution 1% (10, 30 ml), lotion 1% (30 ml)
Econazole (Spectazole)	Apply topically bid × 14 d	Cream 1% (15, 30, 85 g)
Ketoconazole (Nizoral)	Apply topically bid × 14 d	Cream 2% (15, 30, 60 g)
Miconazole (Monistat-Derm, Micatin)	Apply topically bid × 14 d	Ointment 2% (29 g), spray 2% (105 ml), solution 2% (7.39, 30 ml), cream 2% (15, 30, 90 g), powder 2% (90 g), spray powder 2% (90, 100 g), spray liquid 2% (105, 113 ml)
Nystatin (Mycostatin)	Apply topically bid to tid × 14 d	Cream 100,000 U/g (15, 30, 240 g), ointment 100,000 U/g (15, 30 g), powder 100,000 U/g (15 g)

References 189, 190, 191.

(which occurs in colonized patients who are undergoing urologic manipulation or patients with end-organ seeding from candidemia).[173,182] Table 41–5 outlines specific recommendations by clinical syndrome. In every situation, however, certain basic principles apply. First, there is ample evidence that an easy first step, the removal of unnecessary urinary catheters, or even temporary removal with reinsertion of a new urinary catheter, can resolve candiduria nearly half the time.[183–188] Second, the delivery route of each therapy must be considered. Amphotericin bladder washes will not treat or prevent infection in the upper urinary tracts. Fluconazole is ideal, as it is well tolerated and excreted in high concentrations in the urine, but urine levels are low in renal insufficiency. Lundstrom and Sobel suggest that to maintain adequate urinary drug levels in renal failure, it may be necessary to use unadjusted doses of fluconazole.[173] Finally, in every case, care must be taken to correct any reversible host factors that may contribute to the candiduria, such as hyperglycemia or unnecessary treatment with antibacterial antibiotics.

Potential complications of candiduria are many. Emphysematous cystitis or fungal bezoars in the bladder require surgical exploration and drainage to prevent bladder rupture.[174] Emphysematous prostatitis or prostatic abscesses require transurethral drainage. Candidal epididymo-orchitis may require surgical resection and, if a prosthesis is present, removal of the prosthesis. All of these cases require systemic therapy with either fluconazole (at least 400 mg/d) or amphotericin B (at 0.6 mg/kg/d) for 2 to 6 weeks.[178]

Cutaneous Candidiasis

The most common form of candidal infection of the skin is intertrigo, which results in erythema, maceration, and peeling of the skin in the intertriginous areas, most commonly the gluteal folds, interdigital spaces, and the axillae. This is associated with moist and wet skin, particularly in patients with diabetes, the immunocompromised, the critically ill, the incontinent, and neonates (where the syndrome is known commonly as diaper rash or candidal diaper dermatitis).[189,190] Interdigital candidiasis (or *erosio interdigitalis*) is a chronic infection with macerated tissue in the web spaces of the fingers or toes. *Candida* miliaria presents as vesiculopustules on the back of bedridden patients.[191,192] Candidal folliculitis, which presents with pruritus and an erythematous eruption of papules and pustules, is rare but can be associated with intravenous hyperalimentation, antibiotic therapy, or hypothyroidism.[193] Candidal balanitis presents with pain, burning, erythema, and small, irregular, eroded papules on the penis. In patients with diabetes, this can progress to an acute, fulminating, edematous balanoposthitis.[194]

Primary therapy for all of these cutaneous syndromes is topical application for 7 to 14 days, depending upon response (Table 41–5). Moist skin should be kept dry, clean, and aerated, particularly in the cases of intertrigo, interdigital candidiasis, and candidal balanitis. In the case of candidal balanitis a single dose of 150 mg of fluconazole has proven effective.[194] Other cases of cutaneous candidiasis have been successfully treated with two to three doses of once weekly fluconazole at 150 mg.[195] In cases of severe disease, brief courses of oral therapy (fluconazole or itraconazole) can be used, but dosage and duration have not been standardized.[196]

Chronic Mucocutaneous Candidiasis

Chronic mucocutaneous candidiasis is a collection of genetic syndromes associated with a poorly understood impairment of host immune defenses that give rise to debilitating, persistent, and refractory infections of the skin, nails, and mucous membranes with *Candida* spp.[197] Other associated disorders in these syndromes, including hypoadrenalism, hypoparathyroidism, and hypothyroidism, seem to result from autoantibodies against endocrine organs, although other organs may be affected.[198] These patients are also susceptible to multiple other infections, including bacterial (including *nocardia)*, other fungal (such as *Histoplasma*), and disseminated viral diseases.[199] Quality of life has been markedly improved by long-term therapy for many months at a time with the systemic oral azoles.[199] There has been a report of a successful bone marrow transplantation resolving the syndrome.[200] The bone marrow transplant was performed specifically in hopes of curing the patient's chronic cutaneous candidiasis, which had become severe and invasive.

REFERENCES

1. Banerjee SN, Emori TG, Culver DH, et al: Secular trends in nosocomial primary bloodstream infections in the United States, 1980–1989. National Nosocomial Infections Surveillance System. Am J Med 1991;91(3B):86S–89S.
2. Wey SB, Mori M, Pfaller MA, et al: Hospital-acquired candidemia. The attributable mortality and excess length of stay. Arch Intern Med 1988;148:2642–2645.
3. Lecciones JA, Lee JW, Navarro EE, et al: Vascular catheter–associated fungemia in patients with cancer: Analysis of 155 episodes. Clin Infect Dis 1992;14:875–883.
4. Fraser VJ, Jones M, Dunkel J: Candidemia in a tertiary care hospital: epidemiology, risk factors, and predictors of mortality. [See Comments.] [Review] [35 Refs]. Clin Infect Dis 1992;15(3):414–421.
5. Rex JH, Walsh TJ, Sobel JD, et al: Practice guidelines for the treatment of candidiasis. Infectious Diseases Society of America. [See Comments.] Clin Infect Dis 2000;30:662–678.
6. Bates DW, Su L, Yu DT, et al: Mortality and costs of acute renal failure associated with amphotericin B therapy. Clin Infect Dis 2001;32:686–693.
7. Kontoyiannis DP, Bodey GP, Mantzoros CS: Fluconazole vs. amphotericin B for the management of candidaemia in adults: A meta-analysis. Mycoses 2001;44:125–135.
8. Laguna F, Rodriguez-Tudela JL, Martinez-Suarez JV, et al: Patterns of fluconazole susceptibility in isolates from human immunodeficiency virus-infected patients with oropharyngeal candidiasis due to *Candida albicans*. Clin Infect Dis 1997;24:124–130.
9. Pfaller MA, Messer SA, Hollis RJ: Strain delineation and antifungal susceptibilities of epidemiologically related and unrelated isolates of *Candida lusitaniae*. Diagn Microbiol Infect Dis 1994;20:127–133.
10. Yoon SA, Vazquez JA, Steffan PE, et al: High-frequency, in vitro reversible switching of *Candida lusitaniae* clinical isolates from amphotericin B susceptibility to resistance. Antimicrob Agents Chemother 1999;43:836–845.
11. Pfaller MA, Jones RN, Messer SA, et al: National surveillance of nosocomial blood stream infection due to *Candida albicans*: Frequency of occurrence and antifungal susceptibility in the SCOPE Program. Diagn Microbiol Infect Dis 1998;31:327–332.
12. Rex JH, Pfaller MA, Galgiani JN, et al: Development of interpretive breakpoints for antifungal susceptibility testing: Conceptual framework and analysis of in vitro–in vivo correlation data for fluconazole, itraconazole, and *Candida* infections. Subcommittee on Antifungal Susceptibility Testing of the National Committee for Clinical Laboratory Standards. [See Comments.] [Review] [123 Refs]. Clin Infect Dis 1997;24:235–247.
13. Revankar SG, Kirkpatrick WR, Mcatee RK, et al: A randomized trial of continuous or intermittent therapy with fluconazole for oropharyngeal candidiasis in HIV-infected patients: Clinical outcomes and development of fluconazole resistance. Am J Med 1998;105:7–11.
14. White MH, Bowden RA, Sandler ES, et al: Randomized, double-blind clinical trial of amphotericin B colloidal dispersion

vs. amphotericin B in the empirical treatment of fever and neutropenia. [See Comments.] Clin Infect Dis 1998;27:296–302.

15. Hiemenz JW, Walsh TJ: Lipid formulations of amphotericin B: Recent progress and future directions. [Review] [83 Refs]. Clin Infect Dis 1996;22(Suppl-44).

16. Wong-Beringer A, Jacobs RA, Guglielmo BJ: Lipid formulations of amphotericin B: Clinical efficacy and toxicities. [Review] [91 Refs]. Clin Infect Dis 1998;27:603–618.

17. Rex JH, Walsh TJ, Anaissie EJ: Fungal infections in Iatrogenically compromised hosts. [Review] [290 Refs]. Adv Intern Med 1998;43:321–371.

18. Nguyen MH, Peacock JE Jr, Tanner DC, et al: Therapeutic approaches in patients with candidemia. Evaluation in a multicenter, prospective, observational study. Arch Intern Med 1995;155:2429–2435.

19. Rex JH, Bennett JE, Sugar AM, et al: Intravascular catheter exchange and duration of candidemia. NIAID Mycoses Study Group and the Candidemia Study Group. Clin Infect Dis 1995;21:994–996.

20. Edwards JE Jr, Bodey GP, Bowden RA, et al: International Conference for the Development of a Consensus on the Management and Prevention of Severe Candidal Infections. [See Comments.] [Review] [89 Refs]. Clin Infect Dis 1997;25:43–59.

21. Edwards JE Jr, Filler SG: Current strategies for treating invasive candidiasis: Emphasis on infections in nonneutropenic patients. [Review] [72 Refs]. Clin Infect Dis 1992;14(Suppl 13).

22. Rex JH, Bennett JE, Sugar AM, et al: A randomized trial comparing fluconazole with amphotericin B for the treatment of candidemia in patients without neutropenia. Candidemia Study Group and the National Institute. [See Comments.] N Engl J Med 1994;331:1325–1330.

23. Anaissie EJ, Rex JH, Uzun O, Vartivarian S: Predictors of adverse outcome in cancer patients with candidemia. Am J Med 1998;104:238–245.

24. Pfaller MA, Jones RN, Messer SA, et al: National surveillance of nosocomial blood stream infection due to *Candida albicans*: Frequency of occurrence and antifungal susceptibility in the SCOPE Program. Diagn Microbiol Infect Dis 1998;31:327–332.

25. Nguyen MH, Peacock JE Jr, Morris AJ, et al: The changing face of candidemia: Emergence of non-*Candida albicans* species and antifungal resistance. Am J Med 1996;100:617–623.

26. Krçmery V Jr, Mrazova M, Kunova A, et al: Nosocomial candidaemias due to species other than *Candida albicans* in cancer patients. Aetiology, risk factors, and outcome of 45 episodes within 10 years in a single cancer institution. Support Care Cancer 1999;7:428–431.

27. Drutz DJ: In vitro antifungal susceptibility testing and measurement of levels of antifungal agents in body fluids. [Review] [60 Refs]. Rev Infect Dis 1987;9:392–397.

28. Louie A, Kaw P, Banerjee P, et al: Impact of the order of initiation of fluconazole and amphotericin B in sequential or combination therapy on killing of *Candida albicans* in vitro and in a rabbit model of endocarditis and pyelonephritis. Antimicrob Agents Chemother 2001;45:485–494.

29. Rex JH, Pappas PG, Karchmer AW, et al: A randomized and blinded multicenter trial of high-dose fluconazole plus placebo versus fluconazole plus amphotericin B as treatment of candidemia in non-neutropenic patients. 2001. ICAAC 2001.

30. Benoit D, Decruyenaere J, Vandewoude K, et al: Management of candidal thrombophlebitis of the central veins: Case report and review. [Review] [31 Refs]. Clin Infect Dis 1998;26:393–397.

31. Gouello JP, Asfar P, Brenet O, et al: Nosocomial endocarditis in the intensive care unit: An analysis of 22 cases. Crit Care Med 2000;28:377–382.

32. Groll A, Schneider M, Gaida BJ, Hubner K: [Infectious endocarditis from the morphologic viewpoint: on the pathology and clinical aspects of 97 autopsy cases]. [German]. Med Klin 1991;86(2):59–70.

33. Fischer SA, Trenholme GM, Costanzo MR, Piccione W: Infectious complications in left ventricular assist device recipients. Clin Infect Dis 1997;24:18–23.

34. Hogevik H, Alestig K: Fungal endocarditis—a report on seven cases and a brief review. [Review] [40 Refs]. Infection 1996;24:17–21.

35. Mayayo E, Moralejo J, Camps J, Guarro J: Fungal endocarditis in premature infants: Case report and review. [Review] [16 Refs]. Clin Infect Dis 1996;22:366–368.

36. Weems JJ Jr: *Candida parapsilosis*: Epidemiology, pathogenicity, clinical manifestations, and antimicrobial susceptibility. [See Comments.] [Review] [170 Refs]. Clin Infect Dis 1992;14:756–766.

37. Wilson HA, Downes TR, Julian JS, et al: *Candida* endocarditis. A treatable form of pacemaker infection. Chest 1993;103:283–284.

38. Martino P, Micozzi A, Venditti M, et al: Catheter-related right-sided endocarditis in bone marrow transplant recipients. Rev Infect Dis 1990;12:250–257.

39. Fedalen PA, Fisher CA, Todd BA, et al: Early fungal endocarditis in homograft recipients. Ann Thorac Surg 1999; 68:1410–1411.

40. Verghese S, Mullasari A, Padmaja P, et al: Fungal endocarditis following cardiac surgery. Indian Heart J 1998; 50:418–422.

41. Melgar GR, Nasser RM, Gordon SM, et al: Fungal prosthetic valve endocarditis in 16 patients. An 11-year experience in a tertiary care hospital. Medicine 1997;76(2):94–103.

42. Wendt B, Haglund L, Razavi A, Rath R: *Candida lusitaniae*: An uncommon cause of prosthetic valve endocarditis. Clin Infect Dis 1998;26:769–770.

43. Turnier E, Kay JH, Bernstein S, et al: Surgical treatment of *Candida* endocarditis. Chest 1975;67:262–268.

44. Nguyen MH, Nguyen ML, Yu VL, et al: *Candida* prosthetic valve endocarditis: Prospective study of six cases and review of the literature. [Review] [21 Refs]. Clin Infect Dis 1996;22:262–267.

45. Slaughter L, Morris JE, Starr A: Prosthetic valvular endocarditis. A 12-year review. Circulation 1973;47:1319–1326.

46. Baddour LM: Long-term suppressive therapy for *Candida parapsilosis*–induced prosthetic valve endocarditis. Mayo Clinic Proc 1995;70:773–775.

47. Fernandez Guerrero ML, Gadea I: [The treatment of *Candida*-induced endocarditis. The arguments for a medical-surgical focus]. [Spanish] [Review] [44 Refs]. Rev Clin Espanola 1994;194:989–991.

48. Muehrcke DD, Lytle BW, Cosgrove DM III: Surgical and long-term antifungal therapy for fungal prosthetic valve endocarditis. Ann Thorac Surg 1995;60:538–543.

49. Witt MD, Bayer AS: Comparison of fluconazole and amphotericin B for prevention and treatment of experimental *Candida* endocarditis. Antimicrob Agents Chemother 1991;35:2481–2485.

50. Louie A, Liu W, Miller DA, et al: Efficacies of high-dose fluconazole plus amphotericin B and high-dose fluconazole plus 5-fluorocytosine versus amphotericin B, fluconazole, and 5-fluorocytosine monotherapies in treatment of experimental endocarditis, endophthalmitis, and pyelonephritis due to *Candida albicans*. Antimicrob Agents Chemother 1999;43:2831–2840.

51. Witt MD, Imhoff T, Li C, Bayer AS: Comparison of fluconazole and amphotericin B for treatment of experimental *Candida* endocarditis caused by Non-*C. albicans* strains. Antimicrob Agents Chemother 1993;37:2030–2032.

52. Chemlal K, Saint-Julien L, Joly V, et al: Comparison of fluconazole and amphotericin B for treatment of experimental *Candida albicans* endocarditis in rabbits. Antimicrob Agents Chemother 1996;40:263–266.

53. Sanati H, Ramos CF, Bayer AS, Ghannoum MA: Combination therapy with amphotericin B and fluconazole against invasive candidiasis in neutropenic-mouse and infective-endocarditis rabbit models. Antimicrob Agents Chemother 1997;41:1345–1348.

54. Marchetti O, Entenza JM, Sanglard D, et al: Fluconazole plus cyclosporine: A fungicidal combination effective against experimental endocarditis due to *Candida albicans*. Antimicrob Agents Chemother 2000;44:2932–2938.

55. Czwerwiec FS, Bilsker MS, Kamerman ML, Bisno AL: Long-term survival after fluconazole therapy of candidal prosthetic valve endocarditis. Am J Med 1993;94:545–546.

56. Isalska BJ, Stanbridge TN: Fluconazole in the treatment of candidal prosthetic valve endocarditis. BMJ 1988;297(6642):178–179.

57. Zahid MA, Klotz SA, Hinthorn DR: Medical treatment of recurrent candidemia in a patient with probable *Candida parapsilosis* prosthetic valve endocarditis. Chest 1994;105:1597–1598.

58. Bayer AS, Witt MD, Kim E, Ghannoum MA: Comparison of fluconazole and amphotericin B in prophylaxis of experimental *Candida* endocarditis caused by non-*C. albicans* strains. Antimicrob Agents Chemother 1996;40:494–496.

59. Friedland IR: Peripheral thrombophlebitis caused by *Candida*. Pediatr Infect Dis J 1996;15:375–377.

60. Jarrett F, Maki DG, Chan CK: Management of septic thrombosis of the inferior vena cava caused by *Candida*. Arch Surg 1978;113:637–639.

61. Strinden WD, Helgerson RB, Maki DG: *Candida* septic thrombosis of the great central veins associated with central catheters. Clinical features and management. Ann Surg 1985;202:653–658.

62. Ratcliffe FM: Suppurative thrombosis of the superior vena cava: A lethal complication of central venous catheters. Intensive Care Med 1985;11:265–266.

63. Stein JM, Pruitt BA: Suppurative thrombophlebitis. A lethal latrogenic disease. N Engl J Med 1970;282:1452–1455.

64. Munoz Fernandez S, Quiralte J, del Arco A, et al: Osteoarticular infection associated with the human immunodeficiency virus. Clin Exp Rheumatol 1991;9:489–493.

65. Miro JM, Brancos MA, Abello R: Costochondral involvement in systemic candidiasis in heroin addicts: Clinical, scintigraphic, and histologic features in 26 patients. Arthritis Rheum 1988;31:793–797.

66. Miller DJ, Mejicano GC: Vertebral osteomyelitis due to *Candida* species: Case report and literature review. [Review] [48 Refs]. Clin Infect Dis 2001;33:523–530.

67. Swanson H, Hughes PA, Messer SA, et al: *Candida albicans* arthritis one year after successful treatment of fungemia in a healthy infant. [Review] [37 Refs]. J Pediatr 1996;129:688–694.

68. Almekinders LC, Greene WB: Vertebral *Candida* infections. A case report and review of the literature. [Review] [26 Refs]. Clin Orthop 1991;267:174–178.

69. Ferra C, Doebbeling BN, Hollis RJ, et al: *Candida tropicalis* vertebral osteomyelitis: A late sequela of fungemia. Clin Infect Dis 1994;19:697–703.

70. Hennequin C, Bouree P, Hiesse C, et al: Spondylodiskitis due to *Candida albicans*: Report of two patients who were successfully treated with fluconazole and review of the literature. [Review] [18 Refs]. Clin Infect Dis 1996;23:176–178.

71. Sugar AM, Saunders C, Diamond RD: Successful treatment of *Candida* osteomyelitis with fluconazole. A noncomparative study of two patients. Diagn Microbiol Infect Dis 1990;13:517–520.

72. Tang C: Successful treatment of *Candida albicans* osteomyelitis with fluconazole. J Infect 1993;26:89–92.

73. Weers-Pothoff G, Havermans JF, Kamphuis J, et al: *Candida tropicalis* arthritis in a patient with acute myeloid leukemia successfully treated with fluconazole: Case report and review of the literature. [Review] [25 Refs]. Infection 1997;25:109–111.

74. Tunkel AR, Thomas CY, Wispelwey B: *Candida* prosthetic arthritis: Report of a case treated with fluconazole and review of the literature. [Review] [15 Refs]. Am J Med 1993;94:100–103.

75. Dunkley AB, Leslie IJ: *Candida* infection of a silicone metacarpophalangeal arthroplasty. J Hand Surg [Br] 1997;22:423–424.

76. Goodman JS, Seibert DG, Reahl GE Jr, Geckler RW: Fungal infection of prosthetic joints: A report of two cases. J Rheumatol 1983;10:494–495.

77. de Luis D, Aller R, Boixeda D, et al: [Spontaneous peritonitis caused by ascitic fluid with *Candida albicans*]. [Spanish]. Rev Clin Esp 1997;197:500–501.

78. Suarez A, Otero L, Navascues CA, et al: [Ascitic peritonitis due to *Candida albicans*]. [Spanish]. [Review] [15 Refs]. Rev Esp Enferm Dig 1994;86:691–693.

79. Bayer AS, Blumenkrantz MJ, Montgomerie JZ, et al: *Candida* peritonitis. Report of 22 cases and review of the English literature. Am J Med 1976;61:832–840.

80. Levine J, Bernard DB, Idelson BA, et al: Fungal peritonitis complicating continuous ambulatory peritoneal dialysis: Successful treatment with fluconazole, a new orally active antifungal agent. [See Comments.] Am J Med 1989;86(6:Pt 2):825–827.

81. Goldie SJ, Kiernan-Tridle L, Torres C, et al: Fungal peritonitis in a large chronic peritoneal dialysis population: A report of 55 episodes. Am J Kidney Dis 1996;28:86–91.

82. Montenegro J, Aguirre R, Gonzalez O, et al: Fluconazole treatment of *Candida* peritonitis with delayed removal of the peritoneal dialysis catheter. Clin Nephrol 1995;44:60–63.

83. Eisenberg ES, Leviton I, Soeiro R: Fungal peritonitis in patients receiving peritoneal dialysis: Experience with 11 patients and review of the literature. [Erratum appears in Rev Infect Dis 1986;8:839]. [Review] [55 Refs]. Rev Infect Dis 1986;8:309–321.

84. Michel C, Courdavault L, al Khayat R, et al: Fungal peritonitis in patients on peritoneal dialysis. [Review] [28 Refs]. Am J Nephrol 1994;14:113–120.

85. Solomkin JS, Flohr AB, Quie PG, Simmons RL: The role of *Candida* in intraperitoneal infections. Surgery 1980;88:524–530.

86. Calandra T, Bille J, Schneider R, et al: Clinical significance of *Candida* isolated from peritoneum in surgical patients. Lancet 1989;2(8677):1437–1440.

87. Grois N, Mostbeck G, Scherrer R, et al: Hepatic and splenic abscesses—A common complication of intensive chemotherapy of acute myeloid leukemia (AML). A prospective study. Ann Hematol 1991;63:33–38.

88. Thaler M, Pastakia B, Shawker TH, et al: Hepatic candidiasis in cancer patients: The evolving picture of the syndrome. [Review] [38 Refs]. Ann Intern Med 1988;108:88–100.

89. Walsh TJ, Whitcomb PO, Revankar SG, Pizzo PA: Successful treatment of hepatosplenic candidiasis through repeated cycles of chemotherapy and neutropenia. Cancer 1995;76:2357–2362.

90. Lopez-Berestein G, Bodey GP, Frankel LS, Mehta K: Treatment of hepatosplenic candidiasis with liposomal-amphotericin B. J Clin Oncol 1987;5:310–317.

91. Shirkhoda A, Lopez-Berestein G, Holbert JM, Luna MA: Hepatosplenic fungal infection: CT and pathologic evaluation after treatment with liposomal amphotericin B. Radiology 1986;159:349–353.

92. Anaissie E, Bodey GP, Kantarjian H, et al: Fluconazole therapy for chronic disseminated candidiasis in patients with leukemia and prior amphotericin B therapy. Am J Med 1991;91:142–150.

93. Aydin M, Kucukoduk S, Yalin T, et al: Amphotericin B in the treatment of *Candida* meningitis in three neonates. Turk J Pediatr 1995;37:247–252.

94. Alders K, Al Shaman M, Mimic Z, et al: *Candida* meningitis in children: Report of two cases. J Chemother 2000;12:339–344.

95. Hagensee ME, Bauwens JE, Kjos B, Bowden RA: Brain abscess following marrow transplantation: Experience at the Fred Hutchinson Cancer Research Center. 1984–1992. Clin Infect Dis 1994;19:402–408.

96. de Medicos BC, de Medicos CR, Werner B, et al: Central nervous system infections following bone marrow transplantation: An autopsy report of 27 cases. J Hematother Stem Cell Res 2000;9:535–540.

97. Session TF, Flynn HW Jr, Middy WE, et al: Treatment outcomes in a 10-year study of endogenous fungal endophthalmitis. Ophthalmic Surg Lasers 1997;28:185–194.

98. Brod RD, Flynn HW Jr, Clarkson JG, et al: Endogenous Candida endophthalmitis. Management without intravenous amphotericin B. Ophthalmology 1990;97:666–672.

99. Bermig J, Meier P, Retzlaff C, Wiedemann P: [Primary vitrectomy in endophthalmitis]. [German]. Ophthalmologe 1997;94:552–556.

100. Crishna R, Amuh D, Lowder CY, et al: Should all patients with candidemia have an ophthalmologic examination to rule out ocular candidiasis? Abstract 451, IDSA 35th Annual Meeting, 1997.

101. O'Day DM, Head WS, Robinson RD: An outbreak of Candida parapsilosis endophthalmitis: Analysis of strains by enzyme profile and antifungal susceptibility. Br J Ophthalmol 1987;71:126–129.

102. McCray E, Rampell N, Solomon SL, et al: Outbreak of Candida parapsilosis endophthalmitis after cataract extraction and intraocular lens implantation. J Clin Microbiol 1986;24:625–628.

103. Filler SG, Crislip MA, Mayer CL, Edwards JE Jr: Comparison of fluconazole and amphotericin B for treatment of disseminated candidiasis and endophthalmitis in rabbits. Antimicrob Agents Chemother 1991;35:288–292.

104. Akler ME, Vellend H, McNeely DM, et al: Use of fluconazole in the treatment of candidal endophthalmitis. [Review] [59 Refs]. Clin Infect Dis 1995;20:657–664.

105. Sternberg P Jr, Martin DF: Management of endophthalmitis in the post-endophthalmitis vitrectomy study era. [Letter; Comment]. [Review] [18 Refs]. Arch Ophthalmol 2001; 119:754–755.

106. Martinez-Vazquez C, Fernandez-Ulloa J, Bordon J, et al: Candida albicans endophthalmitis in brown heroin addicts: Response to early vitrectomy preceded and followed by antifungal therapy. [See Comments.] Clin Infect Dis 1998; 27:1130–1133.

107. Results of the endophthalmitis vitrectomy study. A randomized trial of immediate vitrectomy and of intravenous antibiotics for the treatment of postoperative bacterial endophthalmitis. Endophthalmitis Vitrectomy Study Group. [See Comments.] Arch Ophthalmol 1995; 113:1479–1496.

108. Fox GM, Joondeph BC, Flynn HW Jr, et al: Delayed onset pseudophakic endophthalmitis. [See Comments.] Am J Ophthalmol 1991;111:163–173.

109. Blumberg HM, Jarvis WR, Soucie JM, et al: Risk factors for candidal bloodstream infections in surgical intensive care unit patients: The NEMIS Prospective Multicenter Study. The National Epidemiology of Mycosis Survey. [See Comments.] Clin Infect Dis 2001;33:177–186.

110. Walsh TJ, Hiemenz J, Pizzo PA: Evolving risk factors for invasive fungal infections—all neutropenic patients are not the same. [Letter; Comment]. Clin Infect Dis 1994;18:793–798.

111. Goodman JL, Winston DJ, Greenfield RA, et al: A controlled trial of fluconazole to prevent fungal infections in patients undergoing bone marrow transplantation. [See Comments.] N Engl J Med 1992;326:845–851.

112. Slavin MA, Osborne B, Adams R, et al: Efficacy and safety of fluconazole prophylaxis for fungal infections after marrow transplantation—a prospective, randomized, double-blind study. J Infect Dis 1995;171:1545–1552.

113. Krçmery V Jr, Sejnova D, Pichnova E: Breakthrough Candida tropicalis fungemia during ketoconazole prophylaxis in cancer patients. Acta Oncolog 1999; 38(5):663–665.

114. Krçmery V Jr, Oravcova E, Spanik S, et al: Nosocomial breakthrough fungaemia during antifungal prophylaxis or empirical antifungal therapy in 41 cancer patients receiving antineoplastic chemotherapy: Analysis of aetiology risk factors and outcome. J Antimicrob Chemother 1998; 41:373–380.

115. Collins LA, Samore MH, Roberts MS, et al: Risk factors for invasive fungal infections complicating orthotopic liver transplantation. J Infect Dis 1994;170:644–652.

116. Hadley S, Samore MH, Lewis WD, et al: Major infectious complications after orthotopic liver transplantation and comparison of outcomes in patients receiving cyclosporine or FK506 as primary immunosuppression. Transplantation 1995;59:851–859.

117. Karchmer AW, Samore MH, Hadley S, et al: Fungal infections complicating orthotopic liver transplantation. Trans Am Clin Climatol Assoc 1994;106:38–47.

118. Kung N, Fisher N, Gunson B, et al: Fluconazole prophylaxis for high-risk liver transplant recipients. [Letter; Comment]. Lancet 1995;345(8959):1234–1235.

119. Tollemar J, Hockerstedt K, Ericzon BG, et al: Liposomal amphotericin B prevents invasive fungal infections in liver transplant recipients. A randomized, placebo-controlled study. Transplantation 1995;59:45–50.

120. Tollemar J, Hockerstedt K, Ericzon BG, et al: Prophylaxis with liposomal amphotericin B (AmBisome) prevents fungal infections in liver transplant recipients: Long-term results of a randomized, placebo-controlled trial. Transplant Proc 1995;27:1195–1198.

121. Linden P, Williams P, Chan KM: Efficacy and safety of amphotericin B lipid complex injection (ABLC) in solid-organ transplant recipients with invasive fungal infections. Clin Transplant 2000;14(4:Pt 1):329–339.

122. Powderly WG, Gallant JE, Ghannoum MA, et al: Oropharyngeal candidiasis in patients with HIV: Suggested guidelines for therapy. [Review] [15 Refs]. AIDS Res Hum Retroviruses 1999;15:1619–1623.

123. Darouiche RO: Oropharyngeal and esophageal candidiasis in immunocompromised patients: Treatment issues. [Review] [83 Refs]. Clin Infect Dis 1998;26:259–272.

124. Arendorf TM, Walker DM: The prevalence and intra-oral distribution of Candida albicans in man. Arch Oral Biol 1980;25:1–10.

125. Epstein JB, Pearsall NN, Truelove EL: Quantitative relationships between Candida albicans in saliva and the clinical status of human subjects. J Clin Microbiol 1980;12:475–476.

126. Shay K, Truhlar MR, Renner RP: Oropharyngeal candidosis in the older patient. [Review] [70 Refs]. J Am Geriatr Soc 1997;45:863–870.

127. Koletar SL, Russell JA, Fass RJ, Plouffe JF: Comparison of oral fluconazole and clotrimazole troches as treatment for oral candidiasis in patients infected with human immunodeficiency virus. Antimicrob Agents Chemother 1990;34:2267–2268.

128. Pons V, Greenspan D, Debruin M: Therapy for oropharyngeal candidiasis in HIV-infected patients: A randomized, prospective multicenter study of oral fluconazole versus clotrimazole troches. The Multicenter Study Group. [See Comments]. J Acquir Immune Defic Syndr 1993;6:1311–1316.

129. Flynn PM, Cunningham CK, Kerkering T, et al: Oropharyngeal candidiasis in immunocompromised children: A randomized, multicenter study of orally administered fluconazole suspension versus nystatin. The Multicenter Fluconazole Study Group. J Pediatr 1995;127:322–328.

130. Pons V, Greenspan D, Lozada-Nur F, et al: Oropharyngeal candidiasis in patients with AIDS: Randomized comparison of fluconazole versus nystatin oral suspensions. Clin Infect Dis 1997;24:1204–1207.

131. Hernandez-Sampelayo T: Fluconazole versus ketoconazole in the treatment of oropharyngeal candidiasis in HIV-infected children. Multicentre Study Group. Eur J Clin Microbiol Infect Dis 1994;13:340–344.

132. De Wit S, Weerts D, Goossens H, Clumeck N: Comparison of fluconazole and ketoconazole for oropharyngeal candidiasis in AIDS. [See Comments.] Lancet 1989;1(8641):746–748.

133. Gritti FM, Raise E, Di Salvo S, et al: [Fluconazole in the treatment of esophageal, bronchial and oral candidiasis in patients with ARC and AIDS]. [Italian]. G Ital Chemioter 1988;35(1-3):61–68.

134. Phillips P, De Beule K, Frechette G, et al: A double-blind comparison of itraconazole oral solution and fluconazole capsules for the treatment of oropharyngeal candidiasis in patients with AIDS. Clin Infect Dis 1998;26:1368–1373.

135. Taillandier J, Esnault Y, Alemanni M: A comparison of fluconazole oral suspension and amphotericin B oral suspension in older patients with oropharyngeal candidosis. Multicentre Study Group. Age Ageing 2000;29:117–123.

136. Fichtenbaum CJ, Powderly WG: Refractory mucosal candidiasis in patients with human immunodeficiency virus infection. [See Comments.] [Review] [88 Refs]. Clin Infect Dis 1998;26:556–565.

137. Phillips P, Zemcov J, Mahmood W, et al: Itraconazole cyclodextrin solution for fluconazole-refractory oropharyngeal candidiasis in AIDS: Correlation of clinical response with in vitro susceptibility. AIDS 1996; 10:1369–1376.

138. Saag MS, Fessel WJ, Kaufman CA, et al: Treatment of fluconazole-refractory oropharyngeal candidiasis with itraconazole oral solution in HIV-positive patients. AIDS Res Hum Retroviruses 1999;15:1413–1417.

139. Fichtenbaum CJ, Zackin R, Rajicic N, et al: Amphotericin B oral suspension for fluconazole-refractory oral candidiasis in persons with HIV infection. Adult AIDS Clinical Trials Group Study Team 295. AIDS 2000;14:845–852.

140. Masci JR: Complete response of severe, refractory oral candidiasis to mouthwash containing lactoferrin and lysozyme. AIDS 2000;14:2403–2404.

141. Jandourek A, Vaishampayan JK, Vazquez JA: Efficacy of melaleuca oral solution for the treatment of fluconazole refractory oral candidiasis in AIDS patients. AIDS 1998;12:1033–1037.

142. Powderly WG, Finkelstein D, Feinberg J, et al: A randomized trial comparing fluconazole with clotrimazole troches for the prevention of fungal infections in patients with advanced human immunodeficiency virus infection. NIAID AIDS Clinical Trials Group. [See Comments.] N Engl J Med 1995;332:700–705.

143. Havlir DV, Dube MP, McCutchan JA, et al: Prophylaxis with weekly versus daily fluconazole for fungal infections in patients with AIDS. [See Comments.] Clin Infect Dis 1998;27:1369–1375.

144. Wilcox CM, Schwartz DA: Endoscopic-pathologic correlates of *Candida* esophagitis in acquired immunodeficiency syndrome. Dig Dis Sci 1996;41:1337–1345.

145. Kim BW, Cho SH, Rha SE, et al: Esophagomediastinal fistula and esophageal stricture as a complication of esophageal candidiasis: A case report. Gastrointest Endosc 2000; 52:772–775.

146. Wilcox CM, Alexander LN, Clark WS, Thompson SE III: Fluconazole compared with endoscopy for human immunodeficiency virus-infected patients with esophageal symptoms. Gastroenterol 1996;110:1803–1809.

147. Barbaro G, Barbarini G, Di Lorenzo G: Fluconazole compared with itraconazole in the treatment of esophageal candidiasis in AIDS patients: A double-blind, randomized, controlled clinical study. Scand J Infect Dis 1995; 27:613–617.

148. Laine L, Dretler RH, Conteas CN, et al: Fluconazole compared with ketoconazole for the treatment of *Candida* esophagitis in AIDS. A randomized trial. [See Comments.] Ann Intern Med 1992;117:655–660.

149. Barbaro G, Barbarini G, Di Lorenzo G: Fluconazole vs itraconazole-flucytosine association in the treatment of esophageal candidiasis in AIDS patients. A double-blind, multicenter placebo-controlled study. The *Candida* Esophagitis Multicenter Italian Study (CEMIS) Group. Chest 1996;110:1507–1514.

150. Wilcox CM, Darouiche RO, Laine L, et al: A randomized, double-blind comparison of itraconazole oral solution and fluconazole tablets in the treatment of esophageal candidiasis. J Infect Dis 1997;176:227–232.

150a. Ally R, Schurmann D, Kreisel W, et al: A randomized, double-blind, double-dummy, multi-center trial of voriconazole and fluconazole in the treatment of esophageal candidiasis in immunocompromised patients. Clin Infect Dis 2001;33:1447–1454.

151. Laine L, Rabeneck L: Prospective study of fluconazole suspension for the treatment of esophageal candidiasis in patients with AIDS. Aliment Pharmacol Ther 1995;9:553–556.

152. Medoff G: Controversial areas in antifungal chemotherapy: Short-course and combination therapy with amphotericin B. [Review] [19 Refs]. Rev Infect Dis 1987;9:403–407.

153. Baddley JW, Smith AM, Moser SA, Pappas PG: Trends in frequency and susceptibilities of *Candida glabrata* bloodstream isolates at a university hospital. Diagn Microbiol Infect Dis 2001;39:199–201.

154. Villanueva A, Gotuzzo E, Arathoon E, et al: The efficacy, safety, and tolerability of caspofungin vs. fluconazole in the treatment of esophageal candidiasis. Abstract 675, 41st Annual ICCAC 2001.

155. Bingham JS: What to do with the patient with recurrent vulvovaginal candidiasis. Sex Transm Infect 1999;75:225–227.

156. Berg AO, Heidrich FE, Fihn SD, et al: Establishing the cause of genitourinary symptoms in women in a family practice. Comparison of clinical examination and comprehensive microbiology. JAMA 1984;251:620–625.

157. Spinillo A, Michelone G, Cavanna C, et al: Clinical and microbiological characteristics of symptomatic vulvovaginal candidiasis in HIV-seropositive women. Genitourin Med 1994;70:268–272.

158. National Guideline for the Management of Vulvovaginal Candidiasis. Clinical Effectiveness Group (Association of Genitourinary Medicine and the Medical Society for the Study of Venereal Diseases). Sex Transm Infect 1999; 75(Suppl-20).

159. Nyirjesy P: Chronic vulvovaginal candidiasis. [Review] [17 Refs]. Am Fam Phys 2001;63:697–702.

160. Fong IW: The value of treating the sexual partners of women with recurrent vaginal candidiasis with ketoconazole. Genitourin Med 1992;68:174–176.

161. Nyirjesy P, Seeney SM, Grody MH, et al: Chronic fungal vaginitis: The value of cultures. Am J Obstet Gynecol 1995;173(3:Pt 1):820–823.

162. Irving G, Miller D, Robinson A, et al: Psychological factors associated with recurrent vaginal candidiasis: A preliminary study. Sex Transm Infect 1998;74:334–338.

163. Sobel JD, Brooker D, Stein GE, et al: Single oral dose fluconazole compared with conventional clotrimazole topical therapy of *Candida* vaginitis. Fluconazole Vaginitis Study Group. Am J Obstet Gynecol 1995;172(4:Pt 1):1263–1268.

164. Sobel JD, Kapernick PS, Zervos M, et al: Treatment of complicated *Candida* vaginitis: Comparison of single and sequential doses of fluconazole. Am J Obstet Gynecol 2001;185:363–369.

165. Bohannon NJ: Treatment of vulvovaginal candidiasis in patients with diabetes. [Review] [62 Refs]. Diabetes Care 1998;21:451–456.

166. Schuman P, Capps L, Peng G, et al: Weekly fluconazole for the prevention of mucosal candidiasis in women with HIV infection. A randomized, double-blind, placebo-controlled trial. Terry Beirn Community Programs for Clinical Research on AIDS. [See Comments.] Ann Intern Med 1997; 126:689–696.

167. Sobel JD, Faro S, Force RW, et al: Vulvovaginal candidiasis: Epidemiologic, diagnostic, and therapeutic considerations. [See Comments.] [Review] [29 Refs]. Am J Obstet Gynecol 1998;178:203–211.

168. Fong IW, Bannatyne RM, Wong P: Lack of in vitro resistance of *Candida albicans* to ketoconazole, itraconazole and clotrimazole in women treated for recurrent vaginal candidiasis. Genitourin Med 1993;69:44–46.

169. Fong IW: The value of prophylactic (monthly) clotrimazole versus empiric self-treatment in recurrent vaginal candidiasis. Genitourin Med 1994;70:124–126.

170. Fisher JF, Chew WH, Shadomy S, et al: Urinary tract infections due to *Candida albicans*. [Review] [107 Refs]. Rev Infect Dis 1982;4:1107–1118.

171. Rivett AG, Perry JA, Cohen J: Urinary candidiasis: A prospective study in hospital patients. Urol Res 1986;14:183–186.

172. Gubbins PO, Piscitelli SC, Danziger LH: Candidal urinary tract infections: A comprehensive review of their diagnosis and management. [Review] [142 Refs]. Pharmacotherapy 1993;13:110–127.

173. Lundstrom T, Sobel J: Nosocomial candiduria: A review. [Review] [44 Refs]. Clin Infect Dis 2001;32:1602–1607.

174. Comiter CV, McDonald M, Minton J, Yalla SV: Fungal bezoar and bladder rupture secondary to *Candida tropicalis*. Urology 1996;47(3):439–441.

175. Ang BS, Telenti A, King B, et al: Candidemia from a urinary tract source: Microbiological aspects and clinical significance. Clin Infect Dis 1993;17:662–666.

176. Bartkowski DP, Lanesky JR: Emphysematous prostatitis and cystitis secondary to *Candida albicans*. J Urol 1988; 139:1063–1065.

177. Greene MH: Emphysematous cystitis due to *Clostridium perfringens* and *Candida albicans* in two patients with hematologic malignant conditions. [Review] [47 Refs]. Cancer 1992;70:2658–2663.

178. Wise GJ, Talluri GS, Marella VK: Fungal infections of the genitourinary system: Manifestations, diagnosis, and treatment. Urol Clin North Am 1999;26:701–718.

179. Roberts JA: Management of pyelonephritis and upper urinary tract infections. [Review] [57 Refs]. Urol Clin North Am 1999;26:753–763.

180. Erden A, Fitoz S, Karagulle T, et al: Radiological findings in the diagnosis of genitourinary candidiasis. Pediatr Radiol 2000;30:875–877.

181. Sanford JP: The enigma of candiduria: Evolution of bladder irrigation with amphotericin B for management—From anecdote to dogma and a lesson from Machiavelli. [See Comments.] Clin Infect Dis 1993;16:145–147.

182. Nassoura Z, Ivatury RR, Simon RJ, et al: Candiduria as an early marker of disseminated infection in critically ill surgical patients: The role of fluconazole therapy. [See Comments.] Trauma 1993;35:290–294.

183. Kauffman CA, Vazquez JA, Sobel JD, et al: Prospective multicenter surveillance study of funguria in hospitalized patients. The National Institute for Allergy and Infectious Diseases (NIAID) Mycoses Study Group. Clin Infect Dis 2000;30:14–18.

184. Gubbins PO, Occhipinti DJ, Danziger LH: Surveillance of treated and untreated funguria in a university hospital. Pharmacotherapy 1994;14:463–470.

185. Sobel JD, Kauffman CA, McKinsey D, et al: Candiduria: A randomized, double-blind study of treatment with fluconazole and placebo. The National Institute of Allergy and Infectious Diseases (NIAID) Mycoses Study Group. [See Comments.] Clin Infect Dis 2000;30:19–24.

186. Leu HS, Huang CT: Clearance of funguria with short- course antifungal regimens: A prospective, randomized, controlled study. Clin Infect Dis 1995;20:1152–1157.

187. Fong IW: The value of a single amphotericin B bladder washout in candiduria. J Antimicrob Chemother 1995; 36:1067–1071.

188. Fan-Harvard P, O'Donovan C, Smith SM, et al: Oral fluconazole versus amphotericin B bladder irrigation for treatment of candidal funguria. Clin Infect Dis 1995;21:960–965.

189. Hay RJ: Antifungal therapy of yeast infections. [Review] [25 Refs]. J Am Acad Dermatol 1994;31(3:Pt 2):S6–S9.

190. Hoppe JE: Treatment of oropharyngeal candidiasis and candidal diaper dermatitis in neonates and infants: Review and reappraisal. [See Comments.] [Review] [72 Refs]. Pediatr Infect Dis J 1997;16(9):885–894.

191. Hay RJ: Fungal skin infections. [Review] [31 Refs]. Arch Dis Child 1992;67:1065–1067.

192. Pazos R, Esteban J, Perez C, Otero JM: [Bilateral hydronephrosis caused by a "fungus ball"]. [Spanish]. Nefrologia 2001;21:319–320.

193. Dekio S, Imaoka C, Jidoi J: *Candida* folliculitis associated with hypothyroidism. Br J Dermatol 1987;117:663–664.

194. Warren JW: Catheter-associated urinary tract infections. [Review] [34 Refs]. Int J Antimicrob Agents 2001;17:299–303.

195. Suchil P, Gei FM, Robles M, et al: Once-weekly oral doses of fluconazole 150 mg in the treatment of tinea corporis/cruris and cutaneous candidiasis. Clin Exp Dermatol 1992;17:397–401.

196. Guidelines for Care of Superficial Mycotic Infections of the Skin: Mucocutaneous candidiasis. Guidelines/Outcome Committee. American Academy of Dermatology. J Am Acad Dermatol 1996;34:110–115.

197. Lilic D, Gravenor I: Immunology of chronic mucocutaneous candidiasis. J Clin Pathol 2001;54:81–83.

198. Kirkpatrick CH: Chronic mucocutaneous candidiasis. [Review] [31 Refs]. J Am Acad Dermatol 1994;31(3:Pt 2):S14–S17.

199. Selby R, Ramirez CB, Singh R, et al: Brain abscess in solid organ transplant recipients receiving cyclosporine-based immunosuppression. Arch Surg 1997;132:304–310.

200. Hoh MC, Lin HP, Chan LL, Lam SK: Successful allogeneic bone marrow transplantation in severe chronic mucocutaneous candidiasis syndrome. Bone Marrow Transplant 1996;18:797–800.

201. Feigal DW, Katz MH, Greenspan D, et al: The prevalence of oral lesions in HIV-infected homosexual and bisexual men: Three San Francisco epidemiological cohorts. AIDS 1991;5:519–525.

202. Van Meter F, Gallo JW, Garcia-Rojas G, et al: A study of oral candidiasis in HIV-positive patients. J Dent Hygiene 1994;68:30–34.

203. Fotos PG, Hellstein JW: *Candida* and candidosis. Epidemiology, diagnosis and therapeutic management. [Review] [130 Refs]. Dent Clin North Am 1992;36:857–878.

204. Epstein JB, Truelove EL, Izutzu KT: Oral candidiasis: Pathogenesis and host defense. [Review] [148 Refs]. Rev Infect Dis 1984;6:96–106.

205. Silverman S, Luangjarmekorn L, Greenspan D: Occurrence of oral *Candida* in irradiated head and neck cancer patients. J Oral Med 1984;39(4):194–196.

206. Guggenheimer J, Moore PA, Rossie K, et al: Insulin-dependent diabetes mellitus and oral soft tissue pathologies: II. Prevalence and characteristics of *Candida* and candidal lesions. Oral Surg Oral Med Oral Pathol Oral Radiol Endod 2000;89:570–576.

207. Maenza JR, Merz WG, Romagnoli MJ, et al: Infection due to fluconazole-resistant *Candida* in patients with AIDS: Prevalence and microbiology. Clin Infect Dis 1997; 24:28–34.

208. Wingard JR: Importance of *Candida* species other than *C. albicans* as pathogens in oncology patients. [Review] [116 Refs]. Clin Infect Dis 1995;20:115–125.

209. Tumbarello M, Caldarola G, Tacconelli E, et al: Analysis of the risk factors associated with the emergence of azole-resistant oral candidosis in the course of HIV infection. Antimicrob Chemother 1996;38:691–699.

210. Maenza JR, Keruly JC, Moore RD, et al: Risk factors for fluconazole-resistant candidiasis in human immunodeficiency virus–infected patients. J Infect Dis 1996;173:219–225.

211. Sobel JD, Ohmit SE, HIV Epidemiology Research Study (HERS) Group: The evolution of *Candida* species and fluconazole susceptibility among oral and vaginal isolates recovered from human immunodeficiency virus (HIV)-seropositive and at-risk HIV-seronegative women. J Infect Dis 2001;183:286–293.

212. Sullivan DJ, Westerneng TJ, Haynes KA, et al: *Candida dubliniensis* sp. nov.: Phenotypic and molecular characterization of a novel species associated with oral candidosis in HIV-infected individuals. Microbiology 1995;141(Pt 7):1507–1521.

213. Boerlin P, Boerlin-Petzold F, Durussel C, et al: Cluster of oral atypical *Candida albicans* isolates in a group of human immunodeficiency virus–positive drug users. J Clin Microbiol 1995;33:1129–1135.

214. Meiller TF, Jabra-Rizk MA, Baqui A, et al: Oral *Candida dubliniensis* as a clinically important species in HIV-seropositive patients in the United States. Oral Surg Oral Med Oral Pathol Oral Radiol Endod 1999;88:573–580.

215. Reef SE, Mayer KH: Opportunistic candidal infections in patients infected with human immunodeficiency virus: Prevention issues and priorities. [Review] [24 Refs]. Clin Infect Dis 1995;21(Suppl 1):S99–S102.

216. King JW, Nguyen VQ, Conrad SA: Results of a prospective statewide reporting system for infective endocarditis. Am J Med Sci 1988;295:517–527.

217. Wilcox CM, Straub RF, Clark WS: Prospective evaluation of oropharyngeal findings in human immunodeficiency virus–infected patients with esophageal ulceration. [See Comments.] Am J Gastroenterol 1995;90:1938–1941.

218. Samonis G, Skordilis P, Maraki S, et al: Oropharyngeal candidiasis as a marker for esophageal candidiasis in patients with cancer. Clin Infect Dis 1998;27:283–286.

219. Chiou CC, Groll AH, Gonzalez CE, et al: Esophageal candidiasis in pediatric acquired immunodeficiency syndrome: Clinical manifestations and risk factors. Pediatr Infect Dis J 2000;19:729–734.

220. Boken DJ, Swindells S, Rinaldi MG: Fluconazole-resistant *Candida albicans*. Clin Infect Dis 1993;17:1018–1021.

221. Bini EJ, Micale PL, Weinshel EH: Natural history of HIV-associated esophageal disease in the era of protease inhibitor therapy. Dig Dis Sci 2000;45:1301–1307.

222. Nelson AL: The impact of contraceptive methods on the onset of symptomatic vulvovaginal candidiasis within the menstrual cycle. Am J Obstet Gynecol 1997; 176:1376–1380.

223. Scudamore JA, Tooley PJ, Allcorn RJ: The treatment of acute and chronic vaginal candidosis. [Review] [29 Refs]. Br J Clin Pract 1992;46:260–263.

224. Spinillo A, Capuzzo E, Acciano S, et al: Effect of antibiotic use on the prevalence of symptomatic vulvovaginal candidiasis. Am J Obstet Gynecol 1999;180(1:Pt 1):14–17.

225. Helfgott A, Eriksen N, Bundrick CM, et al: Vaginal infections in human immunodeficiency virus–infected women. Am J Obstet Gynecol 2000;183:347–355.

226. Minkoff HL, Eisenberger-Matityahu D, Feldman J, et al: Prevalence and incidence of gynecologic disorders among women infected with human immunodeficiency virus. Am J Obstet Gynecol 1999;180:824–836.

227. Walker PP, Reynolds MT, Ashbee HR, et al: Vaginal yeasts in the era of "over the counter" antifungals. Sex Transm Infect 2000;76:437–438.

228. Vazquez JA, Sobel JD, Peng G, et al: Evolution of vaginal *Candida* species recovered from human immunodeficiency virus–infected women receiving fluconazole prophylaxis: The emergence of *Candida glabrata*? Terry Beirn Community Programs for Clinical Research in AIDS (CPCRA). Clin Infect Dis 1999;28:1025–1031.

229. Peer AK, Hoosen AA, Seedat MA, et al: Vaginal yeast infections in diabetic women. S Afr Med J 1993;83:727–729.

230. Spinillo A, Capuzzo E, Gulminetti R, et al: Prevalence of and risk factors for fungal vaginitis caused by non-*albicans* species. [See Comments.] Am J Obstet Gynecol 1997;176(1:Pt 1):138–141.

231. Phillips JR, Karlowicz MG: Prevalence of *Candida* species in hospital-acquired urinary tract infections in a neonatal intensive care unit. Pediatr Infect Dis J 1997;16:190–194.

232. Petraitis V, Petraitiene R, Groll AH, et al: Dosage-dependent antifungal efficacy of V-echinocandin (LY303366) against experimental fluconazole-resistant oropharyngeal and esophageal candidiasis. Antimicrob Agents Chemother 2001;45:471–479.

233. Gubbins PO, McConnell SA, Penzak SR: Current management of funguria. [Review] [27 Refs]. Am J Health Syst Pharm 1999;56:1929–1935.

234. Michigan S: Genitourinary fungal infections. [Review] [85 Refs]. J Urol 1976;116:390–397.

235. Occhipinti DJ, Gubbins PO, Schreckenberger P, Danziger LH: Frequency, pathogenicity and microbiologic outcome of non-*Candida albicans* candiduria. Eur J Clin Microbiol Infect Dis 1994;13:459–467.

236. Voss A, Meis JF, Hoogkamp-Korstanje JA: Fluconazole in the management of fungal urinary tract infections. [Review] [38 Refs]. Infection 1994;22:247–251.

237. Barbaro G, Barbarini G, Calderon W, et al: Fluconazole versus itraconazole for *Candida* esophagitis in acquired immunodeficiency syndrome. *Candida* esophagitis. Gastroenterology 1996;111:1169–1177.

238. Barbaro G, Barbarini G, Di Lorenzo G: Fluconazole vs. flucytosine in the treatment of esophageal candidiasis in AIDS patients: A double-blind, placebo-controlled study. Endoscopy 1995;27:377–383.

239. Fichtenbaum CJ, Koletar S, Yiannoutsos C, et al: Refractory mucosal candidiasis in advanced human immunodeficiency virus infection. Clin Infect Dis 2000;30:749–756.

240. Kontoyiannis DP, Bodey GP, Mantzoros CS: Fluconazole vs. amphotericin B for the management of candidaemia in adults: A meta-analysis. Mycoses 2001;44:125–135.

241. Spinillo A, Colonna L, Piazzi G, et al: Managing recurrent vulvovaginal candidiasis. Intermittent prevention with itraconazole. J Reprod Med 1997;42:83–87.

242. Ringdahl EN: Treatment of recurrent vulvovaginal candidiasis. [Review] [31 Refs]. Am Fam Physician 2000;61:3306–3312.

243. Jacobs LG, Skidmore EA, Freeman K, et al: Oral fluconazole compared with bladder irrigation with amphotericin B for treatment of fungal urinary tract infections in elderly patients. [See Comments.] Clin Infect Dis 1996;22:30–35.

244. Cicalini S, Forcina G, De Rosa FG: Infective endocarditis in patients with human immunodeficiency virus infection. J Infect 2001;42:267–271.

245. Fisher JF, Hicks BC, Dipiro JT, et al: Efficacy of a single intravenous dose of amphotericin B in urinary tract infections caused by *Candida*. J Infect Dis 1987;156:685–687.

246. Nesbit SA, Katz LE, McClain BW, Murphy DP: Comparison of two concentrations of amphotericin B bladder irrigation in the treatment of funguria in patients with indwelling urinary catheters. Am J Health Syst Pharm 1999;56:872–875.

247. Trinh T, Simonian J, Vigil S, et al: Continuous versus intermittent bladder irrigation of amphotericin B for the treatment of candiduria. [See Comments.] J Urol 1995;154:2032–2034.

248. Oliver SE, Walker RJ, Woods DJ: Fluconazole infused via a nephrostomy tube: A novel and effective route of delivery. J Clin Pharm Ther 1995;20:317–318.

249. Bryant K, Maxfield C, Rabalais G: Renal candidiasis in neonates with candiduria. Pediatr Infect Dis J 1999; 18:959–963.

250. Sobel JD, Chaim W: Treatment of *Torulopsis glabrata* vaginitis: Retrospective review of boric acid therapy. Clin Infect Dis 1997;24:649–652.

251. Fong IW: The value of chronic suppressive therapy with itraconazole versus clotrimazole in women with recurrent vaginal candidiasis. Genitourin Med 1992;68:374–377.

252. Guaschino S, De Seta F, Sartore A, et al: Efficacy of maintenance therapy with topical boric acid in comparison with oral itraconazole in the treatment of recurrent vulvovaginal candidiasis. Am J Obstet Gynecol 2001;184:598–602.

chapter 42

Fungal Infections Other Than Candidiasis

DAVID S. MCKINSEY, MD

During the last two decades antifungal treatment options have expanded substantially with the introduction of the azole antifungal compounds, the lipid-based amphotericin B preparations, and the echinocandins. Despite the availability of potent antifungal drugs, however, treatment of the invasive mycoses remains challenging.

This chapter focuses on treatment of the endemic and opportunistic mycoses (with the exception of *Candida* species). Clinical trials of antifungal therapy for these infections have been limited by several factors, including the rarity of the invasive mycoses, their limited geographic distribution, the toxicities of antifungal drugs, and the length of treatment and follow-up required to assess the efficacy of therapy of chronic fungal infections. Because no single medical center encounters enough cases of the endemic or opportunistic mycoses to achieve statistical power in a comparative clinical trial, most published studies either have reported small numbers of patients or have been done at multiple sites, often among heterogeneous patient populations. With few exceptions, most trials of antifungal therapy have not been randomized or placebo controlled, and many have based their conclusions on comparisons with historical control groups. Thus few antifungal drugs have been shown to be superior to other agents, and most clinical decisions must be made on the basis of relatively limited data.

After the diagnosis of a systemic fungal infection is established, the clinician is faced with several questions: Is antifungal therapy warranted, or is the process likely to be self-limited? If systemic antifungal therapy is indicated, can an azole antifungal drug be used, or should intravenous amphotericin B therapy be administered? If an azole drug is to be prescribed, which is preferred, at what dose, and for how long? If amphotericin B therapy is warranted, should one prescribe conventional amphotericin B or a lipid preparation? When should serum concentrations of an antifungal drug be monitored? What is the likelihood of relapse, and when is it necessary to prescribe long-term maintenance therapy? The following review of the available systemic antifungal drugs and the more common endemic and opportunistic mycoses will provide information for the clinician who addresses these questions when managing a patient with a fungal infection.

ANTIFUNGAL DRUGS

Amphotericin B

Amphotericin B is a polyene antifungal drug that was isolated for the first time in 1955 from a soil sample obtained from the bank of the Orinoco River in Venezuela. It binds to ergosterol and thereby increases the permeability of fungal cell membranes,

TABLE 42–1 ■ Antifungal Drugs

Drug	Mechanism of action	Route of administration	Dose
Amphotericin B	Disruption of ergosterol in cell membranes	IV	0.5–1.5 mg/kg/d
Amphotericin B colloidal dispersion	Same	IV	3–6 mg/kg/d
Amphotericin B lipid complex	Same	IV	5 mg/kg/d
Liposomal amphotericin B	Same	IV	3–5 mg/kg/d
Flucytosine	Interferes with pyrimidine synthesis	PO	100 mg/kg/d in 4 divided doses
Ketoconazole	Impairs ergosterol synthesis	PO, topical	200–400 mg qd
Fluconazole	Same	PO, IV	100–800 mg qd
Itraconazole	Same	PO, IV	200 mg qd or bid
Caspofungin	Inhibits α-1.3 glucan synthesis	IV	70-mg loading dose, then 50 mg qd

ultimately causing leakage of intracellullar contents and fungal cell death (Table 42–1). Amphotericin B is fungicidal and has activity against *Blastomyces dermatitidis*, most species of *Candida* (except *C. lusitaneae*), *Coccidioides immitis*, *Cryptococcus neoformans*, *Histoplasma capsulatum*, *Paracoccidioides brasiliensis*, *Penicillium marneffei*, and *Sporothrix schenckii*. It has variable activity against *Aspergillus* spp, *Fusarium* spp, and Mucorales and generally is ineffective against *Pseudallescheria boydii*. After amphotericin B became available for clinical use in the late 1950s, it was the treatment of choice for several invasive mycoses until the oral azole antifungal drugs (which are much less toxic and easier to administer) were introduced into clinical practice. The lipid formulations of amphotericin B, which will be discussed, are less toxic and in some cases may be more effective but are far more expensive. Conventional amphotericin B is still widely used for treatment of life-threatening fungal infections.

Amphotericin B is not well absorbed from the gastrointestinal tract or after intramuscular injection. It is administered intravenously or, in rare situations, as an intravitreal, intraventricular, intracavitary, or intra-articular injection. Peak serum concentrations are attained during the first hour of an intravenous infusion. Serum half-life is between 24 and 48 hours, but there is a terminal phase half-life of up to 2 weeks. Serum concentrations are not affected by either renal insufficiency or hepatic failure. The drug is widely distributed in the body and attains high concentrations in lungs, liver, spleen, and kidney.

Chemical phlebitis occurs after infusion of amphotericin B through peripheral veins, so it is preferable to administer the medication through a central venous catheter. Infusion of amphotericin B frequently causes fever and chills. Although premedication with acetaminophen, diphenhydramine, or methylprednisolone is often prescribed, this practice has not been shown to decrease the frequency of infusion-related toxicities.[1] Meperidine (25 to 50 mg IV) alleviates amphotericin-induced chills. Amphotericin B often causes hypokalemia, hypomagnesemia, and transient renal insufficiency, but the renal

insufficiency usually is completely reversible after discontinuation of the medication. Renal insufficiency can be avoided in some cases by infusing 250 to 500 ml normal saline over 2 hours before amphotericin B administration.[2] If the serum creatinine level rises to 2 mg/dl or higher despite saline infusion, it is prudent either to hold amphotericin B therapy for 1 to 2 days or to change to a lipid-based preparation. Amphotericin B–induced anemia can occur if prolonged (>2 weeks) courses are administered. Other potential toxicities include nausea, anorexia, headache, and renal tubular acidosis. It is recommended that electrolytes and creatinine be monitored daily during amphotericin treatment and that hemoglobin concentrations be checked two to three times a week.

The usual dose of amphotericin B for most fungal infections is 0.5 to 0.7 mg/kg/d, although aspergillosis and mucormycosis should be treated with higher doses, *i.e.* 1 to 1.5 mg/kg/d. Over the years clinicians have developed a wide variety of methods of administering amphotericin B, most of which are based primarily on anecdotal experience. Some authorities have recommended administration of an initial test dose of 1 mg (usually diluted in 50 ml of 5% dextrose in water) over 1 hour to assess for drug-induced anaphylaxis; however, others have suggested that this practice is unnecessary and that frequent monitoring of vital signs during a higher first dose would preclude the inconvenience of a separate test dose.[3] The standard amphotericin B regimen is an initial dose of approximately 0.25 mg/kg/d diluted in 10 ml of 5% dextrose in water per milligram of amphotericin B, which is advanced by about 0.25 mg/kg/d until the target dose is achieved. In more acutely ill patients, however, the target dose can be administered on the first day. It has been a tradition to infuse amphotericin B doses over several hours (approximately 10 mg/h), but infusion of a full dose over 1 hour is safe in most cases.[4]

Lipid-Based Amphotericin B Compounds
Amphotericin B can be combined with various lipid preparations to increase solubility, minimize toxicity, and enhance drug delivery (Table 42–1). There are three approved lipid formulations of amphotericin B in the

United States: amphotericin B colloidal dispersion, amphotericin B lipid complex, and liposomal amphotericin B. The main advantage of the lipid compounds is their ability to transfer amphotericin B from the bloodstream to fungal cells without exposing cholesterol-containing human cells to amphotericin B, thereby decreasing toxicity.[5] Indeed each of the three lipid-based compounds has been shown to be substantially less nephrotoxic than conventional amphotericin B.[5] Liposomal amphotericin B also is far less likely to cause infusion-associated chills than conventional amphotercin B or the other two lipid-based preparations are. The efficacy of the lipid-based preparations appears to be comparable to that of conventional amphotericin B,[6] with two exceptions shown to date. In prospective, randomized, double-blind studies liposomal amphotericin B was more effective than conventional amphotericin B for treatment of severe disseminated histoplasmosis in HIV-infected patients[7] and was associated with a lower incidence of breakthrough fungal infections in febrile neutropenic patients who had received chemotherapy for hematologic malignancies.[8]

Amphotericin B colloidal dispersion is composed of a disklike structure containing amphotericin B and cholesteryl sulfate. These disks are distributed to the organs of the reticuloendothelial system and then dissociate, resulting in the sustained release of free amphotericin B into the bloodstream. The dose is 3 to 6 mg/kg/d, infused at a rate of 1 mg/kg/h. Treatment generally is initiated at the lower dose; if there is an incomplete response to therapy, the dose is increased.

Amphotericin B lipid complex has a ribbonlike structure of a bilayered membrane containing a 7:3 ratio of two phospholipids (dimyristoylphosphatidylglycerol and dimyristoyphosphatidylcholine). It is presumed that activated host cells excrete phospholipases that prompt the release of amphotericin B from the lipid complex. The recommended dose is 5 mg/kg infused over 2 hours.

Liposomal amphotericin B is comprised of a lipid bilayer containing phosphatidylcholine, distearoylphosphatidylglycerol, and amphotericin B, organized into unilamellar vesicles measuring approximately 60 nm in diameter. Liposomal amphotericin B remains intact in the bloodstream and binds with fungal cell membranes; free amphotericin B is then released into fungal cells. The dose is 3 to 5 mg/kg infused over 2 hours. In a prospective, double-blind study, the incidence of infusion-related chills or nephrotoxicity was lower in patients treated with liposomal amphotericin B (either 3 or 5 mg/kg/d) than in those treated with amphotericin B lipid complex (5 mg/kg/d), and there was no apparent difference in the efficacy of the two drugs.[9]

Flucytosine

Flucytosine, a nucleoside analogue that interferes with pyrimidine metabolism, thereby impairing fungal protein synthesis, is selectively toxic to fungi (Table 42–1).

Flucytosine has a limited role in clinical practice: it has in vitro activity against *Candida* species, *Cryptococcus neoformans*, and the organisms that cause chromomycosis, but resistance develops rapidly, so flucytosine should only be used in combination therapy. Its primary role is for treatment of cryptococcal meningitis, in combination with amphotericin B. Flucytosine is available only as an oral preparation. Potential toxicities include bone marrow suppression, elevated hepatocellular enzymes, nausea, diarrhea, and skin rash.[10] The daily dose range is from 100 to 150 mg/kg in four divided doses; toxicity occurs less frequently with the lower dose.[11] Flucytosine is 100% cleared by renal filtration, and the dose should be reduced in patients who have renal insufficiency.

Ketoconazole

Ketonazole, an imidazole drug, is available as a capsule and as a topical cream. It is fungistatic and inhibits C-14α demethylation of lanosterol, which impairs synthesis of ergosterol, a component of the fungal cytoplasmic membrane (Table 42–1). Ketoconazole is best absorbed at an acidic gastric pH, and its absorption is significantly impaired by coadministration of antacids, histamine-2 receptor blocking drugs, or proton pump inhibitors. Ketoconazole is hepatically metabolized and excreted in the bile and does not attain therapeutic concentrations in urine or cerebrospinal fluid. The half-life is approximately 9 hours. Ketoconazole has been shown to be effective treatment for blastomycosis,[12] mucocutaneous candidiasis, coccidioidomycosis,[13] histoplasmosis in nonimmunocompromised hosts,[12] and paracoccidioidomycosis.[14] Ketoconazole is more toxic than the triazole drugs fluconazole and itraconazole, however, and has been largely supplanted by these drugs. Potential adverse events include nausea and vomiting (which occur in more than half of patients treated with doses of 400 mg/d or higher),[12] hypogonadism, adrenal insufficiency,[15] gynecomastia, and hepatic toxicity.[16] Approximately 1 in 15,000 patients treated with ketoconazole has developed drug-induced hepatitis, and some cases have been fatal.[16] The usual dose of ketoconazole is 200 to 400 mg daily; higher doses generally cannot be tolerated because of gastrointestinal side effects.[12]

Fluconazole

Fluconazole was the first triazole antifungal drug to be approved for use in the United States. It has the same mechanism of action as ketoconazole, inhibition of ergosterol synthesis (Table 42–1). In contrast to ketoconazole and itraconazole, fluconazole is highly water soluble and is well absorbed from the gastrointestinal tract regardless of gastric pH.[17] The serum half-life is approximately 28 hours. Fluconazole is excreted unchanged in the urine and attains high concentrations in both urine and cerebrospinal fluid. Fluconazole has been effective for treatment of blastomycosis,[18] mucocutaneous candidiasis,[19] coccidioidomycosis,[20] cryptococcal meningitis,[21] candidemia,[22] histoplasmosis,[23] and sporotrichosis.[24] Resistance is uncommon but has been reported in HIV-infected patients who have received prolonged fluconazole therapy for oropharyngeal candidiasis[25] and in a single HIV-infected patient with histoplasmosis.[26] Fluconazole generally is well tolerated. Reversible alopecia has been reported following administration of high doses for longer than 3 months.[27] Nausea, anorexia, and headache are uncommon side effects. There have been rare reports of fetal malformation after use of fluconazole during pregnancy.[28] The usual dose is 100 to 400 mg daily.

Itraconazole

Itraconazole is a triazole antifungal drug that has enhanced activity against *Aspergillus* and several of the endemic mycoses. Like ketoconazole, itraconazole is a lipophilic agent, is hepatically metabolized, and attains low concentrations in the urine and cerebrospinal fluid (Table 42–1). Itraconazole is available as a capsule, an oral solution, and an intravenous formulation. Absorption of the capsule is better after ingestion of food, whereas the liquid suspension is best absorbed during the fasting state.[29] Serum concentrations of itraconazole may be subtherapeutic in patients treated with the capsule formulation who are receiving histamine-2 blocking agents, proton pump inhibitors, or antacids; absorption is enhanced when oral itraconazole is taken with a cola beverage or fruit juice. After steady state is achieved (which requires approximately 2 weeks), plasma half-life is approximately 20 hours. Itraconazole is effective for treatment of mucocutaneous candidiasis,[30] including cases refractory to fluconazole therapy,[31] blastomycosis,[32] coccidioidomycosis,[33] cryptococcosis,[34] histoplasmosis,[32] paracoccidioidomycosis,[35] and sporotrichosis.[36] In addition, itraconazole is effective prophylaxis against histoplasmosis and cryptococcosis in HIV-infected patients with CD4+ lymphocyte counts below 150/μl.[37] Side effects, which are uncommon, include nausea, diarrhea, skin rash, edema, and hypokalemia. Significant hepatotoxicity and adrenal insufficiency do not appear to accompany itraconazole. The usual dose is 200 mg daily or twice daily. Serum concentrations of itraconazole are decreased by drugs that increase activity of the cytochrome P450 system (e.g., rifampin, isoniazid, phenytoin, fosphenytoin, or carbamazepine). Conversely itraconazole alters the hepatic metabolism of certain drugs and thus increases their serum concentrations; these include digoxin, phenytoin, the sulfonylurea drugs, cyclosporine, tacrolimus, warfarin, and cisapride. Despite itraconazole's long half-life, serum concentrations are higher with a twice-daily dosing regimen than with a once-daily regimen. Dose adjustment is unnecessary in patients who have renal insufficiency. A concentration above 1 μg/ml is considered to be within the therapeutic range. The serum level can be drawn at any point after steady state is achieved; it is not necessary to obtain peak and trough concentrations.

Caspofungin

Caspofungin was the first antifungal drug in the echinocandin class to be licensed for clinical use. Caspofungin inhibits formation of α1,3 glucan in the fungal cell wall[38] (Table 42–1). It has in vitro activity against various *Candida* spp including azole-resistant isolates and also is effective against *Aspergillus* spp, *Pseudallescheria boydii*, and several other fungi uncommonly encountered in clinical practice.[39] Caspofungin is available only as an intravenous preparation. The usual daily dose is 50 mg, following an initial loading dose of 70 mg; each dose should be infused over approximately 1 hour. Caspofungin is metabolized by hydrolysis and N-hydroxylation; less than 2% of a dose is excreted unchanged in the urine. In patients who have moderate hepatic insufficiency the dose should be decreased to 35 mg daily, and caspofungin should not be prescribed for patients who have severe hepatic insufficiency. No dose adjustment is necessary for renal insufficiency, and a supplemental dose is unnecessary following hemodialysis. Caspofungin neither induces nor inhibits the cytochrome P450 system. Caspofungin reduces the area under the curve and the peak serum concentrations of tacrolimus by 20% to 25%, however, so tacrolimus serum concentrations should be monitored in patients treated with both drugs. Furthermore cyclosporine increases the area under the curve of caspofungin by approximately 35%; the manufacturer of caspofungin suggests that the two drugs not be coadministered until further pharmacokinetic and clinical studies have been completed.

Caspofungin therapy generally has been well tolerated; a few cases of skin rash or gastrointestinal toxicity have been reported. The primary role of caspofungin is for the treatment of invasive aspergillosis refractory to amphotericin B, voriconazole, or itraconazole therapy.

FUNGAL INFECTIONS

Cryptococcosis

C. neoformans is an encapsulated yeast that measures 5 to 10 μm in diameter, reproduces by budding, and has a worldwide distribution. There are two varieties of *C. neoformans*: *C. neoformans* var. *neoformans* and *C. neoformans* var. *gattii*, each of which has a unique ecologic niche. *C. neoformans* var. *neoformans* grows in soil, particularly in areas contaminated by pigeon guano. Conversely, *C. neoformans* var. *gattii* is found in the bark of *Eucalyptus camaldulensis* (red river gum) and *Eucalyptus tereticornis* (forest red gum) trees. In tropical and subtropical areas where eucalyptus trees grow, the *gattii* variety predominates, whereas in other parts of the world the *neoformans* variety is more common.[40]

Infection occurs after inhalation of cryptococci from environmental sources. Most infections are asymptomatic, but symptomatic cryptococcal disease can occur in immunocompetent or immunocompromised hosts. Immunocompetent hosts may develop pneumonia, which generally is self-limited; rarely, cryptococcal meningitis results after hematogenous seeding of the meninges, even in previously healthy persons.[41] Impaired cellular immunity substantially increases the risk of symptomatic pulmonary or extrapulmonary cryptococcal infection. Risk factors include AIDS,[42] prolonged systemic corticosteroid therapy, sarcoidosis, chronic lymphocytic leukemia, Hodgkin's disease, reticulum cell sarcoma, hairy cell leukemia,[43] or organ transplantation.

The clinical manifestations of pulmonary cryptococcosis include dry cough, dyspnea, and chest discomfort; severe cases can be associated with respiratory failure. Cryptococcal meningitis is manifested by fever, chronic headaches, cranial nerve palsies, mental status changes, or blindness. Cryptococcal skin lesions (papules, pustules, or ulcers),[44] osteolytic bone lesions,[45] and asymptomatic prostatitis[46] have been documented.

The diagnosis of cryptococcosis is confirmed by smear or by culture of tissue or body fluids positive for *C. neoformans*. Because the airway can be colonized with *C. neoformans*, however, laboratory data should be correlated with the patient's clinical status to confirm the diagnosis of invasive cryptococcal infection rather than asymptomatic colonization. The cryptococcal antigen test is remarkably useful in diagnosing cryptococcal meningitis: the sensitivity of both serum and cerebrospinal fluid cryptococcal antigen testing is greater than 90%. Antigen is detected only in those patients with cryptococcal pneumonia who have either extensive infiltrates or extrapulmonary disease.[47] Serial serum cryptococcal antigen results do not correlate with treatment response in AIDS patients who have cryptococcal meningitis and are not recommended.[48]

The decision about whether to treat a patient with cryptococcal infection is based primarily upon two factors: (1) the presence or absence of extrapulmonary infection and (2) whether the patient has comorbidities resulting in immunosuppression. Treatment is warranted for any case of documented or suspected extrapulmonary infection or for any cryptococcal infection in an immunosuppressed patient. Treatment options for cryptococcosis include amphotericin B, the lipid-based amphotericin B compounds, flucytosine, fluconazole, and itraconazole (Table 42–2).

Clinical trials have focused on the treatment of cryptococcal meningitis. Amphotericin B, with or without concomitant flucytosine, is effective therapy.[49,50] A prospective study of treatment of cryptococcal meningitis in HIV-infected patients compared amphotericin B to fluconazole 200 mg daily. There was no significant difference in outcome in the two arms of the study, but death rate during the first 2 weeks was higher in the fluconazole arm.[21] Accordingly amphotericin B has been recommended as initial therapy for cryptococcal meningitis. The role of adjunctive flucytosine therapy has been debated. A clinical trial in patients with AIDS assessed the efficacy of amphotericin B 0.7 mg/kg/d with or without flucytosine 100 mg/kg/d followed by either fluconazole 400 mg/d or itraconazole 400 mg/d. Although mortality was not significantly different in any of the four arms of the study, there was a trend toward more rapid sterilization of cerebrospinal fluid among patients who received flucytosine.[11] On the basis of the results of these studies, authorities recommend amphotericin B 0.7 mg/kg/d plus flucytosine 25 mg/kg every 6 hours for initial treatment of HIV-infected patients with cryptococcal meningitis.[51] For patients who have persistently elevated cerebrospinal fluid pressure ("intracranial hypertension"), repeated large-volume drainage of cerebrospinal fluid is beneficial.[52]

In HIV-infected patients, long-term maintenance therapy is necessary to prevent relapse of cryptococcal infection after successful induction therapy. In a prospective study the efficacy of maintenance therapy with

TABLE 42–2 ■ Cryptococcosis Treatment

Form	Treatment	Duration
Pneumonia		
Immunocompetent	None	
Immunocompromised or progressive	Fluconazole 400 mg qd	3–6 mo
Meningitis		
HIV seronegative	Amphotericin B 0.7 mg/kg/d or lipid-based amphotericin B plus flucytosine 100 mg/kg/d	2 wk
	Then fluconazole 400 mg/d	3–6 mo
AIDS	Amphotericin B 0.8 mg/kg/d	2 wk
	Then fluconazole 400 mg/d	10 wk
	Then fluconazole 200 mg/d	Indefinitely

fluconazole 200 mg daily was significantly higher than that of amphotericin B 1 mg/kg weekly.[53] A second prospective trial of maintenance therapy demonstrated that fluconazole 200 mg daily was significantly more effective in preventing relapse than itraconazole 200 mg daily; in that study the risk of relapse was lower among patients who had received flucytosine during the induction phase of therapy.[54] Fluconazole 200 mg daily continued indefinitely is the recommended maintenance therapy for HIV-infected patients with cryptococcal meningitis.

Only limited data are available regarding the efficacy of fluconazole for cryptococcal meningitis in HIV-seronegative patients. One small prospective trial compared fluconazole 800 mg/d plus flucytosine 100 mg/kg/d to amphotericin B 0.7 mg/kg/d plus flucytosine 100 mg/kg/d for cryptococcal meningitis. This study was terminated prematurely after it was shown that treatment failure occurred much more frequently among patients who were treated with fluconazole than among those treated with amphotericin B.[55] Although fluconazole might be considered as initial treatment for milder cases of cryptococcosis in patients who are not severely immunocompromised, a combination of amphotericin B 0.7 mg/kg/d and flucytosine 100 mg/kg/d is the treatment of choice for most cases.

The role of the lipid-associated amphotericin B compounds in cryptococcal meningitis treatment remains unclear. One study in HIV-infected patients compared amphotericin B 0.7 to 1.2 mg/kg/d to amphotericin B lipid complex 1.2 to 5 mg/kg/d and showed that the efficacy of the two drugs was similar but that amphotericin B lipid complex was better tolerated.[56] A second study compared amphotericin B 0.7 mg/kg daily to liposomal amphotericin B 4 mg/kg daily. The efficacy of the two amphotericin B preparations was comparable, but cerebrospinal fluid sterilization occurred more rapidly in patients who received liposomal amphotericin B, which also was less nephrotoxic than conventional amphotericin B.[57] Because of the higher expense of the lipid preparations, their use probably should be reserved for patients who have renal insufficiency or who are receiving nephrotoxic medications, for those who are unable to tolerate conventional amphotericin B, or for infections refractory to conventional amphotericin B therapy.

Treatment of cryptococcal pneumonia is indicated for patients who have severe or cavitary lung infiltrates or cellular immunodeficiency secondary to HIV infection, hematologic malignancy, or immunosuppressive therapy. Milder cases in immunocompetent hosts may be self-limited, and in such cases treatment is unnecessary unless the pneumonia progresses or the patient develops extrapulmonary infection. Because there have been no controlled clinical trials assessing treatment of cryptococcal pneumonia, treatment recommendations are extrapolated from the large body of experience with cryptococcal meningitis. For the patient who has cryptococcal pneumonia without concomitant meningitis, amphotericin B and fluconazole are treatment options. Since fluconazole is much easier to administer, it is the recommended first-line treatment. Although the optimal dose of fluconazole for treatment of cryptococcal pneumonia is unknown, in view of its high therapeutic index a daily dose of at least 400 mg is recommended. Treatment should be continued until at least 2 weeks after pulmonary infiltrates resolve.

Although a cryptococcal vaccine has been developed, it has not been tested in humans. Three studies have assessed antifungal drug prophylaxis against cryptococcosis in patients with AIDS (Table 42–3). In one study the incidence of cryptococcosis in HIV-infected patients with CD4+ lymphocyte counts less than 68/μl who were treated with fluconazole 200 mg daily was less than 1%, compared to 4% of historical control patients.[58] A double-blind trial compared treatment with fluconazole 200 mg daily to clotrimazole troches in HIV-infected patients with CD4+ lymphocyte counts less than 200/μl. Cryptococcal infection was documented in 0.9% of fluconazole-treated patients and in 7.1% of those who received clotrimazole; this difference was statistically significant.[59] A placebo-controlled study showed that itraconazole 200 mg daily significantly reduced the incidence of cryptococcosis in patients with CD4+ counts below 150/μl.[37] Despite the clear-cut efficacy of fluconazole and itraconazole prophylaxis, however, such prophylaxis has not been recommended for routine use in view of the declining incidence of cryptococcal infection in Western countries, the high cost of prophylaxis, and the risks of drug toxicity, drug-drug interactions, and emergence of drug-resistant yeast.[60,61]

TABLE 42–3 ■ **Antifungal Prophylaxis**

Infection	Drug	Dose	Recommendation for use
Cryptococcosis, AIDS	Fluconazole	200 mg/d	No
	Itraconazole	200 mg/d	No
Histoplasmosis, AIDS	Itraconazole	200 mg/d	No
Aspergillosis	Itraconazole	200 mg bid	Not routinely; consider if incidence high in individual institution

Histoplasmosis

Histoplasmosis is caused by *H. capsulatum*, a thermal dimorphic fungus that exists as a mycelium at temperatures below 37°C and converts to a yeast at body temperature. Cases of histoplasmosis have occurred on all five continents, but the Ohio and Mississippi River valleys in the United States constitute the major endemic area. Infection occurs after airborne microconidia are inhaled, convert to yeast forms, and spread to contiguous alveoli and then to hilar and mediastinal lymph nodes. Cases can occur sporadically or in outbreaks, which have been reported after such activities as spelunking or cleaning chicken coops or bird roosts.[62,63]

Approximately 99% of *H. capulatum* infections are asymptomatic, but after exposure to a large inoculum of organisms acute pneumonia can occur[64] (Table 42–4). The clinical presentation generally is that of a flulike illness (fever, chills, myalgias, malaise, headache, nonproductive cough), which sometimes is associated with vague substernal discomfort. Milder cases usually resolve spontaneously after a few weeks, but severe cases can cause respiratory failure.[65] Patients who have pulmonary emphysema or chronic bronchitis are at risk for chronic pulmonary histoplasmosis, which causes weight loss, dyspnea, productive cough, and hemoptysis.[66] Disseminated histoplasmosis can occur in patients who have cellular immunodeficiency due to malignancy, immunosuppressive therapy, or advanced age and is seen rarely in previously healthy persons.[67] Since the mid-1980s the most common risk factor for disseminated histoplasmosis has been HIV infection.[68] Typical symptoms of disseminated histoplasmosis include fever, weight loss, nonproductive cough, and diarrhea.

Healed foci of histoplasmosis in the lungs of otherwise healthy persons occasionally cause calcified granulomas known as histoplasmomas. The principal significance of these asymptomatic lesions is that their appearance on chest radiographs can be identical to that of malignant neoplasms. Unusual manifestations of histoplasmosis include mediastinal granuloma (a cystic mediastinal structure composed of coalescent lymph nodes), broncholithiasis (erosion of a granuloma into a bronchus, resulting in expectoration of a stone), and mediastinal fibrosis, an exuberant fibrotic reaction to *H. capsulatum* antigens that eventually can compress the superior vena cava or esophagus.

Useful diagnostic tests include complement fixation and immunodiffusion serology, which usually are positive in acute or chronic pulmonary histoplasmosis; *Histoplasma* polysaccharide antigen, which can be detected in the urine of most patients with disseminated histoplasmosis[69]; cultures of blood, sputum, or other body fluids; and histopathologic studies of tissue specimens. Histoplasmin skin testing is not useful for diagnostic purposes.

Some forms of histoplasmosis either are self-limited or represent host inflammatory responses and do not require antifungal treatment. Most cases of acute pulmonary histoplasmosis are asymptomatic or minimally symptomatic and will resolve spontaneously within a few weeks. Pulmonary histoplasmomas are caused by healed self-contained foci of infection; treatment is unnecessary. Both the rheumatologic presentation of acute histoplasmosis (i.e., erythema nodosum and polyarthritis) and *Histoplasma* pericarditis are caused by inflammatory reactions to the fungus and are best treated with either a nonsteroidal anti-inflammatory drug or prednisone; antifungal therapy is not indicated in these cases.[70] Other forms of histoplasmosis (progressive acute pulmonary histoplasmosis, chronic pulmonary histoplasmosis, and disseminated histoplasmosis) should be treated with a systemic antifungal drug. Treatment options include amphotericin B, one of the lipid amphotericin B preparations, itraconazole, ketoconazole, and fluconazole (Table 42–5).

Acute Pulmonary Histoplasmosis

Although asymptomatic or mildly symptomatic cases generally are self-limited and do not require treatment, in cases of persistent or progressive acute pulmonary histoplasmosis, treatment is warranted. Itraconazole is the most effective of the three available azole drugs. In a clinical trial that assessed the efficacy of itraconazole 200 to 400 mg daily treatment was successful in all seven patients studied.[32] Experience with ketoconazole and fluconazole is limited; a handful of successfully treated cases have been reported, but the efficacy of these drugs has not been established by controlled clinical trials. Because of ketoconazole's unfavorable toxicity profile it has a limited role in the treatment armamentarium. Itraconazole 200 mg once or twice daily is the treatment of choice. Fluconazole therapy should be reserved for situations in which intolerance, impaired absorption, or drug-drug interactions preclude the use of itraconazole. For severe cases of pulmonary histoplasmosis associated with respiratory failure a 10- to 14-day course of amphotericin B 0.5 to 0.6 mg/kg/d is recommended; a brief course of adjunctive systemic corticosteroid therapy may also be beneficial.[65]

TABLE 42–4 ■ **Histoplasmosis Clinical Classification**

Asymptomatic infection
Acute symptomatic infection
  Pulmonary histoplasmosis*
  Pericarditis†
  Arthritis and erythema nodosum†
Chronic pulmonary histoplasmosis‡
Mediastinal fibrosis
Disseminated histoplasmosis‡

*Antifungal treatment indicated for severe cases.
†Antinflammatory treatment.
‡Antifungal treatment indicated for all cases.

TABLE 42-5 ▪ Histoplasmosis Treatment

Type	Treatment	Duration
Acute pulmonary		
Severe	Amphotericin B 0.7 mg/kg/d	2 wk
	Then itraconazole 200 mg qd	10–12 wk
Mild-to-moderate	Itraconazole 200 mg qd or bid	8–12 wk
Chronic pulmonary	Itraconazole 200 mg qd or bid	18–24 mo
Disseminated, HIV negative		
Severe	Amphotericin B 0.7 mg/kg/d	2–4 wk
	Then itraconazole 200 mg bid	6–18 mo
Mild-to-moderate	Itraconazole 200 mg bid	6–18 mo
Disseminated, AIDS		
Severe	Liposomal amphotericin B 3–5 mg/kg/d	2–4 wk
Mild-to-moderate	Itraconazole 200 mg bid	12 wk
Maintenance	Itraconazole 200 mg qd	Lifelong

Chronic Pulmonary Histoplasmosis

Although a few self-limited cases of chronic histoplamosis have been documented, the usual natural history is that of progressive destruction of lung parenchyma. Accordingly antifungal treatment is recommended for all patients with chronic pulmonary histoplasmosis. Amphotericin B was effective in 59% to 100% of patients reported in three series, but relapses occurred in 10% to 15% of these cases even though cumulative doses of 35 to 40 mg/kg were administered.[71–73] Ketoconazole 400 or 800 mg daily was effective in 19 of 23 cases (84%) in one series, but the higher dose was poorly tolerated.[12] The efficacy of itraconazole 200, 300, or 400 mg daily was 80% in a series of 20 cases; however, infection relapsed after completion of therapy in 15% of patients.[32] Five of eleven patients (45%) with chronic pulmonary histoplasmosis responded to fluconazole 200 to 800 mg daily in another prospective study.[23] The treatment of choice is itraconazole 200 mg once or twice daily for 18 to 24 months.

Disseminated Histoplasmosis

In HIV-seronegative patients, untreated disseminated histoplasmosis is fatal in 90% of cases,[74–76] so antifungal therapy is always indicated. Amphotericin B (cumulative doses of 35 to 50 mg/kg) was effective in 68% to 91% of cases reported in three studies; however, post-treatment relapses occurred in 7% to 20% of cases.[76,77] The efficacy of ketoconazole 400 mg/d was 70% in one prospective study, but less than half of patients with underlying immunosuppression responded to therapy.[12] Disseminated histoplasmosis was treated successfully in 71% of patients who received fluconazole in a prospective clinical trial.[23] Itraconazole 200 to 400 mg daily was effective in all 10 patients in another study, and there were no relapses after completion of therapy.[32] Itraconazole is considered the treatment of choice, except for life-threatening cases, for which amphotericin B is indicated.

Disseminated histoplasmosis in patients with AIDS is fatal if not treated, and even after successful initial treatment, relapse occurs in 60% of cases unless long-term maintenance therapy is administered.[78] Accordingly two phases of treatment are necessary: an 8- to 10-week course of induction therapy followed by less-intensive lifelong maintenance therapy. For severe cases a 2-week course of induction amphotericin B therapy should be administered. A recently completed double-blind trial demonstrated that liposomal amphotericin B is more effective and better tolerated than conventional amphotericin B in HIV-infected patients with disseminated histoplasmosis and is associated with improved survival.[7] Thus liposomal amphotericin B 3 to 5 mg/kg/d is the treatment of choice for severe histoplasmosis in HIV-infected patients. For mild to moderately severe cases, oral itraconazole is recommended on the basis of the results of a prospective clinical trial that demonstrated the efficacy of itraconazole 400 mg/d to be 85%.[79] There are several options for long-term maintenance therapy. Amphotericin B 50 mg weekly or bi-weekly was effective in 82% to 97% of cases in two series,[78,80,81] and itraconazole 200 mg once daily prevented relapse in 95%.[82] Fluconazole 100 to 400 mg once daily was effective maintenance therapy for 88% of patients in one retrospective study.[83] In a prospective study, however, relapse was documented in almost one-third of patients who received fluconazole therapy for both induction and maintenance treatment.[84] In a retrospective review ketoconazole maintenance therapy prevented relapse in only 9% of cases.[78] On the basis of the aggregate experience reported in these studies the maintenance therapy of choice is itraconazole 200 mg/d; the second choice is fluconazole 200 to 400 mg/d (which is less effective than amphotericin B but is better-tolerated and easier to administer).

Treatment of soil with 3% formalin solution effectively kills *H. capsulatum* before cleaning or construction work is begun. Because of the potential adverse ecologic impacts of this practice, however, formalin treatment should only be administered by the local or state health departments. There is no effective vaccine against *H. capsulatum*. Among HIV-infected patients the subset at highest risk for histoplasmosis includes those persons who reside in a histoplasmosis endemic area and who have a CD4 lymphocyte count below 150/μl. A reactive histoplasmin skin test, positive *Histoplasma* serology, and radiographic evidence of pulmonary calcifications are not useful markers for high-risk patients.[85] A placebo-controlled trial of itraconazole prophylaxis in HIV-infected patients with CD4 counts below 150/μl showed that itraconazole prevents histoplasmosis (Table 42–3), particularly in the subset of patients with CD4 counts below 100/μl.[37] Because the incidence of histoplasmosis has declined substantially following the advent of highly active antiretroviral therapy, however, prophylaxis is recommended only for persons who reside in communities where histoplasmosis is hyperendemic (i.e., >10 cases per 100 patient-years).[61]

Blastomycosis

Blastomycosis is caused by *B. dermatitidis*, a thermal dimorphic fungus that converts from a mycelium to a yeast at temperatures of 37°C or higher. *B. dermatitidis* measures 2 to 10 μm in diameter, has a highly refractile cell wall, and produces characteristic broad-based buds between parent cells and daughter cells. The endemic area for blastomycosis includes the upper midwestern and southern United States as well as an area along the St. Lawrence River. Cases also have been reported from several Canadian provinces, Poland, Saudi Arabia, Israel, Lebanon, and India. The ecologic niche of *B. dermatitidis* remains poorly characterized, but its environmental reservoir is thought to be in soil.[86] Epidemiologic studies have shown that cases have occurred most frequently in persons who have had intimate exposure to soil in endemic regions.[87,88]

Blastomycosis usually is acquired by inhalation of organisms from an environmental source. In most cases a focal pulmonary infiltrate develops. Hilar lymphadenopathy is noted occasionally, and rarely there is hematogenous spread of organisms to other sites including skin, bones, the genitourinary tract, the central nervous system, the adrenals, or the oropharynx. Disease progression can be noted at one or more of these sites even as pulmonary lesions regress or resolve.

The diagnosis of blastomycosis can be confirmed either by observing organisms in a clinical specimen or by positive culture. Organisms can be visualized in cytology preparations stained with the Papanicolaou smear or in tissue specimens stained with Gomori methenamine silver (GMS) or periodic acid–Schiff (PAS), which also demonstrates the pyogranulomatous reaction that typically occurs in blastomycosis. Unfortunately serologic studies and skin tests are of limited value.

Untreated, blastomycosis typically is a progressive, fatal disease: mortality was 78% in one large series published before the availability of effective antifungal therapy.[89] Even in those patients who appear to have improved spontaneously, extrapulmonary infection can be detected months to years later. On the basis of the natural history of untreated blastomycosis, it is recommended that all

documented cases be treated. Asymptomatic colonization does not occur; a positive smear or a culture result positive for *B. dermatitidis* should be construed as indicative of an active infection and should prompt the initiation of antifungal therapy.

Amphotericin B was the first systemic drug shown to be clinically effective against *B. dermatitides*.[90] In patients who have received cumulative doses of at least 1500 mg, efficacy has been in the 75% to 90% range[90]; lower doses have been associated with a higher risk of relapsed infection.[91] Because there have been no controlled clinical trials of amphotericin B therapy for blastomycosis, the optimal dosage and duration of treatment are not known. Before the availability of the oral azole drugs, it was recommended that patients receive a daily dose of 0.4 to 0.6 mg/kg/d until a cumulative dose of 1500 to 2000 mg was attained.[90] The oral triazole agents, however, have supplanted amphotericin B for treatment of blastomycosis except for severe, life-theatening cases.

Ketoconazole therapy has been assessed in two clinical trials. In one study, efficacy was 79% for patients who were treated with 400 mg daily, and 100% for those who received 800 mg daily; however, the higher dose was poorly tolerated.[12] The second study documented efficacy of 80% in patients who were treated with 400 mg daily for at least 2 weeks.[92]

Although head-to-head comparisons of the azole drugs have not been done, the efficacy of itraconazole appears to be higher than that of ketoconazole. In a prospective trial of 48 patients treated with 200, 300, or 400 mg of itraconazole daily, blastomycosis was cured in 90%; among those patients who adhered to therapy, efficacy was 95%.[32] Toxicity was less than that which had been reported with ketoconazole.[12] Fluconazole therapy has been evaluated in two studies, which assessed daily doses of 200, 400, or 800 mg. Response to therapy was documented in 62% of patients who received 200 mg daily,[18] in 70% to 89% of those treated with 400 mg daily,[18,93] and in 85% who received 800 mg daily.[93]

Because itraconazole has the highest efficacy of the three available azole drugs, it is considered the drug of choice for most cases of blastomycosis (Table 42–6). On the basis of the available data it is unclear whether a daily dose of 400 mg is more effective than a 200-mg daily dose. Accordingly most authorities recommend a starting dose of 200 mg daily; if the clinical response is incomplete, the dose should be increased to 400 mg daily. Immunocompromised patients or those who have diffuse pulmonary infiltrates and respiratory failure should be treated with amphotericin B initially. Another treatment option is intravenous itraconazole, but no data on the use of this formulation for treatment of blastomycosis have been published. After the patient's clinical status improves (typically within 1 to 2 weeks), oral itraconazole therapy can be administered. The typical duration of therapy for pulmonary or disseminated blastomycosis is at least 6 months.[94]

TABLE 42–6 ■ **Miscellaneous Fungal Infection Treatment**

Infection	Drug	Dose	Duration
Blastomycosis	Itraconazole	200 mg qd or bid	>6 mo
Chromomycosis	Itraconazole	100–400 mg qd	Several months
Fusariosis	Lipid-based amphotericin	>5 mg/kg/d	Individualized
Mucormycosis	Lipid-based amphotericin B	>5 mg/kg/d	Individualized
Paracoccidioidomycosis	Itraconazole	100–400 mg qd	>6 mo
Penicilliosis	Amphotericin B	0.6 mg/kg/d	2 wk
	Then itraconazole	200 mg/d	Indefinitely

Two forms of blastomycosis pose particularly difficult treatment problems: meningeal and genitourinary infection. Neither ketoconazole nor itraconazole penetrates the blood-brain barrier well, and they do not attain appreciable concentrations in the urinary tract. Accordingly it is recommended that patients with central nervous system blastomycosis should be treated with amphotericin B. If a patient with genitourinary tract infection is treated with one of the oral azole drugs, a high dose should be used, and the patient should be monitored closely for evidence of treatment failure. Although fluconazole attains much higher concentrations in the urine than either ketoconazole or itraconazole does,[95] its efficacy in the treatment of genitourinary blastomycosis has not been established.

The role of surgery in the management of blastomycosis is limited. Surgical resection of pulmonary masses or infiltrates is not curative since extrapulmonary dissemination of infection occurs in most cases. However, surgery may be necessary for drainage of empyemas or soft-tissue abscesses.

There is no effective vaccine for blastomycosis. In light of the sporadic nature of this disease and the absence of well-defined risk factors, antifungal drug prophylaxis has not been studied.

Coccidioidomycosis

C. immitis is endemic in desert areas in the southwestern United States and in Mexico, Guatemala, Honduras, Colombia, Venezuela, Paraguay, and Argentina. *C. immitis* exists in the environment as a mycelium and is found frequently in the vicinity of rodent burrows. After organisms are inhaled, a complex life cycle is initiated, culminating in the formation of spherules that attain sizes of up to 60 μm.

Coccidioidomycosis is asymptomatic in approximately 60% of cases (Table 42–7). In symptomatic cases of primary pulmonary coccidioidomycosis the clinical presentation usually is nonspecific and is manifested by fever, anorexia, diffuse myalgias, cough, and chest pain.[96,97] Chest radiographs generally show single or multiple patchy pulmonary infiltrates; frank consolidation can occur. Hilar lymphadenopathy is present in approximately 20% of cases. Focal pulmonary nodules

TABLE 42–7 ■ **Coccidioidomycosis Clinical Classification**

Asymptomatic infection
Acute pulmonary coccidioidomycosis*
Pulmonary nodule
Chronic pulmonary coccidioidomycosis†
Coccidioidal meningitis‡
Disseminated coccidioidomycosis†

*Antifungal treatment indicated in some cases.
†Antifungal treatment indicated in all cases.
‡Lifelong antifungal treatment indicated.

develop after resolution of pulmonary coccidioidomycosis in 5% of cases.[98,99] The appearance of such nodules mimics neoplasms. Coccidioidal pulmonary nodules cavitate in about half of cases and can cause hemoptysis, bronchopleural fistula, or empyema. Half of these cavitary lesions close spontaneously within 2 years.[100] In a small subset of patients chronic, progressive pneumonia develops.[101] The clinical findings of chronic pulmonary coccidioidomycosis are similar to those of pulmonary tuberculosis.

Rarely, hematogenous dissemination of coccidioidomycosis occurs; numerous organ systems can be affected, including the skin, bones, joints, central nervous system, lymph nodes, liver, spleen, adrenals, kidneys, eyes, ears, larynx, or genitourinary tract. Although susceptibility to asymptomatic coccidioidomycosis is independent of age, sex, or race, disseminated disease occurs much more commonly in dark-skinned races.[102] Disseminated coccidioidomycosis is particularly common in African Americans and Filipinos, who develop disseminated disease 10 to 15 times more often than whites do,[103] and is more common among pregnant women, Mexicans, Native Americans, and Asians than in the general population. The risk of disseminated infection also is higher among organ transplant recipients,[104] persons receiving immunosuppressive therapy,[105] and patients with advanced HIV infection.[106,107]

The diagnosis can be confirmed by observation of spherules in body fluids or tissue specimens, by positive culture results, or by serology. Although coccidioidin skin testing is mostly of value in epidemiologic studies, it is also useful in assessing prognosis and response to treatment: a nonreactive skin test in a patient with disseminated infection portends an unfavorable prognosis, whereas skin test conversion during treatment indicates a response to therapy.

Primary Coccidioidomycosis

Primary pulmonary coccidioidomycosis often is a self-limited disease, and antifungal therapy is warranted only for severe, progressive cases. The clinical status of patients with primary coccidioidomycosis should be monitored closely, and serial chest radiographs should be obtained. Indications for initiation of therapy include the persistence of symptoms for more than 6 weeks; worsening pulmonary infiltrates; high clinical suspicion of disseminated infection (i.e., paratracheal lymphadenopathy or markedly elevated complement fixation titer); or increased risk for dissemination (dark-skinned race, HIV infection, immunosuppressive therapy, or late stages of pregnancy).

For many years amphotericin B was the standard treatment for symptomatic primary coccidioidomycosis[108,109] (Table 42–8). On the basis of extensive clinical experience a daily dose of 30 to 35 mg has been recommended for adults. The duration of treatment is based on clinical response: in most cases a cumulative dose of 500 to 1000 mg is administered. Although the roles of ketoconazole, itraconazole, and fluconazole in the treatment of primary pulmonary coccidioidomycosis have not been defined by controlled clinical trials, the ease of administration and favorable toxicity profiles of fluconazole and itraconazole have made these drugs appealing options, and both have been used frequently to treat this infection. Early antifungal treatment of coccidioidal pneumonia in patients at high risk for disseminated infection appears to decrease the risk of severe pulmonary or disseminated coccidioidomycosis.[102]

Cavitary pulmonary nodules do not respond to antifungal therapy, and dissemination of infection from such lesions does not occur, so conservative management (i.e., observation) is warranted. Surgical resection of cavities could be considered in certain rare situations, such as recurrent or severe hemoptysis, chronic bacterial superinfection, or bronchopleural fistula.[110,111] Surgical resection, however, may actually induce bronchopleural fistulas or coccidioidal empyema. In those patients who undergo surgical resection, adjunctive antifungal therapy should be administered from approximately 2 weeks before surgery until 2 weeks after surgery, since concomitant small cavities may not be evident. Either amphotericin B or an oral azole antifungal drug could be prescribed.

Chronic Pulmonary Coccidioidomycosis

In untreated cases of chronic coccidioidal pneumonia, apical infiltrates progress over a period of several months, eventually causing pulmonary cavitation and fibrosis. Although amphotericin B therapy is effective, the risk of relapse is high unless a cumulative dose of at least 30 mg/kg is attained.[109] There have been several prospective studies of oral azole therapy for chronic pulmonary coccidioidomycosis. In one study, ketoconazole was effective in 23% of patients treated with 400 mg daily and in 32% of those treated with 800 mg daily; this difference was not statistically significant.[112] In another clinical trial the efficacy of fluconazole therapy (200 mg daily, increased to 400 mg daily if an initial response was not seen) was 86% for patients with skeletal coccidioidomycosis and 76% for those who had soft-tissue infections.[113] Although the median duration of treatment was almost 2 years, infection relapsed after discontinuation of fluconazole in 37% of cases.[113] Itraconazole was effective in 54% of patients with chronic pulmonary coccidioidomycosis treated with either 100, 200, or 400 mg daily in one study,[33] in 57% of patients treated with 50 to 400 mg daily in a second study,[114] and in 94% of patients treated with 400 mg daily in a third clinical trial; however, in the third study 25% of subjects subsequently experienced relapse of infection.[115] The most definitive study of the modern era, which was conducted in a prospective, double-blind fashion, compared itraconazole 200 mg twice daily to fluconazole 400 mg/d; the efficacy

TABLE 42–8 ■ Coccidioidomycosis Treatment

Type	Treatment	Duration
Acute pulmonary		
>6 mo, progressive infiltrates, or risk factors for dissemination	Fluconazole 400 mg qd	3–6 mo
Chronic pulmonary	Fluconazole 400 mg qd OR Itraconazole 200 mg bid	1–2 y
Meningitis	Fluconazole 400–800 mg qd	Lifelong
Disseminated, HIV negative		
Osteoarticular	Itraconazole 200 mg bid	1–2 y
Other sites (nonmeningeal)	Fluconazole 400 mg qd OR Itraconazole 200 mg bid	
Disseminated, AIDS	Amphotericin B 0.5–0.6 mg/kg/d Then itraconazole 200 mg qd	2 wk Indefinite

of itraconazole was 66% for chronic pulmonary coccidioidomycosis and that of fluconazole was 63%.[116] Thus both fluconazole and itraconazole are effective treatment for chronic pulmonary coccidioidomycosis.

Disseminated Coccidioidomycosis

Disseminated coccidioidomycosis is a progressive, life-threatening infection; all cases should be treated. Unfortunately there is a high risk of persistent or recurrent infection even if prolonged treatment is administered. Although amphotericin B usually is effective in the short term when a cumulative dose of 2000 to 4000 mg is given, relapse often occurs after discontinuation of therapy.[109] The azole drugs have been studied for treatment of osteoarticular, genitourinary, and soft tissue infections. In one clinical trial of fluconazole therapy (50 to 100 mg daily) treatment was effective in 86% of patients initially, but in only 29% did infection resolve completely.[20] Another study demonstrated that clinical response rates were higher when doses of 200 to 400 mg daily were used: 86% of patients with skeletal infection and 76% with soft tissue infection improved, but infection subsequently relapsed in 37% of these patients.[113] In the study that compared fluconazole 400 mg/d to itraconazole 200 mg twice daily the efficacy of the two drugs for soft tissue infection was 63% and 66%, respectively, whereas the efficacy for skeletal infections was 37% and 70%, respectively; the latter difference was statistically significant.[116] Accordingly either fluconzole or itraconazole can be used for treatment of all forms of disseminated coccidioidomycosis other than skeletal infection, for which itraconazole is preferred.

Serial complement fixation titers are useful in assessing response to therapy: a declining titer denotes a good response to treatment, whereas a rising titer often indicates treatment failure.[117] Several other parameters can be monitored to assess treatment response: defervescence, resolution of pulmonary infiltrates, declining erythrocyte sedimentation rate or C-reactive protein level, and development of skin test reactivity to coccidioidin. Chronic coccidioidal pneumonia or disseminated coccidioidomycosis may respond to treatment slowly, over a period of months to years. Treatment should not be discontinued until several months after normalization of clinical and laboratory parameters.

Coccidioidal Meningitis

Coccidioidal meningitis is one of the most challenging of all infectious diseases to manage. Fortunately treatment of this life-threatening infection has been revolutionized by the availability of the oral triazole agents. Itraconazole therapy was effective in four of five patients with refractory coccidioidal meningitis who were treated with 300 or 400 mg daily in one study.[118] In an uncontrolled multicenter study, fluconazole 400 mg daily was effective in 79% of cases.[119] Furthermore in a retrospective analysis of 18 patients with prior coccidioidal meningitis in whom

azole therapy was discontinued, relapse occurred in 78%.[120] It is therefore recommended that patients with coccidioidal meningitis receive lifelong azole therapy.[120] Fluconazole is preferred because it penetrates the blood-brain barrier better than itraconazole does.

Coccidioidomycosis in AIDS

There have been no controlled clinical trials of treatment for coccidioidomycosis in patients with AIDS. On the basis of retrospective experience it is recommended that initial treatment consist of amphotericin B 0.5 to 0.6 mg/kg/d.[121] After a 2- to 4-week course of induction amphotericin B therapy, maintenance therapy should be lifelong. The optimal maintenance regimen has not been defined. Because cases of coccidioidomycosis have been reported in HIV-infected patients who were being treated with ketoconazole for candidiasis, however, ketoconazole therapy is not advisable. Most authorities recommend maintenance treatment with either itraconazole 400 mg/d or fluconazole 400 mg/d.

Although a vaccine prepared from killed *C. immitis* spherules was protective in several animal species, it was ineffective in humans.[122] No forms of either immunoprophylaxis or chemoprophylaxis are recommended.

Aspergillosis

Aspergillus spp are molds that grow in decaying organic debris and are ubiquitous in the environment. Airborne *Aspergillus* hyphae are inhaled and then can colonize the airway, elicit a local inflammatory response, or cause potentially lethal invasive infections in immunocompromised hosts. Although all humans frequently are exposed to *Aspergillus* spp, disease generally occurs only in persons who are immunocompromised or who have underlying structural lung disease.

It is important to note that asymptomatic airway colonization with *Aspergillus* commonly is seen in patients who have structurally abnormal airways due to bronchiectasis, emphysema, or other forms of chronic lung disease and does not require treatment. There are three forms of aspergillosis for which medical or surgical treatment may be necessary: allergic bronchopulmonary aspergillosis (ABPA), aspergilloma, and invasive aspergillosis. Since the pathophysiology and the approaches to diagnosis and treatment of these three forms of aspergillosis are distinct, these entities will be discussed separately.

Allergic Bronchopulmonary Aspergillosis

ABPA occurs in persons who have cystic fibrosis or corticosteroid-dependent asthma whose airways become colonized with *Aspergillus* spp. A vigorous allergic response to *Aspergillus* antigens then causes mucus plugs to form in the airways, which exacerbate obstructive lung disease. Several clinical criteria are used to confirm the diagnosis of ABPA: (1) documented asthma, (2) a reactive *Aspergillus* skin test, (3) *Aspergillus*-specific IgE in serum, (4) serum IgE level exceeding 400 IU/ml, (5) *Aspergillus fumigatus*–precipitating antibody in serum, (6) peripheral eosinophilia (absolute eosinophil count >500/mm^3), and (7) a history of unexplained pulmonary infiltrates.[123] Chest radiographs usually reveal atelectasis and pulmonary infiltrates. The diagnosis of ABPA also is suggested when computerized tomographic scanning of the chest reveals central bronchiectasis, which is virtually pathognomonic for ABPA.[124] For many years, long-term prednisone therapy has been the cornerstone of management of ABPA (Table 42–9). The usual dose of prednisone is 50 to 60 mg daily. After pulmonary infiltrates have resolved completely, the dose is tapered over a period of approximately 6 months. There has been long-standing interest in using antifungal therapy to decrease airway colonization with *Aspergillus* and thereby to lessen the inflammatory response to the fungus.[125] A prospective placebo-controlled trial of itraconazole therapy 200 mg twice daily demonstrated that in patients treated with itraconazole the daily corticosteroid requirement decreased significantly.[126] Itraconazole treatment therefore should be considered for patients with symptomatic ABPA.

Aspergilloma

Aspergillomas are saprophytic pulmonary "fungus balls" that arise when pre-existing cavities are colonized with *Aspergillus*. They are seen most commonly in patients who have had tuberculosis. Although most aspergillomas are asymptomatic, some expand into bronchial blood vessels, causing hemoptysis. The diagnosis of aspergilloma can be made when a sputum culture is positive for *Aspergillus* and a characteristic mass lesion within a pulmonary cavity is seen on chest radiograph; the mass lesion sometimes moves with changes in body position. This finding can be confirmed by fluoroscopic examination of the chest.[127] Although aspergillomas generally do not require treatment, resection of the involved portion of lung may be necessary if recurrent or severe hemoptysis occurs.[128,129] In patients who are not surgical candidates, amphotericin B irrigation of the lung cavity via a percutaneously inserted catheter could be considered, although there has been limited clinical experience with this approach.[130] Refractory hemoptysis can be controlled in some cases by bronchial artery embolization.[131]

Invasive Aspergillosis

Invasive aspergillosis is a life-threatening infection that occurs in patients who are severely immunocompromised because of hematologic malignancy, chemotherapy-induced neutropenia, organ transplantation, long-term corticosteroid therapy, or AIDS. Pneumonia is the most common manifestation, but virtually any organ system can be involved. Common clinical manifestations include fever unresponsive to broad-spectrum antibacterial therapy, nonproductive cough, dyspnea, pleuritic chest pain, and hemoptysis (caused by pulmonary infarction due to invasion and occlusion of blood vessels by *Aspergillus* hyphae).[132]

A high index of clinical suspicion for aspergillosis should be maintained for immunocompromised patients who develop pneumonia or unexplained necrotizing infection of the sinuses, skin, bones, or brain. In light of the poor prognosis of invasive aspergillosis, efforts to establish a diagnosis should be undertaken promptly if aspergillosis is suspected. Paradoxically, *Aspergillus* organisms may be difficult to grow in culture specimens from patients who have invasive disease, and a positive sputum culture may reflect colonization rather than invasive infection, particularly in patients with structural lung disease. The only confirmatory diagnostic tests are either tissue biopsy (with demonstration of septated hyphae that branch at 45-degree angles) or positive culture of a tissue specimen; however, in many patients at risk for aspergillosis, invasive procedures such as transbronchial biopsy, fine-needle aspiration, or open lung

---

TABLE 42–9 ■ Aspergillosis Treatment

Form	Treatment	Duration
NONINVASIVE ASPERGILLOSIS		
Allergic bronchopulmonary	Itraconazole 200 mg bid Prednisone if necessary	16 wk
Aspergilloma, recurrent hemoptysis	Surgical resection Bronchial artery embolization Intracavitary amphotericin B	
INVASIVE ASPERGILLOSIS		
Invasive pulmonary	Amphotericin B 1–1.5 mg/kg/d	Individualized; usually several weeks
	Lipid-based amphotericin preparation Itraconazole 200 mg tid 3d Then 200 mg bid Caspofungin 50 mg qd	
Invasive nonpulmonary	Same as above, plus surgical débridement if feasible	

biopsy are relatively or absolutely contraindicated in view of thrombocytopenia or bleeding dyscrasias. In severely immunocompromised patients such as bone marrow transplant recipients, the positive predictive value of a positive sputum culture is high, and treatment is warranted if the clinical presentation is consistent with aspergillosis even if the diagnosis is not confirmed by an invasive procedure.[133]

Serologic tests for aspergillosis have been studied for many years. In Europe a serum assay for *Aspergillus*-specific galactomannan is available; the sensitivity of this test for invasive aspergillosis is 93% and the specificity is 95%.[134] Galactomannan assays have not been approved for use in the United States, however, and there are no readily available, highly accurate polymerase chain reaction tests for aspergillosis. Computed tomography of the chest can be a useful diagnostic test because certain radiographic findings are highly characteristic of aspergillosis, including the so-called halo sign (i.e., decreased attenuation surrounding a rounded mass) or clusters of pulmonary nodules associated with lung cavitation.[135,136]

The most important determinant of prognosis is the rapidity with which either neutropenia or other causes of immunosuppression can be reversed. Nonetheless antifungal therapy plays an important role in management. Available treatment options include amphotericin B, the lipid amphotericin formulations, itraconazole, or caspofungin (Table 42–9). No direct comparisons of these agents have been published. For decades, amphotericin B has been the treatment of choice. Many strains of *Aspergillus* are relatively resistant to amphotericin B, however, so the recommended daily dose is higher—typically 1 to 1.5 mg/kg/d—than would be used for most other fungal infections. The dose of amphotericin B should be increased rapidly so the target daily dose is attained within 2 to 3 days. Typically the cumulative amphotericin B dose is 1000 to 1500 mg. Despite aggressive management, treatment failures are common. In a retrospective review of cases published from 1990 to 2000, only 35% of patients treated with amphotericin B survived.[137] This poor prognosis can be explained by several factors: the severity of comorbidities in patients with invasive aspergillosis, partial or complete resistance of *Aspergillus* to amphotericin B, and limited penetration of the drug into necrotic tissues.

The lipid-based amphotericin preparations are particularly appealing for treatment of invasive aspergillosis, especially for patients who are intolerant of conventional amphotericin B (because of chills or nephrotoxicity) or whose infections are refractory to therapy. To date no prospective comparative trials of amphotericin B vs. a lipid amphotericin B preparation have been published. In one study the efficacy of amphotericin B colloidal dispersion was 49%, compared to 23% for historical control patients who had been treated with conventional amphotericin B.[138] In a compassionate use protocol, 55 of 130 (42%) patients with refractory invasive aspergillosis responded to amphotericin B lipid complex.[139] A prospective blinded study of two doses of liposomal amphotericin B therapy was done; 64% of patients responded to treatment with 1 mg/kg/d, compared to 48% treated with 4 mg/kg/d. The reason for this difference was not apparent.[140] On the basis of these studies there is no clearcut evidence of superiority of one lipid-based amphotericin B preparation over the others, and the optimal doses of these drugs for management of invasive aspergillosis remain unclear.

Itraconazole has in vitro activity against *Aspergillus* spp. In a prospective study the efficacy of itraconazole 100 to 400 mg a day was 39%.[141] There was a complete response to itraconazole therapy in 27% of patients with refractory aspergillosis in another study.[142] No randomized trials comparing itraconazole to amphotericin B for treatment of invasive aspergillosis have been completed. A large retrospective review of patents with invasive aspergillosis reported itraconazole efficacy of 66% and amphotericin B efficacy of 35%.[143] However, these results likely were influenced by selection bias; i.e. investigators probably chose oral itraconazole therapy for their less acutely ill patients.[143] The recommended itraconazole dosing regimen is 200 mg three times a day for 3 days, then 200 mg twice a day; therapy should be continued until at least 6 to 8 weeks after the infection appears to have resolved. In view of the poor absorption of itraconazole capsules in patients who have undergone bone marrow transplantation or who are being treated with histamine-2 blockers or proton pump inhibitors, either the oral solution or the intravenous formulation is recommended. Caspofungin, which has been effective as salvage therapy for aspergillosis (unpublished data) is another treatment option.

In some cases, resection of localized foci of invasive *Aspergillus* infection is indicated, particularly for extrapulmonary infection involving the sinuses, skin, subcutaneous tissues, or bones.[144] Resection traditionally has had a limited role in the management of pulmonary aspergillosis, but recently published data have suggested that early surgical resection of localized pulmonary foci of aspergillosis improves the prognosis.[145] This issue remains unresolved, however, and surgery is recommended only for those cases of pulmonary aspergillosis in which there is radiographic progression of infection despite antifungal therapy.[146]

On the basis of the available data it is recommended that first-line therapy for aspergillosis in immunocompromised patients should consist of conventional amphotericin B, except for those patients who have renal insufficiency or who are receiving potentially nephrotoxic medications, for whom one of the lipid-based amphotericin B preparations should be administered. Oral itraconazole (preferably the solution rather than the capsule formulation) can be used either for step-down therapy for patients who have responded to amphotericin B therapy or for first-line treatment of milder cases.

Caspofungin is recommended for infections refractory to amphotericin B or itraconazole or for patients who are unable to tolerate other antifungal medications. There have been anecdotal reports of the successful use of combinations of a lipid-based amphotericin B compound and an echinocandin, and such a combination could be considered for cases that do not respond to conventional antifungal monotherapy.

There is no vaccine for aspergillosis. High-risk oncology patients often receive fluconazole for antifungal prophylaxis; fluconazole does not have activity against *Aspergillus* spp, and such prophylaxis has not reduced the incidence of aspergillosis.[147] Itraconazole capsules are not reliably absorbed in acutely ill patients who have received chemotherapy. One prospective double-blind trial compared prophylaxis with itraconazole oral solution (2.5 mg/kg twice daily) to amphotericin B capsules and demonstrated that itraconazole decreased the incidence of invasive fungal infections.[148] The routine use of antifungal prophylaxis in neutropenic patients is not recommended,[149] but prophylaxis with itraconazole suspension could be considered if there is a high incidence of aspergillosis in an individual institution and if the patient is not being treated with other medications that have drug interactions with itraconazole (Table 42–3).

Sporotrichosis

Sporotrichosis, caused by the dimorphic fungus *S. schenckii*, has a worldwide distribution, although most cases occur in North and South America. The most common form of sporotrichosis, lymphocutaneous infection, occurs after percutaneous inoculation of *S. schenckii* from an environmental source (such as sphagnum moss or straw) into the skin or subcutaneous tissues. Subsequently, ulcerative or nodular lesions occur, usually on the fingers or wrists, and lymphangitic spread of infection may be seen. Rare manifestations of sporotrichosis include chronic pneumonia or osteoarticular infection. *Sporothrix* pneumonia is associated with low-grade fever, weight loss, and nonproductive cough; hemoptysis occurs in approximately 20% of cases.[150] The diagnosis of sporotrichosis is established when the organism is grown from cultures of body fluids or tissue specimens. Serology studies and skin tests for sporotrichosis are inaccurate and are not useful. Saturated solution of potassium iodide (SSKI) was shown to be effective for treatment of lymphocutaneous sporotrichosis a century ago but is rarely used now because the azole antifungal drugs are more potent and better tolerated. Treatment failures are common with amphotericin B therapy regardless of the cumulative dose administered[150]; accordingly, conventional amphotericin B therapy generally is not recommended for sporotrichosis. Treatment options for sporotrichosis include itraconazole or fluconazole; in rare cases of refractory pulmonary sporotrichosis, surgical resection may be curative. Itraconazole therapy 100 to 600 mg/d was assessed in patients with lymphocutaneous infection or systemic infection; treatment was effective in 81% of cases.[36] Ketoconazole therapy (400 or 800 mg/d) was effective for 73% of cases of cutaneous or osteoarticular sporotrichosis in one study,[151] but treatment of *Sporothrix* pneumonia was unsuccessful in another case.[152] The efficacy of fluconazole therapy, 200 to 800 mg daily, for lymphocutaneous sporotrichosis was 71% in a prospective study, but only 31% of patients with osteoarticular infection responded to treatment.[24] Based on the limited data available, the treatment of choice for sporotrichosis is itraconazole 200 mg twice daily. Treatment should be continued for several months for lymphocutaneous infection and for at least a year for pneumonia.

Paracoccidioidomycosis

Paracoccidioidomycosis (South American blastomycosis) is an endemic mycosis caused by *P. brasiliensis*. This disease occurs in the southern half of Mexico, Central America, and some areas in South America. Infection is thought to result from inhalation of the fungus from an environmental source such as soil. Primary paracoccidioidomycosis usually is asymptomatic, but after a latency period of up to 30 years, chronic pneumonia can occur.[153] Systemic toxicity is uncommon. Cough and sputum production are the most common symptoms of chronic pulmonary paracoccidioidomycosis, and approximately one-quarter of patients also experience hemoptysis or chest pain. About half of patients who develop pneumonia also have extrapulmonary infection with diffuse lymphadenopathy or involvement of the skin or the oral or nasal mucosa. The diagnosis of paracoccidioidomycosis can be established by direct observation of organisms in sputum or purulent drainage, by positive culture results, or by serology tests. Declining complement fixation serology titers correlate with response to therapy, so serial complement fixation titers should be monitored during treatment.

Antifungal therapy is recommended for all patients with documented paracoccidioidomycosis. The oral azole compounds are the drugs of choice for non-life-threatening infection. The efficacy of ketoconazole 400 mg daily for 1 to 3 months followed by 200 mg daily for at least 3 months was 95% in one clinical trial.[14] In another study itraconazole 100 mg daily was as effective as ketoconazole and better tolerated.[35] Fluconazole 200 to 400 mg daily was effective treatment for all five cases reported in a pilot study.[154] Among 250 patients who were treated with amphotericin B for 6 to 8 weeks, 84% responded.[155] Itraconazole 200 mg daily for up to 6 months is considered the treatment of choice (Table 42–6), except for patients with life-threatening infection and those who cannot take oral medications; in these cases, amphotericin B therapy (cumulative dose of 1500 to 2000 mg) is recommended.[155] Because the risk of relapse is high, all patients who are treated with amphotericin B should subsequently receive maintenance therapy for 1 to 2 years.[155] Relapse occurs in 5% to 10% of cases even if maintenance therapy is administered; the risk of relapse is higher with ketoconazole than with itraconazole.[155] Thus itraconazole is the preferred maintenance treatment.

In contrast to other systemic mycoses, paracoccidioidomycosis often responds to sulfadiazine therapy. However, the role of sulfa is limited to maintenance therapy for patients who cannot be treated with oral azole drugs because of intolerance or potential for drug-drug interactions. The typical daily dosage of sulfadiazine is 6 g for adults or 60 to 100 mg/kg for children; sulfa maintenance therapy should be continued for 3 to 5 years.[155] In about 35% of sulfadiazine-treated patients, infection relapsed, often because of emergence of fungal resistance to the drug.[155] Trimethoprim and sulfamethoxazole have synergistic in vitro activity against *P. brasiliensis*, even in strains that are resistant to sulfamethoxazole,[156] but clinical experience with this drug combination is limited.

Pseudallescheriasis

P. boydii has a worldwide distribution in soil and stagnant or polluted fresh water. Infection in immunocompetent hosts can be due to percutaneous inoculation from local trauma or following inhalation or aspiration of organisms; the latter is a well-recognized complication of near drowning. In addition, pseudallescheriasis can cause invasive sinusitis or pneumonia in highly immunocompromised patients including persons with protracted neutropenia, those who have received prolonged corticosteroid therapy, or those who have undergone allogeneic bone marrow transplantation.[157] As is the case with *Aspergillus*, *P. boydii* is an angioinvasive organism that can cause pulmonary infarction. *P. boydii* also is particularly prone to disseminate to the central nervous system, either by local invasion or by hematogenous seeding.

P. boydii is more likely to cause asymptomatic colonization than invasive infection. Positive culture results from nonsterile sites (e.g., sputum, bronchial washings, or wound drainage) do not mandate aggressive treatment unless there is clinical evidence of invasive infection. Treatment of pseudallescheriasis is challenging, since most antifungal drugs have limited efficacy against *P. boydii* and there have been no prospective treatment studies to guide therapeutic decision making. Surgical débridement is recommended for pseudallescheriasis of the paranasal sinuses, soft tissues, bones, joints, or pleural spaces. Amphotericin B does not have in vitro activity against *P. boydii* and generally has been ineffective for treatment of pseudallescheriasis. Miconazole was effective in two of five patients with brain abscesses in one retrospective study[158] and in a single case report[159]; however, miconazole generally is unavailable for clinical use. Three case reports have described successful itraconazole

therapy (in combination with surgical débridement in one case of septic arthritis,[160] with lobectomy in a leukemic patient with pneumonia,[161] and as monotherapy for pneumonia).[162] One patient with disseminated infection and another with a brain abscess have responded to voriconazole therapy.[163,164] Caspofungin has in vitro activity against *P. boydii*, but its effectiveness for treatment of pseudallescheriasis has not been documented. On the basis of the limited data available, no firm treatment guidelines exist, but it is recommended that patients with invasive pseudallescheriasis be treated with itraconazole in combination with aggressive surgical débridement if feasible.

Fusariosis

Fusarium spp can cause skin and soft-tissue infections or osteomyelitis but more commonly are associated with disseminated infection in highly immunocompromised patients, primarily persons with acute leukemia and prolonged neutropenia.[165] The most common clinical manifestations are fever, diffuse myalgias, and necrotic macular or papular skin lesions.[165] Involvement of the digits and toenails has been reported.[166] Fusariosis has a bleak prognosis, with crude mortality in the 50% to 80% range.[165,166] The major determinant of outcome is recovery from neutropenia and remission of malignancy.[165]

No controlled treatment trials have been done. Amphotericin B therapy has been reported to be successful,[166] and there have been case reports describing the efficacy of lipid-based amphotericin preparations,[165,167] which are considered the treatment of choice (Table 42–6). Voriconazole has good in vitro activity against *Fusarium*, but in vivo data are not available.

Mucormycosis

Mucormycosis is an imprecise term that does not describe a single entity but rather is used to characterize those syndromes caused by a number of molds in the order Mucorales. Those most commonly implicated as causes of disease in humans are *Rhizopus* and *Rhizomucor*. These molds are ubiquitous in the environment and grow in decaying organic material, especially in bread. The Mucoraceae do not cause disease in nonimmunocompromised individuals. Major risk factors for infection include hyperglycemia, acidosis, protracted neutropenia, or immunosuppressive therapy for solid organ transplantation.[168] In addition, desferoxamine administration for iron chelation increases the risk of mucormycosis.[169] Infection occurs after spores are inhaled into the respiratory tract. The most common clinical manifestations are rhinocerebral mucormycosis (sinusitis with bony erosion and, occasionally, extension into the brain, cavernous sinus, or internal carotid artery) and pulmonary mucormycosis, which is associated with pulmonary consolidation and cavitation.

The outcome of mucormycosis depends to a large extent on correction of immunodeficiency and débridement of necrotic tissues.[170] Specifically, treatment of ketoacidosis, discontinuation or reduction in the doses of immunosuppressive medications if feasible, and administration of granulocyte colony-stimulating factors may improve the response to antifungal therapy, although data from controlled clinical trials are lacking. The available azole antifungal drugs do not have activity against Mucorales. For years amphotericin B has been the treatment of choice; the usual dose is 1 to 1.5 mg/kg/d. There have been a few case reports describing efficacy of the lipid-based amphotericin B compounds.[171–173] On the basis of these limited anecdotal data and the poor prognosis of mucormycosis, it is recommended that treatment consist of one of the lipid-based amphotericin B preparations at a dose of 5 to 10 mg/kg/d for several weeks (Table 42–6). A few patients with rhinocerebral mucormycosis have been treated with a combination of antifungal therapy and hyperbaric oxygen.[174] Although the efficacy of hyperbaric oxygen has not been confirmed, it could be considered as adjunctive therapy in severe or refractory cases.

Chromomycosis

Chromomycosis is a chronic cutaneous and subcutaneous fungal infection that occurs most frequently among agricultural workers in tropical and subtropical countries. A variety of fungi have been reported to cause chromomycosis including *Fonsecaea pedrosoi* and *Cladosporium carrionii*. Infection occurs after traumatic inoculation of fungi from soil, decaying vegetation, or rotting wood. After an incubation period of several months, single or multiple papules develop at the site of injury. Lesions eventually enlarge and develop a characteristic verrucous, cauliflower-like appearance. Multiple small "black dots" typically are seen on the surfaces of these lesions.

Therapeutic options for chromomycosis include surgical excision, cryosurgery, heat therapy, or antifungal therapy. Surgical excision or cryosurgery may be effective for treatment of smaller lesions, but the larger lesions encountered in clinical practice usually recur unless antifungal therapy is administered. Amphotericin B therapy generally is ineffective and is not recommended. Flucytosine, fluconazole, and itraconazole have been studied for the treatment of chromomycosis. Although flucytosine monotherapy is effective, resistance can develop and lead to relapse.[175] Fluconazole was effective in only one of eight patients in the one clinical trial that has been published, and the infection relapsed after discontinuation of therapy.[154] In two small studies, itraconazole therapy was effective in most cases.[176,177] Thus itraconazole appears to be the most effective treatment for chromomycosis (Table 42–6). Whether concomitant use of flucytosine improves treatment outcome is unknown.

Penicilliosis

P. marneffei infection occurs primarily in HIV-infected persons in southeastern Asia. The endemic area includes Thailand, Indonesia, Vietnam, Singapore, Taiwan, Malaysia, Hong King, Myanmar, and the Guangxi province of China. Patients present with a disseminated infection manifested by fever, weight loss, and nodular or ulcerative skin lesions. Diffuse pulmonary infiltrates are noted in most cases.[178]

Treatment options for penicilliosis include amphotericin B (with or without flucytosine), itraconazole, or fluconazole. In a retrospective study of 86 patients, amphotericin B was effective in 73% of cases, itraconazole in 75%, and fluconazole in 36%.[179] A prospective study in 74 HIV-infected patients assessed the efficacy of amphotericin B 0.6 mg/kg/d for 2 weeks followed by oral itraconazole 200 mg twice daily for 10 weeks; 97% of patients responded to this regimen,[180] which is now considered the treatment of choice (Table 42–6). As is the case with other AIDS-associated opportunistic fungal infections, there is a high risk of relapse, so lifelong maintenance therapy is recommended. After induction therapy, patients should be treated with oral itraconazole 200 mg/d indefinitely for maintenance therapy.[181]

REFERENCES

1. Goodwin SD, Cleary JD, Walawander CA, et al: Pretreatment regimens for adverse events related to the infusion of amphotericin B. Clin Infect Dis 1995;20:755–761.
2. Anderson CM: Sodium chloride treatment of amphotericin B nephrotoxicity. Standard of care? West J Med 1995;162:313–317.
3. Hoeprich P: Clinical use of amphotericin B: Lore, mystique, and fact. Clin Infect Dis 1992;14(Suppl 1):114–119.
4. Cruz JM, Peacock JE Jr, Loomer L, et al: Rapid intravenous infusion of amphotericin B: A pilot study. Am J Med 1992;93:123–130.
5. Walsh T, Heimenz J: Lipid formulations of amphotericin B: Recent developments in improving the therapeutic index of a gold standard. Infect Dis Clin Pract 1998;7(Suppl 1):16–17.
6. Dismukes W: Introduction to antifungal drugs. Clin Infect Dis 2000;30:653–657.
7. Johnson P, Wheat J, Cloud G, et al: Safety and efficacy of liposomal amphotericin B for induction therapy of histoplasmosis in patients with AIDS. Ann Intern Med 2002;137:105–109.
8. Walsh T, Finberg RW, Arndt C, et al: Liposomal amphotericin B for empirical therapy in patients with persistent fever and neutropenia. N Engl J Med 1999;340:764–771.
9. Wingard JP, White MH, Anaissie E, et al: A randomized, double blind comparative trial evaluating the safety of liposomal amphotericin B vs amphotericin B lipid complex in the empirical treatement of febrile neutropenia. Clin Infect Dis 2000;31:1155–1163.
10. Vermes A, Guchelaar H, Dankert J: Flucytosine: A review of its pharmacology, clinical indications, pharmacokinetics, toxicity, and drug interactions. J Antimicrob Chemother 2000;46:171–179.
11. Van der Horst C, Saag M, Cloud G, et al: Treatment of cryptococcal meningitis associated with the acquired immunodeficiency syndrome. N Engl J Med 1997;337:15–21.
12. Dismukes W, Cloud G, Bowles C, et al: Mycoses Study Group. Treatment of blastomycosis and histoplasmosis with

ketoconazole. Results of a prospective randomized clinical trial. Ann Intern Med 1985;103:861–872.

13. Galgiani JN, Stevens DA, Graybill JR, et al: Ketoconazole therapy of progressive coccidioidomycosis. Comparison of 400 and 800 mg doses and observations at higher doses. Am J Med 1988;84:603–610.

14. Negroni R: Ketoconazole in the treatment of paracoccidioidomycosis and histoplasmosis. Rev Infect Dis 1980;2:643–649.

15. Pont A, Graybill JR, Craven PC, et al: High-dose ketoconazole therapy and adrenal and testicular function in humans. Arch Intern Med 1984;144:2150–2153.

16. Lewis JH, Zimmerman HJ, Benson GD, Ishak KG: Hepatic injury associated with ketoconazole therapy. Gastroenterology 1984;86:503–513.

17. Demuria D, Forrest A, Rich J, et al: Pharmacokinetics and bioavailability of fluconazole in patients with AIDS. Antimicrob Agents Chemother 1993;37:2187–2192.

18. Pappas PG, Bradsher RW, Chapman SW, et al: Treatment of blastomycosis with fluconazole: A pilot study. Clin Infect Dis 1995;20:267–271.

19. Laine L, Dretler RH, Conteas CN, et al: Fluconazole compared with ketoconazole for the treatment of *Candida* esophagitis in AIDS. A randomized trial. Ann Intern Med 1992;117:655–660.

20. Catanzaro A, Fierer J, Friedman PJ: Fluconazole in the treatment of persistent coccidioidomycosis. Chest 1990;97:666–669.

21. Saag MS, Powderly WG, Cloud GA, et al: Comparison of amphotericin B with fluconazole in the treatment of acute AIDS-associated cryptococcal meningitis. N Engl J Med 1992;326:83–89.

22. Rex J, Bennett J, Sugar A, et al: A randomized trial comparing fluconazole with amphotericin B for the treatment of candidemia in patients without neutropenia. N Engl J Med 1994;331:1325–1330.

23. McKinsey D, Kaufman C, Pappas P, et al: Fluconazole therapy for histoplasmosis. Clin Infect Dis 1996;23:996–1001.

24. Kauffman C, Pappas P, McKinsey D, et al: Treatment of lymphocutaneous and visceral sporotrichosis with fluconazole. Clin Infect Dis 1996;22:46–50.

25. Rex J, Rinaldi M, Pfaller M: Resistance of *Candida* species to fluconazole. Antimicrob Agents Chemother 1995;39:1–8.

26. Wheat J, Marichal P, Van den Bossche H, et al. Hypothesis on the mechanism of resistance to fluconazole in *Histoplasma capsulatum*. Antimicrob Agents Chemother 1997;41:410–414.

27. Pappas P, Kauffman C, Perfect J, et al: Alopecia associated with fluconazole therapy. Ann Intern Med 1995;354–357.

28. Krçmery V, Huttova M, Masar O: Teratogenicity of fluconazole. Pediatr Infect Dis J 1996;15:841.

29. Stevens D: Itraconazole in cyclodextrin solution. Pharmacotherapy 1999;19:603–611.

30. Wilcox C, Darouiche R, Laine L, et al: A randomized, double-blind comparison of itraconazole oral solution and fluconazole tablets in the treatment of esophageal candidiasis. J Infect Dis 1997;176:227–232.

31. Saag MS, Fessel WD, Kauffman CA, et al: Treatment of fluconazole-refractory oropharyngeal candidiasis in HIV-positive patients. AIDS Res Hum Retroviruses 1999;15:1413–1417.

32. Dismukes WE, Bradsher RW, Cloud GC, et al: Itraconazole therapy for blastomycosis and histoplasmosis. Am J Med 1992;93:489–497.

33. Graybill JR, Stevens DA, Galgiani JN, et al: Itraconazole treatment of coccidioidomycosis. Am J Med 1990;89:282–290.

34. Denning D, Tucker R, Hanson L, et al: Itraconazole therapy for cryptococcal meningitis and cryptococcosis. Arch Intern Med 1989;149:2301–2308.

35. Naranjo MS, Trujillo M, Munera MI et al: Treatment of paracoccidioidomycosis with itraconazole. J Med Vet Mycol 1990;28:67–76.

36. Sharkey-Mathis PK, Kauffman CA, Graybill JR, et al: Treatment of sporotrichosis with itraconazole. Am J Med 1993;95:279–285.

37. McKinsey D, Wheat J, Cloud G, et al: Itraconazole prophylaxis for fungal infections in patients with advanced human immunodeficiency virus infection: Randomized, placebo-controlled, double-blind study. Clin Infect Dis 1999;28:1049–1056.

38. Onishi J, Meinz M, Thompson J, et al: Discovery of novel antifungal (1,3)-beta-glucan synthase inhibitors. Antimicrob Agents Chemother 2000;44:368–377.

39. Arikan S, Lazano-Chiu M, Paetznick V, Rex JH: In vitro susceptibility testing methods for caspofungin against *Aspergillus* and *Fusarium* isolates. Antimicrob Agents Chemother 2001;45:327–330.

40. Levitz SM: The ecology of *Cryptococcus neoformans* and the epidemiology of cryptococcosis. Rev Infect Dis 1991;13:1163–1169.

41. Diamond RD, Bennett JE: Prognostic factors in cryptococcal meningitis: A study in 111 cases. Ann Intern Med 1974;80:176–181.

42. Currie BP, Casadevall A: Estimation of the prevalence of cryptococcal infection among patients infected with the human immunodeficiency virus in New York City. Clin Infect Dis 1994;19:1029–1033.

43. Kaplan MH, Rosen PP, Armstrong D: Cryptococcosis in a cancer hospital: Clinical and pathological correlates in forty-six patients. Cancer 1977;39:2265–2274.

44. Hernandez AD: Cutaneous cryptococcosis. Dermatol Clin 1989;7:269–274.

45. Behrman RE, Masci JR, Nicholas P: Cryptococcal skeletal infections: Case report and review. Rev Infect Dis 1990;12:181–190.

46. Larsen RA, Bozzette S, McCutchan JA et al: Persistent *Cryptococcus neoformans* infection of the prostate after successful treatment of meningitis. Ann Intern Med 1989;111:125–128.

47. Taelman H, Bogaerts J, Batungwanayo J, et al: Failure of the cryptococcal serum antigen test to detect primary pulmonary cryptococcosis in patients infected with human immunodeficiency virus [letter]. Clin Infect Dis 1994;18:119–120.

48. Powderly WG, Cloud GA, Dismukes WE, Saag MS: Measurement of cryptococcal antigen in serum and cerebrospinal fluid: Value in the management of AIDS-associated cryptococcal meningitis. Clin Infect Dis 1994;18:789–792.

49. Bennett JE, Dismukes WE, Duma RJ, et al: A comparison of amphotericin B alone and combined with flucytosine in the treatment of cryptococcal meningitis. N Engl J Med 1979;301:126–131.

50. Dismukes W, Cloud G, Gallis H, et al: Treatment of cryptococcal meningitis with combination amphotericin B and flucytosine for four as compared with six weeks. N Engl J Med 1987;334–341.

51. Saag MS, Graybill JR, Larson RA, et al: Practice guidelines for the management of cryptococcal disease. Clin Infect Dis 2000;30:710–718.

52. Graybill JR, Sobel J, Saag M, et al: Diagnosis and management of increased intracranial pressure in patients with AIDS and cryptococcal meningitis. Clin Infect Dis 2000;30:47–54.

53. Powderly WG, Saag MS, Cloud GC, et al: A controlled trial of fluconazole or amphotericin B to prevent relapse of cryptococcal meningitis in patients with the acquired immunodeficiency syndrome. N Engl J Med 1992;326:793–798.

54. Saag M, Cloud G, Graybill J, et al: A comparison of itraconazole versus fluconazole as maintenace therapy for AIDS-associated cryptococcal meningitis. Clin Infect Dis 1999;28:291–296.

55. Pappas P, Hamill RJ, Kauffman C, et al: Treatment of cryptococcal meningitis in non-HIV infected patients: A randomized comparative trial. In: Abstracts of the Infectious Diseases Society of America 34th Meeting (abstract 73).

56. Sharkey P, Graybill J, Johnson E, et al: Amphotericin B lipid complex compared with amphotericin B in the treatment of cryptococcal meningitis in patients with AIDS. Clin Infect Dis 1996;22:315–321.

57. Leenders AC, Reiss D, Portegies P, et al: Liposomal amphotericin B (AmBisome) compared with amphotericin B followed by oral fluconazole in the treatment of AIDS-associated cryptococcal meningitis. AIDS 1997;11:1463–1471.

58. Nightingale SD, Cal SX, Peterson DM, et al: Primary prophylaxis with fluconazole against systemic fungal infections in HIV-positive patients. AIDS 1992;6:191–194.

59. Goldman M, Cloud G, Smedema M, et al: Does long-term itraconazole prophylaxis result in in vitro azole resistance in mucosal *Candida albicans* isolates from persons with advanced human immunodeficiency virus infection? Antimicrob Agents Chemother 2000;44:1585–1587.

60. Powderly WG, Finkelstein DM, Feinberg J, et al: A randomized trial comparing fluconazole with clotrimazole troches for the prevention of fungal infections in patients with advanced human immunodeficiency virus infection. N Engl J Med 1995;332:700–705.

61. US Public Health Service and Infectious Diseases Society of America: 1999 USPHS/IDSA guidelines for the prevention of opportunistic infections in persons infected with human immunodeficiency virus. MMWR Morb Mortal Wkly Rep 1999;48 (RR10):1–59.

62. Wergin W: Outbreak of histoplasmosis associated with the 1970 Earth Day activities. Am J Med 1973;54:333–342.

63. McKinsey D, Smith D, Driks M, O'Connor M: Histoplasmosis in Missouri: Historical review and current clinical concepts. Mo Med 1994;91:27–32.

64. Wheat LJ: Histoplasmosis—diagnosis and management. Infect Dis Clin Pract 1992;1:287–290.

65. Kataria YP, Campbell PB, Burlingham BT: Acute pulmonary histoplasmosis presenting as adult respiratory distress syndrome: Effect of therapy on clinical and laboratory features. South Med J 1981;74:534–537.

66. Goodwin RA, Owens FT, Snell JD et al: Chronic pulmonary histoplasmosis. Medicine 1976;55:413–452.

67. Goodwin RA, Shapiro JL, Thurman GH, et al: Disseminated histoplasmosis: Clinical and pathological correlations. Medicine 1980;59:1–32.

68. McKinsey D: Histoplasmosis in the acquired immunodeficiency syndrome: Advances in management. AIDS Patient Care STDS 1998;12:775–781.

69. Wheat LJ, Kohler RB, Tewari RP: Diagnosis of disseminated histoplasmosis by detection of *Histoplasma capsulatum* antigen in serum and urine specimens. N Engl J Med 1986;314:83–88.

70. Rosenthal J, Brandt KD, Wheat LJ, Slama T: Rheumatologic manifestations of histoplasmosis in the recent Indianapolis epidemic. Arthritis Rheum 1983;26:1065–1070.

71. Parker J, Sarosi G, Doto I, et al: Treatment of chronic pulmonary histoplasmosis. N Engl J Med 1970;238:225–229.

72. Baum GL, Larkin JC, Sutliff WD: Follow-up of patients with chronic pulmonary histoplasmosis treated with amphotericin B. Chest 1970;58:562–565.

73. Veterans Administration Armed Forces Cooperative Study on Histoplasmosis: Histoplasmosis cooperative study, II. Chronic pulmonary histoplasmosis treated with and without amphotericin B. Am Rev Respir Dis 1964;89:641–650.

74. Sarosi GA, Voth DW, Dahl BA, et al: Disseminated histoplasmosis: Results of long-term follow-up. Ann Intern Med 1971;75:511–516.

75. Rubin H: The course and prognosis of histoplasmosis. Am J Med 1959;27:278–287.

76. Furculow M: Comparison of treated and untreated severe histoplasmosis. JAMA 1963;183:121–127.

77. Reddy P, Gorelick D, Brasher C, Larsh H: Progressive disseminated histoplasmosis as seen in adults. Am J Med 1970;48:629–636.

78. Wheat LJ, Connolly-Stringfield P, Baker RL, et al: Disseminated histoplasmosis in the acquired immune deficiency syndrome: Clinical findings, diagnosis and treatment, and review of the literature. Medicine 1990;69:361–374.

79. Wheat LJ, Hafner R, Korzun AH, et al: Itraconazole treatment of disseminated histoplasmosis in patients with AIDS. Am J Med 1995;98:336–342.

80. McKinsey D, Gupta M, Riddler S, et al: Long-term amphotericin B therapy for disseminated histoplasmosis in patients with AIDS. Ann Intern Med 1989;11:655–659.

81. McKinsey DS, Gupta MR, Driks MR, et al: Histoplasmosis in patients with AIDS: Efficacy of maintenance amphotericin B therapy. Am J Med 1992;92:225–227.

82. Wheat LJ, Hafner RE, Wulfsohn M, et al: Prevention of relapse of histoplasmosis with itraconazole in patients with AIDS. Ann Intern Med 1993;118:610–616.

83. Norris J, Wheat J, McKinsey D, et al: Prevention of relapse of histoplasmosis with fluconazole in patients with AIDS. Am J Med 1994;96:504–508.

84. Wheat J, Mawhinney S, Hafner R, et al: Treatment of histoplasmosis with fluconazole in patients with AIDS. Am J Med 1997;103:223–232.

85. McKinsey D, Spiegel R, Hutwagner L, et al: Prospective study of histoplasmosis in patients with human immunodeficiency virus infection. Incidence, risk factors and pathophysiology. Clin Infect Dis 1997;24:1195–1203.

86. Klein BS, Vergeront JM, Weeks RJ, et al: Isolation of *Blastomyces dermatitidis* in soil associated with a large outbreak of blastomycosis in Wisconsin. N Engl J Med 1986;314:529–534.

87. Armstrong CW, Jenkins SR, Kaufman L, et al: Common source outbreak of blastomycosis in hunters and their dogs. J Infect Dis 1987;155:568–570.

88. Menges RW, Doto IL, Weeks RJ: Epidemiologic studies of blastomycosis in Arkansas. Arch Environ Health 1969;18:956–971.

89. Martin DS, Smith DT: Blastomycosis. I: A review of the literature. Am Rev Tuberc 1939;39:275–304.

90. Parker JD, Doto IL, Tosh FE: A decade of experience with blastomycosis and its treatment with amphotericin B. Am Rev Respir Dis 1969;99:895–902.

91. Lockwood WR, Allison F, Batson BE, et al: The treatment of North American blastomycosis: Ten years' experience. Am Rev Respir Dis 1969;100:314–320.

92. Bradsher RW, Rice DC, Abernathy RS: Ketoconazole therapy for endemic blastomycosis. Ann Intern Med 1985;103:872–879.

93. Pappas PG, Bradsher RW, Kauffman CA, et al: Treatment of blastomycosis with higher doses of fluconazole. Clin Infect Dis 1997;25:200–205.

94. Chapman S, Bradsher R, Campbell D, et al: Practice guidelines for the management of patients with blastomycosis. Clin Infect Dis 2000;30:679–683.

95. Como JA, Dismukes WE: Oral azole drugs as systemic antifungal therapy. N Engl J Med 1994;330:263–272.

96. Kerrick SS, Lungergan LL, Galgiani JN: Coccidioidomycosis at a university health service. Am Rev Respir Dis 1985;131:100–102.

97. Tom PF, Long TJ, Fitzpatrick SB: Coccidioidomycosis in adolescents presenting as chest pain. J Adolesc Health Care 1987;8:365–371.

98. Hyde L: Coccidioidal pulmonary cavitation. Dis Chest 1968;54(Suppl I):273–277.

99. Castellino RA, Blank N: Pulmonary coccidioidomycosis: The wide spectrum of roentgenographic manifestations. Calif Med 1968;109:41–49.

100. Winn WA: A long-term study of 300 patients with cavity-abscess lesions of the lung of coccidioidal origin. Dis Chest 1968;54(Suppl 1):268–272.

101. Sarosi GA, Parker JD, Doto IL, Tosh FE: Chronic pulmonary coccidioidomycosis. N Engl J Med 1970;283:325–329.

102. Rosenstein NE, Emery KW, Werner SB, et al: Risk factors for severe pulmonary and disseminated coccidioidomycosis: Kern County, California, 1995–96. Clin Infect Dis 2001;32:708–715.

103. Pappagianis D, Lindsay S, Beall S, Williams P: Ethnic background and the clinical course of coccidioidomycosis. Am Rev Respir Dis 1979;120:959–961.

104. Calhoun DL: Coccidioidomycosis in recent renal or cardiac transplant recipients. In Einstein HE, Catanzara A (Eds): Proceedings of the 4th International Conference on Coccidioidomycosis. Washington, DC, National Foundation for Infectious Diseases, 1985, pp 312–318.

105. Rutala PJ, Smith JW: Coccidioidomycosis in potentially compromised hosts: The effects of immunosuppressive therapy in dissemination. Am J Med Sci 1978;275:283–295.

106. Bronnimann DA, Adam RD, Galgiani JN, et al: Coccidioidomycosis in the acquired immunodeficiency syndrome. Ann Intern Med 1987;106:372–379.

107. Galgiani JN, Ampel NM: Coccidioidomycosis in human immunodeficiency virus–infected patients. J Infect Dis 1990;162:1165–1169.

108. Winn WA: The use of amphotericin B in the treatment of coccidioidal disease. Am J Med 1959;26:617–635.

109. Drutz DJ: Amphotericin B in the treatment of coccidioidomycosis. Drugs 1983;26:337–346.

110. Salomon NW, Osborne R, Copeland JG: Surgical manifestations and results of treatment of pulmonary coccidioidomycosis. Ann Thorac Surg 1980;30:433–438.

111. Cunningham R, Einstein H: Coccidioidal pulmonary cavities with rupture. J Thorac Cardiovasc Surg 1982;84:172–177.

112. Galgiani JN, Stevens DA, Graybill JR, et al: Ketoconazole therapy of progressive coccidioidomycosis. Comparison of 400- and 800-mg doses and observations at higher doses. Am J Med 1988;84:603–610.

113. Catanzaro A, Galgiani JN, Levin BE, et al: Fluconazole in the treatment of chronic pulmonary and nonmeningeal coccidioidomycosis. Am J Med 1995;98:249–256.

114. Tucker RM, Denning DW, Arathoon EG, et al: Itraconazole therapy for nonmeningeal coccidioidomycosis: Clinical and laboratory observations. J Am Acad Dermatol 1990;23:593–601.

115. Diaz M, Puente R, De Hoyos LA, Cruz S: Itraconazole in the treatment of coccidioidomycosis. Chest 1991;100:682–684.

116. Galgiani J, Catanzaro A, Cloud G, et al: Comparison of oral fluconazole and itraconazole for progressive, nonmeningeal coccidioidomycosis: A randomized, double-blind trial. Ann Intern Med 2000;133:676–686.

117. Smith CE: Serological tests in the diagnosis and prognosis of coccidioidomycosis. Am J Hyg 1950;52:1–21.

118. Tucker RM, Denning DW, Dupont B, Stevens DA: Itraconazole therapy for coccidioidal meningitis. Ann Intern Med 1990;112:1080–1012.

119. Galgiani J, Catanzaro A, Cloud G, et al: Fluconazole therapy for coccidioidal meningitis. Ann Intern Med 1993;119:28–35.

120. Dewsnup DH, Galgiani J, Graybill JR, et al: D. Is it ever safe to stop azole therapy for *Coccidioides immitis* meningitis? Ann Intern Med 1996;124:305–310.

121. Galgiani JN: Coccidioidomycosis: Changes in clinical expression, serological diagnosis, and therapeutic options. Clin Infect Dis 1992;14(Suppl 1):100–105.

122. Pappagianis D, The Valley Fever Vaccine Study Group: Evaluation of the protective efficacy of the killed *Coccidioides immitis* spherule vaccine in humans. Am Rev Respir Dis 1993;148:656–660.

123. Greenberger PS, Patterson R: Allergic bronchopulmonary aspergillosis: Model of bronchopulmonary disease with defined serologic, radiologic, pathologic, and clinical findings from asthma to fatal destructive lung disease. Chest 1987;91(Suppl 6):165–171S.

124. Eaton T, Garrett J, Milne D, et al: Allergic bronchopulmonary aspergillosis in the allergy clinic: A prospective evaluation of CT in the diagnostic algorithm. Chest 2000;118:66–72.

125. Denning DW, Van Wye JE, Lewiston NJ, Stevens DA: Adjunctive therapy of allergic bronchopulmonary aspergillosis with itraconazole. Chest 1991;100:813–819.

126. Stevens DA, Schwartz HJ, Lee J, et al: A randomized trial of itraconazole in allergic bronchopulmonary aspergillosis. N Engl J Med 2000;342:756–762.

127. Glimp R, Bayer A: Pulmonary aspergillomas: Diagnostic and therapeutic considerations. Arch Intern Med 1983;143:303–308.

128. Massard G, Roeslin N, Wihlm JM, et al: Pleuropulmonary aspergilloma: Clinical spectrum and result of surgical treatment. Ann Thoracic Surg 1992;54:1159–1164.

129. Regnard J-F, Icard P, Nicoloso M, et al: Aspergilloma: A series of 89 surgical cases. Ann Thorac Surg 2000;69:898–903.

130. Lee KS, Kim HT, Kim YH, et al: Treatment of hemoptysis in patients with cavitary aspergillosis of the lung: Value of percutaneous instillation of amphotericin B. Am J Roentgenol 1993;161:727–731.

131. Remy J, Arnaud A, Fardou H, et al: Treatment of hemoptysis by embolization of bronchial arteries. Radiology 1977;122:33–37.

132. Denning DW: Invasive aspergillosis. Clin Infect Dis 1998;26:781–803.

133. Horvath J, Dummer S: The use of respiratory tract cultures in the diagnosis of invasive aspergillosis. Am J Med 1996;100:171–178.

134. Denning DW: Early diagnosis of invasive aspergillosis. Lancet 2000;355:423–424.

135. Kuhlman JE, Fishman EK, Siegelman SS: Invasive pulmonary aspergillosis in acute leukemia: Characteristic findings on CT scan, the CT halo sign, and the role of CT in early diagnosis. Radiology 1985;157:611–614.

136. Blum W, Windfuhr M, Buitrago-Tellez C, et al: Invasive pulmonary aspergillosis: MRI, CT, and plain radiographic findings and their contribution for early diagnosis. Chest 1994;106:1157–1167.

137. Lin S-J, Schranz J, Teutsch SM: Aspergillosis case-fatality rate: Systematic review of the literature. Clin Infect Dis 2001;32:358–366.

138. White MH, Anaissie EJ, Kusne S, et al: Amphotericin B colloidal dispersion vs. amphotericin B as therapy for invasive aspergillosis. Clin Infect Dis 1997;24:635–642.

139. Walsh TJ, Hiemenz JW, Seibel NL, et al: Amphotericin B lipid complex for invasive fungal infections: Analysis of safety and efficacy in 556 cases. Clin Infect Dis 1998;626:1383–1396.

140. Ellis M, Spence D, De Pauw B, et al: An EORTC international multicenter randomized trial comparing two dosages of liposomal amphotericin B for treatment of invasive aspergillosis. Clin Infect Dis 1998;27:1406–1412.

141. Denning DW, Lee JY, Hostetler JS, et al: NIAID Mycoses Study Group Multicenter trial of oral itraconazole therapy for invasive aspergillosis. Am J Med 1994;97:135–144.

142. Stevens DA, Lee JY: Analysis of compassionate use itraconazole for invasive aspergillosis by the NIAID Mycoses Study Group criteria. Arch Intern Med 1997;157:1857–1862.

143. Patterson TF, Kirkpatrick WR, White M, et al: Invasive aspergillosis: Disease spectrum, treatment practices, and outcomes. Medicine 2000;79:250–260.

144. Denning DW, Stevens DA: Antifungal and surgical treatment of invasive aspergillosis: Review of 2121 published cases. Rev Infect Dis 1990;12:1147–1201.

145. Caillot D, Casasnovas O, Bernard A, et al: Improved management of invasive pulmonary aspergillosis in neutropenic patients using early thoracic computed tomography scan and surgery. J Clin Oncol 1997;15:139–147.

146. Yeghen T, Kibbler CC, Prentice HG, et al: Management of invasive pulmonary aspergillosis in hematology patients: A review of 87 consecutive cases at a single institution. Clin Infect Dis 2000;31:859–868.

147. Goodman JL, Winston DJ, Greenfield RA, et al: Controlled trial of fluconazole to prevent fungal infections in patients undergoing bone marrow transplantation. N Engl J Med 1992;326:845–851.

148. Harousseau JL, Dekker AW, Stamatoullas-Bastard A, et al: Itraconazole oral solution for primary prophylaxis of fungal infections in patients with hematological malignancy and profound neutropenia: A randomized, double-blind, double-placebo, multicenter trial comparing itraconazole and amphotericin B. Antimicrob Agents Chemother 2000;44:1887–1893.

149. Hughes WT, Armstrong D, Bodey GP, et al: Guidelines for the use of antimicrobial drugs in patients with unexplained fever. Clin Infect Dis 1997;551–573.

150. Pluss JL, Opal SM: Pulmonary sporotrichosis: review of treatment and outcome. Medicine 1986;65:143–153.

151. Calhoun DL, Washkin H, White MP, et al: Treatment of systemic sporotrichosis with ketoconazole. Rev Infect Dis 1991;13:47–51.

152. Dall L, Salzman G: Treatment of pulmonary sporotrichosis with ketoconazole. Rev Infect Dis 1987;9:795–798.

153. Restrepo MA, Robledo M, Gutierrez F, et al: Paracoccidioidomycosis (South American blastomycosis): A study of 39 cases observed in Medellin, Colombia. Am J Trop Med Hyg 1970;19:68–76.

154. Diaz M, Negroni R, Montero-Gei F, et al: A Pan American five-year study of fluconazole therapy for deep mycoses in the immunocompetent host. Clin Infect Dis 1992;14(Suppl 1):S68–S76.

155. Brummer E, Castaneda E, Restrepo A: Paracoccidioidomycosis: An update. Clin Microbiol Rev 1993;6:89–117.

156. Stevens DA, VO PT: Synergistic interaction of trimethoprim and sulfamethoxazole on *Paracoccidioides brasiliensis*. Antimicrob Agents Chemother 1982;21:852–854.

157. Gluckman SJ, Ries K, Abrutyn E: Allescheria (Petriellidium) boydii sinusitis in a compromised host. J Clin Microbiol 1977;5:481–484.

158. Dworzack DL, Clark RB, Borkowski WJ, et al: Pseudallescheria boydii brain abscess: Association with near-drowning and efficacy of high-dose, prolonged miconazole therapy in patients with multiple abscesses. Medicine 1989;68:218–224.

159. Schiess RJ, Coscia MF, McClellan GA. Petriellidium boydii pachymeningitis treated with miconazole and ketoconazole. Neurosurgery 1984;14:220–224.

160. Piper JP, Golden J, Brown D, Broestler J: Successful treatment of Scedosporium apiospermum suppurative arthritis with itraconazole. Pediatr Infect Dis J 1990;9:674–675.

161. Walsh M, White L, Atkinson K, Enno A: Fungal Pseudallescheria boydii lung infiltrates unresponsive to amphotericin B in leukaemic patients. Aust N Z J Med 1992;22:265–268.

162. Nomdedeu J, Brunet S, Martino R, et al: Successful treatment of pneumonia due to Scedosporium apiospermum with itraconazole: Case report. Clin Infect Dis 1993;16:731–733.

163. Girmenia C, Luzi G, Monaco M, Martino P: Use of voriconazole in treatment of Scedosporium apiospermum: Case report. J Clin Microbiol 1998;36:1436–1438.

164. Nesky MA, McDougal EC, Peacock JE: Pseudallescheria boydii brain abscess successfully treated with voriconazole and surgical drainage: Case report and literature review of central nervous system pseudallescheriasis. Clin Infect Dis 2000;31:673–677.

165. Boutati EI, Anaissie EJ: *Fusarium*, a significant emerging pathogen in patients with hematologic malignancy: Ten years' experience at a cancer center and implications for management. Blood 1997;90:999–1008.

166. Hennequin C, Lavarde V, Poirot JL, et al: Invasive *Fusarium* infections: A retrospective survey of 31 cases. J Med Vet Mycol 1997;35:107–114.

167. Wolff MA, Ramphal R: Use of amphotericin B lipid complex for treatment of disseminated cutaneous *Fusarium* infection in a neutropenic patients. Clin Infect Dis 1995;20:1568–1569.

168. Parfrey NA: Improved diagnosis and prognosis of mucormycosis: A clinicopathologic study of 33 cases. Medicine (Baltimore) 1986;65:113–123.

169. Boelaert JR, De Locht M, Van Cutsem J, et al: Mucormycosis during deferoxamine therapy is a siderophore-mediated infection: In vitro and in vivo animal studies. J Clin Invest 1993;91:1979–1986.

170. Kontoyiannis OP, Wessel VC, Bodey GP, Rolston KVI: Zygomycosis in the 1990s at a tertiary care center. Clin Infect Dis 2000;30:851–856.

171. Strasser MD, Kennedy RJ, Adam RD. Rhinocerebral mucormycosis: Therapy with amphotericin B lipid complex. Arch Intern Med 1996;156:337–339.

172. Munckhof W, Jones R, Tosolini FA, et al: Cure of *Rhizopus* sinusitis in a liver transplant recipient with liposomal amphotericin B. Clin Infect Dis 1993;16:183.

173. Ericsson M, Anniko M, Gustafsson H, et al: A case of chronic progressive rhinocerebral mucormycosis treated with liposomal amphotericin B and surgery. Clin Infect Dis 1993;16:585–586.

174. Ferguson BJ, Mitchell TG, Moon R, et al: Adjunctive hyperbaric oxygen for treatment of rhinocerebral mucormycosis. Rev Infect Dis 1988;10:551–599.

175. Lopes CF, Alvarenga RJ, Cisalpino EO, et al: Six years' experience in treatment of chromomycosis with 5-fluorocytosine. Int J Dermatol 1978;17:414–418.

176. Diaz M, Negroni R, Montero-Gei F, et al: A Pan-American 5-year study of fluconazole therapy for deep mycoses in the immunocompetent host. Clin Infect Dis 1992;14(Suppl 1):S68–S76.

177. Restrepo AA, Gonzales A, Gomez I, et al: Treatment of chromoblastomycosis with itraconazole. NY Acad Sci 1988;554:504–516.

178. Duong T: Infection due to *Penicillium marneffei*, an emerging pathogen: Review of 155 cases. Clin Infect Dis 1996;23:125–130.

179. Supparatpinyo K, Nelson G, Merz G, et al: Response to antifungal therapy by human immunodeficiency virus–infected patients with disseminated *Penicillium marneffei* infections and in vitro susceptibilities of isolates from clinical specimens. Antimicrob Agents Chemother 1993;37:2407–2411.

180. Sirisanthana T, Supparatpinyo K, Perriens S, Nelson K: Amphotericin B and itraconazole for treatment of disseminated *Penicillium marneffei* infection in human immunodeficiency virus–infected patients. Clin Infect Dis 1998;26:1107–1110.

181. Supparatpinyo K, Perriens J, Nelson K, Sirisanthana T: A controlled trial of itraconazole to prevent relapse of *Penicillium marneffei* infection in patients infected with the human immunodeficiency virus. N Engl J Med 1998;339:1739–1743.

Index

Note: Page numbers followed by f refer to figures and those followed by t refer to tables.